the calorie carb and fat bible

The UK's Most Comprehensive Calorie Counter

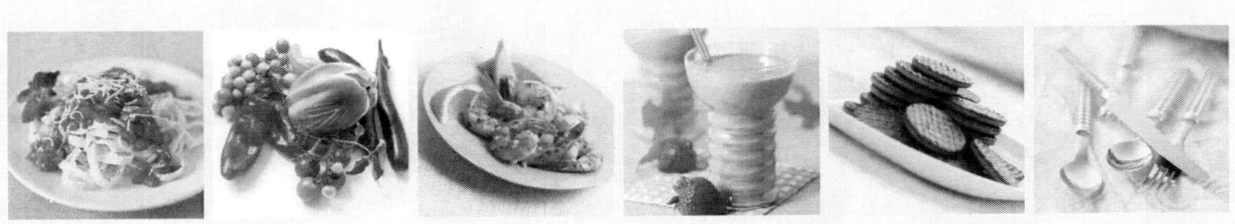

Juliette Kellow BSc RD, Lyndel Costain BSc RD & Rebecca Walton

The Calorie, Carb & Fat Bible

Published by:
Weight Loss Resources Ltd
2C Flag Business Exchange
Vicarage Farm Road
Peterborough
PE1 5TX.

Tel: 01733 345592
www.weightlossresources.co.uk

Companies and other organisations wishing to make bulk purchases of the Calorie, Carb and Fat Bible should contact their local bookstore or Weight Loss Resources direct.

ISBN 978-1-1904512-27-1

Authors: Lyndel Costain BSc RD
Juliette Kellow BSc RD
Rebecca Walton, Weight Loss Resources

Database Editor: Sam Holt

Printed and bound in the UK by Bonacia Ltd
www.bookprintinguk.com

Contents

Losing weight – the easy way

Juliette Kellow BSc RD

PIZZA, curries, chocolate, chips and the odd glass of wine! Imagine being told the best diet to help you lose weight can include all these foods and more. It sounds too good to be true, doesn't it? But the truth is, these are exactly the types of foods you can still enjoy if you opt to lose weight by counting calories.

But you'd be forgiven for not knowing you can still eat all your favourite foods *and* lose weight. In recent years, endless trendy diets have helped to make dieting a complicated business. Added to this, an increasing number of celebrities and so-called nutrition experts have helped mislead us into thinking that dieting is all about restriction and denial. Is it any wonder then that most of us have been left feeling downright confused and miserable about what we should and shouldn't be eating to shift those pounds?

Dieting doesn't have to be a complicated or unhappy experience. In fact, there's really only one word you need to remember if you want to shift those pounds healthily and still eat all your favourite foods. And that's CALORIE!

It's calories that count

When it comes to losing weight, there's no getting away from the fact that it's calories that count. Ask any qualified nutrition expert or dietitian for advice on dropping pounds and you'll receive the same reply: quite simply you need to create a calorie deficit or shortfall. In other words, you need to take in fewer calories than you use up so that your body has to draw on its fat stores to provide it with the energy it needs to function properly. The result: you start losing fat and the pounds start to drop off!

Fortunately, it couldn't be easier to create this calorie deficit. Regardless of your age, weight, sex, genetic make up, lifestyle or eating habits, losing weight is as simple as reducing your daily calorie intake slightly by modifying your diet and using up a few more calories by being slightly more active each day.

Better still, it's a complete myth that you need to change your eating and exercise habits dramatically. You'll notice I've said you need to reduce your calorie intake 'slightly' and be 'slightly' more active. It really is just LITTLE differences between the amount of calories we take in and the amount we use up that make BIG differences to our waistline over time. For example, you only need to consume one can of cola more than you need each day to gain a stone in a year. It's no wonder then that people say excess weight tends to 'creep up on them'.

10 simple food swaps you can make every day *(and won't even notice!)*

Make these simple swaps every day and in just 4 weeks you'll lose 7lb!

SWAP THIS...	FOR THIS...	SAVE...
300ml full-fat milk *(195 calories)*	300ml skimmed milk *(100 calories)*	*95 calories*
1tsp butter *(35 calories)*	1tsp low-fat spread *(20 calories)*	*15 calories*
1tbsp vegetable oil *(100 calories)*	10 sprays of a spray oil *(10 calories)*	*90 calories*
1tsp sugar *(16 calories)*	Artificial sweetener *(2 calories)*	*14 calories*
1tbsp mayonnaise *(105 calories)*	1tbsp fat-free dressing *(10 calories)*	*95 calories*
Regular sandwich *(600 calories)*	Low-fat sandwich *(350 calories)*	*250 calories*
Can of cola *(135 calories)*	Can of diet cola *(1 calorie)*	*134 calories*
Large (50g) packet of crisps *(250 calories)*	Small (25g) packet of crisps *(125 calories)*	*125 calories*
1 chocolate digestive *(85 calories)*	1 small chocolate chip cookie *(55 calories)*	*30 calories*
1 slice thick-cut wholemeal bread *(95 calories)*	1 slice medium-cut wholemeal bread *(75 calories)*	*20 calories*
	TOTAL CALORIE SAVING:	***868 calories***

The good news is the reverse is also true. You only need to swap that daily can of cola for the diet version or a glass of sparking water and you'll lose a stone in a year – it really is as easy as that!

Of course, most people don't want to wait a year to shift a stone. But there's more good news. To lose 1lb of fat each week you need to create a calorie deficit of just 500 calories a day. That might sound like a lot, but you can achieve this by simply swapping a croissant for a wholemeal fruit scone, a regular sandwich for a low-fat variety, a glass of dry white wine for a gin and slimline tonic and using low-fat spread on two slices of toast instead of butter. It is also important to become more active and increase your level of exercise; simply walking a little more will help. Losing 1lb a week, amounts to a stone in 14 weeks, or just under 4 stone in a year!

Taking control of calories

By now you've seen it really is calories that count when it comes to shifting those pounds.

A calorie-controlled diet is one of the few that allows you to include anything, whether it's pizza, wine or chocolate. A healthy diet means including a wide range of foods *(see 'Healthy Eating Made Easy' page 32)*.

And that's where this book can really help. Gone are the days when it was virtually impossible to obtain information about the calorie contents of foods. This book provides calorie information for more than 22,000 different branded and unbranded UK foods so that counting calories has never been easier.

The benefits of counting calories

- *It's guaranteed to help you lose weight providing you stick to your daily calorie allowance*
- *You can include favourite foods*
- *No foods are banned*
- *It's a great way to lose weight slowly and steadily*
- *Nutrition experts agree that it's a proven way to lose weight*

Calorie counting made easy

Forget weird and wacky science, complicated diet rules and endless lists of foods to fill up on or avoid every day! Counting calories to lose weight couldn't be easier. Quite simply, you set yourself a daily calorie allowance to help you lose between ½-2lb (¼-1kg) a week and then add up the calories of everything you eat and drink each day, making sure you don't go over your limit.

To prevent hunger from kicking in, it's best to spread your daily calorie allowance evenly throughout the day, allowing a certain amount of calories for breakfast, lunch, dinner and one or two snacks. For example, if you are allowed 1,500 calories a day, you could have 300 calories for breakfast, 400 calories for lunch, 500 calories for dinner and two snacks or treats of 150 calories each. You'll find more detailed information on p26-31 (Your step-by-step guide to using this book and shifting those pounds).

QUESTION

What affects the calorie content of a food?

ANSWER:

Fat, protein, carbohydrate and alcohol all provide the body with calories, but in varying amounts:

- *1g fat provides 9 calories*
- *1g alcohol provides 7 calories*
- *1g protein provides 4 calories*
- *1g carbohydrate provides 3.75 calories*

The calorie content of a food depends on the amount of fat, protein and carbohydrate it contains. Because fat provides more than twice as many calories as an equal quantity of protein or carbohydrate, in general, foods that are high in fat tend to contain more calories. This explains why 100g of chips (189 calories) contains more than twice as many calories as 100g of boiled potato (72 calories).

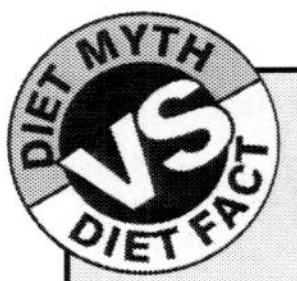

DIET MYTH:
Food eaten late at night stops you losing weight

DIET FACT:
It's not eating in the evening that stops you losing weight. It's consuming too many calories throughout the day that will be your dieting downfall! Providing you stick to your daily calorie allowance you'll lose weight, regardless of when you consume those calories. Nevertheless, it's a good idea to spread your calorie allowance throughout the day to prevent hunger from kicking in, which leaves you reaching for high-calorie snack foods.

Eat for good health

While calories might be the buzz word when it comes to shifting those pounds, it's nevertheless important to make sure your diet is healthy, balanced and contains all the nutrients you need for good health. Yes, you can still lose weight by eating nothing but chocolate, crisps and biscuits providing you stick to your calorie allowance, but you'll never find a nutrition expert or dietitian recommending this. And there are plenty of good reasons why.

To start with, an unbalanced diet is likely to be lacking in essential nutrients such as protein, vitamins, minerals and fibre, in the long term putting you at risk of nutritional deficiencies. Secondly, research proves that filling up on foods that are high in saturated fat and/or salt and sugar can lead to many different health problems. But most importantly, when it comes to losing weight, it's almost impossible to stick to a daily calorie allowance if you're only eating high-calorie foods.

Filling up on lower-calorie foods also means you'll be able to eat far more with the result that you're not constantly left feeling unsatisfied. For example, six chocolates from a selection box contain around 300 calories, a lot of saturated fat and sugar, few nutrients – and are eaten in just six mouthfuls! For 300 calories, you could have a grilled skinless chicken breast (packed with protein and zinc), a large salad with fat-free dressing (a great source of fibre, vitamins and minerals), a slice of wholemeal bread with low-fat spread (rich in fibre and B vitamins) and a satsuma (an excellent source of vitamin C). That's a lot more food that will take you a lot more time to eat! Not convinced? Then put six chocolates on one plate, and the chicken, salad, bread and fruit on another!

Bottom line: while slightly reducing your calorie intake is the key to losing weight, you'll be healthier and far more likely to keep those pounds off if you do it by eating a healthy diet *(see 'Healthy Eating Made Easy' page 32)*.

Eight steps to a healthy diet

1. *Base your meals on starchy foods.*
2. *Eat lots of fruit and vegetables.*
3. *Eat more fish.*
4. *Cut down on saturated fat and sugar.*
5. *Try to eat less salt - no more than 6g a day.*
6. *Get active and try to be a healthy weight.*
7. *Drink plenty of water.*
8. *Don't skip breakfast.*

SOURCE: www.nhs.uk/live-well/eat-well/eight-tips-for-healthy-eating/

Fat facts

Generally speaking, opting for foods that are low in fat can help slash your calorie intake considerably, for example, swapping full-fat milk for skimmed, switching from butter to a low-fat spread, not frying food in oil and chopping the fat off meat and poultry. But don't be fooled into believing that all foods described as 'low-fat' or 'fat-free' are automatically low in calories or calorie-free. In fact, some low-fat products may actually be higher in calories than standard products, thanks to them containing extra sugars and thickeners to boost the flavour and texture. The solution: always check the calorie content of low-fat foods, especially for things like cakes, biscuits, crisps, ice creams and ready meals. You might be surprised to find there's little difference in the calorie content when compared to the standard product.

Uncovering fat claims on food labels

Many products may lure you into believing they're a great choice if you're trying to cut fat, but you need to read between the lines on the labels if you want to be sure you're making the best choice. Here's the lowdown on what to look for:

LOW FAT	by law the food must contain less than 3g of fat per 100g for solids. These foods are generally a good choice if you're trying to lose weight.
REDUCED FAT	by law the food must contain 30 percent less fat than a similar standard product. This doesn't mean the product is low-fat (or low-calorie) though! For example, reduced-fat cheese may still contain 14g fat per 100g.
FAT FREE	the food must contain no more than 0.5g of fat per 100g or 100ml. Foods labelled as Virtually Fat Free must contain less than 0.3g fat per 100g. These foods are generally a good choice if you're trying to lose weight.
LESS THAN 8% FAT	this means the product contains less than 8g fat per 100g. It's only foods labelled 'less than 3% fat' that are a true low-fat choice.
X% FAT FREE	claims expressed as X% Fat Free shall be prohibited.
LIGHT OR LITE	claims stating a product is 'light' or 'lite' follows the same conditions as those set for the term 'reduced'.

10 easy ways to slash fat (and calories)

1	Eat fewer fried foods – grill, boil, bake, poach, steam, roast without added fat or microwave instead.
2	Don't add butter, lard, margarine or oil to food during preparation or cooking.
3	Use spreads sparingly. Butter and margarine contain the same amount of calories and fat – only low fat spreads contain less.
4	Choose boiled or jacket potatoes instead of chips or roast potatoes.
5	Cut off all visible fat from meat and remove the skin from chicken before cooking.
6	Don't eat too many fatty meat products such as sausages, burgers, pies and pastry products.
7	Use semi-skimmed or skimmed milk instead of full-fat milk.
8	Try low-fat or reduced-fat varieties of cheese such as reduced-fat Cheddar, low-fat soft cheese or cottage cheese.
9	Eat fewer high-fat foods such as crisps, chocolates, cakes, pastries and biscuits.
10	Don't add cream to puddings, sauces or coffee.

Getting Ready for Weight Loss Success

Lyndel Costain BSc RD

THIS BOOK not only provides tools to help you understand more about what you eat and how active you are, but guidance on how to use this information to develop a weight loss plan to suit your needs. Getting in the right frame of mind will also be a key part of your weight control journey, especially if you've lost weight before, only to watch the pounds pile back on.

The fact is that most people who want to lose weight know what to do. But often there is something that keeps stopping them from keeping up healthier habits. The same may be true for you. So what's going on? For many it's a lack of readiness. When the next diet comes along with its tempting promises it's so easy to just jump on board. But if you have struggled with your weight for a while, will that diet actually help you to recognise and change the thoughts and actions that have stopped you shifting the pounds for good?

Check out your attitude to weight loss programmes

Before starting any new weight loss programme, including the Weight Loss Resources approach, ask yourself:

Am I starting out thinking that I like myself as a person right now?	(YES or NO)
OR I feel I can only like myself once I lose weight?	(YES or NO)
Do I want to stop overeating, but at the same time find myself justifying it – in other words I want to be able to eat what I want, but with no consequences?	(YES or NO)
Do I believe that I need to take long-term responsibility for my weight?	(YES or NO)
OR Am I relying on 'it' (the diet) to do it for me?	(YES or NO)

Keep these questions, and your replies, in mind as you read through this chapter.

Next Steps

You may have already assessed the healthiness of your weight using the BMI guide on page 37. If not, why not do it now, remembering that the tools are a guide only. The important thing is to consider a weight at which you are healthy and comfortable – and which is realistic for the life you lead *(see opposite - What is a healthy weight?).*

The next step is to have a long hard think about why you want to lose weight. Consider all the possible benefits, not just those related to how you look. Psychologists have found that if we focus only on appearance we are less likely to succeed in the long-term. This is because it so often reflects low self-esteem or self-worth – which can sabotage success – as it saps confidence and keeps us stuck in destructive thought patterns. Identifying key motivations other than simply how you look - such as health and other aspects of physical and emotional well being - is like saying that you're an OK person right now, and worth making changes for. Making healthy lifestyle choices also has the knock on effect of boosting self-esteem further.

Write down your reasons for wanting to lose weight in your Personal Plan *(see page 42)* – so you can refer back to them. This can be especially helpful when the going gets tough. It may help to think of it in terms of what your weight is stopping you from doing now. Here's some examples: to feel more confident; so I can play more comfortably with my kids; my healthier diet will give me more energy; to improve my fertility.

What is a Healthy Weight?

With all the mixed messages in the media it can be easy to get a distorted view about whether your weight is healthy or not. However, as the BMI charts suggest, there is no single 'ideal' weight for anybody. Research also shows that modest amounts of weight loss can be very beneficial to health and are easier to keep off. Therefore, health professionals now encourage us to aim for a weight loss of 5-10%. The ideal rate of weight loss is no more than 1-2 pounds (0.5-1kg) per week – so averaging a pound a week is great, and realistic progress.

The health benefits of modest weight loss include:

- *Reduced risk of developing heart disease, stroke and certain cancers*
- *Reduced risk of developing diabetes and helping to manage diabetes*
- *Improvements in blood pressure*
- *Improvements in mobility, back pain and joint pain*
- *Improvements with fertility problems and polycystic ovarian syndrome*
- *Less breathlessness and sleep/snoring problems*
- *Increased self esteem and control over eating*
- *Feeling fitter and have more energy*

Are You Really Ready to Lose Weight?

When you think of losing weight, it's easy just to think of what weight you'd like to get to. But weight loss only happens as a result of making changes to your usual eating and activity patterns – which allow you to consume fewer calories than you burn *(see 'It's calories that count' page 5)*.

So here comes the next big question. Are you really ready to do it? Have you thought about the implications of your decision? If you have lost weight in the past, and put it all back on - have you thought about why that was? And how confident do you feel about being successful this time?

To help you answer these questions, try these short exercises.

Where would you place yourself on the following scales?

Importance

How important is it to you, to make the changes that will allow you to lose weight?

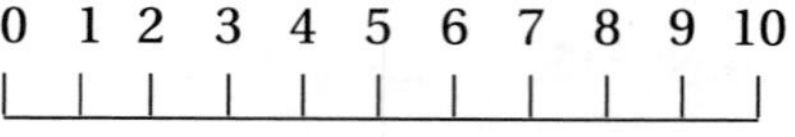

Not at all important *Extremely important*

If you ranked yourself over half way along the scale then move on to the next question. If you were half way or less along the scale, you may not be mentally ready to make the required changes to lose weight. To further explore this, go to *'The Pros and Cons of Weight Loss' (page 17)*.

Confidence

How confident are you in your ability to make the changes that will allow you to lose weight?

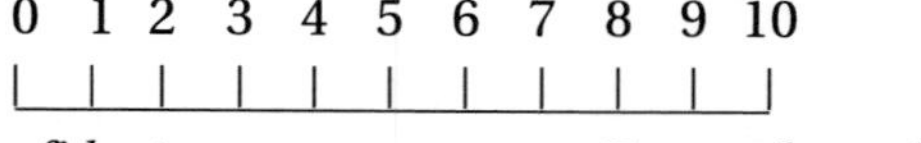

Not at all confident *Extremely confident*

Now ask yourself (regarding your confidence ratings):

1. Why did I place myself here?
2. What is stopping me moving further up the scale (if anything)?
3. What things, information, support would help me move further up the scale? (if not near 10)

If you aren't sure about answers to question 3, then keep reading for some pointers.

The Pros and Cons of Weight Loss

Making lifestyle changes to lose weight is simpler if there are lots of clear benefits or pros, for example, clothes fit again, more energy, helps back pain - but there will also be associated downsides or cons. For example, some may feel it interferes with their social life, or don't have the time to plan meals or check food labels. Or overeating can help, if only temporarily, as a way of coping with unwanted feelings. Being overweight allows some people to feel strong and assertive, or to control their partner's jealousy. So in these cases there are downsides to losing weight, even if the person says they are desperate to do it.

If you are aware of the possible downsides, as well as the pros, you will be better prepared to deal with potential conflicts. Understanding what could be (or were with past weight loss efforts) barriers to success gives you the chance to address them. This boosts confidence in your ability to succeed this time, which in turn maintains your motivation.

Have a go at weighing up the pros and cons using the charts below and on page 18. Some examples are included. If you decide that the pros outweigh the cons, then great. You can also use the cons as potential barriers to plan strategies for *(see page 42)*. If you find it's the other way around, this may not be the best time to actively lose weight. Try the exercise again in a month or so.

Making Lifestyle Changes to Lose Weight Now

CONS *e.g. Must limit eating out, take aways*	**PROS** *e.g. Feel more energetic, slimmer*

Not Making Changes Now – how would I feel in 6 months time?

PROS *e.g. Haven't had to worry about failing; Still able to eat take aways a lot*	**CONS** *e.g. Perhaps gained more weight; Still don't like how I look and feel*

To change your weight, first change your mind

To lose weight you may already have a list of things to change, such as eating more fruit and veg, calculating your daily calorie intake, going for a walk each morning or buying low fat options. Others could also give you tips to try. But knowing what to do isn't the same as feeling motivated or able to do it. To be effective, you have to believe the changes are relevant, do-able and worth it.

What you think, affects how you feel, and in turn the actions you take.

Self-efficacy

In fact, research is telling us that one of the most important factors that influences weight loss success are your feelings of 'self-efficacy'. Self-efficacy is a term used in psychology to describe a person's belief that any action they take will have an effect on the outcome. It reflects our inner expectation that what we do will lead to the results we want. Not surprisingly, high levels of self-efficacy can enhance motivation, and allow us to deal better with uncertainty and conflict, and recovery from setbacks. But low levels, can reduce our motivation. We fear that whatever we do will not bring about our desired goal. This can lead self-defeating thoughts or 'self-talk', which make it hard to deal with set-backs, meaning we are more likely to give up. Here's some examples.

Examples: Low self-efficacy
'No matter how carefully I diet, I don't lose weight . . .'
'I have eaten that chocolate and as usual blown my diet, so I may as well give up now.'
'I had a rich dessert – I have no willpower to say no. I can't stand not being able to eat what I want.'

If you have a strong sense of self-efficacy, your mindset and 'self-talk' will be more like:

Examples: High self-efficacy
'I know from previous weight loss attempts, that if I stay focussed on what I am doing I do lose weight. I have always expected to lose too much too quickly which frustrates me. I know that I will lose weight if I keep making the right changes, and this time it is important to me.'
'The chocolate bar won't ruin my diet, but if I think it has and keep on eating, then my negative self-talk will. So I will get back on track.'
'Losing weight is very important to me, so I ***can*** *make better food choices. After all, the world won't stop if I say no to dessert, and I will feel great afterwards. If I think about it, I am not hungry so would just feel bloated and guilty if I ate it.'*

Willpower is a Skill

Many people feel that they just need plenty of willpower or a good telling off to lose weight. But willpower isn't something you have or you don't have. Willpower is a skill. Like the dessert example on page 19, it's a sign that you've made a conscious choice to do something, because you believe the benefits outweigh any downsides. In reality everything we do is preceded by a thought. This includes everything we eat. It just may not seem like it because our actions often feel automatic *(see 'Look out for trigger eating' page 21)*.

When it comes to weight loss, developing a range of skills – including choosing lower calorie options, coping with negative self-talk and managing things that don't go to plan - will boost your sense of self-efficacy to make the changes you want. This is especially important because we live in such a weight-promoting environment.

Our weight-promoting environment

We are constantly surrounded by tempting food, stresses that can trigger comfort eating and labour-saving devices that make it easy not to be physically active. In other words, the environment we live in makes it easy to gain weight, unless we stop and think about the food choices we make and how much exercise we do. In fact, to stay a healthy weight/maintain our weight, just about all of us need to make conscious lifestyle choices everyday. This isn't 'dieting' but just part of taking care of ourselves in the environment we live in.

It is also true that some people find it more of a challenge than others to manage their weight, thanks to genetic differences in factors such as appetite control, spontaneous activity level and emotional responses to food – rather than metabolic rate, as is often believed. The good news is that with a healthy diet and active lifestyle a healthier weight can still be achieved. But do talk to your doctor if you feel you need additional support.

Coping with Common Slimming Saboteurs

Lyndel Costain BSc RD

Look out for 'trigger' eating

Much of the overeating we do or cravings we have are actually down to unconscious, habitual, responses to a variety of triggers. These triggers can be external, such as the sight or smell of food, or internal and emotion-led, such as a response to stress, anger, boredom or emptiness. Your food diary (see page 43) helps you to recognise 'trigger' or 'non-hungry' eating which gives you the chance to think twice before you eat (see below).

Get some support

A big part of your success will be having someone to support you. It could be a friend, partner, health professional, health club or website. Let them know how they can help you most.

Make lapses your ally

Don't let a lapse throw you off course. You can't be, nor need to be perfect all the time. Doing well 80-90% of the time is great progress. Lapses are a normal part of change. Rather than feel you have failed and give up, look at what you can learn from a difficult day or week and use it to find helpful solutions for the future.

Understand why you eat

When I ask people what prompts them to eat, hunger usually comes down near the bottom of their list of reasons. Some people struggle to remember or appreciate what true hunger feels like. We are lucky that we have plenty of food to eat in our society. But its constant presence makes it harder to control what we eat, especially if it brings us comfort or joy.

If you ever find yourself in the fridge even though you've recently eaten, then you know hunger isn't the reason but some other trigger. The urge to eat can be so automatic that you feel you lack willpower or are out of control. But it is in fact a learned or conditioned response. A bit like Pavlov's dogs. He rang a bell every time he fed them, and from then on, whenever they heard the bell ring they were 'conditioned' to salivate in anticipation of food.

Because this 'non-hungry' eating is learned, you can reprogramme your response to the situations or feelings that trigger it. The first step is to identify when these urges strike. When you find yourself eating when you aren't hungry ask yourself 'why do I want to eat, what am I feeling?' If you aren't sure think back to what was happening before you ate. Then ask yourself if there is another way you can feel better without food. Or you could chat to your urge to eat in a friendly way, telling it that you don't want to give into it, you have a planned meal coming soon, and it's merely a learned response. Whatever strategy you choose, the more often you break into your urges to eat, the weaker their hold becomes.

Practise positive self-talk

Self-talk may be positive and constructive (like your guardian angel) or negative and irrational (like having a destructive devil on your shoulder).

If you've had on-off battles with your weight over the years, it's highly likely that the 'devil' is there more often. 'All or nothing' self-talk for example, 'I ate a "bad food" so have broken my diet', can make you feel like a failure which, can then trigger you into the action of overeating and/or totally giving up *(see 'Diet-binge cycle' page 23)*. One of the most powerful things about it is that the last thoughts we have are what stays in our mind. So if we think 'I still look fat' or 'I will never be slim', these feelings stay with us.

To change your self-talk for the better, the trick is to first recognise it's happening (keeping a diary really helps, *see Keep a Food Diary, page 29*). Then turn it around into a positive version of the same events *(see Self-efficacy, page 18)* where the resulting action was to feel good and stay on track. Reshaping negative self-talk helps you to boost your self-esteem and feelings of self-efficacy, and with it change your self-definition - from someone who can't 'lose weight' or 'do this or that', to someone 'who can'.

And when you believe you can…

The Diet – Binge Cycle

If this cycle looks familiar, use positive self-talk, and a more flexible dietary approach, to help you break free.

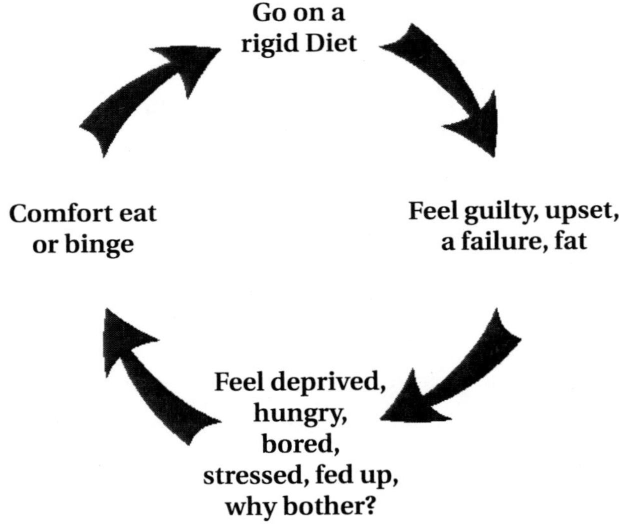

Really choose what you want to eat

This skill is like your personal brake. It also helps you to manage 'trigger/ non-hungry' eating and weaken its hold. It legalises food and stops you feeling deprived. It helps you to regularly remind yourself why you are making changes to your eating habits, which keeps motivation high. But it doesn't just happen. Like all skills it requires practise. Sometimes it will work well for you, other times it won't – but overall it will help. Basically, ask yourself if you really want to eat that food in front of you. This becomes the prompt for you to make a conscious choice, weighing up the pros and cons or consequences of making that choice, and feeling free to have it, reject it or just eat some. Remembering all the while that you can eat this food another time if you want to.

Action Planning

Successful people don't just wait for things to happen. They believe in themselves, plan ahead, take action and then refine their plan until it gets, and keeps on getting the results they want. Successful slimmers use a very similar approach. They don't rely on quick-fixes or magic formulas, but glean information from reliable sources to develop a plan or approach that suits their needs, tastes and lifestyle. Thinking of weight management as a lifelong project, which has a weight loss phase and a weight maintenance phase, is also a route to success.

When the Going Gets Tough - Staying on Track

If things start to go off track, don't panic. Learning new habits takes time. And life is never straightforward so there will be times when it all seems too much, or negative 'self- talk' creeps in to try and drag you back into old ways. So if the going gets tough:

- Value what you've achieved so far, rather than only focus on what you plan to do.
- Look back at your reasons to lose weight and refer to the list often.
- Don't expect to change too much, too quickly. Take things a step at a time.
- Accept difficulties as part of the learning and skill building process.
- Enjoy a non-food reward for achieving your goals (including maintaining your weight).
- Use recipes and meal ideas to keep things interesting.
- Talk to your supporters and get plenty of encouragement. This is really vital!

Strategies of Successful Slimmers

Thanks to research conducted by large studies such as the US National Weight Control Registry and the German Lean Habits Study, we now know more about what works best for people who have lost weight and successfully kept it off. So be inspired!

The key elements of success are to:

- Believe that you can control your weight and the changes involved are really worth it.
- Stay realistic and value what you have achieved rather than dwell on a weight you 'dream' of being.
- Be more active – plan ways to fit activity into your daily life – aim for 1 hour of walking daily.
- Plan ahead for regular meals and snacks, starting with breakfast.
- Choose a balanced, low-fat diet with plenty of fruit and vegetables *(see Healthy Eating Made Easy, page 32)*.
- Watch portion size and limit fast food.
- Sit down to eat and take time over meals, paying attention to what you are eating.
- Have a flexible approach – plan in and enjoy some favourite foods without guilt.
- Recognise and address 'all or nothing' thinking and other negative 'self-talk'.
- Keep making conscious choices.
- Learn to confront problems rather than eat, drink, sleep or wish they would go away.
- Enlist ongoing help and support from family, friends, professionals or websites.
- Regularly (at least once a week but not more than once daily) check your weight.
- Take action before your weight increases by more than 4-5lb (2kg).
- Accept that your weight management skills need to be kept up long-term.
- Take heart from successful slimmers, who say that it gets easier over time.

Your step-by-step guide to using this book and shifting those pounds

Juliette Kellow BSc RD and Rebecca Walton

1. Find your healthy weight

Use the weight charts, body mass index table and information on pages 36-43 to determine the right weight for you. Then set yourself a weight to aim for. Research shows it really helps if you make losing 10% of your weight your first overall target. It also brings important health benefits too *(see 'What is a Healthy Weight?' page 15)*. You can break this down into smaller manageable steps, for example, 3kg/6.5lbs at a time. If 10% is too much, then go for a 5% loss – this has important health benefits too. In fact, just keeping your weight stable is a great achievement these days, because of our weight-promoting environment *(see page 20)*.

Waist Management

In addition to BMI, another important way to assess your weight is by measuring your waist just above belly button level. It is especially useful for men as they tend to carry more excess weight around their bellies, but women should test it out too. Having excess weight around your middle (known as being 'apple-shaped') increases your risk of heart disease and type 2 diabetes. A simple way to stay aware of your waist is according to how well, or otherwise, skirts and trousers fit. Talk to your doctor about any weight and health concerns.

WAIST MEASUREMENT

	Increased Health Risk	High Risk to Health
Women	32-35in (81-88cm)	more than 35in (88cm)
Men	37-40in (94-102cm)	more than 40in (102cm)

2. Set a realistic time scale

With today's hectic lifestyles, everything tends to happen at breakneck speed, so it's no wonder that when it comes to losing weight, most of us want to shift those pounds in an instant. But it's probably taken years to accumulate that extra weight, with the result that it's unrealistic to expect to lose the excess in just a few weeks! Instead, prepare yourself to lose weight slowly and steadily. It's far healthier to lose weight like this. But better still, research shows you'll be far more likely to maintain your new, lower weight.

If you only have a small amount of weight to lose, aim for a weight loss of around 1lb (½kg) a week. But if you have more than 2 stone (28kg) to lose, you may prefer to aim for 2lb (1kg) each week. Remember though, it's better to keep going at 1lb (½kg) a week than to give up because trying to lose 2lb (1kg) a week is making you miserable! The following words may help you to keep your goal in perspective:

'Never give up on a goal because of the time it will take to achieve it – the time will pass anyway.'

Weight Fluctuations

Weight typically fluctuates on a day to day basis. You know that shock/horror feeling when you weigh yourself in the morning then later in the day, or after a meal out, and it looks like youve gained pounds in hours! But this is due to fluid not fat changes. Real changes in body fat can only happen more gradually (remember, to gain 1lb you need to eat 3500 calories more than you usually do). Don't be confused either by seemingly very rapid weight loss in the first week or so.

When calorie intake is initially cut back, the body's carbohydrate stores in the liver and muscles (known as glycogen) are used up. Glycogen is stored with three times its weight in water, meaning that rapid losses of 4.5- 6.6lb (2 -3 kg) are possible. These stores can be just as rapidly refilled if normal eating is resumed. True weight loss happens more gradually and this book helps you to lose weight at the steady and healthy rate of no more than 1-2 lbs per week.

3. Calculate your calorie allowance

Use the calorie tables on pages 39-40 to find out how many calories you need each day to maintain your current weight. Then use the table below to discover the amount of calories you need to subtract from this amount every day to lose weight at your chosen rate. For example, a 35 year-old woman who is moderately active and weighs 12 stone (76kg) needs 2,188 calories a day to keep her weight steady. If she wants to lose ½lb (¼kg) a week, she needs 250 calories less each day, giving her a daily calorie allowance of 1,938 calories. If she wants to lose 1lb (½kg) a week, she needs 500 calories less each day, giving her a daily calorie allowance of 1,688 calories, and so on.

TO LOSE...	Cut your daily calorie intake by	In three months you could lose...	In six months you could lose...	In one year you could lose...
½lb a week	250	6.5lb	13lb	1st 12lb
1lb a week	500	13lb	1st 12lb	3st 10lb
1½lb a week	750	1st 5.5lb	2st 11lb	5st 8lb
2lb a week	1,000	1st 12lb	3st 10lb	7st 6lb

TO LOSE...	Cut your daily calorie intake by	In three months you could lose...	In six months you could lose...	In one year you could lose...
¼kg a week	250	3.25kg	6.5kg	13kg
½kg a week	500	6.5kg	13kg	26kg
¾kg a week	750	9.75kg	19.5kg	39kg
1kg a week	1,000	13kg	26kg	52kg

4. Keep a food diary

Writing down what you eat and drink and any thoughts linked to that eating helps you become more aware of your eating habits. Recognising what is going on helps you feel in control and is a powerful way to start planning change. Keeping a food diary before you start to change your eating habits will also help you identify opportunities for cutting calories by substituting one food for another, cutting portion sizes of high-calorie foods or eating certain foods less often.

Simply write down every single item you eat or drink during the day and use this book to calculate the calories of each item. Then after a few days of eating normally, introduce some changes to your diet to achieve your daily calorie allowance. Remember to spread your daily calorie allowance fairly evenly throughout the day to prevent hunger. You'll find a template for a daily food and exercise diary on page 43.

Top Tip

If you only fill in your main food diary once a day, keep a pen and notepad with you to write down all those little extras you eat or drink during the day – that chocolate you ate in the office, the sliver of cheese you had while cooking dinner and the few chips you pinched from your husband's plate, for example! It's easy to forget the little things if they're not written down, but they can make the difference between success and failure.

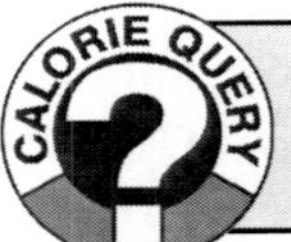

QUESTION: Why are heavier people allowed more calories than those who have smaller amounts of weight to lose?

ANSWER: This confuses a lot of people but is easily explained. Someone who is 3 stone overweight, for example, is carrying the equivalent of 42 small packets of butter with them everywhere they go – up and down the stairs, to the local shops, into the kitchen. Obviously, it takes a lot more energy simply to move around when you're carrying that extra weight. As a consequence, the heavier you are, the more calories you need just to keep your weight steady. In turn, this means you'll lose weight on a higher calorie allowance. However, as you lose weight, you'll need to lower your calorie allowance slightly as you have less weight to carry around.

5. Control your portions

As well as making some smart food swaps to cut calories, it's likely you'll also need to reduce your serving sizes for some foods to help shift those pounds. Even 'healthy' foods such as brown rice, wholemeal bread, chicken, fish and low-fat dairy products contain calories so you may need to limit the amount you eat. When you first start out, weigh portions of foods like rice, pasta, cereal, cheese, butter, oil, meat, fish, and chicken rather than completing your food diary with a 'guesstimated' weight! That way you can calculate the calorie content accurately. Don't forget that drinks contain calories too, alcohol, milk, juices and sugary drinks all count.

6. Measure your success

Research has found that regular weight checks do help. Weighing yourself helps you assess how your eating and exercise habits affect your body weight. The important thing is to use the information in a positive way – to assess your progress - rather than as a stick to beat yourself up with. Remember that weight can fluctuate by a kilogram in a day, for example, due to fluid changes, premenstrually, after a big meal out, so weigh yourself at the same time of day and look at the trend over a week or two.

People who successfully lose weight and keep it off, also tend to continue weighing themselves at least once a week, and often daily (but not in an obsessive way), because they say it helps them stay 'on track'. Probably because they use it as an early warning system. People who weigh themselves regularly (or regularly try on a tight fitting item of clothing) will notice quickly if they have gained a few pounds - and can take action to stop gaining more. Checking your weight less often can mean that you might discover one day that you gained more than you thought. That can be pretty discouraging, and it might trigger you to just give up.

Top Tip

Don't just focus on what the bathroom scales say either – keep a record of your vital statistics, too. Many people find it doubly encouraging to see the inches dropping off, as well as the pounds!

7. Stay motivated

Each time you lose half a stone, or reach your own small goal – celebrate! Treat yourself to a little luxury – something new to wear, a little pampering or some other (non-food) treat. It also helps replace the comfort you once got from food and allows you to take care of yourself in other ways. Trying on an item of clothing that used to be tight can also help to keep you feeling motivated. Make sure you keep in touch with your supporters, and if the going gets tough take another look at the *'Coping with Common Slimming Saboteurs' section on page 21*. Once you've reviewed how well you've done, use this book to set yourself a new daily calorie allowance based on your new weight to help you lose the next half stone *(see point 3 - page 28 - Calculate your calorie allowance)*.

8. Keep it off

What you do to stay slim is just as important as what you did to get slim. Quite simply, if you return to your old ways, you are likely to return to your old weight. The great thing about calorie counting is that you will learn so much about what you eat, and make so many important changes to your eating and drinking habits, that you'll probably find it difficult to go back to your old ways – and won't want to anyway. It's still a good idea to weigh yourself at least once a week to keep a check on your weight. The key is to deal with any extra pounds immediately, rather than waiting until you have a stone to lose *(see page 30)*. Simply go back to counting calories for as long as it takes to shift those pounds and enjoy the new slim you. Page 25 has more information about how successful slimmers keep it off.

QUESTION: Do I need to stick to exactly the same number of calories each day or is it OK to have a lower calorie intake during the week and slightly more at the weekend?

ANSWER: The key to losing weight is to take in fewer calories than you need for as long as it takes to reach your target, aiming for a loss of no more than 2lb (1kg) a week. In general, most nutrition experts recommend a daily calorie allowance. However, it's just as valid to use other periods of time such as weeks. If you prefer, simply multiply your daily allowance by seven to work out a weekly calorie allowance and then allocate more calories to some days than others. For example, a daily allowance of 1,500 calories is equivalent to 10,500 calories a week. This means you could have 1,300 calories a day during the week and 2,000 calories a day on Saturday and Sunday.

Healthy Eating Made Easy

Juliette Kellow BSc RD

HEALTHY EATING doesn't just mean eating salads and smoothies. Eating healthily means we're positively encouraged to eat a wide range of foods, including some of our favourites – it's just a question of making sure we don't eat high fat, high sugar or highly processed foods too often.

Eating a healthy diet, together with taking regular exercise and not smoking, has huge benefits to our health, both in the short and long term. As well as helping us to lose or maintain our weight, a healthy diet can boost energy levels, keep our immune system strong and give us healthy skin, nails and hair. Meanwhile, eating well throughout life also means we're far less likely to suffer from health problems such as constipation, anaemia and tooth decay, or set ourselves up for serious conditions in later life such as obesity, heart disease, stroke, diabetes, cancer or osteoporosis.

Fortunately, it couldn't be easier to eat a balanced diet. To start with, no single food provides all the calories and nutrients we need to stay healthy, so it's important to eat a variety of foods. Meanwhile, most nutrition experts also agree that mealtimes should be a pleasure rather than a penance. This means it's fine to eat small amounts of our favourite treats from time to time.

To help people eat healthily, the NHS recommends eating plenty of different foods from four main groups of foods and limiting the amount we eat from a smaller fifth group. Ultimately, we should eat more fruit, vegetables, starchy, fibre-rich foods and fresh products, and fewer fatty, sugary, salty and processed foods.

The following guidelines are all based on the healthy eating guidelines recommended by health professionals.

Bread, other cereals and potatoes

Eat these foods at each meal. They also make good snacks.

Foods in this group include bread, breakfast cereals, potatoes, rice, pasta, noodles, yams, oats and grains. Go for high-fibre varieties where available, such as wholegrain cereals, wholemeal bread and brown rice. These foods should fill roughly a third of your plate at mealtimes.

TYPICAL SERVING SIZES

- *2 slices bread in a sandwich or with a meal*
- *a tennis ball sized serving of pasta, potato, rice, noodles or couscous*
- *a bowl of porridge*
- *around 40g of breakfast cereal*

Fruit and vegetables

Eat at least five portions every day.

Foods in this group include all fruits and vegetables, including fresh, frozen, canned and dried products, and unsweetened fruit juice. Choose canned fruit in juice rather than syrup and go for veg canned in water without added salt or sugar.

TYPICAL PORTION SIZES

- *a piece of fruit eg: apple, banana, pear*
- *2 small fruits eg: satsumas, plums, apricots*
- *a bowl of fruit salad, canned or stewed fruit*
- *a small glass of unsweetened fruit juice*
- *a cereal bowl of salad*
- *3tbsp vegetables*

Milk, dairy and alternatives

Eat two or three servings a day.

Foods in this group include milk, cheese, yoghurt and fromage frais. Choose low-fat varieties where available such as skimmed milk, reduced-fat cheese and fat-free yoghurt.

TYPICAL SERVING SIZES

- *200ml milk*
- *a small pot of yoghurt or fromage frais*
- *a small matchbox-sized piece of cheese*

Meat, fish and alternatives

Eat two servings a day

Foods in this group include meat, poultry, fish, eggs, beans, nuts and seeds. Choose low-fat varieties where available such as extra-lean minced beef and skinless chicken and don't add extra fat or salt.

TYPICAL SERVING SIZES

- *a piece of meat, chicken or fish the size of a deck of cards*
- *1-2 eggs*
- *3 heaped tablespoons of beans*
- *a small handful of nuts or seeds*

TOP TIP

Healthy Eating on a plate

A simple way to serve up both balance and healthy proportions is to fill one half of your plate with salad or vegetables and divide the other half between protein-rich meat, chicken, fish, eggs or beans, and healthy carbs (potatoes, rice, pasta, pulses, bread or noodles).

Fatty and sugary foods

Eat only small amounts of these foods

Foods in this group include oils, spreading fats, cream, mayonnaise, oily salad dressings, cakes, biscuits, puddings, crisps, savoury snacks, sugar, preserves, confectionery and sugary soft drinks.

TYPICAL SERVING SIZES:

- *a small packet of sweets or a small bar of chocolate*
- *a small slice of cake*
- *a couple of small biscuits*
- *1 level tbsp mayo, salad dressing or olive oil*
- *a small packet of crisps*

Useful Tools

Body Mass Index

The Body Mass Index (BMI) is the internationally accepted way of assessing how healthy our weight is for most people. It is calculated using height and weight. Use the BMI Chart to look up your BMI, and use this table to see which range you fall into.

BMI Under 18.5	*Underweight*
BMI 18.5-25	*Healthy*
BMI 25-30	*Overweight*
BMI 30-40	*Obese*
BMI Over 40	*Severely Obese*

This is what different BMI ranges mean.

- **Underweight:** you probably need to gain weight for your health's sake. Talk to your doctor if you have any concerns, or if you feel frightened about gaining weight.
- **Healthy weight:** you are a healthy weight, so aim to stay in this range (note that most people in this range tend to have a BMI between 20-25).
- **Overweight:** aim to lose some weight for your health's sake, or at least prevent further weight gain.
- **Obese:** your health is at risk and losing weight will benefit your health.
- **Severely obese:** your health is definitely at risk. You should visit your doctor for a health check. Losing weight will improve your health.

Please note that BMI is not as accurate for athletes or very muscular people (muscle weighs more than fat), as it can push them into a higher BMI category despite having a healthy level of body fat. It is also not accurate for women who are pregnant or breastfeeding, or people who are frail.

Body Mass Index Table

HEIGHT IN FEET / INCHES

WEIGHT IN STONES / LBS

	4'6	4'8	4'10	5'0	5'2	5'4	5'6	5'8	5'10	6'0	6'2	6'4	6'6	6'8	6'10
6st 7	22.0	20.5	19.1	17.8	16.7	15.7	14.7	13.9	13.1	12.4	11.7	11.1	10.6	10.0	9.5
7st 0	23.7	22.1	20.6	19.2	18.0	16.9	15.9	15.0	14.1	13.3	12.6	12.0	11.4	10.8	10.3
7st 7	25.4	23.6	22.0	20.6	19.3	18.1	17.0	16.0	15.1	14.3	13.5	12.8	12.2	11.6	11.0
8st 0	27.1	25.2	23.5	22.0	20.6	19.3	18.1	17.1	16.1	15.2	14.4	13.7	13.0	12.3	11.8
8st 7	28.8	26.8	25.0	23.3	21.8	20.5	19.3	18.2	17.1	16.2	15.3	14.5	13.8	13.1	12.5
9st 0	30.5	28.4	26.4	24.7	23.1	21.7	20.4	19.2	18.1	17.2	16.2	15.4	14.6	13.9	13.2
9st 7	32.2	29.9	27.9	26.1	24.4	22.9	21.5	20.3	19.2	18.1	17.1	16.2	15.4	14.7	14.0
10st 0	33.9	31.5	29.4	27.4	25.7	24.1	22.7	21.4	20.2	19.1	18.0	17.1	16.2	15.4	14.7
10st 7	35.6	33.1	30.8	28.8	27.0	25.3	23.8	22.4	21.2	20.0	18.9	18.0	17.0	16.2	15.4
11st 0	37.3	34.7	32.3	30.2	28.3	26.5	24.9	23.5	22.2	21.0	19.8	18.8	17.9	17.0	16.2
11st 7	39.0	36.2	33.8	31.6	29.6	27.7	26.1	24.6	23.2	21.9	20.7	19.7	18.7	17.8	16.9
12st 0	40.7	37.8	35.2	32.9	30.8	28.9	27.2	25.6	24.2	22.9	21.6	20.5	19.5	18.5	17.6
12st 7	42.3	39.4	36.7	34.3	32.1	30.1	28.3	26.7	25.2	23.8	22.5	21.4	20.3	19.3	18.4
13st 0	44.0	41.0	38.2	35.7	33.4	31.4	29.5	27.8	26.2	24.8	23.5	22.2	21.1	20.1	19.1
13st 7	45.7	42.5	39.6	37.0	34.7	32.6	30.6	28.8	27.2	25.7	24.4	23.1	21.9	20.8	19.8
14st 0	47.4	44.1	41.1	38.4	36.0	33.8	31.7	29.9	28.2	26.7	25.3	23.9	22.7	21.6	20.6
14st 7	49.1	45.7	42.6	39.8	37.3	35.0	32.9	31.0	29.2	27.6	26.2	24.8	23.5	22.4	21.3
15st 0	50.8	47.3	44.0	41.2	38.5	36.2	34.0	32.0	30.2	28.6	27.1	25.7	24.4	23.2	22.0
15st 7	52.5	48.8	45.5	42.5	39.8	37.4	35.2	33.1	31.2	29.5	28.0	26.5	25.2	23.9	22.8
16st 0	54.2	50.4	47.0	43.9	41.1	38.6	36.3	34.2	32.3	30.5	28.9	27.4	26.0	24.7	23.5
16st 7	55.9	52.0	48.5	45.3	42.4	39.8	37.4	35.2	33.3	31.4	29.8	28.2	26.8	25.5	24.2
17st 0	57.6	53.6	49.9	46.6	43.7	41.0	38.6	36.3	34.3	32.4	30.7	29.1	27.6	26.2	25.0
17st 7	59.3	55.1	51.4	48.0	45.0	42.2	39.7	37.4	35.3	33.3	31.6	29.9	28.4	27.0	25.7
18st 0	61.0	56.7	52.9	49.4	46.3	43.4	40.8	38.5	36.3	34.3	32.5	30.8	29.2	27.8	26.4
18st 7	62.7	58.3	54.3	50.8	47.5	44.6	42.0	39.5	37.3	35.3	33.4	31.6	30.0	28.6	27.2
19st 0	64.4	59.9	55.8	52.1	48.8	45.8	43.1	40.6	38.3	36.2	34.3	32.5	30.8	29.3	27.9
19st 7	66.1	61.4	57.3	53.5	50.1	47.0	44.2	41.7	39.3	37.2	35.2	33.3	31.7	30.1	28.6
20st 0	67.8	63.0	58.7	54.9	51.4	48.2	45.4	42.7	40.3	38.1	36.1	34.2	32.5	30.9	29.4
20st 7	69.4	64.6	60.2	56.3	52.7	49.4	46.5	43.8	41.3	39.1	37.0	35.1	33.3	31.6	30.1
21st 0	71.1	66.2	61.7	57.6	54.0	50.6	47.6	44.9	42.3	40.0	37.9	35.9	34.1	32.4	30.9
21st 7	72.8	67.7	63.1	59.0	55.3	51.9	48.8	45.9	43.3	41.0	38.8	36.8	34.9	33.2	31.6
22st 0	74.5	69.3	64.6	60.4	56.5	53.1	49.9	47.0	44.4	41.9	39.7	37.6	35.7	34.0	32.3
22st 7	76.2	70.9	66.1	61.7	57.8	54.3	51.0	48.1	45.4	42.9	40.6	38.5	36.5	34.7	33.1
23st 0	77.9	72.5	67.5	63.1	59.1	55.5	52.2	49.1	46.4	43.8	41.5	39.3	37.3	35.5	33.8
23st 7	79.6	74.0	69.0	64.5	60.4	56.7	53.3	50.2	47.4	44.8	42.4	40.2	38.2	36.3	34.5
24st 0	81.3	75.6	70.5	65.9	61.7	57.9	54.4	51.3	48.4	45.7	43.3	41.0	39.0	37.0	35.3
24st 7	83.0	77.2	71.9	67.2	63.0	59.1	55.6	52.3	49.4	46.7	44.2	41.9	39.8	37.8	36.0
25st 0	84.7	78.8	73.4	68.6	64.2	60.3	56.7	53.4	50.4	47.6	45.1	42.8	40.6	38.6	36.7
25st 7	86.4	80.3	74.9	70.0	65.5	61.5	57.8	54.5	51.4	48.6	46.0	43.6	41.4	39.4	37.5
26st 0	88.1	81.9	76.3	71.3	66.8	62.7	59.0	55.5	52.4	49.5	46.9	44.5	42.2	40.1	38.2
26st 7	89.8	83.5	77.8	72.7	68.1	63.9	60.1	56.6	53.4	50.5	47.8	45.3	43.0	40.9	38.9
27st 0	91.5	85.1	79.3	74.1	69.4	65.1	61.2	57.7	54.4	51.5	48.7	46.2	43.8	41.7	39.7
27st 7	93.2	86.6	80.8	75.5	70.7	66.3	62.4	58.7	55.4	52.4	49.6	47.0	44.7	42.4	40.4
28st 0	94.9	88.2	82.2	76.8	72.0	67.5	63.5	59.8	56.4	53.4	50.5	47.9	45.5	43.2	41.1
28st 7	96.5	89.8	83.7	78.2	73.2	68.7	64.6	60.9	57.5	54.3	51.4	48.7	46.3	44.0	41.9
29st 0	98.2	91.4	85.2	79.6	74.5	69.9	65.8	62.0	58.5	55.3	52.3	49.6	47.1	44.8	42.6
29st 7	99.9	92.9	86.6	80.9	75.8	71.1	66.9	63.0	59.5	56.2	53.2	50.5	47.9	45.5	43.3

Weight Chart

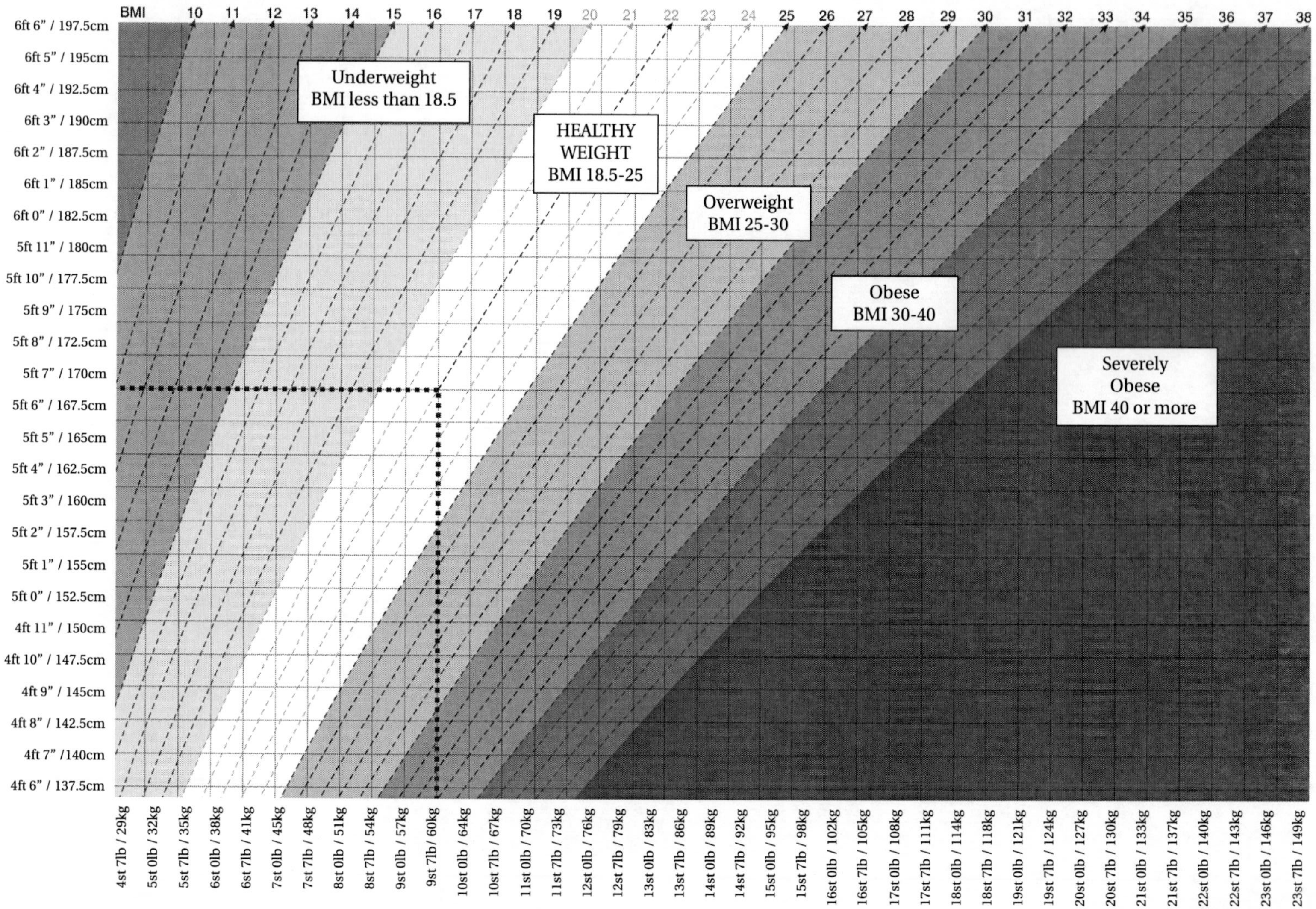

BMI 10 11 12 13 14 15 16 17 18 19 20 21 22 23 24 25 26 27 28 29 30 31 32 33 34 35 36 37 38

6ft 6" / 197.5cm
6ft 5" / 195cm
6ft 4" / 192.5cm
6ft 3" / 190cm
6ft 2" / 187.5cm
6ft 1" / 185cm
6ft 0" / 182.5cm
5ft 11" / 180cm
5ft 10" / 177.5cm
5ft 9" / 175cm
5ft 8" / 172.5cm
5ft 7" / 170cm
5ft 6" / 167.5cm
5ft 5" / 165cm
5ft 4" / 162.5cm
5ft 3" / 160cm
5ft 2" / 157.5cm
5ft 1" / 155cm
5ft 0" / 152.5cm
4ft 11" / 150cm
4ft 10" / 147.5cm
4ft 9" / 145cm
4ft 8" / 142.5cm
4ft 7" /140cm
4ft 6" / 137.5cm

Underweight
BMI less than 18.5

HEALTHY
WEIGHT
BMI 18.5-25

Overweight
BMI 25-30

Obese
BMI 30-40

Severely
Obese
BMI 40 or more

4st 7lb / 29kg
5st 0lb / 32kg
5st 7lb / 35kg
6st 0lb / 38kg
6st 7lb / 41kg
7st 0lb / 45kg
7st 7lb / 48kg
8st 0lb / 51kg
8st 7lb / 54kg
9st 0lb / 57kg
9st 7lb/ 60kg
10st 0lb / 64kg
10st 7lb / 67kg
11st 0lb / 70kg
11st 7lb / 73kg
12st 0lb / 76kg
12st 7lb / 79kg
13st 0lb / 83kg
13st 7lb / 86kg
14st 0lb / 89kg
14st 7lb / 92kg
15st 0lb / 95kg
15st 7lb / 98kg
16st 0lb / 102kg
16st 7lb / 105kg
17st 0lb / 108kg
17st 7lb / 111kg
18st 0lb / 114kg
18st 7lb / 118kg
19st 0lb / 121kg
19st 7lb / 124kg
20st 0lb / 127kg
20st 7lb / 130kg
21st 0lb / 133kg
21st 7lb / 137kg
22st 0lb / 140kg
22st 7lb / 143kg
23st 0lb / 146kg
23st 7lb / 149kg

Calories Required to Maintain Weight
Adult Females

ACTIVITY LEVEL / AGE

WEIGHT IN STONES / LBS	VERY SEDENTARY			MODERATELY SEDENTARY			MODERATELY ACTIVE			VERY ACTIVE		
	<30	30-60	60+	<30	30-60	60+	<30	30-60	60+	<30	30-60	60+
7st 7	1425	1473	1304	1544	1596	1412	1781	1841	1630	2138	2210	1956
8st 0	1481	1504	1338	1605	1629	1450	1852	1880	1673	2222	2256	2008
8st 7	1537	1535	1373	1666	1663	1487	1922	1919	1716	2306	2302	2059
9st 0	1594	1566	1407	1726	1696	1524	1992	1957	1759	2391	2349	2111
9st 7	1650	1596	1442	1787	1729	1562	2062	1996	1802	2475	2395	2163
10st 0	1706	1627	1476	1848	1763	1599	2133	2034	1845	2559	2441	2214
10st 7	1762	1658	1511	1909	1796	1637	2203	2073	1888	2644	2487	2266
11st 0	1819	1689	1545	1970	1830	1674	2273	2111	1931	2728	2534	2318
11st 7	1875	1720	1580	2031	1863	1711	2344	2150	1975	2813	2580	2370
12st 0	1931	1751	1614	2092	1897	1749	2414	2188	2018	2897	2626	2421
12st 7	1987	1781	1648	2153	1930	1786	2484	2227	2061	2981	2672	2473
13st 0	2044	1812	1683	2214	1963	1823	2555	2266	2104	3066	2719	2525
13st 7	2100	1843	1717	2275	1997	1861	2625	2304	2147	3150	2765	2576
14st 0	2156	1874	1752	2336	2030	1898	2695	2343	2190	3234	2811	2628
14st 7	2212	1905	1786	2397	2064	1935	2766	2381	2233	3319	2858	2680
15st 0	2269	1936	1821	2458	2097	1973	2836	2420	2276	3403	2904	2732
15st 7	2325	1967	1855	2519	2130	2010	2906	2458	2319	3488	2950	2783
16st 0	2381	1997	1890	2580	2164	2047	2976	2497	2362	3572	2996	2835
16st 7	2437	2028	1924	2640	2197	2085	3047	2535	2405	3656	3043	2887
17st 0	2494	2059	1959	2701	2231	2122	3117	2574	2449	3741	3089	2938
17st 7	2550	2090	1993	2762	2264	2159	3187	2613	2492	3825	3135	2990
18st 0	2606	2121	2028	2823	2298	2197	3258	2651	2535	3909	3181	3042
18st 7	2662	2152	2062	2884	2331	2234	3328	2690	2578	3994	3228	3093
19st 0	2719	2182	2097	2945	2364	2271	3398	2728	2621	4078	3274	3145
19st 7	2775	2213	2131	3006	2398	2309	3469	2767	2664	4162	3320	3197
20st 0	2831	2244	2166	3067	2431	2346	3539	2805	2707	4247	3366	3249
20st 7	2887	2275	2200	3128	2465	2383	3609	2844	2750	4331	3413	3300
21st 0	2944	2306	2235	3189	2498	2421	3680	2882	2793	4416	3459	3352
21st 7	3000	2337	2269	3250	2531	2458	3750	2921	2836	4500	3505	3404
22st 0	3056	2368	2303	3311	2565	2495	3820	2960	2879	4584	3552	3455
22st 7	3112	2398	2338	3372	2598	2533	3890	2998	2923	4669	3598	3507
23st 0	3169	2429	2372	3433	2632	2570	3961	3037	2966	4753	3644	3559
23st 7	3225	2460	2407	3494	2665	2608	4031	3075	3009	4837	3690	3611
24st 0	3281	2491	2441	3554	2699	2645	4101	3114	3052	4922	3737	3662
24st 7	3337	2522	2476	3615	2732	2682	4172	3152	3095	5006	3783	3714
25st 0	3394	2553	2510	3676	2765	2720	4242	3191	3138	5091	3829	3766
25st 7	3450	2583	2545	3737	2799	2757	4312	3229	3181	5175	3875	3817
26st 0	3506	2614	2579	3798	2832	2794	4383	3268	3224	5259	3922	3869
26st 7	3562	2645	2614	3859	2866	2832	4453	3307	3267	5344	3968	3921
27st 0	3618	2676	2648	3920	2899	2869	4523	3345	3310	5428	4014	3973
27st 7	3675	2707	2683	3981	2932	2906	4594	3384	3353	5512	4060	4024
28st 0	3731	2738	2717	4042	2966	2944	4664	3422	3397	5597	4107	4076
28st 7	3787	2768	2752	4103	2999	2981	4734	3461	3440	5681	4153	4128

Calories Required to Maintain Weight
Adult Males

ACTIVITY LEVEL / AGE

WEIGHT IN STONES / LBS	VERY SEDENTARY			MODERATELY SEDENTARY			MODERATELY ACTIVE			VERY ACTIVE		
	<30	30-60	60+	<30	30-60	60+	<30	30-60	60+	<30	30-60	60+
9st 0	1856	1827	1502	2010	1979	1627	2320	2284	1878	2784	2741	2254
9st 7	1913	1871	1547	2072	2026	1676	2391	2338	1933	2870	2806	2320
10st 0	1970	1914	1591	2134	2074	1724	2463	2393	1989	2955	2871	2387
10st 7	2027	1958	1636	2196	2121	1772	2534	2447	2045	3041	2937	2454
11st 0	2084	2001	1680	2258	2168	1820	2605	2502	2100	3127	3002	2520
11st 7	2141	2045	1724	2320	2215	1868	2677	2556	2156	3212	3067	2587
12st 0	2199	2088	1769	2382	2262	1916	2748	2611	2211	3298	3133	2654
12st 7	2256	2132	1813	2444	2310	1965	2820	2665	2267	3384	3198	2720
13st 0	2313	2175	1858	2506	2357	2013	2891	2719	2322	3470	3263	2787
13st 7	2370	2219	1902	2568	2404	2061	2963	2774	2378	3555	3329	2854
14st 0	2427	2262	1947	2630	2451	2109	3034	2828	2434	3641	3394	2920
14st 7	2484	2306	1991	2691	2498	2157	3106	2883	2489	3727	3459	2987
15st 0	2542	2350	2036	2753	2545	2205	3177	2937	2545	3813	3525	3054
15st 7	2599	2393	2080	2815	2593	2253	3248	2992	2600	3898	3590	3120
16st 0	2656	2437	2125	2877	2640	2302	3320	3046	2656	3984	3655	3187
16st 7	2713	2480	2169	2939	2687	2350	3391	3100	2711	4070	3721	3254
17st 0	2770	2524	2213	3001	2734	2398	3463	3155	2767	4155	3786	3320
17st 7	2827	2567	2258	3063	2781	2446	3534	3209	2823	4241	3851	3387
18st 0	2884	2611	2302	3125	2828	2494	3606	3264	2878	4327	3917	3454
18st 7	2942	2654	2347	3187	2876	2542	3677	3318	2934	4413	3982	3520
19st 0	2999	2698	2391	3249	2923	2591	3749	3373	2989	4498	4047	3587
19st 7	3056	2741	2436	3311	2970	2639	3820	3427	3045	4584	4112	3654
20st 0	3113	2785	2480	3373	3017	2687	3891	3481	3100	4670	4178	3721
20st 7	3170	2829	2525	3434	3064	2735	3963	3536	3156	4756	4243	3787
21st 0	3227	2872	2569	3496	3112	2783	4034	3590	3211	4841	4308	3854
21st 7	3285	2916	2614	3558	3159	2831	4106	3645	3267	4927	4374	3921
22st 0	3342	2959	2658	3620	3206	2880	4177	3699	3323	5013	4439	3987
22st 7	3399	3003	2702	3682	3253	2928	4249	3754	3378	5098	4504	4054
23st 0	3456	3046	2747	3744	3300	2976	4320	3808	3434	5184	4570	4121
23st 7	3513	3090	2791	3806	3347	3024	4392	3862	3489	5270	4635	4187
24st 0	3570	3133	2836	3868	3395	3072	4463	3917	3545	5356	4700	4254
24st 7	3627	3177	2880	3930	3442	3120	4534	3971	3600	5441	4766	4321
25st 0	3685	3220	2925	3992	3489	3168	4606	4026	3656	5527	4831	4387
25st 7	3742	3264	2969	4054	3536	3217	4677	4080	3712	5613	4896	4454
26st 0	3799	3308	3014	4116	3583	3265	4749	4135	3767	5699	4962	4521
26st 7	3856	3351	3058	4177	3630	3313	4820	4189	3823	5784	5027	4587
27st 0	3913	3395	3103	4239	3678	3361	4892	4243	3878	5870	5092	4654
27st 7	3970	3438	3147	4301	3725	3409	4963	4298	3934	5956	5158	4721
28st 0	4028	3482	3191	4363	3772	3457	5035	4352	3989	6042	5223	4787
28st 7	4085	3525	3236	4425	3819	3506	5106	4407	4045	6127	5288	4854
29st 0	4142	3569	3280	4487	3866	3554	5177	4461	4101	6213	5354	4921
29st 7	4199	3612	3325	4549	3913	3602	5249	4516	4156	6299	5419	4987
30st 0	4256	3656	3369	4611	3961	3650	5320	4570	4212	6384	5484	5054

Calories Burned in Exercise

This table shows the approximate number of extra* calories that would be burned in a five minute period of exercise activity.

ACTIVITY	CALORIES BURNED IN 5 MINUTES
Aerobics, Low Impact	*25*
Badminton, Recreational	*17*
Cross Trainer	*30*
Cycling, Recreational, 5mph	*17*
Dancing, Modern, Moderate	*13*
Fencing	*24*
Gardening, Weeding	*19*
Hill Walking, Up and Down, Recreational	*22*
Jogging	*30*
Kick Boxing	*30*
Netball Playing	*23*
Rebounding	*18*
Roller Skating	*30*
Rowing Machine, Moderate	*30*
Running, 7.5mph	*48*

ACTIVITY	CALORIES BURNED IN 5 MINUTES
Situps, Continuous	*17*
Skiing, Moderate	*30*
Skipping, Moderate	*30*
Squash Playing	*39*
Tennis Playing, Recreational	*26*
Toning Exercises	*17*
Trampolining	*17*
Volleyball, Recreational	*10*
Walking, Uphill, 15% Gradient, Moderate	*43*
Walking Up and Down Stairs, Moderate	*34*
Walking, 4mph	*24*
Weight Training, Moderate	*12*
Yoga	*13*

*Extra calories are those in addition to your normal daily calorie needs.

My Personal Plan

Date: ______ **Body Mass Index:** ______

Weight: ______ **Waist Measurement:** ______

Height: ______ **Body Fat % (if known)** ______

10% Weight Loss Goal: ______

Current weight	16stone (224lb)	100kg
- 10% weight	1stone 8½lb (22½lb)	10kg
= 10% loss goal	14stone 5½lb (201½lb)	90kg

My smaller weight targets on the way to achieving my 10% goal will be:

______ ______ ______ ______

Reasons why I want to lose weight:

______

Changes I will make to help me lose weight:

Diet: ______ **Activity:** ______

Potential saboteurs or barriers will be: ______ **Ways I will overcome these:** ______

My supporters will be:

______

I will monitor my progress by:

______

I will reward my progress with:

In the short term: ______ **In the long term:** ______

Food and Exercise Diary

Date:

/ /

Daily Calorie Allowance: (A)

Food/Drink Consumed	*Serving Size*	*Calories*

Total calories consumed (B)

Exercise/Activity	*No. mins*	*Calories*

Calories used in exercise (C)

Calorie balance (D)

You are aiming for your Calorie Balance (Box D) to be as close to zero as possible - ie. you consume the number of calories you need.

Your Daily Calorie Allowance (Box A) should be set to lose ½-2lb (¼-1kg) a week, or maintain weight, depending on your goals.

Daily Calorie Allowance (A) *plus* Extra Calories used in Exercise (C) *minus* Total Calories Consumed (B) *equals* Calorie Balance (D)

A + C - B = D

You can also write down any comments or thoughts related to your eating if you want to.

FOOD & EXERCISE DAILY DIARY AVAILABLE FROM www.weightlossresources.co.uk/shop

Food Information

Nutritional Information

CALORIE AND FAT values are given per serving, plus calorie and nutrition values per 100g of product. This makes it easy to compare the proportions of fat, protein, carbohydrate and fibre in each food.

The values given are for uncooked, unprepared foods unless otherwise stated. Values are also for only the edible portion of the food unless otherwise stated. ie - weighed with bone.

Finding Foods

The Calorie, Carb & Fat Bible has an Eating Out section which is arranged alphabetically by brand. In the General Foods and Drinks A-Z most foods are grouped together by type, and then put in to alphabetical order. This makes it easy to compare different brands, and will help you to find lower calorie and/or fat alternatives where they are available.

This format also makes it easier to locate foods. Foods are categorised by their main characteristics so, for example, if it is bread, ciabatta or white sliced, you'll find it under "Bread".

Basic ingredients are highlighted to make them easier to find at a glance. You'll find all unbranded foods in bold - making the index easier to use, whether it's just an apple or all the components of a home cooked stew.

There are, however, some foods which are not so easy to categorise, especially combination foods like ready meals. The following pointers will help you to find your way around the book until you get to know it a little better.

FILLED ROLLS AND SANDWICHES - Bagels, baguettes, etc which are filled are listed as "Bagels (filled)" etc. Sandwiches are under "Sandwiches".

CURRIES - Popular types of curry, like Balti or Jalfrezi, are listed under their individual types. Unspecified or lesser known types are listed under their main ingredient.

BURGERS - All burgers from fast-food outlets are listed under "Burgers".

CHIPS & FRIES - Are listed separately, depending on the name of the particular brand. All other types of potato are listed under "Potatoes".

SWEETS & CHOCOLATES - Well-known brands, eg. Aero, Mars Bar, are listed under their brand names. Others are listed under "Chocolate" (for bars) and "Chocolates" (for individual sweets).

READY MEALS - Popular types of dishes are listed under their type, eg. "Chow Mein", "Casserole", "Hot Pot", etc. Others are listed by their main ingredient, eg. "Chicken With", "Chicken In", etc.

EATING OUT & FAST FOODS - By popular demand this edition has the major eating out and fast food brands listed separately, at the back of the book. They are alphabetised first by brand, then follow using the same format as the rest of the book, with calories provided per serving.

Serving Sizes

Many ready-meal type foods are given with calories for the full pack size, so that an individual serving can be worked out by estimating the proportion of the pack that has been consumed. For example, if you have eaten a quarter of a packaged pasta dish, divide the calorie value given for the whole pack by 4 to determine the number of calories you have consumed. Where serving sizes are not appropriate, or unknown, values are given per 100g and per 1oz/28g. Serving sizes vary greatly from person to person and, if you are trying to lose weight, it's important to be accurate – especially with high calorie foods such as those that contain a fair amount of fat, sugar, cream, cheese, alcohol etc.

Food Data

Nutrition information for basic average foods has been compiled by the Weight Loss Resources food data team using many sources of information to calculate the most accurate values possible. Some nutrition information for non-branded food records is from The Composition of Foods 6th Edition. Reproduced under licence from The Controller of Her Majesty's Stationary Office. Where basic data is present for ordinary foodstuffs such as 'raw carrots'; branded records are not included.

Nutrition information for branded goods is from details supplied by retailers and manufacturers, and researched by Weight Loss Resources staff. The Calorie Carb & Fat Bible contains data for over 1400 UK brands, including major supermarkets and fast food outlets.

The publishers gratefully acknowledge all the manufacturers and retailers who have provided information on their products.

Calorie & nutrition data for all food and drink items are typical values.

Caution

The information in The Calorie, Carb and Fat Bible is intended as an aid to weight loss and weight maintenance, and is not medical advice. If you suffer from, or think you may suffer from a medical condition you should consult your doctor before starting a weight loss and/or exercise regime. If you start exercising after a period of relative inactivity, you should start slowly and consult your doctor if you experience pain, distress or other symptoms.

Weights, Measures & Abbreviations

ABBREVIATIONS	
kcal	*kilocalories / calories*
prot	*protein*
carb	*carbohydrate*
sm	*small*
med	*medium*
av	*average*
reg	*regular*
lge	*large*
tsp	*teaspoon*
tbsp	*tablespoon*
dtsp	*dessertspoon*
gf	*gluten free*

BRAND ABBREVIATIONS USED	
ASDA	
Good for You	*GFY*
Chosen by You	*CBY*
Good & Counted	*G&C*
MARKS & SPENCER	*M & S*
Count on Us	*COU*
Balanced For You	*BFY*
MORRISONS	
Better For You	*BFY*
SAINSBURY'S	
Be Good to Yourself	*BGTY*
Way to Five	*WTF*
Taste the Difference	*TTD*
TESCO	
Healthy Eating	*HE*
Healthy Living	*HL*
Hearty Food Co	*HFC*
Light Choices	*LC*
WAITROSE	
Perfectly Balanced	*PB*
Cambridge Weight Plan	*CWP*

	Measure INFO/WEIGHT	per Measure KCAL	FAT	Nutrition Values per 100g / 100ml KCAL	PROT	CARB	FAT	FIBRE
ABSINTHE								
Average	***1 Pub Shot/35ml***	***127***	***0***	***363***	***0***	***38.8***	***0***	***0***
ACKEE								
Canned, Drained, Average	***1oz/28g***	***43***	***4.3***	***151***	***2.9***	***0.8***	***15.2***	***0***
ADVOCAAT								
Average	***1 Pub Shot/35ml***	***91***	***2.2***	***260***	***4.7***	***28.4***	***6.3***	***0***
AERO								
Bliss, Milk Chocolate, Aero, Nestle*	1 Piece/8g	46	2.7	545	7.2	56.9	31.6	1.7
Bliss, Praline, Aero, Nestle*	1 Piece/8g	44	2.8	568	6.3	53.2	36.2	1.9
Bliss, Salted Caramel, Aero, Nestle*	1 Piece/8g	43	2.4	537	7.4	58	30.2	1.4
Creamy White Centre, Nestle*	1 Bar/46g	244	13.8	530	7.6	57.4	30	0
Festive Caramel, Sharing Bar, Aero, Nestle*	4 Pieces/14g	74	4.2	532	6.8	57.2	30.1	1.9
Honeycomb, Nestle*	1 Bar/40g	199	10	497	5.9	62.2	25	0
Milk Chocolate, Bubbles, Sharing Bag, Aero, Nestle*	1 Bag/113g	610	34.7	540	6.5	57.8	30.7	0
Milk, Giant, Bar, Nestle*	1 Bar/125g	674	38.6	539	6.6	57.7	30.9	2.2
Milk, Medium, Bar, Nestle*	1 Bar/43g	232	13.3	539	6.6	57.7	30.9	2.2
Milk, Purely Chocolate, Aero*	1 Bar/37g	197	11.2	538	6.8	57.8	30.5	1.9
Milk, Snacksize, Bar, Nestle*	1 Bar/21g	110	6.5	537	6.6	55.9	31.9	2.2
Mint, Bubbles, Aero, Nestle*	1 Bubble/3g	16	0.9	533	4.4	62.7	29.1	0.8
Mint, Nestle*	1 Bar/41g	218	11.9	531	5.4	61.6	28.9	1.1
Mint, Snack Size, Nestle*	1 Bar/21g	112	6.7	548	7.7	55.3	32.8	0.9
Mint, Standard, Aero, Nestle*	1 Bar/43g	233	13.2	542	5.2	60.5	30.8	0.9
Orange, Bubbles, Aero, Nestle*	1 Bubble/3g	16	0.9	538	5.4	60.5	30	1.4
Orange, Nestle*	6 Squares/22g	119	6.8	542	5.1	60.7	30.7	0.9
Peppermint, Bar, Nestle*	1 Bar/37g	199	11.1	537	5.1	61	30	1
ALCOPOPS								
Smirnoff Apple Bite, Frozen, Smirnoff*	1 Pint/568ml	523	0	92	0	15	0	0
Smirnoff Ice, Smirnoff*	1 Bottle/275ml	188	0	68	1.8	12	0	0
ALFALFA SPROUTS								
Raw, Average	***1 Serving/33g***	***8***	***0.3***	***24***	***3***	***3***	***0.9***	***3***
ALLSPICE								
Ground, Schwartz*	1 Tsp/3g	11	0.1	358	6.1	74.3	4	0
ALMONDS								
Blanched, Average	***1 Serving/100g***	***617***	***54.3***	***617***	***25.1***	***6.9***	***54.3***	***8.1***
Candied, Sugared	***1 Serving/100g***	***458***	***16.3***	***458***	***8.4***	***69.2***	***16.3***	***2.2***
Chocolate Covers, Milk, 40%, Hotel Chocolat*	1 Serving/26g	145	9.4	557	10.7	46.3	36.3	4.7
Flaked, Average	***1oz/28g***	***172***	***15.2***	***613***	***24.9***	***6.5***	***54.3***	***7.6***
Flaked, Toasted, Average	***1oz/28g***	***176***	***15.8***	***629***	***24.6***	***5.8***	***56.4***	***7.5***
Grape Tree*	1 Serving/25g	155	14.2	621	21	7	57	12.2
Ground, Average	***1 Serving/10g***	***62***	***5.6***	***625***	***24***	***6.6***	***55.8***	***7.4***
Hickory, Smokey, Co-Op*	1 Pack/40g	254	22	634	24	7.7	55	6.2
Marcona, Average	***1 Serving/100g***	***608***	***53.7***	***608***	***22.1***	***13***	***53.7***	***9.7***
Paste, Roasted, Alnatura*	1 Tsp/5g	30	2.4	607	19	21	47	12
Roasted, Salted, Tesco*	1 Serving/25g	158	13.6	631	25.3	5	54.5	9.7
Toasted, Average	***1oz/28g***	***178***	***15.8***	***634***	***25***	***6.6***	***56.4***	***6.6***
Whole, Average	***1 Serving/20g***	***122***	***11***	***612***	***23.4***	***6.9***	***54.8***	***8.4***
Yoghurt Coated, Holland & Barrett*	1 Pack/100g	536	37	536	10.9	45.3	37	2.8
ALOO								
Bombay, M&S*	1 Serving/100g	81	2.7	81	1.4	11.8	2.7	2
Gobi, Slimming World, Iceland*	1 Pack/350g	150	1.4	43	1.7	7.2	0.4	2.1
Puri, Kazifarms Kitchen*	1 Puri/45g	100	0.5	222	9	43.9	1.2	0
Saag, Gobi, Side, Asda*	½ Pack/148g	114	5.3	77	2.4	7.6	3.6	2.4
Saag, Gobi, Takeaway, Microwaved, Morrisons*	½ Pack/105g	88	3.6	84	2	9.5	3.4	3.9
Saag, Gobi, Waitrose*	½ Pack/150g	129	8.2	86	2	6	5.5	2.4

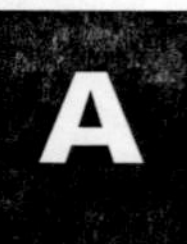

	Measure INFO/WEIGHT	per Measure KCAL	FAT	Nutrition Values per 100g / 100ml KCAL	PROT	CARB	FAT	FIBRE
ALOO								
Saag, Indian, Serves 2, Sainsbury's*	1 Pack/300g	216	10.5	72	2	7	3.5	2.2
Saag, Jane Plan*	1 Pack/300g	270	10.5	90	1.8	11.4	3.5	2.6
Saag, Tesco*	1 Serving/200g	144	7	72	2.1	8	3.5	2
Tikki, Average	***1 Serving/25g***	***48***	***2***	***191***	***4.5***	***25.2***	***8***	***3.5***
AMARANTH								
Seed, Holland & Barrett*	1 Tbsp/15g	56	1	371	14	55	7	6.5
ANCHOVIES								
in Oil, Canned, Drained	***1 Anchovy/4g***	***8***	***0.5***	***195***	***23.4***	***0***	***11.3***	***0***
Marinated, with Peppers, & Kalamata Olives, Tesco*	½ Pack/35g	84	6.7	239	15.1	1	19.2	0.8
ANGEL DELIGHT								
Chocolate Flavour, Kraft*	1 Sachet/67g	305	12.1	455	3.7	69.5	18	0.4
Strawberry Flavour, Kraft*	1 Sachet/59g	286	12.4	485	2.5	71	21	0
Vanilla Ice Cream Flavour, Kraft*	1 Sachet/59g	289	12.7	490	2.5	71.5	21.5	0
ANGEL HAIR								
Pasta, Dry	***1 Serving/50g***	***181***	***1.1***	***362***	***12.4***	***73.6***	***2.2***	***4.4***
ANTIPASTI								
& Olive, Selection, The Deli, Aldi*	½ Pack/85g	122	11.9	144	1.2	1.3	14	3.6
in Oil, Grilled, Cucina, Aldi*	¼ Jar/43g	41	3.7	96	1.1	2.3	8.6	2.2
Mixed, in Olive Oil, Extra Virgin, Drained, M&S*	¼ Jar/40g	76	7	191	1.3	4.8	17.5	4.3
Roasted Aubergine, Mezze, Belazu*	1 Serving/55g	76	7.4	138	0.6	2.9	13.4	1
ANTIPASTO								
Artichoke, Sainsbury's*	1 Serving/70g	141	10.2	202	28	12.5	14.6	4.8
Mixed Mushroom, Sainsbury's*	¼ Jar/72g	70	6.5	97	2.7	1.4	9	3.7
Mixed Pepper, Sainsbury's*	½ Jar/140g	48	1.8	34	1.3	4.2	1.3	3.5
Parma, Salami Milano, Bresaola, Finest, Tesco*	¼ Pack/30g	104	7.9	345	26.4	0.5	26.3	0
Roasted Pepper, Drained, Tesco*	1 Jar /170g	128	9.4	75	0.9	5.5	5.5	4.1
APPLES								
Bites, Average	***1 Pack/118g***	***58***	***0.1***	***49***	***0.3***	***11.6***	***0.1***	***2.2***
Braeburn, Average	***1 Apple/123g***	***58***	***0***	***47***	***0.3***	***12.9***	***0***	***2.9***
Cameo, Average	***1 Apple/125g***	***70***	***0***	***56***	***0***	***13.6***	***0***	***2.4***
Chocolate, Fosters*	1 Apple/140g	51	0.3	36	0	10	0.2	0
Cooking, Baked with Sugar, Flesh Only, Average	***1 Serving/140g***	***104***	***0.1***	***74***	***0.5***	***19.2***	***0.1***	***1.7***
Cooking, Raw, Peeled, Average	***1oz/28g***	***10***	***0***	***35***	***0.3***	***8.9***	***0.1***	***1.6***
Cooking, Stewed with Sugar, Average	***1 Serving/140g***	***104***	***0.1***	***74***	***0.3***	***19.1***	***0.1***	***1.2***
Cooking, Stewed without Sugar, Average	***1 Serving/140g***	***46***	***0.1***	***33***	***0.3***	***8.1***	***0.1***	***1.5***
Cox, English, Average	***1 Apple/123g***	***53***	***0.1***	***43***	***0.4***	***10.2***	***0.1***	***1.8***
Discovery, Average	***1 Apple/182g***	***82***	***0.9***	***45***	***0.4***	***10.6***	***0.5***	***1***
Dried, Average	***1 Pack/250g***	***537***	***0.7***	***215***	***0.8***	***52.8***	***0.3***	***5.9***
Empire, Average	***1 Apple/120g***	***52***	***0.1***	***44***	***0.4***	***10.7***	***0.1***	***1.8***
Fuji	***1 Apple/132g***	***64***	***0.1***	***48***	***0.4***	***11.8***	***0.1***	***1.8***
Gala, Average	***1 Apple/152g***	***66***	***0.2***	***43***	***0.3***	***10.4***	***0.1***	***1.4***
Golden Delicious, Average	***1 Med/102g***	***44***	***0.1***	***43***	***0.3***	***10.1***	***0.1***	***1.6***
Granny Smith, Average	***1 Sm/125g***	***56***	***0.1***	***45***	***0.3***	***10.7***	***0.1***	***1.8***
Green, Raw, Average	***1 Med/182g***	***86***	***0.2***	***48***	***0.4***	***11.3***	***0.1***	***1.8***
Jazz, Tesco*	1 Apple/133g	70	0.1	53	0.4	11.8	0.1	1.8
Kanzi, Tesco*	1 Apple/134g	71	0.1	53	0.4	11.8	0.1	1.8
Mackintosh, Red, Average	***1 Apple/165g***	***81***	***0.5***	***49***	***0.2***	***12.8***	***0.3***	***1.8***
Pink Lady, Average	***1 Apple/125g***	***56***	***0.1***	***45***	***0.4***	***10.6***	***0.1***	***1.9***
Puree, Biona Organic*	1 Serving/100g	48	0.1	48	0.2	10.5	0.1	1.5
Red, Average	***1 Med/149g***	***71***	***0.2***	***48***	***0.3***	***11.8***	***0.1***	***2***
Sliced, Average	***1oz/28g***	***14***	***0***	***49***	***0.4***	***11.6***	***0.1***	***1.8***
APPLETISER*								
Juice Drink, Sparkling, Appletiser, Coca-Cola*	1 Glass/200ml	94	0	47	0	11	0	0.4

	Measure INFO/WEIGHT	per Measure KCAL	FAT	Nutrition Values per 100g / 100ml KCAL	PROT	CARB	FAT	FIBRE
APRICOTS								
Canned, in Syrup, Average	***1oz/28g***	***18***	***0***	***63***	***0.4***	***16.1***	***0.1***	***0.9***
Dried, Average	***1 Apricot/10g***	***17***	***0.1***	***171***	***3.6***	***37.4***	***0.5***	***6.3***
Dried, Soft, Average	***1 Serving/50g***	***104***	***0.2***	***208***	***2.4***	***48.5***	***0.4***	***5.2***
Halves, in Fruit Juice, Average	***1 Can/221g***	***87***	***0.1***	***40***	***0.5***	***9.2***	***0.1***	***1***
Milk Chocolate Coated, Graze*	1 Pack/35g	158	8.6	450	6.1	55.9	24.7	5
Raw, Flesh Only, Average	***1 Apricot/37g***	***19***	***0.2***	***52***	***1.5***	***12***	***0.4***	***2.2***
Raw, Weighed with Stone, Average	***1 Apricot/40g***	***19***	***0.2***	***47***	***1.4***	***10.8***	***0.4***	***1.9***
AQUAFABA								
Average	***1 Tbsp/15ml***	***3***	***0***	***18***	***1***	***2.9***	***0.2***	***0***
ARANCINI								
Mushroom, Chef Select, Lidl*	1 Arancini/29g	70	3.3	242	6.1	27	11.4	2.1
Mushroom, Taste of Italy, Tesco*	1 Arancini/30g	68	2.8	226	5.2	28.9	9.4	2.6
Mushroom, Vegetarian, Waitrose*	1 Arancini/50g	116	5	233	6.2	28.8	9.9	2.1
ARCHERS*								
Aqua, Peach, Archers*	1 Bottle/275ml	206	0	75	0.3	7.7	0	0
Peach (Calculated Estimate), Archers*	1 Shot/35ml	91	0	260	0	0	0	0
ARTICHOKE								
Chargrilled, in Olive Oil, Cooks Ingredients, Waitrose*	1 Serving/30g	54	4.9	134	1.7	2.7	12.3	2.7
Chargrilled, Italian, Drained, Sainsbury's*	1/3 Tub/43g	40	2.7	92	3.1	2.8	6.1	6.5
Fresh, Raw, Average	***1oz/28g***	***13***	***0***	***47***	***3.3***	***10.5***	***0.2***	***5.4***
Hearts, Canned, Drained, Average	***½ Can/117g***	***35***	***0.1***	***30***	***1.9***	***5.4***	***0***	***2.2***
Hearts, Marinated & Grilled, Waitrose*	1 Serving/50g	57	5	114	3	3	10	3
in Oil, Tesco*	1 Piece/15g	17	1.5	115	1.9	2.4	10	4
Marinated, Roasted, M&S*	1 Pack/200g	300	26.6	150	1.9	5	13.3	2.3
ASPARAGUS								
Boiled, in Salted Water, Average	***5 Spears/125g***	***28***	***0.3***	***22***	***2.4***	***4.1***	***0.2***	***2***
British with Butter, Tesco*	1 Serving/50g	26	2	52	2.6	1.6	4	2
Canned, Average	***1 Can/250g***	***41***	***0.4***	***16***	***2***	***1.8***	***0.2***	***1.4***
Trimmed, Raw, Average	***1 Serving/80g***	***20***	***0.4***	***24***	***2.9***	***1.9***	***0.6***	***1.7***
White, Raw, Average	***1 Spear/17g***	***3***	***0***	***17***	***1***	***2.5***	***0.3***	***1***
AUBERGINE								
Baked Topped, M&S*	1 Serving/150g	165	11.6	110	2.4	7.4	7.7	0.9
Bruschetta, Antipasti, Tesco*	½ Jar/95g	200	17.9	210	3.2	5.7	18.8	2.8
Canned, in Tomato Sauce, Palirria*	¼ Can/140g	189	16.2	135	1.3	4.4	11.6	3.3
Fried, Average	***1oz/28g***	***85***	***8.9***	***302***	***1.2***	***2.8***	***31.9***	***2.3***
Marinated & Grilled, Waitrose*	½ Pack/100g	106	10	106	1	3	10	2
Parmigiana di Melanzane, Cook*	1 Pack/310g	477	35.6	154	4.7	6.9	11.5	1.9
Parmigiana, Donald Russell*	1 Pack/300g	657	59.4	219	6.4	4	19.8	1.2
Parmigiana, Gino D'Acampo*	1 Pack/425g	450	28	106	4.2	6.1	6.6	2.1
Parmigiana, M&S*	1 Pack/350g	332	18.6	95	4.6	7.6	5.3	1.1
Raw, Fresh, Average	***1 Sm/250g***	***36***	***1***	***14***	***0.9***	***2.1***	***0.4***	***1.9***
Steaks, Chargrilled, in Asian Sauce, Sainsbury's*	1 Steak/177g	156	7.6	88	1.1	10.3	4.3	2.1
AVOCADO								
Breakfast, Holy Moly*	1 Serving/30g	45	4.5	151	2	9	15	7
Flesh Only, Average	***1 Med/145g***	***276***	***28.3***	***190***	***1.9***	***1.9***	***19.5***	***3.4***
Smash, Morrisons*	1 Pot/150g	222	19.5	148	1.5	3.5	13	5.4
Smashed, Aldi*	1 Serving/100g	213	21	213	1.9	0.6	21	6.6
Smashed, M&S*	½ Pack/100g	140	9.7	140	2.5	9.8	9.7	1.8
Smashed, Pure, Holy Moly*	¼ Pot/40g	64	6.4	160	2	9	16	7
Smashed, Touch of Lime, Tesco*	½ Pot/100g	189	16.7	189	1.5	6.5	16.7	3.6

	Measure INFO/WEIGHT	per Measure KCAL	per Measure FAT	Nutrition Values per 100g / 100ml KCAL	PROT	CARB	FAT	FIBRE
BABY FOOD								
Peaches, & Bananas, Ella's Kitchen*	1 Pouch/120g	75	0.5	62	0.8	13.9	0.4	1.3
BACARDI*								
& Diet Cola, Bacardi*	1 Bottle/275ml	85	0	31	0	1	0	0
37.5% Volume, Bacardi*	1 Pub Shot/35ml	72	0	207	0	0	0	0
40% Volume, Bacardi*	1 Pub Shot/35ml	78	0	222	0	0	0	0
Breezer, Cranberry, Bacardi*	1 Bottle/275ml	154	0	56	0	7.1	0	0
Breezer, Lime, Bacardi*	1 Bottle/275ml	182	0	66	0	9.1	0	0
BACON								
Back, Dry Cured, Average	1 Rasher/31g	77	4.7	250	28.1	0.3	15.1	0.3
Back, Dry Fried or Grilled, Average	1 Rasher/25g	72	5.4	287	23.2	0	21.6	0
Back, Lean, Average	1 Rasher/33g	57	4	174	16.3	0.1	12	0.5
Back, Smoked, Average	1 Rasher/25g	66	5	265	20.9	0	19.9	0
Back, Smoked, Lean, Average	1 Rasher/25g	41	1.2	163	28.2	1.1	5	0.2
Back, Smoked, Rindless, Average	1 Rasher/25g	60	4.3	241	21	0.1	17.4	0
Back, Unsmoked, Average	1 Rasher/32g	78	5.5	242	21.3	0.4	17.3	0
Back, Unsmoked, Rindless, Average	1 Rasher/23g	56	3.9	241	22.5	0	16.9	0
Bits, Average	1oz/28g	75	5.9	268	18.6	0.7	21.2	0.1
Chops, Average	1oz/28g	62	4.2	222	22.3	0	14.8	0
Collar Joint, Lean & Fat, Boiled	1oz/28g	91	7.6	325	20.4	0	27	0
Collar Joint, Lean & Fat, Raw	1oz/28g	81	7.4	290	13.3	0	26.3	0
Collar Joint, Lean Only, Boiled	1oz/28g	53	2.7	191	26	0	9.7	0
Fat Only, Cooked, Average	1oz/28g	194	20.4	692	9.3	0	72.8	0
Fat Only, Raw, Average	1oz/28g	209	22.7	747	4.8	0	80.9	0
Gammon Rasher, Lean Only, Grilled	1oz/28g	48	1.5	172	31.4	0	5.2	0
Lardons, Lean, Oakpark*	1 Pack/130g	169	8.1	130	16.5	1.9	6.2	0.5
Lardons, Smoked, Dry Cured, Free Range, M&S*	1 Serving/100g	312	26.4	312	17.2	1.5	26.4	0.5
Lean Only, Fried, Average	1 Rasher/25g	83	5.6	332	32.8	0	22.3	0
Lean Only, Grilled, Average	1 Rasher/25g	73	4.7	292	30.5	0	18.9	0
Lean, Average	1 Rasher/33g	47	2.2	142	19.6	0.9	6.7	0.2
Loin Steaks, Grilled, Average	1 Serving/120g	229	11.6	191	25.9	0	9.7	0
Medallions, Average	1 Rasher/18g	27	0.6	151	29.4	0.9	3.3	0.1
Middle, Fried	1 Rasher/40g	140	11.4	350	23.4	0	28.5	0
Middle, Grilled	1 Rasher/40g	123	9.2	307	24.8	0	23.1	0
Middle, Raw	1 Rasher/43g	95	7.9	222	14	0	18.4	0
Plant Based, Pieces, Vivera*	½ Pack/88g	83	0.4	95	15	5.9	0.5	4
Plant Based, Smoked, Streaky, Mini, Miami Burger*	1 Serving/25g	42	0.2	167	25	14	1	1
Plant Based, Unsmoked, Naked , Finnebrogue*	2 Rashers/36g	72	4.6	200	10	6.8	12.7	8.9
Rashers, Lean Only, Trimmed, Average	1 Rasher/20g	24	0.8	119	20.6	0	4	0
Smoked, Crispy, Cooked, Average	1 Serving/10g	46	2.7	460	53	2.1	26.9	0
Streaky, Cooked, Average	1 Rasher/20g	68	5.6	342	22.4	0.3	27.8	0
Vegan, Pieces, Vivera*	½ Pack/88g	81	0.4	92	18	1.9	0.4	6
Vegan, Thick Cut, Pan Fried, V Taste, Morrisons*	1 Rasher/12g	40	2.3	339	27	13.1	19.2	2.7
Vegan, Vacon, Smoky, Plant Pioneers, Sainsbury's*	4 Rashers/44g	153	9.3	347	24.5	12.7	21.1	4.2
Vegetarian, Rashers	1 Rasher/16g	33	1.7	206	19.5	8.6	10.4	2.8
BAGUETTE								
Beef, & Horseradish, Freshly Prepared, M&S*	1 Baguette/274g	795	31	290	12.1	37.2	11.3	2
Bistro, Tomate, Fromage, Dr Oetker*	1 Baguette/125g	288	10.9	230	7.3	29	8.7	0
Cheese, & Ham, Average	1 Baguette/203g	593	20.8	292	14	35.9	10.3	1.4
Cheese, & Onion, Asda*	¼ Loaf/42g	154	7.4	366	12	39.8	17.6	1.3
Cheese, & Tomato, Tesco*	1 Baguette/108g	243	8.3	225	9.7	29.3	7.7	1.8
Cheese, Mixed, & Spring Onion, Asda*	1 Pack/190g	629	34.8	331	9.5	32.1	18.3	1.3
Chicken, & Stuffing, Hot, Sainsbury's*	1 Baguette/227g	543	16.3	239	13.7	29.6	7.2	0
Chicken, & Salad, Asda*	1 Serving/158g	326	9.5	206	9	29	6	2.1

	Measure INFO/WEIGHT	per Measure KCAL	FAT	Nutrition Values per 100g / 100ml KCAL	PROT	CARB	FAT	FIBRE
BAGUETTE								
Chicken, Tikka, Asda*	1 Pack/190g	439	17.9	231	10.4	32.8	9.4	1.3
Garlic, & Herb, Reduced Fat, Asda*	¼ Baguette /55g	141	3.2	257	7.9	42	5.9	1.5
Garlic, Essential, Waitrose*	1 Baguette/210g	706	34.9	336	6.8	38.8	16.6	2.4
Ham, & Turkey, Asda*	1 Baguette/360g	774	18.4	215	11.6	30.7	5.1	1.3
Ham, & Cheese, Freshly Prepared, M&S*	1 Baguette/231g	555	11.3	240	13.4	35.9	4.9	2.4
Multi Grain, Rustic, Tesco*	1 Slice/35g	96	1.2	275	11.8	47.8	3.3	3.6
Pepperoni, Pizza, Morrisons*	1 Baguette/120g	272	8.8	227	10.2	28.8	7.3	2.7
Prawn Mayonnaise, Asda*	1 Pack/190g	399	9.3	210	9.1	32.5	4.9	1.3
Salmon, Smoked, & Egg, Freshly Prepared	***1 Baguette/178g***	***455***	***17.3***	***255***	***13.7***	***28.4***	***9.7***	***1.6***
Sourdough, GF, Promise*	1 Baguette /90g	182	1.6	202	5.2	35	1.8	12.7
Steak, & Onion, Snack 'n' Go, Sainsbury's*	1 Baguette/177g	398	8.8	225	14.3	30.6	5	2.2
Stone, Oven Baked, La Boulangere*	½ Baguette/125g	320	1.9	256	8.4	51	1.5	2.6
BAILEYS*								
Almande, Dairy Free, Baileys*	1 Serving/25ml	10	0.2	38	0.6	3.1	0.8	0
Irish Cream, Original, Baileys*	1 Serving/50ml	164	6.5	327	3	25	13	0
BAKE								
Aubergine, & Grain, Moroccan Inspired, Waitrose*	½ Pack/189g	151	8.3	80	1.3	6.9	4.4	3.7
Aubergine, & Mozzarella Cheese, TTD, Sainsbury's*	1 Pack/326g	342	17.3	105	3.3	9.9	5.3	3.4
Broccoli, & Cheese, Asda*	1 Bake/132g	269	15.4	204	5.3	19.3	11.7	2.5
Broccoli, & Cheese, M&S*	1 Pack/400g	480	31.2	120	6.5	5.4	7.8	1.6
Cheese, & Onion, Greggs, Iceland*	1 Bake/141g	437	29.6	310	6.1	23	21	0
Cheese, & Onion, Tesco*	1 Bake/110g	332	17	302	7.8	31.8	15.5	2.3
Chicken, & Ham, M&S*	1 Pack/400g	560	26.8	140	10.3	9.1	6.7	0.9
Chicken, BBQ, Tesco*	1 Bake/131g	348	16	266	9.1	29.2	12.2	1.4
Chicken, Creamy, Morrisons*	1 Bake/125g	367	22.2	294	9.3	23.1	17.8	2
Chicken, Creamy, Tesco*	1 Bake/131g	308	12.3	235	9	27.7	9.4	1.7
Fruit, Strawberry, Bar, Sainsbury's*	1 Bar/35g	127	2.6	362	2.6	67.8	7.4	6.9
Haddock, Average	***1 Serving/400g***	***312***	***9.2***	***78***	***6.4***	***8***	***2.3***	***0.9***
Jackfruit, BBQ, Jackbake, Plant Chef, Tesco*	1 Pack/398g	358	7.2	90	1.9	14.5	1.8	4.3
Lentil, Spiced, Vegetarian, TTD, Sainsbury's*	1 Bake/132g	245	8.4	186	4.8	27.3	6.4	4.2
Mushroom, Rice, Vegetarian, Tesco*	1 Bake/133g	264	11.3	199	5.4	23.6	8.5	3
Steak, Tesco*	1 Bake/131g	296	10.5	226	9.5	28	8	2
Vegetable, Mediterranean, Cooked, CBY, Asda*	1 Bake/120g	279	13.2	232	8.4	22.8	11	4.2
BAKING POWDER								
Average	***1 Tsp/2g***	***3***	***0***	***163***	***5.2***	***37.8***	***0***	***0***
BAKLAVA								
Average	***2 Pieces/50g***	***239***	***14.2***	***478***	***8***	***47.4***	***28.4***	***2.8***
BALTI								
Chicken, Asda*	1 Pack/400g	400	19.6	100	11	2.5	4.9	1.7
Chicken, Canned, Sainsbury's*	½ Pack/200g	192	7.4	96	11	3.3	3.7	2.8
Chicken, Garlic, Chilli, Takeaway, Iceland*	1 Pack/343g	446	24	130	11.1	4.9	7	1.5
Chickpea & Spinach, Cauldron Foods*	1 Pack/400g	356	8	89	2.3	15.5	2	1
Lamb, Bhuna, Tesco*	1 Pack/400g	360	14.8	90	9.2	4.8	3.7	1.1
Prawn, Budgens*	1 Pack/350g	374	24.8	107	5.6	5.2	7.1	1.3
Vegetable, Average	***1 Serving/200g***	***182***	***8.3***	***91***	***1.9***	***11.3***	***4.1***	***1.7***
BAMBOO SHOOTS								
Canned, Average	***1 Sm Can/120g***	***10***	***0.1***	***8***	***1***	***0.8***	***0.1***	***0.8***
BANANA								
Chips, Average	***1oz/28g***	***143***	***8.8***	***511***	***1***	***59.9***	***31.4***	***1.7***
Green, Medium, Average	***1 Sm/101g***	***91***	***0***	***90***	***1***	***23***	***0***	***3***
Raw, Flesh Only, Average	***1 Med/118g***	***105***	***0.4***	***89***	***1.1***	***22.8***	***0.3***	***2.6***
BARLEY								
Canned, in Water, Drained, Napolina*	1 Can/240g	122	0.2	51	1.7	10	0.1	1.9

	Measure INFO/WEIGHT	per Measure KCAL	FAT	Nutrition Values per 100g / 100ml KCAL	PROT	CARB	FAT	FIBRE
BARLEY								
Mix, Pearl, Peas, & Lentils, Cooked, Sainsbury's*	1 Serving/75g	83	0.4	110	6.9	17.3	0.5	5.8
Pot, Raw, Average	***1 Serving/60g***	***212***	***1.4***	***354***	***12.5***	***73.5***	***2.3***	***17.3***
Quick Cook, Wholefoods, Tesco*	1 Portion/83g	291	1.2	351	8	70.7	1.4	11.6
BARS								
Almond, & Cashew, Paleo, Aldi*	1 Bar/45g	203	10.8	451	13	40	24	8.9
Almond, Dark Chocolate, & Sea Salt, Deluxe, Lidl*	1 Bar/40g	219	14.8	548	15.5	34.2	37	6.8
Almond, Madagascan Vanilla, Kind*	1 Bar/40g	203	15.6	507	16	36	39	14
Almond, Nut Butter, Balls, Deliciously Ella*	1 Pack/36g	162	9.7	450	12.5	37.3	27	9.6
Almond, Peanut, & Double Choc, Yes!*	1 Bar/45g	231	15.2	514	22.9	24	33.8	11.2
Almond, Sweet & Nutty, Nature Valley*	1 Bar/30g	143	6.9	475	10	54.3	23	5.4
Apple, & Cinnamon, FattBar*	1 Bar/30g	139	11.1	464	9.1	6.8	37	33
Apple, Fruit & Oat Bakes, Go Ahead*	1 Bar/35g	127	2.7	363	2.7	72.3	7.7	4.3
Apple, Fruit Bake, Go Ahead, McVitie's*	1 Bar/35g	124	2.5	354	2.7	73.8	7.2	1.2
Apple, Fruit Bakes, Crownfield, Lidl*	1 Bar/33g	128	2.6	387	3.8	73.9	8	2
Apple, Granola, McVitie's*	1 Bar/35g	128	3.4	366	6.6	63.1	9.7	4.3
Apricot, & Almond, Eat Natural*	1 Bar/50g	238	13.4	476	6.6	49.7	26.7	5
Apricot, & Almond, Yoghurt Coated, Eat Natural*	1 Bar/50g	233	13.1	476	6.6	49.7	26.7	5
Apricot, & Sultana, Special K, Kellogg's*	1 Bar/27g	104	1.7	385	5.6	74.1	6.3	7.8
Bakewell Tart, Alesto, Lidl*	1 Bar/35g	138	6	394	7.5	50.3	17	4.9
Bakewell Tart, Tru, The Foodie Market, Aldi*	1 Bar/35g	146	6	416	6.7	57	17	5.9
Banana, & Date, Tesco*	1 Bar/26g	88	0.9	340	14	60	3.6	5.6
Banana, Oat, Nom*	1 Bar/40g	177	7.8	443	7.8	54.6	19.6	6.3
Banoffee Pie, Nakd*	1 Bar/35g	129	4.6	368	6.9	53.1	13.2	4.6
Beetroot, & Apple, Yes!*	1 Bar/32g	123	3.7	386	4.8	62.3	11.6	6.6
Beetroot, & Nuts, Snack, Zenb*	1 Bar/32g	140	7.2	438	11.9	40.6	22.5	12.2
Berries & Yoghurt, Protein, Alpen*	1 Bar/34g	124	2.5	364	19	47	7.3	17
Berry Delight, The Foodie Market, Aldi*	1 Bar/35g	141	5.2	402	6.4	57	15	6.8
Berry, & Almond, Seed, Nine*	1 Bar/50g	228	12	456	18.1	39.3	23.9	6.7
Berry, & Nuts, Protein, Special K, Kellogg's*	1 Bar/28g	122	4.5	437	23	47	16	6.5
Berry, & Yoghurt, Giant, Ma Baker*	1 Bar/100g	491	24.5	491	5.7	61.9	24.5	1
Berry, Delight, GF, Nak'd*	1 Bar/35g	135	5.2	385	9	52	15	6
Berry, Energy, High Five*	1 Bar/16g	55	0.7	344	4	70	4.2	0
Berry, Mixed, Moist, Get Fruity*	1 Bar/35g	140	4.6	399	6	61	13	6.3
Berry, Mixed, Trek, Natural Balance Foods*	1 Bar/68g	204	1.5	300	15.6	56.5	2.2	6
Berry, Nut Free, Get Buzzing*	1 Bar/62g	173	8.7	279	3.2	50	14	2.9
Better Brownie, Cherry Bakewell, Vive*	1 Bar/35g	153	8.8	437	15	33	25	13
Better Brownie, Chocolate Berry, Vive*	1 Bar/35g	147	7.7	418	16	34	22	13
Better Brownie, Chocolate Orange, Vive*	1 Bar/35g	150	8.8	429	17	29	25	14
Better Brownie, Coconut Cashew, Vive*	1 Bar/35g	148	8.4	423	15	32	24	16
Birthday Cake, Protein, Battle Bites*	1 Bar/62g	220	8.1	355	33	26	13	13.9
Birthday Cake, Squares, Fibre One*	1 Bar/24g	84	1.5	350	2.8	47.6	6.2	25.1
Biscuit, Chocolate, Chunky, Belmont Biscuit Co, Aldi*	1 Bar/24g	126	6.7	526	6.6	61	28	1.8
Biscuit, Chocolate, Mint, Penguin, McVitie's*	1 Bar/25g	133	6.9	531	5.4	65	27.7	1.5
Biscuit, Chocolate, Orange, Penguin, McVitie's*	1 Bar/25g	133	6.9	531	5.4	65	27.7	1.5
Biscuit, Chocolate, Original, Penguin, McVitie's*	1 Bar/20g	106	5.6	515	5.1	61.4	27.1	2.4
Biscuit, Groovy, Aldi*	1 Bar/27g	123	5.3	457	4.9	64.2	19.7	1.8
Biscuit, Milk Chocolate, M&S*	1 Bar/21g	107	5.5	509	6.4	60	26.4	2.8
Black Forest, Hi-Fi, Slimming World*	1 Bar/20g	71	2	355	3.3	53	10	19
Bliss Balls, Salted Caramel, Tom & Luke*	1 Pack/70g	272	12.7	389	12.9	47.9	18.2	5.9
Blondie, Chocolate Treat, Baileys*	1 Bar/32g	160	8.8	501	4.3	58.3	27.6	0
Blueberry Yoghurt, Amfit*	1 Bar/60g	194	4.8	324	33.3	33.9	8	11.3
Blueberry, Muffin, Fibre, Asda*	1 Bar/24g	86	2.3	359	3.6	54	9.5	22
Breakfast, Blueberry, & Almond, Kind*	1 Bar/50g	220	9	440	6	54	18	10

	Measure INFO/WEIGHT	per Measure KCAL	FAT	Nutrition Values per 100g / 100ml KCAL	PROT	CARB	FAT	FIBRE
BARS								
Breakfast, Golden Grahams, Nestle*	1 Bar/25g	101	3.2	403	7.4	65	13	4.4
Breakfast, Peanut Butter, Kind*	1 Bar/50g	230	11	460	10	44	22	10
Breakfast, Porridge to Go, Cocoa, & Hazelnut, Quaker*	1 Bar/65g	268	8.4	413	8	62	13	9.5
Brownie, Chocolate Orange, Weight Watchers*	1 Bar/18g	63	1.8	346	21	29.6	9.8	27.8
Brownie, Chocolate, Fibre, Asda*	1 Bar/24g	89	2.9	369	5	49	12	23
Brunch, Raisin, Cadbury*	1 Bar/32g	133	4.8	417	5.4	66	15	4.5
Bubbly, White, Tesco*	1 Bar/25g	140	8.4	559	6.4	57.6	33.6	0.1
Cacao Mint, Protein, Energy Ball, Bounce*	1 Ball/42g	176	7.1	422	23	41	17	6.4
Cacao, & Almond, Energy Ball, Deliciously Ella*	1 Ball/40g	173	11.1	433	12.5	35.3	27.8	7.2
Cacao, & Cashew, Quinoa, Perkier*	1 Bar/35g	137	6.3	391	14	39	18	14
Cacao, & Cashew, Rich, Love Vegan*	1 Bar/32g	128	6.5	401	9.6	48	20.2	4.2
Cacao, & Salted Caramel, Perkier*	1 Bar/35g	137	7.4	391	17	26	21	20
Cacao, Coffee, & Ameretto, Love Vegan*	1 Bar/33g	131	6.5	398	9.6	48.2	19.7	4.2
Cacao, Raw Fruit & Nut, Wild Trail*	1 Bar/30g	115	3.3	383	8.6	56	11	11
Cafe Mocha, Keto, Vegan, Youthful Living*	1 Bar/52g	227	17.1	437	16.7	37.2	32.9	28.3
Cake, M&M's, Mars*	1 Bar/26g	126	6.7	485	5.2	59.4	25.6	0
Cake, Red Velvet, Fibre One*	1 Bar/25g	90	3.1	360	3.6	47.2	12.3	22.4
Caramel, Almond, & Sea Salt, Kind*	1 Bar/40g	200	15.6	500	14	39	39	18
Caramel, Chewy, Mini, Sainsbury's*	1 Bar/18g	80	3.3	444	3.5	66.4	18.2	0.5
Caramel, Chocolate, Chewy, Sainsbury's*	1 Bar/36g	167	6.9	464	3.9	68.9	19.2	0
Caramel, Crazy, Tesco*	1 Bar/40g	192	9.2	480	3.9	64	23	1
Caramel, Crispy, Shake That Weight*	1 Bar/58g	212	7	365	25.8	37.4	12.1	6.7
Caramel, Crunchy, Tesco*	1 Bar/21g	98	5.2	467	4.6	56	25	1.4
Caramel, Mega Nuts, Tasti*	1 Bar/40g	213	13.1	533	15.4	41.8	32.7	5.1
Caramel, Minis, Lidl*	1 Bar/22g	101	4	459	3.6	70	18	1.5
Caramel, Nougat, Soft, Shapers, Boots*	1 Bar/25g	86	2.5	343	2.9	60.4	10	0.6
Caramel, Salted, Huel*	1 Bar/49g	200	7.8	408	24	36	16	9
Caramel, Salted, Protein, Ball, Bounce*	1 Ball/40g	170	7	425	1	30	17.5	25
Caramel, Salted, Square, Fibre One*	1 Bar/24g	87	2.8	362	4	49.5	11.7	21.2
Caramel, Skinny Whip*	1 Bar/25g	96	2.3	384	3.6	64	9.2	15.2
Caramel, Wafer, Chewy, Ms Mollys*	1 Bar/18g	88	3.9	489	6.2	66.5	21.6	2
Carrot, Cake, Fibre One*	1 Bar/25g	90	3.4	361	4.2	44	13.4	23.9
Cashew Crush, Raw, Fruit & Nut, Foodie Market, Aldi*	1 Bar/35g	158	8	451	11.7	45.7	22.9	7.7
Cashew, Cookie, Raw Fruit & Nut, GF, Nak'd*	1 Bar/35g	143	8	410	10	46	23	5
Cashew, Crush, Alesto, Aldi*	1 Bar/35g	155	8.2	444	10	46	23.4	4.7
Cereal, & Milk, Nesquik, Nestle*	1 Bar/25g	108	3.7	433	6.2	68.5	14.9	1
Cereal, Apple & Cinnamon, Boka*	1 Bar/30g	88	0.8	293	5.7	58	2.5	19
Cereal, Apple & Sultana, Light, Alpen*	1 Bar/20g	63	0.7	330	4.1	59.4	3.6	21.7
Cereal, Apricot, Almond, & Yoghurt, Tesco*	1 Bar/35g	156	6.8	447	5.9	59.7	19.4	4.9
Cereal, Banana Bonanza, Tesco*	1 Bar/21g	82	1.8	390	6.6	69	8.8	4.3
Cereal, Banoffee, Light, Alpen, Weetabix*	1 Bar/19g	66	1.3	346	4.7	54	7	24
Cereal, Caramel, Boka*	1 Bar/30g	88	0.8	295	6	58	2.7	19
Cereal, Cherry Bakewell, Light, Alpen*	1 Bar/19g	65	1.1	341	5.1	56	5.6	23
Cereal, Choc Chip, Brunch, Cadbury*	1 Bar/32g	137	5.1	427	6.1	65	16	4.7
Cereal, Choco Snaps, Asda*	1 Bar/20g	79	2.2	393	4.6	62	11	13
Cereal, Chocolate & Fudge, Light, Alpen*	1 bar/19g	67	1.3	353	5.6	57	6.7	21
Cereal, Chocolate Chip, Special K, Kellogg's*	1 Bar/21g	84	1.5	401	9	76	7	1.5
Cereal, Chocolate Chunks, & Pecan, Special K, Kellogg's*	1 Bar/36g	170	9	472	25	44.4	25	11.1
Cereal, Chocolate Delight, Dark, Special K, Kellogg's*	1 Bar/24g	97	3.4	404	4.5	57	14	17
Cereal, Chocolate, & Fudge, Asda*	1 Bar/19g	66	1.3	347	4.5	53	6.9	28
Cereal, Chocolate, Double, Asda*	1 Bar/19g	67	1.2	352	5.5	58	6.3	21
Cereal, Chocolate, Double, Benefit, Harvest Morn, Aldi*	1 Bar/19g	62	1	326	6.8	52	5.1	25
Cereal, Chocolate, Double, Light, Alpen*	1 Bar/19g	67	1.2	351	5.6	58	6.3	20

	Measure INFO/WEIGHT	per Measure KCAL	FAT	Nutrition Values per 100g / 100ml KCAL	PROT	CARB	FAT	FIBRE
BARS								
Cereal, Chocolate, Milk, Double, Special K, Kellogg's*	1 Bar/20g	80	2	400	10	65	10	10
Cereal, Chocolate, Mint, Great Shape, Asda*	1 Bar/20g	72	2.2	361	4.6	51	11	20
Cereal, Chocolate, Orange, Great Shape, Asda*	1 Bar/20g	72	2	361	4.7	54	10	18
Cereal, Cranberry & Orange, Weight Watchers*	1 Bar/28g	102	1.1	365	4.5	77.6	4.1	2.3
Cereal, Cranberry & Yoghurt, Harvest Morn, Aldi*	1 Bar/29g	117	2.6	403	6.5	71.9	9	4.1
Cereal, Crunchy Granola, Ginger Nut, Nature Valley*	1 Bar/42g	189	7.1	451	7.9	64.2	16.9	2.3
Cereal, Crunchy Granola, Peanut Butter, Nature Valley*	1 Bar/21g	95	4	452	9.5	64.3	19	4.8
Cereal, Dark Chocolate, & Cranberries, Special K*	1 Bar/27g	100	2.5	372	5.9	68	9.1	10
Cereal, Fruit & Fibre, Asda*	1 Bar/29g	111	2.8	390	6	69	10	4.1
Cereal, Fruit & Nut, Alpen*	1 Bar/28g	109	2.3	390	5.8	73	8.3	2.9
Cereal, Fruit, Average	***1 Bar/34g***	***130***	***3.9***	***382***	***5.9***	***64.7***	***11.5***	***6.5***
Cereal, Fruit, Nuts, & Oats, Raw, W.K Kellogg, Kellogg's*	1 Bar/30g	150	9	500	14	40	30	7
Cereal, Frusli, Blueberry, Jordans*	1 Bar/30g	113	2.1	375	5.2	70.2	7.1	4.9
Cereal, Frusli, Raisin & Hazelnut, Jordans*	1 Bar/30g	117	3.7	390	5.8	64.3	12.2	4.5
Cereal, Hazelnut, Brunch, Cadbury*	1 Bar/35g	160	7.4	460	7	60.5	21.4	2.2
Cereal, Nut & Seed, Organic, Green & Black's*	1 Bar/50g	258	16.3	516	8.4	47.2	32.6	10
Cereal, Oat & Raisin, Basics, Sainsbury's*	1 Bar/25g	98	2.2	391	5.1	72.8	8.8	3.8
Cereal, Oats & Honey, M&S*	1 Bar/30g	110	1.9	367	7.3	63.5	6.3	13.5
Cereal, Red Berries, Frusli, Jordans*	1 Bar/30g	115	1.9	383	6.1	72.7	6.5	4.4
Cereal, Red Berry, Special K, Kellogg's*	1 Bar/22g	85	1.8	387	6	68	8.2	9.9
Cereal, Red Fruit, Chewy & Crispy, Sainsbury's*	1 Bar/23g	82	1.2	358	6	69.4	5.2	10.5
Cereal, Rice Snaps, Asda*	1 Bar/20g	77	2.1	385	3.5	60	10.5	15.5
Cereal, Strawberry with Yoghurt, Alpen*	1 Bar/29g	120	2.9	415	4.8	75	10	2.7
Cereal, Strawberry, Fruit 'n' Grain, Asda*	1 Bar/37g	126	2.6	340	4.2	65	7	4.5
Cereal, Strawberry, Raspberry, & Cranberry, Quaker*	1 Bar/55g	214	3.6	390	5.9	74	6.6	5.9
Cereal, Summer Fruits, Light, Alpen*	1 Bar/19g	65	0.8	341	5.3	60	4.3	20
Cereal, Summer Fruits, Tesco*	1 Bar/19g	66	0.8	350	4.5	65.3	4	17.4
Cherry Bakewell, CWP*	1 Bar/57g	207	6.3	363	23	44	11	4.4
Cherry Bakewell, Porridge Oat, Thins, Stoats*	1 Bar/22g	93	3.3	422	7.2	60.4	15	7.9
Chewy Oat, Toffee Apple, Graze*	1 Bar/23g	97	3.9	422	6.2	59	17	21
Choc Peanut, Skinny Dream*	1 Bar/24g	96	2.7	398	3.9	66.3	11.1	8.6
Choc, Salted Caramel, Tribe*	1 Bar/50g	236	12.5	472	11	48	25	5.6
Chocolate, & Caramel, Rice Krispies Squares, Kellogg's*	1 Bar/36g	155	5	430	4.5	71	14	2
Chocolate, & Peanut, Tracker, Mars*	1 Bar/26g	112	5	432	6.6	50.6	19.1	15.5
Chocolate, Brownie, Average	***1 Bar/68g***	***240***	***4***	***353***	***14.7***	***60.3***	***5.9***	***8.8***
Chocolate, Caramel, & Sea Salt, Nomo*	1 Bar/38g	212	13.7	559	1.9	55	36	0
Chocolate, Caramel, Mini, Mister Choc, Lidl*	1 Bar/22g	100	4.2	453	3.9	66	19	1.1
Chocolate, Caramel, Wacko, Belmont, Aldi*	1 Bar/21g	102	4.6	485	5.3	65	22	1.7
Chocolate, Cosmic Whip, Tesco*	1 Bar/22g	100	3.7	452	3.6	72.4	16.6	0.8
Chocolate, Crispy, Free From, Tesco*	1 Bar/30g	132	4.6	440	4.1	71.2	15.4	0.5
Chocolate, Dark, & Orange, Protein Nut, Trek*	1 Bar/40g	214	14.8	534	26.2	17.5	37.1	12.4
Chocolate, Dark, & Sea Salt, Protein Nut, Trek*	1 Bar/40g	213	14.9	532	25.7	17.3	37.3	12.1
Chocolate, Dark, & Peanut Butter, Deluxe, Lidl*	1 Bar/40g	218	14.6	545	20.2	30.5	36.5	6.8
Chocolate, Dark, & Raspberry, Tesco*	1 Bar/23g	92	2.2	401	7	69	9.8	4.5
Chocolate, Dark, Chewy Delight, Special K, Kellogg's*	1 Bar/24g	97	3.4	404	4.5	57	14	17
Chocolate, Dark, Energy, Jungle*	1 Bar/48g	206	8.4	430	6.5	61	17.4	6.4
Chocolate, Dark, Intense, The Dark One, M&S*	1 Bar/32g	180	10.9	564	9.6	53.1	34.2	2.5
Chocolate, Dark, Mint, Hi-Fi, Slimming World*	1 Bar/20g	70	1.8	351	4	54	8.8	20
Chocolate, Dark, Nuts, & Sea Salt, Kind*	1 Bar/40g	198	14.8	495	14	23	37	17
Chocolate, Double, Snack, Skinny Whip*	1 Bar/25g	96	2.3	385	3.7	64	9.3	15
Chocolate, Fruit & Nut, M&S*	1 Bar/50g	235	12	470	6.5	57.1	24.1	2.5
Chocolate, Fruit & Crunch, NOMO*	1 Bar/32g	160	8	501	3.2	61	25	0
Chocolate, Fudge, Exante Diet*	1 Bar/60g	206	5.9	344	29	38	9.9	8.3

	Measure INFO/WEIGHT	per Measure KCAL	FAT	Nutrition Values per 100g / 100ml KCAL	PROT	CARB	FAT	FIBRE
BARS								
Chocolate, Hazelnut Whip, Fulfil Nutrition*	1 Bar/55g	210	9.9	382	36	27	18	5.5
Chocolate, Hazelnut, High Protein, Misfits*	1 Bar/45g	199	10.8	442	34	15	24	17.7
Chocolate, Hazelnut, Tony's Chocolonely*	1 Bar/47g	262	17	558	8.4	47.8	36.1	0
Chocolate, Hazelnut, Wow Bakes, Graze*	1 Pack/20g	94	5.2	472	6.4	50	26	15
Chocolate, Honeycomb, Bunnycomb, Mini Moos*	1 Bar/25g	143	9.4	571	2.7	59.5	37.6	0
Chocolate, Honeycomb, Hi-Fi, Slimming World*	1 Bar/20g	70	1.8	348	3.6	54	9	1.8
Chocolate, Huel*	1 Bar/49g	200	7.9	406	24	36	16	10
Chocolate, Marshmallow, Rice Krispie Squares, Kellogg's*	1 Bar/36g	158	5	438	3.1	75	14	0.8
Chocolate, Meal Replacement, Ultra Slim, Tesco*	1 Bar/60g	219	6.7	365	28.5	37.3	11.1	8.2
Chocolate, Milk, & Nut, Weight Watchers*	1 Bar/15g	80	5.7	533	13.3	22.7	38	24
Chocolate, Milk, Swiss, M&S*	1 Bar/50g	285	18.4	570	0.2	51	36.8	2
Chocolate, Mint, Club, Mcvitie's*	1 Bar/23g	117	6.1	510	5.7	61.2	26.4	2.3
Chocolate, Mint, Milk, Vitamin & Protein, Fulfil Nutrition*	1 Bar/55g	189	6.9	344	35.9	18.8	12.5	18.8
Chocolate, Mint, Polar, Sainsbury's*	1 Bar/25g	135	7.6	534	4.9	59.9	29.9	2.6
Chocolate, Nutty Nougat, Sainsbury's*	1 Bar/36g	181	9.9	503	9.2	53.6	27.5	2.4
Chocolate, Orange, Huel*	1 Bar/49g	200	7.9	406	24	36	16	10
Chocolate, Orange, Skinny Crunch*	1 Bar/20g	74	2.2	368	4.8	50.2	10.9	24.9
Chocolate, Orange, Whip, Bliss*	1 Bar/25g	98	2.2	393	4.2	71	8.6	6.2
Chocolate, Peanut Butter, Fulfil*	1 Bar/40g	154	6.8	386	37	27	17	5.4
Chocolate, Peanut Butter, Smart, PhD Nutrition*	1 Bar/64g	239	10.2	373	31	38	16	1
Chocolate, Peanut, Almond, Sweet & Salty, Nature Valley*	1 Bar/30g	139	7.2	464	10.1	45.5	24	13
Chocolate, Polar, Sainsbury's*	1 Bar/25g	133	7.2	533	5.5	63	28.6	1.2
Chocolate, Racer, Dairyfine, Aldi*	1 Bar/38g	185	9.5	486	8.6	54	25	4.2
Chocolate, Raspberry Cream, Frys*	1 Bar/49g	203	6.2	414	0	65.3	12.6	0
Chocolate, Reeses Sticks, Hershey*	1 Bar/42g	214	12.8	510	10.3	56	30.4	0
Chocolate, Salted Caramel, Protein, Fulfil Nutrition*	1 Bar/40g	148	6	371	37	28	15	6.2
Chocolate, Sandwich, Seal, Aldi*	1 Bar/25g	131	7	523	5.5	60.6	28.1	3.1
Chocolate, Sour Cherry Chilli, Moser Roth, Aldi*	1 Bar/38g	202	13.7	532	7.6	40	36	9.8
Chocolate, Super Snackers, Graze*	1 Bar/23g	99	4.4	430	6.7	57	19	20
Chocolate, The Milk One, M&S*	1 Bar/32g	174	10.1	545	8.3	56	31.6	1.5
Chocolate, Titan, Aldi*	1 Bar/38g	169	6.8	444	3.5	66	18	0.5
Chocolate, Toffee Biscuit, Sainsbury's*	1 Bar/42g	194	9.7	463	4.6	58.5	23.2	0.9
Chocolate, Toffee Pecan, M&S*	1 Bar/36g	179	9.8	498	4.9	58.3	27.3	0.7
Chocolate, Viennese, Sandwich, Fox's*	1 Bar/14g	76	4.4	542	6.9	57.4	31.6	1.6
Chocolate, Wafer, Blue Riband, Nestle*	1 Bar/18g	92	4.5	513	5	65.8	25.1	1.7
Chocolate, White, Creamy, The White One, M&S*	1 Bar/32g	184	12	574	6.6	51.6	37.5	1.7
Chocolix, Schar*	1 Bar/22g	101	3.9	463	3.6	70	18	4.2
Cinnamon, & Apple, Fruit & Peanut, Asda*	1 Bar/35g	135	5.6	386	12	40	16	16
Club, Fruit, Jacob's*	1 Bar/24g	119	5.9	496	5.9	61.1	24.7	3
Club, Milk Chocolate, Jacob's*	1 Bar/24g	123	6.3	511	5.8	62.6	26.4	2
Club, Mint, Jacob's*	1 Bar/24g	124	6.5	517	5.6	62.5	27.2	1.7
Club, Orange, Crunchies, McVitie's*	1 Bar/24g	115	6.1	481	5.1	59	25.7	1.4
Club, Orange, McVitie's*	1 Bar/23g	116	6	512	5.7	61	26.6	2.3
Coco Pops, & Milk, Kellogg's*	1 Bar/20g	85	2.6	423	7	70	13	1
Cocoa Delight, The Foodie Market, Aldi*	1 Bar/35g	139	5.1	397	7.1	57.1	14.6	7.7
Cocoa Orange, Fruit & Nut, Tru, The Foodie Market, Aldi*	1 Bar/35g	151	6.6	432	8.4	52	19	7
Cocoa, & Hazelnut, Goodness, Go Ahead!*	1 Bar/30g	111	4	369	7.4	56	13.4	7.8
Cocoa, & Hazelnut, Nut Butter, Nature Valley*	1 Bar/38g	191	10	503	7.6	56	26.3	6.1
Cocoa, Crunch, Nak'd*	1 Bar/30g	105	2.6	351	18.4	47.2	8.8	6.3
Cocoa, Delight, Wholefood, GF, Nak'd*	1 Bar/35g	135	5.3	386	9.4	49.4	15.1	6.8
Cocoa, Orange, GF, Nak'd*	1 Bar/35g	145	7	415	11	45.1	20	6.4
Cocoa, Orange, The Foodie Market, Aldi*	1 Bar/35g	151	6.6	432	8.4	52	19	7
Cocoa, Twist, Nak'd*	1 Bar/30g	99	1.7	329	7	59.9	5.6	6

	Measure INFO/WEIGHT	per Measure KCAL	per Measure FAT	KCAL	PROT	CARB	FAT	FIBRE
				Nutrition Values per 100g / 100ml				
BARS								
Coconut & Macadamia, Protein, Energy Ball, Bounce*	1 Ball/40g	178	6.8	445	22	46	17	10
Coconut, & Caramel, Alibi Max*	1 Bar/49g	244	12.7	498	5.5	59	26	0
Coconut, & Chocolate, Saint *	1 Bar/97g	448	17.6	462	4.8	66.7	18.1	7.1
Coconut, & Nuts, Protein, Nature Valley*	1 Bar/40g	198	12.2	495	25.8	22.8	30.5	13.2
Coconut, & Oat, Energy Ball, Deliciously Ella*	1 Ball/40g	145	4.8	362	7.4	56.5	11.9	7.7
Coconut, Chocolate Coated, Nicks*	1 Bar/40g	162	12.8	405	4.8	32.8	32	20.8
Coconut, Chocolate Crisp, Weight Watchers*	1 Bar/25g	89	2.6	356	3.6	71.2	10.4	3.2
Coconut, Cumin, Protein, Balls, Bounce*	1 Ball/40g	184	10	460	22.5	40	25	0
Coconut, Mini, Lidl*	1 Bar/28g	132	7	472	4.4	56	25	5.2
Coconut, Spiral, Aldi*	1 Bar/21g	25	1.6	121	8.8	11	7.7	2.3
Coconut, Tropical, New You Plan *	1 Bar/35g	122	4	349	24	44.9	11.4	0
Coffee, Caramel, Huel*	1 Bar/49g	200	7.9	407	24	36	16	10
Coffee, Espresso, Double, Protein, Primal Pantry*	1 Bar/55g	200	4.7	363	27	43	8.6	3.8
Cookie, Oaty, Maryland*	1 Bar/19g	94	4.6	493	6.8	58.5	24.2	6.1
Cookie, Triple Chocolate, Cream, New You Plan*	1 Bar/35g	139	4.6	397	31.4	40.9	13	2.5
Cranberry, & Dark Chocolate, Yes!*	1 Bar/35g	183	11.9	523	20.3	25.4	34.1	16.5
Cranberry, Crunchy, Meal Replacement, CWP*	1 Bar/55g	214	6.8	389	27.7	42.9	12.3	4.5
Crisp, Chocolate Brownie, Protein, Optimum Nutrition*	1 Bar/65g	213	6.5	327	31	24	10	20
Energy, Cool Mint Chocolate, Cliff*	1 Bar/68g	268	5	394	14	65	7.3	5.9
Fibre Now, Harvest Morn, Aldi*	1 Bar/24g	84	2.5	350	5.4	50	10.4	21.2
Fibre, Chocolate Brownie, Morrisons*	1 Bar/24g	88	3	368	5	48.1	12.6	20.7
Fibre, Lemon Drizzle, Morrisons*	1 Bar/24g	85	2.6	353	3.5	48.7	10.9	23.5
Flapjack, Buttery, Traditional, Organic, Dove's Farm*	1 Bar/40g	173	7.5	432	6.1	59.4	18.8	5.7
Flapjack, Salted Caramel, Protein, Trek*	1 Bar/50g	223	10.2	446	18.5	45.8	20.4	3.7
Flapjack, Slices, Morrisons*	1 Bar/35g	146	5.8	418	7	57	16.7	6
Frosties, & Milk, Kellogg's*	1 Bar/25g	102	2.8	408	7	71	11	1
Frosties, Snack Bar, Kellogg's*	1 Bar/25g	104	2.8	414	7	72	11	1
Fruit & Fibre, Coconut, Apricot, Oats, Spelt, Eat Natural*	1 Bar/40g	165	7	413	6.4	51.6	17.5	6.1
Fruit & Fibre, Plum, Peanut, Oats, Spelt, Eat Natural*	1 Bar/40g	173	7.8	432	10.1	51.1	19.4	6.4
Fruit & Nut, Salted Caramel, & Peanuts, Eat Natural*	1 Bar/45g	223	12.8	496	26	31.3	28.4	5.4
Fruit & Grain, Apple, Harvest Morn, Aldi*	1 Bar/37g	129	3	349	4.2	65	8	4.5
Fruit & Grain, Strawberry, Harvest Morn, Aldi*	1 Bar/37g	130	2.6	349	4.2	65	7	4.5
Fruit & Nut, Apple, Ginger, & Nut, Deluxe, Lidl*	1 Bar/45g	211	11.4	468	7.5	46.9	25.4	11
Fruit & Nut, Cacao & Orange, Raw, Alesto, Lidl*	1 Bar/35g	146	7	417	11	45.1	20	6.4
Fruit & Nut, Dark Chocolate, & Sea Salt, Eat Natural*	1 Bar/45g	197	9.7	438	8.5	49.2	21.5	6.9
Fruit & Nut, Eat Natural*	1 Bar/50g	223	11.2	446	11.6	49.8	22.3	5.3
Fruit & Nut, Raisin, & Hazelnut, Benecol*	1 Bar/40g	174	8.3	435	5.2	52.5	20.8	7.2
Fruit & Nut, with Chocolate, & Orange, Eat Natural*	1 Bar/45g	224	12.8	498	26.1	31.1	28.5	6
Fruit 'n' Fibre, Kellogg's*	1 Bar/25g	95	2.2	380	5	71	9	5
Fruit, & Nut, Apricot, Almond, & Pumpkin Seed, Benecol*	1 Bar/40g	171	8	428	7	52	20	6.8
Fruit, Cacao, & Orange, Natural, Tribe*	1 Bar/42g	178	9.3	424	9	42.9	22.1	7.6
Fruit, GF, Schar*	1 Bar/25g	99	3	396	3.2	65	12	8.2
Fudge Brownie, Carb Killa, Grenade*	1 Bar/60g	220	8.5	366	37.8	25.3	14.1	10.4
Ginger, Bread, GF, Nak'd*	1 Bar/35g	158	10.8	450	10	35	31	9.4
Ginger, Bread, Nak'd*	1 Bar/35g	157	10.7	450	10	35.4	30.8	9.4
Goji, & Coconut, Protein, Balls, Alesto, Lidl*	1 Pack/45g	173	6.3	384	12.9	49.1	14	5.3
Golden Syrup, Morning, Oat So Simple, Quaker*	1 Bar/35g	142	3.5	407	8.2	67.6	10	6.8
Granola, Chocolate & Nut, Crunchy Nut, Kellogg's*	1 Bar/32g	167	10.6	521	12	41	33	6.6
Granola, Coconut, & Chocolate, Tesco*	1 Bar/30g	150	8	500	6.8	54.6	26.8	6.5
Granola, Crunchy, Oats & Chocolate, Nature Valley*	1 Bar/21g	98	4.1	464	8.3	59.8	19.8	7.1
Granola, Honey, Tesco*	1 Bar/30g	146	7.6	485	7.4	53.3	25.5	6.1
Granola, Maple Syrup, Crunchy, Harvest Morn, Aldi*	2 Bars/42g	189	6.7	450	8.2	65	16	5.9
Granola, Oats & Honey, Crunchy, Harvest Morn, Aldi*	2 Bars/42g	191	6.7	455	8.2	66	16	6.2

	Measure INFO/WEIGHT	per Measure KCAL	FAT	Nutrition Values per 100g / 100ml KCAL	PROT	CARB	FAT	FIBRE
BARS								
Granola, Square, Bakery in Store, M&S*	1 Square/60g	275	14.3	455	7.9	53	23.6	5.1
Hazelnut Spirals, Dairyfine, Aldi*	1 Bar/21g	119	7.6	567	8.6	51	36	1.5
Hazelnut, Dark Chocolate Coated, Vive*	1 Bar/50g	227	14	453	21	26	28	13
Hazelnut, Nut Butter, Balls, Deliciously Ella*	1 Pack/36g	164	9.8	455	9.8	42.6	27.1	8
Hazelnut, Wafer, Princessa, Nestle*	1 Bar/34g	188	11.3	552	5.6	57.1	33.1	1.7
Hobnob, Flapjack, Peanut Butter Fudge, McVitie's*	1 Bar/31g	136	5.2	444	5.8	64.5	17.1	4.6
Hobnobs, Choc & Golden Syrup, McVitie's*	1 Bar/31g	129	4	421	6.3	68.2	13.1	4.8
Honey, & Almond, Crunchy, Original, Jordans*	1 Bar/30g	139	6.8	463	8.3	56.7	22.7	6.7
Honey, Almond, & Greek Yoghurt, Atkins*	1 Bar/40g	160	9	400	30	37.5	22.5	22.5
Honeycomb, Caramel, Wow Bakes, Graze*	1 Bar/20g	94	5	470	6.4	52	25	16
Hype, Milk & Cookies, Oatein*	1 Bar/60g	187	4.8	311	29.8	35.1	8	7.6
Hype, Salty Caramel, Oatein*	1 Bar/60g	191	4.9	319	30.1	36.1	8.2	7.7
Jaffa Cake, Benefit, Harvest Morn, Aldi*	1 Bar/66g	228	3.6	346	5.2	58	5.5	22
Jive, Chocolate, Shortcake Finger, Dairyfine, Aldi*	1 Twin Bar/42g	194	9.7	463	4.6	58	23	0.9
Keto Balls, Choc Hazelnut, Boostball*	1 Bag/40g	258	23.7	645	13	10	59.3	11.2
Keto, Keto Vitality*	1 Bar/35g	168	12.1	480	20.9	10	34.6	22.9
Ketone, Ketosource *	1 Bar/60g	220	17	367	9	30.8	28.3	17.3
Kexbar, Nick's*	1 Bars/40g	193	13.8	482	10.5	40.5	34.5	10
LCMs, Choc Chip, Kellogg's*	1 Bar/22g	90	2.2	411	4.1	75.1	9.9	0.7
Lemon Drizzle, Nak'd*	1 Bar/35g	133	5.4	381	6.1	51.8	15.5	5.1
Lemon, Meringue, Flower & White*	1 Bar/24g	99	3.1	421	4	72	13	0
Lemon, Shake That Weight*	1 Bar/58g	212	6.3	365	25	41.7	10.8	6.6
Lemon, Yoghurt, New You Plan*	1 Bar/34g	124	3.6	365	25	41.7	10.6	6.6
Malt Loaf, Soreen*	1 Bar/42g	124	1	295	8.2	57.8	2.3	5.1
Maple Pecan, Salted, The Yes Bar*	1 Bar/40g	220	17	550	12.5	32.5	42.5	7.5
Maple, Glazed Pecan, & Sea Salt, Kind*	1 Bar/40g	213	17.2	532	14	33	43	13
Marshmallow, Rice Krispies Squares, Kellogg's*	1 Bar/28g	119	3.4	424	3	76	12	0.9
Marshmallow, Vanilla Bean, Mallow Puffs*	1 Bar/30g	123	4.2	410	1.4	68	14	0
Marshmallow, Vanilla, Mallow & Marsh*	1 Bar/35g	134	3.7	383	7.1	68.9	10.6	0
Meal Replacement, Chocolate Crunch, Asda*	1 Bar/56g	220	6.7	393	25	44	12	4
Meal Replacement, Nut Fudge, Lighterlife*	1 Bar/46g	155	4.5	338	27	36.8	9.8	8.4
Meal Replacement, Salted Caramel, Lighter Life*	1 Bar/60g	210	6.3	350	24.2	34.2	10.5	16.5
Meal Replacement, Vanilla, & Caramel, Asda*	1 Bar/58g	200	6.4	344	36	29	11	4.7
Meal Replacement, White Chocolate, & Raspberry, Asda*	1 Bar/58g	220	4.2	380	14	26	7.3	2.1
Melto, GF, Schar*	1 Bar/30g	165	9.9	549	6.8	55	33	0
Milk Chocolate, Guylian*	1 Bar/25g	136	8.2	546	9	51	33	0
Milk Slice, Milk & Honey, Ferrero Kinder *	1 Slice/28g	118	7.8	421	7.9	34	27.9	0
Millionaire Crunch, Oatein*	1 Bar/58g	214	10.6	368	26.2	38.2	18.2	0.6
Millionaire, Salted Caramel, Hazelnut, M&S*	1 Bar/62g	285	12	459	2.2	67.1	19.4	3.4
Mint Truffle, M&S*	1 Bar/33g	189	13.1	574	4.4	47.9	39.7	3.5
Mint, & Dark Chocolate, Skinny Whip*	1 Bar/25g	98	2.8	390	2.6	63	11.2	14
Muesli, & Seeds, Bountiful, Aldi*	1 Bar/30g	98	1.4	328	3	53	4.8	18
Muesli, Chocolate, Crownfield, Lidl*	1 Bar/25g	101	2.4	404	7.4	69.1	9.5	6.1
Muesli, Fruit, Morning, Oat So Simple, Quaker*	1 Bar/35g	139	3.2	398	7.7	68.1	9.1	6.6
Muesli, Peanut, No Added Sugar, Crownfield, Lidl*	1 Bar/25g	98	3.3	391	7.9	65.7	13.2	4.7
Munchy, Peanut, Dairyfine, Aldi*	1 Bar/32g	137	6	428	8.1	50	18.8	10.6
Nougat Whip, Morrisons*	1 Bar/22g	102	3.8	464	3.6	72.3	17.3	0.9
Nougat, Chewy, Barratt*	1 Bar/35g	133	1.5	380	4.6	79.2	4.2	2.1
Nougat, Cool Mint, & Dark Chocolate, Shapers, Boots*	1 Bar/25g	81	3.1	324	2.4	48	12.4	1.2
Nougat, Honeycomb, Shapers, Boots*	1 Bar/22g	96	2.9	435	2.8	76	13	1.2
Nougat, Nutty, Treat Size, Sainsbury's*	1 Bar/17g	88	4.6	518	10	57.6	27.1	2.9
Nougat, Summer Strawberry, Shapers, Boots*	1 Bar/23g	83	3	361	2.7	73	13	0.6
Nut, Dark Chocolate, Peanut Butter, Aldi*	1 Bar/40g	213	14.8	533	23	21	37	15

B

	Measure INFO/WEIGHT	per Measure KCAL	per Measure FAT	Nutrition Values per 100g / 100ml KCAL	PROT	CARB	FAT	FIBRE
BARS								
Nut, Feast, Mixed, Eat Natural*	1 Bar/50g	278	20.5	556	18.8	28	41	0
Nutri-Grain, Apple, Kellogg's*	1 Bar/37g	131	3.3	355	4	67	9	4
Nutri-Grain, Apple, Soft & Fruity, Kellogg's*	1 Bar/37g	133	3	359	4	70.3	8.1	4
Nutri-Grain, Blackberry & Apple, Soft & Fruity, Kellogg's*	1 Bar/37g	133	3	359	4	70.3	8.1	4
Nutri-Grain, Blueberry, Kellogg's*	1 Bar/37g	133	3	359	3.5	69	8	3.5
Nutri-Grain, Elevenses, Choc Chip Bakes, Kellogg's*	1 Bar/45g	179	5.8	397	4	66	13	2
Nutri-Grain, Elevenses, Raisin Bakes, Kellogg's*	1 Bar/45g	168	4	374	4.5	68	9	2.5
Nutri-Grain, Strawberry, Kellogg's*	1 Bar/37g	133	3	359	3.5	69	8	3.5
Nutri-Grain, Strawberry, Soft & Fruity, Kellogg's*	1 Bar/37g	133	3	359	4	70.3	8.1	4
Nutty Nougat Caramel, Tesco*	1 Bar/40g	200	11.1	490	8.7	52.7	27.2	3.8
Nutty, Snack Size, Asda*	1 Bar/38g	182	9.5	479	9	54	25	0.9
Oat, Apple & Cinnamon, Nairn's*	1 Bar/40g	169	7.1	422	7	54.7	17.7	8
Oat, Baked, Apple, Raisin, & Cinnamon, Deliciously Ella*	1 Bar/50g	213	8.7	426	5.6	59.2	17.4	5
Oat, Berry & Vanilla, Mini, Graze*	1 Bite/30g	136	6.3	452	12	51	21	5.3
Oat, Chewy, Strawberry, Super Snackers, Graze*	1 Bar/23g	97	3.9	423	6.1	59	17	20
Oat, Choc Chip & Raisin, Mini, Graze*	1 Bite/30g	140	7.6	477	11	53	26	6.2
Oat, Chocolate Chip, Freee, Dove's Farm*	1 Bar/35g	141	6.4	402	6.6	46	18.2	13.6
Oat, Peanut Butter, Deliciously Ella *	1 Bar/50g	230	11.8	460	10.2	50	23.6	5
Oats, Seeds, & Berries, M&S*	1 Bar/30g	128	5.3	427	14.5	47	17.6	11.1
Orange, & Cacao, Dark, Millionaire, Graze*	1 Bar/50g	188	7	376	21	38	14	6.6
Original, Seed, Nine*	1 Bar/40g	221	16	552	16.6	26.7	40.1	9.3
Pea-Nut Square, Choc Berry, My Vegan*	1 Square/50g	233	13.5	466	24	27	27	11
Peach, & Apricot, Special K, Kellogg's*	1 Bar/23g	90	1.4	383	8	75	6	2.5
Peanut Butter, Breakfast, Bounce*	1 Bar/45g	168	7.2	374	22	27	16	16
Peanut Butter, Crunchy, Nature Valley*	1 Pack/42g	204	9	486	10.2	59.7	21.5	6.5
Peanut Chocolish, Nakd*	1 Bar/35g	141	6.9	403	7.5	49.8	19.7	6
Peanut, & Caramel, Tracker, Mars*	1 Bar/26g	113	4.9	436	8.6	51.3	18.9	13
Peanut, & Choco, Minis, Lidl*	1 Bar/22g	108	5.3	491	9.1	58.2	24.1	2.7
Peanut, & Choco, Mister Choc, Lidl*	1 Bar/38g	191	10.6	502	9.5	52	28	0
Peanut, & Dark Chocolate, Tesco*	1 Bar/35g	175	10.4	500	22.2	33	29.7	6
Peanut, & Date, Breakfast, M&S*	1 Bar/40g	171	9.5	428	22.8	19.5	23.8	21.8
Peanut, & Ginger, Snack, Love Vegan*	1 Bar/33g	150	8.9	456	14.3	38.6	26.9	5.4
Peanut, & Milk Chocolate, Flapjack, Pro 2Go, Sci-MX*	1 Bar/50g	176	6.3	352	35	28.3	12.7	9
Peanut, Almond, Dark Chocolate, Protein, Nature Valley*	1 Bar/37g	180	11	486	29.7	32.4	29.7	5.4
Peanut, Caramel, Payday, Hershey*	1 Bar/19g	88	4.8	462	13.5	51.9	25	3.8
Peanut, Crispy, Meal Replacement, CWP*	1 Bar/55g	206	6.9	374	24.3	40.5	12.6	7.8
Peanut, Milk Chocolate, Shake That Weight*	1 Bar/56g	213	6.7	380	24	41	12	10
Peanut, Mr Toms*	1 Bar/40g	210	13	525	20	42.5	32.5	2.5
Peanut, Nature Bake*	1 Bar/30g	182	14	610	26	17	47	7
Peanut, Nutty Crunch, Go Ahead, McVitie's*	1 Bar/20g	94	4.8	483	11	52.8	24.6	3.6
Peanut, Protein, Energy Ball, Bounce*	1 Ball/45g	184	7.2	408	29	37	16	2.4
Peanut, Sweet & Salty Nut, Nature Valley*	1 Bar/30g	143	7.8	478	12.3	43.1	26.1	11
Peanuts, & Pumpkin Seeds, Harvest Morn, Aldi*	1 Bar/30g	136	7.2	452	27	25	24	16
Peanuts, Coconut, & Chocolate, Vegan, Eat Natural*	1 Bar/45g	223	13.5	496	11.9	40.4	30	7.8
Pecan, Pie, GF, Nak'd*	1 Bar/35g	156	10.3	477	7.6	36.4	31.4	8.9
Pineapple, & Cashew Nut, Tropical Wholefoods*	1 Bar/40g	146	3.8	366	5.6	62	9.4	4.7
Popcorn, Peanut Butter, Fibre One*	1 Bar/21g	90	4.3	427	7.6	41.4	20.3	23.9
Popcorn, Peanut, & Sunflower, Asda*	1 Bar/20g	90	4.4	448	8.6	45	22	16
Popcorn, Salted Caramel, Almond, Pretzel, Aldi*	1 Bar/20g	93	4.7	465	8.5	47	23.5	14.5
Porridge, Golden Syrup, Squares, Quaker*	1 Square/55g	216	3.9	393	5.9	73	7.1	6.3
Protein, Caramel Chaos, Carb Killa, Grenade*	1 Bar/60g	214	7.9	357	38.7	22.5	13.2	11.1
Protein, Chocolate Brownie, GF, Quest*	1 Bar/60g	191	7.2	318	33	12	12	25
Protein, Chocolate Caramel, Pas Nutrition *	1 Bar/65g	237	7.2	365	31	29	11	12

	Measure INFO/WEIGHT	per Measure KCAL	FAT	Nutrition Values per 100g / 100ml KCAL	PROT	CARB	FAT	FIBRE
BARS								
Protein, Chocolate Chip Cookie Dough, GF, Quest*	1 Bar/60g	206	9	344	34	12	15	23
Protein, Chocolate Orange, Myprotein*	1 Bar/80g	259	5.9	324	38	30	7.4	13
Protein, Chocolate, Peanut, Asda*	1 Bar/55g	212	10.4	386	33	25	19	6.2
Protein, Cinnamon Roll, GF, Quest*	1 Bar/60g	191	7.2	318	33	16	12	23
Protein, Coconut, Cocoa, & Cashew, Special K, Kellogg's*	1 Bar/28g	118	4.5	423	23	44	16	5.6
Protein, Cookies & Cream, Asda*	1 Bar/60g	221	7.2	368	49	24	12	0
Protein, Cookies & Cream, Barebells*	1 Bar/55g	199	6.7	358	36	30	12	6.1
Protein, Cookies & Cream, Fulfil*	1 Bar/55g	208	9.3	379	36.4	14.9	16.9	20.8
Protein, Cookies & Cream, GF, Quest*	1 Bar/60g	209	9	349	35	12	15	23
Protein, Crispy Coconut, Foodspring*	1 Bar/65g	225	9	346	30.9	30.7	13.9	8.2
Protein, Crunchy Fudge, Barebells*	1 Bar/55g	204	8.2	370	36	33	15	5.1
Protein, Dark Chocolate, & Mint, Carb Killa, Grenade*	1 Bar/60g	214	8.5	357	36.8	22.6	14.2	11.6
Protein, Dark Chocolate, & Raspberry, Grenade*	1 Bar/60g	233	10.2	388	33	31	17	5.6
Protein, Lemon Curd, White Chocolate, Barebells*	1 Bar/55g	205	7.7	372	36	33	14	5.8
Protein, Peanut Butter, Ball, The Protein Ball Co.*	1 Pack/45g	176	7.6	390	23	32	17	13
Pumpkin Seed, & Almond, Tesco*	1 Bar/35g	204	15.8	582	20	21	45	6.6
Quinoa, Goji, & Cranberry, Perkier*	1 Bar/35g	129	3.9	370	12.7	51.1	11.2	10.1
Raisin, & Hazelnut, Protein, Asda*	1 Bar/28g	120	4.8	427	17	48	17	7.7
Raisin, Munch, Tesco*	1 Bar/32g	135	4.1	423	6.2	68	13	4.7
Raisin, Munchy, Dairyfine, Aldi*	1 Bar/32g	132	3.8	413	5.5	69	12	4.2
Raspberry Crisp, Nu+cao*	1 Bar/40g	248	20	621	12.1	27	50.1	6.7
Raspberry Crunch, Protein, Weight Watchers*	1 Bar/23g	68	2.5	297	21.9	49.8	10.9	9.7
Raspberry, & White Chocolate, Tesco*	1 Bar/60g	200	6.6	333	26	43.5	11	4.6
Raspberry, Chocolish, Nakd*	1 Bar/35g	137	6.4	392	6.2	53.9	18.4	5.3
Raspberry, Meringue, Flower & White*	1 Bar/24g	96	3.1	410	4	68	13	0
Raw Choc Brownie, Keto, Boostball *	1 Ball/25g	65	6	258	5.2	4.2	23.7	4.5
Rice Krispies, Snack, Kellogg's*	1 Bar/20g	83	2	415	7	70	10	0.5
Rice Krispies, Squares, Totally Chocolatey, Kellogg's*	1 Bar/36g	156	5.3	439	4.5	72	15	1.5
Rocky Road, M&S*	1 Bar/68g	330	18	486	4.1	56.7	26.5	1.9
Rocky Road, Skinny Dream*	1 Bar/20g	70	1.8	352	4.9	49	8.8	29
Salted Caramel, Dark Chocolate Coated, Vive*	1 Bar/50g	219	13	438	21	28	26	13
Salted Caramel, Exante Diet*	1 Bar/60g	207	6.1	345	26.7	38.3	10.2	9
Salted Caramel, Fruit & Nut, Protein, Deluxe, Lidl*	1 Bar/45g	231	14.3	514	26.7	28.3	31.7	4.2
Salted Caramel, Meringue, Flower & White*	1 Bar/24g	75	1.9	318	4	58	8	0
Salted Caramel, Tru, The Foodie Market, Aldi*	1 Bar/35g	138	4.9	393	7.6	57	14	6.8
Salted Caramel, Whip, Bliss*	1 Bar/25g	97	2.2	389	3.4	66	8.8	18
Salted Peanut, Carb Killa, Grenade*	1 Bar/60g	242	12	403	33	32	20	4.1
Salty Caramel, Nut, Crunchy, Keto Bar*	1 Bar/35g	126	6	360	27.3	19.9	17.1	27.3
Seed, Salted Caramel, Nine*	1 Bar/49g	260	18.6	531	16.8	24.9	38	11.1
Sesame Snaps, Anglo-Dal*	1 Pack/30g	157	8.8	522	12.2	49.4	29.4	0
Sesame Snaps, in Chocolate, Anglo-Dal*	1 Pack/40g	211	11.9	527	9.3	55.6	29.7	0
Shortcake, Caramel, Deluxe, Lidl*	1 Bar/40g	198	11.2	494	4.9	55	28	1.4
Snack, Dreamy Caramel, Tesco*	1 Bar/40g	185	7.8	462	4.3	66.9	19.5	1
Snack, Milk Chocolate, & Golden Syrup, McVitie's*	1 Bar/30g	128	4	420	6.2	68.1	13.2	4.7
Snack, Peanut Butter, Skinny Crunch*	1 Bar/20g	68	2.7	340	7	36	13.5	24.5
Sticky Toffee, Snack, Skinny Crunch*	1 Bar/20g	63	1.8	316	3.8	52.9	8.9	24
Strawberry Sundae, Nakd*	1 Bar/35g	130	4.6	371	7.1	54.4	13	4
Strawberry, & Vanilla, Vitamin & Protein, Fulfil Nutrition*	1 Bar/60g	185	4.9	309	33.4	10.1	8.2	33.1
Strawberry, & Chocolate, Skinny Whip*	1 Bar/25g	96	2.3	385	3.7	64	9.3	15
Strawberry, & Coconut, Porridge Oat, Stoats*	1 Bar/22g	92	3	416	7.5	62.1	13.7	8.8
Strawberry, Fruit & Oat Bakes, Go Ahead*	1 Bar/35g	129	2.7	369	2.8	73.4	7.8	4.2
Strawberry, Fruit Bakes, Go Ahead, McVitie's*	1 Bar/35g	131	3	375	3.5	72	8.5	4
Tiffin, GF, Free From, Co-Op*	1 Bar/62g	321	19.8	518	3.2	53	32	4

B

	Measure INFO/WEIGHT	per Measure KCAL	per Measure FAT	KCAL	PROT	CARB	FAT	FIBRE
				Nutrition Values per 100g / 100ml				
BARS								
Toffee, & Chocolate, Snack, Skinny Whip*	1 Bar/25g	96	2.3	384	3.6	64	9.2	15.2
Tracker, Roasted Nut, Mars*	1 Bar/26g	127	6.6	489	8.1	55	25.3	4.9
Wafer, Hanuta, Ferrero*	1 Slice/44g	238	14	542	7.6	54	31.9	0
Whirly, Asda*	1 Bar/15g	68	2.4	454	3.6	74	16	0.5
BASA								
Fillet, Smoked, Fishmongers Selection, Asda*	1 Fillet/115g	133	3.1	116	23	0	2.7	0
Fillets, Lemon & Herb, Tempura Batter, Gastro, Youngs*	1 Fillet/147g	240	9.7	163	16.3	9.4	6.6	0.3
Fillets, Sea Salt & Cracked Black Pepper, Gastro, Youngs*	1 Fillet/151g	261	12.1	173	14.7	10.5	8	0.3
Fillets, Skinless & Boneless, Aldi*	1 Fillet/120g	140	2.9	117	23.7	0.1	2.4	0
Fillets, Skinless, & Boneless, Raw, Tesco*	1 Fillet/133g	116	2.5	87	17.4	0	1.9	0
Fillets, Smoked, Skinless, Tesco*	1 Fillet/125g	112	2.8	90	17.5	0	2.2	0
Fillets, Southern Fried, Mini, Gastro, Youngs*	½ Pack/115g	238	10.2	207	13.3	17.9	8.9	1.2
Fillets, Tempura, Lemon & Herb, Iceland *	1 Fillet/160g	268	11.3	168	14.3	11.1	7.1	0.9
BASIL								
Dried, Ground	***1 Tsp/1.4g***	***4***	***0.1***	***251***	***14.4***	***43.2***	***4***	***0***
Fresh, Average	***1 Tbsp/5g***	***2***	***0***	***40***	***3.1***	***5.1***	***0.8***	***0***
BATTER MIX								
for Yorkshire Puddings & Pancakes, Tesco*	1 Serving/17g	34	0.3	200	2.3	43.3	1.5	2.5
for Yorkshire Puddings, Baked, Aunt Bessie's*	1 Pudding/13g	48	1.1	356	9.8	34	8.1	2.3
BAY LEAVES								
Dried, Average	***1 Tsp/0.6g***	***2***	***0.1***	***313***	***7.6***	***48.6***	***8.4***	***0***
BEAN SPROUTS								
Mung, Raw, Average	***1oz/28g***	***9***	***0.1***	***31***	***2.9***	***4***	***0.5***	***1.5***
Mung, Stir-Fried in Blended Oil, Average	***1 Serving/90g***	***65***	***5.5***	***72***	***1.9***	***2.5***	***6.1***	***0.9***
Raw, Average	***1 Serving/150g***	***55***	***2.6***	***37***	***2.2***	***3.2***	***1.8***	***1.2***
BEANS								
Aduki, Cooked in Unsalted Water, Average	***1 Tbsp/30g***	***37***	***0.1***	***123***	***9.3***	***22.5***	***0.2***	***5.5***
Aduki, Dried, Raw	***1 Tbsp/30g***	***82***	***0.2***	***272***	***19.9***	***50.1***	***0.5***	***11.1***
Baked, & Sausages, Canned, Morrisons*	1 Can/400g	460	15.6	115	5.5	12.9	3.9	3.1
Baked, & Sausages, in Tomato Sauce, Bramwells, Aldi*	1 Can/400g	412	11.6	103	5.2	12	2.9	3.5
Baked, & Sausages, Vegan, Suma*	½ Can/200g	224	6.6	112	8	10	3.3	5
Baked, Barbecue, Beanz, Heinz*	1 Can/390g	343	0.8	88	4.9	14.6	0.2	3.8
Baked, Cheesy & Sausage, Meal For One, Iceland *	1 Pack/494g	721	30.6	146	6.4	14.3	6.2	3.7
Baked, Curried, Average	***½ Can/210g***	***203***	***1.9***	***96***	***4.8***	***17.2***	***0.9***	***3.6***
Baked, Five, in Tomato Sauce, Heinz*	1 Can/415g	361	0.8	87	5.4	13.6	0.2	4.3
Baked, in Tomato Sauce, Average	***1 Can/400g***	***318***	***1.6***	***80***	***4.6***	***13.9***	***0.4***	***3.7***
Baked, in Tomato Sauce, Reduced Sugar & Salt	***½ Can/210g***	***159***	***0.7***	***76***	***4.6***	***13.6***	***0.3***	***3.8***
Baked, with Sausages, in Tomato Sauce, Corale, Aldi*	1 Can/400g	412	11.6	103	5.2	12	2.9	3.5
Barbecue, Good Grains, Worldwide Foods, Aldi*	1 Pack/256g	264	3.1	103	5.5	15	1.2	5
Black, Cooked, Average	***1 Cup/172g***	***227***	***0.9***	***132***	***8.8***	***23.7***	***0.5***	***8.7***
Borlotti, Canned, Average	***1oz/28g***	***29***	***0.1***	***103***	***7.6***	***16.9***	***0.5***	***4.7***
Borlotti, Dried, Raw, Average	***1 Serving/100g***	***335***	***1.2***	***335***	***23***	***60***	***1.2***	***24.7***
Broad, Canned, Drained, Average	***1 Can/195g***	***136***	***1.1***	***70***	***6.9***	***9.2***	***0.6***	***6.8***
Broad, Dried, Raw, Average	***1oz/28g***	***69***	***0.6***	***245***	***26.1***	***32.5***	***2.1***	***27.6***
Broad, Fresh, without Pod, Boiled, Average	***1 Serving/80g***	***78***	***0.5***	***97***	***7.9***	***11.7***	***0.6***	***6.5***
Broad, Frozen, Average	***1 Serving/80g***	***63***	***0.6***	***79***	***7.6***	***10.8***	***0.7***	***5.3***
Butter, Canned, Drained, Average	***1oz/28g***	***23***	***0.1***	***81***	***6***	***12.8***	***0.5***	***4.3***
Butter, Dried, Boiled, Average	***1oz/28g***	***30***	***0.2***	***106***	***7.2***	***18.6***	***0.6***	***5.2***
Butter, Dried, Raw, Average	***1oz/28g***	***81***	***0.5***	***290***	***19.1***	***52.9***	***1.7***	***16***
Cannellini, Canned, Drained, Average	***1 Portion/80g***	***75***	***0.4***	***94***	***8.7***	***15***	***0.5***	***5.7***
Cannellini, Dried, Tesco*	1 Serving/32g	83	0.3	260	24.8	37.4	0.8	20.9
Chilli, Canned, Average	***1 Can/420g***	***381***	***3.1***	***91***	***5.2***	***15.8***	***0.7***	***4.4***
Edamame, Dry Roasted, with Sea Salt, Hapi*	1 Serving/30g	100	1.4	335	45	13	4.7	0

	Measure INFO/WEIGHT	per Measure KCAL	FAT	Nutrition Values per 100g / 100ml KCAL	PROT	CARB	FAT	FIBRE
BEANS								
Edamame, Sainsbury's*	1 Serving/150g	212	9.6	141	12.3	6.8	6.4	4.2
Five, Canned, in Tomato Sauce, Sainsbury's*	½ Can/200g	168	1	84	4.9	12.4	0.5	5.4
Flageolet, Canned, Average	***1 Can/265g***	***235***	***1.6***	***89***	***6.8***	***14***	***0.6***	***3.5***
Four, Mix, Canned, Delmaine*	1 Can/390g	390	0	100	6.9	13.5	0	0
French, Boiled, Average	***1 Serving/150g***	***38***	***0***	***25***	***2.3***	***3.8***	***0***	***3.7***
French, Raw	***1oz/28g***	***6***	***0.1***	***20***	***1.6***	***2.7***	***0.4***	***1.8***
Green, Cut, Average	***1oz/28g***	***7***	***0.1***	***24***	***1.7***	***3.6***	***0.2***	***2.7***
Green, Fine, Average	***1 Serving/75g***	***18***	***0.3***	***24***	***1.8***	***3.2***	***0.4***	***2.9***
Green, Sliced, Average	***1oz/28g***	***6***	***0.1***	***23***	***1.9***	***3.5***	***0.2***	***2.1***
Green, Sliced, Frozen, Average	***1 Serving/50g***	***13***	***0***	***26***	***1.8***	***4.4***	***0.1***	***4.1***
Green, Whole, Average	***1oz/28g***	***6***	***0.1***	***22***	***1.6***	***3***	***0.4***	***1.7***
Haricot, Canned, Average	***1 Can/400g***	***307***	***2***	***77***	***6.2***	***10.7***	***0.5***	***5.9***
Kidney, Red, Canned, Drained, Average	***½ Can/120g***	***115***	***0.7***	***96***	***7.4***	***20.7***	***0.5***	***5.5***
Kidney, Red, Dried, Boiled in Unsalted Water	***1oz/28g***	***29***	***0.1***	***103***	***8.4***	***17.4***	***0.5***	***6.7***
Kidney, Red, Dried, Raw	***1oz/28g***	***74***	***0.4***	***266***	***22.1***	***44.1***	***1.4***	***15.7***
Kidney, Red, in Chilli Sauce, Sainsbury's*	1 Can/420g	365	1.7	87	5.3	15.6	0.4	4.5
Mixed, Canned, Average	***1 Can/300g***	***300***	***3.5***	***100***	***6.8***	***15.6***	***1.2***	***4.1***
Mixed, in Mild Chilli Sauce, Sainsbury's*	1 Can/420g	328	1.3	78	4.9	13.8	0.3	3.7
Mung, Whole, Dried, Boiled in Unsalted Water	***1oz/28g***	***25***	***0.1***	***91***	***7.6***	***15.3***	***0.4***	***3***
Mung, Whole, Dried, Raw	***1oz/28g***	***78***	***0.3***	***279***	***23.9***	***46.3***	***1.1***	***10***
Pinto, Canned, in Water, Drained, Tesco*	1 Can/236g	238	1.6	101	6.3	13.7	0.7	7.3
Pinto, Dried, Boiled in Unsalted Water	***1oz/28g***	***38***	***0.2***	***137***	***8.9***	***23.9***	***0.7***	***0***
Pinto, Dried, Raw	***1oz/28g***	***92***	***0.4***	***327***	***21.1***	***57.1***	***1.6***	***14***
Refried, Average	***1 Serving/215g***	***162***	***1.5***	***76***	***4.6***	***12.7***	***0.7***	***1.8***
Refried, Mexican, With Chipotle, Gran Luchito*	1 Pouch/430g	473	2.2	110	7	20	0.5	0
Runner, Average	***1 Serving/80g***	***15***	***0.3***	***19***	***1.3***	***2.8***	***0.4***	***2.2***
Soya, Dried, Boiled in Unsalted Water	***1oz/28g***	***39***	***2***	***141***	***14***	***5.1***	***7.3***	***6.1***
Soya, Shelled, Frozen, Raw, Average	***1 Serving/80g***	***99***	***4.3***	***124***	***12.2***	***6.9***	***5.3***	***4.4***
BEEF								
Brisket, Boiled, Lean	***1 Serving/100g***	***225***	***11***	***225***	***31.4***	***0***	***11***	***0***
Brisket, Boiled, Lean & Fat	***1 Serving/100g***	***268***	***17.4***	***268***	***27.8***	***0***	***17.4***	***0***
Brisket, Braised, Lean	***1 Serving/100g***	***280***	***17.4***	***280***	***29***	***0***	***17.4***	***0***
Brisket, Raw, Lean	***1oz/28g***	***39***	***1.7***	***139***	***21.1***	***0***	***6.1***	***0***
Brisket, Raw, Lean & Fat	***1oz/28g***	***60***	***4.4***	***216***	***18.2***	***0***	***15.8***	***0***
Cheeks, Ox, Aberdeen Angus, Waitrose*	1 Serving/100g	123	4.6	123	22	0	4.6	0
Diced, Casserole, Lean, Average	***1oz/28g***	***35***	***1.1***	***126***	***23***	***0***	***3.8***	***0***
Escalope, Healthy Range, Average	***1 Serving/170g***	***233***	***6.7***	***137***	***24.2***	***1.2***	***4***	***0.4***
Flank, Pot-Roasted, Lean	***1oz/28g***	***71***	***3.9***	***253***	***31.8***	***0***	***14***	***0***
Flank, Raw, Lean	***1oz/28g***	***49***	***2.6***	***175***	***22.7***	***0***	***9.3***	***0***
Fore Rib, Lean & Fat, Average	***1oz/28g***	***40***	***1.8***	***144***	***21.7***	***0***	***6.2***	***0.2***
Fore Rib, Raw, Lean	***1oz/28g***	***41***	***1.8***	***145***	***21.5***	***0***	***6.5***	***0***
Fore Rib, Roasted, Lean	***1oz/28g***	***66***	***3.2***	***236***	***33.3***	***0***	***11.4***	***0***
Fore Rib, Roasted, Lean & Fat	***1oz/28g***	***84***	***5.7***	***300***	***29.1***	***0***	***20.4***	***0***
Grill Steak, Average	***1 Steak/170g***	***501***	***39.5***	***295***	***19.3***	***2.1***	***23.2***	***0.1***
Grill Steak, Peppered, Average	***1 Serving/172g***	***419***	***24.4***	***244***	***23.6***	***5.2***	***14.2***	***0.3***
Joint, for Roasting, Average	***1oz/28g***	***38***	***1***	***134***	***24.5***	***1.4***	***3.4***	***0.2***
Joint, Sirloin, Roasted, Lean	***1oz/28g***	***53***	***1.8***	***188***	***32.4***	***0***	***6.5***	***0***
Joint, Sirloin, Roasted, Lean & Fat	***1oz/28g***	***65***	***3.5***	***233***	***29.8***	***0***	***12.6***	***0***
Mince, Cooked, Average	***1 Serving/75g***	***214***	***15.3***	***286***	***24***	***0***	***20.3***	***0***
Mince, Extra Lean, Raw, Average	***1 Serving/100g***	***124***	***5***	***124***	***21.2***	***0.1***	***5***	***0***
Mince, Extra Lean, Stewed	***1oz/28g***	***50***	***2.4***	***177***	***24.7***	***0***	***8.7***	***0***
Mince, Lean, Raw, Average	***1oz/28g***	***48***	***2.8***	***172***	***20.8***	***0***	***10***	***0.1***
Mince, Raw, Average	***1oz/28g***	***68***	***5.1***	***242***	***19.6***	***0.2***	***18.1***	***0***

	Measure INFO/WEIGHT	per Measure KCAL	per Measure FAT	Nutrition Values per 100g / 100ml KCAL	PROT	CARB	FAT	FIBRE
BEEF								
Mince, Raw, Frozen, Average	***1 Serving/100g***	***176***	***10***	***176***	***20.4***	***0***	***10***	***0***
Mince, Steak, Extra Lean, Average	***1oz/28g***	***37***	***1.6***	***131***	***20.5***	***0.4***	***5.6***	***0***
Mince, Steak, Raw, Average	***1 Serving/125g***	***318***	***25***	***254***	***17.2***	***0***	***20***	***0***
Mince, Stewed	***1oz/28g***	***59***	***3.8***	***209***	***21.8***	***0***	***13.5***	***0***
Olive, Skinny, Macaulay's*	1 Olive/88g	127	3.3	144	17	9.5	3.8	2
Olives, As Sold, Halls*	1 Beef Olive/75g	215	15.7	287	11.2	13.6	20.9	0
Peppered, Sliced, Average	***1 Slice/20g***	***26***	***1.1***	***129***	***18.2***	***1.3***	***5.6***	***1***
Potted, Binghams*	1 Serving/30g	76	6.6	254	13.8	1	22	0.6
Roast, Sliced, Average	***1 Slice/35g***	***48***	***1.3***	***136***	***26.1***	***0.4***	***3.6***	***0.2***
Salt, Average	***1 Serving/70g***	***80***	***1.7***	***114***	***21.7***	***1***	***2.5***	***0.1***
Salted, Dried, Raw	***1oz/28g***	***70***	***0.4***	***250***	***55.4***	***0***	***1.5***	***0***
Silverside, Pot-Roasted, Lean	***1oz/28g***	***54***	***1.8***	***193***	***34***	***0***	***6.3***	***0***
Silverside, Pot-Roasted, Lean & Fat	***1oz/28g***	***69***	***3.8***	***247***	***31***	***0***	***13.7***	***0***
Silverside, Raw, Lean	***1oz/28g***	***38***	***1.2***	***134***	***23.8***	***0***	***4.3***	***0***
Silverside, Raw, Lean & Fat	***1oz/28g***	***60***	***4.1***	***213***	***20.2***	***0***	***14.7***	***0***
Silverside, Salted, Boiled, Lean	***1oz/28g***	***52***	***1.9***	***184***	***30.4***	***0***	***6.9***	***0***
Silverside, Salted, Raw, Lean	***1oz/28g***	***39***	***2***	***140***	***19.2***	***0***	***7***	***0***
Silverside, Salted, Raw, Lean & Fat	***1oz/28g***	***64***	***5***	***227***	***16.3***	***0***	***18***	***0***
Sliced, Cooked, From Supermarket, Average	***1 Slice/35g***	***47***	***1.2***	***135***	***23.6***	***2***	***3.5***	***0.5***
Steak, 8oz Rump & Chips	***1 Serving/466g***	***870***	***41.1***	***187***	***10.7***	***16.2***	***8.8***	***0***
Steak, Braising, Braised, Lean	***1oz/28g***	***63***	***2.7***	***225***	***34.4***	***0***	***9.7***	***0***
Steak, Braising, Lean, Raw, Average	***1oz/28g***	***40***	***1.4***	***144***	***24.8***	***0***	***5***	***0***
Steak, Braising, Raw, Lean & Fat	***1oz/28g***	***44***	***2.4***	***158***	***20.5***	***0***	***8.5***	***0***
Steak, Economy, Average	***1oz/28g***	***53***	***2.4***	***190***	***26.9***	***1.2***	***8.7***	***0.4***
Steak, Fillet, Cooked, Average	***1oz/28g***	***54***	***2.4***	***191***	***28.6***	***0***	***8.5***	***0***
Steak, Fillet, Lean, Average	***1oz/28g***	***42***	***2***	***150***	***21***	***0***	***7.3***	***0***
Steak, Fillet, Lean, Cooked, Average	***1oz/28g***	***52***	***2.2***	***186***	***28.6***	***0***	***8***	***0***
Steak, Frying, Average	***1 Steak/110g***	***128***	***2.7***	***116***	***23.7***	***0***	***2.5***	***0***
Steak, Rump, Cooked, Average	***1oz/28g***	***69***	***4***	***246***	***29.1***	***0.5***	***14.1***	***0***
Steak, Rump, Grilled, Rare, Lean	***1 Steak/227g***	***381***	***15.6***	***168***	***26.5***	***0***	***6.9***	***0***
Steak, Rump, Lean, Cooked, Average	***1oz/28g***	***50***	***1.7***	***179***	***31***	***0***	***6.1***	***0***
Steak, Rump, Picanha, Cooked, Average	***1 Serving/100g***	***225***	***14.7***	***225***	***22.5***	***0.5***	***14.7***	***0.5***
Steak, Rump, Raw, Lean & Fat	***1oz/28g***	***49***	***2.8***	***174***	***20.7***	***0***	***10.1***	***0***
Steak, Rump, Raw, Lean, Average	***1 Steak/175g***	***219***	***7.2***	***125***	***22***	***0***	***4.1***	***0***
Steak, Sirloin, Fried, Rare, Lean	***1oz/28g***	***53***	***2.3***	***189***	***28.8***	***0***	***8.2***	***0***
Steak, Sirloin, Fried, Rare, Lean & Fat	***1oz/28g***	***65***	***3.9***	***231***	***26.5***	***0***	***13.9***	***0***
Steak, Sirloin, Grilled, Medium-Rare, Lean	***1oz/28g***	***49***	***2.2***	***176***	***26.6***	***0***	***7.7***	***0***
Steak, Sirloin, Grilled, Medium-Rare, Lean & Fat	***1oz/28g***	***59***	***3.5***	***211***	***24.6***	***0***	***12.5***	***0***
Steak, Sirloin, Grilled, Rare, Lean	***1oz/28g***	***46***	***1.9***	***166***	***26.4***	***0***	***6.7***	***0***
Steak, Sirloin, Grilled, Well-Done, Lean	***1oz/28g***	***63***	***2.8***	***225***	***33.9***	***0***	***9.9***	***0***
Steak, Sirloin, Grilled, Well-Done, Lean & Fat	***1oz/28g***	***71***	***4***	***254***	***31.5***	***0***	***14.3***	***0***
Steak, Sirloin, Raw, Lean & Fat	***1oz/28g***	***56***	***3.6***	***201***	***21.6***	***0***	***12.7***	***0***
Steak, Sirloin, Raw, Lean, Average	***1 Steak/150g***	***202***	***6.8***	***135***	***23.5***	***0***	***4.5***	***0***
Steak, Teriyaki, Sizzle, Ashfield Farm, Aldi*	1 Steak/100g	186	7.9	186	27	1.4	7.9	0.5
Steaks, British, Louisiana Inspired, BBQ, Waitrose*	1 Steak/112g	197	6.3	176	28	3.1	5.6	0.7
Steaks, Meat Free, Quorn*	1 Fillet/95g	106	4.7	112	11.7	5	4.9	5.4
Stewed Steak, Average	***1 Serving/220g***	***258***	***10.1***	***117***	***15.8***	***3.3***	***4.6***	***0***
Stewing Steak, Lean & Fat, Raw, Average	***1 Serving/100g***	***136***	***4.3***	***136***	***24.2***	***0.1***	***4.3***	***0.1***
Stewing Steak, Raw, Lean	***1oz/28g***	***34***	***1***	***122***	***22.6***	***0***	***3.5***	***0***
Stewing Steak, Stewed, Lean	***1oz/28g***	***52***	***1.8***	***185***	***32***	***0***	***6.3***	***0***
Stewing Steak, Stewed, Lean & Fat	***1oz/28g***	***57***	***2.7***	***203***	***29.2***	***0***	***9.6***	***0***
Stir Fry Strips, Raw, Average	***1 Serving/125g***	***149***	***3.8***	***119***	***23***	***0***	***3***	***0.2***
Topside, Lean & Fat, Raw, Average	***1oz/28g***	***55***	***3.6***	***198***	***20.4***	***0***	***12.9***	***0***

	Measure INFO/WEIGHT	per Measure KCAL	FAT	KCAL	PROT	CARB	FAT	FIBRE
				Nutrition Values per 100g / 100ml				
BEEF								
Topside, Raw, Lean	***1oz/28g***	***32***	***0.8***	***116***	***23***	***0***	***2.7***	***0***
Vegetarian, Slices, Peppered Style, Quorn*	¼ Pack/25g	29	0.5	115	14.5	7.6	2.1	4
Wafer Thin Sliced, Cooked, Average	***1 Slice/10g***	***13***	***0.3***	***129***	***24.5***	***0.5***	***3.2***	***0.2***
BEEF BOURGUIGNON								
Aldi*	½ Pack/265g	339	16.7	128	15	2.6	6.3	0.6
and Dauphinoise Potatoes, Charlie Bigham's*	1 Serving/426g	562	30.2	132	8	7.9	7.1	0
Finest, Tesco*	½ Pack/300g	247	7.8	82	9.9	4.8	2.6	0.5
BEEF BRAISED								
& Mash, Mini Meal, Tesco*	1 Pack/241g	251	9.2	104	6.5	10.5	3.8	1.1
Steak, & Mash, British, Meal for One, M&S*	1 Meal/450g	369	11.2	82	6.7	7.3	2.5	1.9
Steak, with Root Vegetable Crush, British, COU, M&S*	1 Pack/380g	243	3.8	64	7.1	5.9	1	1.4
Tender, Pub Specials, Birds Eye*	1 Pack/450g	243	3.6	54	5.5	6.1	0.8	1.8
BEEF DINNER								
Microwaved, Asda*	1 Pack/364g	306	5.8	84	4.8	12	1.6	2.2
Roast with Trimmings	***1 Dinner/840g***	***1310***	***63***	***156***	***6.1***	***17.7***	***7.5***	***2.3***
Roast, Oven Cooked, Morrisons*	1 Pack/380g	361	8.7	95	8.5	9.4	2.3	1.4
BEEF IN								
Black Bean Sauce, Chinese Takeaway, Morrisons*	½ Pack/168g	234	11.3	139	10.3	8.3	6.7	2.3
Black Bean Sauce, Chinese, Tesco*	1 Pack/400g	396	12.4	99	9.1	8.7	3.1	0.5
Black Bean Sauce, M&S*	½ Pack/175g	210	10.2	120	10.9	5.4	5.8	1.4
Gravy, Roast, Birds Eye*	1 Pack/227g	177	3.9	78	13.4	2.2	1.7	0
Gravy, Traditional, Morrisons*	1 Pack/286g	366	10	128	17.9	6	3.5	0.5
Pulled, Bourbon, with Creamy Mash, Finest, Tesco*	1 Pack/369g	579	25.5	157	8.5	14.4	6.9	2
BEEF RAGU								
Superquick, with Penne Pasta, & Spinach, Hello Fresh*	1 Serving/650g	838	26	129	7.5	15.1	4	0
with Rigatoni Pasta, Chianti, BFY, M&S*	1 Pack/370g	492	15.9	133	10.2	12.6	4.3	1.4
BEEF WELLINGTON								
Average	***1 Serving/200g***	***530***	***33.3***	***265***	***12.4***	***17***	***16.6***	***1***
British, Specially Selected, Aldi*	¼ Pack/250g	565	30	226	16	13	12	2.3
Extra Special, Asda*	1 Serving/218g	605	37.1	277	11	20	17	0.9
BEEF WITH								
Black Bean Sauce, Chilli, Sainsbury's*	1 Pack/300g	336	14.4	112	8.7	8.6	4.8	1
Onion, & Gravy, Minced, Princes*	1 Serving/200g	342	24.4	171	9.9	5.5	12.2	0
Peppercorn Sauce, Steak, Rump, M&S*	½ Pack/213g	281	8.7	132	19.4	4.2	4.1	0.1
Vegetables, & Gravy, Minced, Birds Eye*	1 Pack/178g	155	6.1	87	9.1	5.1	3.4	0.6
BEER								
Ale, 1698, Kentish Strong, Shepherd Neame*	1 Bottle/500ml	285	0	57	0.4	4.8	0	0
Ale, American Pale, Low Tide, 0.5%, Shipyard*	1 Bottle/500ml	85	0	17	0.3	3.2	0	0
Ale, Bottled, Old Speckled Hen*	1 Bottle/330ml	124	0.3	38	0.2	1.8	0.1	0.2
Ale, Brown, Alcohol Free, Sam's*	1 Bottle/330ml	69	0	21	0.2	0	0	0
Ale, Gem, 4.1%, Bath Ales*	1 Bottle/500ml	215	1	43	0.4	3.2	0.2	0.5
Ale, Hoppy, Nanny State, Alcohol Free, BrewDog*	1 Bottle/330ml	20	0.3	6	0.1	1.2	0.1	0
Ale, IPA, Punk AF, Alcohol Free, Brewdog *	1 Can/330ml	50	0	15	0	3	0	0
Ale, Low Alcohol, Nanny State, BrewDog*	1 Bottle/330ml	20	0.3	6	0.1	1	0.1	0
Ale, Low Alcohol, Old Speckled Hen*	1 Bottle/500ml	110	0.5	22	0.4	4.1	0.1	0
Ale, Old Peculiar, Theakstons*	1 Serving/500ml	250	0	50	0	4.6	0	0
Ale, Old Speckled Hen*	1 Pint/568ml	185	0.6	32	0.2	1.6	0.1	0.2
Ale, Pale, IPA, Greene King*	1 Pint/568ml	157	0.1	28	0.2	1.6	0	0.1
Ale, Pale, IPA, Innis & Gunn*	1 Bottle/330ml	162	0	49	0.3	4.6	0	0
Ale, Pale, IPA, TTD, Sainsbury's*	½ Bottle/250ml	128	0	51	0.5	4.4	0	0.5
Argus, Lidl*	1 Bottle/250ml	200	0	80	0	0	0	0
Becks Blue Lemon, No Alcohol, Beck & Co*	1 Bottle/1196ml	275	0.1	23	0.2	6	0	0
Bitter, Amber, 3.8%, Banks's*	1 Pint/568ml	170	0	30	0.4	2.4	0	0

B

	Measure INFO/WEIGHT	per Measure KCAL	FAT	Nutrition Values per 100g / 100ml KCAL	PROT	CARB	FAT	FIBRE
BEER								
Bitter, Average	***1 Can/440ml***	***141***	***0***	***32***	***0.3***	***2.3***	***0***	***0***
Bitter, Banks, Marstons PLC*	1 Pint/568ml	193	0.1	34	0.3	3.4	0	0
Bitter, Cask, Draught, London Pride, Fullers*	1 Pint/568ml	201	0	35	0	0	0	0
Bitter, Draught, Average	***1 Pint/568ml***	***182***	***0***	***32***	***0.3***	***2.3***	***0***	***0***
Bitter, Keg, Average	***1 Pint/568ml***	***176***	***0***	***31***	***0.3***	***2.3***	***0***	***0***
Bitter, Low Alcohol, Average	***1 Pint/568ml***	***74***	***0***	***13***	***0.2***	***2.1***	***0***	***0***
Bitter, Strong, Broadside, Adnams*	1 Bottle/500ml	285	0	57	0	0	0	0
Brown Ale, Bottled, Average	***1 Bottle/330ml***	***99***	***0***	***30***	***0.3***	***3***	***0***	***0***
Brune, Leffe*	1 Bottle/330ml	184	0	56	0.5	11.3	0	0
Craft, 3.5% ABV, (Calculated Estimate)	***1 Bottle/330ml***	***102***	***0***	***31***	***0***	***0***	***0***	***0***
Craft, 4% ABV, (Calculated Estimate)	***1 Bottle/330ml***	***116***	***0***	***35***	***0***	***0***	***0***	***0***
Craft, 4.5% ABV, (Calculated Estimate)	***1 Bottle/330ml***	***132***	***0***	***40***	***0***	***0***	***0***	***0***
Craft, 5% ABV, (Calculated Estimate)	***1 Bottle/330ml***	***146***	***0***	***44***	***0***	***0***	***0***	***0***
Craft, 5.5% ABV, (Calculated Estimate)	***1 Bottle/330ml***	***160***	***0***	***49***	***0***	***0***	***0***	***0***
Craft, 6% ABV, (Calculated Estimate)	***1 Bottle/330ml***	***175***	***0***	***53***	***0***	***0***	***0***	***0***
Craft, 6.5% ABV, (Calculated Estimate)	***1 Bottle/330ml***	***189***	***0***	***57***	***0***	***0***	***0***	***0***
Craft, 7% ABV, (Calculated Estimate)	***1 Bottle/330ml***	***204***	***0***	***62***	***0***	***0***	***0***	***0***
Craft, 7.5% ABV, (Calculated Estimate)	***1 Bottle/330ml***	***218***	***0***	***66***	***0***	***0***	***0***	***0***
Craft, 8% ABV, (Calculated Estimate)	***1 Bottle/330ml***	***233***	***0***	***71***	***0***	***0***	***0***	***0***
Craft, 8.5% ABV, (Calculated Estimate)	***1 Bottle/330ml***	***248***	***0***	***75***	***0***	***0***	***0***	***0***
Doom Bar, Ale, 0% Alcohol, Sharps Brewery*	1 Bottle/500ml	65	0.5	13	0.1	3.2	0.1	0
Especial, Modelo*	1 Bottle/355ml	145	0	41	0	1.1	0	0
Guinness* Extra Stout, Bottled	1 Bottle/500ml	215	0	43	4	0	0	0
Guinness*, Draught	***1 Can/440ml***	***158***	***0.2***	***36***	***0.3***	***3***	***0***	***0***
Guinness*, Stout	***1 Pint/568ml***	***205***	***0***	***36***	***0.3***	***3***	***0***	***0***
Hophead, Dark Star*	1 Bottle/500ml	160	0	32	0	0	0	0
Lager, Alcohol Free, Erdinger*	1 Bottle/500ml	125	0.5	25	0.1	5.3	0.1	0
Lager, Alcohol Free, Lost AF, Brewdog *	1 Can/330ml	135	0.3	41	0.1	3	0.1	0
Lager, Unfiltered, 0.5%, Lucky Saint*	1 Bottle/330ml	53	0	16	0.6	3.5	0	0
Low Calorie, Low Carb, Cobra*	1 Bottle/330ml	96	0	29	0.1	1.3	0	0
Mackeson, Stout	***1 Pint/568ml***	***205***	***0***	***36***	***0.4***	***4.6***	***0***	***0***
Mild, Draught, Average	***1 Pint/568ml***	***136***	***0***	***24***	***0.2***	***1.6***	***0***	***0***
Non Alcoholic, Zero, Cobra*	1 Bottle/330ml	79	0	24	0.8	2	0	0
Oak Aged, Original, Innis & Gunn*	1 Bottle/330ml	182	0	55	0.3	4.7	0	0
Pale Ale, Dead Pony Club, Brewdog *	1 Bottle/330ml	116	0	35	0	0	0	0
Pale Ale, Ghost Ship, Adnams*	1 Bottle/500ml	195	0	39	0	0	0	0
Pilsner, Alcohol Free, Kromacher*	1 Bottle/330ml	89	0	27	0	6.4	0	0
Porter, Plum, St Peter's Brewery Co Ltd*	1 Bottle/500ml	230	0.5	46	0.5	4.1	0.1	0
Prohibition Brew, Alcohol Free, Budweiser *	1 Can/330ml	112	0	34	0.2	8	0	0
Stout, Coopers*	1 Pint/375ml	191	0	51	0	2.9	0	0
Stout, Dark Matters, Aldi*	1 Bottle/328ml	128	0	39	0	0	0	0
Ultra, Kingfisher*	1 Bottle/330ml	140	0	42	0	0	0	0
Weissbier, Alcohol Free, Erdinger*	1 Bottle/500ml	125	0	25	0.4	5.3	0	0
Weissbier, Hefe, Franziskaner*	1 Bottle/500ml	225	0	45	0	0	0	0
BEETROOT								
Baby, Pickled, Average	***1 Beetroot/12g***	***5***	***0***	***37***	***1.7***	***7.2***	***0.1***	***1.2***
Cooked, Boiled, Drained, Average	***1 Serving/100g***	***44***	***0.2***	***44***	***1.7***	***10***	***0.2***	***2***
Pickled, in Sweet Vinegar, Average	***1oz/28g***	***16***	***0***	***57***	***1.2***	***12.8***	***0.1***	***1.5***
Pickled, in Vinegar, Average	***1 Serving/50g***	***18***	***0***	***36***	***1.6***	***7.3***	***0.1***	***1.2***
Raw, Unprepared, Average	***1oz/28g***	***8***	***0***	***29***	***1.4***	***5.4***	***0.1***	***1.7***
Rosebud, Sweet Chilli Marinated, M&S*	1 Serving/80g	52	0.2	65	1.5	12.3	0.3	3.6
with Balsamic Vinaigrette, Side Salad, M&S*	1 Pack/225g	146	2.9	65	0.7	12.4	1.3	2.2

	Measure	per Measure		Nutrition Values per 100g / 100ml				
	INFO/WEIGHT	KCAL	FAT	KCAL	PROT	CARB	FAT	FIBRE
BERRIES								
Medley, Grapes, Strawberry, Blueberry, Blackberry, Tesco*	1/ 2 Pack/120g	67	0.2	56	0.6	12.2	0.2	1
Mix, Naturally Wonky, Frozen, Morrisons*	1 Serving/80g	23	0.2	29	0.9	5.6	0.3	0.3
Mixed, Freeze Dried, Albert Heijn*	1 Serving/10g	38	0.2	380	8	75	2	15
Mixed, Fresh, Average	**1 Serving/80g**	**29**	**0.2**	**37**	**0.9**	**8.3**	**0.2**	**3.4**
Mixed, Summer Fruits, Frozen, Tesco*	1 Serving/80g	37	0.4	46	1.1	7.5	0.5	3.9
Summer, Mixed, Frozen, Farmfoods*	1 Serving/80g	37	0	46	0.9	7.6	0	0
BHAJI								
Aubergine, & Potato, Fried in Vegetable Oil, Average	**1oz/28g**	**36**	**2.5**	**130**	**2**	**12**	**8.8**	**1.7**
Cabbage, & Pea, Fried in Vegetable Oil, Average	**1oz/28g**	**50**	**4.1**	**178**	**3.3**	**9.2**	**14.7**	**3.4**
Cauliflower, Fried in Vegetable Oil, Average	**1oz/28g**	**60**	**5.7**	**214**	**4**	**4**	**20.5**	**2**
Mushroom, Fried in Vegetable Oil, Average	**1oz/28g**	**46**	**4.5**	**166**	**1.7**	**4.4**	**16.1**	**1.3**
Okra, Bangladeshi, Fried in Butter Ghee, Average	**1oz/28g**	**27**	**1.8**	**95**	**2.5**	**7.6**	**6.4**	**3.2**
Onion, Fried in Vegetable Oil, Takeaway, Average	**1 Bhaji/70g**	**190**	**10.3**	**270**	**9.8**	**24.6**	**14.7**	**5.6**
Onion, Frozen, Tesco*	1 Bhaji/14g	28	1.4	203	6.3	20.1	9.8	4.5
Potato, & Onion, Fried in Vegetable Oil, Average	**1oz/28g**	**45**	**2.8**	**160**	**2.1**	**16.6**	**10.1**	**1.6**
Potato, Onion & Mushroom, Fried, Average	**1oz/28g**	**58**	**4.9**	**208**	**2**	**12**	**17.5**	**1.5**
Potato, Spinach & Cauliflower, Fried, Average	**1oz/28g**	**47**	**4.2**	**169**	**2.2**	**7.1**	**15.1**	**1.4**
Spinach, & Potato, Fried in Vegetable Oil, Average	**1oz/28g**	**53**	**3.9**	**191**	**3.7**	**13.4**	**14.1**	**2.3**
Spinach, Fried in Vegetable Oil, Average	**1oz/28g**	**23**	**1.9**	**83**	**3.3**	**2.6**	**6.8**	**2.4**
Sweet Potato, & Red Onion, On the Go, Sainsbury's*	1 Pack/64g	157	7.6	245	4.6	25.5	11.8	9
Vegetable, Fried in Vegetable Oil, Average	**1oz/28g**	**59**	**5.2**	**212**	**2.1**	**10.1**	**18.5**	**2.4**
BHUNA								
Chicken, with Rice, Ready Meal, Average	**1 Pack/350g**	**444**	**20.8**	**127**	**9.4**	**8.9**	**5.9**	**1.4**
Lamb, 405, Oakhouse Foods Ltd*	1 Meal/400g	412	14	103	4.8	13	3.5	0.8
Prawn, King, M&S*	1 Pack/400g	308	15.2	77	6.7	3.3	3.8	1.5
Prawn, King, Morrisons*	1 Pack/350g	301	20.6	86	6.5	1.8	5.9	0.5
Prawn, King, Specially Selected, Aldi*	½ Pack/169g	132	6.8	78	5.3	4.4	4	1.4
BILBERRIES								
Fresh, Raw	**1oz/28g**	**8**	**0.1**	**29**	**0.6**	**6.8**	**0.2**	**1.8**
BILTONG								
Average	**1 Serving/25g**	**64**	**1**	**256**	**50**	**0**	**4**	**0**
BIRYANI								
Chicken, Ready Meal, Average	**1 Pack/400g**	**521**	**17.1**	**130**	**7.5**	**15.2**	**4.3**	**1.6**
Chicken, Tikka, Ready Meal, Average	**1 Pack/400g**	**460**	**11.5**	**115**	**7.3**	**14.8**	**2.9**	**1.5**
Chicken, Vegetarian, Linda McCartney*	½ Pack/180g	300	11.7	167	8.6	17	6.5	3.3
Jackfruit, Vegetarian, Waitrose*	1 Pack/375g	386	14.2	103	2.1	12.8	3.8	4.6
Lamb, Average	**1 Serving/200g**	**390**	**19.4**	**195**	**7.3**	**20.9**	**9.7**	**0**
Vegetable, Indian, Waitrose*	1 Pack/450g	626	25.2	139	2.8	17.5	5.6	3.6
Vegetable, Meal for 1, Sainsbury's*	1 Pack/376g	481	19.9	128	2.4	16.6	5.3	2.3
Vegetarian, Chicken Style, Lunch Pot, Quorn*	1 Pot/300g	300	13	100	3.5	10.9	4.4	1.7
BISCUITS								
Abbey Crunch, McVitie's*	1 Biscuit/9g	43	1.6	477	6	72.8	17.9	2.5
Abernethy, Simmers*	1 Biscuit/12g	61	2.7	490	5.7	69.2	21.9	0
Ace Milk Chocolate, McVitie's*	1 Biscuit/24g	122	5.9	510	6.1	66.2	24.5	1.6
All Butter, M&S*	1 Biscuit/8g	42	2.1	505	5.8	63.1	25	2.2
Almond & Chocolate, Biscotti, TTD, Sainsbury's*	1 Biscuit/30g	132	4.8	440	8.4	65.6	16	3.1
Almond, Cantuccini, Italiamo, Lidl*	3 Biscuits/19g	83	2.7	438	9.5	66.7	14	0
Almond, M&S*	1 Biscuit/9g	46	2.4	512	6.9	60.5	26.4	2.3
Almond, Thins, TTD, Sainsbury's*	1 Biscuit/4g	16	0.5	450	6.7	72.8	14.7	3.1
Amaretti, Average	**1 Biscuit/5g**	**22**	**0.8**	**434**	**8.1**	**66.4**	**15.4**	**2.8**
Anzac, Bitesmart*	1 Biscuit/20g	84	4.6	420	5.1	46.8	23	0
Apple & Cinnamon Thins, Finest, Tesco*	1 Biscuit/5g	22	0.8	470	5.9	71.7	17.5	1.5
Apple Crumble, Officially Low Fat, Fox's*	1 Biscuit/23g	85	0.6	365	5.4	80.4	2.4	2.5

	Measure INFO/WEIGHT	per Measure KCAL	per Measure FAT	Nutrition Values per 100g / 100ml KCAL	PROT	CARB	FAT	FIBRE
BISCUITS								
Arrowroot, Thin, Crawfords*	1 Biscuit/7g	35	1.2	450	6.9	71.4	15.2	2.8
Baileys Square, Bahlsen*	1 Square/10g	56	3.5	561	6.4	54	35	0
Baiocchi, Mulino Bianco*	1 Biscuit/9g	46	2.3	511	7.5	60	26	3.3
Baked Bites, Cheddar, Mini, Cathedral City*	1 Pack/22g	115	6.4	521	12.2	51.4	29.2	2.6
Bar, Gold, McVitie's*	1 Bar/18g	95	4.8	519	5.2	64.9	26.4	0.6
Bars, Disco Bits, Oki Doki*	1 Bar/27g	121	5	449	4.9	65.6	18.4	0
Belgian Chocolate Chip, Walkers Shortbread Ltd*	2 Biscuits/25g	124	6.1	494	5.1	63.3	24.5	2.2
Belgian Chocolate, Selection, Finest, Tesco*	1 Biscuit/10g	52	2.7	515	6	62	27	3
Belgian Milk Chocolate, M&S*	1 Biscuit/12g	60	2.5	490	6.2	70.1	20.3	2.5
Billionaire, Salted Caramel, Squares, Moments, McVitie's*	1 Square/41g	194	10.4	473	3.8	56.6	25.4	1.3
Biscoff, Cream, Lotus*	1 Biscuit/10g	52	2.6	522	4.6	66	26	1.2
Biscotti, Chocolate Chip, Kate's Cakes Ltd*	1 Biscotti/36g	134	4.6	372	6.5	57.9	12.7	2.7
Biscotti, Chocolate, Heinz*	1 Biscuit/20g	80	1.7	398	8.5	72	8.7	5.8
Biscotti, Thins, The Artful Baker*	1 Biscotti/5g	25	1	492	11.7	69	19.4	3.7
Bourbon, Average	***1 Biscuit/13g***	***63***	***2.8***	***488***	***5.7***	***68.2***	***21.3***	***2.1***
Brandy Snaps, Average	***1 Biscuit/15g***	***69***	***2.2***	***460***	***2.7***	***79.8***	***14.4***	***0.5***
Brazil Nut, Chocolate, Ringtons*	1 Biscuit/25g	137	8.6	547	6.2	53.2	34.4	1.7
Breakfast, Blueberries, Soft Bakes, Belvita*	1 Biscuit/50g	194	6	388	5.5	63	12	7.5
Breakfast, Blueberry Flaxseeds, Seeds & Berries, Belvita*	1 Biscuit/15g	66	2.1	441	8.4	66	14	7
Breakfast, Choc Chips, Soft Bakes, Belvita*	1 Pack/50g	202	7.5	405	5.7	61	15	6.9
Breakfast, Choco Hazlenut, Tops, Belvita*	1 Pack/50g	230	8	460	7.2	69	16	4.9
Breakfast, Chocolate Chip, Bakes, Genius*	1 Bake/28g	142	7.9	507	5.2	56	28.3	4
Breakfast, Cocoa, Chocolate Chip, Belvita*	1 Pack/50g	220	7.5	440	7.8	66	15	7.1
Breakfast, Golden Grain, Soft Bakes, Belvita*	1 Pack/50g	192	6	385	5.9	63	12	6.7
Breakfast, Honey & Nuts, Belvita*	1 Pack/50g	228	7.5	455	7.6	69	15	4.4
Breakfast, Honey & Oat, Eat Well, M&S*	2 Biscuits/20g	88	3	442	9	65.6	15	4.3
Breakfast, Milk & Cereals, Belvita*	1 Pack/50g	220	7.2	440	7.9	67	14.5	6.5
Breakfast, Oat, Golden, Asda*	1 Pack/45g	210	9	467	6	64	20	5.1
Breakfast, Original, All Bran, Kellogg's*	1 Pack/40g	176	8	440	8	49	20	16
Breakfast, Red Berries, Soft Bakes, Belvita*	1 Pack/50g	190	5.5	380	5.5	65	11	6.6
Breakfast, Strawberry, & Yoghurt, Duo Crunch, Belvita*	2 Biscuits/51g	225	7.1	444	6.9	70	14	4.3
Breakfast, Whole Grain, No Added Sugar, Gullon*	1 Biscuit/9g	37	1.3	410	6.8	65	14	9.8
Butter, Chocolate Brownie, Farmhouse Biscuits*	1 Biscuit/17g	88	5.1	528	5.3	56.1	30.6	0
Butter, Dark Chocolate, Momento, Aldi*	1 Biscuit/14g	69	3.2	491	6.2	63.5	22.6	4.2
Butter, Dark Chocolate, Tesco*	1 Biscuit/14g	72	3.7	511	6.9	58.3	26.7	4.9
Butter, La Trinitaine*	1 Biscuit/10g	48	2.2	500	6.3	66	23	0
Butter, Milk Chocolate, Belmont Biscuit Co, Aldi*	1 Biscuit/14g	69	3.2	492	7.3	63	23	2.8
Butter, Milk Chocolate, Ritter Sport*	1 Biscuit/25g	139	8.5	555	6.1	55	34	0
Butter, Milk Chocolate, Tesco*	1 Biscuit/14g	71	3.6	508	7.8	61	25.4	2.2
Butter, with Dark Chocolate, Belmont Biscuit Co, Aldi*	1 Biscuit/14g	71	3.6	509	6.4	61	26	4.5
Butterli, Migros*	4 Biscuits/28g	130	4.2	463	9.1	72	15	2
Cafe Noir, with Coffee Flavour Icing, McVitie's*	1 Biscuit/6g	27	0.8	458	4.9	76	14	1.7
Cantuccini, with Almonds, Average	***1 Biscotti/30g***	***130***	***5***	***433***	***10***	***60***	***16.7***	***3.3***
Caramel Squares, Thorntons*	2 Biscuits/32g	150	6.4	470	6.2	65	20	2.4
Caramelised, Belmont Biscuit Co, Aldi*	1 Biscuit/8g	40	1.5	480	6.2	72	18	1.2
Caramelised, Biscoff, Lotus*	1 Biscuit/8g	38	1.5	484	4.9	72.7	19	1.3
Cheese Savouries, Sainsbury's*	1 Serving/30g	159	9.4	531	11.3	50	31.3	2.1
Cheese, & Chutney, Delicious, Boots*	1 Pack/134g	290	14.7	217	9	19	11	2.3
Cheese, Baked, Cheddars, Jacob's*	1 Cheddar/4g	20	1.2	525	10.8	47	31.8	2.9
Choc Chip, Paterson's*	1 Biscuit/17g	79	3.6	474	5.6	64	21.6	3.1
Choco Leibniz, Dark Chocolate, Bahlsen*	1 Biscuit/14g	69	3.6	493	6.8	59	26	5.1
Choco Leibniz, Milk, Bahlsen*	1 Biscuit/14g	71	3.5	505	7.5	61	25	2.4
Choco Leibniz, Orange Flavour, Bahlsen*	1 Biscuit/14g	70	3.7	504	7.9	58.5	26.4	0

	Measure INFO/WEIGHT	per Measure KCAL	FAT	Nutrition Values per 100g / 100ml KCAL	PROT	CARB	FAT	FIBRE
BISCUITS								
Choco Leibniz, White, Bahlsen *	2 Biscuits/28g	142	7	508	5.1	65	25	0
Chocolate Fingers, Milk, Cadbury*	1 Biscuit/6g	31	1.6	515	6.8	60.8	27.1	1.7
Chocolate Fingers, Salted Peanut Crunch, Cadbury*	4 Fingers/21g	100	5.5	478	6.6	52.9	26.5	1.4
Chocolate Florentine, M&S*	1 Serving/39g	195	9.7	500	7.4	64.5	24.9	1.7
Chocolate Ginger, Organic, Duchy Originals*	1 Biscuit/12g	64	3.6	518	4.6	59.7	29	2.1
Chocolate Ginger, Thorntons*	1 Biscuit/19g	96	5.3	512	5.9	58.2	28.4	0
Chocolate Kimberley, Jacob's*	1 Biscuit/20g	86	3.4	428	3.9	64.4	17.2	1.1
Chocolate Sandwich Finger, M&S*	1 Biscuit/31g	161	8.8	520	6.2	58.2	28.4	3.2
Chocolate Viennese, Fox's*	1 Biscuit/16g	85	4.9	530	6.7	56.6	30.7	1.7
Chocolate, Breakaway, Nestle*	1 Bar/19g	99	4.9	511	6.1	63.5	25.2	3
Chocolate, Cadbury*	1 Biscuit/20g	102	5	510	5.5	65	25	2.5
Chocolate, Damiler, Sticks, Mikado *	5 Sticks/10g	47	1.8	471	6.5	70	18	3
Chocolate, Dark, & Raspberry, Elizabeth Shaw*	1 Biscuit/16g	72	3.1	450	3.5	62.7	19.4	3.4
Chocolate, Fingers, Average	***1 Biscuit/6g***	***31***	***1.6***	***514***	***6.7***	***61.4***	***26.8***	***1.5***
Chocolate, Golden Crunch, Free From Milk, Tesco*	1 Biscuit/17g	85	4.9	510	4.2	57.2	29.4	4.6
Chocolate, Milk, Special Assortment, Tesco*	1 Biscuit/17g	89	4.6	521	5.6	62.9	27	1.8
Chocolate, Milk, Take Away, Belmont Biscuit Co, Aldi*	1 Biscuit/28g	136	5.9	487	8	65	21	2.5
Chocolatey Orange, Fox's*	1 Biscuit/17g	91	5	536	4.8	62.3	29.5	0.9
Classic, Milk Chocolate, Fox's*	1 Biscuit/13g	67	3.1	517	6.1	64.9	24	1.6
Classico, Gran Cereale*	1 Biscuit/11g	51	2	461	8.3	61.4	18.5	8
Cocoa Cream, Lidl*	1 Biscuit/25g	117	4.5	468	6	69	18	3
Coconut, & Chocolate, Sondey, Lidl*	1 Biscuit/19g	91	5.5	479	6	44	29	9
Coconut, Ring, Average	***1 Biscuit/9g***	***44***	***2***	***490***	***6.1***	***67.4***	***21.8***	***2.6***
Coffee, GF, Barkat*	2 Biscuits/15g	72	2.8	479	2	75	19	0
Cookies & Cream, Belmont Biscuit Co, Aldi*	1 Biscuit/11g	52	2	469	4.9	72	18	2.2
Crispy Fruit Slices, Apple, Sultana, Go Ahead, McVitie's*	1 Slice/13g	50	0.9	388	5.4	74	7.1	2.9
Crispy Fruit Slices, Forest Fruit, Go Ahead, McVitie's*	1 Biscuit/13g	49	0.9	380	5.4	73.7	7	3
Crispy Slices, Raspberry, Crownfield, Lidl*	1 Slice/15g	58	1	399	9.5	73	7	2.8
Crispy Slices, Raspberry, Go Ahead, McVitie's*	1 Slice/13g	50	0.9	385	5.3	74	7	2.8
Croquants de Cordes, No.1, Waitrose*	1 Biscuit/4g	20	0.5	445	10	72.3	12.2	3.2
Crunch Creams, Double Choc, Fox's*	1 Biscuit/15g	77	3.8	511	4.7	65	25	2.7
Crunchers, Salted, Savoury, Crackers, Sainsbury's*	1 Cracker/5g	22	1	448	6.1	59.4	20.4	1.4
Crunchie, Cadbury*	1 Biscuit/13g	64	3.1	495	4.8	65.7	23.6	0.9
Crunchy Caramel, Tesco*	1 Bar/21g	98	5.2	467	4.6	56	25	1.4
Custard Cream, Savers, Morrisons*	1 Biscuit/13g	65	2.9	513	5.8	69.6	22.9	2.4
Custard Creams, Asda*	1 Biscuit/12g	59	2.7	495	5	67	23	2
Custard Creams, Co-Op*	1 Biscuit/12g	60	2.6	497	5.6	68	22	1.5
Custard Creams, M&S*	1 Biscuit/13g	63	2.8	494	5.5	67.2	22	2.4
Custard Creams, Sainsbury's*	1 Biscuit/13g	67	3	514	5.5	70.4	23.4	1.6
Custard Creams, Savers, Morrisons*	1 Biscuit/12g	59	2.5	489	5.6	68.5	21.1	1.4
Custard Creams, Tesco*	1 Biscuit/12g	58	2.4	490	5.7	70.1	20.5	1.1
Custard Creams, Trufree*	1 Biscuit/12g	60	2.8	504	8.7	65	23	1
Dark Chocolate Ginger, M&S*	1 Biscuit/21g	105	5.7	505	5	58.8	27.6	4.2
Dark Chocolate Gingers, Border*	1 Biscuit/17g	74	3.4	445	4.4	61.4	20.1	2.9
Dark Cookie Creams, McVitie's*	4 Biscuits/42g	196	7.5	467	1.5	71	17.8	42.9
Diet Fibre, Gullon*	2 Biscuits/16g	65	2.6	405	6.5	48.7	16.4	23
Digestive with Wheatgerm, Hovis*	1 Biscuit/12g	57	2.4	475	8.3	65	20	3.3
Digestive, Caramels, Milk Chocolate, McVitie's*	1 Biscuit/17g	81	3.7	478	5.6	65.1	21.7	2.3
Digestive, Chocolate	***1 Biscuit/17g***	***84***	***4.1***	***493***	***6.8***	***66.5***	***24.1***	***2.2***
Digestive, Chocolate Chip, Asda*	1 Biscuit/14g	68	3.2	491	6	65	23	2.9
Digestive, Chocolate, Free From, Co-Op*	1 Biscuit/11g	54	2.3	495	6.3	69	21	2.9
Digestive, Chocolate, GF, Just Free, Lidl*	1 Biscuit/13g	64	2.8	482	6.3	66	20.8	3.2
Digestive, Chocolate,Strawberries & Cream, Mcvitie's*	1 Biscuit/15g	74	3.5	495	6.6	62.7	23.4	3

B

	Measure INFO/WEIGHT	per Measure KCAL	FAT	Nutrition Values per 100g / 100ml KCAL	PROT	CARB	FAT	FIBRE
BISCUITS								
Digestive, Dark Choc Chip, Sainsbury's*	1 Biscuit/12g	59	2.6	475	7.1	62.2	20.7	5.5
Digestive, Dark Chocolate, McVitie's*	1 Biscuit/17g	83	4.1	495	6	60.8	24.2	4.2
Digestive, Dark Chocolate, Thins, McVitie's*	1 Biscuit/6g	31	1.5	499	6	60.9	24.7	4.7
Digestive, GF, Schar*	1 Biscuit/10g	48	2.2	483	6.1	62	22	6.2
Digestive, Lemon & Ginger, McVitie's*	1 Biscuit/15g	72	3.1	480	6.7	66.7	20.7	2.7
Digestive, Light, McVitie's*	1 Biscuit/15g	66	2.1	444	7.3	69.5	14.4	3.6
Digestive, Oat, Weight Watchers*	1 Biscuit/11g	50	2.1	457	6	66.3	18.6	6.9
Digestive, Plain Chocolate, Tesco*	1 Biscuit/17g	85	4.1	499	6.2	63.5	24.4	2.8
Digestive, Plain, Average	***1 Biscuit/14g***	***67***	***2.9***	***480***	***7.1***	***65.6***	***20.5***	***3.5***
Digestive, Reduced Fat, McVitie's*	1 Biscuit/15g	70	2.4	467	7.1	72.8	16.3	3.4
Digestive, Sugar Free, Gullon*	1 Biscuit/13g	57	2.1	430	6.2	68	16	6.5
Digestive, Whole Wheat, Organic, Dove's Farm*	1 Biscuit/13g	56	2.4	446	5.9	61.6	19.5	7.8
Digestives, Chocolate Chip Coconut, Twists, McVitie's*	1 Biscuit/9g	47	2.4	505	6.6	57.9	26.1	5.3
Digestives, Dark Chocolate, Asda*	1 Biscuit/18g	84	4	467	6.1	61.1	22.2	2.8
Digestives, Double Chocolate, Mcvitie's*	1 Biscuit/17g	83	4.1	497	6.5	60.9	24.3	3.6
Dorset Knob, Original White, Moores*	1 Biscuit/13g	52	1	398	12	70.5	7.6	0
Double Choc Chip, Trufree*	1 Biscuit/11g	58	3	523	3	67	27	1.8
Elite, Teacake, Jacob's*	1 Biscuit/22g	97	3.7	442	5.3	66	17	1.7
Extremely Chocolatey, Dark Chocolate Rounds, M&S*	1 Biscuit/19g	97	5.6	510	6.2	55.7	29.3	6.3
Extremely Chocolatey, Milk Chocolate, Rounds, M&S*	1 Pack/44g	227	11.7	517	6.4	61.6	26.7	2.3
Fig Roll, Tesco*	1 Biscuit/19g	70	1.6	375	4	69.3	8.8	3.1
Florentines, Milk Chocolate, & Orange, No.1, Waitrose*	1 Florentine/19g	102	6.5	536	7.7	47.7	34.1	3.5
Forest Fruit, Yoghurt, Breaks, Go Ahead, McVitie's*	2 Slices/36g	144	3.6	402	5.4	72.6	10	2.2
Freddo, Face Cakes, Cadbury*	1 Cake/30g	126	5.7	420	6	57	19	1.4
Fruit Shortcake, McVitie's*	1 Biscuit/8g	37	1.5	462	5.6	65.9	18.9	3.1
Fruit Shortcake, Morrisons*	1 Biscuit/8g	38	1.5	469	6.2	68	18.7	1.9
Fruit Shortcake, Tesco*	1 Biscuit/9g	43	1.7	473	5.8	70.1	18.8	1.9
Fruit Shorties, Hill Biscuits Ltd*	1 Biscuit/7g	33	1.3	464	5.7	69	18	2.9
Fruit Slices, Apple, Raisin & Currant, Belmont, Aldi*	1 Biscuit/15g	57	1	379	7	72.8	6.4	1.3
Galaxy, Caramel Secret Centre, Galaxy, Mars*	1 Biscuit/17g	84	4.2	496	5.5	61.8	24.8	0
Galettes Bretonnes, Sondey, Lidl*	1 Biscuit/8g	40	1.6	496	7.4	70.4	20	0
Garibaldi, Asda*	1 Biscuit/10g	39	0.9	375	4.7	68.5	9.1	2.2
Garibaldi, Sainsbury's*	1 Biscuit/9g	34	0.8	378	4.6	67.6	9.2	3.3
Garibaldi, Tesco*	1 Biscuit/10g	40	0.9	400	4.7	74	9.1	2.2
Ginger Crunch Creams, Fox's*	1 Biscuit/15g	77	3.5	501	4.1	68	23	1.6
Ginger, & Lemon, Snaps, Nyakers*	3 Snaps/15g	65	1.8	433	3.3	76.7	11.7	0
Ginger, Belgian Dark Chocolate, Thins, Waitrose*	1 Biscuit/10g	48	2.2	481	6.2	61.2	22.5	4.6
Ginger, Dark Chocolate Coated, Waitrose*	1 Biscuits/23g	122	6.9	530	6.4	56.4	29.8	5.1
Ginger, Scottish, in Dark Chocolate, Lidl*	1 Biscuit/16g	78	4	488	5	58.8	25	3.1
Ginger, Snap, 35% Reduced Fat, Sainsbury's*	1 Biscuit/10g	42	0.9	421	6.8	77.1	9	2.4
Ginger, Thins, Heart Shaped, Ikea*	1 Biscuit/6g	28	1	462	5.4	72	17	0
Gingernut	***1 Biscuit/11g***	***50***	***1.7***	***456***	***5.6***	***79.1***	***15.2***	***1.4***
Gocciole Wild, Pavesi*	1 Biscuit/12g	57	2.5	477	8.2	61	21	5.7
Golden Crunch Creams, Fox's*	1 Biscuit/15g	75	3.8	515	4.7	64.8	26.3	1.2
Hobnobs, Choc Chip, Mcvities*	1 Biscuit/15g	72	3.2	471	7.2	60.5	20.8	6.4
Hobnobs, Chocolate Creams, McVitie's*	1 Biscuit/12g	60	3.1	503	6.7	60.3	26.1	4
Hobnobs, McVitie's*	1 Biscuit/15g	72	3.2	473	7	61.8	20.7	5.4
Hobnobs, Milk Chocolate, McVitie's*	1 Biscuit/19g	92	4.5	479	6.8	60.7	23.3	4.5
Hobnobs, Plain Chocolate, McVitie's*	1 Biscuit/16g	81	3.9	498	6.7	63.3	24.3	4.2
Hobnobs, Vanilla Creams, McVitie's*	1 Biscuit/12g	60	3	501	6.1	62.3	25.2	3.6
Jaffa Cakes, Asda*	1 Cake/12g	43	1	368	4.7	67.5	8.8	1.9
Jaffa Cakes, Belmont Biscuit Co, Aldi*	1 Biscuit/13g	52	1.3	400	3.7	72.8	10.2	1
Jaffa Cakes, Dark Chocolate, M&S*	1 Cake/11g	45	1.5	395	3.7	64.9	13.2	2.8

	Measure INFO/WEIGHT	per Measure KCAL	FAT	Nutrition Values per 100g / 100ml KCAL	PROT	CARB	FAT	FIBRE
BISCUITS								
Jaffa Cakes, Dark Chocolate, Mini, M&S*	1 Cake/5g	20	0.8	410	3.9	62.8	15.8	1.9
Jaffa Cakes, McVitie's*	1 Cake/12g	46	1	380	4.9	70.8	8	2.2
Jaffa Cakes, Mini Roll, McVitie's*	1 Cake/26g	99	2.7	374	3.5	67.1	10.1	2.3
Jaffa Cakes, Sainsbury's*	1 Cake/11g	41	1	373	4.3	69.3	8.8	2
Jaffa Cakes, Smart Price, Asda*	1 Cake/12g	43	1	374	4.3	69	9	2
Jaffa Cakes, Value, Tesco*	1 Cake/12g	45	1.1	388	4.7	70	9.4	2.2
Jam Sandwich Creams, M&S*	1 Biscuit/17g	80	3.7	485	5.7	64.5	22.6	1.8
Jam Sandwich Creams, Sainsbury's*	1 Biscuit/15g	75	3.4	488	4.9	65.6	22.4	2.2
Jam Sandwich Creams, Tesco*	1 Biscuit/15g	72	3.2	482	4.8	67.1	21.4	1.2
Jam, & Creams, Asda*	1 Biscuit/15g	74	3.3	493	5.1	69	22	1.6
Jammie Cart Wheel, Belmont Biscuit Co, Aldi*	1 Wheel/38g	166	5.7	436	4.6	71	15	1.8
Jammie Dodgers, Minis, Burton's*	4 Biscuits/20g	88	2.9	438	4.6	72.2	14.7	2.4
Jammie Dodgers, Minis, Lunchbox, Burton's*	1 Pack/20g	89	3	445	6	70	15.1	2.3
Jammie Dodgers, Original, Burton's*	1 Biscuit/18g	78	2.5	436	5.4	71.3	13.9	1.7
Jammy Wheels, GF, Prewett's*	1 Biscuit/24g	95	5.6	394	5	60.1	23.2	4.7
Lemon Melts, Island Bakery*	1 Biscuit/13g	66	3.6	496	6.2	59	27	0
Lemon, & Chia, Weight Watchers*	1 Biscuit/10g	42	1.5	418	15.4	49.4	15.4	10.2
Lemon, All Butter, Half Coated, Finest, Tesco*	1 Biscuit/17g	84	4.5	505	5.6	60.4	26.9	3.6
Lemon, Farmhouse*	1 Biscuit/19g	104	5.7	545	4.6	63.3	29.9	0
Lion, Caramel, Masterpieces, Godiva*	1 Biscuit/12g	65	3.5	540	8.6	60	29	0
Magretti Cioccolato, Galbusera*	1 Biscuit/5g	22	0.6	441	8.3	72.2	12.5	3
Malted Milk, Average	***1 Biscuit/9g***	***42***	***1.9***	***490***	***7***	***65.6***	***22.2***	***1.8***
Malted Milk, Chocolate, Tesco*	1 Biscuit/10g	52	2.5	500	6.7	64.4	24	1.9
Malted Milk, Milk Chocolate, Sainsbury's*	1 Biscuit/11g	56	2.7	505	6.4	64.4	24.2	2.1
Malted, Moon & Stars, Tesco*	1 Mini Bag/18g	86	3.6	478	7.8	66.1	20	2.2
Maltesers, Mars*	2 Biscuits/22g	112	5.6	509	7.1	61.9	25.3	0
Maple Leaf, M&S*	1 Biscuit/13g	50	1.9	395	5.1	59.8	14.8	2
Maria, Chocolate, Hacendado *	1 Biscuit/10g	47	1.7	466	7.6	69	17	3.2
Maria, Gullon*	1 Biscuit/6g	24	0.7	408	7	75	11	4.5
Marie, Crawfords*	1 Biscuit/7g	33	1.1	475	7.5	76.3	15.5	2.3
Marie, Pingo Doce *	1 Biscuit/6g	26	0.6	430	7.8	76.9	9.6	2.8
Milk Chocolate Digestive, Everyday Value, Tesco*	1 Biscuit/17g	82	3.7	494	7.2	65.4	22.3	1.7
Milk Chocolate, All Butter, M&S*	1 Biscuit/14g	70	3.6	490	7.9	57.4	25.5	1.4
Milk Chocolate, Squares, M&S*	1 Biscuit/14g	70	3.5	498	6.3	61.4	24.8	1.9
Milk, Dark, & White, The Best, Morrisons*	1 Biscuit/17g	88	4.5	517	6.1	62.2	26.6	2.2
Milkshake, Belmont Biscuit Co, Aldi*	1 Biscuit/25g	134	7.5	536	6.4	59	30	1.7
Mint, Viscount*	1 Biscuit/14g	73	4	525	4.5	61.6	28.5	1.8
Moments, Chocolate, Special K, Kellogg's*	1 Bar/25g	96	2.3	383	5.5	72	9.1	2.3
Morning Coffee, Tesco*	1 Biscuit/5g	22	0.7	450	7.6	72.3	14.5	2.4
Nice, Average	***1 Biscuit/8g***	***36***	***1.6***	***484***	***6.3***	***67.3***	***21***	***2.5***
Nut Butter Cups, Almond, Nature Valley*	2 Cups/35g	176	9	503	8.4	56.3	25.8	6
Nut Butter Cups, Cocoa, & Hazelnut, Nature Valley*	2 Cups/35g	178	9.6	510	8.3	54.4	27.3	6.6
Nutella, Ferrero*	1 Biscuit/14g	71	3.4	513	8.4	63.3	24.5	0
Oat Crumbles, Border*	1 Biscuit/15g	66	3.1	443	5.3	58.9	20.7	1.8
Oat Crumbles, Chocolate, Border*	1 Biscuit/15g	71	3.7	475	5.7	56.4	24.7	0
Oat Crumbles, Golden, Border*	1 Biscuit/15g	63	2.9	422	4.9	56.2	19.2	0
Oat, & Chocolate Chip, GF, Breaks, Nairn's*	1 Biscuit/10g	47	2	470	7.6	61.8	20.1	5.5
Oat, & Fruit, GF, Breaks, Nairn's*	1 Biscuit/10g	46	1.9	460	8.4	61.8	18.6	6
Oat, & Stem Ginger, GF, Breaks, Nairn's*	1 Biscuit/10g	46	1.9	463	8.2	62.4	18.8	5.7
Oat, Apple, & cinnamon, Chunky, GF, Breaks, Nairn's*	1 Biscuit/13g	61	2.8	471	8	57	21.7	8
Oat, Beetroot, Nigella, & Three Seed, Waitrose*	1 Biscuit/10g	48	2.4	481	11.9	50.7	23.9	7.7
Oat, Black Sesame & Seaweed, 1, Waitrose*	1 Biscuit/5g	27	1.3	487	10.5	55.5	23.1	7.8
Oat, Dark Chocolate Chip, Nairn's*	1 Biscuit/10g	46	1.7	454	8.1	63.8	16.9	6.7

	Measure INFO/WEIGHT	per Measure KCAL	FAT	Nutrition Values per 100g / 100ml KCAL	PROT	CARB	FAT	FIBRE
BISCUITS								
Oat, Fruit & Spice, Nairn's*	1 Biscuit/10g	43	1.5	425	7.8	65.3	14.7	7.6
Oat, Mixed Berries, Nairn's*	1 Biscuit/10g	43	1.5	427	7.5	64.8	15.3	7.1
Oat, Sweet, Mcallister's*	1 Biscuit/19g	98	5	515	5.6	63.4	26.2	1.5
Oatie Crumble, Asda*	1 Biscuit/14g	69	2.9	476	7	64	20	4.9
Oatie Crumbles, Milk Chocolate, Asda*	1 Biscuit/19g	93	4.4	489	7	62	23	4.6
Oaties, Belmont Biscuit Co, Aldi*	1 Biscuit/20g	95	4.2	476	7.8	62	21	4.8
Oaties, Chocolate, Milk, Aldi*	1 Biscuit/20g	95	4.2	476	7.8	62	21	4.8
Oaties, Chocolate, Orange, & Cranberry, Frank's*	1 Biscuit/38g	171	7.1	456	5	65	19	0
Oaties, GF, Nairn's*	1 Biscuit/10g	48	2.2	480	9	58	22	7
Oaties, Tower Gate, Lidl*	1 Biscuit/15g	74	3.2	491	8.9	63	21	7
Oatmeal Crunch, Jacob's*	1 Biscuit/8g	37	1.5	458	6.8	65.9	18.6	3.6
Oatmeal, Asda*	1 Biscuit/12g	54	2.5	470	6	62	22	6
Oaty, Sugar Free, Siro*	1 Biscuit/16g	75	3.4	466	8	59	21	5.6
Olive Oil, Savoury Ships, Brindisa*	1 Biscuit/8g	33	0.9	409	11.2	63.5	11.6	6
Onion Marmalade, Chilli, & Garlic, Savoury, Co-Op*	2 Biscuits/16g	70	2.3	449	7.7	68	15	5.1
Orange Sultana, Go Ahead, McVitie's*	1 Biscuit/15g	58	1.2	400	5.1	75.7	8.1	3
Oreo, Chocolate Coated, Cadbury, Mondelez*	1 Biscuit/21g	98	4.5	478	5.9	63	22	3
Oreo, Chocolate Cream, Thins, Mondelez*	4 Biscuits/24g	117	4.8	488	5.4	69	20	3.5
Oreo, Thins, Mondelez*	4 Biscuits/24g	118	5.1	490	4.8	69	21	2.6
Oreos, Choc o Brownie, Mondelez*	1 Biscuit/11g	52	2.1	473	5.7	67	19	3.8
Parkin, Westray Bakehouse *	1 Biscuit/22g	95	2.9	433	7	73	13	0
Parmesan Cheese, Sainsbury's*	1 Biscuit/3g	18	1	553	14.7	56.4	29.9	1.8
Party Rings, Iced, Fox's*	1 Biscuit/6g	29	0.9	459	5.1	75.8	15	0
Peanut Butter, American Style, Sainsbury's*	1 Biscuit/13g	63	2.9	504	5.2	68.7	23.1	2.2
Petit Beurre, Stella Artois*	1 Biscuit/6g	26	0.9	440	9	73	15	0
Pink Panther, Home Bargains*	1 Wafer/8g	42	2.2	527	4.6	64	28	1.9
Pink Wafers, Crawfords*	1 Biscuit/7g	36	1.9	521	2.5	68.6	26.5	1.1
Pink Wafers, Eat Me, Aldi*	1 Biscuit/8g	44	2.6	552	4.2	58.4	32.9	2.9
Pink Wafers, Sainsbury's*	1 Biscuit/8g	36	1.8	486	4.6	64.2	23.4	1.7
Praline Squares, Bahlsen*	1 Biscuit/11g	62	4	561	7.7	50	36	0
Raspberry & Cream Viennese, Melts, Fox's*	1 Biscuit/16g	84	4.5	521	4	62.1	28.1	1.7
Raspberry Creams, Bolands*	1 Biscuit/13g	64	3	504	4.6	67.3	23.6	2.2
Raspberry Sandwich Creams, Free From, Morrisons*	2 Biscuits/28g	126	4.3	458	2.9	76.6	15.5	0.1
Raspberry, Yoghurt Breaks, Go Ahead, McVitie's*	1 Pack/35g	143	3.6	408	5.4	73.6	10.2	2.3
Redcurrant Puffs, Eat Well, M&S*	1 Biscuit/7g	32	1.4	470	5.6	67.7	19.8	2
Rich Shorties, Asda*	1 Biscuit/10g	50	2.3	486	6	66	22	2
Rich Tea, Average	***1 Biscuit/10g***	***45***	***1.5***	***451***	***6.8***	***72.8***	***14.5***	***2.5***
Rich Tea, Light, McVitie's*	1 Biscuit/8g	36	0.9	436	7.6	75.3	10.7	3.1
Rich Tea, Reduced Fat, Tesco*	1 Biscuit/9g	40	0.8	424	8.1	76.7	8.7	3.4
Rocky, Chocolate & Caramel, Fox's*	1 Biscuit/21g	107	4.1	507	6.9	60.3	19.3	15.5
Rocky, Chocolate, Fox's*	1 Biscuit/21g	106	5.4	505	5.7	62.4	25.7	2.4
Rounds, Chocolatey, Seriously, Tower Gate, Lidl*	1 Biscuit/17g	84	4	503	5.5	65	24.2	1.5
Rounds, Jammy Shortbread, Festive, Paterson's*	1 Biscuit/24g	112	4.6	470	5.3	67.3	19.5	0
Safari Snacks, Belmont Biscuit Co, Aldi*	1 Bag/22g	108	4.8	492	6.4	65	22	2.8
Savoury, Gluten, Wheat & Dairy Free, Sainsbury's*	1 Biscuit/17g	77	2.9	467	11.7	65.1	17.7	2.4
Shortbread, Salted Toffee, GF, Free From, Sainsbury's*	1 Biscuit/20g	100	4.8	502	4.7	65.8	24.2	0.9
Shortcake Snack, Cadbury*	2 Biscuits/20g	102	5.2	512	6.6	63	26	2.1
Shortcake with Real Milk Chocolate, Cadbury*	1 Biscuit/15g	75	3.5	500	6.3	65.8	23.5	0
Shortcake, Average	***1 Biscuit/11g***	***55***	***3***	***501***	***6.3***	***66.1***	***27.1***	***2.1***
Shortcake, Caramel, Mini, Thorntons*	1 Biscuit/15g	71	4.6	492	4.8	46.3	31.9	0.6
Shortcake, Caramel, Squares, Tesco*	1 Square/54g	274	16.4	507	4.6	54.1	30.4	0.4
Shortcake, Dairy Milk Chocolate, Cadbury*	1 Bar/49g	252	13.5	515	7.5	59.2	27.5	0
Shortcake, Dutch, M&S*	1 Biscuit/17g	90	5.1	540	5.4	59	30.8	2.5

	Measure INFO/WEIGHT	per Measure KCAL	FAT	Nutrition Values per 100g / 100ml KCAL	PROT	CARB	FAT	FIBRE
BISCUITS								
Shortcake, Fruit, Crawfords*	1 Biscuit/8g	34	1.5	419	5.4	55.9	19.3	2.4
Shorties, Fruit, Value, Tesco*	1 Serving/10g	46	1.7	457	5.7	69.3	17.4	3
Shorties, Rich, Tesco*	1 Biscuit/10g	48	2.2	484	6.4	65.6	21.8	2
Shorties, Sainsbury's*	1 Biscuit/10g	50	2.2	500	6.4	69.8	21.8	2
Slices, Forest Fruit, Go Ahead, McVitie's*	1 Slice/15g	55	1	379	5.2	74.8	7	3.6
Snappy, Milk Chocolate Finger, Tesco*	2 Fingers/21g	113	6.1	528	6.5	60.8	28.3	2
Soft Bakes, Choco Hazelnut, Harvest Morn, Aldi*	1 Bar/50g	200	6.5	401	5.5	60	13	8.9
Speculaas, Large, Hema*	1 Biscuit/23g	106	4.8	459	5.4	61.2	20.8	2.6
Speculaas, Sandwich, Fortnum & Mason*	1 Biscuit/22g	111	5.4	504	5.4	63.3	24.7	0
Spekulatius, Chocolate, Tesco*	1 Biscuit/2g	10	0.5	488	6.9	64	22	3.3
Spekulatius, Cinnamon, Tesco*	1 Biscuit/2g	7	0.2	455	6	71.1	15.7	2.5
Spiced, German, Christmas, Favorina, Lidl*	1 Biscuit/10g	47	1.9	472	5.8	70.2	18.7	0
Stem Ginger, Brakes*	1 Biscuit/13g	62	3.1	495	5.6	62.6	24.7	0
Stornoway, Water, Stag Bakeries Ltd*	1 Biscuit/9g	31	1.2	341	6.5	47.9	13.6	1.7
Strawberry, Biscuit Moments, Special K, Kellogg's*	2 Biscuits/25g	98	2	391	5	74	8	1.5
Treacle Crunch Creams, Fox's*	1 Biscuit/13g	65	3.2	502	4.5	65.3	24.8	1.4
Triple Chocolate, Fox's*	1 Biscuit/21g	100	5.2	478	5.7	57.3	25.1	2.5
Twix, Caramel Slice, McVitie's*	1 Slice/29g	142	7.8	491	4.5	57.3	26.8	1.4
Twix, Soft Centre, Mars*	1 Biscuit/18g	83	3.7	462	4.5	64.3	20.4	0
Viennese Finger, Belmont Biscuit Co, Aldi*	1 Biscuit/16g	84	4.7	521	4.8	61	29	1.5
Viennese Shorties, Sugar Free, Farmhouse Biscuits*	1 Biscuit/18g	87	4.5	486	3.4	61.8	24.9	0
Viennese Swirls, All Butter, Waitrose*	1 Biscuit/14g	76	4.7	548	4.9	55.2	33.7	2.1
Viennese Whirl, Fox's*	1 Biscuit/25g	130	7	518	6.7	60.1	27.8	0
Viennese, Chocolate, Melts, Fox's*	1 Biscuit/12g	64	3.4	526	6.1	60.5	28.3	2.4
Viennese, Milk Chocolate, Thins, Tesco*	1 Biscuit/9g	48	2.7	533	5.1	59.7	30.1	1.5
Viennese, Sandwich, Chocolate, M&S*	1 Biscuit/15g	80	4.6	535	7.2	58	30.6	1.7
Viennese, Vanillha, Waitrose*	1 Biscuit/15g	80	4.3	531	6.7	60.9	28.6	1.8
Viennese, with Milk Chocolate Filling	***1 Biscuit/15g***	***81***	***4.5***	***533***	***6.5***	***59.6***	***29.4***	***2.1***
Water, Average	***1 Biscuit/6g***	***24***	***0.7***	***440***	***10.8***	***75.8***	***12.5***	***3.1***
Wheat, Fig, Plum, & Cranberry, 1, Waitrose*	1 Biscuit/10g	40	1.2	399	9.3	62.6	11.8	3
with Sunflower Seeds , For Sa Placa*	1 Biscuit/14g	65	2.8	478	10.7	61	20.5	3.4
Yoghurt Break, Red Cherry, Go Ahead, McVitie's*	1 Slice/18g	72	1.8	407	5.5	73.4	10.1	2.2
Yoghurt Break, Strawberry, Go Ahead, McVitie's*	1 Slice/18g	72	1.8	402	52	72.4	10.3	3.4
Yorkie, Nestle*	1 Biscuit/25g	126	6.2	505	6.1	62.6	24.8	3.2
BISON								
Raw	***1oz/28g***	***31***	***0.5***	***109***	***21.6***	***0***	***1.8***	***0***
BITES								
Blueberry, & Lemon, Oat Squares, Superfood, Graze*	1 Bite/30g	138	7.2	460	6.5	51	24	16
Brookie, Bakers Selection, Asda*	1 Bite/9g	40	1.6	440	4.8	64	18	2.4
Brownie, Chocolate, Tesco*	1 Bite/11g	43	1.6	394	5.3	58	15	30.7
Caramel Crispy, Extremely Chocolatey, Mini, M&S*	1 Bite/11g	50	2	455	4.7	68.2	17.9	2.8
Caramel Shortcake, Mini, Bakers Selection, Asda*	1 Bite/12g	60	3.1	499	5.6	60	26	1.4
Cauliflower, Biryani, Asda*	1 Bite/10g	22	0.8	224	3.5	32	8.5	3.3
Cauliflower, Goan, Gosh!*	1 Bite/22g	44	2.6	199	4.8	22.6	11.6	7.3
Chicken, Breast, Tempura, Cooked, Tesco*	½ Pack/126g	239	8.7	189	17.9	13.7	6.9	0
Chicken, Katsu, with Teri-Mayo, Taiko Foods*	1 Pack/98g	370	30.1	378	13.9	12	30.7	0
Chicken, Meat Free, Plant Based, Asda*	5 Pieces/70g	177	10.5	253	13	14	15	4.7
Chicken, Peperami*	1 Serving/50g	104	5.2	207	22	7.7	10.3	0
Chilli, Cheese, Oven Baked, Asda*	1 Bite/15g	42	2.1	283	8.8	29	14	1.2
Chocolate Cornflake, Mini, M&S*	1 Bite/11.8g	55	2.4	470	6.2	66.3	20.1	3.6
Chocolate Orange, Mini, M&S*	1 Bite/22g	95	4.8	430	5.5	54.6	21.6	1.8
Chocolate, Double, Mini, M&S*	1 Bite/19g	89	4.5	469	5.8	57.2	23.6	2.1
Cocoa & Coconut, Protein Balls, Kit, Asda*	1 Ball/25g	80	2.5	322	17	37	10	6.8

	Measure INFO/WEIGHT	per Measure KCAL	FAT	Nutrition Values per 100g / 100ml KCAL	PROT	CARB	FAT	FIBRE
BITES								
Cornflake Clusters, Morrisons*	1 Cluster/10g	47	1.8	474	6.2	70.4	18.2	2.1
Cornflake, Cluster, Dairy Milk, Cadbury*	1 Bite/11g	54	2.4	493	7	65.6	22.1	2
Cranberry, & Pumpin, Protein, Special K, Kellogg's*	1 Serving/30g	131	4.5	438	19	54	15	5.4
Flapjack, Co-Op*	1 Bite/15g	66	2.8	426	6.1	56	18	6.3
Flapjack, Fruit, & Nut, Tesco*	1 Bite/15g	71	3.4	473	6.3	59.7	22.5	3.2
Flapjack, Mini, M&S*	1 Bite/14g	64	3.1	458	6.1	56.7	21.9	5
Granola, & Yoghurt, Mini, M&S*	1 Piece/10g	49	2.3	492	7.1	62.3	23.4	2
Granola, & Yoghurt, Mini, Sainsbury's*	1 Bite/9g	45	2.1	492	6.8	64.7	22.6	1.4
Granola, Blueberry, The Nature All*	1 Pack/22g	98	4.6	447	11	45	21	17
Granola, Fruit & Seed, Mini, Sainsbury's*	1 Bite/13g	65	3.8	500	8.6	48	29.5	3.9
Hash Brown, Bacon, Farmfoods*	1 Bite/10g	18	0.8	181	2.6	23	7.9	0
Hash Brown, Oven Baked, Asda*	½ Pack/125g	285	13.8	228	2.4	29	11	2.7
Jaffa Cake, Nibbles, McVitie's*	1 Serving/25g	108	4.1	433	4.8	66	16.4	6.3
Jalapeno, Cream Cheese, Tesco*	1 Bite/20g	63	3.9	313	7.2	26.7	19.4	1.6
Lentil, The Foodie Market, Aldi*	1 Pack/20g	89	3.1	445	10	65	15.5	4
Millionaire, Mini, Waitrose*	1 Bite/16g	76	4	484	5.4	57.2	25.6	1.5
Millionaires, Tesco*	1 Bites/12g	60	3.4	500	5.1	55.6	28	2.5
Mozzarella, & Pepperoni, Tesco *	1 Bite/21g	71	4.4	339	10.8	26	20.8	2.2
Nacho, Chicken, Tesco*	1 Bite/12g	27	1.1	225	18.3	16.7	9.2	3.3
Potato, & Vegetable, Spiced, M&S*	1 Pack/96g	162	7.2	169	6.4	16.2	7.5	5.3
Prawn, Asian Prawn Selection, Let's Party, Aldi*	1 Bite/14g	55	3.9	394	10	23	28	3.1
Protein, Honey & Seed, Oat Squares, Graze*	1 Square/30g	140	8.1	465	15	42	27	4.4
Protein, Maple, Graze*	1 Bite/30g	140	7.8	467	16	40	26	5.9
Pumpkin, & Chilli, Sweet, Gosh!*	1 Bite/22g	45	2	203	5.7	28	9.3	7.9
Rocky Road, Mini, M&S*	1 Bite/12g	50	1.6	410	5.2	66.9	13.3	2.5
Rocky Road, Mini, Waitrose*	1 Bite/14g	71	3.8	506	5.2	59	27.1	2.4
Saag Aloo, with Potato, & Spinach, Gosh!*	4 Bites/88g	177	1.1	202	7.1	24	1.3	7.7
Salami, Salamini, Beretta*	1 Bite/5g	24	2	483	28	0.5	41	1.7
Salted Caramel, CWP*	1 Serving/57g	203	5.9	356	23	43	10.4	6.3
Spinach, & Pine Nuts, Gosh!*	4 Bites/88g	207	10.5	236	8.1	27	12	6
Spinach, Oven Cooked, Strong Roots*	3 Bites/75g	202	10	269	4.3	30.5	13.3	5.1
Spinach, Strong Roots*	3 Bites/93g	202	11.2	218	3.4	20.8	12.1	6.4
Strawberry, with a Yoghurt Coating, Tesco*	1 Serving/25g	117	4.7	468	2	72	18.9	0.9
Superfood, The Protein Works*	1 Bite/10g	38	1.8	382	14	41	18	4
BLACK PUDDING								
Average, Uncooked	***1 Serving/40g***	***101***	***6***	***252***	***10.2***	***19***	***14.9***	***0.6***
Clonakilty*	1 Serving/68g	203	13.3	298	11.5	18.8	19.6	6
Wee, Simon Howie*	1 Slice/20g	52	4.1	261	8.3	11.9	20.4	1.8
BLACKBERRIES								
Fresh, Raw, Average	***1 Blackberry/8g***	***3***	***0***	***32***	***0.9***	***5.1***	***0.2***	***3.1***
Frozen, Average	***1 Serving/80g***	***26***	***0.2***	***32***	***0.9***	***5.1***	***0.2***	***3.1***
in Fruit Juice, Average	***½ Can/145g***	***52***	***0.3***	***36***	***0.6***	***7.9***	***0.2***	***1.3***
BLACKCURRANTS								
Dried, Graze*	1 Pack/30g	95	0.3	317	3.3	79	1	0
Fresh, Raw, Average	***1 Serving/80g***	***22***	***0***	***27***	***0.9***	***6.5***	***0***	***3.5***
Stewed with Sugar	***1oz/28g***	***16***	***0***	***58***	***0.7***	***15***	***0***	***2.8***
Stewed without Sugar	***1oz/28g***	***7***	***0***	***24***	***0.8***	***5.6***	***0***	***3.1***
BLUEBERRIES								
Dried, Love Life, Waitrose*	1 Serving/30g	107	0.2	358	1.1	80.1	0.8	3.6
Frozen, Average	***1 Serving/80g***	***41***	***0.2***	***51***	***0.6***	***13.8***	***0.2***	***4.4***
Raw, Average	***50 Berries/68g***	***39***	***0.2***	***57***	***0.7***	***14.5***	***0.3***	***2.4***
BOAR								
Wild, Raw, Average	***1 Serving/200g***	***244***	***6.7***	***122***	***21.5***	***0***	***3.3***	***0***

B

	Measure INFO/WEIGHT	per Measure KCAL	per Measure FAT	KCAL	PROT	CARB	FAT	FIBRE
BOILED SWEETS								
Average	***1 Sweet/7g***	***21***	***0***	***327***	***0***	***87.1***	***0***	***0***
Blackcurrant & Liquorice, Co-Op*	1 Sweet/8g	32	0.4	405	0.9	91	5	0
Cherry Drops, Bassett's*	1 Sweet/5g	18	0	390	0	98.1	0	0
Clear Fruits, Sainsbury's*	1 Sweet/7g	26	0	372	0.1	92.9	0	0
Fruit Drops, Co-Op*	1 Sweet/6g	24	0	395	0.2	98	0	0
Fruit Sherbets, Assorted, M&S*	1 Sweet/9g	35	0.4	405	0.3	91.6	4.3	0.1
Lockets, Mars*	1 Pack/43g	165	0	383	0	95.8	0	0
Pear Drops, Bassett's*	1 Sweet/4g	16	0	390	0	96.4	0	0
Pear Drops, Sugar Free, Sula*	1 Sweet/3g	7	0	235	0.1	97	0.1	0
Soothers, Cherry, Hall's*	1 Pack/45g	165	0	365	0	91.3	0	0
Soothers, Strawberry Flavour, Hall's*	1 Sweet/5g	19	0	385	0	96	0	0
BOK CHOY								
Tesco*	1 Serving/100g	11	0.2	11	1	1.4	0.2	1.2
BOLOGNESE								
Beanfeast, Dry Weight, Batchelors*	1 Pack/120g	408	5.4	340	26	46.2	4.5	5
Mushroom, with Tagliatelle, Cooked, Plant Menu, Aldi*	1 Pack/377g	275	2.6	73	3.1	13	0.7	1.8
Plant Based, Meat Free Mince, Dolmio*	1 Pack/150g	106	2.6	71	5.7	6.9	1.7	2.5
Rigatoni, Allplants*	1 Serving/380g	559	20.1	147	6.1	16	5.3	3.1
Soya, Vegan, Sauce, Fresh, Waitrose*	½ Pot/175g	163	9.4	93	6.2	3.5	5.4	3
Spaghetti, BGTY, Sainsbury's*	1 Pack/400g	364	5.6	91	7.1	12.2	1.4	0.6
Spaghetti, Calorie Controlled, Tesco*	1 Pack/380g	361	7.6	95	6.5	12	2	1.6
Spaghetti, Canned, Asda*	½ Can/197g	142	3.4	72	5.4	8.3	1.7	0.8
Spaghetti, Cook*	1 Serving/390g	491	14.8	126	8.9	14.8	3.8	1.6
Spaghetti, Egg Pasta in Rich Beef Sauce, Waitrose*	1 Pack/400g	404	10.4	101	7.6	11.7	2.6	1
Spaghetti, Italian, Microwaved, Morrisons*	1 Pack/396g	400	9.1	101	6.5	12.7	2.3	1.6
Spaghetti, Meal for One, M&S*	1 Pack/400g	612	31.6	153	7.4	12.3	7.9	1.6
Spaghetti, Microwaved, Iceland*	1 Pack/461g	530	18	115	4.4	14.2	3.9	2.4
Spaghetti, Mini, Oven Cooked, Waitrose*	1 Pack/249g	304	13	122	5.3	13.1	5.2	0.8
Spaghetti, Mushroom, Plant Chef, Tesco*	1 Pack/426g	511	9.8	120	9.1	14.6	2.3	2.4
Spaghetti, Slow Cooked, TTD, Sainsbury's*	1 Pack/400g	474	16.7	125	8	12	4.4	3
Vegetarian, Spaghetti, Quorn*	1 Pack/300g	255	1.8	85	4.4	14.8	0.6	1.5
BOMBAY MIX								
Average	***1oz/28g***	***141***	***9.2***	***503***	***18.8***	***35.1***	***32.9***	***6.2***
Hot, Philon*	1 Sm Bag/47g	228	15.3	485	17.6	43.2	32.6	0
BOOST								
Duo, Cadbury*	2 Bars/68g	391	19	575	5.6	59	28	1.9
Protein, Cadbury*	1 Bar/49g	249	13.3	507	25	42	27	1.2
Standard Bar, Cadbury*	1 Bar/49g	250	13.8	515	5.8	58.6	28.5	1.5
Treat Size, Cadbury*	1 Bar/24g	130	7.4	535	5.3	59.6	30.5	0
BOUILLABAISSE								
Average	***1 Serving/400g***	***556***	***38.8***	***139***	***11.2***	***2***	***9.7***	***0.4***
BOUILLON								
Powder, Miso, Marigold*	1 Tsp/5g	12	0.5	248	7	34	9.3	1.4
Powder, Swiss Vegetable, Green Tub, Marigold*	1 Tsp/5g	12	0.4	245	10.1	30.1	8.5	0
BOUNTY								
Dark, Mars*	1 Funsize/29g	141	7.9	493	3.6	55.8	27.5	0
Milk, Mars*	1 Funsize/29g	139	7.3	487	3.7	58.9	25.7	0
BOVRIL*								
Beef Extract, Drink, Made Up with Water, Bovril*	1 Serving/12g	22	0.1	184	38.9	4.6	1.2	0
Beef, Paste, High Protein, As Sold, Bovril*	1 Serving/12g	25	0.1	206	37	13	1.1	0.8
Chicken Savoury Drink, Bovril*	1 Serving/13g	16	0.2	129	9.7	19.4	1.4	2.1
BRANDY								
37.5% Volume, Average	***1 Pub Shot/35ml***	***72***	***0***	***207***	***0***	***0***	***0***	***0***

Nutrition Values per 100g / 100ml: KCAL, PROT, CARB, FAT, FIBRE

	Measure INFO/WEIGHT	per Measure KCAL	FAT	Nutrition Values per 100g / 100ml KCAL	PROT	CARB	FAT	FIBRE
BRANDY								
40% Volume, Average	***1 Pub Shot/35ml***	***78***	***0***	***224***	***0***	***0***	***0***	***0***
Cherry, Average	***1 Pub Shot/35ml***	***89***	***0***	***255***	***0***	***32.6***	***0***	***0***
BRAWN								
Average	***1 Serving/100g***	***153***	***11.5***	***153***	***12.4***	***0***	***11.5***	***0***
BRAZIL NUTS								
Average	***6 Whole/20g***	***136***	***13.7***	***682***	***15.3***	***2.8***	***68.4***	***5.4***
Carob, Coated, Good Food*	1 Pack/125g	719	51.5	575	5.8	44.3	41.2	0
Milk Chocolate, Tesco*	1 Nut/8g	47	3.5	585	9.9	38	43.7	1.9
BREAD								
50/50, No Crusts, Kingsmill*	1 Slice/23g	49	0.5	214	8.3	38.6	2	4.1
50/50, Wholegrain, No Bits, Medium, 400g, , Kingsmill*	1 Slice/29g	68	0.6	233	9.2	42.2	2	4.9
50/50, Wonderloaf, Med Sliced, Warburton's*	1 Slice/43g	106	1.2	244	8.8	43.4	2.8	4.3
50/50, Wonderloaf, Thick Sliced, Warburton's*	1 Slice/50g	124	1.4	249	10	43.6	2.8	4.2
Ancient Grain, Pave, Bakery, Tesco*	1 Slice/80g	213	3.9	267	9.8	44.1	4.9	3.3
Bagel, Ancient Grain, Fitzgeralds*	1 Bagel/85g	241	3.7	283	11.8	46.6	4.3	5.4
Bagel, Caramelised Onion & Poppy Seed, Tesco*	1 Bagel/85g	221	2.1	260	10.9	47.6	2.5	3.8
Bagel, Cinnamon & Raisin, Tesco*	1 Bagel/85g	230	1.4	270	10.4	51.3	1.7	3.8
Bagel, Cinnamon & Raisin, Warburton's*	1 Bagel/80g	212	1.2	265	10.1	51	1.5	3.6
Bagel, Multi Seed, BFree*	1 Bagel/80g	186	2	232	4.1	51.4	2.5	6.5
Bagel, Multigrain, Sainsbury's*	1 Bagel/113g	293	3.5	259	10	49.6	3.1	2
Bagel, Multiseed, & Cereal, Fitzgeralds*	1 Bagel/85g	228	3.8	268	10.9	50.8	4.5	9.5
Bagel, Onion & Poppy Seed, Average	***1 Bagel/85g***	***225***	***2.8***	***264***	***9***	***50.5***	***3.3***	***3.2***
Bagel, Onion, New York Bagel Co*	1 Bagel/85g	222	1.6	261	10.6	50.4	1.9	3.1
Bagel, Original, Organic, New York Bagel Co*	1 Bagel/85g	221	1	260	9.9	51.5	1.2	1.6
Bagel, Plain, Average	***1 Bagel/78g***	***202***	***1.5***	***259***	***10.1***	***50.4***	***1.9***	***3.1***
Bagel, Plain, Sliced, Warburtons*	1 Bagel/80g	207	1.4	259	10.6	49	1.7	2.7
Bagel, Plain, Thin, Village Bakery, Aldi*	1 Bagel/45g	122	0.8	270	12	51	1.7	2.3
Bagel, Red Onion, & Chive, New York Bakery Co*	1 Bagel/90g	233	1	259	10.6	50.1	1.1	3.3
Bagel, Sesame Seed, Essential, Waitrose*	1 Bagel/85g	243	2.7	286	9.6	54.6	3.2	3.6
Bagel, Sesame, New York Bakery*	1 Bagel/90g	242	2.5	269	10.7	47.8	2.8	4.5
Bagel, Sesame, Sliced, Warburton's*	1 Bagel/80g	214	1.9	268	10.4	50	2.4	2.6
Bagel, Sesame, Sourdough, M&S*	1 Bagel/80g	219	1.8	274	11.1	49.9	2.3	4.4
Bagel, Sourdough, Deli Style, Fitzgeralds*	1 Bagel/85g	235	2.6	277	10.1	49.4	3	4.1
Bagel, Sourdough, M&S*	1 Bagel/75g	205	0.8	273	11	53.3	1	3.6
Bagel, Thins, Plain, New York Bakery Co*	1 Thin/45g	122	0.5	271	11.3	55.5	1.1	3.3
Bagel, Thins, Seeded, Sliced, New York Bakery Co*	1 Thin/45g	129	1.5	286	10	52.1	3.4	3.9
Bagel, Wholemeal, Average	***1 Bagel/90g***	***235***	***2.7***	***261***	***12.7***	***44.6***	***3***	***7.7***
Baguette, Bake At Home, Tesco*	½ Baguette/75g	216	0.9	289	8.6	59.1	1.2	3.5
Baguette, Brioche, Wholemeal, Waitrose*	1 Piece/85g	286	8.2	336	11	49	9.7	4.5
Baguette, French, Tesco*	1 Serving/60g	144	0.7	240	7.8	49.5	1.2	3.4
Baguette, Garlic, & Herb, Asda*	¼ Baguette/55g	189	8.2	345	7.5	44	15	2.1
Baguette, Garlic, Slices, Frozen, CBY, Asda*	1 Slice/26g	92	4.7	355	8.2	38.3	18.1	2.8
Baguette, GF, Schnitzer*	½ Baguette/80g	186	6.2	233	4.7	30	7.8	12
Baguette, Granary, Average	***1 Serving/100g***	***250***	***2.8***	***250***	***20***	***46***	***2.8***	***6***
Baguette, Multiseed, & Cereal, Fitzgeralds*	1 Baguette/125g	326	4.5	261	9.3	46.2	3.6	3.2
Baguette, Multiseed, Mini, GF, Fria*	1 Baguette/70g	203	6	290	3.5	47	8.5	6
Baguette, Part Baked, Baker Street*	½ Baguette/63g	156	0.6	248	8.5	50	1	2.5
Baguette, Part Baked, H.W. Nevill's*	½ Baguette/75g	217	0.9	289	8.6	59.1	1.2	3.5
Baguette, Part Baked, Menissez*	1 Baguette/150g	372	1.8	248	7.5	50.6	1.2	0
Baguette, Ready to Bake, Co-Op*	1/3 Baguette/50g	140	0.4	280	9.2	56	0.8	7.6
Baguette, Ready to Bake, Sainsbury's*	½ Baguette/62g	150	0.8	242	7.8	49.7	1.3	2.8
Baguette, Sourdough, la Brea Bakery*	1 Serving/60g	160	0.4	266	8.8	56.1	0.7	1.8
Baguette, White, Half, Crusty, M&S*	1 Baguette/162g	420	1.8	260	8.4	53.5	1.1	2.3

	Measure INFO/WEIGHT	per Measure KCAL	FAT	Nutrition Values per 100g / 100ml KCAL	PROT	CARB	FAT	FIBRE
BREAD								
Baguette, White, Part Baked, Morrisons*	1 Baguette/150g	422	2	281	9	56.5	1.3	3.7
Baguette, White, Part Baked, Oven Baked, Iceland*	½ Baguette/75g	210	1	280	10.1	55.4	1.3	3.2
Baguette, White, Sainsbury's*	1 Serving/50g	132	0.8	263	9.3	53.1	1.5	2.7
Baguette, White, Sliced, Asda*	1 Baguette/85g	272	6.1	320	9.3	53	7.2	2.9
Baguette,Seeded, Sourdough, Part Baked, Aldi*	1 Baguette/112g	335	3.5	299	9.7	56	3.1	3.7
Baguettine, White, Bakery, Sainsbury's*	½ Baguettine/75g	194	0.7	259	8.6	53.2	0.9	1.7
Banana, Mix, As Prepared, The Skinny Food Co.*	1 Slice/48g	100	4.5	208	9.6	25	9.4	0
Bap, White, Large, Co-Op*	1 Bap/80g	202	3	253	8.1	45.2	3.8	2.6
Bap, White, Medium, Morrisons*	1 Bap/60g	170	3	283	10	46.7	5	0
Bap, White, Soft, Garth Bakery*	1 Bap/75g	171	1.2	228	6.3	50	1.6	0
Bap, Wholemeal, M&S*	1 Bap/56g	134	2.7	239	10.4	35.3	4.8	6.5
Baps, Brown, Large, Asda*	1 Bap/58g	140	0.9	242	10	47	1.6	0
Baps, Brown, Large, G H Sheldon*	1 Bap/64g	169	4.3	264	5.3	47.5	6.7	4
Baps, Cheese Topped, Baker's Soft, Tesco*	1 Bap/65g	176	3.3	268	10.8	43.5	5.1	2.6
Baps, Cheese Topped, G H Sheldon*	1 Bap/70g	197	5.8	282	12.4	38.6	8.3	1.4
Baps, Multigrain, Tesco*	1 Bap/98g	238	3.1	244	8.7	45.1	3.2	1.9
Baps, White, Average	***1 Bap/65g***	***167***	***2.3***	***257***	***9.5***	***47***	***3.5***	***1.9***
Baps, White, Giant, Sainsbury's*	1 Bap/86g	235	3.2	273	8.3	51.7	3.7	3.4
Baps, White, Large, Tesco*	1 Bap/100g	250	1	250	9.2	49.7	1	2.6
Baps, White, Soft, Floured, M&S*	1 Bap/61g	175	3.4	285	11.5	46.6	5.5	2.8
Baps, White, Super Soft, The Bakery, M&S*	1 Bap/60g	161	2.8	268	8.4	46.6	4.7	3
Baps, White, Warburton's*	1 Bap/57g	144	2.5	252	9.8	43.4	4.3	2.7
Baps, Wholemeal, Brace's*	1 Bap/59g	137	2.6	234	10.5	42.5	4.4	4.3
Baps, Wholemeal, Giant, Sainsbury's*	1 Bap/86g	230	3.5	268	9.7	48.1	4.1	7.7
Baps, Wholemeal, Tesco*	1 Bap/46g	104	2.4	227	9.6	41.4	5.3	5.6
Baps, Wholemeal, Waitrose*	1 Bap/80g	191	3.4	238	12	34.8	4.2	6.7
Best of Both, Med Sliced, Eat Well, M&S*	1 Slice/36g	83	0.8	229	9.4	41.2	2.2	3.5
Best of Both, Medium, Hovis*	1 Slice/38g	86	0.8	230	10.2	40.4	2.2	3.9
Best of Both, Thick Sliced, Hovis*	1 Slice/47g	108	1	230	10.2	40.4	2.2	3.9
Black Olive, Finest, Tesco*	1 Slice/72g	184	4.6	255	9.7	39.7	6.4	2.9
Bloomer, Brown, Slices, GF, Made Without Wheat, M&S*	1 Slice/53g	131	2.9	247	4.3	41.4	5.4	7.8
Bloomer, Multi Seed, Sliced, M&S*	1 Slice/54g	150	3.9	280	10.5	43.6	7.2	3.1
Bloomer, Multiseed, Average	***1 Slice/50g***	***120***	***2.4***	***240***	***11.8***	***37.2***	***4.9***	***7.7***
Bloomer, Multiseed, Finest, Tesco*	1 Slice/50g	145	3.8	290	9.8	40.2	7.6	7.4
Bloomer, Multiseed, TTD, Sainsbury's*	1 Slice/50g	119	1.8	239	12	39.7	3.6	8.8
Bloomer, Sunflower Seeded, with Rye, TTD, Sainsbury's*	1 Slice/28g	90	3.4	317	12.6	36	12.1	6.8
Bloomer, White, Crusty, Bakery, Tesco*	1 Slice/50g	122	0.8	244	8.3	47.2	1.7	3.3
Bloomer, White, Sliced, Waitrose*	1 Slice/50g	130	0.9	259	8.5	52.1	1.8	2.6
Bloomer, White, Traditional, Village Bakery, Aldi*	1 Slice/37g	92	0.8	250	9.2	47	2.2	2.7
Both in One, Village Bakery, Aldi*	1 Slice/40g	95	1	237	8.5	43	2.5	4.3
Breadcakes, Big Brown, Morrisons*	1 Cake/63g	154	2.1	245	9	44.6	3.4	4.3
Brioche, Bun, Gourmet, Bundy *	1 Bun/80g	206	2.6	257	9.6	46.2	3.2	2.9
Brioche, Buns, Burger, Sliced, St Pierre*	1 Bun/50g	164	4.1	328	9	53.3	8.2	2.5
Brioche, Burger Bun, Deluxe, Lidl*	1 Bun/50g	170	4.9	339	10.1	51.8	9.8	1.6
Brioche, Burger Bun, M&S*	1 Bun/72g	212	6.1	294	9	43.5	8.5	3.6
Brioche, Burger Buns, Luxury, Specially Selected, Aldi*	1 Bun/50g	159	3.7	317	9.5	52	7.3	3.1
Brioche, Burger Buns, Signature, Morrisons*	1 Bun/55g	156	2.3	284	9.4	51	4.2	2.2
Brioche, Burger Buns, Warburton's*	1 Roll/54g	159	3.2	294	10.2	49.1	6	1.2
Brioche, Loaf, Hand Plaited, Aldi*	1 Slice/50g	178	5.5	355	8.1	50	11	1.7
Brioche, Loaf, Sliced, Bon Appetit*	1 Slice/33g	111	3.3	333	7.3	52	10	2
Brioche, Raisin, Lidl*	1 Slice/35g	104	2.2	296	8.2	50	6.4	0
Brioche, Raisin, Swirls, Sainsbury's*	1 Swirl/45g	130	3.4	288	6.9	47.3	7.5	2
Brioche, Swirl, Bon Appetit, Aldi*	1 Slice/50g	152	5	305	6.1	46	10	1.9

	Measure INFO/WEIGHT	per Measure KCAL	FAT	Nutrition Values per 100g / 100ml KCAL	PROT	CARB	FAT	FIBRE
BREAD								
Brown, Bloomer, Organic, Bakery, Tesco*	1 Slice/80g	193	1.8	241	9	42.8	2.3	6.5
Brown, Danish, Weight Watchers, Warburton's*	1 Slice/20g	48	0.4	233	10.3	40.7	1.8	6.2
Brown, Farmhouse, GF, Newburn, Warburton's*	1 Slice/35g	82	1.9	234	7.8	35.8	5.4	5.7
Brown, Farmhouse, Linwoods*	1 Slice/25g	56	0.4	225	7.3	44.4	1.7	5.8
Brown, Farmhouse, Soft, Sliced, GF, Genius *	1 Slice/36g	92	2.1	256	2.2	44	5.8	9.1
Brown, Malted, Bloomer, Rowan Hill Bakery, Lidl*	1 Slice/57g	155	2.3	272	9.7	46.7	4.1	4.9
Brown, Malted, Farmhouse Gold, Morrisons*	1 Slice/38g	94	0.5	248	8.2	49.6	1.4	3
Brown, Med Slice, Smart Price, Asda*	1 Slice/37g	77	0.6	210	8	41	1.6	6
Brown, Med Sliced	***1 Slice/34g***	***74***	***0.7***	***218***	***8.5***	***44.3***	***2***	***3.5***
Brown, Med Sliced, Asda*	1 Slice/36g	78	0.6	216	8	42	1.8	4.1
Brown, Med Sliced, Bettabuy, Morrisons*	1 Slice/31g	66	0.4	212	8.6	42	1.3	3.6
Brown, Med Sliced, Savers, Morrisons*	1 Slice/30g	78	0.4	260	9.7	50.7	1.3	4
Brown, Mixed Grain, Original, Vogel*	1 Slice/45g	102	0.6	227	9.8	47.1	1.2	6.4
Brown, Multi Grain, Wheat Free, GF	1 Slice/33g	76	1.7	229	5.1	40.8	5.1	5.6
Brown, Oaty Loaf, GF, Made Without Wheat, M&S*	1 Slice/34g	89	1.9	265	5.4	43.2	5.8	9
Brown, Oaty, Super, Sliced, Roberts*	1 Slice/33g	76	0.7	229	8.6	43.6	2.2	3.9
Brown, Premium, Med Sliced, Warburton's*	1 Slice/24g	61	0.9	258	10.6	43.2	3.7	4.3
Brown, Sainsbury's*	1 Slice/34g	81	0.7	239	8.4	46.8	2.1	4.2
Brown, Seeded, GF, Loaf, Made Without Wheat, M&S*	1 Slice/33g	89	3.2	268	4.8	34.5	9.7	11.9
Brown, Sliced, Free From, Tesco*	1 Slice/42g	81	1.7	193	5.3	29.3	4	9.3
Brown, Soda, M&S*	1 Slice/40g	92	1.4	229	9.2	43.6	3.6	4.9
Brown, Soft, Farmhouse , Warburton's*	1 Slice/42g	104	1.1	246	9.9	42.8	2.7	5.3
Brown, Sourdough, Boule, San Francisco Style, Waitrose*	1 Slice/50g	120	0.7	239	9.1	45.5	1.4	3.8
Brown, Super Seeded, Jacksons Of Yorkshire*	1 Slice/45g	130	4	290	13.3	35.5	9	6.9
Brown, Super Seeded, Sliced, Loaf, Extra Special, Asda*	1 Slice/44g	131	4.3	298	12	39	9.7	5.5
Brown, Super Seeds, Kingsmill*	1 Slice/47g	138	2	294	10.9	40	4.2	4.9
Brown, Thick Slice, Tesco*	1 Slice/50g	110	1.2	219	10.3	38.9	2.5	5.3
Brown, Thin Sliced, Sainsbury's*	1 Slice/29g	65	0.5	225	8.2	43.8	1.9	3.9
Brown, Tin Loaf, The Artisan Bread Company*	1 Slice/47g	110	0.7	233	7.1	36.4	1.5	3.9
Brown, Toasted, Average	***1 Slice/24g***	***65***	***0.5***	***272***	***10.4***	***56.5***	***2.1***	***4.5***
Brown, Toastie, Thick Sliced, Kingsmill*	1 Slice/44g	101	1.4	230	9.5	40.5	3.3	4.7
Brown, Very Dark, Albert Heijn*	1 Slice/35g	84	1.4	240	12	35	4	7.4
Bun, Burger, Brioche, The Country Miller*	1 Bun/68g	249	5.4	366	7.3	48.8	7.9	2.8
Buns, Burger Seeded, Sliced, Warburton's*	1 Roll/60g	158	3.2	264	9	43.6	5.3	2.7
Buns, Burger, American Style, Sainsbury's*	1 Bun/50g	131	2.1	261	10.5	45.6	4.1	3.6
Buns, Burger, Brioche, TTD, Sainsbury's*	1 Bun/80g	257	8.2	322	7.8	48.1	10.3	2.6
Buns, Burger, GF, Made Without Wheat, M&S*	1 Bun/80g	201	5	251	4.8	38.9	6.2	10.4
Buns, Burger, Giant, Sainsbury's*	1 Bun/95g	249	4.9	262	8.7	45.2	5.2	2.9
Buns, Burger, M&S*	1 Bun/58g	162	3.3	280	10.1	45.7	5.7	2.5
Buns, Burger, Sainsbury's*	1 Bun/56g	154	2.9	275	9.2	47.8	5.2	4.1
Buns, Burger, Seeded, Large, Tesco*	1 Bun/90g	240	3.2	267	9.5	47.7	3.6	2.9
Buns, Burger, Sesame, American Style, Sainsbury's*	1 Bun/60g	162	3.8	270	7.3	46.2	6.3	2.2
Buns, Burger, Sesame, Sliced, Tesco*	1 Bun/60g	168	4	280	7.9	47.3	6.6	2.1
Buns, White, Burger, Waitrose*	1 Bun/64g	169	2.5	264	10	47.2	3.9	2.7
Buns, White, Stay Fresh, Tesco*	1 Bun/56g	152	3.7	271	7.5	45.5	6.6	0
Butterbread, Nature's Own*	1 Slice/30g	70	0.6	231	11.5	46.2	1.9	0
Challah, Average	***1 Slice/50g***	***143***	***3.6***	***286***	***8.9***	***53.6***	***7.1***	***3.6***
Chapatti, Sainsbury's*	1 Chapatti/99g	287	5	290	8.8	50.5	5	4.1
Cheese, & Garlic, Pizza Style, Sainsbury's*	¼ Bread/63g	199	8.1	318	10.7	39.7	13	2.2
Cheese, & Garlic, Stonebaked, Morrisons*	¼ Bread/69g	228	9.9	331	10.9	39.5	14.4	1.9
Cheese, & Onion, Tear & Share, Sainsbury's*	¼ Bread/71g	202	6.6	285	9.8	40.6	9.3	1.9
Cheese, & Onion, Toastie, Warburton's*	1 Slice/42g	120	5.8	286	7.5	33.1	13.7	0
Cheese, & Tomato, Tear & Share, Sainsbury's*	¼ Bread/72g	211	9.5	293	8	35.7	13.2	1.5

	Measure INFO/WEIGHT	per Measure KCAL	FAT	Nutrition Values per 100g / 100ml KCAL	PROT	CARB	FAT	FIBRE
BREAD								
Cheese, Morrisons*	1 Serving/96g	297	13.6	311	9.9	35.9	14.2	3
Cheese, Onion & Garlic, Tear & Share, Waitrose*	¼ Bread/112g	326	14.6	290	9.4	33.9	13	2.1
Cheese, Tear & Share, Tesco*	¼ Loaf/73g	225	7.8	310	8.8	44	10.7	0.8
Cheese, Three, Bloomer, Bakery, Tesco*	1 Slice/82g	214	5.3	261	13.1	36.7	6.4	2
Chia & Quinoa, GF	1 Slice/40g	80	2.5	200	3.8	26.2	6.2	16.2
Cholla, Average	***1/10 Loaf/154g***	***421***	***14.3***	***274***	***6.9***	***40.8***	***9.3***	***1***
Ciabatta, Black Olive, Bake At Home, Aldi*	¼ Baguette/75g	220	3.1	294	8.9	54	4.1	3.3
Ciabatta, Black Olive, Part Baked, Sainsbury's*	¼ Ciabatta/67g	172	2.5	257	8.8	46.8	3.8	2.4
Ciabatta, Garlic & Parsley, Specially Selected, Aldi*	1 Slice/28g	109	5.2	396	9.5	46	19	2.7
Ciabatta, Garlic, Slices, Tesco*	1 Slice/43g	129	3.2	301	9.6	46.9	7.5	3.6
Ciabatta, Green Olive, Tesco*	¼ Ciabatta/70g	155	3.1	222	7.4	38.2	4.4	1.9
Ciabatta, Half, Handcrafted, TTD, Sainsbury's*	1 Pack/270g	794	12.7	294	11.6	49.8	4.7	3.1
Ciabatta, Half, M&S*	1 Ciabatta/135g	354	5.5	262	10.3	48.1	4.1	2.1
Ciabatta, Half, Organic, Sainsbury's*	½ Ciabatta/63g	152	0.6	241	9.1	48.7	1	2.3
Ciabatta, Half, Part Baked, TTD, Sainsbury's*	¼ Pack/67g	173	3.3	257	8.6	44.6	4.9	3.5
Ciabatta, Half, Tesco*	1 Ciabatta/135g	351	4.7	260	8.9	47.7	3.5	2.2
Ciabatta, Italian Style, Waitrose*	1 Ciabatta/89g	231	1.2	260	10.7	51.2	1.4	2.2
Ciabatta, Loaf, Finest, Tesco*	1 Serving/45g	115	2.1	257	10.1	41.8	4.7	3.3
Ciabatta, Olive & Rosemary, Mini, Tesco*	1 Pack/75g	319	8.2	425	17.8	63	10.9	3.6
Ciabatta, Ready to Bake, Sainsbury's*	½ Ciabatta/66g	172	2.4	260	8.9	47.7	3.7	2.2
Ciabatta, Square, Bake at Home, Part Baked, Asda*	1 Roll/60g	157	2.1	262	8.4	49.1	3.5	2.1
Ciabatta, Sun Dried Tomato & Basil, Tesco*	¼ Ciabatta/75g	193	4.3	257	8.9	42.4	5.7	2.4
Ciabatta, Tomato & Basil, GFY, Asda*	1 Serving/55g	143	1.2	260	9	51	2.2	0
Ciabatta, TTD, Sainsbury's*	¼ Pack/68g	185	4	274	10.4	44.8	5.9	2.7
Ciabatta. Sourdough, Bakery, Waitrose*	¼ Ciabatta/45g	111	0.9	247	12.8	42.5	2	3.8
Cinnamon, & Raisin, Toasty Loaf, Rankin*	1 Slice/40g	113	2	283	6.6	54.2	5	2.5
Cinnamon, Swirl, Asda*	1 Serving/25g	87	3.2	349	6	52	13	1.6
Classic, Family, Brace's*	1 Slice/42g	93	0.7	222	9.5	38.4	1.7	7.5
Cob, Cheese & Chutney, Bakery, Tesco*	1 Slice/50g	124	2.2	249	11.3	39.7	4.4	2.5
Corn, Soft, Old El Paso*	1 Tortilla/42g	121	2	289	8.5	51.8	4.8	2.4
Corn, with Sunflower Seed & Mixed Spice, Bakery, Tesco*	1 Slice/50g	131	2	262	9.9	45	4.1	2.6
Cottage Loaf, Stonebaked, Asda*	1 Serving/67g	155	0.9	232	10	45	1.3	3.2
Cranberry, & Pecan, Tesco *	1 Slice/70g	206	4.8	294	11.3	45.6	6.9	2.9
Crostini, Olive Oil, TTD, Sainsbury's*	1 Roll/4g	16	0.3	409	11.4	72.2	8.3	3.3
Dark, Low Carb, As Prepared, Lizza*	1 Slice/50g	80	3.8	161	13	4.6	7.5	12
Deliciously Seeded, Lower Carb, Hovis*	1 Slice/36g	97	3	269	15.7	27.2	8.3	11.4
Fabulous Fibre, Hovis*	1 Slice/43g	106	1.2	247	11.5	39.2	2.9	9
Farl, Irish Soda, Irwin's Bakery*	1 Farl/150g	334	5.1	223	4	44	3.4	2.3
Farmhouse, Ancient Grains, Sunflower, & Honey, Co-Op*	1 Slice/41g	109	2	267	11	42	4.9	5.4
Farmhouse, Seeded, Sliced, Co-Op*	1 Slice/44g	112	2.5	254	13	34	5.6	7.5
Farmhouse, Wholemeal, Average	***1 Slice/43g***	***94***	***1.4***	***219***	***10.7***	***36.2***	***3.3***	***7.3***
Farmhouse, with Oatmeal, Batch, Finest, Tesco*	1 Slice/44g	110	1.4	240	9.8	43.2	3.1	5.2
Ficelle, Mixed Olive, Waitrose*	1/5 Stick/50g	133	1.4	267	7.5	51.1	2.8	3.4
Fig, & Hazelnut, Loaf, M&S*	1 Serving/100g	285	8.2	285	11	38.9	8.2	5.4
Fig, Almond, Nettorama *	1 Serving/70g	250	4.8	357	6.8	67	6.9	16
Five Seed, Fully Loaded, Aldi*	1 Slice/50g	135	3.3	270	10.9	36.4	6.7	7.9
Flat, Italian, Piada Sfogliata, Italiamo, Lidl*	1 Piece/130g	402	12.5	309	7.9	45.9	9.6	2
Flatbread, Folded, Lge Plain, by, Sainsbury's*	1 Flatbread/65g	192	3.4	295	8.5	51.4	5.3	4.1
Flatbread, Folded, Plain, Sainsbury's*	1 Flatbread/33g	97	1.7	295	8.5	51.4	5.3	4.1
Flatbread, Garlic & Herb, Tear & Share, Sainsbury's*	¼ Bread/68g	201	6.3	297	10.9	42.5	9.3	3.7
Flatbread, Garlic Mushroom, The Best, Morrisons*	1 Flatbread/245g	686	19.8	280	8.7	41.3	8.1	3.6
Flatbread, Garlic, & Cheese, Tesco*	¼ Flatbread/55g	150	4	273	9.9	40.6	7.2	3
Flatbread, Garlic, BGTY, Sainsbury's*	¼ Bread/56g	177	5.7	316	9.6	46.6	10.1	2.7

	Measure INFO/WEIGHT	per Measure KCAL	FAT	Nutrition Values per 100g / 100ml KCAL	PROT	CARB	FAT	FIBRE
BREAD								
Flatbread, Greek Style, Deli Kitchen*	1 Bread/80g	204	3.4	255	11.3	39.7	4.2	6.7
Flatbread, Greek Style, Sainsburys*	1 Flat Bread/77g	212	4	275	12.3	40.9	5.2	7.6
Flatbread, Malted Grain & Seeds, Sliced, Warburton's*	1 Square/66g	174	3.2	264	9.6	45	4.8	4.1
Flatbread, Multiseed, Folded, Tesco*	1 Flatbread/35g	107	2.4	305	10.4	47.8	6.8	5.3
Flatbread, Multiseed, Wholegrain, M&S*	2 Flatbreads/24g	98	2.9	410	13.4	56.7	12.1	10.4
Flatbread, Piadina, Specially Selected, Aldi*	1 Flatbread/75g	220	6.2	294	11	42	8.3	4.1
Flatbread, Plain, Folded, Asda*	1 Flatbread/35g	109	2.4	313	9.6	52	6.8	3.1
Flatbread, Plain, Folded, Luxury, Iceland*	1 Flatbread/35g	113	2.7	323	9.1	53	7.7	2.5
Flatbread, Seeded, Folded, Rowan Hill Bakery, Lidl*	1 Bread/35g	121	3.3	346	10.9	52.6	9.4	4
Flatbread, Seeded, Morrisons*	1 Serving/35g	114	3.8	325	9.9	44.1	10.8	5.7
Flatbread, Super Seeded, Folded, Village Bakery, Aldi*	1 Flatbread/35g	123	4.6	352	9.7	47	13	5.5
Flatbread, Tomato, & Garlic, Sainsbury's*	1/3 Bread/73g	191	4.9	261	8.4	41.7	6.7	3.4
Flatbread, White, Folded, Rowan Hill Bakery, Lidl*	1 Flatbread/35g	112	2.3	320	9.8	54.1	6.5	2.7
Flatbread, White, Folded, Village Bakery, Aldi*	1 Flatbread/35g	106	2.1	303	9.1	51.4	6	2.6
Flatbread, White, Folded, Village Bakery, Aldi*	1 Flatbread/80g	225	3.4	281	8.6	50	4.3	3
Flatbread, White, Sliced, Warburton *	1 Square/63g	173	2.5	275	9.5	49.9	3.9	1
Flatbread, Wholemeal, Folded, Sainsbury's*	1 Flatbread/35g	102	2.4	292	9.5	44	7	7.4
Flatbuns, White, Village Bakery, Aldi*	1 Flatbun/80g	225	3.5	281	8.6	50	4.4	3
Focaccia, Balsamic Onion, & Thyme, Co-Op*	1 Focaccia/60g	155	3.6	258	7.3	41	6	4.9
Focaccia, Cheese, & Tomato, Morrisons*	1 Serving/50g	164	6.5	328	12.7	38.5	13	3
Focaccia, Onion & Herb, Tesco*	½ Pack/190g	547	23.8	288	8.7	35.2	12.5	3.7
Focaccia, Rosemary & Sea Salt, TTD, Sainsbury's*	1 Serving/50g	130	3.5	261	7.4	40.7	7	2.8
Focaccia, Rosemary, & Sea Salt, Tesco*	1 Focaccia/50g	151	4.2	301	9.4	45.5	8.3	3.4
Focaccia, Sliced, Deli Kitchen*	1 Slice/90g	219	5	243	8.7	38.5	5.5	2.3
Focaccia, Sun Dried Tomato, & Olive, Chef Select, Lidl*	1/3 Focaccia/50g	128	3.9	257	7	38.3	7.8	2.6
French, Stick, Average	***1 Serving/60g***	***147***	***0.2***	***245***	***8.7***	***52.2***	***0.4***	***2.1***
Fried, Average	***1 Slice/28g***	***141***	***9***	***503***	***7.9***	***48.5***	***32.2***	***1.6***
Fruit Loaf, & Cinnamon, Finest, Tesco*	1 Slice/37g	134	4.9	363	6.4	54.6	13.2	1.5
Fruit Loaf, Apple & Cinnamon, Soreen*	1 Serving/10g	31	0.4	307	6.9	60.5	4.2	0
Fruit Loaf, Apple, M&S*	1 Slice/39g	100	0.6	255	8.5	51.9	1.5	3.3
Fruit Loaf, Banana, Soreen*	1 Slice/25g	76	1.2	305	7.2	55.6	5	4.4
Fruit Loaf, Cinnamon & Raisin, Soreen*	1/8 Loaf/25g	77	1	308	7.7	54.1	4	4.1
Fruit Loaf, Fruity Five, Snack Pack, Soreen*	1 Pack/45g	148	4	329	7.1	54.9	9	2.7
Fruit Loaf, Plum, Lincolnshire, Soreen*	1 Slice/25g	65	0.8	261	8.4	49.3	3.4	2.1
Fruit Loaf, Sliced, Bakers Selection, Asda*	1 Serving/36g	100	1.5	278	8.2	50	4.2	3.6
Fruit Loaf, Sliced, Rowan Hill Bakery, Lidl*	1 Slice/36g	97	1	271	8.6	51	2.8	3.6
Fruit Loaf, Sliced, Sainsbury's*	1 Slice/40g	104	1.4	260	8.9	47.9	3.6	2.4
Fruit Loaf, Sliced, Tesco*	1 Slice/36g	101	1.3	281	7.9	52.6	3.6	3.2
Fruit Loaf, Sultana & Cherry, Sainsbury's*	1 Slice/50g	178	6.1	357	2.7	59	12.2	1.7
Fruit Loaf, with Cinnamon, & Raisin, Warburton's*	1 Slice/36g	98	1.3	273	7.2	51.1	3.7	3.2
Fruit, & Spice, Extra Thick, Sliced, Vogel*	2 Slices/120g	290	4.1	241	8.3	41.7	3.4	4.9
Fruit, Loaf, Banana, Lunchbox, Soreen*	1 Bar/30g	98	1.7	326	8.1	59.5	5.5	4.6
Fruit, Loaf, Toasted, Cafe Instore, Asda*	1 Slice/33g	89	1.2	269	8	51	3.7	2.9
Fruit, Raisin Swirl, Sun-Maid*	1 Slice/33g	95	1.9	287	8.3	50.4	5.8	2.6
Garlic, & Cheese, Slices, Tesco*	1 Slice/30g	114	5	380	11.7	43.9	16.8	2
Garlic, & Tomato, Pizza, Italiano, Tesco*	½ Bread/140g	405	15.1	289	7.5	40.5	10.8	2.5
Garlic, & Herb, Slices, Reduced Fat, Asda*	1 Slice/33g	91	1.6	277	8.5	49	4.9	1.8
Garlic, & Parsley, Easibake, Iceland*	1 Pack/170g	634	28	373	8.3	46.5	16.5	2.9
Garlic, 30% Less Fat, Morrisons*	1 Serving/80g	231	7.4	289	7.9	43.8	9.2	2.7
Garlic, 50% Reduced Fat, Slices, Morrisons*	2 Slices/52g	122	3.1	235	7.9	36.7	6	1.5
Garlic, Average	***1 Serving/100g***	***327***	***13.8***	***327***	***8.1***	***43.7***	***13.8***	***1.4***
Garlic, Baguette, 50% Reduced Fat, Morrisons*	¼ Baguette/52g	122	3.1	235	7.9	36.7	6	1.5

B

	Measure INFO/WEIGHT	per Measure KCAL	FAT	Nutrition Values per 100g / 100ml KCAL	PROT	CARB	FAT	FIBRE
BREAD								
Garlic, Baguette, Average	***1 Slice/20g***	***66***	***2.8***	***330***	***7.8***	***43.1***	***14.2***	***1.8***
Garlic, Baguette, Free From, Tesco*	¼ Baguette/39g	137	6.2	352	1.2	49.1	15.8	4.4
Garlic, Baguette, HFC, Tesco*	1 Serving/85g	325	18.9	383	6.7	38.2	22.2	1.7
Garlic, Baguette, Italian, Asda*	¼ Baguette/48g	173	9.5	364	7	39	20	3.4
Garlic, Baguette, Italiano, Tesco*	¼ Baguette/53g	186	9.9	355	6.9	39.2	18.8	2.4
Garlic, Baguette, LC, Tesco*	¼ Baguette/52g	130	2.9	250	7	42.2	5.5	2.4
Garlic, Baguette, M&S*	¼ Baguette/52g	172	8.2	330	6.8	38.6	15.8	2.9
Garlic, Baguette, Morrisons*	½ Baguette/95g	316	12.1	333	8	45.9	12.7	1.5
Garlic, Baguette, Sainsbury's*	¼ Baguette/52g	184	7.9	354	8.1	45.2	15.2	2.4
Garlic, Baguette, Slices, Tesco*	1 Serving/60g	187	9.2	312	9.8	33.8	15.3	1.7
Garlic, Baguette, Value, Tesco*	½ Baguette/85g	270	11.1	318	8.1	42	13.1	2.3
Garlic, Cheesy, Slices, M&S*	1 Slice/28g	103	5	368	10.1	40.8	17.7	2.5
Garlic, Ciabatta, & Herb Butter, Sainsbury's*	½ Ciabatta/105g	345	16.3	329	8.5	38.8	15.5	0
Garlic, Ciabatta, Finest, Tesco*	1 Serving/65g	205	8.9	316	8.1	40.1	13.7	2.4
Garlic, Ciabatta, Italiano, Tesco*	1 Ciabatta/65g	211	9.4	324	7.7	40.9	14.4	2.2
Garlic, Ciabatta, Morrisons*	¼ Pack/73g	241	9.6	330	9.6	42.1	13.1	2.7
Garlic, Focaccia, & Rosemary, Sainsbury's*	¼ Focaccia/75g	219	7.4	292	8	43	9.8	2.8
Garlic, Focaccia, & Herb, Italian Style, Morrisons*	1/6 Focaccia/76g	259	10.9	341	8.5	44.7	14.3	2.5
Garlic, Homebake, Tesco*	1 Serving/60g	209	12.3	348	7.1	33.7	20.5	1.5
Garlic, Italian Style Stone Baked, Morrisons*	½ Pack/115g	420	22	365	7.9	40.4	19.1	1.9
Garlic, Pizza Bread, Co-Op*	1 Pizza/240g	756	31.2	315	8	41	13	2
Garlic, Pizza, Cooked, Goodfella's*	¼ Pizza/45g	211	13.2	469	7.5	42.7	29.3	0
Garlic, Slices, Asda*	1 Slice/26g	92	4.7	352	8.2	38	18	2.8
Garlic, Slices, BGTY, Sainsbury's*	1 Slice/33g	98	2.1	299	9.2	50.5	6.3	1.9
Garlic, Slices, Frozen, Co-Op*	1 Slice/26g	94	4.9	362	5.9	41	19	2.9
Garlic, Slices, LC, Tesco*	1 Slice/30g	75	1.7	250	7.3	42.3	5.7	2.9
Garlic, Slices, Morrisons*	1 Slice/32g	109	4.1	341	8.5	46.9	12.9	1.7
Garlic, Stonebaked, M&S*	1 Loaf/85g	314	14.4	369	8.6	44.4	16.9	2.4
Garlic, with Cheese, Asda*	1 Slice/34g	130	6.1	382	11	44	18	0
GF, Cranberry Seedful, Organic, Seedful*	1 Slice/70g	249	18.1	356	8.8	16.5	25.8	0
Glorious Grains, Hovis*	1 Slice/43g	101	1	234	10.4	40.5	2.3	5.1
Grained, Soft, Farmhouse, Warburton's*	1 Slice/42g	109	1.7	258	10.2	44.6	4	5
Grains, & Seeds, Tasty, Warburton's*	1 Slice/38g	100	1.6	264	10.6	45.6	4.3	5.2
Granary, Average	***1 Slice/35g***	***85***	***1***	***242***	***9.8***	***44***	***2.8***	***4.8***
Granary, Baps, Large, Asda*	1 Bap/64g	143	1.4	224	10	41	2.2	4.3
Granary, Loaf, Bakery, Waitrose*	1 Slice/45g	117	1.6	259	8.6	44.8	3.5	6.7
Granary, M&S*	1 Slice/30g	75	0.9	250	9.5	46.4	3.1	3.2
Granary, Malted, Med Brown, Asda*	1 Slice/35g	81	0.9	231	9	43	2.6	3.3
Granary, Med Sliced, 800g, Hovis*	1 Slice/38g	97	0.9	256	10.3	46.4	2.4	3.7
Granary, Sliced, Sm Loaf, Hovis*	1 Slice/33g	84	0.8	256	10.3	46.4	2.4	3.7
Granary, Thick Slice, COU, M&S*	1 Slice/25g	60	0.6	240	10.5	44.1	2.2	6
Granary, Thick, Sliced, 800g, Hovis*	1 Slice/44g	112	1	256	10.3	46.4	2.4	3.7
Granary, Wholemeal, Average	***1 Slice/35g***	***80***	***0.9***	***228***	***10.8***	***38.4***	***2.6***	***6.6***
Half & Half, Medium, Warburton's*	1 Slice/40g	95	0.8	240	8.8	44.2	2	5
Half & Half, Thick Sliced, Warburtons *	1 Slice/47g	118	1.3	248	10	43.6	2.8	4.2
Half & Half, Toastie, Warburton's*	1 Slice/47g	112	0.9	240	8.8	44.2	2	5
Herby, Basket, Snack, Graze*	1 Punnet/20g	101	5	503	8	61	25	3
Herby, Basket, Snack, Retail, Graze*	1 Punnet/18g	90	4.3	500	8.1	61	24	3.5
Heyford, Half Bloomer, Waitrose*	1 Slice/44g	97	1.4	222	10.1	35	3.1	6.6
Irish, Barm Brack, Tesco*	1 Slice/75g	232	5.2	310	16	47.6	6.9	3
Irish, Brown Soda, Tesco*	1 Slice/50g	110	1.9	219	9.2	36.2	3.8	6.4
Irish, Cottage Wheaten, Loaf, Tesco*	1 Slice/50g	116	1.3	231	8.6	41.4	2.6	4.2
Malt Loaf, Fruited, Sliced, Weight Watchers*	1 Slice/23g	68	0.4	294	8.9	60.2	1.9	3.6

	Measure INFO/WEIGHT	per Measure KCAL	FAT	Nutrition Values per 100g / 100ml KCAL	PROT	CARB	FAT	FIBRE
BREAD								
Malt Loaf, Fruity, Sliced, Soreen*	1 Slices/21g	64	0.6	300	8.2	58.2	3	3.9
Malt Loaf, Original, Low Fat, Soreen*	1 Slice/22g	63	0.4	288	7.5	60	1.6	2
Malt Loaf, Rowan Hill Bakery, Lidl*	1 Slice/37g	107	1	289	8.4	55.4	2.6	5.4
Malt Loaf, Seeds & More, Soreen*	1 Slice/52g	174	3.8	336	10.1	54.3	7.4	5.9
Malt Loaf, Strawberry, Lunchbox, Soreen*	1 Loaf/30g	91	0.9	302	8	58.3	3	4.6
Malt Loaf, Tesco*	1 Slice/50g	146	1.4	291	8.6	58	2.7	4.8
Malted Grain, Thick Cut, Loaf, Morrisons*	1 Slice/42g	106	1.1	251	10.1	44.5	2.5	5
Malted, & Seeded, Batch, Organic, Waitrose*	1 Slice/50g	118	2	236	10.9	39.5	3.9	6.2
Malted, Bloomer, Med Sliced, Iceland*	1 Slice/40g	108	1.5	270	9	48	3.8	3.8
Malted, Bloomer, Thick Sliced, Iceland*	1 Slice/51g	136	1.9	269	8.9	48	3.8	3.9
Malted, Brown, Slice, BGTY, Sainsbury's*	1 Slice/22g	53	0.6	239	12.1	41.4	2.8	5.8
Malted, Brown, Thick Sliced, Organic, Tesco*	1 Slice/44g	111	0.9	249	8.9	48.8	2	3.5
Malted, Crusty, Sainsbury's*	1 Slice/42g	109	1.4	259	8.6	48.6	3.3	4.4
Malted, Danish, Weight Watchers, Warburton's*	1 Slice/20g	51	0.3	249	11.8	45.1	1.5	4.2
Malted, Grain, Co-Op*	1 Slice/43g	99	0.9	230	8	46	2	3
Malted, Grain, Good As Gold, Kingsmill*	1 Slice/47g	114	1.2	243	9.5	45.4	2.6	4.2
Malted, Grain, Loaf, Bakery, Tesco*	1 Slice/40g	100	0.4	250	10.5	47.6	0.9	5
Malted, Grain, Loaf, Sliced, Bakery, Tesco*	1 Slice/50g	122	0.7	244	9.1	46.6	1.4	4.3
Malted, Wheat Loaf, Crusty, Finest, Tesco*	1 Slice/50g	115	0.8	230	9.8	44.2	1.5	4.4
Medium, 50/50, Kingsmill*	1 Slice/40g	94	0.9	234	9.4	41.9	2.2	4.7
Multi Grain, Promise*	1 Slice/40g	88	2.9	221	6	26.3	7.3	12.9
Multi Seed, Thick Sliced, Loaf, Morrisons*	1 Slice/40g	119	2.8	297	12.3	37.9	7	7.5
Multi-Seed, Thick Cut, The Best, Morrisons*	1 Slice/42g	114	2.7	272	11.3	39.6	6.4	5.2
Multi-Seeded, Farmhouse, Sliced, Loaf, Waitrose*	1 Slice/33g	96	2.9	291	11.2	38.5	8.8	6.7
Multigrain, & Seed, Warburtons *	1 Slice/31g	83	2.3	268	10	37.1	7.4	6.4
Multigrain, Batch, Sliced, Tesco*	1 Slice/50g	120	0.9	241	9.3	43.7	1.8	6.2
Multigrain, Brown, Farmhouse Baker's, M&S*	1 Slice/51g	115	2.8	225	13	31.2	5.4	5.1
Multigrain, Crusty, Finest, Tesco*	1 Slice/40g	98	1.4	245	9	44.7	3.4	5
Multigrain, Farmhouse, Deluxe, Lidl*	1 Slice/40g	101	1.2	253	10.1	44.3	2.9	4.6
Multigrain, Farmhouse, Loaf, 400g, Waitrose*	1 Slice/33g	83	0.6	253	9.9	47.4	1.7	4.3
Multigrain, GF, Just Free, Lidl*	1 Slice/34g	23	0.4	69	1.6	10.1	1.3	4.6
Multigrain, GF, Sainsbury's*	1 Slice/17g	39	0.8	229	5.1	40.8	5	5.6
Multigrain, Med Sliced, Batch, Tesco*	1 Slice/50g	120	0.9	241	9.3	43.7	1.8	6.2
Multigrain, Soft Batch, Sainsbury's*	1 Slice/44g	106	2.9	242	11.3	34.5	6.5	5.6
Multigrain, Thick Sliced, Tesco*	1 Slice/50g	112	1.2	225	8.4	42.2	2.5	3.9
Multiseed, Farmhouse Batch, Finest, Tesco*	1 Slice/44g	108	1.9	245	9.9	40.4	4.4	7.5
Multiseed, Farmhouse, Finest, Tesco*	1 Slice /50g	135	3.8	270	12.5	37	7.7	5.8
Multiseed, Farmhouse, Loaf, Luxury, Iceland*	1 Slice/44g	125	3.8	282	11.5	37.5	8.6	4.2
Multiseeded, Bloomer, TTD, Sainsbury's*	1 Slice/50g	128	1.8	256	12	39.7	3.6	8.8
Naan, 50% Wholewheat, Garlic & Coriander, Sharwood's*	1 Serving/65g	195	5.1	300	7.6	47.7	7.8	4.3
Naan, 50% Wholewheat, Mini, Sharwoods*	1 Naan/65g	184	3.4	283	8.5	47.7	5.2	5.6
Naan, Asda*	1 Naan/130g	308	2.3	237	7.7	47.4	1.8	2.2
Naan, Average	***1 Naan/130g***	***344***	***5.6***	***264***	***8.3***	***48.5***	***4.3***	***2***
Naan, Bombay Brassiere, Sainsbury's*	1 Naan/140g	372	4.3	266	9.8	49.6	3.1	2.9
Naan, Chicken Tikka, Tandoori, Naanzza*	½ Naan/150g	337	9.6	225	10.9	30.7	6.4	1.3
Naan, Chilli & Mango, Finest, Tesco*	½ Naan/90g	230	5.1	255	8.4	41.9	5.7	3.2
Naan, Currymate*	1 Serving/60g	187	4.5	311	8.6	50.6	7.5	2.9
Naan, Fresh, BGTY, Sainsbury's*	1 Serving/150g	368	4.6	245	9.4	44.9	3.1	2.2
Naan, Garlic & Coriander, Free From, Tesco*	1 Naan/90g	215	6	240	5.1	38.7	6.7	4.9
Naan, Garlic & Coriander, Tesco*	½ Naan/65g	184	3	283	7.5	51.2	4.6	3.3
Naan, Garlic & Coriander, TTD, Sainsbury's*	1 Naan/70g	219	8.4	313	7	44	12	2.9
Naan, Garlic & Coriander, Asda*	1 Naan/165g	473	10.1	287	7.9	48	6.1	5
Naan, Garlic & Coriander, Bilash, Aldi*	1 Naan/130g	333	6.5	256	7.4	44	5	2.2

	Measure INFO/WEIGHT	per Measure KCAL	FAT	Nutrition Values per 100g / 100ml KCAL	PROT	CARB	FAT	FIBRE
BREAD								
Naan, Garlic & Coriander, Clay Oven Bakery*	1 Naan/120g	311	7.8	259	7.6	41.3	6.5	2.3
Naan, Garlic & Coriander, Mini, Asda*	1 Naan/47g	151	3.7	320	8.7	52	7.9	3.4
Naan, Garlic & Coriander, Mini, Sainsbury's*	1 Naan/48g	147	3.4	307	8.3	51.2	7	3
Naan, Garlic & Coriander, Mini, Sharwood's*	1 Naan/65g	196	4.2	302	8	51.5	6.5	2.8
Naan, Garlic & Coriander, Mini, Tesco*	1 Naan/50g	130	2.3	261	7.6	45.9	4.6	3
Naan, Garlic & Coriander, Mini, Weight Watchers*	1 Naan/40g	100	1	250	9.3	47.6	2.5	4.2
Naan, Garlic & Coriander, Patak's*	1 Naan/127g	378	6.9	298	9	52.1	5.4	2.3
Naan, Garlic & Coriander, The Spice Tailor*	1 Naan/110g	366	12.1	333	8.5	49	11	2.2
Naan, Garlic & Coriander, Weight Watchers*	1 Naan/60g	155	2.6	259	8.9	46	4.3	3.4
Naan, Garlic, & Coriander, Pana*	1 Naan/137g	372	11.4	271	7.1	42.1	8.3	2.1
Naan, Garlic, Asda*	1 Naan/160g	410	6.6	256	8.3	46	4.1	1.8
Naan, Indian Meal for One, BGTY, Sainsbury's*	1 Serving/45g	115	1.9	257	10.3	44.2	4.3	2.1
Naan, Meal For Two, Korma/Tikka Masala, Tesco*	1 Naan/97g	291	6.8	300	8.6	49.1	7	3.3
Naan, Ocado*	½ Naan/75g	194	1.7	258	8.4	48.3	2.3	5.3
Naan, Onion & Mint, M&S*	½ Naan/135g	351	11.7	260	8.9	35.8	8.7	2.5
Naan, Onion Bhaji, Sharwood's*	1 Pack/130g	378	9.9	291	7.3	48.4	7.6	2.2
Naan, Peshwari, Apple & Coconut, Mini, Sharwood's*	1 Naan/65g	179	3.1	275	7.5	47.1	4.8	6.7
Naan, Peshwari, Flame Baked, Finest, Tesco*	½ Naan/75g	221	6.2	295	7.2	46.6	8.3	2.5
Naan, Peshwari, Mini, Bilash, Aldi*	1 Naan/58g	212	9.5	366	7	45.1	16.4	4.9
Naan, Peshwari, Sainsbury's*	1 Naan/166g	511	18.3	308	7.1	45.1	11	4.7
Naan, Peshwari, Sharwood's*	1 Naan/130g	334	6.9	257	7.2	45.1	5.3	2.5
Naan, Peshwari, Tesco*	1 Naan/215g	684	26.7	318	7.5	48.9	12.4	4.8
Naan, Plain, As Sold, Asda*	½ Naan/95g	295	7.4	310	8.2	50	7.8	3
Naan, Plain, Average	***1 Naan/160g***	***437***	***10.5***	***273***	***8***	***45.7***	***6.5***	***2.1***
Naan, Plain, Bilash, Aldi*	1 Naan/130g	324	4	249	8.1	46	3.1	2.7
Naan, Plain, Clay Oven Bakery*	1 Pack/180g	418	3.2	232	8.4	44.5	1.8	2.2
Naan, Plain, Co-Op*	1 Naan/130g	361	6.2	278	7.8	49	4.8	4.6
Naan, Plain, Finest, Tesco*	½ Naan/80g	206	4.1	257	8	43.2	5.1	3.1
Naan, Plain, Indian, Mini, Asda*	1 Naan/110g	329	12.6	299	6.6	42.2	11.5	2.1
Naan, Plain, Large, Sainsbury's*	½ Naan/70g	191	4.6	273	7.1	46.2	6.6	3
Naan, Plain, Mini, Asda*	1 Naan/58g	156	2.7	269	8	49	4.6	2.3
Naan, Plain, Mini, BGTY, Sainsbury's*	1 Naan/50g	124	0.6	248	7.6	49.8	1.3	3.3
Naan, Plain, Mini, Weight Watchers*	1 Naan/44g	108	1.1	245	9.1	46.5	2.5	4.9
Naan, Plain, Sainsbury's*	1 Naan/126g	385	11.2	306	7.8	46.9	8.9	3.6
Naan, Plain, Sharwood's*	1 Naan/120g	326	8.9	272	8.5	42.9	7.4	2.4
Naan, Plain, Small, Clay Oven*	½ Naan/50g	116	0.9	232	8.4	44.5	1.8	2.2
Naan, Plain, Tesco*	1 Naan/150g	392	6.9	261	8.4	46.4	4.6	2.3
Naan, Plain, Value, Tesco*	1 Naan/135g	363	9.7	269	8.1	42.9	7.2	1.6
Naan, Santosh*	½ Naan/50g	150	3	300	8	48	6	2
Naan, Smart Price, Asda*	1 Naan/100g	233	1.9	233	8.7	45.3	1.9	2.8
Naan, Take Away, Tesco*	1 Naan/39g	97	1.3	248	8.7	45.6	3.4	1.7
Naan, Tandoori Baked, Waitrose*	1 Naan/140g	372	4.3	266	9.8	49.6	3.1	2.9
Naan, Tandoori, Sharwood's*	1 Naan/130g	330	6.5	254	7.3	45	5	2
Oat, Sunflower, & Pumpkin, Loaf, Irresistible, Co-Op*	1 Slice/50g	152	5.5	304	11	38	11	4.4
Oatmeal, Farmhouse, Soft, M&S*	1 Slice/45g	110	2	245	11.1	39.5	4.4	5.2
Oatmeal, Sliced Loaf, Tesco*	1 Slice/50g	111	1.7	222	7.4	40.5	3.4	2.8
Olive, Kalamata, TTD, Sainsbury's*	1 Slice/50g	121	1.4	242	8.1	44.7	2.8	3
Olive, Waitrose*	1 Slice/28g	86	3	306	9	43.6	10.6	2
Onion, Roasted, M&S*	1 Slice/50g	125	1.6	250	9	46.7	3.3	2.1
Pave, Ancient Grain, Sainsbury's*	1 Slice/50g	128	1.7	255	9.6	44.5	3.4	4
Pave, Ancient Grain, TTD, Sainsbury's*	1 Slice/50g	128	1.7	256	9.6	44.6	3.4	4
Pave, Walnut, Sainsbury's*	1 Slice/50g	140	4.8	280	9	40	9.5	3.5
Pave, Walnut, TTD, Sainsbury's*	1 Slice/50g	138	3.6	277	9.5	41.5	7.3	3.7

	Measure INFO/WEIGHT	per Measure KCAL	FAT	Nutrition Values per 100g / 100ml KCAL	PROT	CARB	FAT	FIBRE
BREAD								
Petit Pain, Homebake, Mini, Tesco*	1 Roll/50g	144	0.6	289	8.6	59.1	1.2	3.5
Petit Pain, Mini, Homebake, Tesco*	1 Roll/45g	110	0.6	245	7.8	49.7	1.3	2.5
Petit Pain, Organic, Tesco*	1 Roll/100g	235	0.8	235	7.8	49.1	0.8	1.2
Petit Pain, Part Bake, Weight Watchers*	1 Roll/50g	111	0.4	223	6.8	43.5	0.9	6.8
Petit Pains, Delifrance*	1 Roll/63g	173	0.6	274	9.3	55.4	0.9	3.3
Pitta, 159, Pride Valley*	1 Pitta/63g	159	1.2	252	10.1	51.2	1.9	2.6
Pitta, Brown, Organic, Waitrose*	1 Pitta/53g	124	0.5	234	8.5	43.9	1	7.4
Pitta, Cohens Bakery*	1 Pitta/78g	162	0.6	208	5.3	45	0.8	2.3
Pitta, Free From, Sainsbury's*	1 Pitta/65g	164	2.5	252	4.1	50	3.9	2.9
Pitta, Garlic, Morrisons*	1 Pitta/60g	149	1.1	249	9.7	51.1	1.8	0
Pitta, Mediterranean Style, Specially Selected, Aldi*	1 Pitta/85g	229	3.5	269	7.9	49	4.1	2.3
Pitta, Mediterranean Style, The Bakery, M&S*	1 Pitta/85g	247	3.7	291	6.7	54.9	4.3	2.8
Pitta, Multi Seed, & Cereal, The Food Doctor*	1 Pitta/60g	150	1.3	250	9.3	51.8	2.1	6.6
Pitta, Pocket, Stone Baked, GF, BFree*	1 Pitta/32g	68	0.6	214	4.9	39.6	1.8	9.8
Pitta, Pockets, Sainsbury's*	1 Pitta/75g	188	0.8	250	8.5	52	1	3.5
Pitta, Sd Tomato, Olive & Oregano, Extra Special, Asda*	1 Pitta/75g	194	0.8	259	7.1	55.2	1.1	1.6
Pitta, Seeded, HL, Tesco*	1 Pitta/60g	153	3.6	255	10.8	39.4	6	12.8
Pitta, Spelt, Albert Heijn*	1 Pitta/80g	196	0.8	245	2.5	48	1	0
Pitta, Spicy Tomato, Herb, & Red Pepper, Finest, Tesco*	1 Pitta/85g	218	3.2	257	8.3	45.7	3.8	3.4
Pitta, Stone Baked, Genius*	1 Pitta/62g	142	3.2	229	2.6	37.1	5.2	11.9
Pitta, White, Average	***1 Pitta/75g***	***191***	***1.1***	***255***	***9.2***	***50.8***	***1.5***	***2.7***
Pitta, White, Carrefour*	1 Pitta/70g	174	0.7	248	8.2	50	1	3.1
Pitta, White, Essential, Waitrose*	1 Pitta/60g	157	0.5	262	9	53.4	0.9	2.3
Pitta, White, Free From, Tesco*	1 Pitta/55g	140	1.2	255	6.5	52.6	2.1	5.5
Pitta, White, Greek Style, Asda*	1 Pitta/50g	126	1	253	8	51	1.9	0
Pitta, White, Hollyland Bakery*	1 Pitta/70g	176	0.8	251	9	53	1.2	3.9
Pitta, White, Large, Tesco*	1 Pitta/80g	220	0.8	275	9.4	54.9	1	4.5
Pitta, White, Mini, Asda*	1 Pitta/18g	44	0.1	245	8.9	49	0.8	3.2
Pitta, White, Mini, Sainsbury's*	1 Pitta/20g	54	0.2	268	8.8	54.6	1.2	2
Pitta, White, Mini, Tesco*	1 Pitta/30g	84	0.6	280	9.8	55.1	2.1	3.4
Pitta, White, Sainsbury's*	1 Pitta/58g	160	0.7	275	9.8	54.7	1.2	3.1
Pitta, White, Speciality Breads, Waitrose*	1 Pitta/60g	149	0.7	249	10.3	49.3	1.2	3.5
Pitta, White, Tesco*	1 Pitta/58g	160	0.6	275	9.4	54.9	1	4.5
Pitta, White, Traditional, Giannis, Aldi*	1 Pitta/45g	110	0.4	245	9.2	50.6	1	0
Pitta, White, Weight Watchers*	1 Pitta/45g	106	0.3	238	8.7	45.9	0.7	6.7
Pitta, Wholegrain, GF, BFree*	1 Pitta/55g	118	1.6	215	5.5	37.7	2.9	8.2
Pitta, Wholemeal, Asda*	1 Pitta/60g	150	0.7	251	10	48	1.2	3.9
Pitta, Wholemeal, Average	***1 Pitta/64g***	***154***	***1.1***	***241***	***11***	***45.8***	***1.7***	***6.4***
Pitta, Wholemeal, Essential, Waitrose*	1 Pitta/60g	159	0.7	264	9.7	50.1	1.2	7.2
Pitta, Wholemeal, Healthy Eating, Co-Op*	1 Pitta/63g	135	1.3	215	12	37	2	9
Pitta, Wholemeal, M&S*	1 Pitta/60g	155	1.6	255	10	45	2.6	5.5
Pitta, Wholemeal, Mini, M&S*	1 Pitta/18g	44	0.4	247	10.3	45.8	2.5	5.6
Pitta, Wholemeal, Mini, Sainsbury's*	1 Pitta/30g	69	0.5	231	10	43.8	1.7	6.2
Pitta, Wholemeal, Mini, Tesco*	1 Pitta/30g	76	0.5	255	11.8	48.2	1.7	4.2
Pitta, Wholemeal, Round, Morrisons*	1 Pitta/93g	249	2.4	268	11.1	46.1	2.6	7.9
Pitta, Wholemeal, Sainsbury's*	1 Pitta/56g	135	0.7	241	10.3	42.3	1.2	9.7
Pitta, Wholemeal, Seeded, Specially Selected, Aldi*	1 Pitta/85g	215	3.5	253	9.6	41	4.1	7.4
Pitta, Wholemeal, Simple & Versatile, As Sold, Tesco*	1 Pitta/58g	145	0.7	250	9.6	46.2	1.2	7.8
Pitta, Wholemeal, So Organic, Sainsbury's*	1 Pitta/60g	140	1	233	9.8	44.8	1.6	8.1
Pitta, Wholemeal, Tesco*	1 Pitta/58g	145	0.7	250	9.6	46.2	1.2	7.8
Pitta, Wholemeal, Waitrose*	1 Pitta/60g	145	0.5	242	12.4	46	0.9	3.1
Potato, Farls, M&S*	1 Farl/55g	79	0.2	144	4.2	33.8	0.4	4.7
Potato, Farls, Slims, Rankin Selection*	1 Farl/60g	80	1.8	134	2.3	24.3	3	1.8

BREAD	Measure INFO/WEIGHT	per Measure KCAL	FAT	Nutrition Values per 100g / 100ml KCAL	PROT	CARB	FAT	FIBRE
Potato, Farls, Sunblest*	1 Farl/100g	156	0.9	156	3.8	33.2	0.9	1.9
Pumpernickel, Average	***1 Slice/50g***	***96***	***0.6***	***191***	***5.5***	***37.9***	***1.1***	***7.8***
Pumpkin Seed, Raisin & Sunflower Seed, Sainsbury's*	1 Slice/30g	76	0.8	255	11.6	45.9	2.8	3.4
Pure Grain, with Prunes, Pure Nature*	1 Slice/50g	169	10.4	338	8	28.3	20.8	9
Raisin, & Pumpkin Seed, Organic, Tesco*	1 Slice/30g	76	1.7	253	9.7	40.6	5.8	3.8
Raisin, with Cinnamon, Warburton's*	1 Slice/36g	96	1.3	267	7.2	51.1	3.7	3.2
Richly Fruited, Loaf, Waitrose*	1 Slice/34g	99	1.5	292	7.5	54.2	4.4	2.8
Roll, Brioche, Chocolate & Custard, Mini, Lidl*	1 Roll/50g	152	4.5	305	7	48	9	2
Roll, Brioche, Chocolate Chip, Tesco*	1 Roll/35g	131	4.4	374	7.6	56.3	12.7	2.1
Roll, Brioche, Sliced, Iceland*	1 Roll/50g	156	3.8	312	9.5	50	7.5	2.5
Roll, Brioche, Sweet, GF, Schar*	1 Roll/50g	146	3.6	293	3.4	52	7.3	3
Roll, Brown, Ciabatta, GF, Dietary Specials*	1 Roll/50g	137	4	274	5.8	36.9	8.1	8.9
Roll, Brown, Deli Sub, Asda*	1 Roll/60g	142	1.9	236	0	35	3.2	0
Roll, Brown, Jackson's Bakery*	1 Roll/74g	203	3.6	274	9	46	4.8	5.1
Roll, Brown, Scotch, Co-Op*	1 Roll/77g	196	1.7	255	9.8	45	2.2	4.1
Roll, Brown, Seeded, Free From, Tesco*	1 Roll/75g	167	5.5	222	6.7	28.8	7.3	7.4
Roll, Brown, Soft, Bakery Select*	1 Roll/70g	176	3.6	252	9.3	41.4	5.1	0
Roll, Cheese & Onion, Bap, Market St, Morrisons*	1 Roll/40g	337	12	842	32.5	100	30	7.5
Roll, Ciabatta, Asda*	1 Roll/90g	230	2.2	256	9.3	48	2.4	2.3
Roll, Ciabatta, Caramelised Onion, Irresistible, Co-Op*	1 Roll/80g	213	4.3	266	9.3	43	5.4	4.2
Roll, Crusty, Iceland*	1 Roll/50g	130	0.8	260	8.7	51.1	1.6	3.3
Roll, Malted Wheat, Bakery, Waitrose*	1 Roll/85g	222	1	262	7.9	52.2	1.2	5.5
Roll, Oatmeal, Deli, M&S*	1 Roll/75g	202	2.8	270	10.9	46.3	3.7	3.7
Roll, Scotch, Sainsbury's*	1 Roll/79g	200	1.9	253	9.2	47	2.4	3.4
Roll, Seeded, Bakers Selection, Asda*	1 Roll/88g	266	6.8	302	10.1	45.9	7.7	0
Roll, Sourdough, Seeded, Gail's*	1 Roll/70g	196	5.5	280	10.2	39.8	7.9	4.6
Roll, Sourdough, White, Irresistible, Co-Op*	1 Roll/73g	176	0.4	241	9	49	0.6	2.6
Roll, Super Seeded, GF, Made Without Wheat, M&S*	1 Roll/75g	170	6.2	227	8	24	8.3	12
Roll, White, Ciabatta, GF, Dietary Specials*	1 Roll/50g	106	0.9	213	4.1	40.9	1.8	8.3
Roll, White, Large, Barm, Jones Village Bakery *	1 Roll/50g	135	2.2	270	8.2	52.5	4.5	2.9
Roll, White, Soft, Warburton's*	1 Roll/55g	146	2.1	265	9.7	46.6	3.9	2.4
Roll, Wholemeal, Bap, Bakers Selection, Asda*	1 Roll/54g	133	2	247	12	38	3.7	6.6
Roll, Wholemeal, Deli, Iceland*	1 Roll/59g	143	1.5	242	9.3	42.4	2.6	5.8
Roll, Wholemeal, Oat Topped, Village Bakery, Aldi*	1 Roll/65g	161	1.8	248	11	41	2.8	7.7
Roll, Wholemeal, Seeded, Love Life, Waitrose*	1 Roll/72g	192	6.3	266	12.6	34.1	8.8	6.4
Rolls, American Style Deli, Tesco*	1 Roll/65g	162	2.2	249	7.8	46.8	3.4	1.6
Rolls, Ancient Grain, Tesco*	1 Roll/80g	231	6.7	289	14.7	34.4	8.4	8.6
Rolls, Ancient Grain, The Best, Morrisons*	1 Roll/72g	198	4.1	275	11.3	41	5.7	7.2
Rolls, Bake at Home, Free From, Tesco*	1 Roll/55g	156	1.9	283	2	57	3.5	7.5
Rolls, Best of Both, Hovis*	1 Roll/62g	148	2.9	239	9.8	39.7	4.6	5
Rolls, Brioche, Asda*	1 Roll/35g	127	4.2	362	7.8	55	12	1.9
Rolls, Brioche, Average	***1 Roll/49g***	***177***	***6.9***	***361***	***8.8***	***50.1***	***14.1***	***1.5***
Rolls, Brioche, Butter, Tesco*	1 Roll/35g	127	4.2	363	7.6	55	12.1	1.9
Rolls, Brioche, Chocolate Chip, Rowan Hill Bakery, Lidl*	1 Roll/35g	134	4.8	384	8.3	55.4	13.8	2.7
Rolls, Brioche, Finest, Tesco*	1 Roll/52g	207	11.6	398	10.8	38.3	22.4	2
Rolls, Brioche, French Milk, Bon Appetit, Aldi*	1 Roll/35g	116	2.7	330	8.3	56	7.8	2.2
Rolls, Brioche, Hot Dog, Specially Selected, Aldi*	1 Roll/45g	142	3.4	316	9.4	52	7.5	2
Rolls, Brioche, Hot Dog, TTD, Sainsbury's*	1 Roll/70g	229	7.3	327	8.3	48.6	10.4	2.8
Rolls, Brioche, La Boulangere, Lidl*	1 Roll/35g	122	3.6	350	8.2	55.5	10.2	1.8
Rolls, Brioche, Plain Chocolate Chip, Sainsbury's*	1 Roll/35g	126	4.5	361	8	52.1	12.9	2.1
Rolls, Brioche, Sainsbury's*	1 Roll/35g	123	3.9	352	8.1	53.5	11.3	1.8
Rolls, Brioche, Tesco*	1 Roll/26g	92	2.9	349	8.5	54	11	0
Rolls, Brotchen, As Prepared, Lizza*	1 Roll/70g	130	4	186	17	6.6	5.7	20

	Measure INFO/WEIGHT	per Measure KCAL	per Measure FAT	Nutrition Values per 100g / 100ml KCAL	PROT	CARB	FAT	FIBRE
BREAD								
Rolls, Brown, Bake at Home, Aldi*	1 Roll/45g	124	0.7	275	9.5	53	1.6	6
Rolls, Brown, Ciabatta, Schar*	1 Roll/50g	138	4.1	274	5.8	40	8.1	8.9
Rolls, Brown, Crusty	***1 Roll/50g***	***128***	***1.4***	***255***	***10.3***	***50.4***	***2.8***	***3.5***
Rolls, Brown, Free From, Tesco*	1 Roll/65g	174	5.3	268	5.4	43.2	8.2	3.6
Rolls, Brown, Large, Asda*	1 Roll/57g	138	0.9	242	10	47	1.6	0
Rolls, Brown, M&S*	1 Roll/105g	242	6.4	230	9.2	37.3	6.1	4.4
Rolls, Brown, Malted Grain, Tesco*	1 Roll/58g	144	1.9	248	8.7	46.2	3.2	1.9
Rolls, Brown, Mini, M&S*	1 Roll/33g	80	2.5	245	9.8	35.5	7.6	3.8
Rolls, Brown, Morning, Farmfoods*	1 Roll/50g	134	1.8	269	12	47	3.7	4.2
Rolls, Brown, Old Fashioned, Waitrose*	1 Roll/63g	152	2.6	241	9.6	41.3	4.1	4.7
Rolls, Brown, Part Baked, Sunnyhills, Aldi*	1 Roll/50g	129	1.5	258	9.3	45.3	3	6.3
Rolls, Brown, Seeded, Organic, Sainsbury's*	1 Roll/70g	166	3.2	237	9.9	39.1	4.6	6.5
Rolls, Brown, Snack, Allinsons*	1 Roll/47g	128	2.5	272	10.2	43.5	5.3	4.9
Rolls, Brown, Soft, Average	***1 Roll/50g***	***134***	***1.9***	***268***	***10***	***51.8***	***3.8***	***3.5***
Rolls, Brown, Soft, Organic, Sainsbury's*	1 Roll/70g	166	3.2	237	9.9	39.1	4.6	6.6
Rolls, Brown, Soft, Tesco*	1 Roll/50g	125	0.5	250	9.2	49.7	1	2.6
Rolls, Cheese Topped, Sandwich, Warburton's*	1 Roll/62g	168	4	270	12.1	40.7	6.5	2.6
Rolls, Cheese, Rustique, Waitrose*	1 Roll/90g	255	3.4	283	11.3	49.7	3.8	2.6
Rolls, Chunky Cheese, Tesco*	1 Roll/80g	219	4.8	274	12.8	41.1	6	2
Rolls, Ciabatta, Cheese Topped, Mini, Finest, Tesco*	1 Roll/30g	85	2.4	282	11.5	40.9	8.1	3.8
Rolls, Ciabatta, Crisp & Floury, Waitrose*	1 Roll/80g	206	2.8	258	8.4	46.5	3.5	3.4
Rolls, Ciabatta, Garlic, Asda*	1 Roll/93g	333	16.7	358	9	40	18	2.3
Rolls, Ciabatta, GF, Schar*	1 Roll/50g	116	1.6	231	4.6	42	3.3	6.8
Rolls, Ciabatta, Mini, Finest, Tesco*	1 Roll/30g	89	2	297	9.9	49.1	6.8	4.1
Rolls, Ciabatta, Sun Dried Tomato, Mini, Finest, Tesco*	1 Roll/30g	79	1.9	262	8.7	42.3	6.4	2.6
Rolls, Ciabatta, Tesco*	1 Roll/100g	295	5.6	295	9.2	50.5	5.6	3
Rolls, Crusty, French, M&S*	1 Roll/65g	159	0.8	245	8.1	50.5	1.2	3.3
Rolls, Finger, Morrisons*	1 Roll/46g	119	0.8	259	10.7	50	1.8	2.3
Rolls, Finger, White, Sainsbury's*	1 Roll/40g	96	1	240	9	45.2	2.6	3.2
Rolls, Focaccia, Amisa*	1 Roll/110g	242	5	220	3.2	39	4.5	0
Rolls, Focaccia, Tesco*	1 Roll/75g	226	7	302	8.7	45.6	9.4	3.8
Rolls, Granary, Average	***1 Roll/70g***	***176***	***2.7***	***251***	***9.6***	***45.2***	***3.9***	***3.3***
Rolls, Granary, Bakers Premium, Tesco*	1 Roll/65g	158	0.8	243	9.9	47.8	1.3	2.3
Rolls, Granary, Mini, Tesco*	1 Roll/34g	92	2.2	271	10	43.5	6.5	3.8
Rolls, Granary, Waitrose*	1 Roll/59g	160	3.8	271	10	47.2	6.4	3.8
Rolls, Green Olive, M&S*	1 Roll/75g	210	4.5	280	11.2	44	6	1.8
Rolls, Half & Half, Warburton's*	1 Roll/55g	144	2.5	261	10.4	42.7	4.5	4
Rolls, Heyford Wholemeal, Soft & Grainy, Waitrose*	1 Roll/75g	164	1.3	219	11.2	36.7	1.7	5.8
Rolls, Hot Dog, Potato, Weis*	1 Roll/57g	160	2	281	8.8	52.6	3.5	1.8
Rolls, Hot Dog, Sliced, Iceland*	1 Roll/50g	130	1.2	261	9.1	49.8	2.3	2.1
Rolls, Hot Dog, Sliced, Sheldon's*	1 Roll/58g	147	1.4	255	9.8	47.2	2.5	1.9
Rolls, Hot Dog, Tesco*	1 Roll/85g	200	2.8	235	7.3	44	3.3	1.9
Rolls, Hot Dog, Value, Tesco*	1 Roll/40g	93	0.8	232	8.7	45	1.9	2.2
Rolls, Hot Dog, White, Warburton's*	1 Roll/55g	142	2.1	259	8.8	46.4	3.9	1.6
Rolls, Low GI, Lidl*	1 Roll/60g	177	5.1	295	14	44.9	8.5	8.4
Rolls, Malted Grain, Sainsbury's*	1 Roll/68g	190	2.9	280	8.7	51.6	4.3	4.2
Rolls, Malted Grain, Submarine, M&S*	1 Roll/109g	300	4.7	275	8.9	53.6	4.3	3
Rolls, Malted, Big Eat, Bakers Selection, Asda*	1 Roll/80g	207	2.5	259	9.7	46	3.1	4.6
Rolls, Malted, Whole Grain Rolls, Batched, Soft, M&S*	1 Roll/80g	180	3.6	225	7.8	38.5	4.5	3.1
Rolls, Mature Cheddar, with Black Pepper, Waitrose*	1 Roll/65g	189	5.7	291	11.3	40.2	8.7	3.1
Rolls, Mini Submarine, M&S*	1 Roll/23g	63	1.1	275	11.4	47.7	4.9	1.1
Rolls, Morning, Scottish, Warburton's*	1 Roll/50g	138	0.4	276	10.9	56.2	0.8	2.1
Rolls, Morning, Tesco*	1 Roll/48g	117	1.2	243	10.4	44.8	2.5	4.7

	Measure INFO/WEIGHT	per Measure KCAL	FAT	Nutrition Values per 100g / 100ml KCAL	PROT	CARB	FAT	FIBRE
BREAD								
Rolls, Multi Seed, Free From, Free From, Tesco*	1 Roll/70g	214	8.3	305	5.4	44.2	11.8	6.3
Rolls, Multigrain, Sourdough, Paul Hollywood*	1 Roll/75g	192	2.5	256	8.4	46.1	3.3	4.2
Rolls, Multigrain, Torpedo, Sainsbury's*	1 Roll/112g	328	7.5	293	10.5	47.7	6.7	6.3
Rolls, Multiseed, Deli, Tesco*	1 Roll/65g	188	4.6	289	10.5	40.7	7.1	10.3
Rolls, Multiseed, Genius*	1 Roll/70g	209	7.8	299	3.9	40.6	11.2	10
Rolls, Oatmeal, Soft, M&S*	1 Roll/83g	224	3.9	270	12.3	43.4	4.7	3.4
Rolls, Olive, Mixed, Waitrose*	1 Roll/90g	240	2.5	267	8.8	50	2.8	3
Rolls, Panini, Sainsbury's*	1 Roll/90g	249	5.6	276	11	44.1	6.2	3
Rolls, Panini, White, Tesco*	1 Roll/85g	232	4.1	273	10.7	44.9	4.8	3.4
Rolls, Part Baked, Iceland*	1 Roll/50g	130	0.8	260	8.7	51.1	1.6	3.3
Rolls, Part Baked, Mini, Tesco*	1 Roll/50g	120	0.6	240	7.8	49.5	1.2	3.4
Rolls, Poppy Seeded Knot, Waitrose*	1 Roll/60g	169	3.2	282	10.3	48.3	5.3	2.2
Rolls, Posh Dog, The Grill, M&S*	1 Roll/64g	195	5.6	305	8.7	45.4	8.8	4.5
Rolls, Pumpkin Seed, Lidl*	1 Roll/80g	271	9	339	15	42.5	11.2	3.8
Rolls, Rustic, Ready to Bake, Paul Hollywood*	1 Roll/75g	199	0.8	265	8.5	54.7	1	1.7
Rolls, Rye, Toasting, Good & Hot*	1 Roll/65g	143	0.7	220	7.3	44.6	1.1	7.1
Rolls, Scotch, Morning, Tesco*	1 Roll/50g	136	0.6	273	11.8	52	1.3	3.2
Rolls, Scottish Morning, Mcghees*	1 Roll/48g	126	0.2	262	10.6	54.6	0.4	5.4
Rolls, Scottish Morning, Morrisons*	1 Roll/60g	157	1.3	261	11.3	51.4	2.2	2.4
Rolls, Seeded, Breakfast, Amisa*	1 Roll/63g	144	5.1	228	4.7	30	8.1	0
Rolls, Seeded, Deli, Rowan Hill Bakery, Lidl*	1 Roll/75g	243	8.2	324	11.4	42.2	11	5.4
Rolls, Seeded, GF, Free From, Morrisons*	1 Roll/75g	166	6.4	222	7.1	20.9	8.5	16.7
Rolls, Seeded, GF, Free From, Waitrose*	1 Roll/75g	183	6.2	244	8	29	8.3	10.5
Rolls, Seeded, Mixed Mini Loaf Pack, M&S*	1 Roll/76g	220	7.3	290	10.6	39.7	9.6	4
Rolls, Seeded, Soft, GF, Newburn, Warburton's*	1 Roll/65g	176	6.2	270	9	33.8	9.5	6.7
Rolls, Snack, Mini, Tesco*	1 Roll/35g	95	2.1	271	19	43	6	4
Rolls, Soft, White, Rowan Hill Bakery, Lidl*	1 Roll/66g	157	1.6	238	8.5	44	2.5	2.8
Rolls, Soft, Wholemeal, Finger, M&S*	1 Roll/66g	145	1.3	220	12.6	38	2	5.8
Rolls, Sourdough, White, No.1, Waitrose*	1 Roll/92g	229	1.7	249	9.8	47.1	1.9	2.2
Rolls, Stone Baked, Bakery Instore, Lidl*	1 Roll/100g	292	1.5	292	9.5	58.4	1.5	3.5
Rolls, Sub, White, Batch, Warburton's*	1 Roll/80g	215	3.5	269	11	45	4.4	2.4
Rolls, Sub, Wholemeal, Warburton's*	1 Roll/94g	231	4.1	246	10.9	40.6	4.4	6.3
Rolls, Submarine, Sainsbury's*	1 Roll/117g	305	4.6	261	9.1	47.4	3.9	2.4
Rolls, Sun Dried Tomato, Homebake, Tesco*	1 Roll/50g	123	1.5	246	11.3	44	3	0
Rolls, Sunflower Seed, Toasting, Good & Hot*	1 Roll/65g	162	3.2	250	8.5	41	5	8
Rolls, Super Seeded, Deli, M&S*	1 Roll/77g	227	6.5	295	12.1	39.4	8.4	6.9
Rolls, Tiger, Crusty, Baked by Us, Morrisons*	1 Roll/63g	143	1.8	227	6.3	46	2.9	2.5
Rolls, Triple Seeded, Genius *	1 Roll/70g	209	7.8	299	3.9	40.6	11.2	10
Rolls, White, 50/50, Soft, Kingsmill*	1 Roll/63g	154	2.4	245	9.3	41.2	3.8	4.4
Rolls, White, BGTY, Sainsbury's*	1 Roll/50g	114	0.5	227	9.1	45.3	1	3
Rolls, White, Cheese Topped, Asda*	1 Roll/46g	121	2	264	10	46	4.4	2
Rolls, White, Cheese Topped, Sainsbury's*	1 Roll/75g	218	6.4	291	12.1	41.6	8.5	2
Rolls, White, Crusty, Average	***1 Roll/50g***	***140***	***1.2***	***280***	***10.9***	***57.6***	***2.3***	***1.5***
Rolls, White, Crusty, Bakery, Tesco*	1 Roll/70g	193	0.6	276	9.3	56.7	0.8	2.6
Rolls, White, Crusty, Home Bake, Tesco*	1 Roll/69g	185	1	270	9.3	54.2	1.4	2.9
Rolls, White, Crusty, Morning, M&S*	1 Roll/65g	176	0.8	270	8.8	53.8	1.3	2.7
Rolls, White, Crusty, Part Baked, Morrisons*	1 Roll/68g	191	0.9	281	9	56.5	1.3	3.7
Rolls, White, Dinner, Village Bakery, Aldi*	1 Roll/70g	183	0.9	262	8.8	52	1.3	3
Rolls, White, Finest, Tesco*	1 Roll/80g	198	2	247	9.3	45.3	2.5	3
Rolls, White, Finger, Smart Price, Asda*	1 Roll/50g	121	0.8	242	9	48	1.6	2.1
Rolls, White, Finger, Tesco*	1 Roll/45g	112	0.4	250	9.2	49.7	1	2.6
Rolls, White, Finger, Value, Tesco*	1 Roll/50g	116	1	232	8.7	45	1.9	2.2
Rolls, White, Floured, Batch, Tesco*	1 Roll/76g	193	2.5	254	8.8	47.3	3.3	2.2

	Measure INFO/WEIGHT	per Measure KCAL	per Measure FAT	KCAL	PROT	CARB	FAT	FIBRE
				Nutrition Values per 100g / 100ml				
BREAD								
Rolls, White, Floury Batch, Sainsbury's*	1 Roll/68g	168	1.9	247	8.3	47.2	2.8	2.2
Rolls, White, Floury, Roberts Bakery*	1 Roll/63g	160	1.6	254	8.4	49.5	2.5	2
Rolls, White, Free From, Co-Op*	1 Roll/65g	80	1.4	123	3.5	19	2.1	6
Rolls, White, Hot Dog, Jumbo, Sainsbury's*	1 Roll/85g	239	5.2	281	7.5	49.1	6.1	2.9
Rolls, White, Hot Dog, Large, Asda *	1 Roll/86g	224	2.1	260	8.7	50	2.4	1.9
Rolls, White, Hot Dog, Tesco*	1 Roll/65g	162	0.6	250	9.2	49.7	1	2.6
Rolls, White, Hot Dog, Tesco*	1 Roll/70g	177	2.5	254	9	45.5	3.6	1.9
Rolls, White, Large, Warburton's*	1 Roll/88g	229	3.1	259	10.2	44.3	3.5	2.5
Rolls, White, Low Price, Sainsbury's*	1 Roll/44g	107	0.7	243	8.9	48.2	1.6	2.1
Rolls, White, Mini, Submarine, M&S*	1 Roll/30g	86	1.5	285	11.4	47.7	4.9	1.1
Rolls, White, Morning, Co-Op*	1 Roll/47g	134	1.4	285	12	53	3	2
Rolls, White, Old Fashioned, Waitrose*	1 Roll/64g	176	2.9	275	8.8	49.8	4.5	2.8
Rolls, White, Organic, Sainsbury's*	1 Roll/65g	170	2	262	8.7	49.9	3	1
Rolls, White, Part Baked, Morrisons*	1 Roll/75g	227	1	303	9.6	63	1.4	2.6
Rolls, White, Sandwich, Sliced, Warburton's*	1 Roll/55g	146	2.1	265	9.7	46.6	3.9	2.4
Rolls, White, Scottish, Tesco*	1 Roll/48g	117	1.2	243	10.4	44.8	2.5	4.7
Rolls, White, Seeded, Sainsbury's*	1 Roll/80g	217	4.7	271	10.9	43.4	5.9	4.8
Rolls, White, Seeded, Soft, M&S*	1 Roll/75g	214	4.3	285	11.7	46.2	5.7	2.8
Rolls, White, Sliced, Morrisons*	1 Roll/59g	157	2.1	266	8.4	48.7	3.5	2.8
Rolls, White, Sliced, Warburton's*	1 Roll/55g	146	2.2	265	9.7	46.6	3.9	2.4
Rolls, White, Snack, Sainsbury's*	1 Roll/67g	159	0.7	237	7.9	49.2	1	2.3
Rolls, White, Soft, Average	***1 Roll/45g***	***114***	***1.5***	***253***	***9.2***	***46.5***	***3.3***	***2.2***
Rolls, White, Soft, Dietary Specials*	1 Roll/75g	130	2.9	172	2.2	29.8	3.8	4.7
Rolls, White, Soft, Hovis*	1 Roll/70g	180	3.1	257	9.5	44.8	4.4	3
Rolls, White, Soft, M&S*	1 Roll/60g	150	1.9	250	10.3	45.2	3.1	2.7
Rolls, White, Soft, Morrisons*	1 Roll/60g	163	1.4	271	8.3	52.8	2.4	2.2
Rolls, White, Soft, Tesco*	1 Roll/55g	137	0.6	250	9.2	49.7	1	2.6
Rolls, White, Softgrain, GFY, Asda*	1 Roll/54g	128	1	237	9	46	1.9	2.9
Rolls, White, Sourdough, Waitrose*	1 Roll/70g	161	0.8	230	9	44.4	1.1	3.1
Rolls, White, Split, Asda*	1 Roll/45g	113	1.5	251	10	45	3.4	2.8
Rolls, White, Submarine, M&S*	1 Roll/109g	300	5.4	275	11	47	5	1
Rolls, White, Super Soft, Bakers Selection, Asda*	1 Roll/64g	173	2.9	272	7.5	49	4.6	2.5
Rolls, White, Super Soft, Village Bakery, Aldi*	1 Roll/63g	154	0.9	245	8.9	48	1.4	2.1
Rolls, White, Tesco*	1 Roll/65g	180	2.5	277	8.7	52	3.8	2.7
Rolls, White, Tesco*	1 Roll/30g	79	0.7	262	9.7	50.5	2.3	2.9
Rolls, White, with Sourdough, Country Miller*	1 Roll/72g	189	0.8	262	9.3	52.3	1.1	2.9
Rolls, Wholemeal	***1 Roll/45g***	***108***	***1.3***	***241***	***9***	***48.3***	***2.9***	***5.9***
Rolls, Wholemeal & White, Kingsmill*	1 Roll/60g	151	2.5	251	9.5	43.7	4.2	3.5
Rolls, Wholemeal, & Oat, Warburton's*	1 Roll/70g	167	2.5	239	10.5	38	3.6	6
Rolls, Wholemeal, Asda*	1 Roll/58g	130	1.6	225	11	39	2.8	6
Rolls, Wholemeal, Deli, Tesco*	1 Roll/65g	156	3.1	240	9	40.2	4.8	5.7
Rolls, Wholemeal, Finest, Tesco*	1 Roll/75g	182	2.6	243	11.3	39	3.4	5.9
Rolls, Wholemeal, Flour Dusted, Sliced, Asda*	1 Roll/60g	135	1.7	225	11	36	2.8	6.6
Rolls, Wholemeal, Floury Batch, Sainsbury's*	1 Roll/68g	152	2.3	223	9.9	37.8	3.4	6.5
Rolls, Wholemeal, Mini, Assorted, Waitrose*	1 Roll/35g	86	2.1	244	9.7	37.9	6	7.3
Rolls, Wholemeal, Morrisons*	1 Roll/67g	155	2.7	231	10.2	38.6	4	6.3
Rolls, Wholemeal, Mothers Pride*	1 Roll/68g	157	1.8	230	8.8	39.2	2.7	6.8
Rolls, Wholemeal, Oat Topped, Deli, Tesco*	1 Roll/65g	170	3.5	260	10.9	38.3	5.3	6.7
Rolls, Wholemeal, Oat Topped, Tesco*	1 Roll/65g	166	2.9	255	11.3	42.2	4.5	5.1
Rolls, Wholemeal, Oaty, Deli Rolls, Morrisons*	1 Roll/65g	153	2	235	10.4	41.3	3.1	6.6
Rolls, Wholemeal, Old Fashioned, Waitrose*	1 Roll/57g	135	2.7	236	11.1	37.2	4.8	6.6
Rolls, Wholemeal, Organic, Sainsbury's*	1 Roll/66g	152	1.8	230	10.7	41	2.7	6.6
Rolls, Wholemeal, Plaited, Morrisons*	1 Roll/100g	195	1	195	6	30	1	6

	Measure INFO/WEIGHT	per Measure KCAL	FAT	Nutrition Values per 100g / 100ml KCAL	PROT	CARB	FAT	FIBRE
BREAD								
Rolls, Wholemeal, Sainsbury's*	1 Roll/65g	153	2.1	236	10.7	40.8	3.3	7.4
Rolls, Wholemeal, Sliced, Sandwich, Warburton's*	1 Roll/56g	130	2.2	233	10.5	35.8	3.9	6.6
Rolls, Wholemeal, Soft, Average	***1 Roll/65g***	***151***	***2.7***	***233***	***10.8***	***37.3***	***4.1***	***6.3***
Rolls, Wholemeal, Soft, Batch Baked, Warburton's*	1 Roll/65g	158	2.1	245	10.7	37.3	3.2	6.1
Rolls, Wholemeal, Soft, Morrisons *	1 Roll/60g	158	1.4	263	9.6	48.1	2.3	5.9
Rolls, Wholemeal, Soft, Sainsbury's*	1 Roll/60g	133	2	221	9.9	37.8	3.4	6.5
Rolls, Wholemeal, Soft, Seeded, Sainsbury's*	1 Roll/75g	193	5.6	257	11.8	35.6	7.4	6.2
Rolls, Wholemeal, Sunflower & Honey, Sainsbury's*	1 Roll/100g	311	8.1	311	10.8	45.9	8.1	5.4
Rolls, Wholemeal, Tasty, Kingsmill*	1 Roll/68g	171	2.5	251	10.7	39.1	3.7	6.5
Rolls, Wholemeal, Tesco*	1 Roll/46g	115	1.8	250	10.9	41.8	4	7.5
Rolls, Wholemeal, The Best, Morrisons*	1 Roll/72g	174	2.1	242	10.5	39.7	2.9	7.6
Rolls, Wholemeal, Village Bakery, Aldi*	1 Roll/63g	144	0.9	228	10	40	1.5	5.3
Rolls, Wholmeal, Deli, Tesco*	1 Roll/65g	156	3.1	240	9	40.2	4.8	5.7
Rolls, York Baps, Adkins Bakery*	1 Roll/100g	264	2.2	264	10.7	53.7	2.2	2.4
Roti, Tesco*	1 Roti/95g	256	5.2	269	8.4	46.4	5.5	3.2
Rukkileib, Rye, Mini Must, Estonia, Fazer*	1 Slice/10g	26	0.1	258	6.7	55.3	1.1	5.4
Russell Hall, Lidl*	1 Slice/50g	119	1	238	8.3	45	2	3.6
Rye Buckwheat, Artisan, Boule, TTD, Sainsbury's*	1 Slice/31g	83	1.2	269	9.7	46.9	4	3.4
Rye, & Flax, Organic, Profusion*	1 Slice/50g	120	4.4	241	20.1	14.4	8.9	11.4
Rye, & Mixed Seed, Dark, Boule, Finest, Tesco*	1 Slice/35g	86	1.2	248	12.1	39.2	3.4	5.9
Rye, Average	***1 Slice/25g***	***55***	***0.4***	***219***	***8.3***	***45.8***	***1.7***	***4.4***
Rye, Dark, Sliced, Trianon*	1 Slice/41g	74	0.6	180	6.5	35	1.5	0
Rye, German Style, Bolletje*	1 Slice/60g	114	1.2	190	6	35	2	9.5
Rye, German Style, Kelderman*	1 Slice/64g	113	0.6	177	6.1	34.4	1	8.3
Rye, German Style, Loaf, Bakery in Store, M&S*	1 Slice/25g	56	0.3	225	9.5	40.8	1.1	6.3
Rye, German, Plichet*	1 Slice/41g	101	2.9	247	8.4	32.3	7.1	9.9
Rye, Half Wheat, The Polish Bakery, Tesco*	1 Slice/40g	93	0.6	233	5.7	51.1	1.5	6.6
Rye, Light, Boule, Bakery, Waitrose*	1 Slice/50g	132	2.1	264	8.5	45.6	4.2	5.2
Rye, Light, Finest, Tesco*	1 Slice/20g	47	0.4	237	10.4	44.3	2	3.7
Rye, Seeded, Organic, The Village Bakery*	1 Slice/50g	107	1.6	214	5	37.8	3.2	7.2
Rye, Sourdough, Part Baked, TTD, Sainsbury's*	1 Slice/30g	70	0.4	233	6.5	45	1.3	7.8
Rye, Stone Baked, Dutch Style , Kelderman*	1 Slice/55g	128	0.5	233	8.1	46	0.9	5.1
Rye, Swedish Style, Kelderman*	1 Slice/50g	92	1.6	185	7.2	31.5	3.2	4.3
Rye, Triple, & Sprouted Grain, Bloomer, Finest, Tesco*	1 Slice/80g	185	0.7	231	8	46.1	0.9	3.4
Rye, Vitality, Organic, Biona*	1 Slice/71g	147	1.4	207	5.3	37	2	9.9
Rye, Whole Grain, Schneiderbrot*	1 Slice/50g	100	0.5	201	5.2	38.9	1	7.7
Rye, Wholegrain , Sliced, Rowan Hill Bakery, Lidl*	1 Slice/56g	118	1	210	5.8	38	1.8	9.3
Rye, Wholegrain, with Sunflower Seeds, Rowan Hill*	1 Slice/56g	126	2.6	225	6.3	35	4.6	9.3
Rye, Wholemeal with Sunflower Seeds, Organic, Biona*	1 Slice/72g	150	2.9	210	7	36	4	6
Rye, Wholemeal, Mestemacher*	1 Slice/72g	165	0.6	229	4.9	44.6	0.9	11.5
Rye, with Sunflower Seeds, Organic, Schneider Brot*	1 Slice/72g	138	2.6	191	6.2	33.4	3.6	7.9
Sandwich Thins, 50/50, Kingsmill*	1 Thin/40g	99	1.1	245	10	43	2.7	4.3
Sandwich Thins, Brown, Warburton's*	1 Thin/40g	100	1.1	252	9.9	45.2	2.8	3.5
Sandwich Thins, Half & Half, Warburtons *	1 Thin/40g	100	1.2	251	10	44.5	2.9	3.6
Sandwich Thins, Multiseed, GF, Warburton's*	1 Thin/50g	142	4	284	6.5	43.1	8.1	6.5
Sandwich Thins, Seeded, Free From, Tesco*	1 Thin/50g	125	3.8	250	7.8	32.3	7.6	10.8
Sandwich Thins, Seeded, GF, Free From, Waitrose*	1 Thin/50g	132	5.1	263	9.3	24.5	10.2	18
Sandwich Thins, Seeded, GF, Warburton's*	1 Thin/43g	122	3.5	284	6.5	43.1	8.1	6.5
Sandwich Thins, Seeded, Kingsmill*	1 Thin/40g	106	1.8	264	9.6	43.6	4.6	4.8
Sandwich Thins, White, CBY, Asda*	1 Thin/42g	105	1.1	250	8	47	2.7	2.3
Sandwich Thins, White, GF, Warburton's*	1 Thin/50g	124	3.2	247	6	38.7	6.3	5.7
Sandwich Thins, White, Kingsmill*	1 Thin/40g	99	1	248	9.4	45.6	2.5	2.9
Sandwich Thins, White, Rowan Hill Bakery, Lidl*	1 Thin /40g	101	0.8	253	9.3	47.7	1.9	3.7

B

	Measure INFO/WEIGHT	per Measure KCAL	FAT	Nutrition Values per 100g / 100ml KCAL	PROT	CARB	FAT	FIBRE
BREAD								
Sandwich Thins, White, Warburton's*	1 Thin/40g	100	1.1	251	9	46.2	2.8	2.5
Sandwich Thins, Wholemeal, Kingsmill*	1 Thin/41g	98	1.2	240	10.3	39.8	3	6.1
Sandwich Thins, Wholemeal, with Pulses, Warburtons*	1 Thin/50g	112	1.8	223	14.7	29.6	3.5	6
Seeded, Batch, Finest, Tesco*	1 Slice/65g	168	4	259	9.3	41.8	6.1	6.1
Seeded, Batch, Hovis*	1 Slice/50g	134	3.4	267	10.9	38.1	6.7	5.6
Seeded, Bloomer, Loaf, Rowan Hill Bakery, Lidl*	1 Slice/57g	166	4.5	292	10.3	42.3	7.9	5
Seeded, Bloomer, Sliced, Co-Op*	1 Slice/57g	153	3.8	268	12	40	6.7	0.5
Seeded, Bloomer, Thick Sliced, Iceland*	1 Slice/57g	152	4.6	267	8.4	36.5	8.1	6.7
Seeded, Farmhouse, GF, Warburton's*	1 Slice/35g	92	3.2	262	8.7	33	9.1	6.5
Seeded, Farmhouse, Loaf, Extra Special, Asda*	1 Slice/44g	92	0.5	207	11	38	1.2	8
Seeded, Free From, Gluten, Wheat, & Milk, Tesco*	1 Slice/42g	95	3.7	227	7	25.7	8.8	8.7
Seeded, GF, Sliced, Cob, Waitrose*	1 Slices/34g	93	2.4	278	5.8	42.7	7.3	9.2
Seeded, GF, Sliced, Free From, Morrisons*	1 Slice/42g	93	3.4	221	6	23.3	8.1	15.2
Seeded, Med Sliced, Average	***1 Slice/44g***	***116***	***2.9***	***262***	***11.3***	***38.6***	***6.5***	***5.6***
Seeded, Mighty, GF, Mini Loaf, Warburton's*	1 Slice/27g	75	2.9	277	7.7	33.5	10.9	7
Seeded, The Really Seeded One, Kingsmill*	1 Slice/44g	118	3.2	268	10.4	37.3	7.3	5.5
Seeded, Triple, Farmhouse, Loaf, GF, Genius*	1 Slice/36g	100	2.9	277	3.5	43.8	8	8
Seeded, Wholesome, Loaf, Schar*	1 Slice/25g	64	1.6	256	4.4	41	6.2	8.7
Six Seeded, Loaf, 400g, Bakery, Waitrose*	1 Slice/30g	82	2.1	275	11.5	37.8	6.9	7.8
Soda	***1oz/28g***	***72***	***0.7***	***258***	***7.7***	***54.6***	***2.5***	***2.1***
Soda Farl, Round, Genesis*	1 Farl/130g	156	0.9	120	4.5	24	0.7	0.8
Soda, Farls, M&S*	1 Farl/110g	267	3	243	9.6	50.1	2.7	2.3
Soda, Farls, Tesco*	1 Farl/142g	325	4.5	229	7.1	42.2	3.2	2.6
Soda, Fruit, M&S*	1 Slice/40g	105	1.9	260	5.9	51.3	4.6	2.5
Soda, M&S*	1 Slice/40g	82	0.6	205	8.7	39.2	1.6	4.2
Softgrain, Mighty White*	1 Slice/36g	81	0.5	224	7.2	45.5	1.5	3.7
Sourdough, 7 Seed, Bake at Home, Promise*	1 Slice/67g	121	1.3	181	7.1	26.6	1.9	14.6
Sourdough, Average	***1 Slice/50g***	***144***	***0.9***	***289***	***11.8***	***56.4***	***1.8***	***2.4***
Sourdough, Chia Seeds, Natural, The Polish Baker*	1 Slice/40g	121	2.1	303	10	58	5.2	5.7
Sourdough, Dark Rye, Specially Selected, Aldi*	1 Slice/58g	140	1	242	7.6	46.6	1.8	4.4
Sourdough, Dark, French, Seasonal, Gail's*	1 Slice/63g	134	0.6	214	7.5	43	0.9	2.4
Sourdough, GF, Loaf, Made Without Wheat, M&S*	1 Slice/39g	86	1.9	223	4.7	36.8	4.9	6.6
Sourdough, Loaf, Finest, Tesco*	1 Slice/33g	86	1.8	262	9.6	41.9	5.5	3.3
Sourdough, London, Watts Farm*	1 Slice/40g	83	0.3	208	7.3	45.6	0.8	2
Sourdough, Malted Wheat, Sliced, Bertinet Bakery*	1 Slice/80g	189	1	236	8.9	45.7	1.2	3.6
Sourdough, Mixed Olive, Bakery, Sainsbury's*	1 Slice/40g	90	3.8	224	6	27	9.5	2.8
Sourdough, Multi Seeded, Sliced, Warburtons *	1 Slice/60g	152	3.7	253	10.2	37.4	6.1	4
Sourdough, Rye, & Mixed Seed, Finest, Tesco*	1 Slice/44g	106	1.6	241	9.1	40.3	3.7	5
Sourdough, Rye, Banneton, Sainsbury's*	1 Slice/50g	115	0.6	230	6.6	46.1	1.1	4.7
Sourdough, Rye, Bloomer, Tesco*	1 Slice/40g	97	0.5	243	8.3	47.2	1.2	4.9
Sourdough, San Francisco, Gail's*	1 Slice/63g	106	0.4	170	6.4	34.6	0.7	1.2
Sourdough, Seeded, Finest, Tesco*	1 Slice/44g	106	1.6	241	9.1	40.3	3.7	5
Sourdough, Seeded, Gail's*	1 Slice/63g	175	4.9	280	10.2	39.8	7.9	4.6
Sourdough, Tomato, Slow Roasted, Irresistible, Co-Op*	1 Slice/50g	110	0.7	219	8.2	41	1.4	4.4
Sourdough, White, Cob, Free From, Tesco*	1 Slice/50g	92	1.4	184	5.1	31	2.7	7.4
Sourdough, White, Sliced, Finest, Tesco*	1 Slice/44g	99	0.9	224	8.4	41	2.1	3.7
Sourdough, White, Sliced, No.1, Waitrose*	1 Slice/50g	115	0.4	230	7.8	46.6	0.7	2.9
Sourdough, Whole Grain, Malted, Gail's*	1 Slice113g	277	6.6	246	9.3	8.7	5.9	5.6
Soya & Linseed, Seeded Loaf, Burgen *	1 Slice/44g	126	4.8	287	15.2	26.9	11	9.8
Soya, & Linseed, Vogel*	1 Slice/42g	95	2.1	227	11.7	34.1	4.9	6.8
Soya, & Linseed, The Best, Morrisons*	1 Slice/44g	116	2.7	264	11.2	37.9	6.1	6.3
Spelt, Soul Bakery*	1 Slice/45g	116	0.8	258	10.4	50	1.7	7.6
Spinach, & Goats Cheese, Twist, Waitrose*	1 Twist/45g	114	2.9	253	11.8	34.7	6.5	4.3

	Measure INFO/WEIGHT	per Measure KCAL	FAT	Nutrition Values per 100g / 100ml KCAL	PROT	CARB	FAT	FIBRE
BREAD								
Sprouted Grain, Ezekiel *	1 Slice/34g	80	0.5	235	11.8	44.1	1.5	0.9
Stoneground, Sm Loaf, Organic, Sainsbury's*	1 Slice/24g	50	0.5	208	10	37.9	2.1	7.9
Stoneground, Wholemeal, Thick, Love Life, Waitrose*	1 Slice/40g	86	1.1	214	10.1	36.5	2.8	7.9
Sunflower, & Pumpkin Seed, So Organic, Sainsbury's*	1 Slice/30g	76	1.6	254	11.4	40	5.4	12.9
Sunflower, & Pumpkin, Cob, Sliced, Finest, Tesco*	1 Slice/40g	120	4.4	299	12.3	34.7	10.9	6.6
Sunflower, Bakers Selection, Asda*	1 Slice/60g	162	5.9	270	11.3	50	9.8	8.3
Sunflower, Seed, Organic, Natural, Mestemacher*	1 Slice/75g	162	3	216	5.6	34.7	4	9.4
Super Seeded, 400g , M&S*	1 Slice/34g	103	3.5	304	12	38.2	10.3	5
Super Seeded, 800g, M&S*	1 Slice/50g	152	5.2	304	12	38.2	10.3	5
Super Seeded, Farmhouse, Loaf, Co-Op*	1 Slice/44g	136	4.8	309	11	39	11	5.3
Super Seeded, Farmhouse, Loaf, Finest, Tesco*	1 Slice/44g	129	4.2	294	11.2	37.9	9.6	5.8
Sweet Potato, with Pumpkin & Sunflower Seeds, BFree*	1 Slice/40g	93	2.5	232	3.5	30.6	6.3	9.2
Tea Loaf, Fruit & Walnut, Organic, Daylesford*	1 Slice/35g	102	2.4	290	4.5	50.2	6.9	0
Tiger Bloomer, Sliced, David Wood Baking*	1 Slice/45g	125	2	277	8.7	48	4.4	4.2
Tiger, Artisan, Bloomer, GF, Warburton's*	1 Slice/50g	120	2.6	241	7.1	38.5	5.3	5.5
Tiger, Baton, Bakery, Tesco*	½ Baton/100g	288	2	288	9.1	57.4	2	2.2
Tiger, Bloomer, Med Sliced, Iceland*	1 Slice/40g	108	1.8	271	9	46.9	4.5	3.5
Tiger, Bloomer, Soft, Warburton's*	1 Slice/38g	94	0.9	251	10.1	46.2	2.4	2
Tiger, Bloomer, The Great, Village Bakery, Aldi*	1 Slice/58g	159	2.6	274	8.8	49	4.4	2.1
Tiger, Bloomer, Thick Sliced, Iceland*	1 Slice/57g	168	4	295	8	48.2	7.1	3.2
Tiger, Loaf, Bloomer, Bakery, Tesco*	1 Slice/50g	133	1.6	266	8.4	49.2	3.2	3.2
Tiger, White, Warburton's*	1 Slice/40g	106	1.3	266	8.4	49.2	3.2	3.2
Toaster, White, Rathbones*	1 Slice/38g	92	0.5	243	9.1	48.6	1.3	2.3
Toastie Pockets, Brown, Easy Fill, Warburtons*	1 Pocket/55g	134	1.6	243	9.8	42.2	3	4.2
Toasties, Low Carb, Lizza*	1 Toastie/55g	135	6.2	246	23	3.1	11.3	20
Tomato, & Chilli, BGTY, Sainsbury's*	¼ Bread/65g	155	3.1	238	11.9	36.9	4.7	2.8
Tomato, & Herb, Tear & Share, Tesco*	¼ Pack/73g	164	3.2	226	6.3	40.2	4.4	2.1
Tortilla, Plain, GF, Free From, Sainsbury's*	1 Tortilla/40g	84	1.8	211	4.3	31	4.4	15.3
Tortilla, Wheat & Corn, Asda*	1 Tortilla/40g	125	1.9	314	9.4	58	4.8	0.6
Walnut, Waitrose*	1/8 Loaf/50g	170	7.6	339	10	40.6	15.2	5.9
Welshcake, Tan Y Castell*	1 Welshcake/40g	159	6.4	398	6.2	55.4	16	3.9
Wheat, Spelt, & Rye, Loaf, Baked by Us, Morrisons*	1 Slice/35g	82	0.7	236	11.3	39.9	2	6.6
Wheaten, Big Slice	***1 Slice/65g***	***139***	***1.7***	***214***	***7.5***	***40.2***	***2.6***	***3.6***
Wheaten, Loaf, Sliced, Genesis*	1 Slice/40g	86	1	214	7.5	40.2	2.6	3.6
Wheaten, M&S*	1 Slice/33g	74	1.2	225	9.3	42.9	3.5	3.9
Wheatgerm, Hovis, Soft, Sliced, M&S*	1 Slice/23g	50	0.7	220	10.1	38.5	3	4.6
White, & Wholemeal, Slimsters Squares, Irish Pride*	1 Square/41g	100	0.4	245	11.6	44	1	7
White, 50/50, Vitamin Boost, Sliced, Kingsmill*	1 Slice/38g	89	0.8	234	9.4	41.9	2.2	4.7
White, Average	***1 Slice/40g***	***94***	***0.8***	***235***	***8.4***	***49.3***	***1.9***	***1.5***
White, Bakers Bloomer, Warburtons *	1 Slice/62g	148	1.5	239	9.2	43.9	2.5	2.4
White, Batch Loaf, Extra Special, Asda*	1 Slice/47g	109	0.9	233	9	45	1.9	2.2
White, Batch, Warburton's*	1 Slice/42g	98	0.9	233	9.8	43.6	2.1	2.7
White, Baton, Part-Baked, TTD, Sainsbury's*	1 Serving/50g	125	0.4	250	7.5	51.4	0.9	3
White, Baton, Sesame Seed, Bakery, Sainsbury's*	1 Serving/50g	139	2	278	11.1	47.9	3.9	3.5
White, Bloomer, Soft, Sliced, Morrisons*	1 Slice/40g	94	0.5	235	8.8	46	1.2	2.8
White, Bloomer, Soft, Warburton's*	1 Slice/48g	120	1.2	249	9.2	45.9	2.6	2.5
White, Classic, Med Sliced, Hovis*	1 Slice/38g	91	0.9	240	11.4	40.3	2.3	2.5
White, Commercially Prepared, Average	***1oz/28g***	***74***	***0.9***	***266***	***7.6***	***50.6***	***3.3***	***2.4***
White, Commercially Prepared, Toasted, Average	***1oz/28g***	***82***	***1.1***	***293***	***9***	***54.4***	***4***	***2.5***
White, Country Maid*	1 Slice/33g	76	0.7	229	8.5	44.1	2.1	3
White, Country, Sliced, Warburtons*	1 Slice/31g	72	0.7	233	9.1	43.1	2.2	2.2
White, Crusty, Fresh, Finest, Tesco*	1 Slice/52g	130	1	250	8.6	48.5	1.9	2.4
White, Crusty, Hovis*	1 Slice/44g	103	1	233	8.8	44.3	2.2	2.1

	Measure INFO/WEIGHT	per Measure KCAL	FAT	Nutrition Values per 100g / 100ml KCAL	PROT	CARB	FAT	FIBRE
BREAD								
White, Crusty, Premium, Warburton's*	1 Slice/31g	77	0.7	254	10.6	46.5	2.3	2.6
White, Crusty, Sliced Loaf, Tesco*	1 Slice/50g	127	0.6	254	9.2	50.1	1.2	3.2
White, Crusty, Split Tin, Bakery, Tesco*	1 Slice/50g	134	0.8	268	9.4	52.6	1.5	3.3
White, Danish Style, Thick Sliced, Light, Tesco*	1 Slice/22g	55	0.6	255	9.4	47.3	2.9	2.7
White, Danish, Lighter, Warburton's*	1 Slice/26g	63	0.3	243	10.5	45.8	1.2	2.6
White, Danish, Med Sliced, Loaf, 400g, Tesco*	1 Slice/22g	57	0.4	258	9.6	48.6	2	3.6
White, Danish, Soft & Light, Thick Cut, Asda*	1 Slice/26g	60	0.4	230	9	45	1.6	2.1
White, Danish, Soft, Weight Watchers, Warburton's*	1 Slice/21g	50	0.3	243	9.8	46.5	1.3	2.9
White, Danish, Thick Sliced, Tesco*	1 Slice/24g	60	0.6	250	9.7	47.4	2.3	2.9
White, Extra Thick Sliced, Kingsmill*	1 Slice/58g	135	1.4	232	8.8	43.8	2.4	2.8
White, Farmhouse Crusty, M&S*	1 Slice/34g	82	0.7	240	8.9	46.6	2.2	3
White, Farmhouse Gold Premium, Morrisons*	1 Slice/38g	90	0.5	236	8.9	47.4	1.2	2.2
White, Farmhouse, Co-Op*	1 Slice/36g	85	0.6	237	8.6	46	1.7	1.9
White, Farmhouse, GF, Newburn, Warburton's*	1 Slice/35g	83	2.1	236	6.8	35.6	6.1	5.5
White, Farmhouse, Hovis*	1 Slice/44g	103	1	234	8.7	44.6	2.3	2.4
White, Farmhouse, Loaf, Co-Op*	1 Slice/50g	118	0.8	237	8.6	46	1.7	1.9
White, Farmhouse, Sliced, Bakery, Tesco*	1 Slice/44g	106	1	240	7.9	46	2.3	2
White, Farmhouse, Sliced, Rowan Hill Bakery, Lidl*	1 Slice/44g	101	0.7	229	8.3	44.4	1.5	2.4
White, Farmhouse, Soft, 400g Loaf, Warburton's*	1 Slice/27g	66	0.7	245	10.1	43.7	2.6	2.8
White, Farmhouse, Soft, 800g Loaf, Warburton's*	1 Slice/43g	104	1.1	243	9	45	2.5	2.3
White, Farmhouse, Soft, Thick Sliced, Waitrose*	1 Slice/34g	86	0.7	253	8.7	47.9	2.2	3.4
White, Fibre, Morrisons*	1 Slice/40g	96	0.7	240	8	48.4	1.7	0.3
White, Fried in Blended Oil	***1 Slice/28g***	***141***	***9***	***503***	***7.9***	***48.5***	***32.2***	***1.6***
White, GF, Sliced, Free From, Co-Op*	1 Slice/38g	70	1	183	4.2	30	2.7	10
White, GF, Sliced, Free From, Morrisons*	1 Slice/42g	84	1.7	200	4.3	31.3	4.1	10.1
White, Gluten & Wheat Free, Free From, Sainsbury's*	1 Slice/89g	189	4.5	212	3.4	32.1	5.1	12.5
White, Loaf, Sliced, Finest, Tesco*	1 Slice/50g	118	0.6	236	8.6	45.5	1.3	4.1
White, Med Slice, Simply, Lidl*	1 Slice/36g	81	0.5	226	8.7	43.1	1.4	2.9
White, Med Sliced, 800g, Sunblest *	1 Slice/40g	95	0.9	238	8.5	44.6	2.2	2.9
White, Med Sliced, Average	***1 Slice/39g***	***93***	***0.6***	***238***	***7.5***	***48.5***	***1.6***	***1.8***
White, Med Sliced, Basics, Sainsbury's*	1 Slice/36g	83	0.5	231	8	46.4	1.5	2.1
White, Med Sliced, Brace's*	1 Slice/42g	104	0.5	248	7.6	50.4	1.3	2.1
White, Med Sliced, Great Everyday, Kingsmill*	1 Slice/40g	93	0.8	232	9	44.6	2	2.7
White, Med Sliced, H.W. Nevill's, Tesco*	1 Slice/42g	99	0.9	238	8	45.3	2.2	2.7
White, Med Sliced, Tesco*	1 Slice/40g	96	0.9	239	8.1	45.6	2.2	2.3
White, Med Sliced, Value, Tesco*	1 Slice/36g	81	0.4	225	7.9	46.1	1	2.1
White, Medium, 400g Loaf, Warburton's*	1 Slice/24g	58	0.5	244	10.3	45.1	1.9	2.4
White, Medium, Warburton's*	1 Slice/40g	98	0.8	244	9.1	46.4	2	2.3
White, Mega Thick, Roberts Bakery*	1 Slice/66g	154	1.2	233	8.3	46.2	1.8	2.2
White, Mighty, GF, Mini Loaf, Warburton's*	1 Slice/27g	67	1.8	249	6.7	37.9	6.5	5.8
White, Milk Roll, Warburton's*	1 Slice/18g	46	0.5	248	9.4	45	2.8	2.4
White, Multiseed, Farmhouse, Sliced, 400g, Waitrose*	1 Slice/33g	96	2.9	291	11.2	38.5	8.8	6.7
White, Multiseed, Med Sliced, Batch, Tesco*	1 Slice/33g	88	2	267	9.9	40.3	6.1	5.5
White, Multiseed, Sainsbury's*	1 Slice/50g	140	3.8	279	11.3	37.4	7.7	7.6
White, Old English, Warburton's*	1 Slice/40g	99	1.2	248	9.8	44.3	2.9	2.8
White, Organic, Bloomer, Bakery, Tesco*	1 Slice/40g	98	0.9	247	9.8	44.8	2.2	4.2
White, Organic, Sainsbury's*	1 Slice/36g	84	0.6	234	8.9	45.5	1.8	2.3
White, Plain, Scottish, Sunblest*	1 Slice/57g	133	1.5	233	10.1	42.3	2.6	2.8
White, Premium, M&S*	1 Slice/40g	95	0.8	235	8.5	45.8	1.9	2.7
White, Sandwich, Bakery, Sainsbury's*	1 Slice/50g	121	0.3	242	10.3	49	0.6	2.9
White, Sandwich, Irish Pride*	1 Slice/38g	89	0.5	233	9.4	44.6	1.4	2.8
White, Scottish Plain, Medium, Mother's Pride*	1 Slice/50g	114	0.8	227	8.7	44.6	1.5	3
White, Seeds, Oats, & Honey, TTD, Sainsbury's*	1 Slice/50g	154	5.4	308	12.1	36.7	10.9	7.1

	Measure INFO/WEIGHT	per Measure KCAL	FAT	Nutrition Values per 100g / 100ml KCAL	PROT	CARB	FAT	FIBRE
BREAD								
White, Sliced, Baker Street*	1 Slice/40g	99	1.6	247	8.8	43	3.9	2.3
White, Sliced, Brennans*	1 Slice/40g	88	0.6	219	8.7	43	1.4	2.8
White, Sliced, GF, Free From, Tesco*	1 Slice/42g	80	1.7	190	5.2	29.7	4	7.3
White, Sliced, Jacksons*	1 Slice/45g	125	3.9	278	10.9	34.5	8.7	9.4
White, Sliced, Roberts Bakery*	1 Slice/35g	87	0.7	249	10	48	2.1	2.5
White, Sm Loaf, Classic, Hovis*	1 Slice/33g	75	0.8	228	11.4	40.3	2.3	6.5
White, Soft Batch, Sliced, Sainsbury's*	1 Slice/44g	102	0.8	232	8.2	45.4	1.9	2.3
White, Soft Crusty, M&S*	1 Slice/25g	64	0.6	256	9.3	49	2.5	2.4
White, Soft, Batch Loaf, Sliced, Tesco*	1 Slice/50g	116	1	233	7.5	46.1	2.1	2.1
White, Soft, Extra Thick, Hovis*	1 Slice/67g	156	1.1	233	8.7	44.6	1.7	2.4
White, Soft, Gold, Kingsmill*	1 Slice/47g	112	1.5	239	8.2	44.5	3.1	2.7
White, Soft, M&S*	1 Slice/47g	105	0.8	225	7.3	46.1	1.7	2.4
White, Soft, Sliced, Hovis*	1 Slice/25g	58	0.6	234	8.7	44.6	2.3	2.4
White, Soft, Thick Sliced, Kingsmill*	1 Slice/44g	105	0.9	238	8	45.6	2	2.7
White, Soft, Toastie, Thick Sliced, Asda*	1 Slice/50g	120	1.1	239	8.1	46	2.2	2.3
White, Sourdough, Country, Oval, la Brea Bakery*	1 Slice/60g	143	0.4	239	8.8	49.4	0.6	1.6
White, Sourdough, M&S*	1 Slice/50g	119	0.8	238	9.3	44.5	1.7	3.6
White, Sourdough, Specially Selected, Aldi*	1 Slice/58g	136	0.5	234	8.4	47	0.8	2.1
White, Sourdough, The Rustik Bakery*	1 Slice/35g	79	0.4	225	9.1	43	1.2	3.9
White, Sourdough, Waitrose*	1 Slice/50g	119	0.6	237	9	45.9	1.2	3.3
White, Sourdough, Yeast Free, Gradz Bakery*	1 Slice/40g	92	0.4	230	8.3	48.7	0.9	3.3
White, Square, Extra Thick Sliced, Hovis*	1 Slice/67g	155	1.3	231	8.5	44.7	2	2.6
White, Square, Med Sliced, Hovis*	1 Slice/40g	92	0.8	231	8.5	44.7	2	2.6
White, Square, Thick Sliced, Hovis*	1 Slice/50g	116	1	231	8.5	44.7	2	2.6
White, Sunflower, & Pumpkin, Soft, TTD, Sainsbury's*	1 Slice/50g	155	5.8	310	12.8	36.5	11.5	4.5
White, Sunflower, & Pumpkin, Cob, Waitrose*	1 Slice/33g	89	2.1	270	11.1	39.3	6.3	5.9
White, Super Seeds, Farmhouse, Sainsbury*	1 Slice/50g	152	5.2	303	11.9	37.9	10.3	5.6
White, Thick Sliced, Brace's*	1 Slice/47g	117	0.6	248	7.6	50.4	1.3	2.1
White, Thick Sliced, Fine Lady*	1 Slice/44g	113	0.5	254	7.8	53.1	1.2	2.3
White, Thick Sliced, Healthy, Warburton's*	1 Slice/38g	84	0.7	222	10.3	41.2	1.8	4.1
White, Thick Sliced, Irwin's Bakery*	1 Slice/42g	95	0.9	226	9.5	41.9	2.1	2.4
White, Thick Sliced, M&S*	1 Slice/42g	96	0.5	228	7.3	46.7	1.3	2.8
White, Thick Sliced, Mighty White*	1 Slice/42g	96	0.8	229	7.4	43.3	1.9	4.6
White, Thick Sliced, Organic, Tesco*	1 Slice/44g	108	0.9	245	8.5	46.8	2.1	3.1
White, Thick Sliced, Sainsbury's*	1 Slice/44g	95	0.8	216	8.7	41.1	1.9	7.1
White, Thick Sliced, Square Cut, Asda*	1 Slice/44g	101	0.7	230	8	46	1.5	2.1
White, Thick Sliced, Sunblest*	1 Slice/40g	91	0.6	228	8	45.7	1.5	2.8
White, Thick Sliced, Super Toastie, Morrisons*	1 Slice/50g	128	1.5	257	8.7	48.9	3	2.1
White, Thick Sliced, Tesco*	1 Slice/44g	106	0.7	240	8.2	47.8	1.5	3
White, Thick, So Organic, Sainsbury's*	1 Slice/44g	102	1	231	8.2	44.6	2.2	3.1
White, Thick, Super Soft, M&S*	1 Slice/48g	120	1.3	249	9	45.3	2.7	3.6
White, Thickest, Warburton's*	1 Slice/58g	137	1.2	239	9.9	43.8	2	2.6
White, Thin Sliced, Sainsbury's*	1 Slice/29g	66	0.4	228	7.1	46.4	1.5	2.8
White, Thin Sliced, Tesco*	1 Slice/30g	68	0.4	228	9.5	44.5	1.3	3.4
White, Tiger, Bloomer, Black Sheep*	1 Slice/57g	168	4	295	8.1	48.2	7	3.2
White, Toasted, Average	***1 Slice/33g***	***87***	***0.5***	***265***	***9.3***	***57.1***	***1.6***	***1.8***
White, Toastie, 400g Loaf, Warburton's*	1 Slice/29g	70	0.5	244	10.3	45.1	1.9	2.4
White, Toastie, GF, Genius*	1 Slice/33g	90	2	272	2.4	47	6.1	9.3
White, Toastie, Loved by Us, Co-Op*	1 Slice/50g	120	1.2	240	7.9	45.4	2.4	2.6
White, Toastie, Thick Cut, Hovis*	1 Slice/50g	115	1	230	8.5	44.8	2	2.5
White, Toastie, Thick, Love to Toast, Kingsmill*	1 Slice/50g	116	1	232	9	44.6	2	2.7
White, Toastie, Warburton's*	1 Slice/47g	116	0.9	244	9.1	46.4	2	2.3
White, Trio of Olive, Bloomer, Bakery, Tesco*	1 Slice/82g	199	4	243	6.8	41.3	4.9	3

	Measure INFO/WEIGHT	per Measure KCAL	FAT	Nutrition Values per 100g / 100ml KCAL	PROT	CARB	FAT	FIBRE
BREAD								
White, Wholesome, Loaf, Sainsbury's*	1 Slice/36g	81	0.7	224	9.4	42.5	1.8	4.4
Whole Meal, Med Sliced, Tesco*	1 Slice/40g	90	0.9	224	10.5	36.8	2.3	6.8
Whole Seed, Cob, Crusty, Bakery, Tesco*	1 Slice/50g	179	6.1	359	13.7	45.7	12.3	5.2
Whole Seed, Loaf, Sliced, Tesco*	1 Slice/40g	109	2.9	272	10.9	38.4	7.2	5.3
Wholegrain, & Rye, Schneider Brot*	1 Slice/50g	98	0.6	197	5.9	36.6	1.2	8.2
Wholegrain, & Oats, Warburton's*	1 Slice/40g	98	1.4	245	11.7	38.8	3.5	5.9
Wholegrain, Average	***1 Slice/44g***	***117***	***1.9***	***265***	***13.4***	***43.3***	***4.2***	***7.4***
Wholegrain, Batch, Finest, Tesco*	1 Slice/44g	112	1.2	254	9.8	47.7	2.7	4.2
Wholegrain, Soft, M&S*	1 Slice/51g	115	2.8	225	13	31.2	5.4	8.2
Wholegrain, Toasted, Average	***1 Slice/40g***	***117***	***1.9***	***288***	***14.5***	***47.1***	***4.6***	***8.1***
Wholemeal & Oat, Loaf, Vogel*	1 Slice/42g	86	0.6	205	8.7	34.3	1.5	9.7
Wholemeal & Tasty Spelt, Sliced, Hovis*	1 Slice/47g	108	1	230	11.1	38.4	2.1	6.7
Wholemeal Loaf, British Farmers, Hovis*	1 Slice/47g	108	1.3	229	10	37.9	2.8	6.8
Wholemeal Oatbran, Sliced, Tesco*	1 Slice/45g	90	0.7	200	10.1	35.3	1.6	7.4
Wholemeal, & Oat Flakes, Gold, Kingsmill*	1 Slice/47g	103	1.6	220	10	37.3	3.4	7
Wholemeal, & Rye, Bloomer, Irresistible, Co-Op*	1 Slice/44g	107	1.7	244	9.8	39	3.8	7.8
Wholemeal, & Rye, Farmhouse, Extra Special, Asda*	1 Slice/50g	112	1.2	225	11	36	2.5	7.3
Wholemeal, & Rye, Cob, Waitrose*	1 Slice/33g	80	0.7	242	11.7	40.5	2.1	6.9
Wholemeal, American Sandwich, Harry's*	1 Slice/43g	110	2.1	259	9	45	5	5
Wholemeal, Average	***1 Slice/40g***	***88***	***1***	***215***	***9.2***	***41.6***	***2.5***	***5.8***
Wholemeal, Baker`s Soft, Medium, Tesco*	1 Slice/40g	94	1.1	235	10.8	37.8	2.8	6.9
Wholemeal, Batch, Sliced, Organic, Duchy, Waitrose*	1 Slice/50g	121	1.2	242	10.2	41.8	2.3	6.8
Wholemeal, Better You, Irwin's Bakery*	1 Slice/29g	55	0.7	188	10	43.3	2.5	7.2
Wholemeal, Bloomer, Heroic, Sliced, Roberts*	1 Slice/37g	87	0.6	236	10.7	41	1.7	6.7
Wholemeal, Brennans*	1 Slice/33g	78	1.4	236	11.2	38.4	4.2	7.7
Wholemeal, Brown, Med Sliced, 400g, Hovis*	1 Slice/29g	64	0.5	221	10	37.8	1.8	6.8
Wholemeal, Classic, Roberts Bakery*	1 Slice/45g	97	0.7	215	10	36.8	1.5	6.9
Wholemeal, Crustless, Kingsmill*	1 Slice/22g	45	0.5	205	10.4	33.1	2.2	5.6
Wholemeal, Crusty, Finest, Tesco*	1 Slice/50g	103	0.8	206	10.8	37	1.7	6.9
Wholemeal, Crusty, Kingsmill*	1 Slice/42g	104	1.8	247	11.2	41.1	4.2	7
Wholemeal, Danish, BFY, Morrisons*	1 Slice/17g	39	0.3	228	11.2	47.9	1.8	6.2
Wholemeal, Farmhouse, Bakery in Store, M&S*	1 Slice/35g	80	1	229	11.4	35.3	3	7.9
Wholemeal, Farmhouse, Med Sliced, Waitrose*	1 Slice/36g	84	0.7	232	10.8	39.1	1.9	7.5
Wholemeal, Farmhouse, Rowan Hill Bakery, Lidl*	1 Slice/47g	102	0.7	218	10.3	37.8	1.4	6.3
Wholemeal, Farmhouse, Sliced, Hovis*	1 Slice/44g	101	1.2	229	10	37.8	2.7	6.8
Wholemeal, Farmhouse, Thick Sliced, 400g, Waitrose*	1 Slice/33g	77	0.6	232	10.8	39.1	1.9	7.5
Wholemeal, Farmhouse, Thick Sliced, Tesco*	1 Slice/37g	82	0.7	222	9.4	38.7	1.9	6.1
Wholemeal, Farmhouse, Thick Sliced, Waitrose*	1 Slice/44g	103	0.8	232	10.8	39.1	1.9	7.5
Wholemeal, Fh, Stoneground, Batch, Finest, Tesco*	1 Slice/50g	108	1.4	215	10.3	36.1	2.8	6.9
Wholemeal, Granary, Med Sliced, Hovis*	1 Slice/47g	111	1.1	236	10.6	39.8	2.4	6.8
Wholemeal, Healthy Range, Pat The Baker*	1 Slice/27g	58	0.5	215	10	36.4	1.8	6.6
Wholemeal, High Protein, High Fibre, Warburton's*	1 Slice/29g	66	1	227	13.5	32	3.3	7.8
Wholemeal, Little Brown Loaf, Unsliced, Hovis*	1 Slice/40g	86	1.1	216	10	37.8	2.7	6.8
Wholemeal, Live Good, Hovis*	1 Slice/26g	67	0.4	258	10	46.9	1.5	6.9
Wholemeal, Loaf, 400g, Kingsmill*	1 Slice/29g	68	0.8	234	10.2	39	2.8	6.2
Wholemeal, Loaf, Sliced, Thick, 800g, Hovis*	1 Slice/47g	104	0.8	221	10	37.8	1.8	6.8
Wholemeal, Longer Life, Thick Slice, Sainsbury's*	1 Slice/45g	101	1.6	224	10.6	37.4	3.6	5.9
Wholemeal, Lower Carb, Hovis*	1 Slice/36g	84	1.3	234	16	27	3.7	14.4
Wholemeal, Med Sliced, 400g Loaf, Asda*	1 Slice/28g	67	0.9	236	12	37	3.3	6.7
Wholemeal, Med Sliced, Essential, Waitrose*	1 Slice/36g	78	0.6	217	10.7	36.2	1.7	7
Wholemeal, Med Sliced, Great Everyday, Kingsmill*	1 Slice/40g	91	1.5	227	10.5	37.7	3.8	6.2
Wholemeal, Med Sliced, H.W. Nevill's, Tesco*	1 Slice/33g	83	0.8	253	9.7	43.8	2.5	8.3
Wholemeal, Med Sliced, Little Big Loaf, Kingsmill*	1 Slice/39g	93	1.5	239	10.5	37.7	3.8	6.2

	Measure INFO/WEIGHT	per Measure KCAL	FAT	Nutrition Values per 100g / 100ml KCAL	PROT	CARB	FAT	FIBRE
BREAD								
Wholemeal, Med Sliced, Loaf, 800g, Village Bakery, Aldi*	1 Slice/40g	90	0.9	225	11	37	2.3	6.2
Wholemeal, Med Sliced, M&S*	1 Slice/40g	80	1.2	200	10.5	32.7	3.1	6.7
Wholemeal, Med Sliced, Morrisons*	1 Slice/33g	72	0.5	216	9.6	38	1.4	6.5
Wholemeal, Med Sliced, Premium, Tesco*	1 Slice/36g	71	0.2	196	9.8	37.8	0.6	7.2
Wholemeal, Med Sliced, Sainsbury's*	1 Slice/36g	77	0.9	214	10.3	37.8	2.4	7.4
Wholemeal, Med Sliced, Sunblest*	1 Slice/40g	94	1.2	235	11.5	36.9	3	7.1
Wholemeal, Med Sliced, Waitrose*	1 Slice/36g	76	0.9	213	10.1	37.6	2.4	7
Wholemeal, Medium, 400g Loaf, Warburton's*	1 Slice/24g	55	0.7	231	10.6	37.8	2.8	6.4
Wholemeal, Medium, 800g Loaf, Warburton's*	1 Slice/45g	103	1.3	231	10.6	37.8	2.8	6.4
Wholemeal, Medium, Sliced, Everyday Essentials, Aldi*	1 Slice/40g	85	0.7	213	10	36	1.7	6.3
Wholemeal, Multigrain, Sliced, Extra Special, Asda*	1 Slice/44g	108	2.2	246	11	35	5	7.7
Wholemeal, Multigrain, Soft Batch, Sainsbury's*	1 Slice/44g	106	2.9	242	11.3	34.5	6.5	5.6
Wholemeal, Multiseed, Batch, So Organic, Sainsbury's*	1 Slice/30g	79	2.2	263	11.8	30.9	7.4	12.9
Wholemeal, Multiseed, Farmhouse, Soft, TTD, Sainsbury's*	1 Slice/50g	140	4.4	280	12.6	33.8	8.8	8.2
Wholemeal, Nimble, Hovis*	1 Slice/22g	50	0.5	226	11.8	37	2.2	6.6
Wholemeal, No Crusts, Kingsmill *	1 Slice/22g	45	0.5	205	10.4	33.1	2.2	5.6
Wholemeal, Oat Topped, TTD, Sainsbury's*	1 Slice/47g	109	1.3	232	10	38.5	2.8	0.3
Wholemeal, Organic, 400g Loaf, Bakery, Sainsbury's*	1 Slice/50g	137	1.2	274	11.3	46.9	2.4	9.7
Wholemeal, Premium, Thick Slice, M&S*	1 Slice/50g	95	1.5	190	9.8	30.8	3	6.4
Wholemeal, Rustic, Tin, Tesco*	1 Slice/37g	92	1.3	249	12.2	44	3.5	3.1
Wholemeal, Seed Sensations, Hovis*	1 Slice/44g	109	2.5	249	11.9	31.4	5.6	12.4
Wholemeal, Seeded Batch, Truly Irresistible, Co-Op*	1 Slice/47g	115	1.9	245	11.5	36.2	4	6.6
Wholemeal, Seeded, Farmhouse, Rowan Hill Bakery, Lidl*	1 Slice/33g	84	2.1	256	12.4	32.7	6.3	9.4
Wholemeal, Seeded, Rowan Hill Bakery, Lidl*	1 Slice/33g	86	1.9	261	12.7	34.9	5.8	9
Wholemeal, Seeded, Signature, Allinson*	1 Slice/46g	118	4	256	11.1	28.9	8.7	8.9
Wholemeal, Seeds & Grains, 400g Loaf, Finest, Tesco*	1 Slice/33g	84	1.6	254	11.7	37.4	5	6.4
Wholemeal, Sliced, Co-Op*	1 Slice/37g	85	0.8	230	11	38	2.1	6.3
Wholemeal, Sliced, Loaf, Average	***1 Slice/40g***	***90***	***0.9***	***224***	***9.9***	***38.8***	***2.4***	***6.9***
Wholemeal, Sliced, McCambridge*	1 Slice/38g	90	0.7	237	7.9	44.7	1.8	0
Wholemeal, Sliced, Medium, Tesco*	1 Slice/40g	93	1.2	234	11.9	36.7	2.9	6.6
Wholemeal, Sliced, Ramsey Bakery*	1 Slice/28g	81	0.8	291	8.5	36	2.9	8.2
Wholemeal, Soft, Medium, 400g, Village Bakery, Aldi*	1 Slice/29g	69	0.9	238	12	38	3	6.2
Wholemeal, Soft, Sliced, Village Bakery, Aldi*	1 Slice/44g	103	1.1	235	12	38	2.6	6.5
Wholemeal, Soft, Thick Sliced, Rowan Hill Bakery, Lidl*	1 Slice/44g	97	0.8	221	10	37.8	1.8	6.8
Wholemeal, Sourdough, Half Bloomer, TTD, Sainsbury's*	1 Slice/40g	103	1.6	258	10.9	42.4	4	4.6
Wholemeal, Square Cut, Thick Sliced, Asda*	1 Slice/44g	91	1	208	10	37	2.2	6
Wholemeal, Stoneground, Batch Baked, Warburton's*	1 Slice/45g	101	1.2	224	10.3	35.7	2.6	6.9
Wholemeal, Stoneground, Organic, Waitrose*	1 Slice/25g	57	0.9	228	10.8	38.2	3.6	7.1
Wholemeal, Stoneground, Thick Sliced, Sainsbury's*	1 Slice/44g	92	0.8	210	10.2	37.9	1.9	7.8
Wholemeal, Supersoft, Eat Well, M&S*	1 Slice/33g	81	1.1	245	10.9	40	3.3	6.7
Wholemeal, Tasty, Medium, Kingsmill*	1 Slice/40g	93	1.1	233	10.2	38.6	2.8	6.3
Wholemeal, Tasty, Thick, Kingsmill*	1 Slice/44g	105	1.7	239	10.5	37.7	3.8	6.2
Wholemeal, The Champion, Batch, Allinson*	1 Slice/46g	108	1.3	234	11	37.8	2.9	6.1
Wholemeal, Thick Slice, Brennans*	1 Slice/27g	69	0.6	257	9.2	45.4	2.1	6.8
Wholemeal, Thick Sliced, Bakers Gold, Asda*	1 Slice/44g	99	1.4	225	12	37	3.2	6
Wholemeal, Thick Sliced, Great Everyday, Kingsmill*	1 Slice/44g	100	1.7	227	10.5	37.7	3.8	6.2
Wholemeal, Thick Sliced, Rathbones*	1 Slice/42g	106	0.9	253	9.5	45.7	2.2	6
Wholemeal, Thick Sliced, Sainsbury's*	1 Slice/44g	103	1.3	234	11.9	36.7	2.9	6.6
Wholemeal, Thick Sliced, So Organic, Sainsbury's*	1 Slice/50g	120	1.6	239	9.6	39.3	3.2	7.2
Wholemeal, Thick Sliced, Tesco*	1 Slice/40g	96	1.1	240	9.5	40.9	2.7	6.8
Wholemeal, Thick Sliced, Toastie, Tesco*	1 Slice/50g	112	1.2	224	10.6	36.8	2.4	6.8
Wholemeal, Thick Sliced, Waitrose*	1 Slice/44g	94	1.1	213	10.1	37.6	2.4	7
Wholemeal, Thick, Weight Watchers, Warburton's*	1 Slice/28g	64	0.6	225	10	38.4	2.2	6

	Measure INFO/WEIGHT	per Measure KCAL	FAT	Nutrition Values per 100g / 100ml KCAL	PROT	CARB	FAT	FIBRE
BREAD								
Wholemeal, Toasted, Average	***1 Slice/26g***	***58***	***0.6***	***224***	***8.6***	***42.3***	***2.2***	***5.8***
Wholemeal, with Rye, Rich & Tasty, Warburton's*	1 Slice/45g	109	1.1	246	9.9	40.6	2.4	7.5
Wholemeal. Medium, Brace's*	1 Slice/42g	95	0.9	226	10.2	44.3	2.2	6
Wholesome, Five Seeded, GF, Genius*	1 Slice/36g	102	3.4	285	3.7	42.3	9.4	7.8
Wholesome, Vitality, GF, Schar*	1 Slice/32g	84	2.9	262	4.5	36	9.2	8.8
Wholewheat, Nature's Own*	1 Slice/28g	66	1	236	14.3	39.3	3.6	10.7
Wholewheat, No Crusts, Harry's*	1 Slice/25g	58	1.1	233	8	40	4.5	5.5
Wholewheat, Soft, Trader Joe's*	1 Slice/37g	70	1	189	10.8	37.8	2.7	5.4
with Walnuts, Pain De Campagne Aux Noix, Carrefour*	1 Slice/33g	88	0.6	266	8	55.6	1.9	0
Wrap, Brown, Soft, Easy Roll, Warburton's*	1 Wrap/65g	190	2.9	292	12	49.3	4.5	3.2
Wrap, Half & Half, Warburton's*	1 Wrap/41g	121	1.8	296	12.8	49.6	4.4	3.8
Wrap, Mediterranean Herb, Soft, Village Bakery, Aldi*	1 Wrap/64g	188	2.6	294	8	54.7	4.1	2
Wrap, Original, Super Soft, Village Bakery, Aldi*	1 Wrap/62g	182	3.2	293	8.3	51	5.2	3.7
Wrap, Seeded, GF, Newburn Bakehouse, Warburton's*	1 Wrap/60g	178	4.5	297	5.5	48.1	7.5	7.4
Wrap, Skinni, Tortilla, Plain, Deli Kitchen*	1 Wrap/31g	94	1.1	302	9	57	3.5	3
Wrap, Tortilla, 8 Pack, Asda*	1 Wrap/50g	143	3	286	8	50	6	1.9
Wrap, Tortilla, 8 Pack, LC, Tesco*	1 Wrap/50g	135	1	270	7.1	53.2	2.1	3.5
Wrap, Tortilla, Ancient Grain, Co-Op*	1 Wrap/40g	123	3	308	9.2	49	7.6	3.4
Wrap, Tortilla, Beetroot, Fibre Fest, Genius*	1 Wrap/40g	83	1.4	208	5.3	32	3.6	13
Wrap, Tortilla, Beetroot, GF, Warburton's*	1 Wrap/45g	131	2.6	292	4.6	52.2	5.8	6.4
Wrap, Tortilla, BGTY, Sainsbury's*	1 Wrap/50g	131	0.8	263	7.3	52.4	1.7	4.3
Wrap, Tortilla, Both in One, Sunnyhills, Aldi*	1 Wrap/64g	184	2.9	287	8.1	52	4.5	3
Wrap, Tortilla, Both Together, Tesco*	1 Wrap/61g	177	3	290	8.5	50	4.9	6
Wrap, Tortilla, Chargrilled, Mission*	1 Wrap/60g	196	4.3	327	8	53.3	7.2	2
Wrap, Tortilla, Coconut, & Black Pepper, Mini, Santa Maria*	1 Wrap/25g	69	1.1	276	7.4	49.8	4.4	3.7
Wrap, Tortilla, Corn & Wheat, Carrefour*	1 Wrap/40g	124	2.9	309	8.2	51	7.3	3
Wrap, Tortilla, Corn, & Wheat, Santa Maria*	1 Wrap/40g	118	2.2	294	7.7	50	5.6	0
Wrap, Tortilla, Corn, Morrisons*	1 Wrap/40g	124	1.8	309	9.1	57.6	4.4	1.5
Wrap, Tortilla, Corn, Soft, Sainsbury's*	1 Wrap/40g	126	1.9	314	9.4	58	4.8	0
Wrap, Tortilla, Deli, Multigrain, Mission Deli*	1 Wrap/61g	202	6.1	330	7.9	50.5	10	3
Wrap, Tortilla, Fibre Fix, The Food Doctor*	1 Wrap/64g	164	2	256	7.5	54	3.2	9.3
Wrap, Tortilla, Flour, Soft, Mini, Stand n Stuff, Old El Paso*	1 Wrap/12g	36	0.6	296	8.5	52.5	5.2	2.7
Wrap, Tortilla, Flour, Soft, Old El Paso*	1 Wrap/41g	123	2.1	299	8.5	53.7	5.2	1.9
Wrap, Tortilla, GF, Lovemore*	1 Wrap/50g	150	4.2	299	1.8	48.1	8.3	4.1
Wrap, Tortilla, Large, Essential, Waitrose*	1 Wrap/64g	190	3.7	297	7.2	52.5	5.8	3.1
Wrap, Tortilla, Low Carb, Carbzone*	1 Wrap/65g	182	8.4	280	18	10	13	26
Wrap, Tortilla, Low Carb, Gerry's Wraps*	1 Wrap/43g	142	3.7	330	6.9	30.3	8.6	31.9
Wrap, Tortilla, Mediterranean Herb, Rowan Hill, Lidl*	1 Wrap/64g	178	2.2	278	7.3	53	3.5	2.5
Wrap, Tortilla, Mediterranean Style, Morrisons*	1 Wrap/64g	177	2.4	277	7.7	51.8	3.7	3
Wrap, Tortilla, Mexican Chilli, & Lime, Mission Deli*	1 Taco/23g	70	1.4	310	8.6	54	6.1	2.6
Wrap, Tortilla, Multigrain, GF, Kelkin*	1 Wrap/42g	92	2.2	219	1.4	35.7	5.2	11
Wrap, Tortilla, Multiseed, Tesco*	1 Wrap/64g	186	4	290	8.6	47.6	6.3	4.4
Wrap, Tortilla, Original, Mini, Mission Deli*	1 Wrap/31g	93	2	299	7.6	50.9	6.6	2.7
Wrap, Tortilla, Plain , Ocado*	1 Wrap/53g	154	4.4	291	6.7	45.7	8.4	3.1
Wrap, Tortilla, Plain, Atkins*	1 Wrap/40g	123	5.2	308	22.5	11	13	25
Wrap, Tortilla, Plain, HL, Tesco*	1 Wrap/64g	182	3.2	284	8.2	49.7	5	3.7
Wrap, Tortilla, Plain, Kids, Mission Deli*	1 Wrap/31g	93	1.8	299	7.1	57	5.8	4
Wrap, Tortilla, Plain, Mini, Asda*	1 Wrap/30g	92	2	307	8.5	52	6.5	2.2
Wrap, Tortilla, Plain, Mini, Morrisons*	1 Wrap/34g	91	1.4	267	8.1	48.9	4	2.8
Wrap, Tortilla, Plain, Ready to Eat, Sunnyhills, Aldi*	1 Wrap/64g	181	2.2	283	7.1	54.5	3.4	3
Wrap, Tortilla, Plain, Rowan Hill Bakery, Lidl*	1 Wrap/64g	204	4.4	319	8.4	55.3	6.8	1.6
Wrap, Tortilla, Plain, Tesco*	1 Wrap/64g	182	3.2	284	8.1	49.7	5	3.8
Wrap, Tortilla, Plain, Village Bakery, Aldi*	1 Wrap/65g	194	4.9	298	7.8	49.6	7.6	2.7

	Measure INFO/WEIGHT	per Measure KCAL	FAT	Nutrition Values per 100g / 100ml KCAL	PROT	CARB	FAT	FIBRE
BREAD								
Wrap, Tortilla, Rice, Mountain Bread*	1 Wrap/25g	68	0.3	272	10	53	1.3	2.6
Wrap, Tortilla, Seeded, Love Life, Waitrose*	1 Wrap/64g	185	3.6	290	8.8	46.6	5.7	4.3
Wrap, Tortilla, Seeded, Mission Deli*	1 Wrap/61g	185	3.8	304	8.6	50.1	6.2	6.2
Wrap, Tortilla, Seeded, Rowan Hill Bakery, Lidl*	1 Wrap/64g	178	3.6	279	9	44.4	5.6	7.3
Wrap, Tortilla, Small, Rapiditas, Bimbo*	1 Wrap/18g	55	1.5	306	8.1	50	8.2	0
Wrap, Tortilla, Soft Flour, Sainsbury's*	1 Wrap/40g	123	2.6	307	8.5	52.5	6.5	2.3
Wrap, Tortilla, Soft Taco, M&S*	2 Tacos/68g	209	5.4	308	9	49.5	7.9	1.5
Wrap, Tortilla, Soft, Flour, Stand n Stuff, Old El Paso*	1 Wrap/24g	75	1.7	312	8.5	52.5	6.9	2.7
Wrap, Tortilla, Soft, M&S*	1 Wrap/64g	186	3.8	290	8	49.7	6	2.5
Wrap, Tortilla, Street Taco, Gran Luchito*	1 Taco/30g	92	2	307	8.5	52.5	6.5	0
Wrap, Tortilla, Sweet Chilli, Tesco*	1 Wrap/64g	184	2.9	288	7.4	53.1	4.5	2.7
Wrap, Tortilla, Sweet Potato, GF, BFree*	1 Wrap/42g	91	0.8	217	5.4	33	1.9	15.2
Wrap, Tortilla, Value, Tesco*	1 Wrap/47g	129	2.4	275	8.5	49.1	5	4.3
Wrap, Tortilla, Wheat & White, Mini, Mission Deli*	1 Wrap/31g	93	2.1	299	7.5	50	6.9	3.6
Wrap, Tortilla, White, Bakers Selection, Asda*	1 Wrap/62g	181	2.9	290	7.9	53	4.6	2.5
Wrap, Tortilla, White, GF, Free From, Tesco*	1 Wrap/40g	84	1.8	211	4.3	31	4.4	15.3
Wrap, Tortilla, White, GF, Warburton's*	1 Wrap/45g	138	2.6	306	3.9	57	5.8	5.3
Wrap, Tortilla, White, Mini, Asda*	1 Wrap/31g	90	1.2	289	8	54	4	2.6
Wrap, Tortilla, White, Mini, Tesco*	1 Wrap/31g	88	1.6	284	8.2	49.7	5	3.7
Wrap, Tortilla, White, Weight Watchers*	1 Wrap/48g	119	0.8	247	6.9	46.3	1.6	9.6
Wrap, Tortilla, Whole & White, HL, Tesco*	1 Wrap/64g	182	1.7	284	8.5	54.1	2.7	4.5
Wrap, Tortilla, Wholemeal , M&S*	1 Wrap/64g	160	2.4	250	11.2	42.5	3.8	6.5
Wrap, Tortilla, Wholemeal, Asda*	1 Wrap/40g	121	3	302	7.7	48	7.4	6.5
Wrap, Tortilla, Wholemeal, Discovery*	1 Wrap/40g	109	3.3	273	9.2	40.4	8.3	6.4
Wrap, Tortilla, Wholemeal, Essential, Waitrose*	1 Wrap/64g	181	4.1	283	9.2	43.4	6.4	7.3
Wrap, Tortilla, Wholemeal, Mini, Asda*	1 Wrap/31g	90	1.4	289	9	49	4.5	8.4
Wrap, Tortilla, Wholemeal, Mini, Tesco *	1 Wrap/31g	86	1.6	279	9	45.7	5.2	6.9
Wrap, Tortilla, Wholemeal, Mission Deli*	1 Wrap/60g	175	5	292	8.4	41.6	8.3	8.8
Wrap, Tortilla, Wholemeal, Weight Watchers*	1 Wrap/50g	118	0.8	236	8.1	52.8	1.5	11
Wrap, Tortilla, Wholewheat, Zanuy*	1 Wrap/40g	131	1.8	327	7.9	60	4.4	8.1
Wrap, White, Soft, Easy Roll, Warburton's*	1 Wrap/65g	192	2.8	296	11.7	51.6	4.3	2
Wrap, Wholegrain, GF, Mini, Warburton's*	1 Wrap/35g	101	2.3	288	9.2	44.7	6.6	6.7
Wrap, Wholemeal, High Protein & Fibre, Warburton's*	1 Wrap/68g	184	3.3	271	15	38.4	4.8	7.3
Wrap. Tortilla, Plain, GF, Genius*	1 Wrap/40g	84	1.8	211	4.3	31	4.4	15.3
Wrap. Tortilla, Wholemeal, Bakers Life, Aldi*	1 Wrap/45g	137	3.7	304	8.2	45.8	8.2	6.4
Wraps, Tortilla, Original, Mini, Soft, Village Bakery, Aldi*	1 Wrap/31g	91	1.6	293	8.3	51	5.2	3.7
Wraps, Tortilla, Sweet Potato, Free From, Sainsbury's*	1 Wrap/40g	73	1.3	182	4.4	26.2	3.2	15.3
BREAD & BUTTER PUDDING								
Average	***1 Serving/250g***	***400***	***19.5***	***160***	***6.2***	***17.5***	***7.8***	***0.3***
BREAD MIX								
Cheddar Cheese, & Onion, Made Up, Wrights*	1 Slice/45g	116	1.1	258	11.6	45.6	2.4	3.5
Ciabatta, Made Up with Water & Olive Oil, Wrights*	1 Slice/45g	113	1.8	251	10	43.6	4	1.8
Crusty White, Made Up, Tesco*	1 Slice/126g	316	2.3	251	9.4	49.3	1.8	2.5
Focaccia, Garlic & Herb, Asda*	1 Serving/125g	385	10	308	11	48	8	3.3
GF, Schar*	1 Serving/100g	345	1.1	345	3.7	77	1.1	6.1
Kornbrot, Saftiges, Made Up, Aurora*	1 Slice/50g	119	0.9	238	8	45	1.8	0
Mixed Grain, Sainsbury's*	1 Serving/45g	103	0.7	228	7.7	46	1.5	4.4
Multiseed, Baked, Sainsbury's*	1 Slice/44g	112	4.3	252	10.8	30.5	9.6	6.8
Multiseed, Crunchy Four Seed, Tesco*	1 Pack/500g	1370	37	274	11.3	38.1	7.4	4.9
Oat & Linseed, Wright's*	1 Slice/45g	110	1.8	244	12.3	41.2	3.9	6.6
Pain De Compagne, Made Up, Francine*	2 Slices/100g	237	2.5	237	9.7	42.3	2.5	0
White Loaf, Asda*	1 Slice/60g	128	0.2	213	7.9	43	0.3	3.5
White, Made Up, Asda*	1 Slice/58g	144	1	248	10	46	1.7	3

B

	Measure INFO/WEIGHT	per Measure KCAL	FAT	Nutrition Values per 100g / 100ml KCAL	PROT	CARB	FAT	FIBRE
BREAD MIX								
White, Premium, Dry Mix, Made Up, Wright's*	1 Slice/45g	112	0.8	248	10.4	46.3	1.7	3
Wholemeal, CBY, Asda*	1 Slice/45g	93	0.3	207	9.6	37.5	0.6	6.5
Wholemeal, Hovis*	1 Serving/65g	148	3.1	227	10	35.8	4.8	6.8
Wholemeal, Made Up, M&S*	1 Loaf/600g	1410	14.4	235	11	42	2.4	5.3
BREADCRUMBS								
Average	***1oz/28g***	***98***	***0.5***	***350***	***10.8***	***74.8***	***1.9***	***2.6***
Panko, Blue Dragon*	1 Serving/30g	81	1.7	270	7.7	46.7	5.7	1.7
Southern Fried, Paxo*	1 Serving/24g	84	0.6	352	11.7	68.2	2.5	4.8
BREADFRUIT								
Raw	***1oz/28g***	***19***	***0.1***	***67***	***0.9***	***16.4***	***0.2***	***0***
BREADSTICKS								
Chive & Onion Twists, Tesco*	3 Twists/24g	115	5.3	480	11.6	57.6	22.1	2.2
Ciabatta, Garlic & Parsley, The Best, Morrisons*	½ Pack/76g	291	13.9	384	9.7	44.1	18.3	2.2
Ciabatta, Garlic, Sainsbury's*	1 Breadstick/36g	147	7.2	412	10.5	45.8	20.1	3.3
Classic, Organico*	1 Breadstick/12g	48	1.3	403	13.4	68.2	10.9	0
Grissini, Black Olive, Crosta & Mollica*	1 Grissini/10g	41	0.9	410	10	69.7	9.4	3.2
Grissini, Italian, Sainsbury's*	1 Breadstick/5g	20	0.4	408	11.6	72.9	7.8	2.9
Grissini, Thin with Olive Oil, Forno Bianco*	1 Stick/5g	21	0.4	420	11	77	7.5	0
Grissini, Waitrose*	1 Breadstick/6g	25	0.4	397	12	72.5	6.2	3.1
Grissini, with Olive Oil, Cypressa*	1 Breadstick/8g	35	1	439	11	68	12.8	3.8
Grissini, with Wholemeal Flour, Faidon*	1 Stick/14g	63	2.3	447	12.8	62.6	16.2	4.5
Italian Original, Tesco*	1 Stick/5.5g	23	0.4	414	11.2	73.1	7.9	2.8
Italian Style, Co-Op*	1 Breadstick/5g	21	0	420	12	74	0	0
Italian, Mini, Morrisons*	1 Breadstick/2g	8	0.2	409	11.5	71.8	7.6	4.2
Mini, Sainsbury's*	1 Breadstick/1g	4	0.1	416	10.4	71.9	8.8	3.8
Mini, Tesco*	1 Breadstick/2g	7	0.1	412	11.1	73.2	7.7	2.9
Parmesan, Torinesi, & Poppy Seed, Crosta & Mollica*	3 Breadsticks/10g	41	0.9	410	13	70	8.8	1
Plain, You Count, Love Life, Waitrose*	1 Breadstick/5g	17	0.1	349	13.4	70.1	1.7	5.6
Sesame Seed Grissini, Sainsbury's*	1 Breadstick/6g	27	0.7	424	13.5	66.2	11	3.1
Sesame, Tesco*	3 Breadsticks/24g	113	4.6	469	15.3	57.2	19.3	2.6
Tomato, & Basil, Mini, Cottage Delight Ltd*	1 Serving/20g	90	3	449	13	64	15	0
BREAKFAST								
All Day, Lunch Bowl, Microwaved, Slimming World*	1 Pack/400g	300	5.6	75	6.9	6.8	1.4	3.5
Bircher, Apple Pie, Allplants*	1 Serving/179g	326	13.6	182	6.1	20	7.6	4.1
Bircher, Blueberry, Nomadic*	1 Pot/150g	225	5.6	150	5	23	3.7	1.9
Bircher, Carrot Cake, Allplants*	1 Serving/183g	307	13.4	168	6	18	7.3	3.6
Cereal, Porridge, Chocolate, Ready Brek, Weetabix*	1 Serving/30g	115	2.4	382	10	64	8	7
Pack, Vegan, Simon Howie*	½ Pack/165g	350	20.3	212	12.8	15.6	12.3	0
Porridge, Apple, & Blueberry, Pot, As Sold, Quaker*	1 Pot/57g	214	2.9	375	14	65	5	5.5
Sausage, Bean, & Potato, Pot, Musclefood*	1 Serving/277g	374	8.6	135	9.5	16	3.1	1.5
Scramble, Amy's*	1 Pack/255g	344	19.1	135	8.6	7.5	7.5	1.6
Shakshuka, Cauliflower, & Aubergine, Spiced, Cook*	1 Pack/365g	219	8.8	60	2.1	9.1	2.4	0
BREAKFAST CEREAL								
Porridge Oats, Protein, Original, Made Up, Quaker*	1 Sachet/38g	235	6.3	623	39.8	76.9	16.7	7.2
Advantage, Weetabix*	1 Serving/30g	105	0.7	350	10.2	72	2.4	9
All Bran, All Bran, Fibre Crunch, Berry Burst, Kellogg's*	1 Serving/45g	176	5	391	7.6	59	11	13
All Bran, Asda*	1 Serving/40g	110	1.4	276	15	46	3.5	27
All Bran, Bran Flakes, & Fruit, Kellogg's*	1 Serving/40g	143	2.4	358	8	68	6	9
All Bran, Bran Flakes, Chocolate, Kellogg's*	1 Serving/30g	106	1.8	354	10	65	6	13
All Bran, Fibre Crunch, Kellogg's*	1 Serving/45g	184	5	409	7.6	63	11	13
All Bran, Fruit 'n' Fibre, Kellogg's*	1 Serving/30g	114	1.8	380	8	69	6	9
All Bran, Golden Crunch, Kellogg's*	1 Serving/45g	182	5	405	8	62	11	13
All Bran, Muesli, Cranberry & Sultana, Kellogg's*	1 Serving/45g	158	2.5	350	10	58	5.5	14

	Measure INFO/WEIGHT	per Measure KCAL	FAT	Nutrition Values per 100g / 100ml KCAL	PROT	CARB	FAT	FIBRE
BREAKFAST CEREAL								
All Bran, Oats, Clusters, Prebiotic, Kellogg's*	1 Serving/40g	166	6.4	414	15	42	16	21
All Bran, Oaty Clusters, Prebiotic, Kellogg's*	1 Serving/45g	186	7.2	414	15	42	16	21
All Bran, Oaty Clusters, Prebiotic, Kellogg's*	1 Serving/45g	175	5.4	388	14	56	12	22
All Bran, Original, High Fibre, Kellogg's*	1 Serving/40g	134	1.4	334	14	48	3.5	27
Almond, Oats & More, Nestle*	1 Serving/40g	162	3.5	404	11	67	8.8	7
Almond, Pecan & Cashew Muesli, Kellogg's*	1 Serving/45g	188	6.3	418	11	62	14	8
Alpen*, Crunchy Bran*	1 Serving/40g	120	1.9	299	11.8	52.3	4.7	24.8
Apple & Cinnamon, Crisp, Sainsbury's*	1 Serving/50g	216	7.4	433	6.2	69.1	14.7	3.4
Apple & Cinnamon Crisp, Tesco*	1 Serving/50g	217	6.6	433	8.7	67.1	13.1	6.1
Apple & Raisin, Additions, Weetabix*	2 Biscuits/43g	149	0.8	344	9.5	66	1.8	13
Apple, & Blueberry, Low Sugar, Aldi*	1 Serving/45g	202	7.2	449	14	57	16	8.3
Apple, & Cinnamon, Crisp, Crownfield, Lidl*	1 Serving/30g	129	3.6	429	8.2	68.5	12	6.9
Apple, & Cinnamon, Flakes, M&S*	1 Serving/30g	113	0.4	377	11.3	78.7	1.3	3
Apricot Wheats, Harvest Morn, Aldi*	1 Serving/30g	101	0.4	337	7.6	72.3	1.4	8
Apricot Wheats, Whole Grain, Tesco*	1 Serving/40g	130	0.6	326	7.6	70.6	1.4	8
Apricot Wheats, Wholegrain, Essential, Waitrose*	1 Serving/45g	151	0.6	335	8	71.3	1.4	8.3
Balance, Oats & Honey, Sainsbury's*	1 Serving/30g	114	0.5	379	7.3	81.4	1.7	4.4
Balance, Sainsbury's*	1 Serving/30g	111	0.4	370	11.4	77.7	1.5	3.2
Banana, Papaya & Honey Oat, Crunchy, Waitrose*	1 Serving/40g	170	4.8	426	9.6	69.8	12	5.5
Beetroot, Apple, Hazelnut, Sainsbury's*	1 Serving/45g	169	3.9	375	10.5	58.5	8.6	11
Benefit Flakes, Original, Harvest Morn, Aldi*	1 Serving/40g	154	0.5	384	12	80	1.3	2.2
Berries, Clusters, & Seeds, Protein, Special K, Kellogg's*	1 Serving/40g	148	1.3	371	12	69	3.2	8.9
Berry Granola, Rude Health*	1 Serving/40g	178	6.4	446	10	61	16	7
Bircher Mix, Almonds, & Honey, Dorset Cereals*	1 Serving/30g	117	3.3	389	10	55	11	8.5
Bircher Muesli, Love Life, Waitrose*	1 Serving/45g	153	3.5	341	8.8	57.7	7.7	6.8
Biscuit, with Coconut & Raisin, Additions, Weetabix*	2 Biscuits/43g	157	2.5	363	9.5	62	5.7	13
Bitesize Wheats, Crownfield, Lidl*	1 Serving/40g	142	0.8	356	10.6	67	1.9	14
Bitesize, Weetabix*	1 Serving/40g	135	0.8	338	11.5	68.4	2	10
Bixies, Wheat Biscuits, Wholegrain, Crownfield, Lidl*	2 Biscuits/40g	145	0.8	362	10.8	70.3	1.9	10
Blueberry Wheaties, Asda*	1 Serving/45g	150	0.6	333	7.9	71	1.4	8.2
Blueberry Wheats, Harvest Morn, Aldi*	1 Serving/45g	150	0.6	333	7.9	71	1.4	8.2
Blueberry Wheats, Sainsbury's*	1 Serving/45g	150	0.6	333	7.9	70.8	1.4	8.2
Blueberry Wheats, Tesco*	1 Serving/50g	168	0.8	336	7.5	71.6	1.5	8.5
Blueberry Wheats, Wholegrain, Essential, Waitrose*	1 Serving/45g	150	0.6	333	7.9	70.8	1.4	8.2
Blueberry, & Banana, with Cultures, GoodBelly, Nestle*	1 Serving/40g	162	4	404	12	61	10	9.8
Bran Flakes, Asda*	1 Serving/30g	108	0.8	360	12	64	2.7	16
Bran Flakes, Free From, Tesco*	1 Serving/30g	107	0.7	358	7.5	69.3	2.3	15
Bran Flakes, Kellogg's*	1 Serving/30g	108	1	359	12	63	3.2	15
Bran Flakes, Sultana Bran, Kellogg's*	1 Serving/40g	138	0.8	344	8	67	2	13
Bran Flakes, Sultana, Dry, Sainsbury's*	1 Serving/30g	98	0.6	325	8.3	68.6	1.9	12.1
Bran Flakes, Tesco*	1 Serving/30g	107	0.7	356	10.8	64.3	2.4	16.8
Bran Flakes, Wholegrain, Essential, Waitrose*	1 Serving/30g	107	0.7	356	10.8	64.7	2.4	16
Bran Flakes, Wholegrain, Sainsbury's*	1 Serving/30g	109	0.9	363	10.1	67.1	3	13.6
Bran Sticks, Organic, BuyWholeFoodsOnline*	1 Serving/30g	85	1.3	283	15	26.9	4.2	38.6
Bran, High Fibre, Morrisons*	1 Serving/30g	102	1	341	13.3	51.6	3.3	25.9
Bran, High Fibre, Tesco*	1 Serving/40g	140	1.6	350	13.7	54	3.9	22.1
Cheerios, Honey Nut, Nestle*	1 Serving/30g	112	1.1	374	7	78.3	3.7	5.2
Cheerios, Honey, Nestle*	1 Serving/50g	184	1.4	369	6.6	79.2	2.8	5.8
Cheerios, Low Sugar, As Sold, Nestle*	1 Serving/30g	120	2.3	399	11.1	67.4	7.6	8.5
Cheerios, Multigrain, Nestle*	1 Serving/30g	114	1.3	380	9.4	72	4.2	8.9
Cheerios, Nestle*	1 Serving/30g	114	1.1	381	8.6	74.5	3.8	7.1
Cheerios, Oat Crisp, Nestle*	1 Portion/40g	154	2.1	385	11	70	5.2	8.5
Cherry, Dark Chocolate, & Almond, Special K, Kellogg's*	1 Serving/30g	129	1.2	430	9	86.7	4	5.3

B

	Measure INFO/WEIGHT	per Measure KCAL	FAT	Nutrition Values per 100g / 100ml KCAL	PROT	CARB	FAT	FIBRE
BREAKFAST CEREAL								
Choc & Nut Crisp, Tesco*	1 Serving/40g	185	8	462	8.3	62.5	19.9	4.8
Choco Crackles, Morrisons*	1 Serving/30g	115	0.7	383	5.5	84.8	2.4	1.9
Choco Squares, Asda*	1 Serving/30g	130	4.2	434	10	67	14	4
Chocolate Chip, Crispy Minis, Weetabix*	1 Serving/40g	154	2	386	10	70	5.1	10
Chocolate Crisp, Tesco*	1 Serving/40g	188	7.8	471	9.3	61.4	19.4	6.9
Chocolate Hoops, Average	***1 Serving/30g***	***116***	***1.3***	***386***	***7.2***	***79.3***	***4.4***	***3.4***
Chocolate Rice, Puffed, Average	***1 Serving/30g***	***117***	***1.2***	***389***	***5.7***	***81***	***4.1***	***3.2***
Chocolate, Smart Food, Futurelife*	1 Serving/50g	174	5.4	348	16	43	10.9	6.1
Chocolatey Squares, Mornflake*	1 Serving/30g	140	5.6	466	6.4	66.7	18.7	2.8
Cinnamon Chips, Harvest Morn, Aldi*	1 Serving/40g	166	4.4	416	6.8	70	11	0
Cinnamon Grahams, Nestle*	1 Serving/40g	164	3.9	411	4.7	76.1	9.8	4.2
Cinnamon Toast, Crunch, Churros, General Mills*	1 Serving/31g	130	3	419	6.4	77.4	9.7	0
Clusters, Honey, & Nut, Harvest Morn, Aldi*	1 Serving/45g	200	6.3	445	9.6	68	14	5.6
Clusters, Nestle*	1 Serving/30g	113	1	377	9	74	3.4	7.9
Coco Pops, Kellogg's*	1 Serving/30g	115	0.6	382	6.3	84	1.9	3
Coco Pops, White, Kellogg's*	1 Serving/30g	116	1	385	6.1	81	3.2	4
Coco Rice, GF, Nestle*	1 Serving/30g	115	0.7	382	6.2	82	2.4	3.1
Coco Snaps, Value, Tesco*	1 Serving/30g	117	0.7	390	7	84.1	2.4	2.4
Cookie Crunch, Nestle*	1 Serving/40g	154	1.1	385	4.6	85.3	2.8	1.8
Cookie Hoops, Asda*	1 Serving/30g	113	0.8	378	9.2	77	2.6	4.9
Corn Flakes, Asda*	1 Serving/30g	111	0.2	370	7	84	0.7	3
Corn Flakes, Crownfield, Lidl*	1 Serving/30g	118	0.1	392	8.6	86.2	0.3	4.8
Corn Flakes, GF, Free From, Morrisons*	1 Serving/30g	114	0.2	380	6.8	86	0.5	2.5
Corn Flakes, Honey Nut, Average	***1 Serving/30g***	***118***	***1.3***	***393***	***7***	***81.4***	***4.3***	***2.4***
Corn Flakes, Kellogg's*	1 Serving/30g	113	0.3	378	7	84	0.9	3
Corn Flakes, Organic, Lima*	1 Serving/50g	178	0.5	355	8.3	77.7	1	6.4
Corn Flakes, Sainsbury's*	1 Serving/25g	93	0.2	371	7.3	83.8	0.7	3
Corn Flakes, Tesco*	1 Serving/30g	116	0.3	386	7.6	85.2	1.1	2.5
Corn Flakes, Value, Tesco*	1 Serving/30g	116	0.3	386	7.6	85.2	1.1	2.5
Cornflakes, Co-Op*	1 Serving/30g	116	0.3	386	7.6	85	1.1	2.5
Cornflakes, Essential, Waitrose*	1 Serving/30g	116	0.3	385	7.4	84.8	1.1	3.1
Cornflakes, GF, Nestle*	1 Serving/30g	115	0.3	384	7.4	84.6	1.1	3.1
Country Crisp with Real Raspberries, Jordans*	1 Serving/50g	214	7.9	429	7.5	64.1	15.8	7.1
Country Crisp with Real Strawberries, Jordans*	1 Serving/50g	214	7.8	428	7.5	64.1	15.7	7.1
Country Crisp, Four Nut Combo, Jordans*	1 Serving/50g	240	12.4	480	8.9	55.4	24.7	6.9
Country Store, Kellogg's*	1 Serving/45g	165	2.3	367	9.1	67	5.2	8
Craze, Chocolate Hazelnut, Harvest Morn, Aldi*	1 Serving/40g	167	4.4	418	7.9	70	11	3.2
Crispy Minis, Banana, Weetabix*	1 Serving/40g	156	2	389	9.3	72	4.9	9.7
Crunchy Bran, Weetabix*	1 Serving/40g	140	1.4	350	11.9	57.6	3.6	20
Crunchy Choco, Crisp & Square, Tesco*	1 Serving/50g	212	7	423	8	66.3	14	6
Crunchy Nut, Clusters, Honey & Nut, Kellogg's*	1 Serving/40g	161	2	402	6	82	5	2.5
Crunchy Nut, Clusters, Milk Chocolate Curls, Kellogg's*	1 Serving/40g	183	7.2	458	8	66	18	4
Crunchy Nut, Clusters, Peanut Butter, Kellogg's *	1 Serving/30g	146	7.5	488	14	49	25	5.5
Crunchy Nut, Clusters, Summer Berries, Kellogg's*	1 Serving/40g	176	6	439	8	68	15	5
Crunchy Nut, Corn Flakes, Kellogg's*	1 Serving/30g	118	1.2	392	6	83	4	2.5
Crunchy Nut, Oat Granola, with Chocolate, Kellogg's*	1 Serving/45g	224	11.2	497	8	57	25	6
Crunchy Weeties, Weetabix*	1 Serving/30g	110	0.5	368	10	73	1.8	10
Curiously Cinnamon, Nestle*	1 Serving/30g	124	3	412	4.9	75.9	9.9	4.1
Digestive Health, Nutri Brex*	1 Serving/40g	142	2.1	356	12	56	5.3	17
Fibre Flakes, GF, Organic, Dove's Farm*	1 Serving/30g	105	0.4	351	7.1	69.7	1.5	15
Fibre Flakes, Red Berry, Asda*	1 Serving/30g	109	0.5	364	10	72	1.8	9.2
Fitness, Chocolate, Nestle*	1 Serving/30g	118	1.9	394	8.5	72.7	6.3	6.2
Fitness, Honey, & Almond, Nestle*	1 Serving/30g	116	1.6	387	9.5	71.8	5.2	7.2

	Measure INFO/WEIGHT	per Measure KCAL	FAT	Nutrition Values per 100g / 100ml KCAL	PROT	CARB	FAT	FIBRE
BREAKFAST CEREAL								
Fitness, Original, Nestle*	1 Serving/30g	110	0.5	368	9.4	74.8	1.8	7.6
Flakes & Grains, Exotic Fruit, BGTY, Sainsbury's*	1 Serving/30g	113	1.5	377	6.8	76.4	4.9	5.9
Frosted Flakes , Asda*	1 Serving/30g	116	0.3	387	6	88	0.9	2
Frosted Flakes, Sainsbury's*	1 Serving/30g	119	0.3	396	5.8	90.1	0.9	1.9
Frosted Flakes, Tesco*	1 Serving/30g	112	0.1	374	4.9	87.8	0.4	2.4
Frosted Wheats, Kellogg's*	1 Serving/30g	104	0.6	346	10	72	2	9
Frosties, Caramel, Kellogg's*	1 Serving/30g	113	0.2	377	5	88	0.6	2
Frosties, Kellogg's*	1 Serving/30g	112	0.2	375	4.5	87	0.6	2
Fruit & Fibre, Flakes, Waitrose*	1 Serving/40g	143	2.5	357	8.2	67.2	6.2	9.9
Fruit & Fibre, Morrisons*	1 Serving/30g	110	2.2	366	8.8	66.5	7.2	8.5
Fruit & Fibre, Value, Tesco*	1 Serving/40g	144	2.2	359	11.4	65.7	5.6	8
Fruit & Nut Crisp, Minis, Weetabix*	1 Serving/40g	148	1.6	371	9.9	69	4.1	9.3
Fruit & Fibre, Asda*	1 Serving/40g	155	2.6	387	8.8	69	6.5	8.8
Fruit & Fibre, Harvest Morn, Aldi*	1 Serving/30g	114	1.8	380	8.4	69	6.1	8
Fruit 'n' Fibre, Kellogg's*	1 Serving/40g	152	2.4	380	8	69	6	9
Fruit Wheats, Raisin, Harvest Morn*	1 Serving/45g	153	0.7	340	8.4	71	1.5	8.4
Fruit Wheats, Raspberry, Morrisons*	1 Serving/45g	150	0.6	333	8	70.8	1.4	8.4
Fruit, Nuts & Flakes, M&S*	1 Serving/30g	117	2.6	391	9.1	69.6	8.5	3.5
GoFree, Honey Flakes, GF, Nestle*	1 Serving/30g	115	0.2	384	5.6	87	0.8	2.3
Golden Grahams, Nestle*	1 Serving/30g	112	0.9	375	6	81	3	3.4
Golden Honey Puffs, Tesco*	1 Serving/30g	115	0.4	382	6.6	86.3	1.2	3
Golden Nuggets, Nestle*	1 Serving/40g	152	0.3	381	6.2	87.4	0.7	1.5
Granola	***1 Serving/45g***	***194***	***8.7***	***430***	***17.5***	***48.8***	***19.4***	***16.8***
Granola, 3 Seed, & Oat, Wholegrain, M&S*	1 Serving/45g	217	9	483	16.1	50.8	20	7.7
Granola, 4 Nut, & Flame Raisin, Wholegrain, M&S*	1 Serving/45g	206	8.3	458	10	59.5	18.5	6.5
Granola, Apple, & Blueberry, Harvest Morn, Aldi*	1 Serving/45g	202	7.2	449	14	57	16	8.3
Granola, Apple, & Cinnamon, Rude Health*	1 Serving/40g	175	5.2	437	10	64	13	7
Granola, Apricot, & Cranberry, The Foodie Market, Aldi*	1 Serving/45g	198	7.2	441	27	44	16	6
Granola, Berry & Orange, Wholegrain, M&S*	1 Serving/45g	178	4.3	396	8.5	65.5	9.6	6.7
Granola, Cherries & Berries, Sainsbury's*	1 Serving/40g	176	5.4	439	10.4	65.1	13.6	7.3
Granola, Cherry Bakewell, 1, Waitrose*	1 Serving/40g	181	4.8	452	12	70	12	8
Granola, Cherry Bakewell, Oat Pantry*	1 Serving/40g	157	6	393	9.5	52	15	7.3
Granola, Chocolate, Dorset Cereals*	1 Serving/40g	206	12	515	8.8	47.2	30	10.5
Granola, Chocolate, Sante *	1 Serving/40g	182	6.8	454	8.8	63	17	6.8
Granola, Cocoa, & Hazelnut, W.K Kellogg, Kellogg's*	1 Serving/35g	157	6.6	449	9	56	19	9.2
Granola, Crunchy Nut Glorious Oat, Kellogg's*	1 Serving/45g	212	9.4	470	7	61	21	4.5
Granola, Crunchy Oat, Raisin, Almond, Harvest Morn, Aldi*	1 Serving/40g	166	4.6	416	8.2	66.9	11.4	6.4
Granola, Crunchy Oat, Tropical Fruits, Harvest Morn, Aldi*	1 Serving/40g	174	5.2	436	9.4	66	13	7.4
Granola, Fruit Mix, Kellogg's*	1 Serving/40g	170	7.3	424	7.8	59	18.2	5.9
Granola, GF, Eat Natural*	1 Serving/30g	148	8.9	494	13.6	40.2	29.6	6.1
Granola, Grain Free, Luxury, No Added Sugar, M&S*	1 Serving/45g	268	21.7	595	18.1	15.7	48.3	12.3
Granola, Grain Free, No Added Sugar, M&S*	1 Serving/45g	267	21.7	594	18.1	15.7	48.3	12.3
Granola, Hazelnuts, & Pecans, Super Goodness, Quaker*	1 Serving/45g	187	5	416	9.6	67	11	8
Granola, High Protein, Lizi's*	1 Serving/40g	180	6.8	450	27	44	17	6.7
Granola, High Protein, Tesco*	1 Serving/50g	211	5.8	422	25.9	50.9	11.5	6.1
Granola, High Protein, Well & Good, Co-Op*	1 Serving/45g	193	4.9	429	28	52	11	6.4
Granola, Honey & Seed, High Protein, Crownfield, Lidl*	1 Serving/45g	202	7.2	448	27.9	45.1	16.1	5.6
Granola, Honey, & Seed, The Foodie Market, Aldi*	1 Serving/20g	92	3.4	461	26	49	17	4.4
Granola, Honey, Dorset Cereals*	1 Serving/40g	204	12	511	13	44	30	7.4
Granola, Low Sugar, Eat Natural*	1 Serving/50g	248	15.7	495	13.7	33	31.4	12.8
Granola, Low Sugar, Make it Your Own, M&S*	1 Serving/45g	197	7	437	13.8	56	15.5	9.1
Granola, Mango, & Coconut, Wholegrain, M&S*	1 Serving/45g	196	6.7	435	10.5	61.3	14.8	7.4
Granola, Maple, & Pecan, Crush*	1 Serving/30g	113	3.9	377	10	52	13	6.7

	Measure INFO/WEIGHT	per Measure KCAL	FAT	Nutrition Values per 100g / 100ml KCAL	PROT	CARB	FAT	FIBRE
BREAKFAST CEREAL								
Granola, Muesli, Fruit & Nut, The Best, Morrisons*	1 Serving/45g	174	4.4	387	8.5	63.2	9.8	6
Granola, Multigrain Nutty, G&B, Asda*	1 Serving/40g	178	7.6	444	12	52	19	7.6
Granola, Nut & Fruit, Lucury, M&S*	1 Serving/45g	205	8.9	455	10.5	55.1	19.8	7
Granola, Nut, Simply Nut, Dorset Cereals*	1 Serving/40g	200	10.8	500	11	48	27	8.3
Granola, Nuts, Pumpkin Seeds, & Fruit, Aldi*	1 Serving/45g	210	8.6	466	27	45	19	5
Granola, Nutty Fruit, 45g, Result Plan*	1 Serving/45g	194	6	431	9.8	62.2	13.3	6.9
Granola, Nutty Fruit, 60g, Result Plan*	1 Serving/60g	258	8	430	10.8	65	13.3	16.7
Granola, Nutty, Dorset Cereals*	1 Serving/45g	223	11.9	496	11.6	49.3	26.4	7.4
Granola, Nutty, with Cinnamon, Troo*	1 Serving/45g	210	10.3	467	15.1	44.7	22.9	20.7
Granola, Oat Clusters, Apple & Cinnamon, Quaker*	1 Pack/48g	193	3.8	403	8	70.2	8	9.4
Granola, Oat, Golden Crunch, 30% Less Fat, Quaker*	1 Serving/45g	193	4.6	429	8.7	71.5	10.3	7.2
Granola, Oat, Simply Oat, Dorset Cereals*	1 Serving/40g	177	6.8	443	8.8	60	17	7.4
Granola, Original, Low Sugar, Crownfield, Lidl*	1 Serving/20g	100	5.1	499	14.2	49.7	25.6	6.5
Granola, Peanut, High Protein, Luxury, M&S*	1 Serving/45g	204	8.1	453	23.1	47.5	18	4.1
Granola, Pink Apple & Cinnamon, Diet Chef Ltd*	1 Pack/40g	193	10.7	483	10.1	49.3	26.8	11.2
Granola, Protein, Eat Natural*	1 Serving/50g	256	16	512	18.4	34.3	32.1	6.5
Granola, Pumpkin & Sunflower, Super Goodness, Quaker*	1 Serving/45g	185	4.5	411	10	67	10	7.6
Granola, Quaker*	1 Serving/48g	210	7	438	10.4	72.9	14.6	6.2
Granola, Raisin, & Almond, Asda*	1 Serving/45g	190	5.4	422	10	65	12	6.5
Granola, Raisin, & Almond, Crownfield, Lidl*	1 Serving/50g	209	5.7	418	9.5	66.9	11.4	5.1
Granola, Raisin, Almond, & Honey, Waitrose*	1 Serving/40g	164	4.4	411	10.6	63.1	11.1	8.3
Granola, Raspberry, Apple, Carrot, W.K. Kellogg's*	1 Serving/45g	191	6.3	425	8.1	62	14	9.4
Granola, Really Nutty, Specially Selected, Aldi*	1 Serving/45g	203	7.4	451	12	60	16.4	7.3
Granola, Salted Caramel, & Popcorn, Finest, Tesco*	1 Serving/50g	230	8	460	8.7	68.3	16	4.1
Granola, Salted Toffee, & Pecan, Co-Op*	1 Serving/80g	358	12	447	13	62	15	6.5
Granola, Simply, Morrisons*	1 Serving/45g	168	2.5	374	11	66	5.6	7.7
Granola, Simply, No Added Sugar, W.K Kellogg, Kellogg's*	1 Serving/40g	172	6	431	8.6	61	15	8.6
Granola, Strawberry, Apple, & Raspberry, Asda*	1 Serving/50g	220	7.5	439	9.4	64	15	7.6
Granola, Strawberry, Crunchy, Weight Watchers*	1 Serving/50g	150	1.4	300	9	57	2.8	24
Granola, Strawberry, Morrisons*	1 Serving/45g	190	5	423	1.2	67.1	11.1	7.1
Granola, Summer Fruits, Pomegranate Infused, M&S*	1 Serving/50g	200	6.4	400	8.6	63.2	12.7	5.8
Granola, Super Berry, Deluxe, Lidl*	1 Serving/45g	201	7	447	10.3	64	15.6	6.8
Granola, Super Berry, Tesco*	1 Serving/45g	195	6	434	9.2	66	13.3	6.5
Granola, Super Fruity, Jordan's*	1 Serving/45g	194	5.6	431	9.5	66.6	12.4	7.5
Granola, Super Nutty, Aldi*	1 Serving/45g	217	9.9	483	11	56	22	7.2
Granola, Super Nutty, Deluxe, Lidl*	1 Serving/45g	211	8.9	469	10.7	58.4	19.8	6.4
Granola, Super Nutty, Finest, Tesco*	1 Serving/50g	229	8.7	457	12.2	59.3	17.4	7
Granola, Super Seedy, with Calming Ginger, Troo*	1 Serving/45g	206	9.6	457	15.7	46.7	21.3	22
Granola, Tropical, Sainsbury's*	1 Serving/45g	194	5.7	431	8.5	68	12.6	62
Granola, Very Berry, Aldi*	1 Serving/45g	191	5.4	424	11	64	12	8.1
Granola, Very Berry, Asda*	1 Serving/45g	187	4.9	417	10	66	11	8
Grape Nuts, Kraft*	1 Serving/45g	158	0.9	350	10.9	81.9	2	11.9
Harvest Crunch, Nut, Quaker*	1 Serving/40g	184	7.8	459	8	62.5	19.5	6
Harvest Crunch, Real Red Berries, Quaker*	1 Serving/50g	224	8.5	447	7	66	17	4.5
High Bran, CBY, Asda*	1 Serving/40g	136	1.5	341	13.6	49.5	3.8	27.1
High Fibre Bran, Co-Op*	1 Serving/40g	110	1.6	275	15	46	4	27
High Fibre Bran, Sainsbury's*	1 Serving/40g	140	1.6	350	13.7	54	3.9	22.1
High Fruit Muesli, BGTY, Sainsbury's*	1 Serving/50g	164	1	328	6.7	71	1.9	6.6
Honey & Nut Crisp, Mini, Weetabix*	1 Serving/40g	150	0.8	375	9.4	75.1	2	9.3
Honey Cheerios with 125ml Semi Skimmed Milk, Nestle*	1 Serving/30g	174	2.9	580	21	99.7	9.7	5.7
Honey Hoops, Harvest Morn, Aldi*	1 Serving/30g	117	1	389	6.5	81	3.4	4
Honey Loops, Kellogg's*	1 Serving/30g	110	0.9	367	8	77	3	6
Honey Nut Clusters, Tesco*	1 Serving/50g	220	7.2	441	9.2	65.7	14.4	6

	Measure INFO/WEIGHT	per Measure KCAL	FAT	Nutrition Values per 100g / 100ml KCAL	PROT	CARB	FAT	FIBRE
BREAKFAST CEREAL								
Honey Nut Crunch , Asda*	1 Serving/40g	176	5.2	441	10	68	13	5.3
Honey Raisin & Almond, Crunchy, Waitrose*	1 Serving/40g	170	4.8	425	10.5	68.8	12	5.7
Honey, Peanut, & Chocolate Crisp, Crownfield, Lidl*	1 Serving/45g	202	6.9	450	8.1	67.4	15.4	4.8
Hoops, Multigrain, Asda*	1 Serving/30g	113	1.2	376	6.5	78.4	4	4.6
Hoops, Multigrain, Tesco*	1 Serving/30g	112	1.1	375	6.5	78.6	3.8	4.6
Hoops, Mutigrain, Harvest Morn, Aldi*	1 Serving/30g	114	1	380	9	75	3.4	7.4
Hot Oat, Aldi*	1 Serving/40g	142	3.3	356	11.6	58.8	8.3	8.9
Hot Oats, Instant, Tesco*	1 Serving/30g	108	2.6	360	11.8	58.4	8.7	7.9
Instant Oats, Dry Weight	***1 Sachet/36g***	***129***	***3.1***	***359***	***11.5***	***59.1***	***8.5***	***8.3***
Jungle Bites, Asda*	1 Serving/30g	112	0.6	375	8	78	2	6.5
Just Right, Kellogg's*	1 Serving/40g	148	0.8	371	7	79	2	4.5
Krave, Chocolate & Hazelnut, Kellogg's*	1 Serving/30g	136	4.8	452	7.2	68	16	3.4
Krave, Milk Chocolate, Kellogg's*	1 Serving/30g	132	3.9	440	7.1	72	13	3.5
Lion, Nestle*	1 Serving/40g	166	3.1	415	7.2	76.9	7.7	4.3
Malted Wheaties, CBY, Asda*	1 Serving/40g	146	0.8	366	10.3	72.7	1.9	8.2
Malted Wheats, Waitrose*	1 Serving/30g	110	0.6	365	10	72.7	1.9	8.5
Malties, Sainsbury's*	1 Serving/40g	146	0.8	366	10.1	71.8	1.9	10.8
Malties, Wholegrain, Aldi*	1 Serving/40g	146	0.8	366	10.1	71.8	1.9	10.8
Malty Flakes with Red Berries, Tesco*	1 Serving/30g	111	0.6	369	9.9	78.1	1.9	3.1
Malty Flakes, Tesco*	1 Serving/40g	148	0.6	371	11	78.4	1.5	4.3
Maple & Pecan Crisp, Sainsbury's*	1 Serving/50g	226	9.8	452	7.9	61.3	19.5	5.4
Maple & Pecan Crisp, Tesco*	1 Serving/50g	215	7.6	430	10.5	62.5	15.2	10.2
Maple & Pecan, Crisp, Asda*	1 Serving/30g	135	5.7	451	8	62	19	6
Maple, & Pecan, Flakes, M&S*	1 Serving/30g	124	2.5	415	11.9	72	8.4	1.9
Mini Bites, Cinnamon, Wholegrain, Be Natural *	1 Serving/30g	106	0.4	354	9.2	69.6	1.3	11.1
Mixed Berry Crisp, Waitrose*	1 Serving/40g	174	5.3	436	9.1	65.9	13.3	8.4
Muesli Base, Wholesome, Waitrose*	1 Portion/50g	125	4.2	250	11.5	31.8	8.4	5
Muesli, 4 Fruit, Almond & Hazelnut, M&S*	1 Serving/45g	162	3.3	360	8.5	61.6	7.3	7.1
Muesli, 8 Fruit, Nut, & Seed, Luxury, M&S*	1 Serving/45g	177	6.3	393	10.2	51.8	14	9.7
Muesli, Base, Four Grain, Hodmedod's*	1 Serving/30g	108	1.8	360	10.9	60.9	5.9	10.1
Muesli, Base, Holland & Barrett*	1 Serving/40g	141	1.3	353	9.9	69	3.3	9
Muesli, Basics, Sainsbury's*	1 Serving/50g	178	2.6	355	11.2	61.5	5.1	9.2
Muesli, Berry, & Cherry, Luscious, Dorset Cereals*	1 Serving/45g	149	0.9	332	7	67	2.1	8.3
Muesli, Bircher, Fruity, The Best, Morrisons*	1 Serving/40g	158	3.6	396	8.8	66.5	9	6.9
Muesli, Bircher, with Apple, & Raspberry, Deliciously Ella*	1 Serving/45g	171	3.3	379	15.2	65.2	7.3	10.5
Muesli, Creamy Tropical Fruit, Finest, Tesco*	1 Serving/80g	283	4.5	354	7.2	68.8	5.6	6.9
Muesli, Crunchy, Organic, Sainsbury's*	1 Serving/40g	168	5.8	420	10.6	62	14.4	9.2
Muesli, Fantastically Fruity, Dorset Cereals*	1 Serving/45g	182	6.8	404	11.6	51.2	15	9
Muesli, Five Grain, with Fruit, Kellogg's*	1 Sachet/45g	166	2.3	369	9.3	67	5.1	9.1
Muesli, Fruchte, Musli-land*	1 Serving/40g	142	1.8	356	9.8	64.6	4.6	8.6
Muesli, Fruit & Nut, 55%, Asda*	1 Serving/40g	151	5.6	378	9	54	14	7
Muesli, Fruit & Nut, Luxury, Co-Op*	1 Serving/40g	150	4	375	8	64	10	6
Muesli, Fruit & Nut, Luxury, Lidl*	1 Serving/57g	205	5.6	360	8	60	9.8	7.5
Muesli, Fruit & Nut, Luxury, Simply Sumptuous, Lidl*	1 Serving/45g	179	6.2	398	8	57.6	13.8	5.8
Muesli, Fruit & Nut, Luxury, Waitrose*	1 Serving/40g	145	3.8	363	9	60.3	9.5	6.5
Muesli, Fruit & Nut, M&S*	1 Serving/40g	128	1.1	320	7.4	74.5	2.8	7.4
Muesli, Fruit & Nut, Organic, M&S*	1 Serving/50g	166	3	333	8.2	61.6	6	7.6
Muesli, Fruit & Nut, Tesco*	1 Serving/50g	190	5.6	380	8.4	60.3	11.3	5.3
Muesli, Fruit & Nut, Whole Wheat, Organic, Asda*	1 Serving/50g	172	3.5	343	10	60	7	7
Muesli, Fruit & Fibre, M&S*	1 Serving/45g	171	4.7	380	8.7	59	10.4	7.6
Muesli, Fruit & Nut, Essential, Waitrose*	1 Serving/45g	173	6.1	384	8.6	51.5	13.5	11
Muesli, Fruit & Nut, Jordans*	1 Serving/50g	180	4.7	361	8	61.2	9.4	7.5
Muesli, Fruit & Nut, Luxury, Sainsbury's*	1 Serving/50g	178	4.6	355	10.3	57.9	9.1	11.3

B

	Measure INFO/WEIGHT	per Measure KCAL	FAT	Nutrition Values per 100g / 100ml KCAL	PROT	CARB	FAT	FIBRE
BREAKFAST CEREAL								
Muesli, Fruit & Nut, Sainsbury's*	1 Serving/30g	114	3.1	379	9.5	58.7	10.3	6.9
Muesli, Fruit & nut, TTD, Sainsbury's*	1 Serving/45g	188	6.3	418	10.8	58.5	13.9	7.9
Muesli, Fruit & Nut, Wholegrain, M&S*	1 Serving/30g	105	1.6	349	9.5	60	5.5	10.8
Muesli, Fruit Nut & Seed, Organic, Dorset Cereals*	1 Serving/70g	251	6.9	358	10.8	56.6	9.8	8.4
Muesli, Fruit, M&S*	1 Serving/40g	145	2.6	362	7.3	64.2	6.4	9.3
Muesli, Fruit, Nut, & Seed, Made Without Wheat, M&S*	1 Serving/45g	170	5.2	377	11.1	51.6	11.6	10.9
Muesli, Fruit, Nut, & Seeds, Classic, Dorset Cereals*	1 Serving/45g	170	3.7	378	10.2	62	8.3	7
Muesli, Fruit, Nuts & Seeds, Dorset Cereals*	1 Serving/45g	172	4	383	10	58	8.9	8.6
Muesli, Fruit, Sainsbury's*	1 Serving/40g	132	1.8	330	8.1	64.3	4.5	9.6
Muesli, Fruit, Waitrose*	1 Serving/30g	101	1.4	338	7.2	66.8	4.7	6.8
Muesli, Fruity, Crownfield, Lidl*	1 Serving/50g	213	7.2	426	7.4	62.6	14.4	8.4
Muesli, Fruity, Sainsbury's*	1 Serving/20g	69	0.5	344	5.9	71.6	2.5	5.7
Muesli, GF, Nature's Harvest, Holland & Barrett*	1 Serving/60g	234	7.8	390	14.1	54.1	13	3.3
Muesli, Golden Sun, Lidl*	1 Serving/40g	144	3.9	360	8	60	9.8	7.5
Muesli, Luxury Fruit, Harvest Morn, Aldi*	1 Serving/50g	179	2.3	358	7.2	69	4.6	5.6
Muesli, Luxury, Finest, Tesco*	1 Serving/50g	197	6.6	394	8.3	60.8	13.1	5.4
Muesli, Natural, Jordans*	1 Serving/40g	142	1.4	354	12	62.6	3.6	11.6
Muesli, Natural, No Added Sugar or Salt, Jordans*	1 Serving/45g	165	1.8	366	10	68	3.9	9.2
Muesli, No Added Sugar Or Salt, Organic, Jordans*	1 Serving/50g	175	4.4	350	9.2	58.4	8.8	9.3
Muesli, No Added Sugar, Crownfield, Lidl*	1 Serving/45g	168	2.7	373	12.4	63.1	6	8.4
Muesli, No Added Sugar, Waitrose*	1 Serving/40g	146	2.5	364	12	64.9	6.3	6.7
Muesli, Orchard Fruit, & Berry, Waitrose*	1 Serving/45g	155	1.5	345	8.4	66.8	3.3	7.3
Muesli, Really Nutty, Dorset Cereals*	1 Serving/70g	253	6.1	362	9.8	61.1	8.7	6.3
Muesli, Really Nutty, Simply Sumptuous, Lidl*	1 Serving/45g	167	3.9	371	9.5	59.2	8.7	8.9
Muesli, Simply Delicious, Dorset Cereals*	1 Serving/45g	166	3.3	368	9.6	61.5	7.3	9
Muesli, Simply Fruity, As Sold, Dorset Cereals*	1 Serving/45g	157	1.3	349	8.6	68.4	2.9	7.3
Muesli, Simply Sumptuous, Luxury Fruit, Lidl*	1 Serving/45g	154	1.5	343	6.5	68.7	3.3	6.2
Muesli, Simply, Sainsbury's*	1 Serving/45g	160	2.3	355	11.2	61.5	5.1	9.2
Muesli, Six Nut, Finest, Tesco*	1 Serving/50g	224	9.6	448	14.2	50.2	19.3	8.4
Muesli, Super Seed, Rude Health*	1 Serving/15g	59	1.9	392	12.7	52.9	12.4	10.5
Muesli, Swiss Style, No Added Salt or Sugar, Sainsbury's*	1 Serving/50g	178	3	357	10.9	64.9	6	6
Muesli, Swiss Style, No Added Sugar or Salt, Asda*	1 Serving/50g	182	3.5	363	11	64	7	8
Muesli, Swiss Style, No Added Sugar, CBY, Asda*	1 Serving/45g	166	2.5	369	11	65	5.6	7.6
Muesli, Swiss Style, No Added Sugar, Lidl*	1 Serving/30g	111	1.8	371	10.9	64.5	6	7.8
Muesli, Swiss Style, No Added Sugar, Tesco*	1 Serving/50g	183	3	367	11.2	62.4	6.1	8.7
Muesli, Swiss Style, Smart Price, Asda*	1 Serving/60g	222	3.6	370	9	70	6	10
Muesli, Swiss Style, Tesco*	1 Serving/50g	189	3.1	378	10.4	67	6.2	6.4
Muesli, Swiss, No Added Sugar or Salt, Tesco*	1 Serving/40g	147	2.4	367	11.2	62.4	6.1	8.6
Muesli, Swiss, Original, Harvest Morn, Aldi*	1 Serving/45g	164	2.1	365	10	65	4.7	10
Muesli, The Ultimate, Organic, Rude Health*	1 Serving/50g	163	4.5	326	10.8	50.5	9	12.3
Muesli, Toasted Spelt, Barley, Oat Flakes, Dorset Cereals*	1 Serving/40g	148	4.5	371	9.5	57.9	11.3	7.4
Muesli, Tropical, Sainsbury's*	1 Serving/50g	182	3.4	365	6.5	69.4	6.8	6.4
Muesli, Waitrose*	1 Serving/45g	172	4.5	383	10	59.6	10	7.4
Muesli, Whole Wheat, No Added Sugar & Salt, Tesco*	1 Serving/40g	154	5	386	9.5	59.1	12.4	7.4
Muesli, Wholewheat, Wholefoods, Morrisons*	1 Serving/30g	110	2.5	366	9.8	59	8.2	8.7
Muesli, with Berries, Swiss, Dry, Love Life, Waitrose*	1 Serving/45g	172	4.3	383	13.5	55.7	9.6	9.8
Multigrain Boulders, Tesco*	1 Serving/30g	112	0.4	375	8.2	82.3	1.3	3.6
Multigrain Flakes with Fruit & Nuts, Aldi*	1 Serving/30g	108	0.7	360	7.5	77.1	2.4	4.5
Multigrain Flakes, with Fruit, Tesco*	1 Serving/40g	147	0.9	367	7.2	77.3	2.2	4.7
Multigrain Hoops, Free From, Tesco*	1 Serving/30g	113	1	376	7.4	77.3	3.2	4.2
Multigrain Hoops, Harvest Morn, Aldi*	1 Serving/30g	109	0.9	364	9.3	69	2.9	12
Multigrain, Fitnesse, Nestle*	1 Serving/30g	109	0.4	363	8	79.8	1.3	5.1
Multigrain, Hoops, Average	***1 Serving/30g***	***112***	***1.1***	***374***	***6.6***	***77.4***	***3.6***	***6.1***

	Measure	per Measure		Nutrition Values per 100g / 100ml				
	INFO/WEIGHT	KCAL	FAT	KCAL	PROT	CARB	FAT	FIBRE
BREAKFAST CEREAL								
Nesquik, Chocolatey Corn & Rice, Nestle*	1 Serving/30g	111	0.5	369	8.4	76	1.7	8.7
Nuts, Clusters, & Seeds, Protein, Special K, Kellogg's*	1 Serving/40g	157	2.8	392	13	65	7	8.3
Oat Bran, Fine Cut, Dry Weight, Whites*	1 Serving/30g	108	1.5	361	11.8	65	5	8.7
Oat Bran, Hodgson Mill*	1 Serving/40g	48	1.2	120	6	23	3	6
Oat Clusters, Triple Chocolate Crunch, M&S*	1 Serving/45g	212	8.9	471	8.5	61.9	19.8	5.6
Oat Granola, Quaker*	1 Serving/50g	206	4.4	411	8.6	73	8.8	5.2
Oat Granola, Raisin, Quaker*	1 Serving/45g	188	4.1	418	8	70.9	9.1	6.9
Oatbran 100%, Pure & Simple, Mornflake*	1 Serving/40g	146	3.8	364	13.4	47.3	9.4	18.2
Oatbran Flakes, Nature's Path*	1 Serving/30g	124	1.4	414	8.7	83	4.7	6.7
Oatbran Sprinkles, Mornflake*	1 Serving/40g	146	3.8	364	13.4	47.3	9.4	18.2
Oatbran, Original Pure, Mornflake*	1 Serving/30g	104	2.9	345	14.8	49.7	9.7	15.2
Oatibix Flakes, Red Berries, Oatibix*	1 Serving/30g	121	2.5	403	11	67	8.3	8.1
Oatibix, Flakes, Weetabix*	1 Serving/50g	190	2.8	381	9.5	73.2	5.6	3.5
Oatibix, Original, Bitesize, Weetabix*	1 Serving/36g	133	2.4	370	10.6	66.5	6.8	10.1
Oatibix, Weetabix*	2 Biscuits/48g	189	3.8	394	12.5	64.3	8	7.3
Oatmeal, Raw	***1oz/28g***	***112***	***2.4***	***401***	***12.4***	***72.8***	***8.7***	***6.8***
Oats, Apple, Cinnamon, Amisa*	1 Serving/40g	141	2.2	352	11.6	59.7	5.5	8.6
Oats, Easy, Original, Sachet, As Prepared, Sainsbury's*	1 Sachet/27g	190	5.4	704	35.2	90	20	10.7
Oats, Golden Syrup Flavour, Instant, Hot, Waitrose*	1 Serving/39g	153	2.3	393	7.8	77.4	5.8	6
Organic, Weetabix*	2 Biscuits/38g	134	0.7	358	11.5	68.6	2	10
Pillows, Choco Nut, Free From, Tesco*	1 Serving/30g	136	4.7	453	6.4	70.8	15.6	2.1
Porage Oats, Old Fashioned, Dry, Scotts*	1 Serving/40g	142	3.2	355	11	60	8	9
Porage Oats, Original, Dry, Scotts*	1 Serving/40g	142	3.2	355	11	60	8	9
Porage Oats, Original, So-Easy, Dry, Scotts*	1 Sachet/30g	109	2.6	364	11	60	8.5	9
Porage Oats, Syrup Swirl, So-Easy, Dry, Scotts*	1 Sachet/37g	135	2.2	366	8	70	6	6.5
Porridge Oats, & Bran, Co-Op*	1 Serving/40g	141	2.8	353	12.5	60	7	12
Porridge Oats, Banana, Oat So Simple, Quaker*	1 Sachet/35g	134	2.3	385	9.1	67.6	6.5	7.4
Porridge Oats, Co-Op*	1 Serving/40g	144	3.2	360	12	61	8	9
Porridge Oats, Cocoa, Banana, Allplants*	1 Serving/172g	255	8.4	148	4.7	19	4.9	3.2
Porridge Oats, Dry Weight, Value, Tesco*	1 Serving/50g	180	4	359	11	60.4	8.1	8.5
Porridge Oats, Everyday Essentials, Aldi*	1 Serving/40g	162	2.6	405	12	70	6.4	8.9
Porridge Oats, GF, Sachets, Made Without Wheat, M&S*	1 Sachet/32g	116	1.6	362	12	63.8	4.9	7.1
Porridge Oats, Golden Syrup, Asda*	1 Sachet/36g	137	2.1	381	9.3	70	5.7	6.8
Porridge Oats, Mornflake*	1 Serving/40g	147	3.4	367	12.1	56.1	8.4	9.1
Porridge Oats, Organic, Kavanagh's, Aldi*	1 Serving/40g	148	2.1	370	12	64	5.3	8.6
Porridge Oats, Organic, Tesco*	1 Serving/50g	184	4.2	368	12.1	56.1	8.4	10
Porridge Oats, Original, Asda*	1 Sachet/27g	101	2	375	12	61	7.4	8.4
Porridge Oats, Original, Big Pot, As Sold, Quaker*	1 Pot/67g	251	3.9	374	15	62.4	5.8	6.4
Porridge Oats, Raspberry, Chia, & Pumpkin, Moma Foods*	1 Pack/35g	132	3.9	378	13	51.8	11.1	9.9
Porridge Oats, Rolled, Tesco*	1 Serving/50g	180	4	359	11	60.4	8.1	8.5
Porridge Oats, Scottish, Hamlyns*	1 Serving/40g	154	3.1	384	11.2	63.2	7.7	8.7
Porridge Oats, Scottish, Organic, Sainsbury's*	1 Serving/45g	172	2.2	383	10	74.4	5	7.9
Porridge Oats, Scottish, Tesco*	1 Serving/50g	180	4	359	11	60.4	8.1	8.5
Porridge, Almond Butter, & Pomegranate, Dry, Quaker*	1 Sachet/33g	124	2.1	377	8.9	67	6.5	7.3
Porridge, Apple & Blueberry, Dry, Oat So Simple, Quaker*	1 Sachet/36g	136	2.2	378	8.6	68	6.2	7.2
Porridge, Apple, & Blueberry, Made Up, Quaker*	1 Sachet/36g	221	4.9	614	26.7	91.7	13.6	7.2
Porridge, Apple, Sultana & Cinnamon, M&S*	1 Sachet/40g	144	3	360	10.3	62.3	7.5	8.6
Porridge, Basis, Alnatura*	1 Serving/30g	114	2.6	380	13	58	8.5	9.9
Porridge, Berry Burst, Wholegrain, Instant , M&S*	1 Pot/70g	252	3.3	360	12.6	62.7	4.7	8.4
Porridge, Blueberry, Cranberry, Guava, Made Up, Quaker*	1 Serving/35g	128	2.3	365	9	63	6.7	9.1
Porridge, Blueberry, Frozen, Tesco*	1 Pack/250g	202	4.4	81	3.5	12	1.8	1.7
Porridge, Carrot Cake, Oat Pantry*	1 Serving/40g	159	5.2	398	11	57	13	7.5
Porridge, Cherry Bakewell, Oat Pantry*	1 Serving/40g	157	6	393	9.5	52	15	7.3

	Measure INFO/WEIGHT	per Measure KCAL	FAT	Nutrition Values per 100g / 100ml KCAL	PROT	CARB	FAT	FIBRE
BREAKFAST CEREAL								
Porridge, Chocolate Orange, Oat Pantry*	1 Serving/40g	162	4.8	404	9.8	60	12	7.8
Porridge, Cinnamon, Protein, Dry, Oat So Simple, Quaker*	1 Sachet/46g	177	2.9	384	20	59	6.2	5.8
Porridge, Coconut, & Chia, Dry, Moma Foods*	1 Serving/55g	222	8.6	403	10.6	55.1	15.6	9.3
Porridge, Coconut, Rice, & Grain, Pot, Waitrose*	1 Pot/250g	258	12.5	103	2	10.8	5	2.8
Porridge, Coconut, Sachet, Asda*	1 Sachet/36g	135	2.2	375	11	65	6.1	7.9
Porridge, Coconut, with Lime, Pot, As Sold, Wolfy's*	1 Pot/110g	456	12.8	415	8.6	66	11.6	6.6
Porridge, Complete Protein, Bulk Powders*	1 Serving/50g	188	3.1	377	29.9	47	6.2	6.5
Porridge, Cranberry & Raisin, Dry, Moma Foods*	1 Serving/70g	248	2.7	355	13.9	63.6	3.9	6.2
Porridge, Fastpot, As Sold, Lighter Life*	1 Pot/43g	153	3.6	355	30	33.4	8.4	12.7
Porridge, Fresh, Double Cream, & Demerara Sugar, M&S*	1 Pot/200g	244	13.6	122	3.9	10.8	6.8	1.2
Porridge, GF, Oat So Simple, Quaker*	1 Sachet/35g	130	2.5	370	13.2	58.5	7.2	9.2
Porridge, Gingerbread, Pot, Made Up, Sainsbury's*	1 Pot/226g	215	2.5	95	3.4	17.2	1.1	1.1
Porridge, Golden Honey, Oatibix, Weetabix*	1 Serving/40g	145	2.6	363	9.2	66.7	6.6	7
Porridge, Golden Syrup, Dry, Oat So Simple, Quaker*	1 Sachet/36g	143	2.7	398	8.7	71	7.4	5.9
Porridge, Golden Syrup, High Protein, Pot, Fuel 10K*	1 Pot/70g	258	4.1	369	18.6	57.6	5.9	6.3
Porridge, Golden Syrup, Instant, As Consumed, Slim Fast*	1 Sachet/29g	99	1.3	340	17.4	53.2	4.6	7.9
Porridge, Golden Syrup, Made Up, Quaker*	1 Sachet/36g	228	5.8	633	26.7	94.4	16.1	5.8
Porridge, Golden Syrup, Pot, As Sold, Quaker*	1 Pot/57g	213	2.9	373	14	66	5.1	5.5
Porridge, Golden Syrup, Prepared, Oatilicious, Lidl*	1 Sachet/39g	140	1.5	358	8.8	69	3.9	6
Porridge, Honey & Vanilla, Dry, Oat So Simple, Quaker*	1 Sachet/34g	129	2.2	381	8.8	68	6.4	7.2
Porridge, Instant, Sweet Cinnamon, Harvest Morn, Aldi*	1 Pot/57g	211	2.6	371	15	64	4.5	7.8
Porridge, Made with Semi Skimmed Milk, Waitrose*	1 Serving/50g	277	7.5	554	24.6	80.4	15	8.6
Porridge, Maple & Pecan, Dry, Oat So Simple, Quaker*	1 Sachet/35g	133	2.3	376	8.4	67	6.5	6.9
Porridge, Maple Syrup Flavour, Pot, As Sold, M&S*	1 Pot/70g	260	2.6	371	11.6	70.7	3.7	4.3
Porridge, Mince Pie, Dry, Sainsbury's*	1 Sachet/36g	135	2.1	375	10.5	66	5.9	7.8
Porridge, Mince Pie, Instant, Pot, Made Up, Sainsbury's*	1 Pot/228g	214	3.2	94	3.4	66	1.4	1.6
Porridge, Multi-Grain, Apple, Raisin, Dry, Quaker*	1 Sachet/35g	131	2.5	374	11	62	7.1	9.3
Porridge, Multigrain, Jordans*	1 Serving/40g	134	2.2	335	10.4	60.9	5.5	10
Porridge, Oat, & Barley, Instant, M&S*	1 Pot/70g	257	4.3	367	11.4	62.2	6.1	9.4
Porridge, Oats, Apple & Blueberry, Instant, Pot, Tesco*	1 Pot/205g	210	2.9	102	3.6	18.1	1.4	1.5
Porridge, Oats, Berry & Cherry, Instant, Pot, Tesco*	1 Pot/225g	207	2.9	92	3.2	16.2	1.3	1.4
Porridge, Oats, Berry, Instant, Free From, Asda*	1 Sachet/27g	98	1.1	364	10	68	4.1	7.6
Porridge, Oats, Cinnamon, Instant, Pot, Tesco*	1 Pot/225g	212	3.2	94	3.3	16.4	1.4	1.4
Porridge, Oats, Dry, Smart Price, Asda*	1 Serving/50g	186	4	372	11	60	8	8
Porridge, Oats, Golden Syrup, Instant, Pot, Tesco*	1 Pot/55g	210	2.7	380	11.4	70	4.9	5.5
Porridge, Oats, Golden Syrup, Sainsbury's*	1 Sachet/39g	143	2.1	367	6.3	73.6	5.3	6.7
Porridge, Oats, Instant, Dry Weight, Essential, Waitrose*	1 Sachet/27g	99	1.6	365	11.9	61.6	5.9	8.9
Porridge, Oats, Irish, Multi Seed, Flahavans*	1 Serving/40g	166	5.3	415	14	55.4	13.3	9
Porridge, Oats, Jumbo, 100% Whole Grain, Dry, Quaker*	1 Serving/40g	150	3.2	374	11	60	8	9
Porridge, Oats, No Added Sugar, Love Life, Waitrose*	1 Pot/60g	224	3.8	373	17.5	57.8	6.4	7.2
Porridge, Oats, Original, Big Bowl, Dry, Quaker*	1 Sachet/39g	142	3	370	11	58	7.7	9
Porridge, Oats, Original, Big Bowl, Made Up Quaker*	1 Sachet/39g	254	7.1	660	31.2	88.3	18.4	9.1
Porridge, Oats, Original, Instant, Pot, Tesco*	1 Pot/256g	208	3.3	81	3.1	13.5	1.3	1.6
Porridge, Oats, Rolled, 100% Whole Grain, Dry, Quaker*	1 Serving/40g	150	3.2	374	11	60	8	9
Porridge, Oats, Twice the Fibre, M&S*	1 Portion/60g	230	3.5	384	10.4	62.6	5.9	19.5
Porridge, Oats, Whole, Chunky, Traditional, Jordans*	1 Serving/40g	143	2.7	358	6.7	63.6	6.8	7.9
Porridge, Original, Diet Chef Ltd*	1 Sachet/40g	157	2.5	392	12	67	6.3	9.8
Porridge, Original, Dry, Oat So Simple, Quaker*	1 Sachet/27g	100	2.1	370	11	59	7.7	9
Porridge, Original, Express, Sachet, Sainsbury's*	1 Pack/27g	100	2.2	370	11	58	8	10.8
Porridge, Original, High Protein, Pot, M&S*	1 Pot/70g	241	3.6	344	24.3	46.3	5.2	7.6
Porridge, Original, Instant, Pot, Made Up, Aldi*	1 Pot/220g	187	2.9	85	4	14	1.3	1.3
Porridge, Original, Made Up, Oat So Simple, Quaker*	1 Sachet/27g	180	5	667	33	88.9	18.5	10.4
Porridge, Original, Pot, As Sold, Oat So Simple, Quaker*	1 Pot/45g	164	2.6	365	17	57	5.8	7

	Measure INFO/WEIGHT	per Measure KCAL	FAT	Nutrition Values per 100g / 100ml KCAL	PROT	CARB	FAT	FIBRE
BREAKFAST CEREAL								
Porridge, Original, Pot, M&S*	1 Pot/70g	250	2.9	357	16.7	59.4	4.2	7.5
Porridge, Original, Pot, Made Up, Asda*	1 Pot/221g	199	2.7	90	3.3	16	1.2	2.1
Porridge, Original, Pot, Made Up, Morrisons*	1 Pot/225g	205	2.7	91	3.5	16	1.2	1.1
Porridge, Original, Ready Brek, Weetabix*	1 Serving/40g	149	3.5	373	11.7	57.9	8.7	7.9
Porridge, Original, Simply, Sachet, Asda*	1 Sachet/27g	96	2.2	356	11	60	8	8
Porridge, Peanut Butter, & Chia Seeds, Oat Pantry*	1 Serving/40g	181	7.5	452	16.8	52	18.8	9
Porridge, Plain, Dry, Moma Foods*	1 Serving/65g	232	2.9	357	18.3	58.3	4.5	6.8
Porridge, Plain, Pot, As Sold, Moma Foods*	1 Pot/70g	250	3.2	357	18.3	58.3	4.5	6.8
Porridge, Protein 360, The Protein Works*	1 Serving/50g	190	3.8	380	27	54	7.5	6.5
Porridge, Raspberry, Apple, & Acai, Dry, Quaker*	1 Sachet/36g	131	2.3	367	9.1	64	6.4	8.8
Porridge, Rice & Buckwheat, Free From, Sainsbury's*	1 Serving/50g	179	0.4	358	6.8	81.1	0.7	1.4
Porridge, Salted Caramel, Protein, Pot, Fuel 10K*	1 Pot/70g	258	4.3	369	18.6	56.6	6.1	6
Porridge, Spiced Sultana, Diet Chef Ltd*	1 Pack/37g	148	2.5	400	9.6	70.8	6.7	8.8
Porridge, Strawberry, Raspberry & Cranberry, Dry, Quaker*	1 Sachet/33g	127	2.2	379	8.9	67.4	6.6	7.3
Porridge, Sultana, Raisin, Cranberry, & Apple, Dry, Quaker*	1 Sachet/39g	143	2.2	371	8.4	68.2	5.7	6.9
Porridge, Sweet Cinnamon, Dry, Oat So Simple, Quaker*	1 Sachet/33g	125	2.2	379	9	67.2	6.6	7.4
Porridge, Traditional, Scottish, Pot, As Sold, Stoats*	1 Pot/60g	216	3.6	361	17.6	59	6	6.6
Porridge, Vanilla, & Blueberry, Made Up, Quaker*	1 Sachet/33g	210	5.3	633	27.7	93.4	16	9.6
Protein Crunch, Chocolate, Weetabix*	1 Serving/30g	114	1	379	20	64	3.2	7
Protein Crunch, Weetabix*	1 Serving/30g	114	0.8	379	20	66	2.5	6.1
Puffed Rice, Average	***1 Serving/30g***	***115***	***0.8***	***382***	***7.1***	***82.2***	***2.8***	***3***
Puffed Rice, Organic, Natural, Kallo*	1 Bowl/25g	92	0.5	370	7	81	2	3
Puffed Wheat, Quaker*	1 Serving/15g	49	0.2	328	15.3	62.4	1.3	5.6
Puffed Wheat, Tesco*	1 Serving/28g	104	0.9	373	13.9	72.2	3.2	5.7
Rainbow Hoops, Asda*	1 Serving/30g	115	0.4	383	10	80	1.5	4.2
Raisin & Almond, Crunchy, Jordans*	1 Serving/45g	186	5.7	412	9.9	61.6	12.6	6.6
Raisin Wheats, Essential, Waitrose*	1 Serving/45g	153	0.7	340	8.4	71.2	1.5	8.4
Raisin Wheats, Kellogg's*	1 Serving/45g	104	0.6	345	9	69	2	9
Raisin, Bran Flakes, Asda*	1 Serving/50g	166	1.5	331	7	69	3	10
Raisin, Oats & More, Nestle*	1 Serving/30g	112	1.4	373	8.9	73.7	4.7	5.8
Raspberry Wheaties, Asda*	1 Serving/45g	150	0.6	333	8	71	1.4	8.4
Red Berries, Additions, Weetabix*	2 Biscuits/43g	152	0.8	350	9.8	67	1.9	13
Red Berries, Special K, Kellogg's*	1 Serving/30g	113	0.4	376	8.9	79	1.5	5.3
Red Berry Benefit, Harvest Morn, Aldi*	1 Pack/50g	186	0.2	372	7.2	82	0.5	3.3
Red Berry, & Almond, Luxury Crunch, Jordans*	1 Serving/40g	176	7.4	441	8.2	60.5	18.5	6.6
Rice & Wheat Flakes, Toasted, Love Life, Waitrose*	1 Serving/30g	115	0.4	382	11.7	79.7	1.3	2.2
Rice Krispies, Kellogg's*	1 Serving/30g	116	0.4	387	7	86	1.2	2
Rice Krispies, Multi-Grain, Shapes, Kellogg's*	1 Serving/30g	111	0.8	370	8	77	2.5	8
Rice Pops, GF, Nestle*	1 Serving/30g	116	0.4	385	7.5	85	1.2	1.5
Rice Snaps, Asda*	1 Serving/28g	105	0.4	376	7	84	1.3	1.5
Rice Snaps, Everyday Value, Tesco*	1 Serving/30g	115	0.3	380	7.5	84.5	0.9	1.4
Rice Snaps, Free From, Tesco*	1 Serving/30g	112	0.3	373	6	84	1	2
Right Balance, Morrisons*	1 Serving/50g	181	1.1	362	6.9	78.6	2.2	5.3
Shredded Wheat, Average	***2 Biscuits/45g***	***157***	***0.8***	***348***	***9***	***77***	***1.8***	***10***
Shredded Wheat, Bitesize, Nestle*	1 Serving/40g	148	0.9	369	11.8	69.6	2.2	11.8
Shredded Wheat, Honey Nut, Nestle*	1 Serving/40g	151	2.6	378	11.2	68.8	6.5	9.4
Shreddies, Coco Orange Flavoured, Nestle*	1 Serving/40g	150	0.8	374	8.5	76.2	2	8.6
Shreddies, Cocoa, Nestle*	1 Serving/40g	148	0.8	371	9.2	75	1.9	9.3
Shreddies, Crunchy Cranberry & Oat Granola, Nestle*	1 Serving/45g	181	3.1	403	13	68	7	7.2
Shreddies, Frosted, Nestle*	1 Serving/45g	166	0.7	370	9.2	76	1.5	9
Shreddies, Frosted, Variety Pack, Nestle*	1 Pack/45g	163	0.6	363	6.7	81.1	1.3	6.8
Shreddies, Honey, Nestle*	1 Serving/45g	169	0.7	375	8.2	78.1	1.5	8.1
Shreddies, Malt Wheats, Tesco*	1 Serving/45g	169	0.9	375	10.3	73.8	2	8.2

	Measure INFO/WEIGHT	per Measure KCAL	per Measure FAT	Nutrition Values per 100g / 100ml KCAL	PROT	CARB	FAT	FIBRE
BREAKFAST CEREAL								
Shreddies, Nestle*	1 Serving/30g	111	0.6	371	10	73.7	1.9	9.9
Special Flakes, Gluten, Wheat, & Milk, Free From, Tesco*	1 Serving/30g	115	0.6	382	6.5	83	2	3
Special Flakes, Honey, Oats, & Almonds, Tesco*	1 Serving/30g	116	0.7	385	7.2	82.5	2.2	3.1
Special Flakes, Peach & Apricot, Morrisons*	1 Serving/30g	112	0.3	373	7	82.3	1.1	3.1
Special Flakes, Red Fruits, Asda*	1 Serving/30g	115	0.4	382	7.1	84	1.3	2.7
Special Flakes, Tesco*	1 Serving/20g	74	0.3	371	11	78.4	1.5	4.3
Special Flakes, with Red Berries, Crownfield, Lidl*	1 Serving/30g	113	0.5	377	6.5	81	1.6	6.4
Special K, Bliss, Strawberry & Chocolate, Kellogg's*	1 Serving/30g	115	0.9	383	13	76	3	2.5
Special K, Kellogg's*	1 Serving/30g	114	0.4	379	14	76	1.5	2.5
Special K, Oats & Honey, Kellogg's*	1 Serving/30g	114	0.9	381	9	77	3	5
Special K, Peach & Apricot, Kellogg's*	1 Serving/30g	112	0.3	373	14	77	1	2.5
Special K, Protein Plus, Kellogg's*	1 Serving/29g	100	3	345	34.5	31	10.3	17.2
Special K, Purple Berries, Kellogg's*	1 Serving/30g	112	0.3	374	13	77	1	3.5
Start, Kellogg's*	1 Serving/30g	117	1	390	8	79	3.5	5
Strawberry Crisp, Asda*	1 Serving/33g	140	3.3	425	9.5	70	10	6.8
Strawberry Crisp, Crownfield, Lidl*	1 Serving/45g	197	5.2	438	9.3	71.9	11.6	4.2
Strawberry, & Raspberry, Crisp, Morrisons*	1 Serving/45g	194	5.2	431	8.5	70.3	11.5	6
Strawberry, Alpen*	1 Serving/40g	144	1.9	359	9.4	69.5	4.8	7.9
Sultana Bran, Asda*	1 Serving/40g	140	0.8	351	9.5	67	2.1	13
Sultana Bran, Co-Op*	1 Serving/40g	130	1.2	325	9	66	3	11
Sultana Bran, HL, Tesco*	1 Serving/30g	98	0.6	325	8.2	68	1.9	12
Sultana Bran, Morrisons*	1 Serving/30g	98	0.9	325	8.8	65.8	3	11.4
Sultana Bran, Waitrose*	1 Serving/30g	97	0.6	324	8.2	68.6	1.9	11.6
Triple Chocolate Crisp, Co-Op*	1 Serving/40g	170	5	425	8	67.5	12.5	4.8
Triple Chocolate Crunch, Made Without Wheat, M&S*	1 Serving/45g	209	8	465	8.6	65.1	17.8	5.2
Twinkies, Post*	1 Serving/30g	139	5.4	462	2.6	74.4	17.9	2.6
Weet-Bix, Blends, Multi-Grain, Sanitarium*	2 Biscuits/48g	185	2.1	385	10.7	70.2	4.4	8.9
Weetabix, Banana, Weetabix*	1 Serving/44g	157	0.9	357	10	70.4	2	9.8
Weetabix, Chocolate, Weetabix*	2 Biscuits/45g	166	1.8	368	10.1	67.9	4	10
Weetaflakes, Weetabix*	1 Serving/30g	102	0.4	340	8.9	72.9	1.4	11
Weetos, Chocolate, Weetabix*	1 Serving/30g	113	1.5	378	8.4	75.1	4.9	5.8
Wheat Biscuits, Average	***2 Biscuits/38g***	***130***	***0.8***	***347***	***11.7***	***68.4***	***2.2***	***9.9***
Wheat Biscuits, Banana, Fruit Bowl*	2 Biscuits/40g	153	2	382	10.9	69.5	5	7.5
Wheat Bisks, Chocolate, Asda*	2 Biscuits/43g	158	1.5	367	10	69	3.4	10
Wheat Puffs, Honey Monster*	1 Serving/30g	107	0.5	357	7.1	74	1.8	8.4
Wheat Shreds, Bitesize, Crownfield, Lidl*	1 Serving/40g	142	0.8	356	10.6	67	1.9	14
Wheat Shreds, Harvest Morn, Aldi*	2 Shreds/45g	156	0.8	346	13	64	1.8	13
Wheaties, Choco, Harvest Morn, Aldi*	1 Serving/40g	149	0.7	372	10.5	72.5	1.8	0
Wheats, Mince Pie, Sainsbury's*	1 Serving/45g	138	0.6	307	7.8	65.5	1.4	8.5
Whole O's, Natures Path*	1 Serving/40g	160	2	400	6.7	83	5	10
Wholegrain Hoops, Goldenvale, Aldi*	1 Serving/30g	111	0.8	371	6.9	74	2.6	10.7
Wholegrain Wheats, Classic, Organic, Kellogg's*	1 Serving/40g	148	1	371	14	68	2.5	10
Wholegrain, Apricot, Wheats, Sainsbury's*	1 Serving/45g	151	0.6	335	8	71.3	1.4	8.3
Wholegrain, Fruit & Fibre, Sainsbury's*	1 Serving/40g	149	2.3	372	9.3	66.1	5.7	9.4
Wholegrain, Mini Wheats, Sainsbury's*	1 Serving/40g	144	0.7	359	11.8	68.2	1.8	11.2
Wholegrain, Minis, Weetabix*	1 Serving/40g	149	0.8	372	10.2	73.2	2	10
Wholesome Crunch, Granola, Pecan & Brazil Nut, Quaker*	1 Serving/45g	189	5	420	11.1	61.8	11.1	13.2
Wholesome Crunch, Granola, Goji & Blueberry, Quaker*	1 Serving/45g	181	3.6	402	11	64.5	7.9	13.5
Yoghurt & Raspberry, Crisp, Sainsbury's*	1 Serving/45g	191	6.7	424	7.5	65.2	14.8	6.4
BRESAOLA								
Average	***1 Serving/28g***	***51***	***1***	***181***	***33.6***	***0.4***	***3.7***	***0.2***
BROCCOLI								
Green, Boiled, Average	***1 Serving/80g***	***19***	***0.6***	***24***	***3.1***	***1.1***	***0.8***	***2.3***

	Measure INFO/WEIGHT	per Measure KCAL	FAT	Nutrition Values per 100g / 100ml KCAL	PROT	CARB	FAT	FIBRE
BROCCOLI								
Green, Raw, Average	***1 Serving/80g***	***24***	***0.7***	***30***	***3.7***	***1.6***	***0.8***	***2.5***
Purple Sprouting, Boiled, Average	***1 Serving/80g***	***15***	***0.5***	***19***	***2.1***	***1.3***	***0.6***	***2.3***
Purple Sprouting, Raw	***1oz/28g***	***10***	***0.3***	***35***	***3.9***	***2.6***	***1.1***	***3.5***
Steamed, Average	***1 Serving/100g***	***24***	***0.8***	***24***	***3.1***	***1.1***	***0.8***	***2.3***
Tenderstem, Average	***1 Serving/80g***	***28***	***0.4***	***35***	***4.1***	***2.9***	***0.6***	***2.3***
BROWNIES								
Average	***1 Brownie/60g***	***243***	***10.1***	***405***	***4.6***	***0***	***16.8***	***0***
Billionaire, Fingers, Thorntons*	1 Finger/21g	87	4.1	423	5.8	54.5	19.7	0
Chocolate Chip, Cadbury*	1 Brownie/25g	116	7.2	465	4.8	46	29	3
Chocolate Chip, Free From, Morrisons*	1 Slice/30g	143	8	478	6	52.5	26.5	2.9
Chocolate, Average	***1 Serving/100g***	***446***	***22.3***	***446***	***5.9***	***55.6***	***22.3***	***2.2***
Chocolate, Chunky, Belgian, M&S*	1 Brownie/55g	242	11.2	440	6.2	57.7	20.3	2.5
Chocolate, Double, Bites, Amaze, Cadbury*	1 Bite/14g	65	3.3	470	5.3	56.7	24.1	3.1
Chocolate, Double, Mini Bites, Sainsbury's*	1 Serving/18g	73	3.1	406	5.5	55.9	17.2	2.6
Chocolate, Double, Weight Watchers*	1 Dessert/86g	174	3.5	202	4.5	35.9	4.1	1.9
Chocolate, Fudge, Mini, Thorntons*	1 Bite/14g	61	2.8	435	5.6	57.4	20	0
Chocolate, Fudgy, M&S*	1 Brownie/87g	400	21.9	460	4.8	56.9	25.2	3
Chocolate, Mini Bites, Asda*	1 Brownie/15g	62	3	420	5	55	20	1.4
Chocolate, Orange, Organic, The Village Bakery*	1 Brownie/30g	126	6.7	421	5	50.5	22.2	0.9
Chocolate, Wheat & GF, Mrs Crimble's*	1 Slice/48g	180	9.6	379	4.2	47.9	20.3	1.5
Chocolate, Wicked Kitchen, Tesco*	½ Brownie/110g	406	21.1	369	6.5	41.1	19.2	3
Fudge, Organic, Honeyrose Bakery*	1 Brownie/55g	241	9.9	439	5.3	62.1	18	3.5
Mini, The Skinny Bakery*	1 Brownie/17g	38	1.4	230	6.4	34.6	8.5	5.2
Oreo, Creme Filled, Nabisco*	½ Brownie/43g	180	8	419	4.6	60.5	18.6	0
Salted Caramel, Costa*	1 Slice/85g	398	23.7	468	5.4	47.6	27.9	0
BRUSCHETTA								
Cheese & Tomato, Asda*	1 Bruschetta/38g	68	1.7	180	8.6	26	4.6	2.9
Garlic, & Parsley, Valentina*	1 Bruschetta/10g	55	3.1	538	8.4	56.9	30.4	0
Red Pepper & Onion, Brunchetta, Golden Vale*	1 Pack/90g	266	17.1	296	14.6	17	19	1.3
Toasted, Olive Oil & Sea Salt, Tesco*	1 Serving/30g	126	4.6	420	11.5	58.7	15.5	4.5
Tomato, & Oregano, Valentina*	1 Piece/10g	47	2.2	473	9.8	58	21.5	0
Tomato, Tesco*	¼ Jar/48g	31	1.4	65	1.7	6.5	3	2.5
BRUSSELS SPROUTS								
& Sweet Chestnuts, Asda*	1 Serving/100g	73	1.7	73	3.1	11	1.7	4.2
& Bacon, Oven Baked, Iceland*	¼ Pack/83g	85	3.5	103	4.2	10	4.3	3.8
Boiled, Average	***1 Serving/80g***	***27***	***1***	***33***	***3***	***3***	***1.2***	***3.3***
Button, Raw, Average	***1 Serving/80g***	***28***	***1***	***36***	***3.3***	***2.8***	***1.3***	***3***
Canned, Drained	***1oz/28g***	***5***	***0.2***	***17***	***1.6***	***1.5***	***0.6***	***1.6***
Raw, Average	***1 Serving/80g***	***28***	***0.8***	***35***	***3.3***	***3.1***	***1***	***2.9***
Steamed, Average	***1 Serving/100g***	***35***	***1.3***	***35***	***3.1***	***3.2***	***1.3***	***3.5***
with Bacon, Smoked, & Chestnuts, M&S*	1/5 Pack/175g	219	8.2	125	5.1	13.9	4.7	3.5
with Chestnuts, & Bacon, Tesco*	1 Serving/100g	151	6.6	151	4.7	14.4	6.6	7.7
BUBBLE & SQUEAK								
Fried in Vegetable Oil	***1oz/28g***	***35***	***2.5***	***124***	***1.4***	***9.8***	***9.1***	***1.5***
BUCKWHEAT								
Average	***1oz/28g***	***102***	***0.4***	***364***	***8.1***	***84.9***	***1.5***	***2.1***
Puffed, GF, Holland & Barrett*	1 Serving/30g	112	1.2	375	9.7	78	3.9	5.1
BULGUR WHEAT								
& Quinoa Mix, Cooked, Tesco*	1 Serving/80g	122	1.1	153	5.2	28.3	1.4	3.1
& Quinoa Mix, Dry Weight, Tesco*	1 Serving/30g	122	1.1	407	14	75.3	3.7	8.3
Dry Weight, Average	***1oz/28g***	***99***	***0.5***	***353***	***9.7***	***76.3***	***1.7***	***8***
Green Lentils & Barley, Wholefoods, Tesco*	½ Pack/125g	225	2.8	180	7.5	29.9	2.2	5.2
Lemon, & Coriander, Steamers, Waitrose*	1 Sachet/140g	162	2.2	116	4.1	18.9	1.6	4.8

B

	Measure INFO/WEIGHT	per Measure KCAL	per Measure FAT	Nutrition Values per 100g / 100ml KCAL	PROT	CARB	FAT	FIBRE
BUNS								
Assorted, Cottage Bakery *	1 Bun/25g	104	4.7	416	4.1	57.7	18.9	0
Bao, Chicken, Morrisons*	1 Bun/17g	38	0.9	224	8.8	32.9	5.3	2.4
Bao, M&S*	3 Buns/84g	213	1.3	253	6.4	52.5	1.5	2.1
Bao, no Filling, M&S*	3 Buns/84g	213	1.3	253	6.4	52.5	1.5	2.1
Bath, Tesco*	1 Bun/80g	262	8.9	328	8	48.9	11.1	5.8
Belgian, Asda*	1 Bun/133g	464	19.9	350	4.8	49	15	2.2
Belgian, Co-Op*	1 Bun/118g	413	15.3	350	5	54	13	2
Belgian, Iced, Essential, Waitrose*	1 Bun/89g	292	7.6	328	5.7	56	8.5	2.2
Belgian, Sainsbury's*	1 Bun/110g	398	11.3	362	6.1	61.3	10.3	1.9
Belgian, Tesco*	1 Bun/123g	438	15.7	356	5.2	54.9	12.8	2.2
Brioche, Gourmet, Bundys*	1 Bun/80g	207	3.4	259	9.2	47.6	4.2	3.1
Brioche, Sliced, The Best, Morrisons*	1 Roll/54g	163	3.3	302	9.4	51.4	6.2	1.7
Burger Building, Roberts*	1 Bun/90g	274	3.2	304	8.9	59.1	3.6	2.8
Burger, Avoca-Dough, M&S*	1 Bun/60g	161	3.2	268	8.6	44.5	5.3	4
Burger, Brioche, Mega, Baker Street*	1 Bun/75g	279	11.7	372	10.5	45.8	15.6	3.3
Burger, Brioche, Seeded, Sliced, Specially Selected, Aldi*	1 Bun/50g	160	4.5	320	9.2	50	9	2.6
Burger, Brioche, Vegan, Specially Selected, Aldi*	1 Bun/62g	193	4.3	311	9.6	52	6.9	2.1
Burger, GF, Schnitzer*	1 Bun/63g	132	3	210	3	36	4.8	5.4
Burger, Maitre Jean Pierre, Lidl*	1 Bun/46g	129	2.5	280	9.7	46.1	5.5	0
Burger, Mega, Baker Street*	1 Bun/75g	221	4.1	295	9.3	50.2	5.5	3.7
Burger, Plain, Rowan Hill Bakery, Lidl*	1 Bun/51g	143	2.8	280	9.7	46.1	5.5	3.5
Burger, Seeded, Village Bakery, Aldi*	1 Roll/76g	204	3	268	10.7	46	4	4
Burger, Sesame Seed, Sliced, Bundy's*	1 Bun/50g	136	2.5	271	9.3	46	5	2.5
Burger, with Sesame, Dulcesol*	1 Bun/139g	385	7	277	9.5	47	5	3.2
Butterfly, GF, Free From, Asda*	1 Bun/37g	159	7.7	434	3.2	58	21	0.5
Cha-Siu, Superior Food*	1 Bun/50g	120	2.6	240	9.2	39.2	5.2	1.4
Chelsea	***1 Bun/78g***	***285***	***10.8***	***366***	***7.8***	***56.1***	***13.8***	***1.7***
Choux, Caramel, Asda*	1 Bun/189g	745	51	394	4.3	33.5	27	1.3
Choux, Chocolate, Tesco*	1 Bun/74g	259	18.1	350	7.3	24.4	24.5	1.2
Choux, Fresh Cream, Tesco*	1 Bun/95g	340	23.7	358	4.9	28.5	24.9	0.9
Choux, M&S*	1 Bun/78g	247	17.3	317	5.4	25.6	22.2	0.3
Cinnamon, Bakers Selection, Asda*	1 Bun/97g	348	13.6	359	6.3	51	14	1.7
Cinnamon, Kit, Bakedin*	1 Bun/52g	186	0.5	357	8.2	78	0.9	0
Currant	***1 Bun/60g***	***178***	***4.5***	***296***	***7.6***	***52.7***	***7.5***	***0***
Finger, Iced, Essential, Waitrose*	1 Bun/40g	139	3.5	347	6.7	59.2	8.7	2.6
Fruit, Waitrose*	1 Bun/54g	155	2.3	287	8.1	54	4.3	1.6
Fruited, Iced & Spiced, M&S*	1 Bun/85g	270	4.6	318	4.9	61.3	5.4	2.2
Hamburger, Kaiser, Gourmet, Bundys*	1 Bun/70g	192	2.5	274	9.3	48.9	3.6	2.9
Hot Cross	***1 Bun/50g***	***156***	***3.5***	***312***	***7.4***	***58.5***	***7***	***1.7***
Hot Cross, Asda*	1 Bun/60g	190	3.8	317	10	55	6.3	3.3
Hot Cross, BGTY, Sainsbury's*	1 Bun/70g	186	2	266	7.1	51.7	2.8	2.7
Hot Cross, Bramley Apple & Cinnamon, Waitrose*	1 Bun/70g	194	2.7	277	7.7	52.2	3.8	1.5
Hot Cross, Bramley Apple, & Cinnamon, Finest, Tesco*	1 Bun/70g	191	3.7	273	7.5	47.4	5.3	3
Hot Cross, Chilli, & Cheese, M&S*	1 Bun/65g	179	6.4	275	11.3	34.2	9.8	2.2
Hot Cross, Chocolate, & Orange, Waitrose*	1 Bun/70g	217	6.2	310	10.6	45.1	8.9	3.3
Hot Cross, Chocolate, Free From, Sainsbury's*	1 Bun/70g	202	8.4	288	3.7	36.4	12	9.6
Hot Cross, Co-Op*	1 Bun/60g	174	3.3	290	8.2	51	5.5	2.5
Hot Cross, Extra Fruity, Finest, Tesco*	1 Bun/80g	205	2.2	256	7.2	48.9	2.7	3.7
Hot Cross, Free From, Tesco*	1 Bun/70g	161	2.6	231	4.2	41.2	3.7	7.8
Hot Cross, Fruity, Free From, Sainsbury's*	1 Bun/70g	195	6.2	279	3.3	41.4	8.8	10.2
Hot Cross, GF, Free From, Morrisons*	1 Bun/68g	148	2.7	217	4.3	37.3	3.9	7.6
Hot Cross, GF, M&S*	1 Bun/70g	206	4.1	294	2.9	54.1	5.9	6.1
Hot Cross, Jackson's of Yorkshire*	1 Bun/78g	221	2.6	285	8.2	57.2	3.3	2.8

	Measure INFO/WEIGHT	per Measure KCAL	FAT	Nutrition Values per 100g / 100ml KCAL	PROT	CARB	FAT	FIBRE
BUNS								
Hot Cross, Luxury, Rowan Hill Bakery, Lidl*	1 Bun/75g	204	3.5	272	8.3	47	4.7	4
Hot Cross, Made Without Wheat, M&S*	1 Bun/65g	185	3.5	284	2.7	52.1	5.4	8.3
Hot Cross, Mini, M&S*	1 Bun/41g	110	1.4	265	7.8	51.4	3.4	3.7
Hot Cross, Morrisons*	1 Bun/72g	178	1.4	247	7.4	49.9	2	3.3
Hot Cross, Richly Fruited, Bakery, Waitrose*	1 Bun/31g	89	1.4	288	7.8	52.1	4.6	3.3
Hot Cross, Richly Fruited, Tesco*	1 Bun/70g	180	2.2	257	8.8	56.7	3.1	3.3
Hot Cross, Salted Caramel, & Chocolate Chip, Tesco*	1 Bun/72g	205	4.5	284	8.1	47.1	6.2	3.8
Hot Cross, St Clements, Waitrose*	1 Bun/70g	188	1.9	268	7.7	51.6	2.7	3.1
Hot Cross, Sticky Toffee, The Best, Morrisons*	1 Bun/77g	222	3.5	288	6.8	52.8	4.6	4
Hot Cross, Triple Berry, Specially Selected, Aldi*	1 Bun/70g	185	1.5	264	6.9	53	2.1	3.3
Hot Cross, Triple Chocolate, Lidl*	1 Bun/70g	201	5.3	287	9	44.1	7.6	3.1
Hot Cross, White, Sainsbury's*	1 Bun/70g	199	3.4	284	7.9	50.6	4.8	3.4
Hot Cross, Wholemeal, Asda*	1 Bun/70g	182	4.2	262	9	43	6	6
Hot Cross, Wholemeal, Waitrose*	1 Bun/66g	176	3.2	267	9.6	43.2	4.9	5.7
Iced Finger, Average	***1 Bun/40g***	***130***	***3.1***	***325***	***7.2***	***57***	***7.7***	***2.3***
Mushroom, Steamed, M&S*	1 Bun/25g	58	1.2	231	5.5	40	4.9	2.4
Original, Bundys*	1 Bun/50g	130	1.7	261	9.2	47.4	3.4	2.3
Schoggi-Weggli, Co-Op*	1 Bun/72g	294	10.8	409	9.5	59	15	0
Vanilla Iced, Soft, M&S*	1 Bun/39g	125	3.1	320	7.6	54.9	8	2.9
BURGERS								
& Chips, Heat Me, Eat Me*	1 Pack/203g	440	17.6	217	7.5	26	8.7	2.3
American Style, Tesco*	1 Burger/125g	250	9.1	200	13	20.4	7.3	3.9
Aubergine, & Feta, Aromatic & Minty, Waitrose*	1 Burger/101g	238	12.9	235	5.2	22.3	12.7	5.3
BBQ, Gourmet, Flame Grilled, Rustlers*	1 Burger/215g	593	27.7	276	14.6	24.7	12.9	0
Bean, BBQ, Monterey Jack, Oven Baked, Tesco*	1 Burger/131g	312	16.4	238	6.1	22.4	12.5	5.6
Bean, Chilli, Crisp & Spicy, Frozen, Cooked, Waitrose*	1 Burger/95g	226	8.3	238	5.8	31	8.7	6.1
Bean, Mexican Style, Meat Free, Tesco*	1 Burger/106g	214	9.6	202	4.8	22	9.1	6.4
Bean, Mexican, Spiced, Free From, Sainsbury's*	1 Burger/114g	227	10	199	5.6	21.2	8.8	6.1
Bean, Nacho, Spicy, Iceland*	1 Burger/140g	326	16.5	233	6.9	20.1	11.8	4.4
Bean, Spicy Veg, with Chipotle Chilli, Good Life*	1 Burger/108g	227	10.5	210	5.8	20	9.7	8.9
Bean, Spicy, BGTY, Sainsbury's*	1 Burger/113g	223	11.2	197	4.5	19.6	9.9	5.7
Bean, Spicy, Cauldron Foods*	1 Burger/88g	203	9.8	232	5.4	27.4	11.2	6.2
Bean, Spicy, in Herby Nacho Crumb, Morrisons*	1 Burger/102g	185	8.1	181	5.2	19.5	7.9	5.5
Bean, Spicy, Quarter Pounder, Mae's Kitchen, Aldi*	1 Burger/105g	287	13.6	274	5.4	30	13	9.7
Bean, Spicy, Vegetarian, Tesco*	1 Burger/106g	214	9.6	202	4.8	22	9.1	6.4
Beef, 100%, Average	***1 Burger/52g***	***148***	***11.6***	***286***	***20.5***	***0.6***	***22.3***	***0.1***
Beef, 3%, M&S*	1 Burger/100g	122	2.8	122	18.8	5.5	2.8	0.5
Beef, 97%, Grilled, Heck*	1 Burger/113g	246	12.5	217	26.9	3.4	11	0
Beef, Aberdeen Angus, Asda*	1 Burger/112g	249	13.3	222	22.2	6.7	11.8	0.9
Beef, Aberdeen Angus, Fresh, Waitrose*	1 Burger/113g	269	21	238	16.4	1.2	18.6	0
Beef, Aberdeen Angus, Grilled, Finest, Tesco*	1 Burger/88g	266	18.7	302	26.4	0.5	21.3	1
Beef, Aberdeen Angus, Scotch, Deluxe, Lidl*	1 Burger /170g	430	30.4	253	21.9	0.7	17.9	0.6
Beef, Angus, Quarter Pounder, Grilled, Gold, Ocado*	1 Burger/90g	208	11.7	231	26	1.5	13	1.3
Beef, Applewood Smoke, Grilled, Waitrose*	1 Burger/80g	215	13.9	269	23.7	4	17.4	0.6
Beef, Barbecue, Tesco*	1 Burger/114g	295	22.7	260	15.6	3.5	20	0.5
Beef, Best, Cheese, Gherkin, Tomato, & Mustard, M&S*	1 Burger/167g	414	32.2	248	15.4	3.2	19.3	0.1
Beef, BGTY, Sainsbury's*	1 Burger/110g	177	6	161	20.8	7.1	5.5	1.1
Beef, Black Premium*	1 Burger/125g	290	22.5	232	17	0.5	18	0
Beef, British, Grilled, Finest, Tesco*	1 Burger/88g	266	18.7	302	26.4	0.5	21.3	1
Beef, British, Grilled, Sainsbury's*	1 Burger/67g	174	12.5	258	20	2.4	18.6	0.5
Beef, British, Organic, Duchy, Waitrose*	1 Burger/65g	152	9.4	234	22.8	2.9	14.4	0.9
Beef, British, Organic, Waitrose*	1 Burger/85g	226	16.6	266	19	3.5	19.5	1
Beef, British, Quarter Pounder, Grilled, Finest, Tesco*	1 Burger/99g	206	11.6	208	21.5	3.9	11.7	0.5

	Measure INFO/WEIGHT	per Measure KCAL	FAT	Nutrition Values per 100g / 100ml KCAL	PROT	CARB	FAT	FIBRE
BURGERS								
Beef, British, Quarter Pounders, 5% Fat, Morrisons*	1 Burger/114g	157	5.4	138	20.4	3.3	4.7	0.5
Beef, British, Quarter Pounders, Grilled, Fire Pit, Tesco*	1 Burger/92g	212	13.3	231	19.9	4.4	14.5	1.6
Beef, British, Waitrose*	1 Burger/113g	279	21	247	18.6	1.2	18.6	0
Beef, Butter, British, Grilled, Luxury, Iceland*	1 Burger/89g	224	15.3	251	22.1	1.9	17.1	0.5
Beef, Caramelised Onion, Grilled, Finest, Tesco*	1 Burger/88g	196	11.4	223	19.1	7.4	12.9	0.5
Beef, Carrot, & Onion, Tesco*	1 Burger/96g	154	7.3	160	15.3	6.4	7.6	2.3
Beef, Chargrill, Tesco*	1 Burger/114g	246	18.4	217	17	0.8	16.2	2.5
Beef, Cheddar Cheese, Hereford, Waitrose*	1 Burger/85g	220	14.7	259	23.2	2.3	17.3	0.6
Beef, Double Cheese, Iceland*	1 Burger/113g	221	14.3	196	16.4	3.9	12.6	0.4
Beef, Frozen, Tesco*	1 Burger/44g	117	8.4	266	18.9	4.6	19.1	0
Beef, Hereford, Peppered, Waitrose*	1 Burger/90g	219	13.8	243	23.7	2.2	15.3	1
Beef, Irish, Grilled, Fire Pit, Tesco*	1 Burger/76g	175	11	231	19.9	4.4	14.5	1.6
Beef, Lean, Grilled, The Butchers Market, Iceland*	1 Burger/70g	125	4.3	179	26.8	3.3	6.2	1.2
Beef, Morrisons*	1 Burger/57g	169	14.3	298	12.3	5.5	25.2	0.6
Beef, Nedal*	1 Burger/100g	208	14.8	208	17.3	1.3	14.8	0.2
Beef, Organic, Super Value*	1 Burger/151g	228	11.2	151	19.6	1.4	7.4	0
Beef, Original, & Best, Birds Eye*	1 Burger/46g	115	8.9	252	14.1	5.1	19.5	0.4
Beef, Original, with Onion, Grilled, Birds Eye*	1 Burger/38g	110	9.5	287	13.4	2.6	24.8	0.3
Beef, Our Best Ever, M&S*	1 Burger/170g	450	36.4	265	16.5	1.7	21.4	0
Beef, Quarter Pounder, British, Grilled, Sainsbury's*	1 Burger/94g	249	17.1	264	22.3	2.6	18.1	0.5
Beef, Quarter Pounder, Reduced Fat, Grilled, Asda*	1 Burger/94g	178	8	189	20	6.9	8.5	1.6
Beef, Quarter Pounders, 5% Fat, Ashfield Farm, Aldi*	1 Burger/78g	119	3.8	152	21	6.2	4.9	0.5
Beef, Quarter Pounders, Chilled, Morrisons*	1 Burger/115g	228	13.9	198	17.2	4.4	12.1	0.2
Beef, Quarter Pounders, Grilled, Oakhurst, Aldi*	1 Burger/85g	248	17	292	27.1	1.2	20	0
Beef, Quarter Pounders, Morrisons*	1 Burger/114g	338	28.6	298	12.3	5.5	25.2	0.6
Beef, Quarter Pounders, Original, Birds Eye*	1 Burger/85g	251	21.2	296	15	2.7	25	0.5
Beef, Quarter Pounders, Premium, Birds Eye*	1 Burger/71g	238	20.7	333	16	1.9	29	0.3
Beef, Quarter Pounders, Red Fat, Tesco*	1 Burger/95g	171	12.4	180	14	1.8	13	0.8
Beef, Quarter Pounders, Scotch, Sainsbury's*	1 Burger/114g	255	15.4	225	22.2	3.5	13.6	0.5
Beef, Quarter Pounders, Scotch, The Best, Morrisons*	1 Burger/97g	223	13.9	230	21	4	14.3	0.5
Beef, Quarter Pounders, with Onion, BGTY, Sainsbury's*	1 Burger/83g	171	7.8	205	26.6	3.8	9.3	0.9
Beef, Red Onion & Cheese, Butchers Selection, Asda*	1 Burger/114g	243	13.7	213	21	5	12	0.5
Beef, Rump, British, Grilled, Waitrose*	1 Burger/110g	262	15.1	238	24.2	4.1	13.7	0.6
Beef, Scotch, Ultimate, TTD, Sainsbury's*	1 Burger/119g	265	15.8	223	25.3	0.5	13.3	1
Beef, Sea Salt, & Black Pepper, Grilled, Asda*	1 Burger/88g	166	7.9	188	21	5.4	9	0.5
Beef, Skinny, Less than 3% Fat, Sainsbury's*	1 Burger/76g	120	2.1	157	26.5	6.3	2.8	0.5
Beef, Skinny, Reduced Fat, Birchwood Farm, Lidl*	1 Burger/84g	112	2.3	133	21.9	5	2.7	0.5
Beef, Steak, 5oz, As Sold, Birds Eye*	1 Burger/142g	476	41.2	335	17	1.4	29	0.5
Beef, Steak, Aberdeen Angus, As Sold, Deluxe, Lidl*	1 Burger/131g	285	19.8	217	18.7	1.1	15.1	0.5
Beef, Steak, Aberdeen Angus, Extra Special, Asda*	1 Burger/170g	362	20.4	213	23	3.2	12	0.5
Beef, Steak, British, Cooked, TTD, Sainsbury's*	1 Burger/110g	276	19.2	250	21.6	1.8	17.4	0.5
Beef, Steak, Mini, Waitrose*	1 Burger/45g	107	6.2	238	24.2	4.1	13.7	0.6
Beef, with Onion, Sainsbury's*	1 Burger/42g	102	6.2	243	20.7	6.9	14.8	1
Beef, with West Country Cheddar, TTD, Sainsbury's*	1 Burger/112g	252	13.7	225	26.4	2.3	12.2	0
Beetroot, & Root Vegetable, Vegetarian, Asda*	½ Pack/107g	158	8.8	148	3.7	11	8.2	7.2
Beetroot, & Bean, Vegan, As Sold, Strong Roots*	1 Burger/75g	148	6.3	198	4.7	22	8.4	8
Beetroot, BBQ, Tesco*	1 Burger/96g	137	1	143	5	26.3	1	4.6
Broad Bean, & Bulgur Wheat, Vegetarian, Waitrose*	1 Burger/100g	159	9	159	6.6	10.2	9	5.1
Cheese, Halloumi, Asda*	1 Burger/63g	202	15.8	320	22	2.3	25	0
Cheese, Triple, Ultimate, Specially Selected, Aldi*	1 Burger/121g	311	20.6	257	23	3.4	17	0.5
Cheese, with Bacon, & Rosemary Fries, Gousto*	1 Serving/499g	1138	55.9	228	11	21.6	11.2	1.9
Cheeseburger	***1 Burger/275g***	***706***	***29***	***257***	***13.7***	***25.6***	***10.6***	***1.8***
Cheeseburger, Bacon with Bun, Chargrilled, Tesco*	1 Burger/265g	726	42.1	274	13	19.6	15.9	1

	Measure INFO/WEIGHT	per Measure KCAL	FAT	Nutrition Values per 100g / 100ml KCAL	PROT	CARB	FAT	FIBRE
BURGERS								
Cheeseburger, Double Stack, Flame Grilled, Feasters*	1 Burger/202g	545	30.7	270	14.7	17.5	15.2	0
Cheeseburger, Quarter Pounder, Rustlers*	1 Burger/190g	505	25.1	266	13.6	22.4	13.2	0
Cheeseburger, with Sesame Seed Bun, Tesco*	1 Burger/275g	644	32.2	234	12.2	20.1	11.7	2
Chicken, 100% Breast, Golden Wholegrain, Birds Eye*	1 Burger/49g	119	5.9	243	13	20	12	1.4
Chicken, Average	***1 Burger/46g***	***111***	***5.6***	***242***	***14.9***	***18.7***	***12.1***	***1***
Chicken, Cajun Spiced, Tesco*	1 Burger/90g	207	8.9	230	19.5	15.7	9.9	0
Chicken, Cajun, Fillets, Birds Eye*	1 Pack/180g	275	8.8	153	21.5	5.8	4.9	0.3
Chicken, Fillet, Southern Fried, Asda*	1 Burger/91g	192	7	210	20	14	7.7	1.6
Chicken, Italia, Grilled, Heck*	1 Burger/105g	161	5.9	153	20.5	4.7	5.6	0
Chicken, Sizzler, Fillet, Chicken Shop, Birds Eye*	1 Burger/115g	255	13.8	222	16	12	12	0.8
Chicken, Southern Fried, Rustlers*	1 Burger/142g	410	18.3	289	10	32.3	12.9	0
Chicken, Style, Vegetarian, Quorn*	1 Burger/60g	122	5.1	205	12.1	16.5	8.6	6.6
Chicken, Thigh, Oakhurst, Aldi*	1 Burger/138g	324	15.2	235	17	16	11	0.7
Chicken, Truffle, Grilled, Luxury, Iceland*	1 Burger/125g	258	14.8	207	16.7	7.9	11.9	0.5
Chilli, Hot, M&S*	1 Burger/114g	293	22.6	258	15.3	4	19.9	0.6
Cod, Fish Fillet, Breaded, Birds Eye*	1 Burger/118g	241	8.6	204	13	21	7.3	1
Duck, Hoisin, M&S*	1 Burger/131g	290	14.7	221	17.6	11.9	11.2	1.1
Fish, Fillet, Ultimate, Birds Eye *	1 Burger/117g	266	15.2	227	14	13	13	0.9
Halloumi, Specially Selected, Aldi*	1 Burger /70g	209	15.4	298	18	7.2	22	1.1
Hemp, Vegetarian, Bean Supreme*	1 Burger/85g	148	5.8	174	9.3	15.2	6.8	7.3
Hot & Spicy, Vegan, Quorn*	1 Burger/66g	139	5.7	211	11.1	20.3	8.7	3.4
Jackfruit, Vegan, Plant Menu, Aldi*	1 Burger/114g	197	8.1	173	2.5	23	7.1	3.5
Kale, & Quinoa, Vegetarian, Strong Roots*	1 Burger/80g	165	8.4	206	4.5	21.9	10.5	2.7
Kale, Curly, & Hemp, Vegan, Biona Organic*	1 Burger/80g	198	10.2	247	6.8	23	12.8	6.4
Lamb, & Apricot, Spiced, Waitrose*	1 Burger/84g	180	9.7	215	17.1	9.6	11.6	2.1
Lamb, & Mint, Quarter Pounder, Grilled, TTD, Sainsbury's*	1 Burger/85g	204	13.3	240	23.6	1.2	15.7	0
Lamb, Firecracker, Grilled, Shazans*	1 Burger/102g	191	9.5	187	17.4	8.2	9.3	0.6
Lamb, Minted, Average	***1 Burger/56g***	***125***	***7.4***	***223***	***20.6***	***5.5***	***13.2***	***0.2***
Lamb, Minted, Grilled, Specially Selected, Aldi*	1 Burger/92g	223	14.7	242	17	6.4	16	0.5
Lamb, Minted, Quarter Pounder, Grilled, Iceland*	1 Burger/85g	231	17	271	18	3	19.9	1.9
Lamb, Waitrose*	1 Burger/67g	99	4.7	148	15.7	5.4	7	0.9
Lentil, & Spinach, Quarter Pounder, Indian, Sainsbury's*	1 Burger/114g	222	11.9	196	4.2	18.9	10.5	4.5
Manhattan, Amy's Kitchen*	1 Burger/68g	88	2.9	129	3.8	18	4.2	1.8
Mc2, No Beef, The Vegetarian Butcher*	1 Burger/80g	135	6.5	169	15.2	8	8.1	1.5
Meat Free, Average	***1 Burger/113g***	***195***	***8.8***	***172***	***17.5***	***7.9***	***7.8***	***3***
Meat Free, Green Cuisine, Birds Eye*	1 Burger/100g	238	17	238	14	3.9	17	6.5
Meat Free, Grilled, Plant Based, Asda*	1 Burger/112g	167	10.8	149	5.9	5.7	9.6	8
Meat Free, Grilled, Plant Chef, Tesco*	1 Burger/95g	182	6.3	192	11.8	17.8	6.6	7.4
Meat Free, Quarter Pounders, Move Over Meat*	1 Burger/113g	279	17	246	17	11	15	1.4
Meat Free, Sainsbury's*	1 Burger/45g	67	1.8	149	19.1	6.4	4	5.6
Meat Free, Spicy, Bean & Nacho, Cooked, Asda*	1 Burger/113g	247	9.6	218	5.3	27.7	8.5	4.7
Meat Free, The Meatless Farm Co*	1 Burger/114g	231	12	203	21.8	3.3	10.5	4.5
Meat Free, Traditional, Fry's*	1 Burger/80g	119	4.5	148	14	7.4	5.6	6.2
Meat Free, Veggie Kitchen, Farmfoods*	1 Burger/48g	86	4.1	180	18	4.9	8.5	5.9
Mix, Vegetarian, Slim & Save*	1 Serving/38g	140	4.5	371	30.8	31.9	12	6.1
Mushroom, & Chestnut, Oven Cooked, Waitrose*	1 Burger/113g	166	5	147	4.8	19.3	4.4	5.8
Mushroom, Vegan, Biona Organic*	1 Burger/80g	215	13.6	269	5.2	21	17	4.5
Mushroom, with Lentil, & Butter Bean, Gosh!*	1 Burger/125g	174	3.9	139	6	25	3.1	6.6
No Beef, Vegan, Mae's Kitchen, Aldi*	1 Burger/109g	268	16.4	246	17	11	15	1.4
No Beef, Vegetarian, Plant Kitchen, M&S*	1 Burger/160g	339	22.7	212	11.2	73	14.2	5.3
No Chicken, Plant Menu, Aldi*	1 Burger/96g	251	13	261	14.6	17.7	13.5	2.4
Nut, Jumbo, Veggie Chef*	1 Burger/60g	194	13.3	323	18.8	10.5	22.2	3
Nut, with Carrot, & Parsnip, Oven Baked, Goodlife*	1 Burger/80g	197	11.8	246	5.3	22.1	14.8	2.2

	Measure INFO/WEIGHT	per Measure KCAL	per Measure FAT	Nutrition Values per 100g / 100ml KCAL	PROT	CARB	FAT	FIBRE
BURGERS								
Ostrich, Quarter Pounder, Oslinc*	1 Burger/113g	132	1.5	117	22.9	3.5	1.3	1.1
Patties, American Style, Stateside Diner*	1 Pattie/50g	82	5.1	164	10.6	7.2	10.2	0.6
Pesto, Supergreen, Oven Baked, Goodlife*	1 Burger/105g	163	7.6	155	8.5	11.6	7.2	5
Plant Based, Beyond Burger, Vegan, Beyond Meat*	1 Patty/114g	318	21.1	280	21.5	6.6	18.6	0.5
Plant Based, Patties, Without Meat, Lidl*	1 Burger/114g	258	16.2	226	17.9	4.8	14.2	3.5
Plant Based, Plant To Plate*	1 Burger/113g	157	5.4	139	14.4	7.1	4.8	4.7
Plant Based, The Big Fry, Vegan, Fry's*	1 Burger/112g	161	4.5	144	17.7	8	4	3.1
Plant, Ultimate, Plant Pioneers, Sainsbury's*	1 Burger/86g	184	10	213	16.2	7.8	11.6	6.3
Plant, Vegan, Vivera *	1 Burger/100g	161	5.1	161	17	8.9	5.1	6
Pork, Free Range, Waitrose*	1 Burger/115g	306	19.9	266	19.3	7.7	17.3	1
Pork, & Apple, Quarter Pounder, Grilled, Asda*	1 Burger/80g	147	6.4	184	23.9	4.1	8	0.5
Pork, & Chorizo, Quarter Pounders, Tesco*	1 Burger/88g	240	15.8	273	21.1	5.9	18	1.3
Pork, Pulled, Quarter Pounder, Grilled, Linda McCartney*	1 Burger/97g	150	4.5	154	16.1	11.1	4.6	2
Pumpkin, & Spinach, Vegetarian, Strong Roots*	1 Burger/80g	162	7.5	202	3.9	24.6	9.3	2.3
Pumpkin, & Sweet Potato, Vegetarian, Vivera*	1 Burger/99g	98	3	99	5.1	10.3	3	5.4
Quarter Pounder, Loved by Us, Co-Op*	1 Burger/114g	301	23.9	265	19	0.5	21	0
Quarter Pounder, Mozzarella, Vegetarian, Linda McCartney*	1 Burger/98g	238	13.5	243	18.2	10.3	13.8	2.3
Quarter Pounder, Quorn*	1 Burger/114g	170	6.8	150	14.4	7.7	6	4
Quarter Pounder, Steak, Deluxe, Lidl*	1 Burger/98g	237	17.6	242	18	2.1	18	0
Quarter Pounder, Vegan, Vivera*	1 Burger/113g	251	15.8	222	15	5.7	14	5.2
Quinoa, Sweet Potato, & Lentil, Vegetarian, Sainsbury's*	1 Burger/88g	168	8.2	192	4.7	19.3	9.4	5.8
Red Lentil, & Sunflower Seed, Vegan, Biona Organic*	1 Burger/80g	207	8.8	259	7.8	29	11	6.8
Salmon, Lemon & Herb, Mini, Waitrose*	1 Burger/55g	114	5.7	208	23	4.9	10.3	1.6
Salmon, Quarter Pounders, Tesco*	1 Burger/114g	145	2.7	128	15.9	10.6	2.4	1.2
Salmon, Smoky BBQ, The Grill, M&S*	1 Burger/90g	175	8.4	194	16.4	10.3	9.3	1.7
Salmon, Thai, Grilled, Waitrose*	1 Burger/83g	161	8.4	194	18.6	6.7	10.1	1
Sausage, Plant Based, Moving Mountains*	1 Burger/114g	285	16	250	11	6.6	14	6.1
Soya, Chunky, Vegan, Waitrose*	1 Burger/101g	161	6.5	160	18.8	3.2	6.5	7.1
Soya, Quarter Pounders, Meat Free Butcher, Aldi*	1 Burger/108g	297	18.4	275	13	16	17	3.6
Steak, Peppered, M&S*	1 Burger/114g	310	24.4	272	18.8	0.8	21.4	0.7
Sweet Potato, & Edamame, Meat Free, Morrisons*	1 Burger/88g	144	8	164	6.4	10.6	9.1	7.2
Sweet Potato, & Black Bean, Tesco*	1 Burger/97g	145	1.5	150	5.3	25.6	1.6	5.8
Sweet Potato, & Quinoa, Vegetarian, Waitrose*	1 Burger/91g	222	11.8	244	5.1	23.8	13	5.4
Sweet Potato, Buckwheat, Vegan, Biona Organic*	1 Burger/80g	198	9.6	248	5.2	27	12	3.5
Sweet Potato, Chickpea, Carrot, Red Pepper, Aldi*	1 Burger/115g	172	2.6	150	4.2	25	2.3	6.1
Turkey, British, Grilled, Sainsbury's*	1 Burger/97g	171	6.5	176	24.6	4.1	6.7	0.5
Turkey, Cheese, & Jalapeno, Tesco*	1 Burger/114g	174	7.8	153	17.5	5	6.8	0.7
Turkey, Mini, Mexican, Result Plan*	1 Serving/221g	314	8	142	11	16	3.6	0.6
Turkey, Sea Salt & Pepper, Butchers Selection, Asda*	1 Burger/96g	141	4.4	147	23	3.2	4.6	0.5
Veg, Crunchy, Gro, Co-Op*	1 Burger/140g	304	18.2	217	2.6	21	13	2.1
Vegan, Onion Bhaji, Frozen, As Consumed, Tesco*	1 Burger/117g	167	8.5	143	3.5	12.3	7.3	7.1
Vegan, Quarter Pounder, Gro, Co-Op*	1 Burger/113g	189	11.3	167	10	3.7	10	9
Vegan, Ultimate, Pan Fried, Heck*	1 Burger/103g	179	10.5	174	4.6	11.2	10.2	9.7
Vegan, Vivera*	1 Burger/100g	169	7.3	169	18.5	4.8	7.3	5
Vegetable, Average	***1 Burger/56g***	***100***	***4.5***	***179***	***4.4***	***22.4***	***8***	***2.3***
Vegetable, Frozen, Oven Baked, Asda*	1 Burger/106g	204	8.4	192	3.9	25	7.9	3.6
Vegetable, Organic, Tesco*	1 Burger/90g	108	3.9	120	2.6	17.6	4.3	2.1
Vegetable, Quarter Pounders, Crisp & Golden, Waitrose*	1 Burger/113g	236	8.8	209	4.8	28.2	7.8	3.4
Vegetable, Quarter Pounders, Meat Free, Vegan, Tesco*	1 Burger/106g	229	10.6	216	3.7	25.8	10	3.9
Vegetable, Quarter Pounders, Sainsbury's*	1 Burger/102g	225	10.1	221	4.8	26	9.9	4.4
Vegetable, Spicy, Asda*	1 Burger/56g	108	6.2	193	3.4	20	11	0
Vegetarian, Average	***1 Std Patty/60g***	***112***	***5.3***	***187***	***17.2***	***2.9***	***8.8***	***3.3***
Vegetarian, Frozen, Grilled, Quorn*	1 Burger/44g	77	3.6	174	15.7	7.4	8.1	4.7

	Measure INFO/WEIGHT	per Measure KCAL	FAT	Nutrition Values per 100g / 100ml KCAL	PROT	CARB	FAT	FIBRE
BURGERS								
Vegetarian, Quarter Pounders, Grilled, Linda McCartney*	1 Burger/105g	232	12.5	220	17.3	9.8	11.9	2.4
Veggie, Frozen, Birds Eye*	1 Burger/125g	222	5.5	181	4.2	23	4.5	2.1
Veggie, Katsu Curry, Goodlife*	1 Burger/99g	154	7.3	156	7	13.4	7.4	4.3
Veggie, Moroccan, Macro*	1 Burger/125g	270	7.8	216	5.7	31.5	6.2	5.1
Veggie, Vegan, Co-Op*	1 Burger/140g	304	18.2	217	2.6	21	13	2.1
Veggie, with Seitan, & Quinoa, Lidl*	1 Burger/80g	149	4.2	186	17.8	15.6	5.3	2.4
Venison, & Pork, Grilled, Sainsbury's*	1 Burger/64g	130	6.1	203	22.6	6	9.6	0.8
Venison, As Sold, Outlanddish*	1 Burger/113g	149	5.4	132	18	4.4	4.8	0
Venison, Finnebrougue Estate*	1 Burger/142g	170	7	120	19.9	4.2	4.9	0.5
Zebra, Cooked, Kezie*	1 Burger/110g	160	3.8	145	25.3	2.2	3.5	0
BURRITO								
Bean, & Rice, Mexican, GF, Amy's Kitchen*	1 Burrito/158g	234	6	148	4.5	24	3.8	3.2
Beef	***1 Serving/225g***	***536***	***20.2***	***238***	***12***	***27***	***9***	***2.2***
Beef, Chilli, As Consumed, Morrisons*	½ Pack/200g	368	16	184	8.9	17.7	8	2.7
Beef, Chilli, Inspired Cuisine, Aldi*	1 Pack/400g	748	26.4	187	6.8	24	6.6	2.6
Beef, Naked, Slimming World*	1 Pack/398g	366	3.2	92	8.2	11.3	0.8	3.3
Beef, Spicy, Tex Mex, Tesco*	1 Burrito/192g	326	8.4	170	6.5	24.8	4.4	2.6
Chicken, BBQ, Morrisons*	1 Burrito/18g	35	1.1	194	10	25	6.1	1.7
Chicken, Core Food Plan*	1 Pack/400g	397	7.1	99	12	7.2	1.8	0
Hot, Wicked Kitchen, Tesco*	1 Burrito/356g	695	22.1	195	5	27.7	6.2	4.1
Pork, Pulled, BBQ, Scratch, Waitrose*	½ Pack/404g	654	18.6	162	10.1	18.2	4.6	0
BUTTER								
Brandy, Average	***1 Serving/10g***	***56***	***3.8***	***556***	***0.2***	***46.2***	***38.4***	***0.1***
Creamery, Average	***1 Serving/10g***	***74***	***8.1***	***736***	***0.5***	***0.4***	***81.4***	***0***
French, with Sea Salt Crystals, Waitrose*	1 Thin Spread/7g	51	5.6	727	0.7	1	80	0
Fresh, Average	***1 Thin Spread/7g***	***51***	***5.7***	***735***	***0.6***	***0.4***	***81.3***	***0***
Garlic, Crushed, Lurpak*	1 Serving/10g	69	7.5	692	1.3	3.7	75	0
Goat's, St Helen's Farm*	1 Thin Spread/7g	56	6.2	794	0.5	0	88	0
Guernsey Dairy*	1 Thin Spread/7g	53	5.8	755	0.6	0.6	83.4	0
Pure, Irish, Lakeland Dairies*	1 Thin Spread/7g	52	5.7	738	0.6	0.8	81.4	0
Reduced Fat, Fresh, Average	***1 Thin Spread/7g***	***26***	***2.8***	***368***	***2.3***	***1.2***	***39.4***	***0.2***
Salted, Average	***1 Thin Spread/7g***	***51***	***5.7***	***729***	***0.4***	***0.3***	***81.1***	***0***
Spreadable, Fresh, Average	***1 Thin Spread/7g***	***51***	***5.7***	***730***	***0.4***	***0.3***	***80.8***	***0***
Spreadable, Reduced Fat, Average	***1 Thin Spread/7g***	***38***	***4.2***	***540***	***0.5***	***0.5***	***60***	***0***
Unsalted, Tesco*	1 Thin Spread/7g	52	5.8	745	0.6	0.6	82.2	0
West Country, Specially Selected, Aldi*	1 Thin Spread/7g	52	5.7	745	0.6	0.6	82	0.5
with Hill Farm Rapeseed Oil, The Butter Works*	1 Thin Spread/7g	48	5.2	681	0.3	0.8	75	0
with Olive Oil, Lighter, Spreadable, Lurpak*	1 Thin Spread/7g	38	4.2	543	0.3	0.4	60	0
with Rapeseed Oil, The Butterworks*	1 Thin Spread/7g	48	5.2	681	0.3	0.8	75	0
with Sea Salt Crystals, Finest, Tesco*	1 Thin Spread/7g	51	5.7	734	0.6	0.6	81	0
BUTTERMILK								
Average	***1 Mug/400ml***	***177***	***1.3***	***44***	***4.2***	***5.9***	***0.3***	***0***
BUTTERNUT SQUASH								
Chips, Crinkle Cut, Cooked, Sainsbury's*	½ Pack/95g	66	0.9	70	2.2	11.7	0.9	3.1
Chunks, Frozen, Four Seasons, Aldi*	1 Serving/80g	30	0.4	37	0.9	7.4	0.5	1.4
Chunks, Roast, Strong Roots*	1 Serving/106g	113	6.5	107	1.1	11	6.1	1.5
Frozen, Tesco*	1 Serving/80g	29	0.2	36	1	6.1	0.2	2.7
Noodles, Ready Prepared, Sainsbury's*	½ Pack/152g	50	0.8	33	1.1	5.8	0.5	1.4
Winter, Boiled, Flesh Only	***1 Serving/80g***	***27***	***0.1***	***34***	***0.7***	***8.8***	***0.1***	***2.6***
Winter, Butternut, Baked, Average	***1 Serving/100g***	***32***	***0.1***	***32***	***0.9***	***7.4***	***0.1***	***1.4***
Winter, Butternut, Raw, Prepared, Average	***1 Serving/80g***	***29***	***0.1***	***36***	***1.1***	***8.3***	***0.1***	***1.6***
Winter, Butternut, Raw, Unprepared, Average	***1 Serving/80g***	***24***	***0.1***	***30***	***0.9***	***6.8***	***0.1***	***1.3***

	Measure INFO/WEIGHT	per Measure KCAL	FAT	Nutrition Values per 100g / 100ml KCAL	PROT	CARB	FAT	FIBRE
BUTTONS								
Chocolate, Giant, Free From, Tesco*	10 Buttons/23g	125	8	544	2.5	48.4	35	12.5
Chocolate, Orange, Free From, Asda*	1 Bag/25g	140	8.8	562	2.4	58	35	2.6
Milk Chocolate, Asda*	1 Bag/70g	368	21	526	7	57	30	1.5
Milk Chocolate, Giant, Dairy Milk, Cadbury*	1 Button/2g	11	0.6	530	7.6	56.5	30.5	0.7
Milk Chocolate, M&S*	1 Pack/75g	375	19	500	8.6	59.8	25.3	1.9
Milk Chocolate, Tesco*	1 Bag/70g	359	19.3	513	7.1	59.1	27.6	2.1
Mixed, White & Milk, Dairy Milk, Cadbury*	¼ Bag/28g	150	8.4	536	3.6	60.7	30	1.1
White Chocolate, Co-Op*	½ Pack/35g	186	9.8	530	7	64	28	0
White Chocolate, Dairy Milk, Cadbury*	1 Pack/32g	174	9.5	540	4.7	63	29.5	0
White Chocolate, Milkybar, Nestle*	1 Bag/30g	164	9.5	546	7.5	58.1	31.6	0
White Chocolate, Tesco*	1 Bag/70g	388	23.4	554	5.1	58	33.5	0

	Measure INFO/WEIGHT	per Measure KCAL	FAT	Nutrition Values per 100g / 100ml KCAL	PROT	CARB	FAT	FIBRE
CABBAGE								
& Leek, Ready Sliced, Sainsbury's*	1 Pack/240g	53	1.2	22	1.1	2.2	0.5	2.1
& Leek, Sliced, Tesco*	1/3 Pack/100g	32	0.6	32	2.1	3.4	0.6	2.6
Boiled, Average	***1 Serving/90g***	***14***	***0.3***	***15***	***1***	***2.2***	***0.3***	***1.7***
Creamed, Cooked, Sainsbury's*	½ Pack/150g	95	6.8	67	2	2.6	4.8	2.5
Duo, Tesco*	½ Pack/103g	72	4.8	70	2.5	3.1	4.7	2.8
Greens, Trimmed, Average	***1oz/28g***	***8***	***0.1***	***28***	***2.9***	***3***	***0.5***	***3.4***
Raw, Average	***1 Serving/100g***	***21***	***0.4***	***21***	***1.3***	***3.2***	***0.4***	***1.8***
Red, Average	***1 Serving/90g***	***19***	***0.2***	***21***	***1***	***3.7***	***0.3***	***2.2***
Red, Braised with Red Wine, M&S*	½ Pack/150g	180	7.2	120	1.4	17.1	4.8	1
Red, Braised, with Bramley Apples, M&S*	½ Pack/150g	126	3	84	1	14	2	2.8
Red, Pickled, Average	***1 Serving/50g***	***13***	***0.1***	***26***	***0.9***	***4.6***	***0.2***	***1.6***
Red, Spiced, Steamer, Sainsbury's*	½ Pack/150g	105	3.3	70	1	10.5	2.2	2.9
Red, with Apple, Bramley, British, Sainsbury's*	1 Pack/300g	213	1.5	71	1.2	14.9	0.5	2.3
Red, with Apple, Finest, Tesco*	½ Pack/150g	177	8.8	118	1.6	14.7	5.9	4.6
Red, with Apple, Red Wine & Cranberries, Waitrose*	1/3 Pack/97g	116	5.7	120	1.4	14.2	5.9	2.6
Red, with Apple, Tesco*	½ Pack/144g	118	3	82	1.4	12.5	2.1	4.1
Savoy, Boiled in Salted Water, Average	***1 Serving/90g***	***15***	***0.4***	***17***	***1.1***	***2.2***	***0.5***	***2***
Savoy, Raw, Average	***1 Serving/90g***	***24***	***0.4***	***27***	***2.1***	***3.9***	***0.5***	***3.1***
Spring Greens, Boiled, Average	***1 Serving/80g***	***16***	***0.6***	***20***	***1.9***	***1.6***	***0.7***	***2.6***
Spring Greens, Raw, Average	***1 Serving/80g***	***22***	***0.7***	***28***	***2.5***	***2.6***	***0.8***	***2.9***
Steamed, Average	***1 Serving/100g***	***15***	***0.3***	***15***	***1***	***2.2***	***0.3***	***1.7***
Sweetheart, Raw	***1 Serving/100g***	***26***	***0.6***	***26***	***2.1***	***3.2***	***0.6***	***2.8***
Trio, with Pancetta, Finest, Tesco*	½ Pack/91g	79	5	87	4.4	3.4	5.5	3.4
White, Raw, Average	***1oz/28g***	***8***	***0.1***	***27***	***1.4***	***5***	***0.2***	***2.1***
CACAO								
Berry, Clean Paleo*	1 Serving/50g	310	25.8	620	17.6	17.6	51.6	16
Butter, Organic, Sevenhills Wholefoods*	1 Button/2g	18	2	896	0.2	0	99.5	0.3
Nibs, Organic, Naturya*	1 Tbsp/15g	95	8.4	633	13	15	56	10
Nibs, Organic, So Cacao, Holland & Barrett*	1 Serving/100g	632	52	632	12	30	52	23
Nibs, Raw, Hatton Hill*	1 Tbsp/15g	70	6.4	464	14	36	43	0
Powder, El Canario*	2 Scoops/40g	136	1.1	340	5.5	72.1	2.9	3.1
Powder, Green Origins*	1 Tsp/5g	18	0.6	353	25	21	11	35
Powder, Natural, 100%, Food Thoughts*	1 Tsp/5g	21	1	418	28.1	14.5	21	31
CAKE								
Almond, Slices, Mr Kipling*	1 Slice/35g	144	6.5	411	6	54.2	18.5	1.8
Almond, Slices, Sainsbury's*	1 Serving/27g	120	7.1	444	5.9	45.9	26.3	1.5
Angel Slices, 30% Less Sugar, Mr Kipling*	1 Slice/24g	98	4.8	410	3.5	53	19.9	2.5
Angel, Average	***1 Slice/44g***	***175***	***7.9***	***397***	***4.2***	***54.9***	***17.9***	***0.8***
Apple Crumble, Rowan Hill Bakery, Lidl*	1 Serving/50g	190	6.6	381	4	60.2	13.2	2.6
Apple, Bramley, & Blackberry Crumble, M&S*	1/8 Cake/56g	221	10	395	4.4	54.1	17.9	1.5
Apple, Home Style, M&S*	1 Cake/54g	189	7.9	350	5.3	49.4	14.7	1.5
Apple, Slices, Delightful, Mr Kipling*	1 Slice/29g	92	1.1	317	4.4	66.2	3.9	1.3
Apple, Sticky Toffee, Finest, Tesco*	1 Slice/51g	247	9.2	487	3	52.7	18.1	0.6
Bakewell, Cherry, Co-Op*	1 Cake/47g	205	8	435	3.7	67.2	16.9	1.8
Bakewell, Cherry, Delightful, Mr Kipling*	1 Cake/45g	176	5.8	390	3.9	66.4	12.9	1.2
Bakewell, Cherry, M&S*	1 Cake/44g	185	7.8	420	4.5	61.7	17.7	1
Bakewell, Cherry, Mini, Sainsbury's*	1 Cake/27g	101	3.3	370	3.4	62.2	12	0.4
Bakewell, Cherry, Slices, GFY, Asda*	1 Slice/29g	98	0.7	337	3.4	75.4	2.4	0.7
Bakewell, Cherry, Waitrose*	1 Cake/44g	184	8.5	419	3.8	57.4	19.3	2.1
Bakewell, Lemon, Average	***1 Cake/42g***	***173***	***6.4***	***411***	***3.7***	***64.6***	***15.2***	***1.3***
Bakewell, Slices, Mr Kipling*	1 Slice/35g	146	6.2	414	4.1	59.2	17.6	1
Bakewell, Slices, Weight Watchers*	1 Slice/26g	84	0.6	324	3.7	71	2.4	2
Banana, Bread, Brilliant, Graze*	1 Cake/23g	72	3.6	312	5.2	40.4	15.6	3

C

	Measure INFO/WEIGHT	per Measure KCAL	FAT	Nutrition Values per 100g / 100ml KCAL	PROT	CARB	FAT	FIBRE
CAKE								
Banana, J. Donald*	1 Slice/25g	38	4	152	2	0	16	0
Banana, Loaf, Tesco*	1 Slice/40g	152	6.9	380	5.3	50.3	17.2	1.6
Banana, Loaf, The Best, Morrisons*	1 Serving/75g	273	13.4	364	5.7	44.1	17.9	2
Banana, Loaf, Waitrose*	1 Slice/70g	236	7.5	337	5	55.2	10.7	1.7
Banana, with An Afternoon Tea Infusion, Graze*	1 Punnet/18g	55	2.5	307	5	39	14	3
Bara Brith, Tan Y Castell*	1 Serving/100g	261	1	261	4	58.8	1	1.5
Battenberg, Mini, Mr Kipling*	1 Cake/32g	128	3.2	399	3.8	72.9	10	1.2
Battenberg, Mr Kipling*	1 Serving/38g	161	4.6	421	5	73.3	12	1.6
Birthday, M&S*	1 Serving/60g	240	7.1	400	2.3	70.9	11.9	0.8
Birthday, Piece of Cake, M&S*	1 Serving/85g	395	24.4	465	4.3	39.7	28.7	0.9
Birthday, Present, Tesco*	1 Serving/79g	347	13.9	439	3.5	66.6	17.6	0.4
Blueberry, Fitbakes*	1 Cake/17g	36	1	206	11	47	6	0
Butterfly, Mr Kipling*	1 Cake/29g	114	6.4	392	4.4	43.4	22.2	0.6
Caramel, Salted, The Best, Morrisons*	1/6 Cake/63g	262	12.2	416	3.9	56.2	19.4	0.5
Carrot, & Orange, Finest, Tesco*	1/8 Cake/50g	205	10.2	410	4.6	51.2	20.5	2.1
Carrot, & Orange, Waitrose*	1/6 Cake/47g	164	7.4	350	5.3	46.8	15.7	1.8
Carrot, & Walnut, Aldi*	¼ Cake/100g	409	23	409	5.1	44	23	2.2
Carrot, & Walnut, Layered, Asda*	1 Serving/42g	172	8	409	4.6	55	19	1
Carrot, & Walnut, Mini Classics, Mr Kipling*	1 Cake/39g	172	9.8	440	4.5	48.6	25.2	1
Carrot, Average	***1 Slice/56g***	***211***	***10.4***	***377***	***4.6***	***47.6***	***18.6***	***1.4***
Carrot, Fitbakes*	1 Cake/15g	49	2.6	322	16	50	17	5
Carrot, Free From, Finest, Tesco*	1 Slice/67g	288	17.7	429	3	43.3	26.3	3.5
Carrot, GF , Finest, Tesco*	1 Serving/50g	204	10.4	407	3.4	50.4	20.9	1.9
Carrot, Iced, Tesco*	1 Serving/61g	246	12	404	3.1	53.7	19.6	1.6
Carrot, TTD, Sainsbury's*	1 Slice/72g	287	13.7	398	4.5	51.1	19	2.5
Carrot, with Cream Cheese Icing, On the Go, Sainsbury's*	1 Cake/64g	251	11.9	392	4.3	51.5	18.6	1
Carrot, with Walnuts, M&S*	1 Pack/75g	290	13.5	387	4.5	50.6	18	2.4
Celebration Rose, Mary Berry*	1 Slice/100g	410	14.5	410	2.9	66.6	14.5	0
Cherry & Almond Slices, GF, Free From, Sainsbury's*	1 Slice/33g	144	7.9	442	6.5	48.7	24.3	1
Cherry Bakewell, Asda*	1 Cake/46g	189	6.9	411	3.8	63	15	2.1
Cherry Bakewell, Mr Kipling*	1 Bakewell/46g	200	8	435	3.4	65.5	17.4	1.4
Cherry Crumble, Rowan Hill Bakery, Lidl*	1 Slice/50g	196	7	392	3.4	62.6	13.9	1.6
Chocolate	***1oz/28g***	***128***	***7.4***	***456***	***7.4***	***50.4***	***26.4***	***1.7***
Chocolate Chip, Co-Op*	1/6 Cake/63g	275	16.9	440	5	44	27	0.5
Chocolate Chip, Slices, Mr Kipling*	1 Slice/25g	109	5.1	442	6.2	57.4	20.5	1.6
Chocolate Slices, Mr Kipling*	1 Slice/32g	132	6	411	3.4	56.3	18.7	1.7
Chocolate, & Blood Orange, Bars, Lunchbox, Soreen*	1 Bar/30g	105	2.5	349	8.9	57.5	8.2	5.2
Chocolate, & Madeira, Marble Loaf, M&S*	1/6 Cake/88g	380	20.4	430	5	50	23.1	1
Chocolate, & Orange, Rolls, M&S*	1 Cake/60g	228	17	380	3.6	27	28.4	1.3
Chocolate, & Salted Caramel, Delice, TTD, Sainsbury's*	1 Serving/65g	207	12.3	319	3.6	32.5	19	1.9
Chocolate, Crispy Clusters, Mini, Tesco*	1 Cluster/8g	37	1.5	470	7	67.8	18.7	2.5
Chocolate, Free From, Finest, Tesco*	1 Slice/64g	279	16.1	438	4.1	46.9	25.3	3.2
Chocolate, Fudge	***1 Serving/110g***	***415***	***19.1***	***377***	***4.4***	***50.4***	***17.4***	***1.4***
Chocolate, Jumbo bakery *	1/8 Cake/90g	373	20.5	414	5	46.4	22.8	3.7
Chocolate, Large, Happy Birthday, Tesco*	1/14 Cake/63g	291	16	462	4.2	53.4	25.4	1.7
Chocolate, Log, Mini, Free From, Sainsbury's*	1 Slice/45g	202	10.8	450	5.6	51	24	3
Chocolate, Mini Roll, Bites, Tesco*	1 Bite/18g	78	3.6	435	6	58	19.8	1.9
Chocolate, Mousse, Galaxy, Mars*	1 Serving/71g	250	15.5	354	5.3	33	22	0
Chocolate, Orange, Sponge, Asda*	1 Serving/70g	298	18.2	425	4.9	42.9	26	3
Chocolate, Rice Crispy, Knightsbridge, Lidl*	1 Cake/24g	88	4.2	368	3.9	48.7	17.5	0.1
Chocolate, Roll, Triple, Cadbury*	1 Serving/40g	165	6.7	410	4.3	60.1	16.6	1.5
Chocolate, Sponge, Tesco*	1 Serving/37g	129	3.6	358	5.1	60.8	10.1	1.7
Chocolate, Sponge, Victoria, Co-Op*	1 Slice/61g	201	9.8	330	5	42	16	1

	Measure INFO/WEIGHT	per Measure KCAL	FAT	Nutrition Values per 100g / 100ml KCAL	PROT	CARB	FAT	FIBRE
CAKE								
Chocolate, Triple Layer, Celebration, Tesco*	1/24 of cake/79g	345	18.8	430	5	47.7	23.4	2.8
Chocolate, Truffle, Mini, Finest, Tesco*	1 Cake/28g	125	6.6	448	5.9	52.9	23.7	0.3
Chocolate, Vegan, Just Love Food*	1 Slice/61g	249	13.4	409	3.4	48.4	22	0
Chocolate, White, 885g, Waitrose*	1/12 Cake/74g	332	16.2	448	3.2	59.3	21.9	0
Chocolate, White, Party, Asda*	1 Slice/100g	424	22	424	3.1	52	22	1.4
Chocolate, White, Triple Layer, Party Cake, Asda*	1 Slice/68g	306	15.6	450	2.9	57	23	1.1
Chocolate, Wiggles The Caterpillar, Mini, Sainsbury's*	1 Cake/30g	139	6.7	462	4.8	59.9	22.2	1.8
Chocolate, Wiggles The Caterpillar, Sainsbury's*	1 Slice/40g	170	7.6	425	5.2	57.3	19	1.9
Chocolate, with Butter Icing, Average	***1oz/28g***	***135***	***8.3***	***481***	***5.7***	***50.9***	***29.7***	***0***
Christmas, Connoisseur, M&S*	1 Slice/60g	216	5.5	360	4.1	64.7	9.2	3.3
Christmas, Fruit, Iced, Bar, Bakers Selection, Asda*	1 Serving/67g	233	5.3	349	3.8	64	7.9	2.5
Christmas, Fully Iced, M&S*	1/12 Cake/72g	261	5.1	362	2.6	71.3	7.1	1.3
Christmas, Iced Rich Fruit, Finest, Tesco*	1/8 Cake/50g	183	4.3	366	4.3	66.4	8.6	3.3
Christmas, Iced, Slices, Tesco*	1 Slice/45g	168	4.4	369	2.9	67.6	9.6	1.2
Christmas, Rich Fruit, Free From, Tesco*	1/12 Cake/75g	284	6.4	376	3	71	8.5	1.6
Christmas, Rich Fruit, Organic, Tesco*	1 Serving/76g	282	7.6	374	3.9	67.1	10	2
Christmas, Rich Fruit, Tesco*	1 Serving/75g	261	7.2	348	3.8	60.6	9.6	2.1
Christmas, Slices, Mr Kipling*	1 Slice/43g	159	3.8	368	3	68.4	8.8	1.4
Christmas, Top Iced, Rich Fruit , Essential, Waitrose*	1 Slice/75g	278	5.8	368	3.6	69.6	7.7	2.9
Coconut	***1 Slice/70g***	***304***	***16.7***	***434***	***6.7***	***51.2***	***23.8***	***2.5***
Coconut, & Raspberry, M&S*	1 Serving/52g	231	13.9	445	5	45.5	26.8	2.3
Coconut, & Raspberry, Loaf, Tesco*	1/6 Cake/46g	178	7.4	388	5.2	54.5	16.1	1.9
Coconut, Snowball, Bobby's*	1 Cake/18g	80	4	436	2.2	57.3	22.1	0
Coconut, Snowball, Tunnock's*	1 Cake/30g	134	6.2	446	4.2	56.7	20.8	3.6
Coconut, Sponge, Mini Classics, Mr Kipling*	1 Cake/38g	155	8.7	409	3.7	47	22.9	0.9
Coffee, & Walnut Slices, HE, Tesco*	1 Slice/23g	69	0.5	301	4.4	65.7	2.3	2.8
Colin the Caterpillar, M&S*	1 Slice/60g	234	12.8	390	5.3	57.2	21.3	1.3
Cookies & Cream, Fitbakes*	1 Cake/78g	173	7	221	12	40	9	0
Cornflake, Average	***1 Cake/18g***	***83***	***3.7***	***464***	***5.2***	***64.6***	***20.4***	***2***
Cornflake, Chocolate Clusters, Asda*	1 Cake/14g	64	2.6	460	8.2	65.2	18.5	2.7
Cornflake, Chocolate, Mini Bites, Tesco*	1 Bite/14g	62	2.5	446	7.1	64.1	17.9	5.9
Cream Sponge, Morrisons*	1 Serving/46g	138	6.4	302	3.8	39.8	13.9	1.2
Cream, Oysters, M&S*	1 Cake/72g	227	15.3	315	3.6	27.5	21.2	3
Cream, Slices, M&S*	1 Slice/80g	310	18.3	387	2.3	45.7	22.9	0.6
Date, & Walnut Loaf, Sainsbury's*	1/10 Slice/40g	148	8.2	371	6.7	40.1	20.4	1
Eccles, All Butter, M&S*	1 Cake/86g	345	14.8	400	4.5	57.4	17.2	3.2
Eccles, Fresh Baked	***1 Cake/45g***	***171***	***7.6***	***381***	***4.3***	***56.3***	***17***	***1.5***
Fairy, Average	***1 Cake/23g***	***96***	***4.6***	***416***	***5.1***	***53***	***20.2***	***1.5***
Fairy, Chocolate, Ms Mollys*	1 Cake/23g	95	4.9	413	4.2	49.7	21.4	2.5
Fairy, Iced, Average	***1 Cake/23g***	***91***	***3.4***	***394***	***4.2***	***60.8***	***14.8***	***0.9***
Fairy, Lemon Iced, Average	***1 Cake/23g***	***90***	***3.1***	***393***	***4.4***	***63.2***	***13.6***	***1.1***
Fairy, Plain, Average	***1 Cake/23g***	***95***	***4.6***	***413***	***5.5***	***51.1***	***20.2***	***1.5***
Fairy, Strawberry Iced, Tesco*	1 Cake/24g	94	3.2	392	4.9	62.9	13.4	1.4
Fairy, Vanilla Iced, Average, Tesco*	1 Cake/23g	89	2.8	388	4.4	65.1	12.2	1.2
Fondant Fancies, Sainsbury's*	1 Cake/28g	103	2.5	373	2.7	69.7	9.1	0.7
Fondant, Dark Chocolate, Graze*	1 Pack/40g	157	5.8	393	3.5	66.2	14.5	0
Fondant, with Chocolate, Mini, Delhaize*	1 Cake Mini/20g	88	6.2	440	4.6	36.3	30.8	3.8
French Fancies, Average	***1 Cake/27g***	***100***	***2.5***	***371***	***2.7***	***69.6***	***9.1***	***0.8***
French Fancies, Lemon, Average	***1 Cake/28g***	***106***	***2.7***	***378***	***2.5***	***69.9***	***9.8***	***0.5***
French Fancies, Strawberry, Mr Kipling*	1 Cake/28g	106	2.7	379	2.5	70.6	9.6	0.4
Fruit, & Cherry, Loaf, Cakebasket*	1 Slice/30g	118	5.5	395	4.3	55.4	18.2	0
Fruit, Iced, Slices, Tesco*	1 Slice/50g	171	2.9	342	2.8	68	5.8	3.3
Fruit, Iced, Topped, Bar, Holly Lane, Aldi*	1 Slice/50g	176	3.4	353	3.7	69	6.7	0.5

	Measure INFO/WEIGHT	per Measure KCAL	FAT	Nutrition Values per 100g / 100ml KCAL	PROT	CARB	FAT	FIBRE
CAKE								
Fruit, Petit Cakes Aux Fruits, Bonne Maman*	1 Cake/25g	102	5.2	407	5.4	48	21	0
Fruit, Plain, Average	***1 Slice/90g***	***319***	***11.6***	***354***	***5.1***	***57.9***	***12.9***	***0***
Fruit, Rich, Average	***1 Slice/70g***	***225***	***8.8***	***322***	***4.9***	***50.7***	***12.5***	***1.7***
Fruit, Rich, Iced	***1 Slice/70g***	***249***	***8***	***356***	***4.1***	***62.7***	***11.4***	***1.7***
Fruit, Rich, Iced, Bar, Finest, Tesco*	1 Serving/100g	360	10.7	360	3.8	61.3	10.7	4.2
Fruit, Rich, Slices, Free From, Sainsbury's*	1 Slice/40g	144	5	361	4.5	57.4	12.6	3.7
Fruit, Slice, Lazy Day Foods*	1 Slice/50g	134	2.8	269	3	51.8	5.6	3
Genoa, Tesco*	1 Serving/44g	150	3.9	340	3.7	59.1	8.8	3.1
Ginger, & Syrup, Tesco*	1 Serving/32g	134	7	420	4.5	51.4	21.8	0.7
Ginger, Drizzle, Iced, Co-Op*	1/6 Cake/64g	226	7.7	350	3	58	12	1
Ginger, Jamaica, McVitie's*	1/9 Cake/26g	92	2.6	362	3.7	63.1	10.4	1.6
Ginger, Loaf , Stem, Waitrose*	1 Slice/35g	134	4.8	384	3.7	60.1	13.7	2.6
Granola, Square, All Butter, Finest, Tesco*	1 Square/72g	322	16.1	447	7.8	50.7	22.4	5.9
Granola, Square, M&S*	1 Square/72g	330	18.1	464	7.9	49.3	25.5	5
Hazelnut Choc, Fitbakes*	1 Cake/14g	40	1.5	284	14	43	11	0
Hazelnut Choc, Fitbakes*	1 Cake/14g	40	1.5	284	14	43	11	0
Jaffa Chocolate, Fitbakes*	1 Cake/65g	169	5.2	259	13	43	8	0
Lebkuchen, Chocolate, Dark, Mini, M&S*	1 Cake/9g	34	1.1	378	5.6	62.2	12.2	2.2
Lemon Drizzle, Fitbakes*	1 Cake/77g	154	4.6	199	10	48	6	0
Lemon Slices, Mr Kipling*	1 Slice/24g	100	4.5	416	3.5	58.2	18.6	0.9
Lemon, & Orange, Finest, Tesco*	1 Serving/53g	216	10.7	410	4.5	52.4	20.3	1.1
Lemon, & Lime, Drizzle, No.1, Waitrose*	1/12 Cake/52g	209	9.2	402	3.1	57.5	17.6	0.8
Lemon, & Poppy Seed, Slices, Weight Watcher*	1 Slice/19g	69	2.1	364	3.7	60.9	11.3	1.9
Lemon, Average	***1 Slice/81g***	***320***	***14.5***	***396***	***4.1***	***54.8***	***18***	***0.6***
Lemon, Drizzle Cake, Asda*	1 Serving/50g	150	6	299	2.8	45	12	0.4
Lemon, Drizzle, Classic, M&S*	1 Serving/100g	333	13.6	333	4	47.5	13.6	2.2
Lemon, Drizzle, Finest, Tesco*	1 Slice/68g	266	11.2	391	3.6	56.3	16.5	1.6
Lemon, filled with Lemon Curd, TTD, Sainsbury's*	1 Slice/73g	299	13.5	407	3.9	56.1	18.4	0.7
Lemon, Hand Finished, Irresistible, Co-Op*	1/16 Cake/64g	241	9.6	377	3.9	57	15	0.6
Lemon, Iced, Asda*	1/8 Cake/36g	142	5.4	393	4.1	60	15	0.9
Lemon, Loaf, M&S*	1 Slice/47g	190	8.8	400	2.1	55.8	18.6	0.6
Lemon, Slice, GF, Free From, Sainsbury's*	1 Slice/35g	169	10.1	477	6.5	47.6	28.6	1.8
Lemon, Slices, Free From, Tesco*	1 Slice/38g	156	6.6	410	3	59.5	17.5	1
Lemon, Slices, Iced, Tesco*	1 Slice/29g	114	4.9	394	3	56.1	17.1	2
Lemon, Slices, Low Fat, Weight Watchers*	1 Slice/26g	79	0.5	303	3.1	68.1	2	2.2
Lemon, Slices, Sainsbury's*	1 Slice/30g	130	6.3	432	4.1	56	20.9	1.7
Leo the Lion, Birthday, Asda*	1 Slice/81g	325	12.9	402	2.6	62	16	0.5
Madeira	***1 Slice/40g***	***157***	***6.8***	***393***	***5.4***	***58.4***	***16.9***	***0.9***
Madeira, Cherry, Sainsbury's*	1 Slice/34g	117	2.6	349	4	64.8	7.9	1.3
Madeira, Cherry, Tesco*	1 Serving/38g	135	4.2	357	4.6	58.9	11	1.8
Madeira, Iced, Asda*	1/8 Cake/36g	141	5.1	388	3.9	61	14	1
Madeira, Iced, Tesco*	1 Slice/40g	157	5.8	393	3.8	60.7	14.6	1.7
Madeira, Lemon Iced, Co-Op*	1 Cake/290g	1131	52.2	390	4	53	18	0.6
Madeira, Lemon Iced, Tesco*	1 Slice/40g	169	7.4	418	4.9	58.1	18.2	1.1
Madeleine, Bonne Maman*	1 Madeleine/25g	114	6.8	456	6.3	46	27	2.1
Madeleine, with Lemon, Bonne Maman*	1 Madeleine/25g	100	5.5	402	5.6	45	22	0
Madeleines, Classic, French, GF, Mrs Crimbles*	1 Cake/30g	136	7.8	453	4.7	49	26	0
Madeleines, Tesco*	1 Cake/25g	122	7.3	486	4.8	50.5	29.1	1.5
Manor House, Mr Kipling*	1 Serving/69g	277	13.8	400	5.3	49.7	20	1.4
Marble, Half Moon, Bobby's*	1 Pack/350g	1572	73.5	449	5.1	60	21	0
Marble, Tesco*	1/8 Cake/45g	184	8.4	410	4.4	55.9	18.7	1.5
Mini Rolls, Cadbury*	1 Roll/26g	117	6.1	450	4.8	56.3	23.5	2.3
Mini Rolls, Chocolate, Average	***1 Cake/27g***	***122***	***6.2***	***453***	***4.8***	***56.9***	***22.9***	***0.9***

CAKE	Measure INFO/WEIGHT	per Measure KCAL	FAT	Nutrition Values per 100g / 100ml KCAL	PROT	CARB	FAT	FIBRE
Mini Rolls, Jaffa, Average	***1 Cake/29g***	***111***	***3.3***	***382***	***3.5***	***67.2***	***11.2***	***1.4***
Mini Rolls, Jam, Average	***1 Cake/29g***	***115***	***4.5***	***395***	***3.8***	***59.8***	***15.6***	***1.8***
Orange, Marmalade, M&S*	1 Slice/50g	195	9.2	390	3.6	53.2	18.3	1.8
Pandoro, Italian	***1/8 Cake/87g***	***357***	***18.2***	***408***	***7.1***	***47.2***	***20.8***	***1.6***
Panettone, Average	***1 Portion/90g***	***345***	***15.3***	***383***	***8***	***52***	***17***	***0***
Panettone, Free From, Tesco*	1 Pack/100g	299	10.8	299	3.8	42.9	10.8	7.6
Panettone, Prosecco Maron Glace, TTD, Sainsbury's*	1 Slice/85g	328	14.6	386	6.6	50.1	17.2	2.2
Pineapple, Alba Bakeries*	1 Serving/63g	258	9.4	410	1.5	66	15	2.6
Plum, & Ginger, Crumble, Graze*	1 Punnet/33g	119	9.1	361	6.2	35.1	27.6	3.3
Pumpkin, Patch, Cadbury*	1 Cake/31g	149	7.1	480	5.3	61.7	22.9	2.4
Punschrulle Punsch Roll, Delicato*	1 Roll/40g	173	8	433	5	59	20	0
Raisin, Fruit Slab, Basics, Sainsbury's*	1 Slice/50g	183	6.2	367	5.3	57.3	12.5	1.9
Raspberry Chocolate, Lava, Allplants*	1 Pot/93g	329	14.9	354	5.5	44	16	3.4
Raspberry Ripple, Layer, Lewis & Green*	1/8 Cake/32g	119	3.5	373	3.9	65	11	0.9
Raspberry, & Passion Fruit, Irresistible, Co-Op*	1/6 Cake/61g	242	10.4	396	3.2	56	17	1
Raspberry, Rockin' Raspberry, Slices, Mr Kipling*	1 Slice/21g	85	4.2	397	4.3	50.6	19.5	1
Raspberry, Slice, Dairy Milk, Cadbury*	1 Slice/29g	122	5.7	420	4.6	55	19.6	1.8
Raspberry, Sponge, Value, Tesco*	1 Slice/39g	130	4.6	334	3.4	53.4	11.9	0.7
Red Velvet, The Best, Morrisons*	1/6 Cake/63g	277	13.2	440	3.7	58.8	20.9	0.8
Red Velvet, TTD, Sainsbury's*	1 Slice/71g	302	16	428	2.8	52.8	22.7	0.8
Rock	***1 Sm Cake/40g***	***158***	***6.6***	***396***	***5.4***	***60.5***	***16.4***	***1.5***
Salted Caramel, Hand Finished, Specially Selected, Aldi*	1/6 Cake/58g	241	11.6	415	4.1	54	20	0.8
Salted Caramel, Layered, Finest, Tesco*	1 Slice/75g	341	17	455	2.6	57.2	22.7	0.5
Shrek Birthday, Tesco*	1/16 Cake/72g	248	8.8	344	3.3	64	12.2	0.5
Snowballs, Sainsbury's*	1 Snowball/18g	80	4.1	445	2.5	55.6	23	3.6
Snowballs, Tesco*	1 Snowball/18g	79	4	432	2.5	55.8	22.1	5.4
Sponge	***1 Slice/53g***	***243***	***13.9***	***459***	***6.4***	***52.4***	***26.3***	***0.9***
Sponge, Fatless	***1 Slice/53g***	***156***	***3.2***	***294***	***10.1***	***53***	***6.1***	***0.9***
Sponge, Jam Filled	***1 Slice/65g***	***196***	***3.2***	***302***	***4.2***	***64.2***	***4.9***	***1.8***
Sponge, Roll, Chocolate, M&S*	¼ Cake/66g	251	12.1	380	3.9	50.5	18.4	1.8
Sponge, with Butter Icing	***1 Slice/65g***	***318***	***19.9***	***490***	***4.5***	***52.4***	***30.6***	***0.6***
Sticky Pudding, Golden Syrup, Lyle's, McVitie's*	1 Slice/30g	108	3.3	361	3.8	61.5	11	1.6
Stollen, Bites, Finest, Tesco*	1 Bite/17g	68	3.2	398	5	50.9	18.8	4.4
Stollen, Bites, Waitrose*	1 Bite/18g	71	3.1	395	4.6	54.5	17.1	2.2
Stollen, Chocolate & Rum, Finest, Tesco*	1/8 Cake/68g	262	9.5	381	5.3	57	13.8	3.9
Stollen, Marzipan Butter, Mini, Favorina, Lidl*	1 Stollen/18g	81	4.2	452	9.5	49.2	23.3	0
Stollen, Slices, Average	***1 Slice/42g***	***160***	***6.3***	***381***	***5.5***	***55.8***	***15***	***3.1***
Strawberry, & Clotted Cream, Cornish, M&S*	1/6 Slice/68g	277	12.9	410	3.9	55.5	19.1	0.5
Strawberry, Sponge Roll, M&S*	1/6 Cake/49g	160	4.6	330	2.8	58	9.5	0.8
Sultana, & Cherry, M&S*	1 Slice/50g	180	5.8	360	0	59.5	11.5	2
Sultana, Fair Trade, Co-Op*	1/8 Cake/45g	155	4	345	5	60	9	1
Swiss Roll, Apricot, Co-Op*	1 Serving/44g	158	3.7	357	2.9	67	8.3	1
Swiss Roll, Average	***1oz/28g***	***77***	***1.2***	***276***	***7.2***	***55.5***	***4.4***	***0.8***
Swiss Roll, Chocolate, Individual	***1 Roll/26g***	***88***	***2.9***	***337***	***4.3***	***58.1***	***11.3***	***0***
Swiss Roll, Lemon, Tesco*	1 Slice/32g	118	3	371	3.7	67.4	9.4	1
Swiss Roll, Raspberry, Average	***1 Slice/35g***	***107***	***1.2***	***305***	***3.8***	***64.8***	***3.5***	***0.6***
Swiss Roll, Strawberry & Cream, Tesco*	1 Slice/32g	113	2.5	353	3.5	66.6	7.8	1.4
Swiss Roll, Strawberry & Vanilla, Jumbo, Ms Mollys*	1/12 Roll/33g	120	3.1	364	4.2	65.2	9.3	1.5
Tea Loaf, Rowan Hill Bakery, Lidl*	1 Slice/50g	135	0.4	270	3.8	63.3	0.9	3.4
Tiffin, Chocolate, Sainsbury's*	1 Cake/61g	184	11.6	301	2.7	29.8	19	1.3
Toffee, & Pecan Slices, M&S*	1 Slice/36g	160	8.5	445	4.7	54	23.7	1.3
Toffee, Apple, McVitie's*	1 Slice/26g	95	2.9	363	3.8	61.5	11	1.6
Toffee, Iced, Tesco*	1 Serving/35g	132	5.2	376	3.3	57.2	14.9	1.6

C

	Measure INFO/WEIGHT	per Measure KCAL	FAT	Nutrition Values per 100g / 100ml KCAL	PROT	CARB	FAT	FIBRE
CAKE								
Toffee, Terror Whirls, Mr Kipling*	1 Whirl/28g	141	7.9	509	3.9	58.3	28.7	1.2
Vanilla, Sponge, Fresh Cream, Sainsbury's*	1 Slice/50g	152	5.1	304	7.5	45.6	10.2	0.4
Victoria Sandwich, Average	***1 Slice/68g***	***267***	***12.9***	***392***	***4.4***	***50.9***	***19***	***1***
Victoria Sponge, Free From, Finest, Tesco*	1 Slice/61g	238	11.8	393	2.9	51.3	19.4	0.8
Victoria Sponge, Lemon, Co-Op*	1 Slice/42g	151	8	360	4	44	19	0.7
Victoria Sponge, Mini, Bobby's*	1 Cake/35g	164	9.6	469	4	51.3	27.5	0.2
Victoria Sponge, Mini, Mr Kipling*	1 Cake/36g	152	6.9	420	3.9	58.5	19	0.8
Victoria Sponge, Mini, Weight Watchers*	1 Cake/30g	103	2.5	343	5.7	57.2	8.3	8.4
Viennese, Whirl, Average	***1 Cake/28g***	***131***	***6.9***	***467***	***4.1***	***56.7***	***24.8***	***1.1***
Viennese, Whirl, Chocolate, Mr Kipling*	1 Whirl/28g	134	7.8	484	4.6	53.1	28	2.1
Viennese, Whirl, Lemon, Mr Kipling*	1 Cake/28g	115	4.5	409	4.2	62.2	15.9	0.7
Walnut, Holly Lane, Aldi*	1/8 Cake/38g	154	6.8	404	6.2	54	18	1.4
Walnut, Sandwich, Sainsbury's*	1/8 Cake/48g	182	8.3	379	5.4	53.8	17.3	1.3
Welsh, Average	***1oz/28g***	***121***	***5.5***	***431***	***5.6***	***61.8***	***19.6***	***1.5***
Winter Whirl, Mr Kipling*	1 Whirl/28g	145	8.1	515	3.6	59.4	28.7	2.4
Yorkshire Parkin, Bakers Delight*	1oz/28g	111	4.1	395	5.1	60.3	14.8	1.5
CAKE BAR								
Caramel, Tesco*	1 Cake/26g	103	4.9	395	5.1	50.8	19	8.2
Carrot, Tesco*	1 Bar/68g	239	12.6	351	4.7	41.4	18.5	2.4
Chocolate & Orange, Go Ahead, McVitie's*	1 Cake/33g	109	2	330	4.3	64.9	6	1
Chocolate Chip, Average	***1 Cake/28g***	***120***	***6***	***428***	***6.3***	***51.9***	***21.6***	***1.6***
Chocolate Dream, Go Ahead, McVitie's*	1 Bar/36g	141	4.8	391	4.6	63.2	13.4	0.9
Chocolate, Average	***1 Cake/28g***	***125***	***6.2***	***446***	***5.6***	***56.3***	***22.1***	***1.9***
Double Chocolate, Free From, Sainsbury's*	1 Cake/50g	196	7.9	391	4.2	58.2	15.7	1
Double Chocolate, Free From, Tesco*	1 Serving/45g	190	9.1	425	4.2	55.6	20.3	4.1
Flake, Cadbury*	1 Cake/25g	120	6.2	470	4.8	56.5	24.4	1.9
Galaxy, Salted Caramel, Festive, Galaxy, Mars*	1 Bar/26g	113	5.3	438	5.6	58.7	20.4	0
Golden Syrup, McVitie's*	1 Cake/33g	127	4.8	385	3.6	60.2	14.4	1.2
Jaffa Cakes, Spooky, McVitie's*	1 Bar/25g	96	3.5	390	3.2	62.1	14.2	2.7
Jaffa, McVitie's*	1 Bar/25g	96	3.5	395	3.1	62.9	14.5	2.5
Jamaica Ginger, McVitie's*	1 Cake/33g	128	4.9	388	3.5	60.2	14.7	1.2
Milk Chocolate, Cadbury*	1 Bar/25g	110	5.6	445	4.9	53.8	22.8	2.9
Milky Way, McVitie's*	1 Cake/26g	124	6.2	476	5.1	58.5	23.6	1.2
Peanut, High Fibre, Squares, Tesco*	1 Square/24g	92	3.1	383	6	49	13	23
Vanilla, & Raspberry, Mini Rolls, Ms Mollys*	1 Roll/20g	74	2.2	368	4.7	62	11	1.2
CALLALOO								
Leaves, Raw, Unprepared	***1 Cup/28g***	***6***	***0.1***	***23***	***2.5***	***4***	***0.3***	***0***
CANAPES								
Aegean Tomato, Finest, Tesco*	1 Canape/15g	45	2.2	300	7.2	34.3	14.7	2.1
Salmon & Dill, Finest, Tesco*	1 Canape/15g	47	2.4	315	9.2	32.7	16.1	1.9
Salmon, Smoked, Tesco*	1 Canape/8g	20	1.5	241	14.7	4.1	18.3	0.5
Smoked Salmon, Youngs*	1 Canape/10g	21	1.5	210	15.9	2	15.2	0.7
CANNELLONI								
Beef, As Prepared, Waitrose*	1 Pack/360g	501	26.7	139	6.2	11.5	7.4	1
Beef, Meal for One, M&S*	1 Pack/400g	572	30.8	143	6.7	10.7	7.7	2.1
Bolognese, Pingo Doce*	¼ Pack/250g	405	21.2	162	7.9	13	8.5	1.1
Mushroom, Italian, Sainsbury's*	1 Pack/450g	598	31	133	5.2	12.5	6.9	0.5
Spinach, & Ricotta, Fresh, Ready Meal, Average	***1 Serving/300g***	***393***	***22***	***131***	***5***	***10.8***	***7.4***	***1.2***
Spinach, & Ricotta, Low Fat, COU, M&S*	1 Pack/400g	340	7.6	85	4.8	11.4	1.9	1.7
Spinach, & Ricotta, Ready Meal, Average	***1 Serving/300g***	***426***	***22***	***142***	***5.6***	***13.3***	***7.3***	***1.4***
Tubes, Dry, Average	***1oz/28g***	***101***	***1***	***361***	***12.5***	***69.1***	***3.6***	***1.2***
Vegetarian, Tesco*	1 Pack/400g	552	34.4	138	5.3	9.8	8.6	1.5

C

	Measure INFO/WEIGHT	per Measure KCAL	FAT	Nutrition Values per 100g / 100ml KCAL	PROT	CARB	FAT	FIBRE
CAPERS								
in Vinegar, Average	***1 Tsp/5g***	***2***	***0***	***34***	***1.7***	***3***	***0.6***	***0***
CAPPELLETTI								
Ham, & Cheese, Cooked, Tesco*	½ Pack/150g	288	7.5	192	8.8	27.2	5	1.6
Jambon Cru, Rana La Famiglia*	1 Serving/125g	376	9.5	301	13	44	7.6	0
Parma Ham, Fresh, Waitrose*	½ Pack/125g	368	11.5	294	14.1	38.6	9.2	2.2
with Parma Ham, M&S*	½ Pack/125g	342	9.1	274	15.7	35.4	7.3	1.8
CAPRI SUN								
Blackcurrant, No Added Sugar, Capri-Sun*	1 Pouch/200ml	10	0	5	0	0.9	0	0
Orange	***1 Pouch/200ml***	***90***	***0***	***45***	***0***	***11***	***0***	***0***
Orange, 100%, Juice	***1 Pouch/200ml***	***75***	***0***	***38***	***0.5***	***9.2***	***0***	***0.1***
CARAMAC								
Nestle*	1 Bar/31g	173	10.4	559	6.2	57.9	33.7	0
CARBONARA								
Chicken, & Bacon, BFY, M&S*	1 Pack/375g	476	11.2	127	10.1	14.4	3	0.8
Chicken, & Bacon, Calorie Counted, Asda*	1 Pack/324g	311	4.9	96	7.5	12	1.5	1.5
Chicken, Mushroom, & Ham, Spaghetti, Asda*	1 Pack/700g	686	14	98	10	10	2	1.5
Chicken, Slimming World, Iceland*	1 Bowl/550g	556	3.8	101	10.2	12.5	0.7	2.2
Creamy, As Prepared, Pot Pasta*	1 Pot/260g	275	11.5	105	2.9	13	4.4	0.5
Mushroom, Vegan, Love Your Veg!, Sainsbury's*	1 Pack/400g	420	15.6	105	3.3	13.2	3.9	1.9
Mushroom, Vegan, Waitrose*	1 Pack/380g	437	19.4	115	2.3	14	5.1	2
Pasta, Taste of Italy, Oven Baked, Iceland*	¼ Pack/281g	346	12.1	123	5.4	15.1	4.3	1.2
Penne, Taste of Italy, Tesco*	½ Pack/400g	604	18.5	151	7.9	19	4.6	0.9
Rigatoni, Allplants*	1 Serving/390g	534	23	137	6	14	5.9	2.3
Spaghetti, BGTY, Sainsbury's*	1 Pack/400g	392	7.6	98	5.9	14	1.9	0.7
Spaghetti, COU, M&S*	1 Pack/330g	346	7.2	105	6.1	15.7	2.2	0.8
Spaghetti, Extra Special, Asda*	1 Pack/350g	578	25.9	165	7.9	16	7.4	0.8
Spaghetti, Heated, HL, Tesco*	1 Pack/365g	372	5.1	102	6	16	1.4	0.8
Spaghetti, Italian Quisine, Microwaved, Aldi*	1 Pack/400g	669	33.4	174	7.1	16	8.7	1.5
Spaghetti, M&S*	1 Pack/400g	656	29.2	164	7.5	16.6	7.3	0.7
Spaghetti, M&S*	1 Pack/400g	560	27.2	140	5.2	14	6.8	0.9
Spaghetti, Ready Meal, Average	***1 Pack/400g***	***524***	***21.5***	***131***	***5.9***	***14.4***	***5.4***	***1.1***
Spaghetti, Smoked Bacon, & Parmigian, TTD, Sainsbury's*	1 Pack/345g	583	28.3	169	8.1	15	8.2	1.2
Tagliatelle, Ready Meal, Average	***1 Serving/400g***	***460***	***13.4***	***115***	***5.5***	***15.8***	***3.3***	***1***
CARDAMOM								
Black, Ground, Average	***1 Tsp/2g***	***6***	***0.1***	***311***	***10.8***	***68.5***	***6.7***	***28***
CAROB POWDER								
Average	***1 Tsp/2g***	***3***	***0***	***159***	***4.9***	***37***	***0.1***	***0***
CARP								
Fillet, Raw, Average	***1 Fillet/218g***	***244***	***10.2***	***112***	***17.5***	***0***	***4.7***	***0***
CARROT & SWEDE								
Diced, for Mashing, Average	***½ Pack/250g***	***58***	***0.7***	***23***	***0.6***	***4.7***	***0.3***	***1.9***
Mash, From Supermarket, Average	***1 Serving/150g***	***138***	***7.5***	***92***	***1.3***	***10.4***	***5***	***1.3***
Mash, Healthy Range, Average	***1 Serving/150g***	***98***	***4.2***	***66***	***1.3***	***8.6***	***2.8***	***2.1***
Mash, with Potato, British, Sainsbury's*	½ Pack/199g	143	3	72	1.3	12.2	1.5	2.1
CARROTS								
& Peas, Sainsbury's*	1 Serving/200g	100	1	50	3.3	8.3	0.5	3.8
Baby, Canned, Average	***1 Can/195g***	***40***	***0.5***	***21***	***0.5***	***4.2***	***0.3***	***2.1***
Baby, Fresh, Average	***1 Serving/80g***	***28***	***0.1***	***35***	***0.6***	***8.2***	***0.1***	***2.9***
Batons, Fresh, Average	***½ Pack/150g***	***41***	***0.4***	***28***	***0.6***	***5.7***	***0.3***	***2.6***
Boiled, Average	***1oz/28g***	***6***	***0.1***	***22***	***0.6***	***4.4***	***0.4***	***2.3***
Canned, Average	***1oz/28g***	***6***	***0.1***	***20***	***0.5***	***4***	***0.2***	***1.9***
Chantenay, Cut, Frozen, Tesco*	1 Serving/80g	24	0.3	29	0.6	4.3	0.4	3.1
Chantenay, Wood Farm, Raw, Aldi*	1 Serving/80g	34	0.4	42	0.6	7.9	0.5	2.4

	Measure INFO/WEIGHT	per Measure KCAL	FAT	Nutrition Values per 100g / 100ml KCAL	PROT	CARB	FAT	FIBRE
CARROTS								
Raw, Average	***1 Med/61g***	***25***	***0.1***	***41***	***0.9***	***9.6***	***0.2***	***2.8***
Raw, Scrubbed, Average	***1 Serving/80g***	***24***	***0.4***	***30***	***0.7***	***6***	***0.5***	***2.4***
Sliced, Canned, Average	***1 Serving/180g***	***36***	***0.2***	***20***	***0.7***	***4.1***	***0.1***	***1.5***
Sliced, Fresh, Average	***1 Serving/60g***	***17***	***0.2***	***28***	***0.7***	***5.7***	***0.3***	***2***
Sticks, & Houmous, Reduced Fat, M&S*	1 Pack/130g	157	9.9	121	3.3	7.8	7.6	3.9
Whole, Raw, Peeled, Average	***1 Carrot/75g***	***21***	***0.2***	***29***	***0.6***	***6.4***	***0.3***	***2.2***
CASHEW NUTS								
& Jumbo Raisins, Iceland*	1 Serving/30g	123	5.4	411	8.5	52.2	18.1	2.5
Cheese Flavour, Graze*	1 Pack/26g	140	10.8	540	15.3	35.7	41.5	0
Cracking Black Pepper, Graze*	1 Punnet/36g	216	16.6	600	19	26	46	4
Plain, Average	***½ Pack/25g***	***146***	***12.2***	***584***	***15.7***	***18.8***	***48.9***	***3.4***
Roasted & Salted, Average	***1 Serving/50g***	***306***	***25.6***	***612***	***18.8***	***19.6***	***51.1***	***3.1***
Roasted, Tamari, Organic, Clearspring*	1 Pack/30g	162	11.7	539	17	29	39	2.7
Wasabi, Roasted, Vitasia, Lidl*	1 Serving/30g	185	14.6	616	17.5	25.6	48.6	0
CASSAVA								
Baked, Average	***1oz/28g***	***43***	***0.1***	***155***	***0.7***	***40.1***	***0.2***	***1.7***
Boiled in Unsalted Water, Average	***1oz/28g***	***36***	***0.1***	***130***	***0.5***	***33.5***	***0.2***	***1.4***
Gari, Average	***1oz/28g***	***100***	***0.1***	***358***	***1.3***	***92.9***	***0.5***	***0***
CASSEROLE								
Beef	***1 Serving/336g***	***490***	***23***	***146***	***16.3***	***4.6***	***6.8***	***0.6***
Beef, & Ale, Average	***1 Serving/300g***	***251***	***6.8***	***84***	***9.4***	***6.5***	***2.2***	***1.3***
Beef, & Red Wine, Average	***1 Serving/350g***	***290***	***7.3***	***83***	***7.2***	***8.2***	***2.1***	***1.5***
Beef, Low & Slow, Slimming World, Iceland*	1 Serving/175g	88	1.2	50	6.6	3.7	0.7	0.9
Beef, with Dumplings, Ready Meal, Average	***1 Serving/350g***	***464***	***21.1***	***132***	***9.5***	***10.1***	***6***	***1.5***
Beef, with Herb Potatoes, Ready Meal, Average	***1 Serving/475g***	***504***	***17.1***	***106***	***6.8***	***11.5***	***3.6***	***1.6***
Chicken, & Asparagus, HL, Tesco*	1 Serving/450g	342	10.3	76	6.3	8.3	2.3	0.5
Chicken, & Dumplings, Sainsbury's*	1 Serving/450g	612	24.8	136	9.1	12	5.5	1.2
Chicken, & Vegetable, Ready Meal, Healthy Range	***1 Serving/330g***	***265***	***11.9***	***80***	***4.7***	***7.6***	***3.6***	***1.1***
Chicken, & Bacon, Shake That Weight*	1 Pack/275g	256	12.4	93	11.2	2.4	4.5	1
Chicken, & Dumpling, M&S*	1 Pack/450g	612	28.4	136	10.2	9	6.3	1.3
Chicken, & Dumplings, Parsley Box*	1 Pack/270g	254	4.6	94	8.3	11	1.7	1
Chicken, & Mushroom, Slim Cook, Tesco*	1 Pack/495g	193	2	39	5.6	2.6	0.4	1.6
Chicken, Leek & Mushroom, Tesco*	1 Pack/350g	382	22	109	4.5	8.6	6.3	1
Chicken, Meal Kit, Aldi*	¼ Pack/165g	288	18.1	175	18	1.4	11	0.6
Chicken, Spanish, Ready Set Cook!, Aldi*	¼ Pack/169g	417	28.7	247	22	2.2	17	0.5
Chicken, Spanish, with Peppers, Waitrose*	¼ Pack/150g	237	12	158	19.4	1.9	8	0.6
Lamb, & Rosemary, Eat Well, M&S*	1 Pack/380g	325	11	86	7.6	7	2.9	2.2
Pork, Apple, & Cider, Asda*	1 Pack/360g	443	15.5	123	14	6.3	4.3	1.1
Pork, Normandy Style, Finest, Tesco*	1 Pack/450g	405	21.6	90	7.6	4.1	4.8	2.3
Rabbit, Average	***1oz/28g***	***29***	***1.4***	***102***	***11.6***	***2.6***	***5.1***	***0.4***
Red Lentil, & Mixed Bean, Cook*	1 Serving/290g	218	4.4	75	4.5	14.2	1.5	6.6
Sausage, & Potato, M&S*	1 Serving/200g	190	11.8	95	3.3	7.5	5.9	0.9
Sausage, & Bean, Steam Fresh, Farmfoods*	1 Pack/350g	336	11.2	96	5	9.7	3.2	0
Sausage, CBY, Asda*	1 Pot/400g	240	15.2	60	3.6	1.9	3.8	2.1
Steak, & Ale, Average	***1 Serving/275g***	***324***	***14.4***	***118***	***9***	***8.8***	***5.2***	***1***
Steak, & Mushroom, Average	***1 Serving/275g***	***274***	***15.5***	***100***	***6.2***	***6***	***5.6***	***1***
Vegetable, Root, & Kale, Waitrose*	1 Pack/357g	343	15	96	1.9	11.6	4.2	2.1
Vegetables, Mix, Frozen, Boiled, Iceland*	1 Serving/80g	20	0.2	25	0.7	4.1	0.3	1.7
Veggie, Meal for One, M&S*	1 Pack/450g	436	16.6	97	2.2	12.5	3.7	2.3
CASSEROLE MIX								
Beef & Ale, Colman's*	1 Pack/45g	144	0.9	320	9.2	66.3	2	2.3
Beef, Recipe, Colman's*	1 Pack/42g	142	0.5	338	9.1	13.1	1.1	4
Beef, Recipe, Schwartz*	1 Pack/43g	123	0.9	287	7	56.6	2.1	6.6

	Measure INFO/WEIGHT	per Measure KCAL	FAT	Nutrition Values per 100g / 100ml KCAL	PROT	CARB	FAT	FIBRE
CASSEROLE MIX								
Chicken Chasseur, Asda*	1 Pack/80g	273	0.8	341	9	74	1	1.4
Chicken, Authentic, Schwartz*	1 Serving/66g	210	0.7	318	14	62.1	1	2.1
Chicken, Recipe, As Sold, Colman's*	1 Pack/40g	131	1	328	6.2	68.2	2.6	3.1
Game, No.1, Waitrose*	1 Pack/250g	308	5.2	123	25.2	0.6	2.1	0.5
Lamb, Authentic, Schwartz*	1 Pack/35g	116	1.2	332	7.7	68	3.3	1.3
Peppered Beef, Schwartz*	1 Pack/40g	129	2	323	7	62.9	4.9	7.3
Sausage, As Sold, Colman's*	1 Pack/39g	136	1	350	10	70	2.5	6
Sausage, Classic, Schwartz*	1 Pack/35g	96	0.9	275	12.4	50.1	2.7	14.9
CATFISH								
Cooked, Steamed, Weighed with Bone, Average	**1 Serving/100g**	**101**	**3.1**	**101**	**18.2**	**0**	**3.1**	**0.7**
CAULIFLOWER								
Bang Bang, Love Your Veg!, Sainsbury's*	½ Pack/62g	129	6	208	2.5	26.3	9.7	2.7
Bang Bang, Waitrose *	½ Pack/88g	214	14.9	243	2.2	19.4	16.9	2.4
BBQ, Bites, Tesco*	½ Pack/128g	83	1.1	65	2.3	10.9	0.9	2.2
Bites, Buffalo, Tesco*	½ Pack/115g	163	7.5	142	2.6	16.5	6.5	3.7
Boiled, Average	**1 Serving/80g**	**22**	**0.7**	**28**	**2.9**	**2.1**	**0.9**	**1.6**
Cous Cous, Ready to Cook, As Sold, Morrisons*	1 Pack/330g	129	3	39	3.6	2.8	0.9	2.6
Grills, Tesco*	1 Grill/96g	236	13.7	246	5.6	22	14.3	3.2
Popcorn, Vegan, Plant Based, Asda*	¼ Pack/75g	113	4.6	150	2.2	20	6.1	3
Popcorn, with Spicy Buffalo Dip, Plant Kitchen, M&S*	½ Pack/113g	213	12.7	189	2.3	18.7	11.3	1.6
Raw, Average	**1 Serving/80g**	**25**	**0.7**	**31**	**3.2**	**2.7**	**0.8**	**1.6**
Spiced, Roasted, Tesco*	½ Pack/70g	59	4.4	84	2.2	3.9	6.2	1.8
Spiced, Roasting, Sainsbury's*	1 Serving/107g	62	3	58	2.3	4.8	2.8	2.2
Steamed, Average	**1 Serving/100g**	**28**	**0.9**	**28**	**2.9**	**2.1**	**0.9**	**1.6**
Wing, Bites, BBQ, Fire Pit, Tesco*	½ Pack/126g	146	2.5	116	6	16.6	2	4
CAULIFLOWER CHEESE								
& Broccoli, Average	**1 Serving/200g**	**127**	**6.4**	**64**	**3.8**	**4.6**	**3.2**	**2**
Average	**1 Meal/400g**	**362**	**23.3**	**90**	**4.5**	**4.6**	**5.8**	**1.3**
Frozen, Iceland*	1 Serving/200g	190	12	95	4	5.5	6	1.6
Frozen, Oven Baked, Asda*	½ Pack/150g	187	10.6	125	5.9	8.3	7.1	1.9
Made with Semi-Skimmed Milk	**1oz/28g**	**28**	**1.8**	**100**	**6**	**5.2**	**6.4**	**1.3**
Made with Skimmed Milk	**1oz/28g**	**27**	**1.7**	**97**	**6**	**5.2**	**6**	**1.3**
Made with Whole Milk	**1oz/28g**	**29**	**1.9**	**105**	**6**	**5.2**	**6.9**	**1.3**
with Wexford Mature Cheddar, M&S*	½ Pack/225g	263	17.6	117	6.7	4.3	7.8	1.3
CAVIAR								
Average	**1oz/28g**	**25**	**1.3**	**89**	**11.6**	**0.5**	**4.6**	**0**
Salmon, Elsinore*	1 Jar/50g	120	6.5	240	30	0.5	13	0
Trout, Caspian Tradition *	1 Tsp/8g	16	0.6	194	28	2.6	7.9	0
CELERIAC								
Boiled in Salted Water, Average	**1oz/28g**	**5**	**0.1**	**18**	**0.9**	**1.9**	**0.4**	**3.2**
Raw, Average	**1 Serving/80g**	**17**	**0.3**	**21**	**1**	**1.9**	**0.4**	**3.2**
Remoulade, Waitrose *	1 Serving/110g	335	32.6	304	1.2	7.3	29.6	1.6
CELERY								
Boiled in Salted Water	**1 Serving/50g**	**4**	**0.2**	**8**	**0.5**	**0.8**	**0.3**	**1.2**
Raw, Trimmed, Average	**1 Stalk/40g**	**3**	**0.1**	**7**	**0.5**	**0.9**	**0.2**	**1.1**
CHAMPAGNE								
Average	**1 Glass/125ml**	**95**	**0**	**76**	**0.3**	**1.4**	**0**	**0**
CHANNA MASALA								
M&S*	1 Pack/225g	360	23.7	160	5.6	11.2	10.5	8.2
Potato, Gunpowder, Co-Op*	1 Pack/350g	396	11.9	113	2.7	17	3.4	1.9
Waitrose*	1 Pack/300g	300	18.3	100	3.7	7.4	6.1	7.9
CHAPATIS								
Brown Wheat Flour, Waitrose*	1 Chapati/42g	128	3.4	305	8.6	49.4	8	4.6

	Measure INFO/WEIGHT	per Measure KCAL	FAT	Nutrition Values per 100g / 100ml KCAL	PROT	CARB	FAT	FIBRE
CHAPATIS								
Elephant Atta*	1 Chapati/45g	129	2.9	287	7.5	53.1	6.4	3.2
Indian Style, Asda*	1 Chapati/43g	95	0.4	221	8	45	1	2.9
Loyd Grossman*	1 Chapatti/60g	179	2.8	298	9	52.4	4.7	5
Made with Fat	***1 Chapati/60g***	***197***	***7.7***	***328***	***8.1***	***48.3***	***12.8***	***0***
Made without Fat	***1 Chapati/55g***	***111***	***0.6***	***202***	***7.3***	***43.7***	***1***	***0***
Morrisons*	1 Chapati/40g	108	2.8	269	8.6	49.8	6.9	0
Plain, Original, Wrap, Patak's*	1 Chapati/42g	115	3.2	273	9.4	48.8	7.5	0
Sainsbury's*	1 Chapatti/95g	306	7	322	8.9	52.8	7.4	4.1
White, Dina Foods Ltd*	1 Chapatti/50g	120	1.4	240	7.4	45.1	2.8	1.5
Wholemeal, Patak's*	1 Chapati/42g	130	4	310	11.2	44.9	9.5	9
CHARD								
Average	***1 Serving/80g***	***15***	***0.2***	***19***	***1.4***	***3.3***	***0.2***	***0.8***
Silverbeet, Fresh, Steamed	***1 Serving/100g***	***15***	***0***	***15***	***1.9***	***1.3***	***0***	***3.3***
Swiss, Boiled in Unsalted Water	***1oz/28g***	***6***	***0***	***20***	***1.9***	***4.1***	***0.1***	***2.1***
Swiss, Raw	***1oz/28g***	***5***	***0.1***	***17***	***1.7***	***3.4***	***0.2***	***1.5***
CHEDDARS								
Baked, Mini, Blue Cheese, Jacob's*	1 Pack/25g	132	7.9	530	8.8	50.3	31.8	2.5
Baked, Mini, Pepper Jack, Jacob's*	1 Pack/25g	128	7	511	9.3	53.5	28	2.7
Cheese & Ham, Baked, Mini, McVitie's*	1 Bag/30g	160	8.9	534	11	55.5	29.8	2
Cheese, Baked, Mini, Original, Jacobs*	1 Bag/25g	129	7.2	516	9.2	53.2	28.8	2.8
Chilli Beef, Baked, Mini, Jacob's*	1 Pack/50g	262	15	522	9	52.2	29.9	2.7
Mini, Average	***1 Bag/26g***	***134***	***7.8***	***516***	***11.2***	***50.8***	***29.9***	***2.4***
Mini, BBQ, Jacob's*	1 Pack/25g	131	7.6	525	9.3	51.6	30.3	2.6
Mini, Monterey Jack, Jacob's*	1 Bag/25g	128	7	511	9.3	53.5	28	2.7
Red Leicester, Baked, Mini, Jacob's*	1 Pack/25g	132	7.9	530	8.7	50.2	31.8	2.5
Stilton, Baked, Mini, Jacob's*	1 Pack/25g	132	7.9	530	8.8	50.3	31.8	2.5
CHEESE								
& Nuts, Salt & Pepper, Fridge Raiders, Mattessons*	1 Pack/40g	163	10.4	407	25	17	26	0
Babybel, Cheddar Variety, Mini, Fromageries Bel*	1 Cheese/20g	75	6.2	375	24	0	31	0
Babybel, Cheddar, Light, Mini, Fromageries Bel*	1 Mini/20g	59	4.4	296	24	0.5	22	0
Babybel, Emmental, Fromageries Bel*	1 Serving/20g	63	4.9	316	23	1	24.5	0
Babybel, Light, Mini, Fromageries Bel*	1 Babybel/20g	42	2.4	208	25	0	12	0
Babybel, Organic, Fromageries Bel*	1 Cheese/20g	59	4.6	293	21.5	0	23	0
Babybel, Original, Mini, Fromageries Bel*	1 Cheese/20g	61	4.8	304	22	0.1	24	0
Beechwood, Smoked, Slices, Tesco*	1 Slice/25g	75	6	299	20.7	0	24	0
Belegen, 48+, Slices, Beemster*	1 Slice/25g	97	8	387	25.2	0	31.8	0
Bites, Mini, Sainsbury's*	1 Serving/20g	65	4.7	323	25.3	3.1	23.3	0
Blue, Castello, Soft, Castello*	¼ Pack/37g	162	15.6	432	14	0.5	41.5	0
Blue, French, CBY, Asda*	1 Serving/30g	90	7.4	301	20	0	24.5	0
Blue, Rich & Creamy, St Agur*	1 Serving/30g	108	9.9	361	16	0.5	33	0
Blue, Shropshire, The Delicatessen, Tesco*	1 Serving/30g	123	10.5	410	23.7	0.1	35	0
Blue, Yorkshire, Artisan, Shepherds Purse*	1 Serving/30g	122	10.7	405	19.5	1.3	35.7	0.5
Brie, Average	***1 Serving/25g***	***74***	***6***	***296***	***19.7***	***0.3***	***24***	***0***
Brie, Breaded, Bites, Frozen, Tesco*	1 Bite/17g	54	3.4	319	8.6	24.2	20.2	2.8
Brie, Cornish, Lactofree, Arla*	1 Serving/30g	105	9.3	351	17	1.7	31	0
Brie, Reduced Fat, Average	***1 Serving/50g***	***99***	***5.7***	***198***	***23***	***0.8***	***11.4***	***0***
Burrata, 1, Waitrose*	1 Serving/30g	67	5.6	222	13.4	0.2	18.6	0
Burrata, Organic , Murgella *	1 Serving/30g	67	5.7	222	10	2.8	19	0
Caerphilly, Average	***1 Serving/50g***	***187***	***15.6***	***374***	***23***	***0.1***	***31.3***	***0***
Cambazola, Tesco*	1 Serving/30g	128	12.3	425	13.5	0.5	41	0
Camembert, Average	***1 Serving/50g***	***141***	***11.1***	***283***	***20.5***	***0.1***	***22.2***	***0***
Camembert, Breaded, Average	***1 Serving/90g***	***307***	***20.9***	***342***	***16.6***	***14.2***	***23.2***	***0.4***
Camembert, Caramelised Red Onion, Deluxe, Lidl*	1 Serving/30g	85	6.1	282	15.4	9	20.4	0.5

	Measure INFO/WEIGHT	per Measure KCAL	FAT	Nutrition Values per 100g / 100ml KCAL	PROT	CARB	FAT	FIBRE
CHEESE								
Cantal, French, Sainsbury's*	1 Serving/30g	106	8.7	353	23	0.1	29	0
Cheddar, & Mozzarella, Grated, M&S*	1 Serving/30g	101	8.3	337	22	0.1	27.6	0.1
Cheddar, & Mozzarella, Grated, Morrisons*	1 Serving/30g	108	8.4	360	25.4	2.8	28	0
Cheddar, & Mozzarella, Grated, Waitrose*	1 Serving/30g	103	7.8	342	24.9	2.1	26	0
Cheddar, Average	***1 Serving/30g***	***123***	***10.3***	***410***	***25***	***0.1***	***34.4***	***0***
Cheddar, Canadian, Average	***1 Serving/30g***	***123***	***10.3***	***409***	***25***	***0.1***	***34.3***	***0***
Cheddar, Cracked Peppercorn, Isle Of Man Creamery*	1 Serving/30g	121	9.7	402	23	4.1	32.3	0.5
Cheddar, Davidstow, Mature, Average	***1 Serving/28g***	***115***	***9.6***	***410***	***25***	***0.1***	***34.4***	***0***
Cheddar, Extra Mature, Average	***1 Serving/30g***	***123***	***10.3***	***410***	***25.1***	***0.1***	***34.4***	***0***
Cheddar, Grated, Average	***1 Serving/50g***	***206***	***17.2***	***413***	***24.4***	***1.5***	***34.3***	***0***
Cheddar, Mature, Average	***1 Serving/30g***	***123***	***10.3***	***410***	***25***	***0.1***	***34.4***	***0***
Cheddar, Mature, Grated, Average	***1 Serving/28g***	***113***	***9.3***	***404***	***24.7***	***1.6***	***33.2***	***0***
Cheddar, Mature, Lactose Free, Cathedral City*	1 Serving/30g	125	10.5	416	25.4	0.1	34.9	0
Cheddar, Mature, Reduced Fat, Average	***1 Serving/25g***	***68***	***4.2***	***271***	***30***	***0.1***	***16.7***	***0***
Cheddar, Medium, Average	***1 Serving/30g***	***123***	***10.4***	***411***	***24.9***	***0.2***	***34.5***	***0***
Cheddar, Mild, Average	***1 Serving/30g***	***123***	***10.3***	***409***	***25***	***0.1***	***34.3***	***0***
Cheddar, Reduced Fat, Average	***1 Serving/30g***	***76***	***4.2***	***255***	***32.2***	***0.1***	***14***	***0***
Cheddar, Smoked, Average	***1 Serving/30g***	***123***	***10.3***	***411***	***25.2***	***0.1***	***34.4***	***0***
Cheddar, Vintage, Tickler, Castello*	1 Serving/30g	125	10.8	417	24	0.5	36	0
Cheddar, White, Vintage, Finest, Tesco*	1 Serving/30g	125	10.5	416	25.4	0.1	34.9	0
Cheddar, with Caramelised Onion, Tesco*	1 Serving/50g	183	14	366	21.4	7.1	28	0.4
Cheddar, with Mixed Peppers, Sliced, Mexicana *	1 Slice/20g	79	6.3	396	23.7	4.7	31.3	0
Cheddar, with Onion & Chives, Davidson*	1 Serving/25g	100	8.3	400	24.3	0.6	33.3	0
Cheddar, with Pickled Onions, & Chives, Asda*	1 Serving/30g	104	8.4	347	20	4.6	28	0.6
Chedds, Bricks, Cathedral City, Dairy Crest Ltd*	1 Brick/18g	75	6.3	416	25.4	0.1	34.9	0
Cheedar, & Mozzarella, Grated, Mix, Sain*	1 Serving/30g	100	7.5	333	22.3	4.9	24.9	0.5
Cheshire	***1oz/28g***	***106***	***8.8***	***379***	***24***	***0.1***	***31.4***	***0***
Cinco Lanzas, 16 Month, The Best, Morrisons*	1 Serving/30g	131	11.1	437	23.7	1	37	2.4
Compte Aop, No.1, Waitrose*	1 Slice/30g	128	9.7	428	28.4	4.8	32.4	1.8
Cottage, Low Fat, 2% Fat, Natural, Average	***1 Serving/75g***	***68***	***1.4***	***90***	***13.7***	***3.6***	***1.9***	***0***
Cottage, Onion & Chive, Fat Free, Sainsbury's*	1 Serving/30g	22	0.2	75	11.8	6.4	0.5	0.5
Cottage, Onion, & Chive, Fat Free, Emporium, Aldi*	1 Serving/30g	18	0.2	59	11	3.3	0.5	0.5
Cottage, Pineapple, Fat Free, Emporium, Aldi*	1 Serving/30g	25	0.2	82	12	7.6	0.5	0.5
Cottage, Pineapple, Low Fat, Morrisons*	1 Serving/30g	23	0.3	76	9	7.8	1	0
Cottage, Plain, Average	***1 Tbsp/20g***	***19***	***0.7***	***93***	***12***	***3.3***	***3.5***	***0.1***
Cottage, Plain, Reduced Fat, Average	***100g***	***85***	***1.9***	***85***	***12.3***	***4.4***	***1.9***	***0.1***
Cottage, Virtually Fat Free, Average	***1 Tbsp/20g***	***16***	***0.2***	***79***	***13***	***4.5***	***1***	***0***
Cottage, Whole Milk, Natural, Average	***1 Serving/75g***	***77***	***3.4***	***103***	***12.5***	***2.7***	***4.5***	***0***
Cottage, with Black Pepper, HE, Tesco*	1 Pot/125g	101	2.2	81	12.1	4	1.8	0
Cottage, with Onion & Chive, GFY, Asda*	¼ Tub/75g	50	1	66	9.3	3.8	1.4	0.5
Cottage, with Onion & Chive, Asda *	¼ Pot/76g	44	0.4	58	9.3	4.6	0.5	0.5
Cottage, with Onion, & Chive, Rowan Glen*	1/3 Pot/100g	78	1.6	78	10.5	5	1.6	0.6
Cottage, with Onion, & Chive, Spelga*	1 Serving/30g	28	1.2	94	10.2	4	4.1	0
Cottage, with Pineapple, Fat Free, Tesco*	1 Serving/30g	22	0.1	73	8.8	8.6	0.4	0
Cream, Average	***1 Portion/30g***	***132***	***14.2***	***439***	***3.1***	***0***	***47.4***	***0***
Cream, Garlic & Herbs, Boursin*	1 Serving/30g	119	11.7	396	8.5	3	39	0
Cream, Garlic & Herbs, Light, Boursin*	1 Portion/20g	26	1.8	131	8	4.5	9	0
Cream, Garlic, & Herbs, Velvety, Boursin*	1 Serving/25g	78	7.6	311	6.5	2.5	30.5	0
Cream, Marmite, M&S*	1 Spread/15g	42	3.4	283	8.1	10.9	22.8	0.7
Cream, Reduced Fat, Average	***1 Serving/20g***	***23***	***1.1***	***117***	***13***	***4***	***5.3***	***0.1***
Dairylea, Light, Slices, Kraft*	1 Slice/25g	44	1.9	177	16	8.2	7.6	1.6
Danish Blue, Average	***1 Serving/30g***	***106***	***8.7***	***352***	***20.8***	***0***	***29.1***	***0***
Demi Pont L'eveque, Finest, Tesco*	1 Serving/46g	138	10.6	301	21.1	0.4	23	0

C

	Measure INFO/WEIGHT	per Measure KCAL	FAT	Nutrition Values per 100g / 100ml KCAL	PROT	CARB	FAT	FIBRE
CHEESE								
Dolcelatte, Average	1 Serving/30g	110	9.7	366	17.8	0.4	32.3	0.4
Double Gloucester, Average	1 Serving/30g	121	10.2	404	24.5	0.1	34	0
Doux De Montagne, Average	1 Serving/25g	88	7.1	352	22.9	1.5	28.3	0
Edam, Average	1 Serving/10g	33	2.5	326	25.3	0	24.9	0
Edam, Dutch, Garlic & Herb Wedge, Asda*	1 Serving/60g	197	15	329	26	0	25	0
Edam, Slices, Average	1 Slice/30g	96	7.2	320	25	0.4	24.1	0
Emmental, Average	1 Serving/10g	37	2.8	368	28.4	0	28.4	0
Emmental, Light, Slices, President*	1 Slice/20g	60	3.6	298	34	0	18	0
Feta, & Tomato Sauce, Eridanous, Lidl*	1 Serving/15g	40	3.4	265	3.9	8.4	22.9	0
Feta, Apetina, Light, 10 % Fat, Arla*	1 Serving/30g	52	3	173	18.4	0.6	10.1	0
Feta, Average	1 Serving/30g	79	6.4	262	16.3	1	21.5	0
Feta, Lactose Free, Greco*	1 Serving/30g	81	6.8	270	16.4	0.4	22.5	0
Fiery, Blend, Grated, Asda*	1 Serving/30g	107	8.1	358	24	4.6	27	0.5
Fondue, Swiss, Easy Cook, Tesco*	¼ Pack/100g	235	17	235	15.5	4	17	0
Fontina, Average	1 Serving/28g	109	9	389	25	0	32.1	0
for Pizza, Grated	1 Serving/50g	163	12.2	326	25	1.6	24.4	0
Four, Mix, Grated, Sainsbury's*	1 Serving/30g	112	8.8	373	22.2	5.3	29.2	0.5
German, Smoked, with Jalapeno, Milbona, Lidl*	1 Slice/20g	66	5.3	332	19.5	3.5	26.6	0.5
Goats, Average	1 Tsp/10g	26	2.1	262	13.8	3.8	21.2	0
Goats, Blue, Beacon, Finest, Tesco*	1 Serving/30g	100	8.6	333	19	0.1	28.5	0
Goats, Breaded, Bites, Sainsbury's*	1 Bite/25g	84	6.2	337	13	15.1	25	0.8
Goats, French, Mild, Average	1 Serving/30g	49	3.5	163	11.2	3	11.8	0
Goats, Honey & Ginger, Welsh, Emporium, Aldi*	1 Serving/30g	85	5.7	284	13	16	19	0.5
Goats, Premium, Average	1 Serving/30g	98	7.8	327	20.5	0.6	26.1	0
Goats, Soft, Average	1 Serving/30g	79	6.3	262	16.7	1.8	20.8	0.5
Goats, Tomato, Chipotle, Herbs, World Deli, Waitrose*	½ Pack/45g	156	13	347	14.9	6.1	28.9	1.1
Gorgonzola, Average	1 Serving/30g	100	8.1	334	20	0	27	0
Gouda, Average	1 Serving/30g	113	9.4	376	24	0	31.5	0
Gouda, Light, Slices, Milbona, Lidl*	1 Slice/17g	42	2.7	250	23	3.5	16	0.5
Gouda, Popped, Crunchy, Cheesies*	1 Serving/20g	119	9.4	593	40	0	47	0
Gouda. & Chorizo, Rollitos, Tesco*	2 Rollitos/22g	81	6.6	369	22.4	1.8	29.9	1.6
Gran Padano, Reserva, Deluxe, Lidl*	1 Serving/10g	39	2.8	388	33	0	28.4	0
Grana Padano, Grated, Emporium, Aldi*	1 Serving/30g	119	8.7	398	33	0	29	0
Grana Padano, Italian Cheese, Waitrose*	1 Serving/14g	54	4	388	33	0	28.4	0
Greek Style, Salad Cheese, Everyday Value, Tesco*	1 Serving/30g	80	6.2	270	17.2	1.9	21	0
Greek Style, Salad, Light, Essential, Waitrose*	1 Serving/30g	57	3.6	190	20	0.6	12	0
Gruyere	1oz/28g	115	9.3	409	27.2	0	33.3	0
Halloumi, Average	1 Serving/80g	253	19.7	316	20.8	1.6	24.7	0
Halloumi, Chilli, Morrisons*	1 Serving/30g	94	7.2	313	21.5	1.7	24.1	1.8
Halloumi, Light Average	1 Serving/100g	245	15.3	245	24.7	1.7	15.3	0
Halloumi, Pesto, The Grill, M&S*	½ Pack/113g	318	23.6	283	19.8	3.2	21	1.1
Halloumi, with Chilli, Burger Slices, Aldi*	1 Slice/50g	168	13.5	335	23	1.2	27	0.5
Hard, Grated, Asda*	1 Serving/10g	51	3.6	509	43	3.1	36	0.5
Havarti, Sliced, M&S*	1 Slice/23g	77	6	336	24	1.4	26	0
Healthy Range, Average	1 Slice/20g	39	2.1	197	20.6	5.2	10.4	0
Healthy Range, Slices, Average	1 Slice/25g	45	2.2	180	19.5	5.4	9	0
Iberico, TTD, Sainsbury's*	1 Serving/30g	117	9.6	390	23.8	1	32.1	1
Italian, Hard, Dairy Free, Shredded, Follow Your Heart*	1 Tbsp/10g	34	2.6	344	0	29	26	0
Jarlsberg, Slices, Average	1 Slice/15g	54	4	360	27	0	27	0
Kvarg, Coconut, Lindahls, Nestle*	1 Serving/30g	18	0.1	60	11	3.4	0.2	0
Kvarg, Raspberry, Lindahls, Nestle*	1 Pot/150g	90	0.3	60	11.3	3.4	0.2	0
Kvarg, Stracciatella, Lindahls, Nestle*	1 Pot/150g	94	0.9	63	11	3.4	0.6	0
Kvarg, White Chocolate, Lindahls, Nestle*	1 Serving/50g	32	0.1	63	11	3.4	0.2	0

	Measure INFO/WEIGHT	per Measure KCAL	FAT	Nutrition Values per 100g / 100ml KCAL	PROT	CARB	FAT	FIBRE
CHEESE								
Kvarg, White Chocolate, Nestle*	1 Pot/151g	95	0.3	63	11	3.4	0.2	0
Lactose Free, Arla*	1 Serving/30g	103	8.1	344	25.3	1	27	0
Lancashire	***1oz/28g***	***104***	***8.7***	***373***	***23.3***	***0.1***	***31***	***0***
Le Fleuret, Waitrose*	1 Serving/30g	74	5.8	245	14.9	2.8	19.3	0
Leerdammer, Lighter, Sliced, M&S*	1 Slice/23g	62	3.9	271	29.5	0.1	17	0
Leerdammer, Original, Sliced, Leerdammer*	1 Slice/20g	71	5.5	356	27	0.1	27.5	0
Manchego	***1 Serving/70g***	***340***	***30.8***	***485***	***22.2***	***0.1***	***44***	***0***
Mascarpone, 30% Lighter, Morrisons*	1 Tbsp/15g	45	4.2	299	8.3	3.5	28	0
Mascarpone, Average	***1 Serving/30g***	***131***	***13.1***	***437***	***5.6***	***4.1***	***43.6***	***0***
Mature, Half Fat, Average	***1 Serving/25g***	***66***	***3.9***	***265***	***29.9***	***0.4***	***15.6***	***0.1***
Mild, Reduced Fat, Grated, Average	***1 Serving/30g***	***70***	***3.3***	***235***	***31.5***	***2.2***	***11.1***	***0***
Mini Roule, with Garlic & Herb, Emporium, Aldi*	1 Serving/30g	99	9.3	329	9	2.5	31	1.3
Mozzarella, & Tomatoes, Marinated, Italian, M&S*	1 Serving/30g	75	6.1	249	10.9	5.3	20.3	0.9
Mozzarella, Average	***½ Ball/63g***	***172***	***12.9***	***275***	***21.2***	***1.2***	***20.6***	***0***
Mozzarella, Marinated, Italian, M&S*	1 Serving/30g	85	6.9	282	16.9	1.1	23.1	1.2
Mozzarella, Reduced Fat, Average	***½ Ball/63g***	***115***	***6.4***	***184***	***21.2***	***1***	***10.2***	***0***
Mozzarella, Sticks, Free From, Tesco*	2 Sticks/25g	75	4.5	301	15.3	18.6	18	1.7
Mozzarella, Sticks, Melting, Crispy Golden Crumb, M&S*	½ Pack/75g	269	18.1	359	18.2	16.4	24.1	1.8
NeufchÃ‚Â¢tel, Soft, Average	***1 Serving/30g***	***76***	***6.9***	***253***	***9***	***3.6***	***23***	***0***
Norvegia, Sliced Light, Tine*	1 Slice/10g	27	1.6	272	32	0	16	0
Ossau-Iraty, Average	***1 Serving/30g***	***120***	***10.2***	***400***	***22.3***	***0.2***	***34***	***0***
Parmesan, Average	***1 Tbsp/10g***	***42***	***2.8***	***422***	***40***	***2***	***28.5***	***0***
Protein, Eatlean*	1 Serving/30g	51	0.9	169	37	0.5	3	0.5
Provolone, Salami & Cheese Selection, The Deli, Aldi*	2 Slices/5g	16	1.2	318	22	2.2	24	0.9
Quark, Average	***1 Serving/20g***	***13***	***0***	***66***	***11.9***	***4***	***0.2***	***0***
Quark, with Mixed Berry, Glenisk*	1 Serving/30g	16	0	53	8.3	5	0	1.3
Raclette, Richsmonts*	1 Slice/28g	100	8	357	25	0	28.6	0
Reblochon	***1 Serving/30g***	***95***	***8***	***318***	***19.7***	***0***	***26.6***	***0***
Red Leicester, Average	***1 Serving/30g***	***120***	***10.1***	***400***	***23.8***	***0.1***	***33.7***	***0***
Red Leicester, Reduced Fat, Average	***1 Serving/30g***	***78***	***4.6***	***261***	***30.2***	***0.1***	***15.4***	***0***
Ricotta, Average	***1 Serving/50g***	***67***	***4.8***	***134***	***9.3***	***2.9***	***9.5***	***0***
Roquefort, Average	***1oz/28g***	***105***	***9.2***	***375***	***19.7***	***0***	***32.9***	***0***
Roule, French, Sainsbury's*	1 Serving/30g	96	9.2	321	8.5	3	30.5	0
Roule, Garlic, & Herb, Lidl*	1 Serving/30g	90	8.4	301	7.3	5	28	0
Sage Derby	***1oz/28g***	***113***	***9.5***	***402***	***24.2***	***0.1***	***33.9***	***0***
Salad, 40% Less Fat, Asda*	1 Serving/30g	56	3.6	188	19	1	12	0
Salad, Greek Style, Simply, Lidl*	1 Serving/30g	78	6	259	18.2	0.5	20	0
Shropshire, Blue, Average	***1 Serving/50g***	***196***	***17.1***	***391***	***21***	***0***	***34.2***	***0***
Skyrella, Milbona, Lidl*	1 Serving/30g	36	0.8	119	22.5	1.5	2.6	0
Slices, Average	***1 Slice/23g***	***82***	***6.6***	***358***	***24***	***0.8***	***28.6***	***0***
Slices, Smoked with Ham, Aldi*	1 Slice/21g	66	5.2	313	21	1	25	0.1
Soft, Extra Light, Average	***1 Serving/20g***	***25***	***1.2***	***125***	***14.3***	***3.6***	***5.9***	***0.1***
Soft, Full Fat, Average	***1 Serving/50g***	***156***	***15.2***	***312***	***8.2***	***1.7***	***30.3***	***0***
Soft, Full Fat, Original, Lactose Free, Kraft*	1 Serving/30g	84	8.2	280	4.5	2.7	27.5	0.3
Soft, Garlic & Herb, Philadelphia*	1 Serving/30g	44	3.3	148	7.1	5.4	11	0.4
Soft, Garlic & Herb, Roulade, M&S*	1 Portion/100g	295	27.3	295	7.8	4.1	27.3	1.3
Soft, Garlic, & Herb, Lighter, Sainsbury's*	1 Serving/30g	49	3.3	163	9.6	6.4	11	0
Soft, Herbs, Lightest, Philadelphia*	1 Serving/30g	26	0.8	87	11	4.9	2.5	0.4
Soft, Jalapeno, Philadelphia *	1 Serving/30g	40	2.8	134	6.6	5.1	9.3	0.7
Soft, Kefir, Red Pepper, & Cumin, Bio-tiful Dairy*	1 Serving/30g	30	0.3	100	16.7	6.4	0.9	0
Soft, Light & Herbs, with Breadsticks, Philadelphia*	1 Pack/41g	86	3.7	212	8.8	23	9	2.3
Soft, Light, Average	***1 Tbsp/30g***	***54***	***3.9***	***179***	***12.1***	***3.2***	***13.1***	***0***
Soft, Light, with Breadsticks, Philadelphia*	1 Serving/43g	103	4.7	242	7.9	26	11	1.2

C

	Measure INFO/WEIGHT	per Measure KCAL	per Measure FAT	KCAL	PROT	CARB	FAT	FIBRE
				Nutrition Values per 100g / 100ml				
CHEESE								
Soft, Med Fat, Average	***1 Serving/30g***	***62***	***5.4***	***207***	***8.4***	***3***	***17.9***	***0***
Soft, Med Fat, with Chives, Philadelphia*	1 Serving/30g	44	3	146	7.4	5.1	10	0.6
Soft, Mediterranean Herbs, Full Fat, Philadelphia*	1 Serving/30g	64	5.7	213	5	4.1	19	0.3
Soft, Salmon & Dill, Light, Med Fat, Philadelphia*	1 Serving/20g	28	2	142	7.3	5.1	10	0.5
Soft, Sheeps, Ewe's Milk, Flower Marie*	1 Serving/30g	103	8.7	344	18.8	3	29	0
Soft, Sweet Chilli, Light, Med Fat, Philadelphia*	1 Serving/20g	30	2	148	6.8	7.3	10	0.5
Soft, White, Lactofree, Arla*	1 Serving/30g	59	5	197	8.6	3	16.5	0
Soft, with Black Pepper, Light, Sainsbury's*	½ Pack/100g	205	16.5	205	11	3	16.5	0
Soft, with Chocolate, Milka, Philadelphia*	1 Serving/30g	86	3.9	285	6.3	34	13	1.7
Soft, with Garlic & Herbs, Full Fat, Deli, Boursin*	1 Serving/28g	84	8.3	299	3.5	5	29.5	0
St Felicien, Du Dauphine, Finest, Tesco*	1 Serving/30g	80	7.2	266	12	0.5	24	0
Stilton, Average	***1 Serving/30g***	***123***	***10.6***	***410***	***22.4***	***0.1***	***35.5***	***0***
Stilton, Blue, Average	***1 Serving/30g***	***124***	***10.7***	***412***	***22.8***	***0.1***	***35.7***	***0***
Stilton, White, Average	***1oz/28g***	***101***	***8.8***	***362***	***19.9***	***0.1***	***31.3***	***0***
Taleggio D.o.p., Finest, Tesco*	1 Serving/30g	89	7.5	297	18	0	25	0
Tallegio, Waitrose*	1 Serving/30g	94	7.9	315	19	0.9	26.2	0
Twisted, Cheestrings*	1 String/20g	61	4.5	305	23	2.5	22.5	0
Vacherin Badoz, Waitrose*	1 Serving/30g	87	7.2	289	17.6	0.7	24	0
Wensleydale, Average	***1 Serving/25g***	***92***	***7.8***	***369***	***22.4***	***0.1***	***31***	***0***
Wensleydale, with Blueberries, M&S*	1 Portion/30g	111	7.9	370	18.7	13.4	26.4	0.9
Wensleydale, with Cranberries, Sainsbury's*	1 Serving/50g	180	13.9	359	20.7	6.4	27.8	0
CHEESE ALTERNATIVE								
Block, Original, Vegan, Waitrose*	1 Serving/30g	89	7	297	0.5	18.4	23.4	5.2
Blue Cheese, Free From, Asda*	1 Serving/30g	98	8.1	327	0.5	19	27	4.7
Camembert Style, Mouse's Favourite*	1 Serving/30g	130	10.4	432	14.7	15.2	34.7	0
Cheddar Style, Coconut Based, Sainsbury's*	1 Serving/30g	91	6.9	304	0.7	21.7	22.9	4
Cheddar, Coconut Base, Free From, Morrisons*	1 Serving/30g	97	7	323	1.7	26	23.2	1.5
Cheddar, Dairy Free, Koko*	1 Serving/30g	95	7.9	318	0.7	22.5	26.3	1.5
Cheddar, Mature, Free From, Asda*	1 Serving/30g	86	6.3	285	0.5	21	21	5.1
Cheddar, Mature, Sliced, Free From, Asda*	1 Slice/20g	57	4.2	285	0.5	21	21	5.1
Cheddar, V Taste, Morrisons*	1 Serving/30g	97	7	323	1.7	26	23.2	1.5
Cheezly, Feta Style in Oil, The Redwood Co*	1 Serving/25g	119	11.8	475	2.5	10.6	47	0
Coconut Oil, Jalapeno, & Chilli, Free From, Tesco*	1 Serving/30g	88	6.2	294	0.5	23.3	20.8	5.7
Edam, Slices, V Taste, Morrisons*	1 Slice/22g	67	5.2	305	1.1	21.4	23.8	0.5
Greek Style, V Taste, Morrisons*	1 Serving/30g	90	7.2	301	0.1	20.1	24.1	1.6
Greek, White, Block, Violife*	1 Serving/30g	92	8.7	305	0	11	29	0
Hard, Italian Style, Free From, Tesco*	1 Serving/30g	92	5.9	306	1.2	29.5	19.6	3.6
Mediterranean Style, Block, Violife*	1 Slice/100g	260	15	260	1.2	30	15	0
Mozzarella, Grated, Free From, Asda*	1 Serving/30g	94	7.8	313	0.5	18	26	3.2
Mozzarella, Grated, Free From, Tesco*	1 Serving/30g	94	7.8	313	0	18.3	26	3.2
Mozzarella, Slices, Dairy Free	***1 Slice/19g***	***80***	***6***	***420***	***10.5***	***10.5***	***31.5***	***0***
Natural, Almond, Spread, Nush Foods*	1 Serving/30g	64	5.4	215	7	5.9	18	0
Red Leicester Style, Vegan, Scheese*	1 Serving/30g	89	6.7	298	0.5	21.4	22.2	5.5
Red Leicester, Slices, V Taste, Morrisons*	1 Slice/22g	72	5.2	329	2.1	24.5	23.8	4
Smoked, Gouda Style, Slices, Follow Your Heart*	1 Slice/20g	57	4.6	285	0	20	23	0
Smoky, Vegan, Applewood*	1 Serving/30g	92	7.4	305	1.5	19.4	24.6	0.5
Soft, Coconut Based, Garlic & Herb, Sainsbury's*	1 Serving/30g	83	7.9	277	6.6	2.2	26.3	2.5
Soft, Cream Cheese, Koko*	1 Serving/30g	60	5.6	199	0.4	7.6	18.7	0.9
Soft, Garlic & Herb, Free From, Asda*	1 Serving/15g	40	3.8	266	5.8	2.4	25	2.2
Soft, Garlic, & Herb, Free From, Tesco*	1 Serving/30g	75	7.5	250	0.3	5.4	25	1.2
Soft, V Taste, Morrisons*	1 Serving/30g	73	7.3	244	0.2	5.8	24.3	0.7
Treenut, Organic, Nutcrafter Creamery*	1 Serving/30g	163	16.3	543	27.7	7.4	54.3	6.7
Vegetarian, Average	***1 Serving/30g***	***110***	***8.4***	***368***	***28.2***	***0***	***28.1***	***0***

	Measure INFO/WEIGHT	per Measure KCAL	FAT	Nutrition Values per 100g / 100ml KCAL	PROT	CARB	FAT	FIBRE
CHEESE PUFFS								
Average	***1 Bag/25g***	***129***	***7.4***	***517***	***7.8***	***54.8***	***29.5***	***1.5***
CHEESE SPREAD								
Average	***1 Serving/30g***	***76***	***6.4***	***254***	***9.4***	***5.9***	***21.4***	***0.1***
Cheese & Ham, Primula*	1 Serving/20g	43	2.9	214	12.8	7.8	14.6	0
with Chives, Primula*	1 Serving/30g	65	4.5	217	12.5	8.2	15	4.5
with Prawn, Primula*	1 Squeeze/25g	48	3.6	190	12.5	3.3	14.4	3.6
CHEESE STRAWS								
All Butter, Finest, Tesco*	1 Straw/13g	73	5.2	587	17.9	33.7	41.8	2.1
Cheddar, M&S*	1 Straw/11g	59	3.8	535	14.9	40.1	34.9	2.4
Cheese Twists, Tesco*	1 Twist/8g	40	2.1	507	13.8	52.1	26.4	2.8
Finest, Tesco*	1 Straw/7g	39	2.6	558	13.3	41.5	37.6	1.5
Homemade or Bakery, Average	***1 Straw/41g***	***173***	***12.6***	***422***	***12***	***24.2***	***30.7***	***0.7***
Selection, Sainsbury's*	1 Straw/7g	41	2.9	558	16.6	34.5	39.3	2.8
CHEESE TRIANGLES								
Average	***1 Triangle/14g***	***33***	***2.2***	***238***	***10.3***	***14.2***	***15.6***	***0.2***
Dairylea, Light, Kraft*	1 Triangle/16g	26	1.4	167	15	6.3	9	0.4
Light, Extra, The Laughing Cow, Fromageries Bel*	1 Triangle/18g	19	0.4	108	17	5.5	2	0
Light, with Blue Cheese, The Laughing Cow*	1 Triangle/16g	24	1.4	151	13	5.5	8.5	0
Lighter, Valley Spire, Lidl*	1 Triangle/17g	24	1.3	141	12	6	7.5	0.5
Reduced Fat, Average	***1 Triangle/18g***	***27***	***1.2***	***154***	***15.4***	***7***	***7***	***0***
CHEESE TWISTS								
Parmesan & Garlic, Sainsbury's*	1 Twist/8g	38	2	493	13.8	51	25.3	2.8
Parmesan, All Butter, TTD, Sainsbury's*	1 Serving/8g	38	2	487	13.8	51	25.3	2.8
Pre Packed, Average	***1 Twist/8g***	***41***	***2.2***	***515***	***13.7***	***47.9***	***27.7***	***2.3***
CHEESECAKE								
Average	***1 Slice/115g***	***490***	***40.8***	***426***	***3.7***	***24.6***	***35.5***	***0.4***
Berry, Autumn, Waitrose*	1 Slice/92g	316	20.3	343	4.4	31.5	22.1	2
Berry, Red, Waitrose*	1 Slice/101g	350	22.5	346	4.6	31.3	22.2	1.4
Blackcurrant, Average	***1 Serving/90g***	***237***	***11.9***	***263***	***3.6***	***32.3***	***13.2***	***2.4***
Blackcurrant, Healthy Range, Average	***1 Serving/90g***	***182***	***4.7***	***203***	***4.7***	***33.6***	***5.3***	***2.1***
Blueberry, & Vanilla, TTD, Sainsbury's*	1 Serving/95g	353	24.8	372	5.4	28.9	26.1	2.1
Caramel, Salted, Frozen, Tesco*	1 Serving/75g	241	10.6	321	6.5	41.5	14.1	0.9
Caramel, Salted, Mini, Iceland*	1 Cake/22g	85	4.7	380	3.2	44.5	20.9	0.6
Caramel, Swirl, Cadbury*	1 Slice/91g	373	23.5	410	6	40.1	25.8	0
Cherry, Healthy Range, Average	***1 Serving/90g***	***172***	***3***	***191***	***3.7***	***36.4***	***3.3***	***1.1***
Chocolate, & Honeycomb, Slice, Sainsbury's*	1 Slice/98g	333	20.3	340	3.7	33.7	20.7	2.4
Chocolate, & Irish Cream Liqueur, Tesco*	1 Serving/93g	385	28	414	5	30.7	30.1	0.8
Chocolate, & Vanilla, Reduced Fat, M&S*	1 Serving/114g	319	13.7	280	7	37.9	12	1.5
Chocolate, & Vanilla, Tesco*	1 Serving/90g	330	19.4	365	5.2	37.1	21.5	1.6
Chocolate, & Vanilla, Free From, Gu*	1 Pot/82g	320	21.3	390	2.9	36.4	26	1.5
Chocolate, Average	***1 Serving/75g***	***265***	***15.7***	***353***	***5.7***	***35.6***	***20.9***	***1.9***
Chocolate, Triple, Slices, M&S*	1 Slice/92g	377	21.5	410	4.3	44.2	23.4	1.7
Citrus, Good Choice, Mini, Iceland*	1 Cake/111g	198	4.7	178	3.5	31.6	4.2	0.4
Cookies & Cream, The Best, Morrisons*	1 Slice/90g	368	24.7	409	5	35.1	27.4	1
Fruit, Average	***1 Serving/75g***	***207***	***10.9***	***276***	***5.3***	***32.3***	***14.5***	***1.6***
Irish Cream, McVitie's*	¼ Slice/190g	616	36.9	324	4.4	33	19.4	0.4
Key Lime, Slices, Finest, Tesco*	1 Slice/90g	314	17.1	349	4.1	39.6	19	1.4
Lemon, & Blueberry, Light, Gu*	1 Pud/77g	150	8.5	195	2.6	21	11	0.5
Lemon, Average	***1 Serving/90g***	***307***	***19.5***	***341***	***4.1***	***33***	***21.6***	***1.8***
Lemon, Free From, Gu*	1 Ramekin/92g	327	19.3	355	1.8	40	21	0.6
Lemon, Meringue, Tesco*	1 Slice/94g	352	25	375	3.8	30.1	26.6	0.3
Madagascan Vanilla, Slices, Finest, Tesco*	1 Slice/90g	367	23.4	408	5.4	37.9	26	0.3
Mandarin, Morrisons*	1 Serving/135g	335	16.9	248	3.8	32.2	12.5	0.8

	Measure INFO/WEIGHT	per Measure KCAL	FAT	Nutrition Values per 100g / 100ml KCAL	PROT	CARB	FAT	FIBRE
CHEESECAKE								
Millionaires, Pot, Tesco*	1 Pot/100g	274	14	274	3.8	32.9	14	0.6
New York, Baked, Waitrose*	1/12 Cake/83g	317	22.6	380	5.1	28.3	27.1	1.2
New York, Mini, Iceland*	1 Cake/22g	86	5.1	385	3.6	40.7	23	0.5
Pink Gin, Slice, Asda*	1 Slice/95g	331	20.9	349	4.5	33	22	0.9
Raspberry, & Mascarpone, Best, Morrisons*	1 Cake/84g	257	14	306	3.9	34.8	16.7	1
Raspberry, & Strawberry, M&S*	1 Slice/105g	340	21.1	325	3.9	33.4	20.2	1.2
Raspberry, & Vanilla, Slices, M&S*	1 Slice/100g	300	17.5	300	4.4	30.4	17.5	1.7
Raspberry, & Blackcurrant, Light, Gu*	1 Pud/77g	151	7.7	196	2.6	23	10	0.8
Raspberry, Rapture, Slices, Tesco*	1 Slice/110g	341	20.4	310	4.2	30.8	18.5	1.8
Raspberry, Ripple, Sainsbury's*	1 Portion/95g	355	21.8	373	4.5	37	22.9	0.9
Salted Caramel, Free From, Gu*	1 Ramekin/83g	287	16.6	346	1.6	39	20	0.5
Salted Caramel, Gu*	1 Pot/92g	333	21.3	362	3.7	34.5	23.1	0.7
Salted Caramel, Vegan, Gu*	1 Ramekin/83g	287	16.6	346	1.6	39	20	0.5
Strawberry, & Cream, Finest, Tesco*	1 Serving/104g	325	22.4	312	4.3	25.3	21.5	0.5
Strawberry, & Rhubarb, Slice, M&S*	1 Pack/100g	377	23.8	377	4.3	35.7	23.8	1.3
Strawberry, & Vanilla, Light, Gu*	1 Pud/77g	153	9.2	199	4.3	19	12	0.5
Strawberry, Devonshire, McVitie's*	1/6 Cake/66g	192	10.7	291	4.4	31.8	16.2	3.6
Strawberry, Finest, Tesco*	1 Slice/113g	383	25.1	339	4.8	30.1	22.2	0.9
Strawberry, Free From, Tesco*	1 Serving/77g	228	12.1	296	1.6	36.4	15.7	1.3
Strawberry, Frozen, Sainsbury's*	1/6 Cake/84g	277	14.2	332	4.3	40.4	17	2.3
Strawberry, Individual, Tesco*	1 Pot/100g	231	7.7	231	2.5	37.4	7.7	1
Strawberry, Slice, Asda*	1 Slice/95g	326	19.9	344	4.2	34	21	0.9
Strawberry, Somerset Valley, Sainsbury's*	1 Pot/90g	194	8.3	215	3.2	29.1	9.2	1.3
Strawberry, Swirl, Ms Mollys*	1/5 Cake/75g	242	11.2	323	5.2	41.7	14.9	0.6
Tiramisu, Allplants*	1 Serving/95g	338	24.7	356	9	20	26	3.9
Toffee, & Pecan, Wedge, Sainsbury's*	1 Serving/75g	296	21.8	395	5.4	28.1	29	3.1
Toffee, Lidl*	1 Pot/100g	275	12.3	275	3	37.6	12.3	1
Toffee, M&S*	1 Serving/105g	357	22.6	340	5.2	37.2	21.5	0.9
Toffee, Mini, Asda*	1 Cake/20g	57	2.4	286	4.6	40	12	2.1
Toffee, Tesco*	1 Serving/100g	265	12.9	265	4.3	33.1	12.9	0.8
Vanilla	***1 Serving/100g***	***395***	***26.2***	***395***	***5.3***	***42.8***	***26.2***	***1.1***
Vanilla Berry, Allplants*	1 Serving/95g	299	20	315	7.5	22	21	3.5
Vanilla, Creamy, New York, Slices, Tesco*	1 Slice/90g	314	21.4	349	5.1	28.3	23.7	0.8
Vanilla, New York, Slices, M&S*	1 Slice/105g	361	23.6	344	4.5	30.1	22.5	1.5
White Chocolate, & Mixed Berry, Finest, Tesco*	1 Serving/70g	246	13.7	353	4.5	38.9	19.6	1.3
Zillionaires, Gu*	1 Pot/92g	362	22	396	3.6	42	24	1.3
CHERRIES								
Black in Syrup, Average	***1 Serving/242g***	***160***	***0***	***66***	***0.6***	***16***	***0***	***0.7***
Black, Fresh, Average	***1 Serving/80g***	***41***	***0.1***	***51***	***0.9***	***11.5***	***0.1***	***1.6***
Glace, Average	***1oz/28g***	***79***	***0***	***280***	***0.4***	***71.2***	***0.2***	***1.1***
Picota, Average	***1 Serving/80g***	***42***	***0.1***	***52***	***0.9***	***11.4***	***0.1***	***1.2***
Raw, Average	***1oz/28g***	***14***	***0***	***49***	***0.9***	***11.2***	***0.1***	***1.4***
Stewed without Sugar, Average	***1oz/28g***	***12***	***0***	***42***	***0.8***	***10.1***	***0.1***	***0.8***
CHESTNUTS								
Average	***1 Serving/100g***	***174***	***2.3***	***174***	***2.9***	***31***	***2.3***	***8.9***
Candied, Marrons Glace, Wholefoods Online*	1 Piece/20g	65	0.2	325	0.8	76.4	0.8	4.8
Roasted, Peeled, Average	***1 Nut/10g***	***17***	***0.3***	***170***	***2***	***36.6***	***2.7***	***4.1***
CHEWING GUM								
Airwaves, Sugar Free, Wrigleys*	1 Pack/15g	23	0	155	0	62	0	0
Doublemint, Wrigleys*	1 Stick/3g	10	0	370	0	74.1	0	0
Extra, Cool Breeze, Wrigleys*	1 Piece/2g	3	0	153	0	64	0	0
Extra, Peppermint, Sugar Free, Wrigleys*	1 Piece/2g	3	0	155	0	39	0	0
Peppermint, Sugar Free, Active, Aldi*	2 Pieces/3g	4	0	146	0	61	0	0

	Measure INFO/WEIGHT	per Measure KCAL	FAT	Nutrition Values per 100g / 100ml KCAL	PROT	CARB	FAT	FIBRE
CHEWING GUM								
Spearmint, Extra, Wrigleys*	1 Piece/1g	1	0	143	0	64.3	0	0
Spearmint, Wrigleys*	1 Piece/3g	9	0	295	0	73	0	0
CHICK PEAS								
Bombay, Hearty Tomato Curry, Tasty Bite*	½ Pack/142g	179	7.4	126	4.8	13	5.2	3.7
Canned, Drained, Average	***1 Can/240g***	***276***	***6***	***115***	***7.4***	***15.2***	***2.5***	***4.6***
Curried, Canned, East End*	½ Can/200g	258	11	129	5.7	11.9	5.5	4.4
Curried, Incredible, Jamie Oliver*	½ Pack/125g	169	5.4	135	6.1	15.6	4.3	4.5
Curried, Worldwide Foods, Aldi*	½ Pack/125g	172	4.8	138	7.3	15	3.8	6.5
Dried, Average	***1 Serving/100g***	***319***	***5.4***	***319***	***21.7***	***47.4***	***5.4***	***8***
Dried, Boiled, Average	***1 Serving/75g***	***85***	***1.7***	***114***	***7.3***	***16.4***	***2.2***	***2.6***
in Salted Water, Canned, Average	***1 Can/179g***	***204***	***5.2***	***114***	***7.2***	***14.9***	***2.9***	***4.1***
in Water, Canned, Average	***1 Can/250g***	***282***	***6.6***	***113***	***7.2***	***15.3***	***2.6***	***4.8***
Roasted, Curry, Cheeky P's*	1 Pack/50g	215	5	430	22	63	10	15
Roasted, Dark Choc, Brave*	1 Serving/30g	129	5.4	430	14	47	18	13
CHICKEN								
& Stuffing, Slices, Iceland*	1 Pack/70g	88	2.7	125	20.7	1.4	3.9	0.9
Arrabbiata, Inspired Cuisine, Aldi*	1 Pack/375g	458	9.8	122	7.8	16	2.6	1.3
Arrabbiata, M&S*	1 Pack/350g	360	4.6	103	8.5	13.5	1.3	1.4
BBQ, & Sweet Potato, Memphis, Co-Op*	1 Pack/350g	284	3.9	81	6.1	10	1.1	2.6
Bites, Breaded, Sainsbury's*	1 Bite/22g	63	3.6	288	15.5	18.9	16.4	1.1
Bites, Finest Quality, Delicatessen*	3 Bites/50g	114	8	227	13	7.3	16	0
Bites, Hot & Spicy, Tesco*	1 Pack/110g	143	1.8	130	18.9	9.6	1.6	2.5
Bites, Slow Roasted, Mini, Fridge Raiders, Mattessons*	1 Mini Bag/23g	43	2.2	190	21	3.2	10	0
Bites, Southern Fried, Tesco*	4 Bites/38g	93	5.2	247	17.8	11.9	13.8	1.9
Bites, Southern Style, Mini, Fridge Raiders, Mattessons*	1 Pack/23g	37	2.1	166	17	4.2	9.2	0
Bites, Tikka, Average	***1 Serving/50g***	***96***	***5.3***	***193***	***20.7***	***3.8***	***10.5***	***1.9***
Breast, BBQ, Sweet & Smokey, Slices, Sainsbury's*	1 Serving/89g	116	1.5	130	22.6	4.9	1.7	0.5
Breast, Butter Roast, Sliced, Extra Special, Asda*	2 Slices/79g	90	0.9	114	26	0.5	1.1	1.5
Breast, Chargrilled, Premium, Average	***1 Piece/10g***	***13***	***0.3***	***134***	***25.9***	***0.6***	***2.6***	***0.3***
Breast, Chargrilled, Sliced, Average	***1 Slice/19g***	***24***	***0.5***	***124***	***24.4***	***0.5***	***2.7***	***0.4***
Breast, Cheese & Bacon Wrapped, Iceland*	½ Pack/158g	291	19.4	184	16.6	1.2	12.3	0.9
Breast, Cooked, Lemon, & Herb, Tesco*	½ Pack/90g	115	1.4	128	22	6.6	1.5	0.2
Breast, Diced, Average	***1 Serving/188g***	***242***	***4.4***	***129***	***26.9***	***0.1***	***2.4***	***0.1***
Breast, Extra Tasty, Protein Pot, Asda*	1 Pot/80g	102	0.9	127	27	2.3	1.1	0
Breast, Fillet, Mini, Southern Fried, British, Waitrose*	½ Pack/131g	278	10.1	212	18	17.1	7.7	1
Breast, Fillet, Pesto Breaded, Finest, Tesco*	½ Pack/151g	293	10.9	194	21.5	10.5	7.2	0.5
Breast, Fillet, Strips, Barbecue, Oven Baked, Iceland*	1 Serving/100g	237	9.4	237	16.1	21.3	9.4	1.3
Breast, Fillet, with Cheese Sauce, & Crumb, Sainsbury's*	½ Pack/158g	219	7.4	139	21.9	2	4.7	0.7
Breast, Fillets, Bacon Wrapped, Hunter Style, Sainsbury's*	½ Pack/189g	293	8.7	155	25	3.4	4.6	0
Breast, Fillets, Bacon, & Brie, Morrisons*	1 Fillet/183g	306	14.1	167	21.7	2.2	7.7	1.1
Breast, Fillets, Breaded, Average	***1 Fillet/112g***	***246***	***11.6***	***220***	***17.6***	***14***	***10.4***	***1.3***
Breast, Fillets, Cajun, Average	***1 Fillet/93g***	***124***	***2.6***	***134***	***23.6***	***3.5***	***2.8***	***0.3***
Breast, Fillets, Chargrilled, Average	***1 Serving/100g***	***120***	***1.1***	***120***	***27.3***	***0.3***	***1.1***	***0.3***
Breast, Fillets, Chilli & Lime, Mini, Sainsbury's*	½ Pack/134g	175	4.3	131	24.7	0.8	3.2	0.5
Breast, Fillets, Coronation, Oven Baked, Asda*	½ Pack/141g	194	4.8	138	22	4.2	3.4	0.9
Breast, Fillets, Fajita Cooked, Mini, Tesco*	½ Pack/85g	100	0.8	118	19.5	7.5	1	0.4
Breast, Fillets, Garlic & Herb, Mini, Tesco*	½ Pack/86g	96	0.9	112	22.8	3.2	1	0
Breast, Fillets, Ginger, Coriander, & Lime, Waitrose*	½ Pack/103g	163	5.3	158	27.7	0.5	5.1	0.5
Breast, Fillets, Hunters, Morrisons*	½ Pack/172g	274	8.6	159	22.7	5.6	5	0.5
Breast, Fillets, Korma Style, Average	***1 Serving/100g***	***132***	***2.8***	***132***	***27.4***	***0.8***	***2.8***	***0.6***
Breast, Fillets, Mini, Moroccan Style, Asda*	1/3 Pack/66g	78	0.6	118	23	3.8	0.9	0.6
Breast, Fillets, Mini, Raw, Average	***1oz/28g***	***34***	***0.4***	***121***	***26.9***	***0.2***	***1.5***	***0.1***
Breast, Fillets, Organic, Average	***1 Serving/150g***	***153***	***1.1***	***102***	***24***	***0***	***0.8***	***0***

C

	Measure INFO/WEIGHT	per Measure KCAL	FAT	Nutrition Values per 100g / 100ml KCAL	PROT	CARB	FAT	FIBRE
CHICKEN								
Breast, Fillets, Skinless & Boneless, Raw, Average	***1 Breast/100g***	***129***	***2***	***129***	***27.7***	***0***	***2***	***0***
Breast, Grilled, Average	***1 Breast/130g***	***174***	***2.8***	***134***	***29***	***0.1***	***2.2***	***0***
Breast, Hot & Spicy, Slices, Everyday Essentials, Aldi*	1 Serving/80g	109	1.9	136	28	0.5	2.4	0.5
Breast, in Breadcrumbs, GF, Sainsbury's*	1 Fillet/150g	294	12.6	196	18	11.5	8.4	1.3
Breast, Joint, & Stuffing, Tesco*	1 Serving/128g	197	11.4	154	13.1	5	8.9	0.7
Breast, Joint, Rotisserie, with Sticky Marinade, M&S*	½ Pack/233g	319	13	137	20.5	1	5.6	0.1
Breast, Meat & Skin, Raw, Average	***1 Serving/145g***	***249***	***13.4***	***172***	***20.8***	***0***	***9.2***	***0***
Breast, Meat & Skin, Weighed with Bone, Raw, Average	***1oz/28g***	***39***	***2.1***	***138***	***16.7***	***0***	***7.4***	***0***
Breast, Meat Only, Fried	***1 Serving/50g***	***68***	***1.7***	***137***	***24.4***	***0.4***	***3.4***	***0***
Breast, Nacho Toppers, Iceland*	1 Topper/96g	199	9.9	208	12.8	15.1	10.3	1.7
Breast, Pieces, Chunky, Cooked, Smart Price, Asda*	1 Serving/120g	152	1.7	127	28	0.5	1.4	0
Breast, Pieces, Tikka, Average	***1 Serving/100g***	***154***	***3.4***	***154***	***28.2***	***2.8***	***3.4***	***0.4***
Breast, Piri Piri, Fillets, Cooked as per Instructions, Tesco*	1 Breast/141g	251	9.4	178	28.8	0.5	6.7	0.1
Breast, Piri Piri, Pieces, Cooked, Ready to Eat, Tesco*	1 Serving/90g	117	2.2	130	24	2.8	2.4	0.6
Breast, Roast, Sliced, From Supermarket, Average	***1 Slice/13g***	***17***	***0.4***	***139***	***25***	***1.8***	***3.5***	***0.2***
Breast, Roast, without Skin, Average	***1oz/28g***	***41***	***1.3***	***146***	***24.8***	***1***	***4.6***	***0.2***
Breast, Schnitzel, Oven Baked, Iceland*	1 Schnitzel/194g	541	24.6	279	16.7	28.3	12.7	2.2
Breast, Skewers, Mini, Asda*	1 Skewer/12g	17	0.3	140	24	5.5	2.5	0
Breast, Slices, Flame Grilled, Ready to Eat, Aldi*	½ Pack/90g	120	2.2	133	27	0.5	2.4	0.5
Breast, Slices, Piri Piri, Simply, Lidl*	½ Pack/120g	150	1.6	125	26.3	1.6	1.3	1
Breast, Smoked, Sliced, Average	***1 Slice/20g***	***22***	***0.5***	***110***	***20.7***	***0.9***	***2.6***	***0.1***
Breast, Steaks, Cajun Style, Oven Cooked, Morrisons*	1 Steak/90g	138	2.7	153	28.1	2.8	3	0.9
Breast, Steaks, Garlic, & Herb, Tesco*	1 Steak/142g	201	4	142	26.6	2.7	2.8	0
Breast, Strips, Raw, Average	***1 Serving/280g***	***358***	***5.7***	***128***	***27.1***	***0.4***	***2***	***0.3***
Breast, Stuffed, M&S*	½ Pack/53g	78	2.5	147	23.5	2.3	4.7	0.5
Breast, Sweet Chilli, Fiery & Delicious, Maggi*	1 Breast/150g	164	3.3	109	9.3	12.3	2.2	1.3
Breast, Tandoori Style, Average	***1 Serving/180g***	***237***	***6.8***	***132***	***22.3***	***2.3***	***3.8***	***1***
Breast, Tikka, Chunks, Ready to Eat, Sainsbury's*	½ Pack/125g	171	2.7	137	26.7	2.4	2.2	0.5
Breast, Tikka, Sliced, Average	***1oz/28g***	***34***	***0.5***	***120***	***24.9***	***2***	***1.7***	***0.6***
Breasts, with Tomato Pesto, & Parmigian, Sainsbury's*	½ Pack/199g	282	10.1	142	23.3	0.6	5.1	0.5
Chargrill, Sweet & Sticky, As Sold, Birds Eye*	1 Grill/88g	148	7.2	168	17	6.6	8.2	0.5
Chargrills, BBQ, Asda*	1 Chargrill/85g	146	7.2	172	20	3.4	8.5	0.7
Chargrills, BBQ, Sweet & Sticky, Birds Eye*	1 Chargrill/87g	146	7.3	167	16	7.1	8.3	0
Chunks, Crispy, Oven Baked, Iceland*	5 Chunks/100g	219	8.8	219	15.3	19.2	8.8	1.2
Coronation, Morrisons*	1 Serving/100g	176	9.3	176	11.9	11.1	9.3	0.5
Coronation, Slimming World*	1 Pot/400g	380	4.8	95	10.1	10.4	1.2	1.5
Crown, Garlic & Herb, Aldi*	1 Pack/740g	1088	32.6	147	26	0.5	4.4	0.5
Curried, Coconut, & Lime, Slices, Ashfield Farm, Aldi*	1 Pack/180g	202	4.3	112	21	0.8	2.4	1.3
Diet Cola, Microwaved, Slimming World, Iceland*	1 Pack/550g	358	3.8	65	9.8	4.4	0.7	0.9
Dippers, Crispy, Average	***5 Dippers/93g***	***231***	***14.3***	***249***	***13.2***	***14.4***	***15.4***	***0.6***
Drumsticks, BBQ Flavour, Average	***1 Serving/200g***	***348***	***16***	***174***	***22.6***	***3.1***	***8***	***0.4***
Drumsticks, Breaded, Fried, Average	***1oz/28g***	***66***	***3.9***	***237***	***18.7***	***9.4***	***13.9***	***0.6***
Drumsticks, Chinese Style, Average	***1 Serving/100g***	***178***	***8.1***	***178***	***22.6***	***3.6***	***8.1***	***0.7***
Drumsticks, Meat & Skin, Weighed with Bone, Raw	***1 Serving/133g***	***188***	***11***	***141***	***15.7***	***0.1***	***8.3***	***0***
Drumsticks, Meat Only, no Skin, Boneless, Raw	***1 Serving/100g***	***106***	***3.3***	***106***	***19.2***	***0***	***3.3***	***0***
Drumsticks, Meat Only, Weighed with Bone, Raw	***1 Serving/122g***	***159***	***9.3***	***130***	***14.4***	***0.1***	***7.6***	***0***
Drumsticks, Meat Only, Weighed with Bone, Roast	***1 Serving/100g***	***116***	***5.5***	***116***	***16***	***0.3***	***5.5***	***0.1***
Drumsticks, Pulled, Tandoori, Sainsbury's*	½ Pack/115g	202	8.4	175	22.3	4.9	7.3	0.5
Drumsticks, with Skin, Average	***1 Piece/125g***	***268***	***16.6***	***215***	***22.1***	***1.8***	***13.3***	***0.3***
Escalope, Breaded, Average	***1 Escalope/128g***	***361***	***21.6***	***282***	***13.4***	***19.1***	***16.9***	***0.7***
Escalope, Plain, Breast, Average	***1 Serving/100g***	***110***	***2.2***	***110***	***22.3***	***0.7***	***2.2***	***0.5***
Fillets, Battered, Average	***1 Fillet/90g***	***199***	***10.4***	***221***	***16.1***	***13.3***	***11.5***	***0.5***
Fillets, Breaded, Average	***1 Piece/98g***	***214***	***10.5***	***219***	***14.2***	***15.9***	***10.7***	***1.9***

	Measure INFO/WEIGHT	per Measure KCAL	FAT	Nutrition Values per 100g / 100ml KCAL	PROT	CARB	FAT	FIBRE
CHICKEN								
Fillets, Breaded, Salt & Pepper, Mini, Waitrose*	½ Pack/144g	317	13	220	17	17.4	9	0.9
Fillets, Cajun, Ashfield Farm, Aldi*	1 Fillet/122g	161	3.3	132	26	0.7	2.7	0.5
Fillets, Chinese Style, Average	***1oz/28g***	***37***	***0.5***	***132***	***24.4***	***4.6***	***1.8***	***0.5***
Fillets, Honey & Mustard, Average	***1 Serving/100g***	***138***	***3.7***	***138***	***18.4***	***7.5***	***3.7***	***0.8***
Fillets, Hot & Spicy, Average	***1oz/28g***	***58***	***3.1***	***206***	***16.4***	***10.5***	***11***	***1.1***
Fillets, in Tempura Batter, Crispy, Birds Eye*	1 Fillet/89g	229	12.5	257	13	19	14	1.4
Fillets, Mini, Mango, Coconut, & Lime, Tesco*	½ Pack/150g	230	2.8	153	26	7.9	1.9	0
Fillets, Mini, Salt & Chilli, Tesco*	½ Pack/146g	337	13	231	19.1	18.7	8.9	0
Fillets, Mini, Sweet & Smokey, Eat Well, M&S*	½ Pack/60g	70	0.2	117	25.5	2.9	0.4	0.1
Fillets, Red Thai, Mini, Average	***1oz/28g***	***36***	***0.6***	***128***	***21.7***	***5.4***	***2***	***0.6***
Fillets, Southern Fried, Meat Only, Average	***1 Piece/100g***	***222***	***12***	***222***	***16.4***	***12.2***	***12***	***1.1***
Fillets, Tandoori Style, Mini, Average	***1 Serving/100g***	***128***	***2***	***128***	***24.7***	***2.6***	***2***	***0.4***
Fillets, Tikka, Average	***1 Serving/100g***	***141***	***5***	***141***	***22.4***	***1.7***	***5***	***1.1***
Fillets, Tikka, Mini, Average	***1oz/28g***	***35***	***0.6***	***124***	***25.1***	***1.3***	***2.2***	***1.2***
Fingers, Average	***1 Serving/75g***	***188***	***9.9***	***250***	***13.7***	***18.8***	***13.2***	***1.2***
Flatties, Coronation, M&S*	½ Pack/183g	322	15.6	176	19	5.4	8.5	1
Goujons, Breaded, Average	***1 Serving/114g***	***293***	***17.1***	***258***	***15.8***	***15.2***	***15***	***1***
Goujons, Breast, Fresh, Average	***1oz/28g***	***36***	***0.5***	***127***	***28***	***0***	***1.6***	***0***
Goujons, British, GF, Made Without Wheat, M&S*	¼ Pack/105g	236	13.4	225	11.2	15.6	12.8	1.5
Goujons, Chipotle, Meat Free, Quorn*	1 Serving/83g	156	3.6	188	12.2	20.7	4.3	8.9
Goujons, Southern Fried, Co-Op*	1 Pack/245g	657	44.1	268	13	13	18	2
Goujons, Southern Fried, Coopers, Lidl*	3 Pieces/68g	187	9.5	275	18	19	14	0.7
Hunters, & Potato Wedges, COU, M&S*	1 Pack/360g	299	3.6	83	9.3	8.3	1	1.6
Hunters, Hasselback, Easy to Cook, Waitrose*	½ Pack/159g	251	7.5	158	23.9	5	4.7	0
in Mushroom Sauce, Calorie Controlled, Tesco*	1 Pack/360g	281	7.9	78	7.8	6.2	2.2	1.3
in Szechuan Sauce, Waitrose *	½ Pack/175g	177	6.5	101	9.5	7	3.7	1
Joint, Butter Basted, with Salt & Pepper, M&S*	1 Serving/100g	156	5.5	156	20.4	6.2	5.5	0.1
Kebab, Sweet Chilli, On the Go, Sainsbury's*	1 Pack/80g	163	6.1	204	20.9	12.6	7.6	1
Leg or Thigh, Hot & Spicy, Average	***1oz/28g***	***50***	***3***	***179***	***19.4***	***1***	***10.8***	***0.4***
Leg Portion, Roast, weighed with Bone, without Skin	***1 Portion/114g***	***175***	***11***	***153***	***30.9***	***0***	***9.6***	***0***
Leg Portion, Roasted Dry, with Skin, without Bone	***1 Portion/120g***	***188***	***11.8***	***156***	***16.7***	***0.2***	***9.8***	***0.2***
Leg, Meat Only, Cooked, Stewed, Average	***1 Serving/60g***	***111***	***4.8***	***185***	***26***	***0***	***8***	***0***
Leg, Meat Only, Raw, Average	***1oz/28g***	***34***	***1.1***	***120***	***20.1***	***0***	***3.8***	***0***
Leg, Meat Only, Raw, Weighed with Skin & Bone	***1oz/28g***	***21***	***0.7***	***76***	***12.8***	***0***	***2.4***	***0***
Leg, Meat Only, Stewed with Bone & Skin, Average	***1oz/28g***	***31***	***1.4***	***111***	***15.8***	***0***	***4.8***	***0***
Leg, with Skin, Raw, Average	***1 Serving/250g***	***430***	***26***	***172***	***19.1***	***0***	***10.4***	***0***
Leg, with Skin, Roasted, Weighed with Bone, Average	***1oz/28g***	***47***	***3.3***	***166***	***15.3***	***0.1***	***11.6***	***0***
Legs, Slow Cooked in Mushroom Sauce, M&S*	½ Pack/310g	505	33.8	163	14.6	1.4	10.9	0.6
Lemon, & Herb, Cook*	1 Pack/280g	300	4.8	107	6.3	18.1	1.7	2.9
Light Meat, Roasted	***1oz/28g***	***43***	***1***	***153***	***30.2***	***0***	***3.6***	***0***
Meat & Skin Portions, Deep Fried, Average	***1oz/28g***	***73***	***4.7***	***259***	***26.9***	***0***	***16.8***	***0***
Meat & Skin, Roasted, Average	***1oz/28g***	***60***	***3.9***	***216***	***22.6***	***0***	***14***	***0***
Meat Free, Nuggets, Tex-Mex, Oven Cooked, Quorn*	4 Nuggets/80g	191	8.8	239	11	21	11	6.5
Meat Free, Southern Fried, Green Cuisine, Birds Eye*	3 Strips/83g	227	14.1	274	9.6	19	17	3.1
Meat Free, Style Pieces, Plant Pioneers, Sainsbury's*	5 Pieces/48g	122	8	254	17.1	5.8	16.6	6.6
Meat Free, with Patatas Bravas, & Aioli, Gousto*	1 Serving/396g	538	24.9	136	6	14.3	6.3	3.6
Meat, Roasted, Average	***1oz/28g***	***47***	***1.9***	***167***	***25***	***0***	***6.6***	***0***
Mexican Chilli, Sliced, Eat Well, M&S*	1 Pack/130g	169	3.4	130	25.9	0.8	2.6	0.5
Mexican, Tray Bake, Tesco*	½ Pack/179g	315	14	176	16.7	9.1	7.8	1.2
Middle Eastern, with Spiced Mixed Grains, Cook*	1 Pack/320g	362	11.5	113	10.2	11.4	3.6	2.8
Mince, Average	***1oz/28g***	***39***	***1.7***	***140***	***20.9***	***0.1***	***6***	***0.2***
Nuggets, Battered, Average	***1 Nugget/20g***	***50***	***2.9***	***251***	***13.5***	***16.9***	***14.4***	***0.9***
Nuggets, Breaded, Average	***1 Nugget/14g***	***37***	***2***	***263***	***14.8***	***19.8***	***13.8***	***1.9***

C

	Measure INFO/WEIGHT	per Measure KCAL	FAT	Nutrition Values per 100g / 100ml KCAL	PROT	CARB	FAT	FIBRE
CHICKEN								
Nuggets, Free From Gluten & Wheat, Sainsbury's*	1 Nugget/19g	47	2.5	251	13.4	19.7	13.2	0.8
Nuggets, Frozen, M&S*	1 Serving/150g	346	17.7	231	14.4	16.3	11.8	1.2
Nuggets, Vegan, Crispy, Quorn*	4 Nuggets/76g	144	6.3	190	9.4	17	8.3	4.5
Parmigiana, Finest, Tesco*	½ Pack/225g	326	14.8	145	17	3.7	6.6	1.3
Parmigiana, Tomato & Basil Sauce, Waitrose*	½ Pack/177g	257	11.9	145	16.2	4.6	6.7	0.8
Pieces, Boneless, Breaded, Fried, From Restaurant	***1 Piece/17g***	***51***	***3.3***	***301***	***17***	***14.4***	***19.4***	***0***
Pieces, Veggie Kitchen, Farmfoods*	5 Pieces/48g	122	8	254	17.1	5.8	16.6	6.6
Piri Piri, The Gym Kitchen*	1 Pack/400g	348	4.4	87	8.9	8.4	1.1	3.8
Plant-Based, This Isn't, This*	1 Serving/100g	152	3.8	152	22.7	8	3.8	0
Poke, Bowl, with Katsu Dressing, M&S*	1 Bowl/280g	392	8.7	140	5.3	22.2	3.1	1.1
Poppers, Ready to Eat, Tesco*	1 Popper/10g	27	1.6	273	11.5	19.9	16.2	0.7
Poppets, Boneless Bucket, SFC*	1 Box/190g	426	21.8	224	15.4	16.2	11.5	1.6
Rashers, Oak Park*	1 Rasher/25g	25	0.6	100	19.6	0.5	2.2	0.5
Roast, Stuffing Topped, Slices, Specially Selected, Aldi*	1 Slice/68g	82	1.4	121	24	1.6	2	0
Roast, Wafer Thin, Slices, Birchwood Farm, Lidl*	1 Serving/50g	68	2.8	136	18.9	2.3	5.6	0.5
Roll, Breast, Average	***1 Slice/10g***	***17***	***1***	***167***	***16.1***	***3.2***	***10***	***0.2***
Salted Chilli, Crispy, Richardsons*	1 Serving/100g	277	16.7	277	16.4	15.5	16.7	1.1
Satay, Skewers, Lidl*	1 Skewer/10g	23	1.3	233	19.1	4.1	12.6	0
Schnitzel, As Prepared, Easy to Cook, Waitrose*	½ Pack/99g	168	5.4	170	27	2.4	5.5	1.3
Sizzlers, Mediterranean, Ashfield Farm, Aldi*	1 Pack/300g	501	19.2	167	27	0.6	6.4	0.5
Skewers, Satay, Iceland*	1 Skewer/16g	30	1.2	187	20.3	8.9	7.7	0.3
Skewers, Satay, Tesco*	1 Skewer/15g	27	1.3	177	19.5	5	8.6	0.8
Skewers, Smokey Chipotle, Aldi*	1 Skewer/80g	107	3	134	18.6	6	3.8	0
Skewers, Sticky, with Sesame Seeds, Iceland*	1 Skewer/22g	33	0.1	152	21.7	14.4	0.5	1.4
Skewers, Thigh, Yakitori, M&S*	½ Pack/69g	167	6.7	242	5	13.6	9.7	0
Skewers, Tikka, Crestwood, Aldi*	1 Skewer/43g	99	6	231	19	7.8	14	1.1
Skin, Dry, Roasted or Grilled, Average	***1 Serving/100g***	***501***	***46.1***	***501***	***21.5***	***0***	***46.1***	***0***
Skin, Moist, Roasted or Grilled, Average	***1 Serving/100g***	***452***	***42.6***	***452***	***17***	***0***	***42.6***	***0***
Sliced, Cooked, Average	***1 Slice/15g***	***18***	***0.4***	***118***	***22.4***	***1.6***	***2.4***	***0.1***
Slices, Lemon, Garlic, & Herb, Morrisons*	¼ Pack/50g	66	0.6	132	25.1	4.4	1.3	1
Southern Fried, Chunks, Waitrose*	5 Chunks/70g	135	4.9	193	15	16.8	7	1.5
Spatchcock, Piri Piri, Cooked as per Instructions, Tesco*	¼ Pack/178g	329	17.4	185	23.1	1	9.8	0.1
Spatchcock, Poussin, Sainsbury's*	1 Serving/122g	168	6.6	138	21.1	0.1	5.4	0.2
Steak, Piri Piri, Fire Pit, Tesco*	1 Steak/61g	80	0.8	131	26.2	3.4	1.3	0.5
Steaks, Average	***1 Serving/100g***	***205***	***9.4***	***205***	***21.1***	***9***	***9.4***	***0.7***
Steaks, Breaded, Co-Op*	1 Steak/125g	309	20	247	16	9.6	16	1.5
Steaks, Breaded, Frozen, Morrisons*	1 Steak/95g	220	11.5	232	15.6	14.5	12.1	1.1
Steaks, Breaded, Garlic, Tesco*	1 Steak/84g	234	14.5	278	14.4	15.3	17.3	1.5
Steaks, Breaded, Morrisons*	1 Steak/112g	318	18.7	284	15.6	16.9	16.7	1.7
Steaks, Mango, & Coconut, Waitrose*	1 Steak/47g	81	1.6	172	31	4.1	3.5	0.5
Steaks, Southern Fried, Sainsbury's*	1 Steak/95g	233	13.7	245	15.3	13.1	14.4	0.6
Strips, Mexican, Sliced, M&S*	½ Pack/70g	77	0.4	110	24.3	2.3	0.6	0.5
Supreme, Weight Watchers, Heinz*	1 Pack/350g	350	3.5	100	5.9	16.6	1	0.7
Tandoori, with Roasted Vegetable, Tesco*	1 Pack/351g	390	6	111	8.6	14.3	1.7	2.1
Tandoori, with Spiced Pilau Rice, BFY, M&S*	1 Pack/360g	396	12.6	110	9.2	9.5	3.5	1.7
Tenders, Crispy, Buttermilk, M&S*	3 Pieces/150g	320	17.2	213	15.6	11	11.5	1.5
Tenders, Hot & Spicy, Farmfoods*	1 Serving/200g	398	18.2	199	16	14.4	9.1	2.3
Tenders, Premium, No Dips, Foxwood*	1 Serving/100g	224	8.1	224	20.8	16.5	8.1	1.1
Thigh, Chops, Lemon & Herb, Iceland*	1 Chop/101g	220	12.5	218	24.7	1.6	12.4	0
Thigh, Fillet, Buttermilk, Morrisons*	1 Thigh/114g	245	13.1	215	16.4	11.4	11.5	0
Thigh, Fillet, Jerk Spiced, Waitrose*	1 Thigh/70g	136	6.3	194	24.1	4	9	0.5
Thigh, Fillets, Tandoori, Ready to Eat, Morrisons*	½ Pack/75g	119	4.6	159	22.4	2.7	6.2	1.4
Thigh, Meat & Skin, Casseroled, Average	***1oz/28g***	***65***	***4.6***	***233***	***21.5***	***0***	***16.3***	***0***

	Measure INFO/WEIGHT	per Measure KCAL	FAT	Nutrition Values per 100g / 100ml KCAL	PROT	CARB	FAT	FIBRE
CHICKEN								
Thigh, Meat & Skin, Raw, Average	***1 Serving/100g***	***218***	***14.7***	***218***	***21.4***	***0***	***14.7***	***0***
Thigh, Meat & Skin, Weighed with Bone, Raw, Average	***1 Serving/100g***	***186***	***14.1***	***186***	***13.8***	***0.2***	***14.1***	***0***
Thigh, Meat Only, Diced, Casseroled	***1oz/28g***	***50***	***2.4***	***180***	***25.6***	***0***	***8.6***	***0***
Thigh, Meat Only, Raw, Average	***1 Thigh/90g***	***144***	***9***	***160***	***18.5***	***0***	***10***	***0***
Thigh, Roast, Average	***1 Serving/100g***	***238***	***15.6***	***238***	***23.8***	***0.4***	***15.6***	***0***
Thigh, Smoky Paprika, M&S*	½ Pack/311g	678	51.3	218	16	1.3	16.5	0
Thighs, Southern Fried, Boneless, Oven Baked, Iceland*	2 Pieces/84g	176	8.5	210	17.1	12.2	10.1	0.9
Thighs, Stuffed, Pork & Apple, Waitrose*	1 Thigh/85g	198	12.2	233	23.9	1.9	14.3	0.3
Thins, Flame Grilled, Tesco*	½ Pack/90g	130	2.8	145	28.6	0.5	3.1	0
Tikka, Thigh Flatties, The Grill, M&S*	½ Pack/206g	333	18.5	162	18.7	1.5	9	0
Vegan, Fillets, Southern Fried, Plant Chef, Tesco*	1 Fillet/123g	268	12.8	218	17.4	11.7	10.4	4.1
Vegan, Goujons, Breaded, Plant Chef, Tesco*	3 Goujons/89g	213	7.7	239	13.7	24.9	8.6	3.5
Vegan, Slices, Deli Style, Quorn*	½ Pack/50g	47	1.2	94	11	4.1	2.3	6.2
Vegan, Strips, No Chick, V Taste, Morrisons*	1 Strip/35g	119	6.3	341	15.7	27	18	3.9
Vegetarian, Bucket, Linda McCartney*	½ Pack/172g	449	25.8	261	14.6	14.8	15	4.6
Vegetarian, Chicken Style, Strips, Meat Free, Fry's*	1 Serving/95g	226	12.3	238	20.4	10	13	5.6
Vegetarian, Fillets, Crispy, Quorn*	1 Fillet/100g	192	8.5	192	12.5	14.2	8.5	4
Vegetarian, Pieces, Chicken Style, Chilled, Quorn*	½ Pack/175g	173	4.6	99	13.8	1.7	2.6	7.1
Vegetarian, Pieces, Chicken Style, Frozen/Chilled, Quorn*	1 Serving/100g	113	2.8	113	15.3	3.9	2.8	5.3
Vegetarian, Roast Style, Quorn*	1/5 Roast/91g	96	1.8	106	15	4.5	2	4.9
Vegetarian, Roast, Family, Frozen, Cooked, Quorn*	1 Serving/80g	91	2.2	114	16.7	3	2.7	5
Vegetarian, Southern-Style, Linda McCartney*	4 Pieces/101g	267	15.9	265	16.9	11.2	15.8	5.1
Veggie, Dippers, Plant Menu, Aldi*	1 Dipper/26g	60	2.9	228	3.7	27	11	5.5
Wafer Thin, Average	***1 Slice/10g***	***12***	***0.4***	***120***	***19***	***2.8***	***3.6***	***0.2***
Whole, Roast, Average	***½ Chicken/685g***	***910***	***57.7***	***133***	***13.4***	***0.9***	***8.4***	***0.1***
Wing Quarter, Meat Only, Casseroled	***1oz/28g***	***46***	***1.8***	***164***	***26.9***	***0***	***6.3***	***0***
Wing, Breaded, Fried, Average	***1oz/28g***	***77***	***4.8***	***273***	***17.1***	***13***	***17.2***	***0.4***
Wing, Meat & Skin, Cooked, Average	***1 Wing/85g***	***216***	***14.3***	***254***	***23.8***	***0***	***16.9***	***0***
Wing, Meat Only, Cooked, Average	***1 Wing/21g***	***43***	***1.7***	***203***	***30.5***	***0***	***8.1***	***0***
Wing, Meat Only, Raw, Average	***1 Wing/29g***	***37***	***1***	***126***	***22***	***0***	***3.5***	***0***
Wings, BBQ Flavour, Average	***3 Wings/150g***	***330***	***18.7***	***220***	***20.3***	***6.6***	***12.4***	***0.6***
Wings, Chinese Style, Average	***1oz/28g***	***72***	***4.3***	***256***	***24.2***	***5.1***	***15.5***	***0.6***
Wings, Hot & Spicy, Average	***1oz/28g***	***65***	***3.8***	***231***	***21.8***	***5.2***	***13.6***	***0.8***
Wings, Meat & Skin, Raw, Average	***1 Wing/150g***	***286***	***19.3***	***191***	***17.5***	***0***	***12.8***	***0***
Wings, Meat Free, The Vegilantes, Morrisons*	½ Pack/120g	284	11.6	237	20	16	9.7	3
Wings, Salt, & Chilli, Oven Cooked, Tesco*	1 Pack/167g	389	22.4	233	24.7	2.4	13.4	1.8
CHICKEN &								
Black Bean Sauce, with Egg Fried Rice, Ready Meal	***1 Serving/400g***	***390***	***6.1***	***97***	***6.5***	***14.5***	***1.5***	***0.8***
Cashew Nuts, Chinese, Ready Meal, Average	***1 Serving/400g***	***497***	***24***	***124***	***9.2***	***7.5***	***6***	***1.2***
Chorizo Paella, Go Cook, Asda*	½ Pack/475g	591	10.5	124	10.2	15.9	2.2	2.6
Fries, Southern Fried Style, Tesco*	1 Pack/500g	930	40	186	11.5	16	8	1.4
King Prawn Special Fried Rice, Finest, Tesco*	1 Pack/450g	734	32	163	7.7	17	7.1	0.7
Mushroom with Rice, Egg Fried, Average	***1 Serving/400g***	***421***	***10.1***	***105***	***6.3***	***14.4***	***2.5***	***0.8***
Pineapple, Chilled, Tesco*	1 Pack/350g	364	8.4	104	9.6	11.1	2.4	5.5
Roasted Potatoes, Spanish, Charlie Bigham's*	½ Pack/387g	479	25.9	124	7.2	9.8	6.7	0
CHICKEN ARRABIATA								
Arrabbiata, COU, M&S*	1 Pack/360g	396	6.7	110	8.5	14.5	1.9	1.3
COU, M&S*	1 Meal/360g	396	6.5	110	8.4	14.5	1.8	1.3
Italian Kitchen, Tesco*	1 Pack/414g	492	11.6	119	8.3	14.2	2.8	1.8
M&S*	1 Pack/396g	436	6.7	110	8.5	14.5	1.7	1.3
Meal for One, M&S*	1 Pack/400g	528	20.8	132	7.9	12.5	5.2	1.9
Morrisons*	1 Pack/400g	488	8.8	122	8.2	16.6	2.2	1.5

C

	Measure INFO/WEIGHT	per Measure KCAL	FAT	Nutrition Values per 100g / 100ml KCAL	PROT	CARB	FAT	FIBRE
CHICKEN CHASSEUR								
Average	***1 Serving/400g***	***363***	***9.2***	***91***	***12.2***	***4.9***	***2.3***	***0.9***
CHICKEN CHILLI								
Sweet, Battered, Chinese Favourites Box, M&S*	½ Pack/120g	220	4.9	183	11	24.9	4.1	1.1
Sweet, CBY, Asda*	½ Pack/170g	253	6.8	149	19.1	8.9	4	0.7
Sweet, Pieces, Morrisons*	1 Pack/200g	282	5	141	25.5	4.1	2.5	0.5
Sweet, With Noodles, Ready Meal, Average	***1 Serving/400g***	***404***	***5.8***	***101***	***6.5***	***15.5***	***1.4***	***1.4***
CHICKEN CHINESE								
Balls, M&S*	1 Ball/16g	45	2.2	280	10.8	29.2	13.6	2.1
Stir Fry, Morrisons*	1 Serving/319g	341	5.4	107	5.7	17	1.7	1.5
with Ginger & Spring Onion, Tesco*	1 Serving/350g	299	10.1	85	7.6	7.3	2.9	0.6
CHICKEN DINNER								
Cooked, Eat Smart, Morrisons*	1 Pack/355g	245	4.3	69	8.2	4.4	1.2	4.1
Morrisons*	1 Pack/379g	375	6.1	99	7.4	12.7	1.6	1.9
Roast Potatoes, Peas, Carrots, & Stuffing, HFC, Tesco*	1 Pack/382g	368	9.1	96	9	8.8	2.4	2
Roast, 104, Oakhouse Foods Ltd*	1 Meal/400g	368	8.4	92	8.2	9.4	2.1	1.5
Roast, Calorie Controlled, Tesco*	1 Pack/381g	274	3	72	8.1	7.2	0.8	1.8
Roast, Frozen, Inspired Cuisine, Aldi*	1 Pack/400g	404	11.6	101	8.3	9.3	2.9	1.9
Roast, Mini Meals, Tesco*	1 Pack/218g	234	7	108	6.9	12	3.2	1.7
Roast, Morrisons*	1 Pack/379g	375	6.1	99	7.4	12.7	1.6	1.9
Roast, Oven Baked, Asda*	1 Pack/384g	449	11.5	117	11	11	3	1.2
Roast, Sainsbury's*	1 Pack/351g	400	13.7	114	10.7	8.4	3.9	1.3
Roast, Taste The World, Aldi*	1 Pack/500g	500	15.5	100	6.8	10	3.1	1.6
Roast, What's Cooking, Lidl*	1 Pack/400g	360	7.2	90	7.7	10.4	1.8	0.6
CHICKEN EN CROUTE								
& Bacon, Gastropub, M&S*	1 En Croute/220g	645	41.8	293	12.1	17.9	19	1.1
Just Cook, Sainsbury's*	1 En Croute/180g	481	27.2	267	16.8	15.9	15.1	0.4
CHICKEN IN								
Barbeque Sauce, Breasts, COU, M&S*	1 Pack/350g	420	6.7	120	8.5	20.6	1.9	0.6
BBQ Sauce, Breast, Sainsbury's*	1 Serving/170g	199	1.2	117	14.5	13.1	0.7	1.3
BBQ, Smoky, SlimWell, Aldi*	1 Pack/500g	331	4.3	70	10	3.2	0.9	3.4
Black Bean Sauce, Sainsbury's*	1 Pack/465g	484	7.9	104	5	17.3	1.7	0.3
Dijon, with Rice, TTD, Sainsbury's*	1 Pack/368g	552	11.4	150	8	21.9	3.1	0.9
Gravy, Breast, Sainsbury's*	1 Box/200g	124	1	62	11.8	2.9	0.5	0.2
Hunter's BBQ Sauce, Asda*	½ Pack /190g	348	14.1	183	19.1	10.3	7.4	0
Mushroom, Sauce, Tesco*	1 Pack/370g	289	8	78	7.8	6.2	2.2	1.3
Oyster Sauce & Mushrooms, Tesco*	1 Pack/350g	252	5.6	72	8	6.3	1.6	0.7
Peppercorn Sauce, Counted, Morrisons*	1 Pack/353g	364	7.8	103	8.2	11.8	2.2	1.8
Prosecco Sauce, Finest, Tesco*	½ Pack/181g	245	10.9	135	17.7	2.3	6	0.6
Red Wine, Gastropub, M&S*	½ Pack/233g	296	11.9	127	17	3	5.1	0.5
Sweet Chilli Sauce, Breast, Fresh Tastes, Asda*	½ Pack/180g	288	9	160	18.4	10.3	5	0.5
Teriyaki Sauce, with Noodles, Wat Kitchen*	1 Box/250g	352	7.2	141	3.7	24.6	2.9	1.4
Tomato & Basil Sauce, Breast Fillets, Morrisons*	½ Pack/171g	231	7.5	135	21.3	2.5	4.4	1.4
Tomato & Basil Sauce, Breast, GFY, Asda*	1 Pack/392g	447	13.3	114	12	9	3.4	1.5
White Sauce, Canned, 200g, Sainsbury's*	1 Can/200g	280	16	140	13.2	3.4	8	0.6
White Sauce, Canned, Princes*	½ Can/82g	109	6.6	133	10.4	4.5	8.1	0.5
CHICKEN LEMON								
Battered, Cantonese, Sainsbury's*	1 Pack/350g	560	19.6	160	10.7	16.6	5.6	0.9
Battered, Chinese Meal for Two, Tesco*	½ Serving/175g	294	13	168	6.6	18.8	7.4	2
Cantonese, Sainsbury's*	½ Pack/140g	218	8.8	156	11	13.9	6.3	0.6
COU, M&S*	1 Pack/150g	150	1.4	100	17.9	5.6	0.9	0.8
CHICKEN MOROCCAN								
Harissa Spiced, Cook*	1 Pack/315g	350	12.9	111	11.5	7.8	4.1	1.6
Style, Sainsbury's*	½ Pack/269g	334	7	124	14.7	10.4	2.6	3.1

	Measure INFO/WEIGHT	per Measure KCAL	FAT	Nutrition Values per 100g / 100ml KCAL	PROT	CARB	FAT	FIBRE
CHICKEN PASANDA								
Microwaved, Luxury, Iceland*	1 Pack/360g	562	34.9	156	12.5	4.1	9.7	1.3
Sainsbury's*	1 Serving/200g	368	24.8	184	14.7	3.4	12.4	2.3
with Pilau Rice, HL, Tesco*	1 Pack/440g	466	11	106	5.7	15.2	2.5	0.9
CHICKEN SUPREME								
Breast, Sainsbury's*	1 Serving/187g	421	29.5	225	20.6	0.3	15.8	0.6
with Rice, Asda*	1 Pack/450g	616	31.5	137	15	3.4	7	1.1
with Rice, HE, Tesco*	1 Pack/400g	384	6.4	96	4.9	15.6	1.6	1.5
CHICKEN SZECHUAN								
Tesco*	1 Pack/350g	385	10.5	110	7.2	13.6	3	0.3
with Noodles, Sainsbury's*	1 Pack/450g	423	14	94	6	10.4	3.1	0.9
CHICKEN TANDOORI								
& Basmati Rice, Aromatic, Asda*	1 Pack/380g	399	8	105	7.5	12	2.1	3.7
Breast, Fillets, with Creamy Sauce, Morrisons*	1 Fillet/144g	220	7.8	153	21.3	4.4	5.4	0.8
Fresh Tastes, Asda*	1 Pack/400g	356	5.6	89	6.4	12.7	1.4	2.1
Oven Baked, Asda*	½ Pack/141g	186	5.9	132	20	3.6	4.2	0.6
Sizzler, Sainsbury's*	1 Pack/400g	536	29.2	134	12.8	4.3	7.3	1.7
Sizzler, Tesco*	1 Serving/175g	243	11.6	139	10	10	6.6	1
with Rice, City Kitchen, Tesco*	1 Pack/385g	597	21.2	155	6.7	19.6	5.5	1.8
CHICKEN TERIYAKI								
& Noodles, Asda*	½ Pack/340g	445	8.8	131	9	18	2.6	0.9
Noodles, HL, Tesco*	1 Pack/367g	282	1.8	77	6.4	10.5	0.5	2.3
Teriyaki, Japanese, Sainsbury's*	1 Pack/380g	486	11.4	128	7.4	16.8	3	2.1
Teriyaki, Japanese, Street Kitchen*	1 Pack/255g	398	4.1	156	1.6	31	1.6	0
CHICKEN TIKKA								
& Lemon Rice, Deli Meal, M&S*	1 Pack/360g	342	7.2	95	9.8	10.2	2	0.7
& Cauliflower Rice, Spiced, BFY, M&S*	1 Pack/400g	276	8	69	8.4	3.3	2	1.9
Less Than 3% Fat, BGTY, Sainsbury's*	1 Pack/303g	373	3.6	123	6	21.3	1.2	1
Masala, & Pilau Rice, Charlie Bigham's*	½ Pack/403g	737	43.9	183	6.9	15.3	10.9	0
Masala, with Rice, Weight Watchers, Heinz*	1 Pack/310g	333	7.4	108	5.4	15.8	2.4	0.7
Takeaway	***1 Serving/350g***	***421***	***15***	***120***	***20.3***	***0***	***4.3***	***0.3***
The Gym Kitchen*	1 Pack/392g	384	6.7	98	8.5	10	1.7	3.5
with Cauliflower Rice, Lighter For You, Lidl*	1 Pack/523g	314	7.3	60	7.4	3.3	1.4	2.3
with Pilau Rice, GFY, Asda*	1 Pack/450g	382	2.7	85	7	13	0.6	1.8
CHICKEN WITH								
a Sea Salt & Black Pepper Crust, Breasts, Asda*	1 Serving/154g	186	4.3	121	19	5	2.8	0
a Sticky Honey & Chilli Sauce, Breast, Asda*	1 Serving/175g	247	5.6	141	20	8	3.2	0
Caesar Melt & Prosciutto, Breast, M&S*	1 Pack/375g	488	18.8	130	19.6	1.3	5	1
Chips, & Peas, Goujons, Breaded, Wiltshire Farm Foods*	1 Pack/340g	507	20.4	149	7.2	15	6	0
Coconut, Bowl, with Spinach, & Brown Rice, BFY, M&S*	1 Pack/300g	351	11.1	117	9.7	10.6	3.7	1
Cous Cous, Lemon & Herb, Finest, Tesco*	1 Pack/370g	492	18.5	133	10.5	11.5	5	0.9
Leek & Bacon, M&S*	½ Pack/183g	239	12.8	131	15.3	1.2	7	0.9
Leeks, & White Wine Sauce, Finest, Tesco*	½ Pack/180g	258	10.3	143	20.9	1.5	5.7	1.2
Lime & Coriander, Easy, Waitrose*	½ Pack/168g	203	7.9	121	18.9	0.7	4.7	0.5
Lyonnaise Potatoes, M&S*	½ Pack/260g	286	8.1	110	12.6	8	3.1	0.9
Mediterranean Style, with Couscous, Iceland*	1 Serving/373g	328	6	88	7.6	9.9	1.6	1.4
Mushroom & Bacon, Fillets, M&S*	½ Pack/188g	225	11.2	120	15.5	0.5	6	1.7
Pork Stuffing, Breast, Roast, M&S*	1 Serving/100g	165	6.5	165	24.1	3	6.5	0
Rice, Jamaican Jerk, Healthier Choice, Co-Op*	1 Pack/406g	365	9.3	90	7.8	9.8	2.3	3.4
Sage & Onion Stuffing, Breast, Roast, Sliced, M&S*	1 Slice/17g	27	1.1	165	24.1	3	6.5	0
CHICORY								
Fresh, Raw, Average	***1 Head/150g***	***30***	***0.9***	***20***	***0.6***	***2.8***	***0.6***	***0.9***
CHILLI								
& Rice, Bowl, BFY, M&S*	1 Pack/300g	318	6.9	106	8	12.2	2.3	2.4

C

	Measure INFO/WEIGHT	per Measure KCAL	FAT	Nutrition Values per 100g / 100ml KCAL	PROT	CARB	FAT	FIBRE
CHILLI								
& Rice, Calorie Controlled, Tesco*	1 Pack/385g	393	6.5	102	6.2	13.2	1.7	4.7
3 Bean, Chipotle, Hi Five*	1 Pack/467g	355	8.4	76	3.2	12.8	1.8	2.7
Bean, 3, Inspired Cuisine, Aldi*	1 Pack/380g	312	2.3	82	2.5	16	0.6	2.4
Bean, Bowl, Microwaved, Quorn*	1 Bowl/297g	300	1.2	101	5.1	17	0.4	4.4
Bean, Mixed, Chipotle, with Wild Rice, Eat Well, M&S*	1 Pack/300g	312	5.7	104	3.9	15.9	1.9	3.9
Bean, Nacho, Allplants*	1 Serving/451g	487	17.1	108	4.1	12	3.8	4
Bean, Smoky, Jane Plan*	1 Pack/220g	246	7.5	112	3.7	15	3.4	2.9
Bean, Three, & Rice, As Consumed, Counted, Morrisons*	1 Pack/390g	386	4.7	99	3.5	17	1.2	3.1
Bean, Three, Slim Choice, Sainsbury's*	1 Pack/465g	437	2.8	94	3.7	16.1	0.6	4.9
Bean, Triple, Plant Chef, Tesco*	1 Pack/390g	417	6.6	107	3.2	17.9	1.7	3.4
Beef with Rice, GFY, Asda*	1 Serving/402g	354	6	88	4.7	14	1.5	0.9
Beef, & 3 Bean, with Wild Rice, Inspired Cuisine, Aldi*	1 Pack/377g	369	6.4	98	5.7	14	1.7	2
Beef, & Rice, HL, Tesco*	1 Pack/370g	370	5.9	100	5	13.7	1.6	5.5
Beef, & Rice, Tex Mex, Tesco*	1 Pack/450g	604	13	134	5.4	20.4	2.9	2.5
Beef, Asda*	½ Pack/200g	190	7.8	95	7	8	3.9	1.2
Beef, Chunky, Slimming World*	1 Pack/550g	418	6.6	76	8.8	5.9	1.2	3.1
Beef, Chunky, Slow Cooked, M&S*	½ Pack/268g	289	8.3	108	15.3	3.6	3.1	2.1
Con Carne & Rice, Tex Mex, M Kitchen, Morrisons*	1 Pack/450g	580	22.9	129	0.5	14.9	5.1	0.5
Con Carne & Sweetcorn Mash, Fuller Longer, M&S*	1 Pack/400g	380	13.2	95	8.5	7.4	3.3	3.9
Con Carne with Rice, GFY, Asda*	1 Serving/400g	456	6.4	114	6	19	1.6	0.9
Con Carne with Rice, Healthy Choice, Asda*	1 Pack/400g	412	8.4	103	6	15	2.1	0.9
Con Carne with Rice, Morrisons*	1 Pack/400g	328	5.2	82	5.3	12.2	1.3	1.4
Con Carne, & Mexican Rice, Charlie Bigham's*	½ Pack/421g	589	25.2	140	7.2	14.1	6	0
Con Carne, & Rice, Fiesta, Aldi*	1 Pack/450g	648	24.3	144	6.7	16	5.4	2.3
Con Carne, Asda*	1 Can/392g	376	13.7	96	7	9	3.5	0
Con Carne, Beef, Slim Cook, Tesco*	1 Pack/476g	376	7.1	79	5.4	9.6	1.5	3.1
Con Carne, Canned, Morrisons*	1 Can/392g	368	11.8	94	8.8	8	3	2.4
Con Carne, Canned, Sainsbury's*	½ Can/200g	162	4.2	81	6.6	8.9	2.1	2.5
Con Carne, Classic, Canned, Stagg*	½ Can/200g	260	10	130	7	13	5	4.5
Con Carne, From Restaurant, Average	***1 Serving/253g***	***256***	***8.3***	***101***	***9.7***	***8.7***	***3.3***	***0***
Con Carne, Frozen, Co-Op*	1 Pack/340g	306	3.4	90	6	15	1	1
Con Carne, M&S*	1 Pack/285g	285	10.5	100	8.7	7.4	3.7	2
Con Carne, Medium, Canned, Bramwells, Aldi*	1 Can/400g	408	17.6	102	8.8	4.7	4.4	4
Con Carne, Microwaved, Asda*	1 Pack/400g	532	15.2	133	5.9	18	3.8	1.5
Con Carne, Mild, Canned, Princes*	1 Can/392g	576	34.9	147	6.5	9.1	8.9	2
Con Carne, Recipe Mix, Colman's*	1 Pack/27g	84	2.1	312	12.3	37.8	7.7	22.9
Con Carne, with Long Grain Rice, COU, M&S*	1 Pack/390g	394	6.6	101	5.4	15	1.7	2.2
Con Carne, with Rice, BGTY, Sainsbury's*	1 Pack/374g	385	8.6	103	6.3	13.4	2.3	2.1
Con Carne, with Rice, Classic, Co-Op*	1 Pack/400g	464	13.6	116	5.9	14	3.4	2.7
Con Carne, with Rice, Counted, Morrisons*	½ Pack/158g	150	2.4	95	5.9	13.5	1.5	1.6
Con Carne, with Rice, Iceland*	1 Meal/375g	431	17.2	115	5.7	12.2	4.6	1.1
Con Carne, with Rice, Meal for One, M&S*	1 Pack/450g	536	12.2	119	5.5	18	2.7	0.5
Con Carne, with Rice, PB, Waitrose*	1 Pack/400g	404	7.2	101	5.8	15.3	1.8	1.7
Con Carne, with Rice, Tesco*	1 Pack/400g	468	8.4	117	6.1	17.6	2.1	2
Con Carne, with White Rice, Sainsbury's*	1 Pack/400g	469	13.6	117	5.1	16	3.4	1.2
Mixed Vegetable, Tesco*	1 Pack/400g	352	11.6	88	3.9	11	2.9	3.2
Quick, with Basmati Rice, & Soured Cream, Hello Fresh*	1 Serving/660g	812	27.1	123	6.5	14	4.1	0.2
Quorn, Full of Beans, Microwaved, Quorn*	1 Pack/385g	366	4.2	95	4.7	15.2	1.1	2.6
Smoky, Soul, Allplants*	1 Serving/430g	555	17.2	129	5.1	16	4	3.9
Vegan, Two Bean, Waitrose*	1 Pack/368g	254	5.9	69	3.1	9.4	1.6	2.4
Vegetable	***1oz/28g***	***16***	***0.2***	***57***	***3***	***10.8***	***0.6***	***2.6***
Vegetable & Rice, BGTY, Sainsbury's*	1 Pack/450g	410	5	91	3.5	16.7	1.1	3.5
Vegetable, Retail	***1oz/28g***	***20***	***0.6***	***70***	***4***	***9.4***	***2.1***	***0***

	Measure INFO/WEIGHT	per Measure KCAL	FAT	Nutrition Values per 100g / 100ml KCAL	PROT	CARB	FAT	FIBRE
CHILLI								
Vegetarian with Rice, Tesco*	1 Pack/500g	575	13	115	4	19	2.6	1.8
Vegetarian, Mexican, Chef's Selection, Quorn*	½ Pack/170g	143	4.3	84	6.6	6.5	2.5	4.5
Vegetarian, Soya Mince, & Rice, Waitrose*	1 Pack/402g	442	8.4	110	5.4	14.9	2.1	5.4
Vegetarian, with Rice, Ready Meal, Average	***1 Serving/400g***	***434***	***6***	***108***	***3.8***	***20***	***1.5***	***1.3***
Veggie, Packed, with Brown Rice, Hello Fresh*	1 Serving/739g	525	14.8	71	3	10	2	0
Veggie, Smoky, Jamie Oliver*	1 Serving/125g	111	2.6	89	4.6	10	2.1	5.1
CHILLI POWDER								
Average	***1 Tsp/4g***	***16***	***0.7***	***405***	***12.3***	***54.7***	***16.8***	***34.2***
CHIPS								
American Style, Oven, Co-Op*	1 Serving/150g	255	9	170	2	26	6	3
American Style, Thin, Oven, Tesco*	1 Serving/125g	210	8.1	168	2.7	24.6	6.5	2.1
Chip Shop, Fishnchickn*	1 Portion/311g	734	38.6	236	3.2	27.9	12.4	0
Chunky Oven, Harry Ramsden's*	1 Serving/150g	184	5.4	123	2.8	19.9	3.6	1.6
Chunky, Chilled, Waitrose*	1/3 Pack/150g	237	5.6	158	2.8	26.5	3.7	3.8
Chunky, COU, M&S*	1 Serving/150g	158	2.4	105	2.1	20.5	1.6	2.3
Chunky, Gastropub, M&S*	1 Pack/400g	520	12.4	130	2.6	22.4	3.1	2.3
Chunky, in Light Crisp Batter, M&S*	1 Serving/100g	119	2.9	119	2.1	19.6	2.9	3.2
Chunky, M&S*	½ Pack/200g	292	7.6	146	2	24.7	3.8	2.6
Chunky, Maris Piper, Oven Cooked, The Best, Morrisons*	½ Pack/176g	267	6.1	152	2.3	26.5	3.5	2.7
Chunky, Oven Cooked, Finest, Tesco*	1 Pack/387g	546	14.7	141	2.8	22.6	3.8	2.7
Chunky, Ready to Bake, M&S*	1 Serving/200g	310	8.4	155	2.2	26.8	4.2	2
Chunky, Skin On, Oven Baked, Tesco*	¼ Pack/125g	104	0.3	83	2.9	16.4	0.2	2.1
Crinkle Cut, Frozen, Fried in Corn Oil	***1 Serving/125***	***362***	***20.9***	***290***	***3.6***	***33.4***	***16.7***	***2.2***
Fine Cut, Frozen, Fried in Blended Oil	***1oz/28g***	***102***	***6***	***364***	***4.5***	***41.2***	***21.3***	***2.4***
French Fries, Crispy, Oven Baked, McCain*	1 Serving/100g	231	7.7	231	3.1	35.5	7.7	3.3
Fried, Average	***1 Serving/130g***	***266***	***10.9***	***204***	***3.2***	***29.6***	***8.4***	***1.2***
Fried, Chip Shop, Average	***1 Sm/100g***	***239***	***12.4***	***239***	***3.2***	***30.5***	***12.4***	***2.2***
Frites, M&S*	1 Sm Pack/100g	161	4.5	161	3.2	25.8	4.5	2.3
Fry or Oven, Oven Cooked, Smart Price, Asda*	1 Serving/125g	192	4.3	153	2.1	26.9	3.4	3.3
Home Chips, Crinkle Cut, Oven Baked, McCain*	1 Serving/100g	197	7.7	197	2.4	28	7.7	2.8
Home Chips, Straight Cut, Baked, McCain*	1 Serving/150g	312	10.8	208	3.3	31	7.2	2.9
Home, Straight Cut, Lighter, Reduced Fat, Baked, McCain*	1 Serving/100g	181	3.4	181	3.2	33	3.4	3.3
Homemade, Fried in Blended Oil, Average	***1oz/28g***	***53***	***1.9***	***189***	***3.9***	***30.1***	***6.7***	***2.2***
Homemade, Fried in Corn Oil, Average	***1oz/28g***	***53***	***1.9***	***189***	***3.9***	***30.1***	***6.7***	***2.2***
Homemade, Fried in Dripping, Average	***1oz/28g***	***53***	***1.9***	***189***	***3.9***	***30.1***	***6.7***	***2.2***
Homestyle Oven, Sainsbury's*	1 Serving/125g	206	5.4	165	2.4	29.2	4.3	2.1
Homestyle, BFY, Morrisons*	1 Serving/88g	175	5.2	199	2.8	32.1	5.9	3.6
Homestyle, Crispy & Fluffy, Oven Cooked, Aunt Bessie's*	1 Serving/100g	157	5.1	157	2.8	23	5.1	3.4
Homestyle, Crispy, Ovenbaked, Asda*	1 Serving/125g	249	7.4	199	2.8	32	5.9	3.6
Homestyle, Frozen, Aunt Bessie's*	1 Serving /125g	155	4.4	124	2.4	20	3.5	1.9
Homestyle, Harvest Basket, Lidl*	1 Serving/150g	202	5.8	135	2.4	21.5	3.9	2.3
Homestyle, Oven, Straight Cut , Tesco*	1 Serving/125g	218	5.1	174	2.1	30.9	4.1	2.5
Maris Piper, Oven, Chunky, Extra Special, Asda*	1 Serving/125g	211	4.4	169	2	31	3.5	2.7
Microwave, Cooked	***1oz/28g***	***62***	***2.7***	***221***	***3.6***	***32.1***	***9.6***	***2.9***
Oven, Frozen, Baked	***1 Serving/125g***	***202***	***5.2***	***162***	***3.2***	***29.8***	***4.2***	***2***
Oven, Steak Cut, Asda*	1 Serving/100g	153	4.1	153	2	27	4.1	2.5
Oven, Steak Cut, Sainsbury's*	1 Serving/165g	266	7.8	161	2.6	27.1	4.7	2.8
Oven, Steak Cut, Waitrose*	1 Serving/165g	218	5.6	132	2.7	22.7	3.4	1.7
Oven, Straight Cut, 5% Fat, Sainsbury's*	1 Serving/165g	280	8.1	170	3.4	28	4.9	2.5
Oven, Straight Cut, Asda*	1 Serving/100g	199	5	199	3.5	35	5	3
Oven, Straight Cut, BFY, Morrisons*	1 Serving/165g	249	5.8	151	2.8	27.1	3.5	2.1
Oven, Straight Cut, Crispy, Oven Baked, Iceland*	1 Serving/100g	210	7	210	3.2	31.5	7	3.7
Oven, Straight Cut, Less Than 3% Fat, Baked, Asda*	1 Serving/121g	162	2.9	134	2.7	24	2.4	2.5

	Measure INFO/WEIGHT	per Measure KCAL	FAT	Nutrition Values per 100g / 100ml KCAL	PROT	CARB	FAT	FIBRE
CHIPS								
Oven, Straight Cut, Naked, Oven Baked, McCain*	1 Serving/100g	162	3.9	162	2.3	28	3.9	2.1
Oven, Straight Cut, Reduced Fat, Tesco*	1 Serving/100g	127	3	127	2.3	22.7	3	2.1
Oven, Straight Cut, Waitrose*	1 Serving/165g	219	6.1	133	2	23	3.7	1.7
Oven, Sweet Potato, Cooked, Tesco*	¼ Pack/87g	153	4.8	175	3	26.2	5.5	4.5
Oven, Thick Cut, Frozen, Baked	***1 Serving/125g***	***196***	***5.5***	***157***	***3.2***	***27.9***	***4.4***	***1.8***
Oven, Thin Cut, American Style, Asda*	1 Serving/100g	240	10	240	3.4	34	10	3
Oven, Thin Fries, Morrisons*	1 Serving/100g	161	6.1	161	2.9	23.6	6.1	1.2
Potato, Lights, Reduced Fat, Lay's*	1 Serving/25g	118	5.5	470	7.5	60	22	5
Proper, Frozen, Strong Roots*	1 Serving /125g	150	3.8	120	1.9	20	3	2.7
Salt & Pepper, Crinkle, Tesco*	1 Serving/112g	179	5.7	160	2.3	24.6	5.1	3.4
Salt & Pepper, Iceland*	1 Serving/100g	231	7.6	231	4.1	34.1	7.6	4.6
Steak Cut, Frying, Asda*	1 Serving/97g	181	6.8	187	2.9	28	7	2.8
Steak Cut, Harvest Basket, Lidl*	1 Serving/100g	155	4	155	2.7	26.6	4	1.2
Steak Cut, Iceland*	1 Serving/100g	156	4.1	156	3.3	24.6	4.1	3.6
Steak Cut, Morrisons*	1 Serving/125g	171	3.9	137	2.1	23.7	3.1	3.1
Steak Cut, Oven, Cooked, Tesco*	1/7 Pack/138g	247	6.3	179	3.7	29.3	4.6	3.2
Steak, Cut, Oven, Frozen, Essential, Waitrose*	1 Serving/180g	241	6.5	134	2.4	22.1	3.6	1.7
Steakhouse, Fry, Tesco*	1 Serving/125g	278	15.1	222	3.1	25.2	12.1	2
Straight Cut, Frozen, Fried in Blended Oil	***1 Serving/125g***	***341***	***16.9***	***273***	***4.1***	***36***	***13.5***	***2.4***
Straight Cut, Frozen, Fried in Corn Oil	***1 Serving/125g***	***341***	***16.9***	***273***	***4.1***	***36***	***13.5***	***2.4***
Thick Cut, Frozen, Fried in Corn Oil, Average	***1 Serving/125g***	***292***	***12.7***	***234***	***3.6***	***34***	***10.2***	***2.4***
Triple Cooked, Beef Dripping, Harvest Basket, Lidl*	1 Serving/150g	344	19.8	229	2.7	23	13.2	3.5
Triple Cooked, Finest, Tesco*	½ Pack/178g	262	6.8	147	2.6	24.1	3.8	3
Triple Cooked, Gastro, Frozen, McCain*	1 Serving/187g	379	22.2	203	1.9	21	11.9	2.2
Triple Cooked, Gastro, Oven Baked, McCain*	1 Serving/135g	379	20.5	281	2.9	31.6	15.2	3
Vegetable, Fries, Aldi*	1 Serving/100g	192	11	192	2.5	18	11	6.7
CHIVES								
Fresh, Average	***1 Tsp/2g***	***0***	***0***	***23***	***2.8***	***1.7***	***0.6***	***1.9***
CHOC ICES								
Chocolate, Real Milk, Sainsbury's*	1 Choc Ice/41g	126	8	311	3	29.9	19.8	0.6
Dark, Morrisons*	1 Choc Ice/70g	150	10.2	214	1.7	18.7	14.6	0.7
Dark, Sainsbury's*	1 Choc Ice/41g	115	7.2	283	2.7	27.2	17.8	1.5
Dark, Sainsbury's*	1 Choc Ice/41g	115	7.2	283	2.7	27.2	17.8	1.5
Dark, Tesco*	1 Choc Ice/43g	132	8.7	305	3.5	28	20	0.1
Essential, Waitrose*	1 Choc Ice/70g	124	8.4	177	1.7	15.4	12	0.7
Everyday, Value, Tesco*	1 Choc Ice/31g	95	6.3	300	2.3	26.7	19.9	1
Plain, Co-Op*	1 Choc Ice/42g	123	8	293	3.1	26	19	0
CHOCOLATE								
100% Cocoa, M&S*	1 Square/10g	62	5.4	620	12.5	13.2	54	15.6
Acorns, Salted Caramel, M&S*	1 Chocolate/22g	112	6.1	508	4.6	59.2	27.7	1.6
Advent Calendar, Dairy Milk, Cadbury*	1 Chocolate/4g	22	1.3	525	7.5	56.6	30.1	0.7
Advent Calendar, Maltesers, Mars*	1 Chocolate/4g	21	1.2	537	6.8	57.9	30.9	0
Almond Butter, Cup, Dark, Pip & Nut*	1 Cup/17g	102	7.9	599	11.2	30.3	46.6	0
Almond, Orange, Organic, Vivani *	1 Bar/35g	199	12.8	568	3.6	54.9	36.6	0
Alpine Milk , Milka*	1 Serving/25g	132	7.4	530	6.6	58.5	29.5	1.8
Balls, Protein, Exante Diet*	1 Pack/158g	713	27.8	451	42.9	28.9	17.6	2.9
Bar, Animal, Nestle*	1 Bar/19g	97	5	513	5.8	63.6	26.1	0
Bar, Bliss Truffle, Cadbury*	1 Bar/40g	226	14.9	565	6.6	48.8	37.3	2.8
Bar, Bubbly, Milk, Tesco*	1 Bar/25g	138	8.2	554	6.1	57.7	32.8	1.9
Bar, Cappuccino, Thorntons*	1 Bar/38g	201	13.2	529	5.2	49.7	34.7	0.5
Bar, Chocolate Cream, Fry's*	1 Piece/10g	42	1.3	415	2.8	70.8	13.2	1.2
Bar, Chopped Nuts, Dairy Milk, Cadbury*	6 Chunks/24g	130	7.8	547	7.9	52	33	2.5
Bar, Cookies & Cream, Hello, Lindt*	1 Square/10g	56	3.7	565	7	52	37	0

	Measure INFO/WEIGHT	per Measure KCAL	FAT	Nutrition Values per 100g / 100ml KCAL	PROT	CARB	FAT	FIBRE
CHOCOLATE								
Bar, Dark, Thorntons*	1 Sm Bar/48g	250	17.7	521	7.3	39.9	36.9	10.9
Bar, Deliciously, Free From, Sainsbury's*	1 Bar/35g	190	12.2	543	2.5	48.2	35	12.4
Bar, Duplo, Ferrero*	1 Bar18g	101	6.1	555	6.1	56	33.5	5
Bar, Free From, Asda*	1 Bar/35g	194	12.1	563	2.5	58	35	2.8
Bar, Fruit & Nut, Free From, Sainsbury's*	2 Squares/21g	120	7.7	573	4	54.3	36.8	4.1
Bar, Hazel Nut & Cashew, Dairy Milk, Cadbury*	3 Chunks/18g	96	6	540	8.8	50.6	33.5	1.8
Bar, Mandolin, Cadbury*	1 Bar/28g	139	4.6	495	3.5	66.5	16.5	0.6
Bar, Milk, Thorntons*	1 Sm Bar/50g	269	16	538	7.5	54.8	32	1
Bar, Salted Caramel, Aldi*	1 Bar/26g	138	7.8	532	5.1	57	30	5.4
Bar, Soft & Whippy, Sainsbury's*	1 Bar/22g	100	3.5	455	3.6	73.6	15.9	0
Bar, Truffle, M&S*	1 Bar/35g	168	11.4	480	5.9	41.7	32.5	8.3
Bar, White, Thorntons*	1 Bar/50g	274	15.6	547	6.5	59.5	31.3	0
Bars, Chocolate, Strawberry, Lindt*	1 Bar/100g	470	22.8	470	4.5	61.6	22.8	0
Bars, Milk Chocolate, Galaxy, Mars*	1 Bar/42g	229	13.6	546	6.7	56	32.4	1.5
Bars, Milk Chocolate, Gold, Lindt*	1 Bar/300g	1605	92.9	535	6.6	58.7	31	0
Bars, Milk Chocolate, Hazelnut, Lindt*	1 Bar/100g	570	38.8	570	8.5	47	38.8	0
Bars, Milk Chocolate, Lindt*	1 Bar/100g	622	47	622	4.6	44	47	0
Bars, Milk Chocolate, Raisin & Hazelnut, Lindt*	1 Bar/100g	530	31.6	530	3.1	54.7	31.6	0
Bars, Milk, Bubblies, Treat Size, Asda*	1 Bar/10g	53	3	528	7.1	57	30	0.6
Batons, Dark, 85%, Hotel Chocolat*	1 Baton/9g	56	4.6	625	9.4	22	51	19
Batons, Nutmilk, Hotel Chocolat*	1 Baton/8g	38	2.8	474	2.6	36.3	35.3	3.7
Batons, Supermilk, 65%, Hotel Chocolat*	3 Batons/24g	136	10.7	568	10.3	28.6	44.5	9.7
Beans, Coffee, Dark, Solid, M&S*	1 Serving/10g	53	3.8	532	4.7	42.4	37.6	11.6
Bear, Lindt*	1 Bear/11g	60	3.6	572	7.5	57.7	34.6	0
Belgian Milk, TTD, Sainsbury's*	1 Piece/10g	55	3.5	549	9.6	48.3	35.3	2
Belgian, Milk, Mini Eggs, M&S*	1 Egg/8g	43	2.5	535	7	55.8	31.7	2.7
Bittermints, Bendicks*	1 Mint/18g	77	3	428	3.5	62.8	16.8	0
Bloc, Hazelnut, Green & Black's*	1 Bloc/20g	116	8	578	6.8	43	40	7.4
Block, Orange Crisp, Thorntons*	1 Serving/100g	530	30	530	6.6	57	30	0
Blueberry Intense, Excellence, Lindt*	1 Serving/40g	200	12.4	500	6	50	31	0
Bubbly Santa, M&S*	1 Santa/23g	124	7.3	540	7	55.8	31.7	2.7
Bubbly, Dairy Milk, Cadbury*	1 Bar/35g	185	10.5	525	7.7	56.9	29.7	0.7
Bunny, Easter, Mars*	1 Bunny/29g	155	9.2	535	6.2	56.2	31.7	0
Bunny, Kit Kat, Nestle*	1 Bunny/29g	156	9.1	537	6.2	55.6	31.4	2.9
Bunny, Lidl*	1 Rabbit/125g	676	38.9	541	7.2	57.1	31.1	1.9
Bunny, Lindt*	1 Bunny/11g	60	3.6	572	7.5	57.5	34.6	0
Buttons, Bournville, Cadbury*	1 Serving/25g	128	6.8	510	3.9	60	27	6.2
Buttons, Caramel Crunch, Galaxy, Mars*	1 Serving/31g	161	8.4	519	6.5	62	27	0
Buttons, Caramel Filled, M&S*	6 Buttons/25g	127	7	509	5.7	57.6	28.1	1.3
Buttons, Dairy Milk, Cadbury*	1 Bag/30g	160	9	535	7.3	57	30	2.1
Buttons, Free From, Tesco*	1 Bag/25g	136	8.8	544	2.5	48.4	35	12.5
Buttons, Giant, Orange, Dairy Milk, Cadbury*	1 Serving/25g	133	7.5	533	7.4	57	30	2.1
Buttons, Gigantic, M&S*	1/5 Pack/125g	704	40.8	563	7.7	58.8	32.6	1.6
Buttons, Maltesers, Mars*	1 Bag/32g	166	8.6	518	7.4	60	27	0
Buttons, Orange, Dairy Milk, Cadbury*	10 Buttons/25g	133	7.5	533	7.4	57	30	2.1
Buttons, White, Free From, Tesco*	1 Pack/25g	132	8.1	528	0.4	51.7	32.5	13.3
Buttons, White, Giant, Cadbury*	1 Serving/25g	134	7.2	535	4.8	63	29	0
Caramel & Sea Salt, Pure, Moser Roth, Aldi*	1 Tablet/25g	133	7.5	533	4.7	58	30	5.7
Caramel, & Sea Salt, Vegan, Galaxy*	½ Bar/50g	290	19.4	581	3	53.4	38.9	0
Caramel, Bar, Dairy Milk, Cadbury*	1 Serving/37g	179	8.9	485	5.1	61	24	0.4
Caramel, Choceur, Aldi*	4 Squares/33g	158	7.6	479	5.1	62	23	2.7
Caramel, Chunk, Dairy Milk, Cadbury*	1 Chunk/33g	158	7.6	480	5	63	23	0
Caramelised Hazelnut, Vegan, Galaxy *	4 Squares/29g	173	12	596	3.4	50.8	41.5	0

C

	Measure INFO/WEIGHT	per Measure KCAL	FAT	Nutrition Values per 100g / 100ml KCAL	PROT	CARB	FAT	FIBRE
CHOCOLATE								
Caramelles, Mister Choc, Lidl*	1/5 Pack/25g	120	5.1	482	4.2	69	20.5	2.2
Chips, Dark, Tesco*	1 Serving/25g	134	8	536	6.7	51.3	32.2	7.3
Chips, Dark, The Pantry, Aldi*	1 Serving/25g	126	6.5	505	3.8	60	26	6.1
Chips, Milk, Tesco*	¼ Pack/25g	141	8.8	563	5.9	55.1	35	1.9
Chocolat Noir, Lindt*	1/6 Bar/17g	87	5.4	510	6	50	32	0
Chocolate Favourites, Tesco*	½ Box/227g	1015	43.6	447	4.2	64.3	19.2	0.3
Chocowafer, Milka*	1 Biscuit/30g	159	8.8	530	7.2	57.7	29.5	0
Chomp, Cadbury*	1 Bar/24g	112	4.8	465	3.3	67.9	20	0.2
Chomp, Treat Size, Cadbury*	1 Bar/12g	56	2.4	466	2.8	68	20	0.7
Christmas Tree Decoration, Average	***1 Chocolate/12g***	***63***	***3.6***	***522***	***7.6***	***56.4***	***29.9***	***0.4***
Chunk Bar, Dairy Milk, Cadbury*	1 Chunk/7g	35	2	525	7.5	57	29.8	0.1
Cocoa Fudge, Hotel Chocolat*	1 Bar/45g	170	6.3	378	1.8	62.1	13.9	2.1
Coconut, White, Excellence, Lindt*	1 Square/10g	61	4.4	610	6	48	44	0
Coins, Marzipan, & Cherry , Favorina, Lidl*	1 Serving/30g	132	5.7	439	5.3	58	19	3.3
Cranberry, Almond, & Hazelnut, Dark, Excellence, Lindt*	1 Pack/100g	518	29	518	5.1	55	29	0
Crispies, Chunk, Dairy Milk, Cadbury*	1 Chunk/31g	158	8.5	510	7.6	58.6	27.4	0
Crispies, Dairy Milk, Cadbury*	1 Bar/49g	250	13.4	510	7.6	58.6	27.4	0
Crispy, Sainsbury's*	4 Squares/19g	99	5.4	521	9.1	56.9	28.5	2.1
Dairy Milk with Oreo, Dairy Milk, Cadbury*	3 Chunks/15g	85	5.4	560	6.1	53.5	35.5	0.7
Dairy Milk, 30% Less Sugar, Dairy Milk, Cadbury*	1 Sm Bar/35g	176	10.8	503	5.8	42	31	18
Dairy Milk, Cadbury*	1 Bar/45g	242	13.6	534	7.3	57	30	2.1
Dairy Milk, Oreo, Mint, Dairy Milk, Cadbury*	3 Chunks/15g	84	5.2	557	5.9	54	35	1.5
Dark Cherry Tart, Graze*	1 Pack/40g	182	10.4	454	4.6	53	26	5.4
Dark with Chilli, Thorntons*	4 Squares/20g	107	7.9	533	7.2	36.3	39.5	10.4
Dark, Finest, 85% Cocoa, Moser Roth, Aldi*	1 Bar/25g	152	12.8	608	11	18	51	15
Dark, 60%, Amazonas, Lidl*	1 Square/13g	75	5.2	574	5.7	44	40	7.5
Dark, 64%, Almonds, Popped Quinoa, Moser Roth, Aldi*	1 Square /10g	57	4.1	573	8.7	39	41	8.4
Dark, 70% Cocoa Solids, Extra Fine, Lindt*	1 Square/10g	54	4.1	537	8	33	41	12.2
Dark, 70% Cocoa Solids, Organic, Green & Black's*	1 Serving/18g	104	7.5	580	9.1	36	42	10
Dark, 70% Cocoa Solids, Organic, Morrisons*	½ Bar/50g	266	20.6	531	7.9	31.6	41.1	11
Dark, 70%, with Raspberries, Divine Chocolate*	1 Square/5g	29	2.2	584	6.7	32.2	45	11.3
Dark, 70%, Irresistible, Co-Op*	2 Squares/20g	115	8.4	575	8.5	36	42	10
Dark, 70%, No Added Sugar, Live Cultures, Ohso*	1 Bar/14g	63	4.9	466	5.1	27.1	35.9	26.1
Dark, 70%, Peruvian, Moser Roth, Aldi*	1 Square/10g	58	4.3	584	9.1	35	43	9.3
Dark, 70%, Velvet, Green & Black's*	1 Bar/90g	557	44.1	619	6.1	33	49	9.7
Dark, 70%, with Salted Caramel Pieces, J D Gross, Lidl*	1 Square/13g	68	4.6	543	7.1	41.7	36.5	9.6
Dark, 72%, Pure, Godiva*	1 Square/10g	57	4.2	567	9.1	32	42	0
Dark, 72%, Swiss, Aldi*	4 Squares/17g	98	7.4	591	6.9	35.8	44.3	0
Dark, 75%, Madagascan, Single Origin, No.1, Waitrose*	1 Square/10g	58	4.3	585	9.3	33.4	43.8	10.5
Dark, 85% Cocoa, Excellence, Lindt*	1 Serving/40g	212	18.4	530	11	19	46	16.3
Dark, 85% Cocoa, J D Gross, Lidl*	1 Square/12g	69	5.6	579	10.8	21.4	46.8	14.5
Dark, 85% Cocoa, TTD, Sainsbury's*	1 Serving/25g	149	12.8	596	9.6	16.8	51.4	14.1
Dark, 85%, J D Gross, Lidl*	1 Square/13g	75	6.1	579	10.8	21.4	46.8	14.5
Dark, 90% Cocoa, Lindt*	1 Square/10g	59	5.5	592	10	14	55	0
Dark, 95% Cocoa, Arriba, J D Gross, Lidl*	1 Square/13g	75	6.5	594	12.5	12.7	51.1	16.7
Dark, Almond, & Sea Salt, Tony's Chocolonely*	1 Bar/180g	970	63	539	7.4	44	35	0
Dark, Basics, Sainsbury's*	3 Pieces/20g	103	5.8	516	4.4	56.1	29	6.3
Dark, Baton, 100%, Hotel Chocolat*	1 Baton/8g	47	4.2	586	11.9	0	52.9	29.3
Dark, Belgian, Extra Special, Asda*	2 Squares/20g	102	8	508	11	26	40	16
Dark, Belgian, Luxury Continental, Sainsbury's*	1 Bar/100g	490	38.7	490	11.1	24.2	38.7	7.4
Dark, Belgian, Rich, Intense, Waitrose*	1 Square/18g	98	7	547	10.6	30	39.1	16.1
Dark, Belgian, with Raisins, & Almonds, Waitrose*	1 Square/18g	92	5.5	510	7.7	45.9	30.8	9.3
Dark, Bournville, Classic, Cadbury*	1 Bar/45g	238	13.5	530	3.8	59.5	29.9	5.5

	Measure INFO/WEIGHT	per Measure KCAL	FAT	Nutrition Values per 100g / 100ml KCAL	PROT	CARB	FAT	FIBRE
CHOCOLATE								
Dark, Buttons, Giant, Bourneville, Cadbury*	1 Serving/25g	128	6.8	510	3.9	60	27	6.2
Dark, Chilli, Excellence, Lindt*	1 Serving/40g	202	12.8	506	5.4	49	32	0
Dark, Choco-Low, Dairyfine, Aldi*	2 Squares/20g	103	7.8	514	8.3	40	39	9.6
Dark, Classic, 74% Cocoa, Tesco*	1 Square/10g	56	4.1	561	9.7	32	41	12.7
Dark, Classic, Bourneville, Cadbury*	4 Squares/25g	125	6.8	505	4.7	58.8	27.3	2
Dark, Co-Op*	1 Bar/50g	252	14.5	505	4	57	29	6
Dark, Discs, Extra Fine, M&S*	1 Disc/5g	29	2.3	589	7.7	31.3	45.6	11.2
Dark, Everyday Essentials, Aldi*	½ Pack/50g	258	15	517	7.2	50	30	7.3
Dark, Fair Trade, Co-Op*	1 Bar/45g	214	13	475	4	49	29	6
Dark, Finest, 74% Cocoa, Fin Carre, Lidl*	1 Square/10g	57	4.2	571	9.9	32	42	12.6
Dark, Fudge, Salty, Johnny Doodle*	1 Block/13g	63	3.5	504	5	56	28	0
Dark, Ganache, Belgian, Godiva*	1 Piece/8g	48	3.1	582	6.7	53	37	0
Dark, Ginger, & Turmeric, 75% Cocoa, No.1, Waitrose*	1 Square/10g	57	4	568	8.3	38.5	40.3	9.2
Dark, Ginger, & Mandarin, Peruvian, Moser Roth, Aldi*	2 Squares//20g	108	6.8	539	7	48	34	7.2
Dark, Hazelnut Crisp, Mini Bar, Mister Choc, Lidl*	1 Mini Bar/18g	102	6.8	566	7.7	46.2	37.9	4.4
Dark, Honeycomb, Excellence, Lindt*	1 Serving/20g	106	6	529	5.4	56	30	0
Dark, Intense, 85% Cocoa, Tesco*	1 Square/10g	58	4.7	585	11.2	22	47	14.7
Dark, Lovetts*	3 Pieces/20g	101	5.9	507	1.2	56.5	29.3	6.3
Dark, Madagascan, 70%, J D Gross, Lidl*	1 Square/10g	56	4.1	562	8.5	33.5	41.2	11.5
Dark, Madagascan, 80%, TTD, Sainsbury's*	2 Pieces/20g	118	9.1	592	9.4	30.6	45.5	10.8
Dark, Mint, Intense, Lindt*	1 Square/10g	53	3.2	529	5	51	32	0
Dark, No Added Sugar, Red*	1 Bar/26g	74	6.2	286	4.7	33	24	0
Dark, Orange & Almond, Moser Roth, Aldi*	1 Serving/25g	133	8	532	5.9	51	32	7.9
Dark, Orange, Zesty, Tesco*	2 Squares/20g	111	7.1	554	5.7	50	35.3	6.9
Dark, Peruvian, 85%, Organic, Moser Roth, Aldi*	2 Squares/20g	119	9.6	597	11	24	48	13
Dark, Plain, Average	***1oz/28g***	***143***	***7.8***	***510***	***5***	***63.5***	***28***	***2.5***
Dark, Pure, Artisan, Raw, Raw Halo Ltd*	1 Bar/33g	201	16.9	610	7.7	30.1	51.1	0
Dark, Raspberry, Velvet Fruit, Green & Black's*	8 Pieces/26g	129	7.4	490	4.3	51	28	8.1
Dark, Rich, Tesco*	1 Serving/20g	98	6.1	491	5.8	60	30.4	11.5
Dark, Roasted Hazelnut, Excellence, Lindt*	1 Square/10g	55	3.5	546	6	47	35	0
Dark, Rum & Raisin, Old Jamaica, Bourneville, Cadbury*	4 Chunks/23g	105	5.3	465	4.2	59.6	23.4	2
Dark, Salted Caramel, Nespresso*	1 Piece/5g	27	1.7	543	7.9	48.4	33.7	7.3
Dark, Seriously Rich, 65%, Waitrose*	1 Sm Bar/30g	169	11.6	562	8.2	40.3	38.6	10.4
Dark, Simply, Lidl*	3 Squares/20g	98	5.6	491	4.6	51	28	8.1
Dark, Smooth, Bar, Galaxy, Mars*	1 Bar/125g	651	42	521	6.2	48	33.6	9.3
Dark, Smooth, No Added Sugar, Sainsbury's*	1 Piece/10g	53	4.2	529	8.2	34.3	42.2	11
Dark, Spiced Orange, Single Origin, No.1, Waitrose*	1 Square/10g	54	3.5	540	6.1	45.4	35.3	8.2
Dark, Sugar Free, Amul*	1 Serving/11g	52	3.7	475	6	57.3	33.7	0
Dark, Tiddly Pot, Hotel Chocolat*	1 Serving/58g	311	22.4	537	13.9	30.5	38.7	8.7
Dark, Whole Nut, Tesco*	1 Serving/13g	67	4.5	539	6.1	48.3	35.7	6.5
Dark, with Almonds, Green & Black's*	1 Lrg Bar/90g	560	45	622	9.2	29	50	9.4
Dark, with Blood Orange, Godiva*	2 Pieces/15g	76	4.4	509	5.4	60	29	0
Dark, with Mint, Velvet, Green & Black's*	1 Square/9g	56	4.4	619	6.1	33	49	9.7
Dark, with Orange, Co-Op*	2 Squares/20g	108	6.8	540	6.6	47	34	7.3
Dark, with Salted Caramel, Velvet, Green & Black's*	1 Lrg Bar/90g	540	40.5	600	5.2	39	45	8.2
Dark, with Sea Salt, Velvet, Green & Black's*	1 Lrg Bar/90g	554	44.1	616	6.1	33	49	9.7
Darker Milk, Galaxy, Mars*	1 Serving/22g	119	7	542	6.1	55	32	0
Darkmilk, Cadbury*	1 Bar/35g	197	13	562	5.8	49	37	4.8
Darkmilk, Salted Caramel, Cadbury*	3 Chunks/14g	77	4.9	551	5.2	52	35	4.3
Darkmilk, with Roasted Almonds, Cadbury*	3 Chunks/14g	79	5.3	567	7.2	45	38	5.3
Dessert, Milka*	3 Square/20g	112	7.4	562	6.6	48	37	4.3
Desserts, Collection, Lily O'briens*	1 Chocolate/12g	61	3.8	505	5.3	57.9	31.6	2.6
Discovery Collection, Box, Lir Chocolates Ltd*	1 Chocolate/10g	52	3.2	517	5.7	50.2	31.6	4.6

	Measure INFO/WEIGHT	per Measure KCAL	FAT	Nutrition Values per 100g / 100ml KCAL	PROT	CARB	FAT	FIBRE
CHOCOLATE								
Domes, Raspberry Crunch, Godiva*	1 Dome/10g	51	3	511	6.9	50	30	0
Double, Caramel, Cups, Deliciously Ella*	1 Pack/36g	162	8.4	450	7.3	50.2	23.4	5.1
Ferrero Rocher, Ferrero*	1 Chocolate/13g	75	5.3	603	8.2	44.4	42.7	0
Ferrero Rocher, Heart, Ferrero*	1 Chocolate/13g	75	5.3	603	8.2	44.4	42.7	0
Fingers, Milk, Mister Choc, Lidl*	1 Finger/18g	104	6.9	579	6.2	51.7	38.4	0.9
Freddo, Caramel, Dairy Milk, Cadbury*	1 Freddo/19g	93	4.7	490	5.5	60.5	24.8	0.5
Freddo, Dairy Milk, Cadbury*	1 Freddo/18g	95	5.4	530	7.5	57	29.8	0.7
Freddo, Rice Crisps, Dairy Milk, Cadbury*	3 Squares/25g	131	7.1	523	7.4	58.6	28.3	0
Fruit & Nut, Dark, Tesco*	4 Squares/25g	124	7	494	5.8	54.8	27.9	6.5
Fruit & Nut, Dairyfine, Aldi*	4 Squares/25g	131	8	525	8.1	50	32	4.2
Galaxy, Crispy, Galaxy, Mars*	1 Portion/20g	111	6.6	546	6.4	56.7	32.2	0
Golden Biscuit Crunch, Dairy Milk, Cadbury*	4 Chunks /25g	135	8.2	545	6.2	55.5	33	0.8
Golf Balls, Milk Chocolate, Lindt*	1 Pack/110g	619	39.5	563	6.5	53.6	35.9	0
Hazelnut Crunch, Choceur, Aldi*	1 Serving/40g	226	14.4	564	9.2	49.7	36	2.4
Honeycomb, & Nuts, Dairy Milk, Cadbury*	1 Serving/11g	58	3.3	525	7.3	59.1	29.5	0
Honeycomb, Asda*	1 Serving/35g	173	7.7	495	4.3	69	22	2.1
Honeycomb, Cone, M&S*	1 Cone/73g	210	11.2	287	3.9	32.9	15.4	0.5
Jazzies, Mini, Asda*	1 Jazzie/1g	4	0.1	449	3.4	81	12	0.6
Kinder Bueno, Bar, Ferrero*	1 Bar/21g	122	8	572	8.6	49.5	37.3	0
Kinder Maxi, Ferrero*	1 Bar/21g	116	7.1	550	10	51	34	0
Kinder Surprise, Ferrero*	1 Egg/20g	110	6.8	552	8.1	52.3	34.2	0
Kinder, Bar, Small, Ferrero*	1 Bar/13g	71	4.4	566	8.7	53.5	35	0
Kinder, Bueno, Bar, White, Ferrero*	1 Piece/20g	111	7	572	8.8	53	35.9	0
Kinder, Riegel, Ferrero*	1 Bar/21g	117	7.1	558	10	53	34	0
Kirsch, Lindt & Sprungli*	1 Bar/21g	98	4.8	467	4.5	57	23	0
Little Bars, Dairy Milk, Cadbury*	1 Bar/18g	96	5.4	534	7.3	57	30	2.1
Mars, Bites, Mars*	4 Bites/20g	90	3.3	449	4.1	70.2	16.6	0
Matchmakers, Mint, Cool, Quality Street, Nestle*	4 Sticks/17g	84	3.6	495	3.7	70.6	21.3	2.4
Matchmakers, Mint, Nestle*	1 Stick/4g	20	0.8	477	4.3	69.7	20.1	0.9
Matchmakers, Orange, Nestle*	4 Sticks/17g	84	3.6	492	3.7	70	21.3	2.4
Matchmakers, Yummy Honeycomb, Nestle*	4 Sticks/15g	72	3.1	495	3.7	70.6	21.3	2.4
Medley, Dark, Biscuit & Fudge, Dairy Milk, Cadbury*	1 Piece/9g	52	3.2	555	5.9	54.5	34	2
Mikado, Daim, Mikado *	11 Biscuits/25g	119	4.5	474	6.5	70	18	3.1
Milk for Baking, Value, Tesco*	½ Bar/50g	265	14.5	530	6.7	60	29	2.2
Milk with Honey & Almond Nougat, Swiss, Toblerone*	1 Piece/8g	42	2.4	525	5.4	59	29.5	2.2
Milk with Whole Almonds, Organic, Green & Black's*	1 Lrg Bar/90g	520	38	578	11.8	37.7	42.2	5.2
Milk, & White, Alpine, Sweet Winter, Milka*	¼ Bar/25g	133	7.4	531	6.2	59.5	29.5	1.6
Milk, 41%, Honeycomb, Love Cocoa*	1 Block/75g	432	27.2	576	5.7	54.9	36.2	1.9
Milk, 55% Cocoa, Bar, Lindt*	1 Bar/80g	483	37.6	604	8.8	33	47	0
Milk, 65%, Cocoa Excellence, Lindt*	1 Square/8g	51	4.3	635	8.9	24	54	0
Milk, Almond, Choceur, Aldi*	1 Square/29g	171	12.2	589	13	38	42	3.5
Milk, Almond, Fin Carre, Lidl*	2 Squares/13g	78	5.4	603	11.8	42.8	41.7	5
Milk, Average	***1oz/28g***	***146***	***8.6***	***520***	***7.7***	***56.9***	***30.7***	***0.8***
Milk, Bars, M&S*	1 Bar/40g	214	12.8	535	7.8	54	32	1.9
Milk, Belgian, No Added Sugar, Chocologic*	4 Squares/13g	64	4.8	484	7.9	33.7	36.2	17
Milk, Biscuit Sticks, Mikado, Kraft*	1 Stick/2.3g	11	0.5	475	7.8	67	19.8	3.1
Milk, Bubbly, Mister Choc, Lidl*	4 Squares/17g	89	5.3	538	7.9	53.5	32	2.4
Milk, Bubbly, Swiss, M&S*	1 Serving/40g	218	13.7	545	8	52	34.3	2.5
Milk, Caramel Sea Salt, Tony's Chocolonely*	1 Piece/30g	161	9.5	537	7	54.3	31.7	0
Milk, Creamy, Organic, Green & Black's*	1 Bar/90g	504	32	560	9.1	50.3	35.5	1.6
Milk, Everyday Essentials, Aldi*	1 Serving/25g	130	6.5	519	6	64	26	1.9
Milk, Extra Au Lait, Milch Extra, Lindt*	½ Bar/50g	268	15.5	535	6.5	57	31	0
Milk, Extra Creamy, Excellence, Lindt*	1 Bar/100g	560	37.1	560	6	51.1	37.1	0

	Measure INFO/WEIGHT	per Measure KCAL	FAT	Nutrition Values per 100g / 100ml KCAL	PROT	CARB	FAT	FIBRE
CHOCOLATE								
Milk, Extra Fine, Swiss, M&S*	1 Serving/25g	141	9.2	565	7.2	50.9	36.7	2.3
Milk, Fair Trade, Tesco*	1 Serving/45g	236	13.3	524	7.6	56.7	29.6	2
Milk, Figures, Hollow, Dairyfine, Aldi*	1 Serving/11g	58	3.2	523	5.5	59.9	29	3.1
Milk, Fin Carre, Lidl*	1 Serving/17g	88	5	528	6.8	57.2	29.7	2.1
Milk, Fruit & Nut, Fin Carre, Lidl*	4 Pieces/17g	83	4.5	499	6.4	56.7	26.7	3.4
Milk, Fruit & Nut, Tesco*	2 Sqaures/18g	95	5.9	528	9.9	47.4	32.6	2.5
Milk, Giant Buttons, M&S*	1 Button/8g	44	2.7	550	7.1	52.3	34.2	0.4
Milk, Latte Macchiato, Mini Bar, Mister Choc, Lidl*	1 Mini Bar/18g	106	7.4	588	7.7	46.2	41.2	2.8
Milk, Lindor, Lindt*	1 Square/11g	68	5.2	615	4.7	43	47	0
Milk, Mint, Truffle Balls, Mini, Lindt*	3 Balls/15g	92	6.8	612	5.4	45	45	0
Milk, Orange, Bubbly, Mister Choc, Lidl*	1 Serving/17g	92	5.4	541	6.6	56.1	31.9	1.3
Milk, Organic, Tesco*	1 Serving/25g	140	9.1	558	6.3	51.4	36.3	2.3
Milk, Rich Coffee, Bar, Tesco*	2 Squares/20g	109	6.4	547	6.6	56.6	32.3	1.7
Milk, Sainsbury's*	4 Squares/25g	133	7.7	533	9.2	54.6	30.8	2.2
Milk, Salted Butterscotch, Extra Special, Asda*	1/5 Bar/20g	110	7	552	6.9	52	35	2.7
Milk, Salted Caramel, Godiva*	1 Square/10g	53	3	524	7.1	57	30	0
Milk, Salted Caramel, Thin, Organic, Green & Black's*	1 Square/12g	67	4.1	550	8.4	51.5	33.5	2.6
Milk, Santa, Lolly, Dairyfine, Aldi*	1 Lolly/15g	81	4.5	541	6.3	60	30	2.2
Milk, Santas, Tesco*	1 Bag/90g	433	21.8	481	4.5	61.4	24.2	1.4
Milk, Strawberry Yogurt, Mini Bar, Mister Choc, Lidl*	1 Mini Bar/18g	102	6.5	566	6	52.8	36.3	2.8
Milk, Swiss, Cooking, Menier*	1 Serving/17g	89	5	538	7.3	57.4	30.4	2.8
Milk, Swiss, Diabetic with Fruit & Nuts, Boots*	½ Bar/21g	97	6.7	462	7	55	32	2.7
Milk, Swiss, Finest, Tesco*	2 Squares/20g	112	7	558	8.5	50.6	35.2	2.3
Milk, Tesco*	1 Serving/25g	133	7.7	533	9.5	54.7	30.7	2.2
Milk, Tony's Chocolonely*	1 Sm Bar/50g	272	16.6	545	7.7	51.9	33.2	0
Milk, Value, Tesco*	1/6 Bar/16g	83	4.5	520	6.8	60	28	2.3
Milk, Whole Nut, Tesco*	1 Serving/25g	129	8.4	517	8.7	53.4	33.8	9
Milk, Wholenut, with Hazelnuts, Dairyfine, Aldi*	4 Squares/25g	144	9.5	574	8.3	47	38	4.2
Milk, Winnie the Pooh, Solid Shapes, M&S*	1 Chocolate/6g	32	1.9	540	8.1	54.1	32.4	1.3
Milk, with Orange, Divine Chocolate*	1 Sm Bar/35g	189	11	541	6.2	57.3	31.4	1.7
Milk, with Salted Pistachio, Thorntons*	1 Pack/80g	434	25.6	543	7.9	55	32	0
Milky Bar, Giant Buttons, Mars*	1 Sweet/2g	11	0.6	546	7.5	57.7	31.6	0
Millionaire, Crispy, Stackers, Free From, Co-Op*	1 Stacker/30g	149	7.8	498	4.1	60	26	3.3
Mini Eggs, Aero, Nestle*	8 Eggs/24g	129	7.3	537	6.8	57.7	30.4	2.1
Mini Eggs, Belgian, Doubly Divine, Moser Roth, Aldi*	1 Egg/11g	57	3.2	516	6.2	55	29	4.5
Mini Eggs, Cadbury*	1 Egg/3g	16	0.7	495	4.6	69.5	21.5	1.3
Mini Eggs, Caramel, Cadbury*	1 Mini Egg/11g	55	2.9	485	5.7	59	25.7	0.4
Mini Eggs, Daim, Cadbury*	1 Egg/11g	60	3.4	535	6.9	56.5	30.5	1.8
Mini Eggs, Lindor, Lindt*	3 Eggs/15g	92	6.8	611	5.4	45	45	0
Mini Eggs, Oreo, Cadbury*	1 Egg/10g	58	3.7	565	5.9	53.5	36	1.3
Mini, Toblerone*	1 Serving/6g	32	1.8	525	5.6	57.5	30	3.5
Mint Chips, Dairy Milk, Cadbury*	1 Bar/49g	247	12.8	505	6.6	61.6	26.1	0.6
Mint Creme, Sainsbury's*	1 Serving/20g	93	4.9	467	2.8	62.7	24.5	2.1
Mint Crisps, M&S*	1 Mint/8g	40	2.4	494	5.4	54.8	29.6	3.1
Mint, Bar, Lindor, Lindt*	1 Bar/38g	232	17.1	611	5.3	45	45	0
Mint, Bubbly, Dairyfine, Aldi*	6 Squares/25g	137	7.8	547	5.7	60	31	0.5
Mint, Fondant Thins, Dark Chocolate, Sainsbury's*	1 Thin/10g	48	2	478	4.9	67.5	19.9	4.6
Mint, Thins, Mister Choc, Lidl*	7 Thins/25g	133	7.8	533	7.6	51.5	31.3	7.6
Mint, Waves, Choceur, Aldi*	7 Waves/25g	129	7	516	6.4	56	28	6
Mints, Christmas, Cadbury*	1 Mint/13g	72	5	552	6.7	45	38.7	0
Mistletoe Kisses, Mars*	1 Pack /42g	209	11.5	498	5.3	57	27.3	0
Mix Mps, Milkybar, Nestle*	1 Pack/33g	175	10.2	538	10	53.2	31.3	1.2
Mountain Bar, Dark, M&S*	1 Bar/100g	572	41.9	572	7.4	36.2	41.9	10.3

	Measure INFO/WEIGHT	per Measure KCAL	FAT	Nutrition Values per 100g / 100ml KCAL	PROT	CARB	FAT	FIBRE
CHOCOLATE								
Mountain Bar, Fruit & Nut, M&S*	1 Bar/100g	551	34.3	551	7	52.4	34.3	2.5
Mountain Bar, Milk, M&S*	1 Bar/100g	552	33.9	552	6.9	53.8	33.9	2.1
Mountain Bar, White, M&S*	1 Bar/100g	574	36.9	574	6.3	54.1	36.9	0.2
Natural Orange, Excellence, Lindt*	1 Bar/100g	560	37	560	7	50	37	0
Natural Vanilla, Excellence, Lindt*	1 Bar/100g	590	40	590	6	51	40	0
Nuts About Caramel, Cadbury*	1 Bar/55g	272	15.1	495	5.8	56.6	27.4	0
Nutty Nougat, Bite Sized, Sainsbury's*	1 Bar/23g	111	5.5	481	7.6	59	23.8	0.6
Operetta, M&S*	1 Chocolate/12g	71	5	589	9	40	42	0
Orange Cream, Fry's*	1 Bar/50g	210	6.8	420	2.8	72.3	13.7	0
Orange, Bar, Terry's*	1 Bar/40g	210	11.7	530	7.3	58	29.5	2.1
Orange, Dark, Terry's*	1 Segment/9g	45	2.6	511	4.3	57	29.3	6.2
Orange, Milk, Mini Segments, Minis, Terry's*	1 Segment/4g	21	1.1	520	5.8	59.5	28	2.4
Orange, Milk, Terry's*	1 Orange/157g	816	44	520	5.8	59.5	28	2.4
Orange, Mini Eggs, Terry's*	6 Eggs/23g	118	6	514	6.6	64	26	1
Orange, Plain, Terry's*	1 Orange/157g	801	43.2	510	5.2	55.5	27.5	7.6
Orange, Segsations, Terry's*	1 Segsation/7g	36	2	520	6.9	58.5	28.5	2.8
Orange, Tangs, Hotel Chocolat*	1 Piece/5g	19	0.6	381	2.4	62	12	4.5
Orange, Tuile, Lindt*	1 Tuile/3g	18	1	513	5	54	29	9.6
Oreo, Bar, Dairy Milk, Cadbury*	1 Bar/41g	226	13.7	550	6	55	33.5	1.6
Oreo, Bites, Dairy Milk, Cadbury*	1 Serving/25g	138	8.2	551	5	57	33	1.5
Oreo, Peanut Butter, Dairy Milk, Cadbury*	1 Chunk/5g	28	1.8	558	5.9	54	35	1.5
Panna Cotta & Raspberry, M&S*	1 Bar/36g	190	12.1	528	4.7	51.4	33.6	0.3
Peanut Butter Cup, Big Cup, Reese's, Hershey*	1 Cup/39g	210	12	538	10.3	53.8	30.8	2.6
Peanut Butter Cup, Mini, Reeses, Hershey*	2 Mini Cups/7g	38	2.1	542	8.8	58.3	30.5	0
Peanut Butter Cup, Miniature, Reese's, Hershey*	1 Cup/9g	44	2.6	500	9.1	59.1	29.6	2.3
Peanut Butter Cup, Reese's, Hershey*	1 Cup/21g	105	6.5	500	11.9	57.1	31	5.9
Peanut Butter Cups, Dark, Hershey*	1 Pack/39g	202	12.7	519	10.6	50.7	32.5	0
Peanut Butter Cups, Sugar Free, Reese's, Hershey*	1 Cup/11g	45	3.3	409	6.8	61.4	29.6	13.6
Peanut Butter Cups, Super Nature*	1 Cup/20g	119	9.4	597	8	31	47	0
Peanut Butter, Buttercup, LoveRaw*	1 Cup/17g	100	7.3	590	15	32	43	0
Peanut Caramel Crisp, Big Taste, Dairy Milk, Cadbury*	1 Chunk/12g	63	3.9	547	9.8	49	34	2.5
Pen Pals, Hotel Chocolat*	1 Animal/40g	235	16.4	588	7.5	46.2	40.9	1.5
Peppermint Cream, Fry's*	1 Bar/51g	217	7.9	425	2.6	68.8	15.4	0
Peppermint, Ritter Sport*	1 Bar/100g	483	26	483	3	60	26	0
Pingui, Kinder, Ferrero*	1 Serving/30g	135	8.9	450	7	37.8	29.7	0
Plain with Hazelnuts, Tesco*	4 Squares/25g	135	8.9	539	6.1	48.3	35.7	6.5
Plain, 72% Cocoa Solids, Finest, Tesco*	1 Square/10g	60	4.4	603	7.7	44	44	3.7
Plain, Belgian, Organic, Waitrose*	1 Bar/100g	505	37.6	505	9.6	32	37.6	5.6
Plain, Couverture, Belbake, Lidl*	1 Serving/25g	133	8	531	6.9	49	32	0
Plain, Dark, Fruit & Nut, Rich, Sainsbury's*	4 Squares/25g	122	7	489	5.2	53.9	27.9	5.7
Plain, Ms Mollys*	1 Bar/100g	520	31	520	5.7	51	31	7
Plain, Whole Nut, Belgian, Waitrose*	4 Squares/25g	135	9.5	540	6.3	45.4	38	7.8
Plain, with Mint, Tesco*	2 Squares/20g	111	7	557	6.7	50.2	35.2	6.7
Pocket Coffee, Ferrero*	1 Pocket/13g	55	2.6	440	3.5	58.8	20.5	0
Praline, Dizzy, Hotel Chocolat*	1 Chocolate/13g	74	5.4	589	8.3	42.2	43.2	3.9
Praline, M&S*	1 Bar/34g	185	12	545	7.3	49.6	35.2	3.1
Pretzel, Salted, Choceur, Aldi*	1 Rectangle/29g	151	8.1	520	8.4	58	28	2.5
Probiotic, Bar, Ohso*	1 Bar/14g	72	5	514	5	47	36	15.5
Rafaello, Roche, Ferrero*	1 Sweet/10g	60	4.7	600	9.7	35.4	46.6	0
Raspberry Intense, Lindt*	2 Squares/20g	102	6.2	510	5	51	31	0
Raspberry, Intense, Excellence, Lindt*	1 Square/10g	52	3.1	522	5.2	51	31	0
Reese's Pieces, Bite Size, Minis, Hershey*	11 Pieces/39g	200	12	513	7.7	59	30.8	2.6
Reese's, Fast Break, Candy Bar, Hershey*	1 Bar/56g	260	12	464	8.9	62.5	21.4	3.6

	Measure INFO/WEIGHT	per Measure KCAL	FAT	Nutrition Values per 100g / 100ml KCAL	PROT	CARB	FAT	FIBRE
CHOCOLATE								
Reindeer, Baileys*	1 Reindeer/80g	440	27.2	550	7.7	52.2	34	2.2
Reindeer, Lindt*	1 Reindeer/107g	588	35.3	550	7.2	55	33	0
Rocky Road, Clusters, Tesco*	1 Bite/11g	52	2.2	470	5.6	65.2	20.3	2.1
Salted Butterscotch, Milk, The Best, Morrisons*	2 Squares/20g	112	7.1	558	6.2	53.1	35.3	1.6
Salted Caramel, Crunchy, Choceur, Aldi*	5 Squares/33g	181	10.6	548	6.6	57	32	1.3
Sesame Grille, Lindt*	1 Square/10g	52	3.2	525	7.1	50	32	0
Sharing Block, Smarties, Nestle*	3 Pieces/17g	88	4.8	529	6.6	59.6	28.9	1.8
Smooth Praline, Choceur, Aldi*	1 Square/5g	27	1.6	544	7.8	52	33	3.9
Snack Bar, Kinder*	1 Bar/21g	116	7.1	554	10	52	34	0
Snack Size, Dairy Milk, Cadbury*	1 Bar/30g	159	9	530	7.8	57.1	29.9	0
Snickers, More Nuts, Snickers*	1 Bar/58g	299	17.3	515	10.1	52.8	29.8	0
Snowman, Mousse, Dairy Milk, Cadbury*	1 Snowman/29g	162	10.2	560	6.7	54.5	35	0.4
Tasters, Dairy Milk, Cadbury*	1 Bag/45g	238	13.7	530	7.6	56.4	30.5	0
Tasting Selection, Green & Black's*	1 Piece/15g	85	5.8	567	9	41	39	6.7
Tiffin, Honeycomb, Hare-Brained, McVitie's*	1 Slice/41g	197	9.3	480	4.2	64	22.6	2
Tiffin, Limited Edition, Dairy Milk, Cadbury*	6 Chunks/24g	120	6	502	6.7	60	25	2.1
Toffifee, Storck*	1 Sweet/8g	43	2.4	516	5.9	58.5	28.7	0
Treatsize, Dairy Milk, Cadbury*	1 Bar/14g	73	4.2	525	7.5	57	29.8	0.7
Triple Choc Sensation, Big Taste, Dairy Milk, Cadbury*	2 Triangles/21g	116	6.6	541	6.1	57	31	2.1
Truffle, Bomb, Giunduja, Hotel Chocolat*	1 Truffle/10g	60	4.9	595	9.6	26.1	48.8	11.7
Turkish Delight, Dairyfine, Aldi*	3 Squares/25g	119	6	475	3.4	62	24	0.5
Turkish Delight, Lge Bar, Dairy Milk, Cadbury*	1 Square/8g	35	1.6	470	5.6	63.2	21.4	0.5
Twirl, Bites, Cadbury*	1 Bite/2g	11	0.6	530	7.7	56.5	30.3	0.8
Vanilla, Madagascan, Moser Roth, Aldi*	1 Bar/25g	148	10.2	590	8.3	48	41	0.5
Wafer, Bar, Time Out, Cadbury*	1 Bar/21g	111	6.1	527	6.7	60	29	2.1
Whips, Double Chocolate, M&S*	1 Whip/29g	140	7.3	485	6.6	57.8	25.3	1
White with Honey & Almond Nougat, Toblerone*	1 Serving/25g	132	7.2	530	6.2	60.5	29	0.2
White with Strawberries, Divine*	1 Piece/3g	16	0.9	534	7.6	59.9	29.3	0.1
White, 0% Sugar, Blanco, Torras*	1 Piece/13g	60	4.2	464	5	57	32	4
White, Average	***1oz/28g***	***148***	***8.7***	***529***	***8***	***58.3***	***30.9***	***0***
White, Bar, Sainsbury's*	1 Strip/25g	144	9.5	578	7.1	51.4	38.2	0.5
White, Buttons, Smarties, Nestle*	6 Buttons/15g	77	3.9	515	7.9	61.8	26.1	0.5
White, Creamy Vanilla, Green & Black's*	1 Lge Bar/90g	516	32.9	573	7.4	53.5	36.6	0.1
White, Mice, Morrisons*	¼ Pack/18g	95	5	529	4.8	63.9	28	1
White, Tiny, Toblerone*	1 Tiny/8g	43	2.4	535	6.1	62	29.5	0.2
White, Toblerone*	1 Triangle/33g	177	9.6	537	6.1	62	29	0.2
White, with Oreo, Dairy Milk, Cadbury*	1 Bar/41g	227	13.5	554	4.5	60	33	0.6
Whole Nut, Dairy Milk, Cadbury*	1 Bar/49g	270	17.4	550	8.9	49.5	35.4	1.7
Whole Nut, Sainsbury's*	4 Chunks/25g	142	9.4	566	8.5	48.5	37.6	2.6
Wildlife Bar, Cadbury*	1 Bar/21g	109	6.2	520	7.8	56.8	29.3	0
Winter Gingerbread, Dairy Milk, Cadbury*	3 Pieces/15g	82	5	549	6.1	56	33	1.8
Wispa, Bitsa Wispa, Cadbury*	¼ Bag/43g	238	14.7	550	7.3	53	34	0.9
with Crunchie Bits, Dairy Milk, Cadbury*	1 Bar/200g	1000	48.8	500	6.2	63.3	24.4	0
with Hazelnuts, Whole, Milka*	2 Squares/15g	83	5.3	554	8.1	50	35.5	2
with Shortcake Biscuit, Dairy Milk, Cadbury*	1 Square/6g	31	1.7	520	7.5	59	28	0
CHOCOLATE RAISINS								
Milk Chocolate Coated, Average	***1 Serving/50g***	***207***	***7.7***	***415***	***4.4***	***64.6***	***15.4***	***2***
CHOCOLATE SPREAD								
& Caramel, Gu*	1 Serving/25g	153	11.5	613	4.2	45	46	2
& Hazelnut, Smooth, Nutsy*	1 Serving/25g	136	7.6	542	1.6	66	30.2	0
Average	***1 Tsp/12g***	***68***	***4.5***	***569***	***4.1***	***57.1***	***37.6***	***0***
Caramel, Morrisons*	1 Tsp/5g	27	1.5	535	6.1	58.9	30.4	0.8
Chocaholic, The Skinny Food Co.*	1 Tsp/5g	25	2	505	0	53	39	0

	Measure INFO/WEIGHT	per Measure KCAL	FAT	Nutrition Values per 100g / 100ml KCAL	PROT	CARB	FAT	FIBRE
CHOCOLATE SPREAD								
Crunchie, Cadbury*	1 Tsp/5g	28	1.7	554	3.4	58	34	1.5
Crunchy, Hazelnut, Vego*	1 Tbsp/15g	84	5.4	563	6.1	51	36	5.5
Hazelnut, Jim Jams*	1 Tbsp/15g	74	5.5	494	6.4	49.4	36.6	0
Hazelnut, No Added Sugar, Tesco*	1 Tbsp/15g	75	5.6	502	6.3	49.5	37.5	2.8
Hazelnut, Nutella, Ferrero*	1 Tbsp/15g	80	4.6	533	6.6	56.4	31	3.5
Hazelnut, Nutoka, Aldi*	1 Tsp/5g	27	1.7	549	5.9	54	34	3.2
Hazelnut, Sainsbury's*	1 Serving/12g	67	4.2	555	6	53.5	34.5	3
Hazelnut, Smooth, Plant Kitchen, M&S*	1 Tbsp/15g	85	5.6	569	4.2	51.6	37.1	6
Hazelnut, Weight Watchers*	1 Serving/15g	50	1.8	333	4.7	45.3	12	12
La Crema, Vegan, Valsoia*	1 Serving/15g	77	4.2	514	5.2	57	28	6.8
Nussa, Lidl*	1 Serving/20g	112	7.1	558	6.1	51.8	35.5	3.5
with Nuts	***1 Tsp/12g***	***66***	***4***	***549***	***6.2***	***60.5***	***33***	***0.8***
CHOCOLATES								
All Gold, Dark, Terry's*	1 Serving/30g	152	8.7	505	4	57.5	29	4.3
All Gold, Milk, Terry's*	1 Serving/30g	158	9.2	525	4.8	58	30.5	1.5
Alpini, Thorntons*	1 Chocolate/13g	70	4.2	538	7	54.6	32.3	2.3
Bites, Maltesers*	1 Bag/32g	166	8.6	518	7.4	60	27	0
Buttons, Mint, Maltesers, Mars*	1 Serving/34g	176	9.2	517	7.42760		27	0
Buttons, White Chocolate, Dairyfine, Aldi*	1 Pack/70g	386	22.4	551	4.4	61	32	0.5
Caramels, Sainsbury's*	1 Sweet/12g	57	2.6	490	3.5	69	22.2	0.2
Celebrations, Mars*	1 Sweet/8g	40	2	497	5.6	61.7	25	1.7
Champagne Truffles, Milk, The Best, Morrisons*	1 Truffle/12g	57	2.9	479	5.2	57.9	24.8	1.4
Chocolatiers Selection, Gift Wrapped Box, M&S*	1 Serving/20g	109	7	545	5.1	51	35.2	2.7
Coconut, Lindor, Lindt*	1 Ball/13g	79	6	632	5.4	42	48	0
Coffee Cream, Average	***1 Chocolate/12g***	***54***	***2***	***446***	***3.3***	***70.4***	***17***	***2.4***
Continental, Belgian, Thorntons*	1 Chocolate/13g	67	3.9	514	5.8	53.5	30.3	2.9
Continental, Thorntons*	1 Chocolate/15g	76	4.4	506	5.6	54.5	29.3	2.7
Cookies n Creme, Drops, Hershey's*	½ Pack/40g	205	10.4	512	6	63.9	26.1	0
Country Caramel, Milk, Thorntons*	1 Chocolate/9g	45	2.4	500	4.6	62.2	26.7	0
Creme, Wafer Curls, Galaxy, Mars*	1/3 Pack/30g	151	6.9	502	8.4	64	23	0
Crunchie Rocks, Cadburys *	4 Pieces/24g	115	4.6	478	4.7	71	19	2
Dairy Box, Milk, Nestle*	1 Piece/11g	50	2.1	456	4.4	65.9	19.4	0.7
Dark Milk, Buttons, Giant, Cadbury*	1 Serving/25g	140	9.2	562	5.8	49	37	4.8
Dark, Rondnoir, Ferrero*	1 Ball/12g	67	4.2	555	6.2	51.4	35	0
Dark, Rose & Violet Creams	***1 Chocolate/13g***	***55***	***1.6***	***422***	***2.2***	***76.1***	***12.5***	***1.7***
Dark, Swiss Thins, Lindt*	1 Pack/125g	681	46.2	545	4.8	49.2	37	0
Filled, Average	***1 Chocolate/13g***	***58***	***2.8***	***447***	***4.9***	***62.9***	***21.3***	***1.3***
Hazelnut & Ginger, Hotel Chocolat*	1 Chocolate/13g	72	5.3	555	8	34	40.7	9.7
Heroes, Cadbury*	1 Sweet/8g	38	1.8	480	4.8	65.1	22.4	0.4
Italian Collection, Amaretto, M&S*	1 Chocolate/13g	60	3.1	480	4.4	59.7	25.1	2.3
Italian Collection, Favourites, M&S*	1 Chocolate/14g	74	4.7	530	5.7	50.4	33.7	1.6
Italian Collection, Panna Cotta, M&S*	1 Chocolate/13g	70	4.7	545	5.3	49.4	36.4	0.1
Jingly Bells, Hazelnut, Cadbury*	2 Balls/16g	93	5.9	565	6.8	51	36	2.8
Jingly Bells, Noisette, Dairy Milk, Cadbury*	1 Jingly Bell/8g	45	2.7	547	8	53	33	2.7
Liqueurs, Brandy, Asda*	1 Chocolate/8g	34	1.4	409	4	60	17	0.8
Liqueurs, Brandy, Favorina, Lidl*	1 Keg/12g	53	2.6	444	1.7	54.3	21.4	0
Liqueurs, Cherry, Mon Cheri, Ferrero*	1 Chocolate/11g	50	2.2	455	3	52.8	20.3	0
Liqueurs, Cognac Truffle, Thorntons*	1 Chocolate/14g	65	3.8	464	7.3	40	27.1	2.9
Liqueurs, Cointreau, Plain, Barrels	***1 Chocolate/10g***	***44***	***1.8***	***435***	***3.5***	***57***	***18***	***0***
Milk Tray, Cadbury*	1 Chocolate/9g	47	2.4	495	4.7	61.5	25.8	0.7
Milk, Mini Eggs, Green & Black's*	1 Mini Egg/8g	42	2.7	562	8.6	48.3	35.5	3.8
Milk, Swiss Thins, Lindt*	1 Pack/125g	688	43.3	550	5.8	53.6	34.6	0
Mini Eggs, Mix, Cadbury*	1 Pack/276g	1419	74.5	514	1.6	60	27	1.6

	Measure INFO/WEIGHT	per Measure KCAL	per Measure FAT	Nutrition Values per 100g / 100ml KCAL	PROT	CARB	FAT	FIBRE
CHOCOLATES								
Mini Eggs, Orange, Smarties, Nestle*	4 Eggs/69g	335	13.2	486	4	73.9	19.1	1
Mini Eggs, with Soft White Truffle Centre, M&S*	1 Egg/6g	33	2	550	6.5	56.3	33.9	1.4
Mint Batons, After Dinner, M&S*	¼ Pack/31g	165	8.8	531	3.5	63.2	28.5	3.6
Mint Creams, Dark, Smooth & Fragrant, Waitrose*	1 Sweet/10g	42	0.9	410	3	77.9	9.1	2.4
Mint Crisp, Bendicks*	1 Mint/8g	38	2.3	494	5.2	55	29.9	0
Mint Crisp, Dark, Elizabeth Shaw*	1 Chocolate/6g	27	1.2	458	1.9	68	20.7	0
Mint, Selection, Sainsbury's*	1 Chocolate/10g	48	2.3	484	3.4	64.9	23.1	1.5
Mint, Thins, After Eight, Nestle*	1 Chocolate/8g	35	1.1	428	2.3	74.1	12.9	2.7
Mints, After Eight, Dark, Nestle*	1 Sweet/7g	32	0.9	461	5	63	12.9	2
Mints, After Eight, Straws, Nestle*	1 Sweet/5g	24	1.4	526	5.1	56.6	31	4
Misshapes, Assorted, Cadbury*	1 Chocolate/8g	41	2.3	515	5.2	57.5	29.1	0
Moments, Thorntons*	1 Chocolate/7g	37	2	511	5.4	59.9	27.8	1.9
Mousse au Chocolat, Hotel Chocolat*	1 Chocolate/15g	76	5.2	505	7.2	38	34.9	7.1
Orange Cream, Average	***1 Chocolate/12g***	***53***	***2***	***440***	***3.2***	***69.3***	***16.7***	***0***
Peppermint Bliss, Sharing Box, Aero, Nestle*	3 Chocolates/25g	136	8	546	7.4	56.4	31.8	1.7
Peppermint Cream, Average	***1 Chocolate/12g***	***50***	***1.4***	***418***	***1.9***	***76.4***	***11.4***	***1.6***
Pinecones, Salted Caramel, M&S*	1 Pinecone/21g	107	5.8	508	4.6	59.2	27.7	1.6
Praline, Coffee, Thorntons*	1 Chocolate/7g	37	2.4	529	7	47.1	34.3	2.9
Praline, Hazelnut, Thorntons*	1 Chocolate/5g	27	1.8	540	7	48	36	4
Praline, Marzipan, Thorntons*	1 Chocolate/14g	63	3	450	5.9	58.6	21.4	2.1
Praline, Roast Hazelnut, Thorntons*	1 Chocolate/13g	70	4.4	538	6	51.5	33.8	3.1
Pralines, Mini, Lindt*	1 Chocolate/5g	26	1.6	530	7.5	54	31	0
Quality Street, Nestle*	1 Sweet/9g	44	1.9	470	3.5	67.3	20.5	1.5
Rainbow Buttons, Morrisons*	1/3 Pack/23g	114	4.9	496	2.5	73.5	21.2	0.5
Roses, Cadbury*	1 Chocolate/9g	41	1.9	480	3.3	66	22.5	1.3
Sea Shells, Belgian, Guylian*	1 Chocolate/14g	78	5	555	7.7	50	36	0
Seashells, Milk & White, Belgian, Waitrose*	1 Serving/15g	77	4.6	511	5	53.1	31	2.8
Stars, Mini Wishes, Truffle Centre, Cadbury*	1 Star/13g	70	4.1	540	6.9	55.6	31.8	1.3
Strawberries & Cream, Thorntons*	1 Chocolate/12g	64	3.9	533	5.1	54.2	32.5	0.8
Truffle, & Caramel, Selection, Vegan, M&S*	1 Chocolate/10g	51	3.1	506	5.4	46.7	31.3	8.1
Truffle, Amaretto, Thorntons*	1 Chocolate/14g	66	3.6	471	5.5	55	25.7	2.9
Truffle, Balls, Swiss Milk Chocolate, Waitrose*	1 Chocolate/13g	78	5.8	621	4.1	47	46	1.4
Truffle, Belgian Milk, Waitrose*	1 Truffle/14g	74	4.8	525	5.8	52.9	34.1	1.2
Truffle, Caramel Milk Chocolate, Aldi*	1 Truffle/12g	76	5.8	633	5.8	42.5	48.3	4.2
Truffle, Champagne, Premier, Thorntons*	1 Chocolate/17g	88	5.6	518	6.9	45.3	32.9	2.4
Truffle, Dark, Balls, Lindor, Lindt*	1 Ball/12g	76	6.2	630	3.4	38.5	51.4	0
Truffle, Filled, Swiss, Balls, Finest, Tesco*	3 Balls/37g	240	19	640	5	40.7	50.8	1.5
Truffle, French Cocoa Dusted, Sainsbury's*	1 Truffle/10g	57	4.5	570	4	37	45	0
Truffle, Hazelnut, Balls, Lindor, Lindt*	1 Ball/12g	76	6.1	632	5	39.1	50.6	0
Truffle, Lemon, White, Thorntons*	1 Chocolate/14g	63	3.5	450	4.6	64.3	25	0.7
Truffle, Milk Chocolate, Balls, Lindor, Lindt*	1 Ball/12g	75	5.6	623	4.9	44	47	2.8
Truffle, Mini Milk Chocolate Balls, Lindor, Lindt*	3 Balls/15g	90	7	600	6.7	40	46.7	0
Truffle, Rum, Average	***1 Truffle/11g***	***57***	***3.7***	***521***	***6.1***	***49.7***	***33.7***	***1.9***
Truffle, Selection, Tesco*	1 Chocolate/14g	75	4.2	539	5.1	62	29.8	0.5
Truffle, Seville, Thorntons*	1 Chocolate/14g	76	4.7	543	7.1	53.6	33.6	1.4
Truffle, Thorntons*	1 Chocolate/7g	33	1.9	471	6	48.6	27.1	1.4
Truffle, Vanilla, Thorntons*	1 Chocolate/13g	64	3.5	492	4.8	57.7	26.9	1.5
Truffle, Viennese, Dark, Thorntons*	1 Chocolate/10g	53	3.6	530	5.9	47	36	3
Truffle, Viennese, Milk, Thorntons*	1 Chocolate/10g	56	3.6	560	4.9	54	36	0
Truffle, White Chocolate, Balls, Lindor, Lindt*	1 Ball/12g	76	5.9	636	3.7	45	49	0
Truffles, Orange , Galaxy, Mars*	1 Truffle/21g	116	7.2	552	5.3	53.4	34.5	0
Truffles, Salted Caramel, Plant Kitchen, M&S*	1 Truffle/12.5g	61	3.8	489	6.9	43.7	30.6	5.8

C

C

	Measure INFO/WEIGHT	per Measure KCAL	per Measure FAT	Nutrition Values per 100g / 100ml KCAL	PROT	CARB	FAT	FIBRE
CHOW MEIN								
Beef, Ready Meal, Average	***1 Serving/400g***	***422***	***12.2***	***106***	***6***	***13.4***	***3***	***1***
Chicken, & Vegetable, Fuller Longer, M&S*	1 Pack/380g	266	4.9	70	6.3	8.7	1.3	2.1
Chicken, & Vegetable, COU, M&S*	1 Pack/380g	262	3.8	69	6.6	7.4	1	1.9
Chicken, & Vegetable, Slim Cook, Tesco*	1 Pack/490g	304	2.5	62	5.9	7.6	0.5	1.9
Chicken, Ready Meal, Average	***1 Serving/400g***	***375***	***9.4***	***94***	***6.5***	***11.5***	***2.4***	***1.2***
Chicken, with Peppers, & Green Beans, Hello Fresh*	1 Serving/403g	616	16.1	153	10	18	4	0
Pork, PB, Waitrose*	½ Pack/310g	332	2.8	107	7.6	17.2	0.9	1.6
Prawn, Takeaway, Chinese	***1 Portion/550g***	***792***	***60***	***144***	***5.6***	***6.1***	***10.9***	***2.8***
Special, Ready Meal, Average	***1 Serving/400g***	***383***	***9.7***	***96***	***6.5***	***12.1***	***2.4***	***1***
Vegetable, Ready Meal, Average	***1 Serving/400g***	***337***	***6.7***	***84***	***4.2***	***12.8***	***1.7***	***2***
CHRISTMAS PUDDING								
Alcohol Free, 450g, Sainsbury's*	1 Serving/114g	330	3.5	290	2.7	61.3	3.1	3.2
Average	***1oz/28g***	***81***	***2.7***	***291***	***4.6***	***49.5***	***9.7***	***1.3***
GF, Made Without Wheat, M&S*	1 Pack/100g	336	6.7	336	2.2	64.5	6.7	4.6
Gluten & Wheat Free, Finest, Tesco*	1 Pudding/100g	305	7.1	305	3.3	55.1	7.1	3.7
Hidden Clementine, Heston, Waitrose*	1 Serving/114g	352	7.7	310	2.9	57.8	6.8	3.1
Luxury	***1 Serving/114g***	***416***	***18.8***	***365***	***2.5***	***48.6***	***16.4***	***1***
Nut Free & Alcohol Free, Tesco*	1 Serving/114g	395	7.6	347	2.2	68.2	6.7	2.6
Plant Kitchen, M&S*	1 Pudding/100g	341	6.9	341	2.2	65.4	6.9	4.2
CHUTNEY								
Albert's Victorian, Baxters*	1 Serving/25g	40	0.1	159	1.1	37.9	0.3	1.5
Apple & Pear, TTD, Sainsbury's*	1 Serving/20g	39	0.2	193	0.6	45	0.8	1.7
Apple & Walnut, Waitrose*	1 Serving/20g	49	0.5	243	12	53.8	2.6	3.8
Apple, & Pear, Spiced, M&S*	1 Tbsp/15g	34	0	230	0.8	55.5	0.2	1.6
Apricot, Sharwood's*	1 Tsp/16g	21	0	131	0.6	32	0.1	2.3
Beetroot, & Orange, Extra Special, Asda*	1 Tbsp/15g	20	0.1	136	0.5	32	0.5	1.6
Bengal Spice Mango, Sharwood's*	1 Tsp/5g	12	0	236	0.5	58	0.2	1.2
Caramelised Onion, Sainsbury's*	1 Serving/25g	28	0.4	111	1.1	23.5	1.4	1.1
Caramelised Red Onion, Loyd Grossman*	1 Serving/10g	11	0	111	0.5	27.2	0	0.5
Caramelised Red Onion, Shaws*	1 Tbsp/15g	28	0	186	0.9	44.5	0.1	0
Fig, Plum, & Date, Specially Selected, Aldi*	1 Tbsp/15g	30	0.1	202	1.4	46	0.9	2.9
Gooseberry, Hot, Tiptree, Wilkin & Sons*	1 Tbsp/15g	39	0	263	0	63	0	0
Indian Appetisers, Pot, Waitrose*	1 Pot/158g	330	2.2	209	1.8	47.3	1.4	1.8
Lime & Chilli, Geeta's*	1 Serving/25g	63	0.3	253	1.9	57.5	1.3	1.7
Mango with Hint of Chilli & Ginger, Waitrose*	1 Serving/20g	52	0	259	0.5	64.2	0	0.7
Mango, Hot & Spicy, Waitrose*	1 Serving/20g	46	0.1	230	0.6	51.6	0.3	1.8
Mango, Spicy, Mild, M&S*	1 Tsp/5g	11	0.1	217	0.4	49.3	1.7	1.6
Mango, Spicy, Sainsbury's*	1 Tbsp/15g	33	0.1	222	0.5	53.8	0.5	1.9
Mango, Sweet	***1 Tsp/16g***	***30***	***0***	***189***	***0.7***	***48.3***	***0.1***	***0***
Mixed Fruit	***1 Tsp/16g***	***25***	***0***	***155***	***0.6***	***39.7***	***0***	***0***
Onion, Vitasia, Lidl*	1 Tbsp/15g	40	0.1	266	0.9	63.1	0.9	0
Peach, Spicy, Waitrose*	1 Serving/20g	43	0.3	215	1	49	1.5	1.5
Ploughman's, M&S*	1 Tbsp/15g	22	0	150	0.8	34.6	0.3	2.9
Plum, Ploughman's, Tesco*	1 Tsp/5g	8	0	154	1	34.1	0.4	5.3
Red Onion, Tiptree, Wilkin & Sons*	1 Tbsp/15g	45	0.2	301	2.3	63	1.5	0
Spicy Fruit, Baxters*	1 Serving/15g	22	0	146	0.6	35.4	0.2	0
Sticky Fig & Balsamic Chutney, M&S*	1 Servin/25g	57	0.3	228	1.6	49.8	1.3	5.4
Sweet Mango, Patak's*	1 Tbsp/15g	39	0	259	0.3	67.4	0.1	0.7
Tomato	***1 Tsp/16g***	***20***	***0***	***128***	***1.2***	***31***	***0.2***	***1.3***
Tomato & Chilli, Specially Selected, Aldi*	1 Tbsp/15g	21	0.1	138	12	32	0.5	1.3
Tomato & Red Pepper, Baxters*	1 Jar/312g	512	1.2	164	2	38	0.4	1.5
Tomato, Mediterranean, Branston*	1 Tbsp/15g	23	0.1	155	1.5	34.6	0.6	1.8
Tomato, Sundried, & Garlic, Woolliss & Sons Ltd*	1 Tbsp/15g	17	0	113	1.4	25.2	0.2	1.3

	Measure INFO/WEIGHT	per Measure KCAL	FAT	Nutrition Values per 100g / 100ml KCAL	PROT	CARB	FAT	FIBRE
CIDER								
Apple, Low Alcohol, Sainsbury's*	1 Glass/250ml	75	0.4	30	0.5	5.4	0.2	0
Basics, Sainsbury's*	1 Glass/250ml	200	0	80	0	0	0	0
Berries, & Cherries, 4%, Old Mout*	1 Bottle/500ml	270	0	54	0	7.8	0	0
Berry, Irish, Magner's*	1 Bottle/500ml	215	0	43	0	4.3	0	0
Classic, Low Alcohol, Sheppy's*	1 Serving/200ml	56	0	28	0	0	0	0
Cyder, Organic, Aspall*	1 Serving/200ml	120	0.2	60	0.1	3.1	0.1	0
Cyder, Perronelle's Blush, Aspall*	1 Serving/200ml	122	0.2	61	0.1	5.4	0.1	0.5
Cyder, Premier Cru, Aspall*	1 Serving/200ml	120	0	60	0	3.1	0	0
Cyder, Suffolk, Medium, Aspall*	1 Serving/200ml	134	0	67	0.1	4.4	0	0
Dry, Average	***1 Pint/568ml***	***205***	***0***	***36***	***0***	***2.6***	***0***	***0***
Dry, Strongbow*	1 Bottle/375ml	161	0	43	0	3.4	0	0
Founder's Reserve, Symonds*	1 Serving/200ml	72	0	36	0	2.6	0	0
Gold, Thatchers*	1 Bottle/500ml	230	0	46	0	4.5	0	0
Haze, Cloudy, Thatchers*	1 Bottle/500ml	245	0	49	0	2.4	0	0
Irish, Alcohol Free, Magner's*	1 Bottle/330ml	66	1.6	20	0.5	5.1	0.5	0
K, K Cider*	1 Can/500ml	230	0	46	0	0	0	0
Laid Back, 2.5%, M&S*	1 Can/330ml	125	0	38	0	0	0	0
Light, Bulmers*	1 Can/500ml	140	0	28	0	0.8	0	0
Low Alcohol	***1 Pint/568ml***	***97***	***0***	***17***	***0***	***3.6***	***0***	***0***
Low Carb, Stowford*	1 Bottle/500ml	140	0	28	0	0.2	0	0
Magner's*	½ Pint/284ml	105	0	37	0	2	0	0
Nordic Berries, Alska*	1 Bottle/500ml	195	0	39	0	1.1	0	0
Organic, Westons*	1 Serving/200ml	96	0	48	0	3.1	0	0
Original, Bulmers*	1 Serving/250ml	105	0	42	0	4	0	0
Original, Gaymers*	1 Bottle/330ml	148	0	45	0	4.7	0	0
Passionfruit, Rekorderlig*	1 Bottle/500ml	315	0	63	0	8.5	0	0
Pear, Bulmers*	1 Serving/200ml	86	0	43	0	3.6	0	0
Pear, Magner's*	1 Bottle/568ml	179	0	32	0	0	0	0
Scrumpy, Average	***1 Serving/200ml***	***93***	***0***	***46***	***0***	***2.3***	***0***	***0***
Strawberry & Lime, Non Alcoholic, Kopparberg*	1 Bottle/500ml	205	2.5	41	0.5	10.1	0.5	0
Strawberry, & Pomegranate, 4%, Old Mout*	1 Bottle/500ml	265	0	53	0	7.4	0	0
Sweet, Average	***1 Pint/568ml***	***239***	***0***	***42***	***0***	***4.3***	***0***	***0***
Vintage	***1 Pint/568ml***	***574***	***0***	***101***	***0***	***7.3***	***0***	***0***
CINNAMON								
Ground, Average	***1 Tsp/3g***	***8***	***0.1***	***261***	***3.9***	***55.5***	***3.2***	***0***
Stick, Average	***1 Stick/1g***	***3***	***0***	***246***	***3.9***	***77***	***1.5***	***53.1***
CLAMS								
in Brine, Average	***1oz/28g***	***22***	***0.2***	***79***	***16***	***2.4***	***0.6***	***0***
in Tomato Sauce, Italiamo, Lidl*	1 Pack/350g	290	25.2	83	3.6	1	7.2	0
Raw, Average	***20 Sm/180g***	***133***	***1.7***	***74***	***12.8***	***2.6***	***1***	***0***
CLEMENTINES								
Raw, Weighed with Peel, Average	***1 Med/61g***	***22***	***0.1***	***35***	***0.6***	***9***	***0.1***	***1.3***
Raw, Weighed without Peel, Average	***1 Med/46g***	***22***	***0.1***	***47***	***0.8***	***12***	***0.2***	***1.7***
COCKLES								
Boiled	***1 Cockle/4g***	***2***	***0***	***53***	***12***	***0***	***0.6***	***0***
Bottled in Vinegar, Drained	***1oz/28g***	***8***	***0.1***	***28***	***6.3***	***0***	***0.3***	***0***
COCKTAIL								
Alcoholic, Juice Based, Average	***1 Glass/200ml***	***464***	***29.2***	***232***	***6.4***	***18.7***	***14.6***	***1.4***
Bloody Mary, Average	***1 Glass/250ml***	***86***	***0***	***42***	***0***	***2.3***	***0***	***0.6***
Bucks Fizz, Premixed, M&S*	1 Glass/250ml	152	0	61	0	9	0	0
Bucks Fizz, Tesco*	1 Serving/200ml	100	0	50	0	0	0	0
Cherry, & Amaretto, Fizz, M&S*	1 Glass/125ml	75	0	60	0	0	0	0
Cosmo, Skinny Brands*	1 Can/250ml	90	0.2	36	0	1.3	0.1	0

	Measure INFO/WEIGHT	per Measure KCAL	per Measure FAT	Nutrition Values per 100g / 100ml KCAL	PROT	CARB	FAT	FIBRE
COCKTAIL								
Cosmopolitan, Canned, M&S*	1 Serving/200ml	456	0	228	0	22	0	0
Daiquiri, Strawberry, Frozen, Average	***1 Glass/250ml***	***132***	***0***	***53***	***0***	***14.1***	***0***	***0***
Grenadine, Orange Juice, Pineapple Juice	***1 Serving/200ml***	***158***	***0.3***	***79***	***0.5***	***19.2***	***0.1***	***0.2***
Long Island Iced Tea, Average	***1 Glass/250ml***	***282***	***0***	***113***	***0***	***13.6***	***0***	***0***
Mai Tai, Average	***1 Serving/200ml***	***209***	***0.1***	***105***	***0.2***	***13.9***	***0.1***	***0.1***
Mix, Bloody Mary, Bloody Ben's*	1 Serving/25ml	17	0	67	1.3	14.2	0.1	0.8
Mixer, Espresso Martini, Tipplesworth*	1 Serving/50ml	61	0	122	0.3	29.1	0.1	0
Mojito, Canned, M&S*	1 Can/250ml	208	0	83	0	8.9	0	0
Pina Colada	***1 Glass/250ml***	***592***	***20***	***237***	***1***	***28***	***8***	***0***
COCOA								
Nibs, Naturya*	1 Serving/10g	58	5	578	13	18.2	50.3	13.4
COCOA POWDER								
Cadbury*	1 Tbsp/16g	52	3.3	322	23.1	10.5	20.8	0
Dark, Fine, Dr Oetker*	3 Tbsp/25g	89	5.2	357	20	8.9	21	28
Dry, Unsweetened, Average	***1 Tbsp/5g***	***11***	***0.7***	***229***	***19.6***	***54.3***	***13.7***	***33.2***
Fairtrade, Co-Op*	1 Tbsp/15g	58	3.3	390	19	12	22	37
Hazelnut, Hotel Chocolat*	1 Pack/35g	37	2	105	4.8	8.7	5.6	0.5
Organic, Green & Black's*	1 Tsp/4g	16	0.8	405	22	19	21	27
Organic, Naturya*	1 Tbsp/15g	56	1.8	370	27	26	12	26
The Pantry, Aldi*	1 Tsp/5g	18	1	357	20	8.7	21	28
COCONUT								
Creamed, Average	***1oz/28g***	***186***	***19.2***	***666***	***6***	***6.7***	***68.4***	***7***
Creamed, Block, Biona Organic*	1 Serving/100g	711	69	711	7	7.4	69	16.3
Desiccated, Average	***1oz/28g***	***169***	***17.4***	***604***	***5.6***	***6.4***	***62***	***13.7***
Flaked, Neal's Yard*	1 Serving/30g	181	18.6	604	5.3	44.4	62	13.7
Flakes, Unsweetened, Dr Goerg*	1 Serving/100g	686	67	686	7	6	67	15.6
Fresh, Flesh Only, Average	***1oz/28g***	***69***	***7.1***	***246***	***2.2***	***2.6***	***25.2***	***5.1***
Ice, Average	***1oz/28g***	***104***	***3.6***	***371***	***1.7***	***66.7***	***12.7***	***2.6***
Milk, Kefir, Organic, CoYo*	1 Serving/250ml	315	30	126	0.8	4.3	12	0
Rolls, Kiddylicious*	1 Pack/7g	37	2	529	2.9	64.7	27.9	1.5
Water, with Pressed Coconut, Vita Coco*	1 Serving/200ml	50	1	25	0	5	0.5	0
COD								
Baked, Average	***1oz/28g***	***27***	***0.3***	***96***	***21.4***	***0***	***1.2***	***0***
Beer Battered, TTD, Sainsbury's*	1 Fillet/180g	356	17.1	198	11.5	16.4	9.5	0.5
Dried, Salted, Average	***1oz/28g***	***82***	***0.7***	***290***	***62.8***	***0***	***2.4***	***0***
Fillet, Bites, M&S*	1 Serving/95g	189	7.6	199	13.7	17.5	8	1.1
Fillet, in Florentine Sauce, Ocean Trader, Lidl*	½ Pack/155g	183	7.1	118	13.5	5.2	4.6	0.7
Fillet, in Mornay Sauce, 568, Wiltshire Farm Foods*	1 Serving/400g	312	10.4	78	6.3	6.8	2.6	0
Fillet, Lightly Dusted, Salt & Pepper, Sainsbury's*	1 Serving/116g	189	8.3	163	14.3	10	7.2	0.5
Fillets, Battered, Average	***1 Fillet/125g***	***219***	***10.2***	***176***	***12.6***	***13***	***8.2***	***1***
Fillets, Breaded, Average	***1 Fillet/125g***	***258***	***12.2***	***206***	***13***	***16.7***	***9.8***	***1***
Fillets, Breaded, Chunky, Average	***1 Piece/135g***	***204***	***8***	***151***	***13.7***	***10.9***	***5.9***	***1.4***
Fillets, Breaded, Light, Healthy Range, Average	***1 Fillet/135g***	***209***	***6.9***	***154***	***13.6***	***13.3***	***5.1***	***1.2***
Fillets, Broccoli Mornay, Cooked, Ocean Trader*	½ Pack/155g	142	5.4	92	12	2.4	3.5	1.2
Fillets, Chunky, Average	***1 Fillet/198g***	***267***	***7.3***	***135***	***17.1***	***8.2***	***3.7***	***0.8***
Fillets, Skinless & Boneless, Raw, Average	***1 Fillet/140g***	***137***	***2.4***	***98***	***17.8***	***0***	***1.8***	***0.4***
Fillets, Smoked, Average	***1 Serving/150g***	***152***	***2.4***	***101***	***21.6***	***0***	***1.6***	***0***
Fillets, Tempura, Battered, Crispy, Gastro, Youngs*	1 Fillet/131g	252	12.1	192	12.9	14.1	9.2	0.8
Fillets, Wild, in Tomato & Rosemary Sauce, Birds Eye*	1 Fillet/136g	184	10.9	135	15	0.8	8	0.5
Filltes, Breaded, GF, Free From, Tesco*	1 Fillet/135g	263	10.4	195	12.7	18	7.7	1.5
Loins, Average	***1 Serving/145g***	***116***	***1.2***	***80***	***17.9***	***0.1***	***0.8***	***0.2***
Mornay, with Mash & Peas, HL, Tesco*	1 Pack/364g	335	9.1	92	7.7	8.6	2.5	2
Poached, Average	***1oz/28g***	***26***	***0.3***	***94***	***20.9***	***0***	***1.1***	***0***

	Measure INFO/WEIGHT	per Measure KCAL	FAT	Nutrition Values per 100g / 100ml KCAL	PROT	CARB	FAT	FIBRE
COD								
Smoked, Raw, Average	***1oz/28g***	***22***	***0.2***	***78***	***18.1***	***0***	***0.6***	***0***
Steaks, Battered, Chip Shop Style, Average	***1 Serving/150g***	***321***	***18***	***214***	***12.5***	***14.3***	***12***	***1.1***
Steaks, in Butter Sauce, Youngs*	1 Serving/137g	111	3.2	81	9.8	5.1	2.3	0.2
Steamed, Average	***1oz/28g***	***23***	***0.3***	***83***	***18.6***	***0***	***0.9***	***0***
COD IN								
Butter Sauce, Ross*	1 Serving/150g	126	5.8	84	9.1	3.2	3.9	0.1
Butter Sauce, Sainsbury's*	1 Serving/150g	198	13.5	132	10.6	2	9	0.1
Butter Sauce, Steaks, Birds Eye*	1 Pack/170g	185	9.4	109	9.8	5	5.5	0.1
Butter Sauce, Steaks, Frozen, Asda*	1 Pouch/152g	163	4	107	16	5	2.6	0.8
Butter Sauce, Tesco*	1 Pack/150g	123	5.4	82	9.4	2.9	3.6	0.5
Cheese Sauce, BGTY, Sainsbury's*	1 Serving/170g	144	4.1	85	12.8	3.1	2.4	0
Mushroom Sauce, BGTY, Sainsbury's*	1 Serving/170g	112	2.9	66	9.9	2.8	1.7	0.1
Parsley Sauce, Pre Packed, Average	***1 Serving/150g***	***123***	***4.7***	***82***	***10.1***	***3.3***	***3.1***	***0.5***
Red Pepper Sauce, Sweet, Fillets, GFY, Asda*	½ Pack/170g	143	2.7	84	15	2.3	1.6	0.1
COD WITH								
Fish Pesto, Fillets, COOK!, M&S*	½ Pack/165g	210	5.1	127	16.4	8.4	3.1	4.2
Roasted Vegetables, M&S*	1 Serving/280g	238	10.6	85	8	4.9	3.8	1.7
Sweet Chilli, COU, M&S*	1 Pack/400g	360	2	90	7.7	13.1	0.5	1.6
COFFEE								
3 in 1, Kenco*	1 Sachet/20g	83	2.1	415	2.5	80	10.5	0
Americano, Azera, Made up, Nescafe*	1 Cup/200ml	2	2	1	0.1	3	1	0.3
Americano, Decaf, Pod, Kenco*	1 Pod/17g	0	0	1	0.2	0.1	0	0
Azera, Barista Style Instant, Nescafe*	1 Serving/200ml	2	0	1	0.1	0	0	0
Black, Average	***1 Mug/270ml***	***5***	***0***	***2***	***0.2***	***0.3***	***0***	***0***
Cafe Hazelnut, Nescafe*	1 Sachet/17g	73	2.4	428	9.3	66	14.1	0
Cafe Irish Cream, Cafe Range, Nescafe*	1 Sachet/23g	98	3.2	425	8.2	65.2	14.1	1.2
Cafe Latte, Instant, Made Up, Maxwell House*	1 Serving/13g	53	1.7	424	6.4	68	13.6	0
Cafe Latte, Velvetiser, Dry Weight, Hotel Chocolat*	1 Sachet/35g	196	15.4	561	7.3	34.6	43.9	2.5
Cafe Latte, Vita Coco*	1 Carton/330g	132	3.3	40	1.7	6	1	0
Cafe Mocha, Cafe Range, Nescafe*	1 Sachet/22g	92	2.9	418	8.5	66.6	13.1	0
Cafe Vanilla, Latte, Cafe Range, Nescafe*	1 Sachet/19g	73	1.6	395	9.2	68.3	8.5	4.1
Cappuccino, Cafe Mocha, Dry, Maxwell House*	1 Serving/23g	100	2.5	434	4.3	78.2	10.8	0
Cappuccino, Cafe Specials, Dry, M&S*	1 Serving/14g	55	1.6	395	14	59	11.5	0.7
Cappuccino, Cappio, Iced, Kenco*	1 Can/200ml	138	6	69	3	7	3	0
Cappuccino, Decaff, Instant, Made Up, Nescafe*	1 Mug/200ml	68	2.3	34	1	5	1.2	0
Cappuccino, Decaff, Nescafe*	1 Sachet/16g	68	2.3	428	11.6	62.6	14.6	0
Cappuccino, Decaff, Unsweetened, Dry, Gold, Nescafe*	1 Tbsp/15g	60	2.3	398	13.3	48.3	15.2	5.3
Cappuccino, Decaff, Unsweetened, Nescafe*	1 Sachet/16g	70	3.1	437	14.5	51.2	19.4	4.3
Cappuccino, Dry, Maxwell House*	1 Mug/15g	52	1.4	350	12	64	9.6	0.4
Cappuccino, Dry, Waitrose*	1 Sachet/13g	58	2.3	439	15.1	56	17.2	4.4
Cappuccino, for Filter Systems, Kenco*	1 Sachet/6g	22	0.8	375	19	44	13.5	0
Cappuccino, Gold, Hazelnut Flavour, Mokate*	1 Sachet/13g	56	1.2	428	5.1	80	9.4	0
Cappuccino, Gold, Nescafe*	1 Sachet/100g	60	1.3	60	1.4	10.3	1.3	0.7
Cappuccino, Iced, Cowbelle, Aldi*	1 Serving/250ml	169	4.5	68	3.3	9.6	1.8	0.3
Cappuccino, Instant, Aldi*	1 Sachet/13g	49	1.7	393	12.5	55.1	13.6	0
Cappuccino, Instant, Asda*	1 Sachet/15g	60	2.3	399	13	53	15.2	0.9
Cappuccino, M&S*	1 Serving/164g	66	2.6	40	1.5	4.4	1.6	0
Cappuccino, Made Up, Dolce Gusto, Nescafe*	1 Serving/240ml	84	3.7	35	1.6	4	1.5	0.3
Cappuccino, Original, Sachets, Nescafe*	1 Sachet/18g	80	3.1	444	11.7	60.3	17.4	0
Cappuccino, Semi Skimmed Milk, Average	***1 Serving/200ml***	***63***	***2.3***	***31***	***2.2***	***3.2***	***1.2***	***0***
Cappuccino, Skinny, Sachets, Gold, Nescafe*	1 Sachet/15g	54	0.8	371	22.9	55	5.7	5
Cappuccino, Unsweetened, Gold, Nescafe*	1 Sachet/14g	55	1.8	392	12.9	52.5	13	5.7
Capuccino, Alcafe, Aldi*	1 Sachet/135ml	61	1.6	45	0.5	8.2	1.2	0.4

	Measure INFO/WEIGHT	per Measure KCAL	FAT	Nutrition Values per 100g / 100ml KCAL	PROT	CARB	FAT	FIBRE
COFFEE								
Chococino, Made up, Dolce Gusto, Nescafe*	1 Serving/210g	147	5.4	70	2.3	9.4	2.6	0.7
Coconut, Caffe, Alpro*	1 Carton/250ml	88	2.8	35	0.2	5.2	1.1	0.9
Columbian, Nescafe*	1 Serving/2g	2	0	111	16.7	11.1	0	5.6
Compliment*	1 Serving/14ml	20	1.8	143	1.4	6.4	12.9	0
Cortado, Capsule, Dolce Gusto, Nescafe*	1 Capsule/80ml	23	1.1	29	1.5	1.9	1.4	1
Espresso, Instant, Nescafe*	1 Tsp/2g	2	0	118	7.8	3.1	0.2	34.1
Espresso, Made Up, Dolce Gusto, Nescafe*	1 Serving/60ml	1	0.1	2	0.1	0	0.2	0.3
Flat White, Duo, Instant, Made Up, Kenko*	1 Serving/22g	92	3.8	417	18.5	46.3	17.1	0
Flat White, Pods, As Sold, Dolce Gusto, Nescafe*	1 Pod/12g	50	2.3	425	19.7	36.8	19.7	4.3
Flat White, Tassimo, Kenco*	1 Cup/235ml	73	4.7	31	0.3	2.5	2	0.1
Gold Blend, Nescafe*	1 Cup 200ml/5g	3	0	63	7	9	0.2	27
Ground, Made Up with Water, Average	***1 Serving/200ml***	***2***	***0***	***1***	***0***	***0***	***0***	***0***
Hazlenut, Caffe, Alpro*	1 Serving/250ml	78	2.2	31	0.2	5.2	0.9	1
Infusion, Avg with Semi-Skimmed Milk	***1 Cup/220ml***	***15***	***0.4***	***7***	***0.6***	***0.7***	***0.2***	***0***
Infusion, Avg with Single Cream	***1 Cup/220ml***	***31***	***2.6***	***14***	***0.4***	***0.3***	***1.2***	***0***
Instant, Alta Rica, Nescafe*	1 Tsp/2g	2	0	98	13.8	10	0.3	21
Instant, Decaffeinated, Nescafe*	1 Tsp/2g	2	0	101	14.9	10	0.2	8.4
Instant, Fine Blend, Nescafe*	1 Tsp/2g	1	0	63	7	9	0.2	27
Instant, Made with Skimmed Milk	***1 Serving/270ml***	***15***	***0***	***6***	***0.6***	***0.8***	***0***	***0***
Instant, Made with Water & Semi Skimmed Milk	***1 Serving/350ml***	***24***	***0.7***	***7***	***0.4***	***0.5***	***0.2***	***0***
Instant, Made with Water, & Whole Milk	***1 Cup/220ml***	***18***	***0.9***	***8***	***0.5***	***0.6***	***0.4***	***0***
Instant, Original, Nescafe*	1 Tsp/2g	2	0	118	7.8	3.1	0.2	34.1
Instant, Smooth, Dry Weight, Kenco*	1 Tsp/2g	2	0	100	7.5	15	0	0
Instant, Smooth, Made Up, Kenco*	1 Serving/200ml	4	0	2	0.2	0.3	0	0
Instant, with Skimmed Milk, Costa Rican, Kenco*	1 Mug/300ml	17	0.1	6	0.6	0.8	0	0
Irish Latte, Gold, Nescafe*	1 Mug/22g	90	2.2	411	8.3	70.6	9.9	2.6
Latte Macchiato, Made Up, Dolce Gusto, Nescafe*	1 Serving/220g	89	4.2	40	2	4.1	1.9	0.3
Latte, Cafe, M&S*	1 Serving/190g	142	5.3	75	4.3	8.3	2.8	0
Latte, Caramel, As Prepared with Water, Gold, Nescafe*	1 Mug/227ml	68	1.6	30	0.7	5	0.7	0.2
Latte, Caramel, Instant, Sachets, Sainsbury's*	1 Sachet/17g	70	1.7	412	8.2	71.2	10	0
Latte, Chai, Instant, Sainsbury's*	3 Spoons/30g	22	0.6	73	3.9	9.7	2	0.5
Latte, Costa, Made Up, Tassimo*	1 Cup/325ml	72	4.4	22	0.2	1.8	1.4	0.1
Latte, Double Shot, L'or, Tassimo*	1 Cup/336ml	74	4.7	22	0.3	1.8	1.4	0.1
Latte, Duo, Instant, Kenco*	1 Sachet/23g	97	3.9	423	18	50	17	0
Latte, Duo, Kenko*	1 Serving/224ml	99	3.9	44	1.8	5.4	1.7	0
Latte, Honest, Honest Organic Coffee*	1 Bottle/250ml	112	4.5	45	0	4.9	1.8	0
Latte, Iced, Salted Caramel, Dry Weight, Kenco*	1 Sachet /21g	83	1.5	391	7	75	7	0.4
Latte, Light, Dry Weight, Alcafe, Aldi*	1 Sachet/19g	75	0.9	395	22.1	63.2	4.7	2.6
Latte, Oat, Sachets, Dry, Gold, Nescafe*	1 Sachet/16g	68	2.4	414	3.3	64.8	14.5	4.7
Latte, Praline, Gold, Nescafe*	1 Mug/200ml	75	1.9	38	0.8	6.4	1	0.2
Latte, Sachet, Gold, Nescafe*	1 Sachet/19g	78	2.2	403	14.2	58.8	11.4	3.4
Latte, Skinny, Nescafe*	1 Sachet/20g	72	1.1	359	24.1	54.3	5.3	1.1
Latte, Skinny, Sachets, Made Up, Tesco*	1 Serving/219g	72	1.3	33	1.7	5.2	0.6	0.2
Latte, Smooth & Silky, Sachet, Kenco*	1 Sachet/20g	79	2.2	397	7	68	11	0
Latte, Soya, Caramel, Chilled, Alpro*	1 Serving/200ml	84	24	42	2.1	5.2	12	1.3
Latte, Toffee Nut, As Sold, Gold, Nescafe*	1 Serving/8g	34	0.8	409	8.8	68.8	10.2	2.1
Latte, Toffee Nut, Dolce Gusto, Nescafe*	1 Pack/200ml	76	3	38	1.5	4.3	1.5	0.2
Latte, Vanilla, Costa, Tassimo*	1 Cup/310ml	79	3.9	25	0.2	3.2	1.3	0.1
Macchiato, Caramel, Iced, Pre-made, Starbucks*	1 Cup/220ml	136	3.5	62	2.8	9.1	1.6	0
Made with 1% Milk, Average	***1 Mug/250ml***	***15***	***0.2***	***6***	***0.5***	***0.8***	***0.1***	***0***
Mocha, Double Chocolate, Gold, Nescafe*	1 Sachet/23g	93	2.3	403	9.4	66.3	9.8	5.1
Mocha, Made Up, Dolce Gusto, Nescafe*	1 Serving/210g	117	5.1	56	2.4	6.1	2.4	0.6
Mocha, Sachet, Gold, Nescafe*	1 Mug/22g	88	2	402	8	70.2	8.9	3.8

	Measure INFO/WEIGHT	per Measure KCAL	FAT	Nutrition Values per 100g / 100ml KCAL	PROT	CARB	FAT	FIBRE
COFFEE								
Mocha, Sainsbury's*	1 Serving/22g	84	3	383	14	51	13.7	1.3
COFFEE WHITENER								
Alcafe, Aldi*	1 Tsp/5g	39	2.4	553	2	57	35	0.5
Light, Tesco*	1 Tsp/3g	12	0.2	406	1	85.5	6.7	0
Lighter, Sainsbury's*	1 Serving/3g	12	0.2	387	12	81.1	6.4	0.5
Original, Coffee Mate, Nestle*	1 Tsp/3.5g	19	1.2	547	2.4	56.7	34.4	0
Sainsbury's*	1 Serving/3g	16	0.9	528	2	62.5	30	0
Tesco*	1 Tsp/3g	16	0.9	533	1.2	61.3	31.4	0
COGNAC								
40% Volume	***1 Pub Shot/35ml***	***78***	***0***	***222***	***0***	***0***	***0***	***0***
COLA								
Average	***1 Can/330ml***	***135***	***0***	***41***	***0***	***10.9***	***0***	***0***
Coke, Cherry, Coca-Cola*	1 Bottle/500ml	225	0	45	0	11.2	0	0
Coke, Cherry, Zero, Coca-Cola*	1 Can/330ml	1	0	0	0	0	0	0
Coke, Diet with Cherry, Coca-Cola*	1 Bottle/500ml	5	0	1	0	0	0	0
Coke, Diet, Caffeine Free, Coca-Cola*	1 Can/330ml	1	0	0	0	0.1	0	0
Coke, Mango, Exotic, Diet, Coca-Cola*	1 Bottle/500ml	2	0	0	0	0	0	0
Coke, Strawberry, Diet, Twisted, Coca-Cola*	1 Bottle/500ml	2	0	0	0	0	0	0
Coke, Vanilla, Coca-Cola*	1 Bottle/500ml	215	0	43	0	10.6	0	0
Coke, with Vanilla, Diet, Coca-Cola*	1 Glass/200ml	1	0	0	0	0.1	0	0
Diet, Average	***1 Serving/200ml***	***1***	***0***	***1***	***0***	***0***	***0***	***0***
Light, 0% Sugar, Harboe*	1 Serving/200ml	2	1	1	0.5	0.5	0.5	0
Pepsi Max, Ginger, Pepsi*	1 Can/250ml	1	0	0	0	0	0	0
Pepsi Max, Raspberry, Pepsi*	1 Serving/250ml	1	0	0	0.1	0.1	0	0
Zero, Caffeine Free, Coca-Cola*	1 Glass/200ml	0	0	0	0	0	0	0
Zero, Coca-Cola*	1 Can/330ml	1	0	0	0	0	0	0
COLESLAW								
& Potato Salad, Baby, Finest, Tesco*	1 Serving/50g	105	9.6	210	1.4	7.2	19.2	1.4
Apple, Raisin & Walnut, TTD, Sainsbury's*	1 Serving/75g	212	19.6	283	2.3	8	26.2	2.8
Asian, Slaw, Moorish*	1 Serving/25g	24	1.6	95	2.6	7.4	6.4	2.7
Basics, Sainsbury's*	1 Serving/25g	27	2.4	107	1	3.7	9.8	1.6
Cheese, Deli Style, Waitrose*	¼ Tub/75g	247	24.3	330	3.8	5.1	32.5	0.9
Cheese, M&S*	1 Serving/57g	185	19.1	325	4.2	2	33.5	1.7
Cheese, Sainsbury's*	1 Serving/75g	184	16.8	246	3.8	6.5	22.4	1.4
Coronation, Sainsbury's*	¼ Pot/75g	145	11.6	193	1	11.4	15.5	1.9
COU, M&S*	½ Pack/125g	75	3.4	60	1.3	7.4	2.7	1.7
Creamy, Asda*	1 Serving/25g	62	6	248	0.9	7	24	1.8
Creamy, Co-Op*	1 Serving/30g	68	6.6	228	0.9	5.7	22	1.3
Creamy, Farmfoods*	1 Serving/50g	84	7.4	167	1	6.8	14.8	0
Creamy, LC, Tesco*	1/3 Pot/100g	105	8.8	105	1.2	4.9	8.8	1.6
Creamy, Meadow Fresh, Lidl*	1 Serving/50g	91	8.5	182	0.9	5.5	17	1.8
Creamy, Morrisons*	1 Serving/50g	112	10.9	224	0.7	5.4	21.8	1.5
Creamy, Tesco*	1 Serving/75g	142	13.4	190	1	5.5	17.8	1.5
Deli Salad, Tesco*	1 Serving/50g	91	8.5	183	0.9	5.5	17.1	1.6
Deli Style, M&S*	1 Serving/50g	103	9.6	206	1.6	5.5	19.1	2.7
Eastmans, Tesco*	1 Serving/50g	58	5	116	0.9	4.7	10	1.4
Essential, Waitrose*	1 Tbsp/20g	50	4.9	248	0.8	5.4	24.6	1.2
Extra Special, Asda*	1 Serving/50g	106	10.5	213	1.1	3.5	21	3.9
Four Seasons, Woolworths*	1 Serve/100g	23	0.9	23	1.2	2.8	0.9	0
From Restaurant, Average	***3/4 Cup/99g***	***147***	***11***	***148***	***1.5***	***12.9***	***11.1***	***0***
Fruit, Celery, & Nut, Sainsbury's*	1 Serving/75g	143	11.6	191	2.1	96	15.5	2.4
Fruity, Waitrose*	1 Serving/90g	217	20.9	241	0.9	6.6	23.2	1.4
Half Fat, Waitrose*	1 Serving/100g	38	2.7	38	0.6	2.9	2.7	1.2

C

	Measure INFO/WEIGHT	per Measure KCAL	per Measure FAT	Nutrition Values per 100g / 100ml KCAL	PROT	CARB	FAT	FIBRE
COLESLAW								
Iceland*	1 Serving/50g	80	6.9	160	0.8	6.9	13.8	2.3
Jalapeno, Sainsbury's*	1 Serving/75g	142	13.4	190	0.9	5.6	17.9	1.6
Lite, Butlers*	1 Serving/50g	75	7	150	1.1	4.2	14	2.7
Luxury, Asda*	1 Serving/50g	108	10.5	217	0.9	6	21	0
Luxury, Lidl*	1 Serving/50g	102	9.7	203	0.9	5.9	19.4	0
Luxury, Rich & Creamy, TTD, Sainsbury's*	1 Serving/50g	123	11.8	246	1.8	5.9	23.6	1.5
Pink, Pickled, Tangy, Sainsbury's*	½ Pot/100g	43	0.5	43	0.9	8.7	0.5	1.5
Premium, Co-Op*	1 Serving/50g	160	17	320	1	3	34	2
Rainbow, Finest, Tesco*	¼ Pack/84g	192	18.7	229	1.3	4.9	22.3	1.7
Red, Tesco*	½ Pack/70g	53	1	76	1	13.5	1.5	2.4
Reduced Fat, Average	***1 Tbsp/20g***	***23***	***1.9***	***113***	***1***	***6.4***	***9.3***	***2***
Slaw, Pickled, Sainsbury's*	½ Pot/100g	43	0.5	43	0.9	8.7	0.5	1.5
Traditional, Reduced Fat, M&S*	1 Serving/50g	82	7.2	164	1	6.5	14.5	1.7
TTD, Sainsbury's*	¼ Med Pot/75g	185	17.7	246	1.8	5.9	23.6	1.5
Vegan, Deli Style, Sainsbury's*	1 Serving/50g	83	7.7	166	1	5	15.4	1.6
Vegan, Gro, Co-Op*	1 Serving/50g	100	9	199	1	7	18	1
Vegan, Plant Chef, Tesco*	1 Serving/50g	96	8.8	192	1.1	6	17.7	2.3
Vegan, Plant Kitchen, M&S*	½ Pack/112g	161	14.2	143	1	5.3	12.6	2.4
with Real Mayonnaise, Hellmann's*	1 Serving/50g	134	13.4	268	1.2	4.6	26.9	0
with Reduced Calorie Dressing, Retail	***1 Serving/40g***	***27***	***1.8***	***67***	***0.9***	***6.1***	***4.5***	***1.4***
Yoghurt Dressed, The Best, Morrisons*	1 Serving/50g	66	5.4	132	1.4	6.4	10.8	1.7
COLEY								
Portions, Raw, Average	***1 Serving/92g***	***65***	***0.6***	***71***	***15.9***	***0***	***0.6***	***0***
Steamed, Average	***1oz/28g***	***29***	***0.4***	***105***	***23.3***	***0***	***1.3***	***0***
CONCHIGLIE								
Cooked, Average	***1 Serving/185g***	***247***	***1.6***	***134***	***4.8***	***26.6***	***0.8***	***0.6***
Dry Weight, Average	***1 Serving/100g***	***352***	***1.7***	***352***	***12.5***	***71.6***	***1.7***	***2.6***
Shells, Dry, Average	***1 Serving/100g***	***346***	***1.5***	***346***	***12.3***	***70.4***	***1.5***	***3***
Whole Wheat, Dry Weight, Average	***1 Serving/75g***	***237***	***1.5***	***316***	***12.6***	***62***	***2***	***10.7***
CONSERVE								
Apricot, Average	***1 Tbsp/15g***	***37***	***0***	***244***	***0.5***	***59.3***	***0.2***	***1.5***
Blackberry, Bramble, & Gin, M&S*	1 Tbsp/15g	35	0.2	233	0.8	54.2	1.1	1.4
Blackcurrant, Average	***1 Tbsp/15g***	***37***	***0***	***245***	***0.6***	***60***	***0.1***	***1.9***
Blueberry, M&S*	1 Tbsp/15g	31	0	206	0.3	51.1	0.1	1.3
Cherry, Black, Bonne Maman*	1 Tbsp/15g	36	0	243	0.7	59	0.2	1.1
Fig, Bonne Maman*	1 Tbsp/15g	36	0	240	0.5	59	0	1
Ginger, Tiptree, Wilkin & Sons*	1 Tbsp/15g	40	0	270	0	66	0	0
Hedgerow, TTD, Sainsbury's*	1 Tbsp/15g	41	0	276	0.5	68.2	0.1	0.5
Morello Cherry, Waitrose*	1 Tbsp/15g	39	0	258	0.4	64.2	0	1.4
Peach, Bonne Maman*	1 Tbsp/15g	36	0	241	0.4	59	0.1	1.3
Plum, Damson, Bonne Maman*	1 Tbsp/15g	36	0	241	0.4	59	0.1	1.3
Plum, Mirabelle, Bonne Maman*	1 Tbsp/15g	36	0	241	0.4	59	0.1	1.4
Plum, TTD, Sainsbury's*	1 Tbsp/15g	36	0.1	243	0.5	59.6	0.5	0.9
Raspberry, Average	***1 Tbsp/15g***	***37***	***0.1***	***249***	***0.6***	***61***	***0.3***	***1.3***
Rhubarb & Ginger, M&S*	1 Tbsp/15g	29	0	194	0.3	47.9	0.1	1
Rhubarb, & Ginger, The Best, Morrisons*	1 Tbsp/15g	37	0	248	0.4	60.8	0.2	1.1
Rhubarb, & Strawberry, Bonne Maman*	1 Tbsp/15g	36	0	241	0.3	59	0.1	1.2
Strawberry, Average	***1 Tbsp/15g***	***37***	***0***	***250***	***0.4***	***61.6***	***0.1***	***0.5***
CONSOMME								
Average	***1oz/28g***	***3***	***0***	***12***	***2.9***	***0.1***	***0***	***0***
Beef, Canned, Sainsbury's*	1 Can/415g	46	0	11	2	0.7	0	0
Beef, Luxury, with Sherry, Baxters*	1 Can/415g	62	0	15	2.7	1	0	0

	Measure INFO/WEIGHT	per Measure KCAL	FAT	Nutrition Values per 100g / 100ml KCAL	PROT	CARB	FAT	FIBRE
COOKIE MIX								
Chocolate, Mug Mix, Bakedin*	1 Mug/100g	388	6	388	5.8	76	6	0
Dough, Milk Choc Chip, Asda*	1 Serving/125g	615	28.8	492	5.7	65	23	1.6
COOKIES								
All Butter, Almond, Italian Style, M&S*	1 Cookie/23g	120	6.4	515	6.7	59.4	27.6	3.6
All Butter, Ginger Bread, M&S*	1 Cookie/23g	102	5	445	4.3	57.5	21.8	2.4
Almond, Ose*	1 Cookie/10g	46	1.4	456	8.4	74	14	0
Apple & Raisin, Go Ahead, McVitie's*	1 Cookie/15g	66	1.9	443	5.3	76.8	12.7	3.4
Bounty, Mars*	1 Cookie/46g	215	9.6	468	5.7	63.4	20.9	0
Brazil Nut, Prewett's*	1 Cookie/50g	122	7.4	244	2.6	25.2	14.8	1
Butter & Sultana, Sainsbury's*	1 Cookie/13g	61	2.6	473	4.5	68.4	20.1	1.6
Butter, Danesita*	1 Cookie/9g	45	2	529	5.9	67.6	23.5	2.9
Carrot Cake, Soft Bake, Asda*	1 Cookie/20g	88	3.4	440	5.4	64	17	2.1
Cheesecake, New York, Desserts, Maryland*	1 Cookie/10g	51	2.3	485	5.9	64.9	22.2	1.6
Choc Chip & Coconut, Maryland*	1 Cookie/10g	55	2.5	512	5.1	62.9	23.7	0
Choc Chip & Hazelnut, Maryland*	1 Cookie/11g	55	2.7	513	6.3	65.3	25	0
Choc Chip, Big, Treats, Maryland*	1 Cookie/16g	85	4.6	531	5.1	61.2	29	3.2
Choc Chip, Mini, Good to Go, Waitrose*	1 Bag/25g	127	6.6	508	6	60.4	26.4	2.4
Choc Chunk, Finest, Tesco*	1 Cookie/80g	355	14.1	445	5.7	65.3	17.7	1.8
Chocolate & Orange, COU, M&S*	1 Cookie/26g	90	0.7	350	5.7	77.2	2.6	3.2
Chocolate Chip & Hazelnut, Extra Special, Asda*	1 Cookie/25g	130	8.1	516	6	51	32	2.5
Chocolate Chip, Average	***1 Cookie/10g***	***49***	***2.5***	***489***	***5.5***	***64.1***	***24.7***	***2.9***
Chocolate Chip, Free From, Tesco*	1 Cookie/12g	59	2.6	488	5.2	65.6	22	3.4
Chocolate Chip, GF, Organic, Dove's Farm*	1 Cookie/17g	77	3.1	451	4.3	66.9	18.5	0
Chocolate Chunk & Hazelnut, Tesco*	1 Cookie/22g	118	6.7	538	6.2	60.2	30.3	1.9
Chocolate Chunk & Hazelnut, TTD, Sainsbury's*	1 Cookie/25g	132	7.7	527	6.7	54.2	30.8	3.3
Chocolate Chunk, All Butter, M&S*	1 Cookie/24g	120	6	500	5.2	62.4	25.2	2.9
Chocolate Chunk, Cadbury*	1 Cookie/22g	119	6.9	540	6.5	58	31.2	0
Chocolate Fruit & Nut, Extra Special, Asda*	1 Cookie/25g	125	7.1	509	6	56	29	2
Chocolate Orange, Half Coated, Finest, Tesco*	1 Cookie/22g	107	5.6	488	4.9	59.6	25.5	1.2
Chocolate, Belgian, Extra Special, Asda*	1 Cookie/26g	138	8	535	6	58	31	2
Chocolate, Dark, & Ginger, Free From, Finest, Tesco*	1 Cookie/19g	92	4.2	485	4.6	66	22	2.1
Chocolate, Double, Sainsbury's*	1 Cookie/45g	202	8.5	450	5.8	63.1	18.9	2
Chocolate, Double, Tesco*	1 Cookie/42g	187	8.1	447	5.8	60.8	19.4	3.2
Chocolate, Milk, Belgian, Puddle, Finest, Tesco*	1 Cookie/35g	171	8.5	488	6.3	60.2	24.2	1.9
Chocolate, Milk, Free From, Tesco*	1 Cookie/20g	100	6.1	500	5.6	50.4	30.7	4.1
Chocolate, Quadruple, Finest, Tesco*	1 Cookie/25g	128	6.9	512	6.3	58.3	27.5	3
Chocolate, Triple, Chunkie, Fox's*	1 Cookie/23g	115	5.8	500	4.9	63	25	3.4
Chocolate, Triple, Half Coated, Finest, Tesco*	1 Cookie/25g	131	7.3	525	5.7	58.7	29.3	2.3
Chocolate, Triple, Irresistible, Co-Op*	1 Cookie/19g	97	5.1	511	6.8	57.9	26.8	4.2
Chocolate, Triple, Wheat, & GF, Finest, Tesco*	1 Cookie/19g	97	5	508	5.8	60.4	26.2	3.5
Christmas, Selection, Waitrose*	1 Cookie/25g	124	6.3	496	6	60.3	25.1	2.5
Chunkie Extremely Chocolatey, Fox's*	1 Cookie/26g	130	6.8	506	6.2	61	26.3	2.6
Cocoa, Sandwich, No Added Sugar, Gullon*	1 Cookie/11g	43	1.8	408	5	65	17	9
Coconut & Raspberry, GF, Sainsbury's*	1 Cookie/20g	102	5.9	511	5.9	56	29.3	6.7
Coconut, Gluten-Free, Sainsbury's*	1 Cookie/20g	103	6.1	516	5.6	54.4	30.7	4.1
Coconut, Sugar Free, Free'ist*	1 Cookie/17g	78	5.6	461	4.8	35.2	32.7	0
Cranberry & Orange, Finest, Tesco*	1 Cookie/26g	125	5.8	490	4.1	67.4	22.6	3.2
Cranberry, & White Chocolate, Lean, Myprotein*	1 Cookie/50g	194	3	387	50	32	6	2
Dairy Milk, with Chocolate Chunks, Dairy Milk, Cadbury*	1 Cookie/45g	210	9.3	467	6	63.6	20.6	1.4
Danish Butter, Tesco*	1 Cookie/26g	133	6.6	516	4.7	66.7	25.6	1.3
Dark Chocolate Chunk & Ginger, The Best, Morrisons*	1 Cookie/25g	126	6.4	503	4.6	63.7	25.5	2.8
Double Choc Chip, Mini, M&S*	1 Cookie/22g	108	5.2	490	5.3	63.6	23.7	1.8
Double Choc Chip, Tesco*	1 Cookie/11g	55	2.7	500	4.2	65.3	24.7	3

C

	Measure INFO/WEIGHT	per Measure KCAL	per Measure FAT	KCAL	PROT	CARB	FAT	FIBRE
COOKIES								
Double Choc, Maryland*	1 Cookie/10g	51	2.6	510	5.2	64.4	25.7	0
Double Choc, Minis, Maryland*	1 Mini Bag/20g	100	5	503	5.7	62.3	24.9	3.6
Double Chocolate & Walnut, Soft, Tesco*	1 Cookie/25g	116	6.4	463	5.8	52.1	25.7	4.7
Double Chocolate Chip, Co-Op*	1 Cookie/17g	87	4.6	510	5	63	27	2
Double Chocolate Chip, Organic, Waitrose*	1 Cookie/18g	96	5.6	535	5.1	58.6	31	1.9
Eton Mess, Finest, Tesco*	1 Cookie/66g	281	9.7	426	5.1	67.6	14.7	1.4
Finest White Chocolate & Honeycomb, Bakery, Tesco*	1 Cookie/65g	290	11.2	446	5.3	67.1	17.2	0.9
Flapjack, All Butter, Waitrose*	1 Cookie/25g	121	5.8	484	4.6	62.1	23.4	2.7
Flapjack, Fruity, Truly Irresistible, Co-Op*	1 Cookie/25g	116	5.1	464	5.2	64	20.4	2.4
Fortune, Average	***1 Cookie/8g***	***30***	***0.2***	***378***	***4.2***	***84***	***2.7***	***1.6***
Frui & Nut, Half Coated, Belmont Biscuit Co, Aldi*	1 Cookie/25g	122	6	488	6	61	24	2.5
Fruit, & Oat, All Butter, The Best, Morrisons*	1 Cookie/25g	110	4.4	441	5.7	63	17.6	3.9
Fudge Brownie American Cream, Sainsbury's*	1 Cookie/12g	60	2.8	499	4.8	67.9	23.2	2.2
Galaxy, Galaxy, Mars*	1 Cookie/46g	207	8	451	5.6	67.3	17.4	0
Ginger & Choc Chip, BGTY, Sainsbury's*	1 Cookie/17g	69	3.2	415	5.8	55.3	19	12.1
Hazelnut, Heart, Sondey, Lidl*	1 Cookie/25g	129	6.8	515	5.7	60.1	27.3	3.2
Honey, Lemon & Ginger, Nothing Naughty*	1 Cookie/60g	246	9	410	2.9	64.4	15	0
Lemon Zest, GF, Organic, Dove's Farm*	1 Cookie/17g	79	3	463	3.8	70.9	17.9	1.3
Maple Syrup, & Pecan, Finest, Tesco*	1 Biscuit/25g	127	6.6	507	6.7	59.9	26.4	1.7
Milk Chocolate Chunk, Average	***1 Cookie/25g***	***129***	***6.9***	***515***	***6.6***	***60***	***27.6***	***1.6***
Milk Chocolate, Classic, Millie's Cookies*	1 Cookie/45g	190	10.2	422	5.1	49.3	22.7	1.3
Milk Chocolate, Hazelnut, Waitrose*	1 Cookie/21g	112	6.6	533	6.6	54.9	31.4	2.1
Mince PIe, Finest, Tesco*	1 Cookie/23g	104	4	453	4.1	68.7	17.5	2.1
Oat & Treacle, TTD, Sainsbury's*	1 Cookie/25g	121	5.9	482	5.7	61.8	23.6	3.7
Oat & Raisin, Bites, Tesco*	1 Cookie/5g	25	1	458	6.1	65.2	18.5	2.9
Oat & Sultana, Free From, Sainsbury's*	1 Cookie/19g	87	3.7	462	6.2	62.6	19.8	4.2
Oat, & Raisin, Free From, Finest, Tesco*	1 Cookie/19g	80	2.8	422	6.2	63	15	5.1
Oatflake & Raisin, Waitrose*	1 Cookie/17g	80	3.8	469	5.8	61.7	22.1	4.7
Oreo, Mini, Oreo*	1 Pack/25g	120	4.8	480	4.8	70	19.2	2.4
Oreo, Nabisco*	1 Cookie/11g	52	2.1	474	5.4	68	19	2.7
Pecan, & Caramel, Co-Op*	1 Cookie/25g	123	5.5	493	6	67	22	1.5
Pineapple, Coconut & White Chocolate, M&S*	1 Cookie/23g	119	5.7	518	5.1	56.7	24.9	2.9
Pistachio & Almond, All Butter, M&S*	1 Cookie/25g	132	8	528	10.7	46.9	32.1	4.5
Raisin & Cinnamon, Low Fat, M&S*	1 Cookie/22g	78	0.9	355	6.2	73	4.1	3.2
Raspberry, & Chocolate, Wonders, Maryland*	1 Cookie/18g	90	4.6	502	4.7	60.5	25.9	3.3
Red Velvet, Filled, Bakery, Tesco*	1 Cookie/42g	170	5.5	405	4.6	66.6	13.1	1.3
Salted Caramel, M&S*	1 Cookie/25g	124	5.8	496	5.2	65.6	23.2	1.6
Stem Ginger, Aldi*	1 Cookie/13g	58	2.4	463	3.6	68.5	19.4	0
Stem Ginger, All Butter, Deluxe, Lidl*	1 Cookie/17g	80	3.6	468	5.1	62	21	5.4
Stem Ginger, Co-Op*	1 Cookie/25g	118	4.8	473	5	69	19	1.2
Stem Ginger, Deluxe, Lidl*	1 Cookie/17g	80	3.6	468	5.1	62	21	5.4
Stem Ginger, Reduced Fat, Waitrose*	1 Cookie/17g	75	2.7	448	4.5	71	16.2	1.6
Stem Ginger, Tesco*	1 Cookie/20g	98	4.8	489	4.2	64	24	2
Stem Ginger, The Best, Morrisons*	1 Cookie/25g	110	3.8	441	5.4	69	15.4	2.5
Stem Ginger, TTD, Sainsbury's*	1 Cookie/25g	124	6.2	496	4.9	62.3	24.7	2.2
Sticky Toffee, Finest, Tesco*	1 Cookie/63g	258	9.4	410	4.5	63.5	15	1.5
Sugar Free, Maryland*	1 Cookie/22g	94	4.8	433	6.1	60.6	22.3	3.6
Sultana, & Oat, Tesco*	1 Cookie/20g	91	3.9	454	5.5	61.6	19.7	4.4
Sultana, All Butter, Reduced Fat, M&S*	1 Cookie/17g	70	2.4	420	4.9	68.6	14.2	2.6
Sultana, Deluxe, Lidl*	1 Cookie/17g	77	3.2	453	5.3	64.7	18.8	2.9
Sultana, Soft & Chewy, Sainsbury's*	1 Cookie/25g	104	3.5	414	4.4	67.8	13.9	2.5
Triple Chocolate, Belgian, Bakery, Finest, Tesco*	1 Cookie/65g	310	14.9	478	6.1	60.1	23	2.9
Triple Chocolate, TTD, Sainsbury's*	1 Cookie/72g	344	16.5	478	5.8	61.2	22.9	2

	Measure INFO/WEIGHT	per Measure KCAL	FAT	Nutrition Values per 100g / 100ml KCAL	PROT	CARB	FAT	FIBRE
COOKIES								
White Chocolate & Raspberry, Finest, Tesco*	1 Cookie/76g	304	9.6	400	5.2	66.3	12.6	2.4
White Chocolate, Chunk, Average	***1 Cookie/25g***	***124***	***6.2***	***498***	***5.5***	***62.8***	***24.8***	***1***
COQ AU VIN								
658, Oakhouse Foods Ltd*	1 Serving/400g	728	39.6	182	14	7.9	9.9	2.8
Chicken, Parsley Box*	1 Pack/270g	221	6.8	82	14	0.9	2.5	0.4
Diet Chef Ltd*	1 Pack/300g	285	13.2	95	7.7	6.1	4.4	2.2
Donald Russell*	1 Pack/250g	230	7.2	92	10.7	3.5	2.9	0.4
CORDIAL								
Apple & Mango, Hi Juice, As Prepared, Morrisons*	1 Serving/250ml	69	0	28	0	6.7	0	0.1
Apple, & Blackcurrant, Diluted, Diet Rite*	1 Serving/250ml	7	0	3	0	0.7	0	0
Blackcurrant, New Zealand Honey Co*	1 Serving/30ml	109	0.3	363	1	88	1	0
Cherry, Sour, Super Concentrated, Optima*	1 Serving/30ml	78	0.1	260	1.5	63	0.2	0
Elderflower, Undiluted, Waitrose*	1 Serving/20ml	22	0	110	0	27.5	0	0
Lemon & Lime, High Juice, M&S*	1 Glass/250ml	75	0	30	0	7	0	0
Lime Juice, 30%, Mexican, Diluted, Waitrose*	1 Serving/200ml	4	0	2	0.1	0.5	0	0
Lime Juice, Concentrated	***1 Serving/20ml***	***22***	***0***	***112***	***0.1***	***29.8***	***0***	***0***
Lime Juice, Diluted	***1 Glass/250ml***	***55***	***0***	***22***	***0***	***6***	***0***	***0***
Lime, Crushed, & Mint, Diluted, Robinson's*	1 Serving/200ml	34	0	17	0	4.1	0	0
Lime, with Sweetener, No Added Sugar, Diluted, Co-Op*	1 Serving/200ml	4	1	2	0.5	0.5	0.5	0.5
Pear, & Elderflower, Pressed, Diluted, Robinsons*	1 Serving/200ml	36	0	18	0	4.2	0	0
Pear, & Ginger, Undiluted, Urban Cordial*	1 Serving/10ml	10	0	100	0	24	0	0
Summer Fruits, Sun Quench, Aldi*	1 Serving/25ml	4	0.1	15	0.5	2	0.5	0.5
CORIANDER								
Leaves, Dried, Average	***1oz/28g***	***78***	***1.3***	***279***	***21.8***	***41.7***	***4.8***	***0***
Leaves, Fresh, Average	***1 Bunch/20g***	***5***	***0.1***	***23***	***2.1***	***3.7***	***0.5***	***2.8***
CORN								
Baby, Average	***1 Serving/80g***	***21***	***0.3***	***26***	***2.5***	***3.1***	***0.4***	***1.7***
Baby, Canned, Drained, Average	***1 Serving/80g***	***18***	***0.3***	***23***	***2.9***	***2***	***0.4***	***1.5***
Cobs, Boiled, Weighed with Cob, Average	***1 Ear/200g***	***78***	***1.7***	***39***	***1.5***	***6.8***	***0.8***	***0.8***
Cobs, with Butter, From Restaurant, Average	***1 Ear/146g***	***155***	***3.4***	***106***	***3.1***	***21.9***	***2.4***	***0***
Creamed Style, Green Giant*	1 Can/418g	238	2.1	57	1.2	11.9	0.5	3
Roasted, & Salted, Sunburst Snacks*	1 Serving/20g	90	2.2	449	7.8	79.3	11.2	0
Roasted, Smokehouse BBQ, Crunch, Alesto, Lidl*	1 Serving/31g	130	3.2	419	8.9	69	10.4	7
Snack, Salt & Vinegar, Love Corn*	1 Pack/45g	194	5.7	430	7.1	68.3	12.7	7
CORN CAKES								
& Lentil, Lightly Salted, Tesco*	1 Lentil Cake/8g	31	0.2	383	19	68.5	2.7	4.4
Harvest Morn, Aldi*	1 Corn Cake/7g	26	0	375	8.6	84	0.5	2.3
Organic, Kallo*	1 Corn Cake/7g	26	0.1	383	7.6	83.6	1.1	7.2
Slightly Salted, Mrs Crimble's*	1 Pack/28g	104	0.9	380	7.9	80	3.4	5.4
The Best, Morrisons*	1 Corn Cake/7g	29	0.2	390	7.7	80.1	3.3	4.4
Unsalted, M&S*	1 Corn Cake/8g	30	0	381	6.5	87	0.3	1.9
with Chai Seeds, Kallo*	1 Corn Cake/7g	27	0.2	389	8	81	2.4	0
CORNED BEEF								
Average	***1 Slice/35g***	***75***	***4.3***	***214***	***25.9***	***0.7***	***12.2***	***0***
Lean, Healthy Range, Average	***1 Slice/30g***	***57***	***2.6***	***191***	***27***	***1***	***8.7***	***0***
Reduced Salt, Canned, Princes*	1 Can/340g	741	44.2	218	24.8	0.5	13	0
Sliced, Premium, Average	***1 Slice/31g***	***69***	***3.9***	***222***	***26.6***	***0.5***	***12.6***	***0***
CORNFLOUR								
Average	***1 Tsp/5g***	***18***	***0.1***	***355***	***0.6***	***86.9***	***1.2***	***0.1***
COURGETTE								
Baby, Raw, Average	***1 Courgette/29g***	***6***	***0.1***	***22***	***2***	***2***	***0.5***	***1.2***
Courgetti, Italian, Tomato, Pot, Bol*	1 Pot/380g	441	18.2	116	2.5	15	4.8	1.4
Fried, Average	***1oz/28g***	***18***	***1.3***	***63***	***2.6***	***2.6***	***4.8***	***1.2***

	Measure INFO/WEIGHT	per Measure KCAL	FAT	Nutrition Values per 100g / 100ml KCAL	PROT	CARB	FAT	FIBRE
COURGETTE								
Raw, Average	***1 Whole/224g***	***40***	***0.9***	***18***	***1.8***	***1.8***	***0.4***	***0.9***
Spaghetti, Waitrose*	½ Pack/80g	16	0.3	20	1.8	1.8	0.4	1.2
Spirals, Tomato, & Basil, Vegetable Pot, Tesco*	1 Pot/230g	94	0.8	41	2.5	5.4	0.4	3
COUS COUS								
Cooked, Average	***1 Tbsp/15g***	***24***	***0.3***	***158***	***4.3***	***31.4***	***1.9***	***1.3***
Cooked, From Restaurant, Average	***1 Cup/157g***	***176***	***0.3***	***112***	***3.8***	***23.2***	***0.2***	***1.4***
Coriander & Lemon, As Consumed, Sainsbury's*	½ Pack/140g	195	1	139	4.8	27.5	0.7	1.9
Dry, Average	***1 Serving/50g***	***178***	***0.7***	***356***	***13.7***	***72.8***	***1.5***	***2.6***
Giant, Cooked, Sainsbury's*	1 Serving/130g	126	2.1	97	3.6	16.2	1.6	1.7
Giant, Dry, Sainsbury's*	1 Serving/38g	126	2.1	332	12.4	55.5	5.5	5.8
Giant, Wholewheat, Lightly Toasted, Merchant Gourmet*	1 Serving/50g	198	0.8	396	12.3	76.9	1.7	11.9
Lemon, & Coriander, As Prepared, Morrisons*	½ Pack/139g	212	1.4	152	5.8	29.4	1	0.9
Lemon, & Coriander, As Prepared, Tesco*	½ Pack/140g	207	1.7	148	5.6	27.5	1.2	2.3
Mediterranean Inspired, As Prepared, Tesco*	½ Pack/141g	204	1.7	145	5.8	26.7	1.2	2.3
Mediterranean, Morrisons*	½ Pack/140g	204	1.5	146	5.6	27.7	1.1	1.4
Moroccan Spiced, Fruity, Waitrose*	1 Serving/78g	146	3.7	187	4.5	29.2	4.8	4.4
Moroccan, Medley, Ainsley Harriott*	½ Sachet/130g	178	2	137	5.4	25.4	1.5	2.2
Moroccan, Style, Fruity, M&S*	1 Serving/200g	370	5.4	185	3.4	36.7	2.7	3.4
Moroccan, Style, TTD, Sainsbury's*	¼ Pot/100g	203	4.7	203	5.1	33.1	4.7	3.7
Moroccan, Twist'd Flavour Co.*	½ Pack/130g	177	2	136	4.9	24.9	1.5	1.8
Roasted Vegetable, As Prepared, Sainsbury's*	½ Pack/140g	211	2	151	4.5	29.2	1.4	1.5
Roasted Vegetable, Newgate, Lidl*	1 Serving/135g	186	2	138	4.6	26.2	1.5	2.2
Roasted Vegetable, Worldwide Foods, Aldi*	1 Serving/130g	182	1.5	140	5.1	26.2	1.2	1.9
Tomato, Mediterranean, GFY, Asda*	½ Pack/141g	192	1.3	136	5	27	0.9	1.7
Tomato, Sun Dried, CBY, Asda*	1 Pack/310g	515	12.1	166	4.6	26.2	3.9	4
Vegetable, Chargrilled, Smoky, Finest, Tesco*	½ Pack/125g	194	5.6	156	4.3	23.2	4.5	2.6
Vegetable, Roasted, Dry, Ainsley Harriott*	½ Sachet/50g	180	2	360	14.6	66.4	4	6.8
Vegetable, Roasted, Fresh, Meadow Fresh, Lidl*	½ Pack/140g	211	7.3	151	4.6	20	5.2	0
Vegetable, Roasted, Made Up, Ainsley Harriott*	½ Pack/130g	177	1.6	136	4.8	25.5	1.2	1.9
Vegetable, Roasted, Snack Salad Pot, HL, Tesco*	1 Pack/60g	213	2.4	355	15.1	64.6	4	4.2
Vegetable, Roasted, Waitrose*	1 Serving/200g	328	13.2	164	3.9	22	6.6	0.9
Vegetable, Spicy, GFY, Asda*	½ Pack/55g	71	0.6	129	4.7	25	1.1	2
Vegetable, Spicy, Morrisons*	1 Pack/110g	187	5.5	170	5.1	26.2	5	2.9
CRAB								
Boiled, Meat Only, Average	***1 Tbsp/40g***	***51***	***2.2***	***128***	***19.5***	***0***	***5.5***	***0***
Cornish 50/50, Seafood & Eat It*	1 Pot/100g	144	5.8	144	21.6	1.2	5.8	0.5
Cornish Potted, Seafood & Eat It*	1 Pack/100g	235	17.5	235	15	5.1	17.5	0.8
Crab, Classic, Shippam's Foods*	1 Jar/75g	74	1.4	98	15.2	4.7	1.8	0
Dressed, Average	***1 Can/43g***	***66***	***3.4***	***154***	***16.8***	***4.1***	***7.9***	***0.2***
Lump, Meat, Kingfisher*	1 Can/105g	84	0.5	80	17.1	1.5	0.5	0
Meat in Brine, Average	***½ Can/60g***	***41***	***0.2***	***69***	***15.6***	***0.8***	***0.4***	***0.1***
Meat, Jumbo, Canned, in Brine, Drained, Kingfisher*	1 Can/120g	96	0.6	80	17	1.5	0.5	0
Meat, Raw, Average	***1oz/28g***	***28***	***0.2***	***100***	***20.8***	***2.8***	***0.6***	***0***
CRAB CAKES								
Goan, M&S*	1 Pack/190g	228	7.6	120	8	12.9	4	1.8
Iceland*	1 Serving/18g	52	3.2	288	7.2	25.6	18	1.3
Shetland Isles, Dressed, TTD, Sainsbury's*	1 Cake/75g	130	8.3	174	12.4	6	11.1	0.5
Tesco*	1 Serving/130g	281	16	216	11	15.4	12.3	1.1
Thai Style, TTD, Sainsbury's*	1 Cake/141g	297	14.1	210	8.7	20.5	10	1.8
CRAB STICKS								
Average	***1 Stick/15g***	***14***	***0***	***94***	***9.1***	***13.9***	***0.3***	***0***
CRACKERBREAD								
Original, Ryvita*	1 Cracker/5g	20	0.2	390	10.5	77.5	3.7	2.5

	Measure INFO/WEIGHT	per Measure KCAL	FAT	Nutrition Values per 100g / 100ml KCAL	PROT	CARB	FAT	FIBRE
CRACKERBREAD								
Quinoa, Red, & Sesame, Protein, Ryvita*	1 Slice/10g	37	0.5	368	20.7	53.2	4.9	14.1
Wholegrain, Ryvita*	1 Cracker/5g	19	0.2	379	11.3	70.9	3.9	7.3
CRACKERS								
All Butter, Cheese, Oat, Nibbles, Finest, Tesco*	1 Oat Nibble/7g	39	2.6	563	13.1	43.3	36.9	2.8
Baked Bites, Olive Oil, & Grana Padano, Ritz*	1 Serving/25g	115	4.2	460	12	63	17	4.1
Bath Oliver, Jacob's*	1 Cracker/12g	52	1.6	432	9.6	67.6	13.7	2.6
Beetroot, & Seed, Finest, Tesco*	2 Crackers/15g	75	3.7	497	12.2	53.1	24.8	6.4
Beetroot, Apple, & Chilli, Specially Selected, Aldi*	1 Cracker/4g	17	0.4	423	8.7	70	11	4.3
Black Olive, M&S*	1 Cracker/4g	20	1	485	8.3	59.4	23.5	4.3
Black Pepper for Cheese, Ryvita*	1 Cracker/7g	27	0.2	384	13.2	72.9	2.9	6.8
Black Pepper, Savoury, Gourmet, Specially Selected, Aldi*	1 Cracker/5g	24	1.1	490	8.6	62	22	3.2
Bran, Jacob's*	1 Cracker/7g	32	1.3	454	9.7	62.8	18.2	3.2
Buckwheat & Chia, Rude Health*	1 Cracker/7g	29	0.7	388	14	56	8.8	15
Butter Puff, Sainsbury's*	1 Cracker/10g	54	2.7	523	10.4	60.7	26.5	2.5
Butter Puffs, Jacob's*	1 Cracker/11g	55	2.7	502	9.3	59	24.8	3.1
Caramelised Onion, Ciabatta, Jacob's*	1 Cracker/10g	43	1	426	12.5	68.6	10.3	4.3
Cheese & onion, Triangles, Eat Well, M&S*	1 Bag/30g	128	3.3	425	9.8	69.4	11	4.7
Cheese Thins, Asda*	1 Cracker/4g	21	1.3	532	12	49	32	0
Cheese Thins, Co-Op*	1 Cracker/4g	21	1.3	530	12	49	32	3
Cheese Thins, Oven Baked, Rivercote, Lidl*	1 Cracker/4g	21	1.3	534	10.9	45.8	33.6	2.3
Cheese Thins, Savour Bakes, Aldi*	1 Thin/4g	19	0.8	475	15	62.5	20	0
Cheese Thins, Tesco*	1 Biscuit/4g	20	1.2	543	11.3	47.5	33.7	2.5
Cheese Thins, Waitrose*	1 Cracker/4g	21	1.2	545	11.9	52.6	31.9	2.5
Cheese, Cheddar, Crispies, TTD, Sainsbury's*	1 Thin/4g	21	1.5	576	14.2	39	40.4	2.2
Cheese, GF, Made Without Wheat, M&S*	1 Cracker/6g	26	0.8	425	5	72.5	12.5	5
Cheese, Oat Bakes, Nairn's*	1 Bag/30g	130	4.7	432	15	57.4	15.8	1.3
Cheese, Ritz*	1 Cracker/4g	17	0.9	486	10.1	55.9	24.7	2.2
Christmas, Festive, Extra Special, Asda*	¼ Pack/79g	144	8.7	182	11.9	7.9	11	1.8
Ciabatta, Sundried Tomato & Basil, Jacobs*	1 Cracker/10g	42	1	424	12.4	68.5	10.2	4.3
Corn Thins, 97% Fat Free, Real Foods*	1 Cracker/6g	23	0.2	378	10.2	81.7	3	8.6
Cream Cheese & Onion Flavour, Bakefuls, Ritz*	1 Bag/23g	109	4.8	474	7	63	21	2.7
Cream, Average	***1 Cracker/7g***	***31***	***1.1***	***440***	***9.5***	***68.3***	***16.3***	***2.2***
Cream, Light, Jacob's*	1 Cracker/8g	31	0.5	388	10.6	72.2	6.3	4.1
Crispy Cheese, M&S*	1 Cracker/4g	20	1	470	9.4	58.1	22.1	3
Crispy Chickpea, M&S*	¼ Pack/25g	99	1.4	396	17.6	67.8	5.5	2.5
Digestive, Savour Bakes, Aldi*	1 Cracker/11g	51	2.1	467	8.1	62	19	6.1
Emmental, Netto*	1 Serving/25g	130	7	520	13	53	28	3.1
Extra Wheatgerm, Hovis*	1 Serving/6g	27	1.1	447	10.2	60	18.5	4.4
Flatbread, Multigrain, Carr's*	1 Cracker/10g	42	0.7	411	11	73.8	6.8	5.3
Flatbread, Multigrain, Jacob's*	1 Cracker/10g	42	0.7	411	11	73.8	6.8	5.3
Garlic & Herb, Jacob's*	1 Cracker/10g	45	1.7	450	10	68.3	16.7	3.3
Garlic, CBY, Asda*	2 Biscuits/12g	58	2.6	483	7	63.3	21.5	4.2
Garlic, Rivercote, Lidl*	1 Cracker/6g	27	1.2	488	8	63.4	21.5	4.4
Harvest Grain, Sainsbury's*	1 Cracker/6g	27	1.1	458	8.5	64.5	18.4	4.1
Herb, & Onion, Free From, Morrisons*	1 Cracker/7g	31	0.9	448	1.7	78.6	12.8	5.7
Herbs & Spice Selection, Jacob's*	1 Cracker/6g	27	0.9	451	9.5	68	15.7	2.7
Japanese Beef Teriyaki, Sensations, Walkers*	1 Serving/24g	118	6.3	490	1.4	62	26	3.5
Light & Crispy, Sainsbury's*	1 Cracker/11g	42	1.2	384	11.3	61	10.5	13
Lightly Salted, Crispy, Sainsbury's*	1 Cracker/5g	25	1.3	533	7.8	62.6	27.9	2.1
Lightly Salted, Italian, Jacob's*	1 Cracker/6g	26	0.8	429	10.3	67.6	13	2.9
Lightly Salted, Savoury Bakes, Aldi*	7 Crackers/25g	128	6.2	511	7.7	62	25	2.1
Luxury, Selection, Lidl*	1 Cracker/5g	22	0.7	437	9.8	67.5	13.2	4.3
Matzos, Flame Baked, Rakusen's*	1 Cracker/21g	75	0.2	357	10	79	1	4.3

	Measure INFO/WEIGHT	per Measure KCAL	FAT	Nutrition Values per 100g / 100ml KCAL	PROT	CARB	FAT	FIBRE
CRACKERS								
Matzos, Tea, Flamed Baked, Round, Rakusen's*	1 Cracker/5g	19	0	382	9.9	85.7	0.8	3.7
Mini, Savoury, Huntley & Palmers*	1 Serving/25g	127	6.5	508	6	62	26	0
Mixed Grain, Lunch Bakes, Jacobs*	1 Cracker/10g	49	1.5	489	9.6	75.8	15.3	4.8
Mixed Seed, Lunch Bakes, Jacobs*	1 Cracker/9g	45	1.6	497	10.6	71.1	18	4.3
Mixed Seed, Multi Grain, Asda*	1 Cracker/6g	28	1.1	445	11	62	17	4.4
Multi Seed, Thins, Ryvita*	1 Thin/9g	39	1.3	434	16.4	56.2	14.1	8.1
Multi-grain, Aldi, Savour Bakes, Aldi*	1 Cracker/5g	20	0.8	404	8.3	55	16.8	5.1
Multigrain, Choice Grain, Jacobs*	1 Cracker/8g	34	1.1	429	8.8	63.9	14.2	5.5
Multigrain, Morrisons*	10 Crackers/20g	76	2.2	379	8.8	61.3	11	5.1
Multigrain, Savour Bakes, Aldi*	1 Cracker/5g	23	1.1	491	9.9	58	23	5.5
Multigrain, Tesco*	1 Cracker/5g	24	1	477	8.8	60.8	20.8	5.7
Naan, Multiseed, Tesco*	1 Cracker/3g	14	0.6	477	11.4	61.2	20	3.2
Naan, Tandoori, Tesco*	1 Cracker/2g	11	0.4	451	10.9	65.8	15.4	2.9
Oat & Wheat, Weight Watchers*	4 Crackers/20g	74	0.5	370	10.5	75	2.5	4
Olive Oil & Oregano, Mediterreaneo, Jacob's*	1 Cracker/6g	25	0.7	412	12.4	65.5	11.2	6
Oriental, Asda*	1 Serving/30g	115	6	383	1.7	49	20	4.3
Original, Breaks, Ritz*	1 Cracker/6g	29	1.1	460	8.4	65	18	3.5
Original, Ritz*	7 Crackers/25g	122	5.8	490	7.2	62	23	2.2
Paprika, & Nigella Seed, The Best, Morrisons*	1 Cracker/7g	31	1.2	448	10	61.4	16.9	4.9
Pizza Flavour, Mini, Sainsbury's*	1 Serving/25g	113	4	454	7.6	68.7	15.9	2.7
Plain, Free From, Morrisons*	1 Cracker/6g	27	0.8	443	1.5	77.9	12.7	5.4
Poppy & Sesame Seed, Sainsbury's*	1 Cracker/4g	20	1	482	9.5	57	23	4.2
Poppy Oat, Cracker Selection, TTD, Sainsbury's*	1 Cracker/4g	19	0.7	467	9.8	65	17.7	4.1
Poppy Seed, Savour Bakes, Aldi*	1 Cracker/4g	19	0.7	463	13	61	18	2
Poppy, & Sesame Seed, Thins, M&S*	1 Thin/4g	19	0.9	487	10.5	57.9	22.8	4
Pops, Multigrain, Onion Flavour, Slim's*	1 Cracker/5g	15	0	300	20	60	0	0
Pumpkin Seed, & Cheese, Bettabuy, Morrisons*	1 Cracker/23g	97	3	421	20.8	51.7	13	6.9
Rosemary, Free From, Morrisons*	1 Cracker/6g	27	0.8	455	1.3	80.7	12.7	6.4
Rosemary, Rivercote, Lidl*	1 Cracker/6g	30	1.4	493	8.1	61.2	23.3	2.9
Rosemary, Sainsbury's*	1 Cracker/6g	30	1.4	502	7.8	65.1	22.7	3.1
Rye Cakes, Lightly Salted, Ryvita*	1 Cake/6g	23	0.1	363	8.9	69.9	2	13.7
Salt & Black Pepper, Jacob's*	1 Cracker/6g	27	1	457	9.5	67.5	16.5	2.7
Salt & Black Pepper, Eat Well, M&S*	1 Pack/25g	106	3.7	422	9.6	62.9	14.7	5.1
Salt & Pepper, Sainsbury's*	1 Cracker/6g	29	1.3	504	8.1	65.8	22.5	3.2
Salt & Pepper, Tesco*	1 Cracker/6g	30	1.4	499	8.2	62.5	23.4	2.7
Salt, & Pepper, Asda*	1 Cracker/6g	30	1.4	497	8.2	63	23	2.7
Saltine, Wholewheat, Savour Bakes, Aldi*	1 Cracker/4g	19	0.9	478	10	58	22	5.6
Sea Salt & Vinegar Flavour, Bakefuls, Ritz*	1 Bag/23g	108	4.8	471	7	61	21	2.8
Sea Salt, & Black Pepper, Free From, Co-Op*	1 Cracker/6g	25	0.4	424	2.6	84	6.5	10
Sea Salt, Asda*	1 Serving/24g	123	5.8	508	8.1	65	24	2.8
Sea Salt, Gourmet, Savour Bakes, Aldi*	1 Cracker/3g	15	0.6	454	11	60	18	6.1
Sea Salt, Gourmet, Specially Selected, Aldi*	4 Crackers/20g	94	4	471	8.7	63	20	4.1
Sea Salt, Tesco*	5 Crackers/30g	149	7	496	8.1	61.8	23.5	2.8
Seeded, Gail's*	1 Cracker/10g	40	2.2	396	12	33.2	22.2	7.6
Selection, Finest, Tesco*	1 Serving/30g	136	4.3	452	9.6	71	14.4	0
Sesame & Poppy Thins, Tesco*	1 Cracker/4g	20	1	485	9.9	57.6	23.5	4.4
Smokehouse BBQ Crunch, Graze*	1 Box/31g	137	4.7	441	10	62	15	5.4
Snackers, Tesco *	1 Cracker/3g	14	0.6	471	8.1	65.8	18.9	2.9
Sourdough, Rosemary, No.1, Waitrose*	1 Cracker/4g	15	0.2	379	10.4	69.5	4.5	9.2
Spicy Indonesian Vegetable, Waitrose*	1 Pack/60g	295	16.3	492	1.2	60.6	27.2	2.2
Spicy, Asda*	¼ Pack/25g	126	6.5	504	0.9	65	26	2
Sweet Chilli, Dipping, Tesco*	1 Cracker/3g	12	0.5	470	9.3	63.2	19.6	2
Sweet Chilli, Oat Bakes, Nairn's*	1 Bag/30g	128	4	426	8.1	68.4	13.3	7.2

	Measure INFO/WEIGHT	per Measure KCAL	FAT	Nutrition Values per 100g / 100ml KCAL	PROT	CARB	FAT	FIBRE
CRACKERS								
Sweet Chilli, Thins, Ryvita*	1 Thin/8g	31	0.1	382	12	77.5	1.5	5.2
Tapas, Quely*	1 Cracker/6g	25	0.9	451	9.1	66	16	3.2
Tarallini with Fennel Seeds, Crosta & Mollica*	1 Cracker/4g	21	0.9	529	8.2	67.5	22	4.2
Thai Spicy Vegetable, Sainsbury's*	1 Pack/50g	231	10.4	462	7.2	61.5	20.8	2.6
The British Barbecue, Graze*	1 Punnet/25g	127	8	508	17.4	36.8	32.2	7.4
Thins, Thai Sweet Chilli, Crisps, Jacob's*	1 Pack/25g	119	4.8	476	8.2	65.6	19.3	3.1
Tuc, Cheese Sandwich, Jacob's*	1 Cracker/14g	72	4.3	531	8.4	53.8	31.4	0
Tuc, Cheese, Mini, Jacobs*	¼ Pack/50g	242	11.5	485	9.2	59	23	2.4
Tuc, Jacob's*	1 Cracker/5g	25	1.4	518	6.9	54.2	29.9	2.6
Tuc, Mini with Sesame Seeds, Jacob's*	1 Biscuit/2g	10	0.5	523	9.7	63.1	25.8	3.9
Tuc, Original, Jacob's*	1 Cracker/4g	17	0.7	478	8.3	67	19	2.4
Veggie, Chickpea, & Paprika, Deliciously Ella*	1 Pack/30g	129	2.4	430	6.5	81	8	4.3
Water Biscuits, High Bake, M&S*	1 Cracker/5g	22	0.4	409	9.8	75.1	6.8	3.9
Wheat, Tesco*	6 Crackers/30g	139	5.6	464	11.2	60.2	18.8	4.6
Wheaten, M&S*	1 Cracker/4g	20	0.9	450	10.2	57	20.2	5
CRANBERRIES								
& White Chocolate, Shot, Asda*	1 Pack/25g	94	2	375	2.8	71	8.1	3
Dried, Sweetened, Average	**1 Serving/10g**	**34**	**0.1**	**335**	**0.3**	**81.1**	**0.8**	**4.4**
Fresh, Raw, Average	**1oz/28g**	**4**	**0**	**15**	**0.4**	**3.4**	**0.1**	**3**
Frozen, Sainsbury's*	1 Portion/80g	18	0.1	22	0.4	3.4	0.1	3
Yoghurt Coated, Wilko*	1 Serving/25g	117	4.8	469	1.5	71.4	19	3
CRAYFISH								
Raw	**1oz/28g**	**19**	**0.2**	**67**	**14.9**	**0**	**0.8**	**0**
CREAM								
Aerosol, Average	**1oz/28g**	**87**	**8.7**	**309**	**1.8**	**6.2**	**30.9**	**0**
Aerosol, Reduced Fat, Average	**1 Serving/55ml**	**33**	**3**	**60**	**0.6**	**2**	**5.4**	**0**
Brandy, Extra Thick, TTD, Sainsbury's*	1 Serving/30ml	131	12.3	436	1.4	10.4	40.8	0.5
Brandy, Really Thick, Finest, Tesco*	½ Pot/125ml	579	49.5	463	1.3	19.7	39.6	0
Chantilly, TTD, Sainsbury's*	2 Tbsp/30g	136	14	455	1.4	6.9	46.8	0
Clotted, Fresh, Average	**1 Serving/28g**	**162**	**17.5**	**579**	**1.6**	**2.3**	**62.7**	**0**
Double, Average	**1 Tbsp/15ml**	**68**	**7.3**	**452**	**1.6**	**2.4**	**48.4**	**0**
Double, Brandy, Waitrose*	1 Serving/30ml	138	12.4	460	1.3	14.4	41.4	0
Double, Reduced Fat, Average	**1 Serving/30g**	**73**	**7**	**243**	**2.7**	**5.6**	**23.3**	**0.1**
Oat Alternative, Dairy Free, Oatly*	1 Carton/250ml	375	32.5	150	1	6	13	0.8
Pistachio, Petit Pot, La Laitiere, Nestle*	1 Pot/100g	184	10.3	184	4.6	18.8	10.3	0
Real Dairy, Lighter, Spray, Tesco*	1 Spray/13g	29	2.4	221	2.5	11	18.6	0
Real Dairy, Spray, Tesco*	1 Portion/13g	44	4.4	338	2.2	5.9	34	0
Single, Average	**1 Tbsp/15ml**	**28**	**2.7**	**188**	**2.6**	**3.9**	**18**	**0.1**
Single, Extra Thick, Average	**1 Serving/38ml**	**72**	**6.9**	**192**	**2.7**	**4.1**	**18.4**	**0**
Single, Soya, Fresh, Plant Based, Cuisine, Alpro*	1 Tbsp/15g	18	1.5	122	2	4.5	10.2	0.4
Single, Soya, UHT, Plant Based, Cuisine, Alpro*	1 Tbsp/15g	23	2.2	151	2	1.2	15	0.3
Soured, Fresh, Average	**1 Tsp/5ml**	**10**	**0.9**	**191**	**2.7**	**3.9**	**18.4**	**0**
Soured, Reduced Fat, Average	**1 Tsp/5ml**	**6**	**0.4**	**119**	**5.2**	**6.7**	**8.6**	**0.4**
Soured, Squeezy, Old El Paso*	1 Tbsp/15g	20	1.7	130	0.7	6.8	11	0.5
Whipping, Average	**1 Tbsp/15ml**	**52**	**5.5**	**348**	**2.1**	**3.2**	**36.4**	**0**
CREAM ALTERNATIVE								
Double, Light, Elmlea*	1 Serving/30g	73	7.2	243	2.7	4.1	24	0
Double, Vegan, Plant, Elmlea*	1 Serving/25ml	72	7.8	289	0.6	2	31	0
Single, Oatly*	½ Carton/125ml	188	16.2	150	1	6	13	0.7
Single, Vegan, Plant, Elmlea*	1 Serving/25ml	38	3.8	153	1.5	2.4	15.4	0
Whipped, Vegan, Heavenly, Food Heaven*	1 Squirt/10ml	20	1.6	203	0	15	16	0
CREAM SODA								
American with Vanilla, Tesco*	1 Glass/313ml	75	0	24	0	5.9	0	0

	Measure INFO/WEIGHT	per Measure KCAL	FAT	Nutrition Values per 100g / 100ml KCAL	PROT	CARB	FAT	FIBRE
CREAM SODA								
Barr's*	1 Can/330ml	33	0	10	0.5	2.2	0	0
Diet, Sainsbury's*	1 Serving/250ml	2	0	1	0	0	0	0
Shapers, Boots*	1 Bottle/300ml	3	0	1	0	0	0	0
Traditional Style, Tesco*	1 Can/330ml	139	0	42	0	10.4	0	0
CREME BRULEE								
Average	***1 Serving/100g***	***313***	***26***	***313***	***3.8***	***15.7***	***26***	***0.2***
Reduced Fat, M&S*	1 Serving/89g	186	13.1	210	4.9	14.2	14.8	0.5
CREME CARAMEL								
Average	***1 Serving/128g***	***140***	***2.8***	***109***	***3***	***20.6***	***2.2***	***0***
CREME EGG								
Cadbury*	1 Egg/40g	177	6	440	3.2	73	15	0.4
Minis, Cadbury*	1 Egg/12g	50	1.9	435	4.2	67	16.5	0.5
CREME FRAICHE								
Average	***1 Pot/295g***	***1067***	***112.2***	***362***	***2.2***	***2.6***	***38***	***0***
Half Fat, Average	***1 Tbsp/15g***	***27***	***2.4***	***181***	***3.1***	***5.5***	***16.2***	***0***
Low Fat, Average	***1 Tbsp/30ml***	***43***	***3.6***	***143***	***3.3***	***5.6***	***12.1***	***0.1***
Oat, Creamy, Oatly*	1 Tbsp/15ml	27	2.2	177	1	9.1	15	1
CREPES								
Chocolate Filled, Saint Albert *	1 Crepe/30g	143	6.6	478	6.1	60	22	0
Chocolate Filled, Tesco*	1 Crepe/32g	137	5.2	429	5.9	63.5	16.2	3
Duc De Coeur, Lidl*	1 Crepe/50g	78	3.5	156	5.6	17	7	0
Galette, Buckwheat, Average	***1 Serving/100g***	***161***	***1.7***	***161***	***5.8***	***30.2***	***1.7***	***1***
Mushroom, M&S*	1 Pack/186g	195	4.5	105	5.7	17.1	2.4	2.5
CRISPBAKES								
Cheddar & Onion, Cooked, Free From, Tesco*	1 Bake/125g	291	15.1	232	7.1	22.8	12.1	2
Cheddar Style, & Spring Onion, Free From, Sainsbury's*	1 Bake/110g	259	16.2	235	3.4	21.5	14.7	1.8
Cheese & Onion, Tesco*	1 Bake/116g	233	12.6	201	5.4	18.6	10.9	3.3
Cheese & Onion, Meat Free, Morrisons*	1 Bake/136g	282	13.8	207	1.5	23.5	10.1	4.9
Cheese & Onion, Ovenbaked, Iceland*	1 Bake/77g	145	5.3	189	4.8	25.9	6.9	2.3
Cheese, & Onion, British Classic, Sainsbury's*	1 Bake/110g	272	17.5	247	7	18.2	15.9	1.4
Cheese, & Bacon, Crestwood, Aldi*	1 Bake/114g	316	19.3	278	6.9	23	17	2
Cheese, & Onion, Asda*	1 Bake/130g	315	14.3	242	7.6	28	11	1.6
Cheese, Spring Onion & Chive, Sainsbury's*	1 Bake/107g	232	10.2	216	6.4	25.1	9.5	2.2
Dutch, Asda*	1 Bake/8g	31	0.3	388	14.7	74.9	3.3	4.2
Dutch, Co-Op*	1 Bake/10g	38	0.4	375	16	69.6	3.5	6.5
Dutch, HL, Tesco*	1 Bake/8g	30	0.2	385	14.7	74.9	2.7	4.2
Dutch, Original, Van Der Meulen*	1 Bake/8g	30	0.2	386	14.4	73.4	3.1	3.4
Dutch, Sainsbury's*	1 Bake/10g	38	0.5	392	14.5	72.3	5	5.8
Dutch, Tesco*	1 Bake/10g	40	0.5	397	13.6	71.7	5.3	4.2
Minced Beef, M&S*	1 Bake/113g	226	12.3	200	10	15.6	10.9	1.5
Minced Beef, M&S*	1 Bake/114g	218	10.2	192	9.2	17.6	9	1.9
Roast Vegetable & Basil, Cauldron Foods*	1 Bake/115g	242	11	210	3.5	26	9.6	2.9
Vegetable, Crunchy, Vegetarian, Waitrose*	1 Bake/113g	234	10.4	207	4.5	27.5	9.2	3.5
Vegetable, M&S*	1 Bake/114g	200	10.3	175	2.5	19.2	9	2.6
CRISPBREAD								
3 Grain 3 Seed, Foodie Market, Aldi*	1 Crispbread/25g	109	4.2	436	15	52	17	8.8
3 Seed, Classic, Gourmet, Dr Karg*	1 Crispbread/25g	108	4.9	430	16.5	46.6	19.7	10.9
Apple & Cinnamon, Ryvita*	1 Crispbread/15g	54	0.2	356	7.2	72.5	1.6	11.8
Chia Seed, & Buckwheat, Protein, Ryvita*	1 Crispbread/10g	38	0.4	371	21.5	56.9	3.7	12
Cracked Black Pepper, Thins, Ryvita*	1 Crispbread/10g	35	0.2	344	8.8	66.6	1.6	14.5
Currant, Seed, & Oat, Fruit Crunch, Ryvita*	1 Crispbread/15g	54	0.8	358	8.3	61.8	5.4	14.9
Dark Rye, Ryvita*	1 Crispbread/10g	34	0.1	342	8.5	66.5	1.2	15.2
Dill, Ikea*	1 Crispbread/25g	100	1.9	399	14	69	7.5	0

	Measure INFO/WEIGHT	per Measure KCAL	FAT	Nutrition Values per 100g / 100ml KCAL	PROT	CARB	FAT	FIBRE
CRISPBREAD								
Fibre Plus, Wholegrain with Sesame, Wasa*	1 Crispbread/10g	35	0.7	350	13	47	7	24
Fruit Crunch, Ryvita*	1 Crispbread/12g	45	0.7	358	8.3	61.8	5.4	14.9
GF, Average	***1 Serving/8g***	***25***	***0.1***	***331***	***6.4***	***72.9***	***1.5***	***0***
Mixed Grain, Jacobs*	1 Crispbread/10g	41	1.3	436	9.1	66.7	13.9	4.2
Multigrain, Rye, Crunchy, Ryvita*	1 Crispbread/10g	37	0.5	354	12.8	55.7	5.1	17.2
Multigrain, Ryvita*	1 Crispbread/11g	41	0.8	370	11.2	56	7.2	18.3
Original Rye, Thin, Finn Crisp*	1 Crispbread/6g	22	0.2	339	10	59	2.6	20
Original, Ryvita*	1 Crispbread/10g	35	0.2	350	8.5	66.9	1.7	16.5
Protein Punch, GF, Genius*	1 Crispbread/24g	120	7.7	501	17	27	32	21
Pumpkin Seeds & Oats, Ryvita*	1 Crispbread/13g	46	0.8	366	13.5	54.7	6.6	16.8
Rye, Original, Tesco*	1 Crispbread/9g	32	0.3	357	11.6	62.4	2.8	18
Scan Bran, Slimming World*	1 Crispbread/10g	31	0.5	310	14.9	29	5.3	42.1
Sesame & Rye, Tesco*	1 Crispbread/9g	34	0.8	385	12.5	55.6	8.7	17.2
Sesame, Ryvita*	1 Crispbread/10g	37	0.7	373	10.5	58.3	7	17.5
Sesame, Savour Bakes, Aldi*	1 Crispbread/9g	31	0.5	344	10	57.8	5.6	15.6
Sesame, Simply, Ryvita*	1 Crispbread/10g	40	0.7	383	13.4	57.5	6.9	18.5
Sourdough, Original, Peter's Yard*	1 Crispbread/3g	11	0.1	381	12.9	68.3	4.1	9.5
Sweet Onion, Ryvita*	1 Crispbread/12g	43	0.2	356	9	70.6	1.4	12.6
Wheat, Morrisons*	1 Crispbread/8g	28	0.3	377	11.5	73.1	3.4	4.2
with Chives, Lunch Bakes, Jacob's*	1 Crispbread/10g	49	1.5	487	9.6	75.2	15.3	4.7
CRISPS								
American Hot Pizza, Walkers*	1 Serving/25g	124	6.8	496	5.8	55	27	5
Apple, Eat Smart, Morrisons*	1 Pack/20g	68	0.1	338	1.9	75.3	0.7	11.4
Apple, Thyme & Sage, M&S*	1 Bag/55g	253	13.4	460	5.5	55.3	24.3	6.1
Bacon Bites, Asda*	1 Bag/25g	126	6.2	502	6.6	62	25	2
Bacon Rashers, M&S*	1 Pack/18g	72	1.4	398	8.4	72.1	7.8	3.1
Bacon, Crispies, Sainsbury's*	1 Bag/25g	117	5.7	468	19.9	45.8	22.8	4.8
Bacon, Rashers, BGTY, Sainsbury's*	1 Pack/10g	34	0.2	340	10.8	70.3	1.6	3.5
Bacon, Rashers, COU, M&S*	1 Pack/20g	72	0.6	360	9.4	77.5	2.9	3.5
Bacon, Rashers, Iceland*	1 Bag/75g	330	13.2	440	8.3	61.9	17.6	2.9
Bacon, Rashers, Snackrite, Aldi*	1 Bag/18g	89	4.3	496	5.6	63	24	1.7
Bacon, Rice Bites, Asda*	1 Bag/30g	136	4.8	452	7	70	16	0.4
Bacon, Shapers, Boots*	1 Bag/23g	99	3.4	431	8	66	15	3
Bacon, Sizzler, Ridge Cut, McCoys*	1 Bag/32g	165	9.7	516	7.1	53.6	30.3	3.9
Bacon, Sizzler, Ridged, Snackrite, Aldi*	1 Pack/30g	160	9.3	532	7.2	55	31	3.9
Bacon, Smith's, Walkers*	1 Bag/23g	113	5.3	488	7.5	62	23	1.3
Bacon, Smoky, BGTY, Sainsbury's*	1 Bag/25g	118	5.9	472	6.5	58.5	23.6	5.7
Bacon, Smoky, Select, Tesco*	1 Bag/25g	134	8.7	536	6.4	49	34.9	4.3
Bacon, Smoky, Snackrite, Aldi*	1 Bag/25g	130	7.2	522	6	57	29	3.3
Bacon, Smoky, Sunseed Oil, Walkers*	1 Bag/35g	183	11.4	530	6.5	51	33	4
Bacon, Smoky, Tayto*	1 Bag/35g	184	11.9	526	7.6	47.3	34	4.5
Baked, Average	***1 Bag/25g***	***93***	***1.5***	***374***	***6.5***	***73.5***	***5.9***	***5.8***
Barbecue, Corn Chips, Popchips*	1 Bag/17g	73	2.9	430	6	65	17	1.6
Barbecue, Pirato*	1 Pack/29g	156	8.4	539	6.5	56	29	0
Barbecue, Pop Outs, Passions, Aldi*	1 Pack/100g	422	13	422	5.8	69	13	3
Barbecue, Potato Crisps, Popchips*	1 Pack/23g	97	3.4	420	5.7	62	15	3.9
BBQ Rib, Double Crunch, Max, Walkers*	1 Serving/30g	145	7.4	483	7.7	55.3	24.7	5.7
BBQ, Double, Max, Walkers*	1 Serving30g	146	7.4	485	7.7	55.3	24.6	5.8
BBQ, Popped Chips, Asda*	1 Serving/21g	91	3.2	432	6.2	67	15	4.5
BBQ, Southern Style, Bugles, Walkers*	1 Pack/20g	105	6	525	6.5	56	30	3.5
BBQ, Spicy, Popped Chips, Co-Op*	1 Pack/23g	92	1.4	399	6.7	77	6.3	3.5
BBQ, Stackers, Snackrite, Aldi*	1 Serving/25g	134	8.5	538	3.1	53	34	4
Beasty Bites, Pickled Onion, Asda*	1 Bag/22g	111	5.5	505	6.2	64	25	0.5

C

C

	Measure INFO/WEIGHT	per Measure KCAL	FAT	Nutrition Values per 100g / 100ml KCAL	PROT	CARB	FAT	FIBRE
CRISPS								
Beef Wellington, M&S*	1 Pack/40g	203	11.4	507	7.3	51.6	28.5	7.4
Beef, & Onion Flavour, Average	***1 Bag/25g***	***131***	***8.3***	***524***	***6.5***	***50***	***33.1***	***4.3***
Beef, & Red Wine, Specially Selected, Aldi*	1 Serving/25g	130	7.3	519	5.1	59	29	2.5
Beef, Barbecue, Select, Tesco*	1 Pack/25g	134	8.7	536	6.4	49.2	34.8	4.4
Beef, Chinese Sizzling, McCoys*	1 Bag/35g	177	10.6	506	6.9	51.8	30.2	4
Beef, Maize & Potato, Happy Shopper*	1/3 Pack/23g	120	6.7	520	7.3	58	29	1.6
Beef, Roast, Monster Claws, Snackrite, Aldi*	1 Pack/17g	87	4.4	511	6.3	62	26	1.2
Beef, Space Raiders, KP Snacks*	1 Pack/13g	64	2.9	495	6.5	65.3	22.8	1
Beefy, Smiths, Walkers*	1 Bag/25g	133	9.2	531	4.3	45.2	37	0
Beetroot, Eat Smart, Morrisons*	1 Pack/20g	63	0.1	313	15.1	52	0.4	20.5
Beetroot, with Sweet Chilli Jam, Baked with Veg, Walkers*	1 Pack/23g	100	3.2	434	7.2	67	14	3.4
Black Truffle, & Olive Oil, M&S*	1 Serving/30g	148	8.1	493	4.3	54.7	27	8.3
Cheddar, & Chive, Mature, Tyrrells*	1 Serving/30g	134	6.9	447	6.9	53.7	23.1	2.4
Cheddar, & Onion, Crinkles, Walkers*	1 Pack/28g	150	9.3	538	6	51.5	33.3	3.5
Cheddar, & Red Onion Chutney, Sensations, Walkers*	1 Bag/40g	198	11.2	495	6.5	54	28	4.5
Cheddar, & Red Onion, Mature, Finest, Tesco*	1 Bag/40g	208	8.3	519	5.1	58.6	20.8	2.5
Cheddar, & Jalapeno, Popchips*	1 Pack/85g	351	12.8	413	6.4	64	15	4.2
Cheddar, & Onion, Double Crunch, Max, Walkers*	1 Serving/30g	146	7.5	486	7.7	55	24.9	5.8
Cheddar, & Onion, McCoys*	1 Pack/25g	132	7.5	530	7.4	54	30	4.3
Cheddar, & Red Onion, Specially Selected, Aldi*	1 Pack/25g	126	7	504	9	50	28	6.6
Cheddar, Mature, & Onion, Hand Cooked, Spar*	1 Serving/22g	109	5.4	495	8	58.4	24.7	3.6
Cheddar, Mature, & Red Onion, Hand Cooked, M&S*	1 Pack/40g	206	11.7	515	7.8	52.5	29.2	5.6
Cheese & Onion, 30% Less Fat, Sainsbury's*	1 Pack/25g	115	5.4	459	7.5	58.1	21.8	5.4
Cheese & Onion, Crinkle Cut, Low Fat, Waitrose*	1 Bag/25g	122	5.8	490	7.7	62.6	23.2	4.7
Cheese & Onion, GFY, Asda*	1 Pack/26g	122	5.7	470	7	61	22	4.2
Cheese & Onion, M&S*	1 Bag/25g	134	8.9	535	5.5	48.8	35.5	5
Cheese & Onion, Max, Walkers*	1 Pack/50g	266	16.4	533	6.8	51	32.9	2.9
Cheese & Onion, Organic, Tesco*	1 Bag/25g	128	8.2	514	5.2	49.9	32.6	7
Cheese & Onion, Sainsbury's*	1 Bag/25g	132	8.7	527	4.6	48.8	34.8	3.9
Cheese & Onion, Squares, Walkers*	1 Bag/25g	108	4.5	430	6.5	61	18	5.5
Cheese & Onion, Value, Tesco*	1 Bag/20g	108	7.2	541	6	48.3	36	4.8
Cheese & Onion, Walkers*	1 Pack/22g	95	3.5	430	5	66	16	5
Cheese & Onion Flavour, Asda*	1 Bag/25g	130	7.8	519	5.6	53.6	31.4	3.7
Cheese & Onion, Baked, Walkers*	1 Bag/32g	164	5.1	436	6.7	68.6	13.6	6.2
Cheese & Onion, Crinkle, Seabrook*	1 Pack/32g	170	10.5	536	5.9	51.1	33.1	5.2
Cheese & Onion, Discos, KP Snacks*	1 Pack/28g	146	8.2	520	5.1	59.1	29.3	2.5
Cheese & Onion, Golden Wonder*	1 Bag/25g	132	8	530	6.1	53	31.9	3
Cheese & Onion, Oven Baked, Asda*	1 Bag/25g	95	2	380	5.1	72	8	3.3
Cheese & Onion, Oven Baked, Tesco*	1 Bag/25g	102	1.6	410	5.3	74.7	6.6	7.7
Cheese & Onion, Pom Bear, Intersnack Ltd*	1 Bag/19g	95	5.3	498	3.8	58.1	27.8	3.2
Cheese & Onion, Pom Bear, KP Snacks*	1 Bag/13g	68	3.6	521	3.9	63	28	2.4
Cheese & Onion, Pop, Protein, Corners*	1 Pack/85g	343	7.7	403	27.4	47.7	9.1	10.5
Cheese & Onion, Smiths*	1 Pack/25g	130	10.1	518	6.2	52.9	40.4	4.2
Cheese & Onion, Snackrite, Aldi*	1 Pack/25g	137	8.2	548	7.2	55	33	1.5
Cheese & Onion, Sunseed Oil, Walkers*	1 Bag/33g	171	10.7	525	7	50	33	4
Cheese & Onion, Tesco*	1 Pack/25g	135	8	535	5.4	54.8	31.8	3.2
Cheese & Onion, Walkers*	1 Multi Bag/25g	124	6.7	495	5.6	55.9	26.7	4.4
Cheese Balls, Free From, Tesco*	1/6 Pack/25g	123	5.8	492	5.6	65.1	23.1	0.4
Cheese Curls, Morrisons*	1 Bag/17g	95	6.1	557	3.1	54.8	35.6	2.6
Cheese Curls, Sainsbury's*	1 Pack/16g	87	5.5	546	3.3	55.6	34.1	1.9
Cheese Curls, Snaktastic, Lidl*	1 Pack/12g	65	4.2	545	3.4	54.1	34.6	1.8
Cheese Curls, Tesco*	1 Bag/14g	75	4.5	520	4.5	54.4	31.1	1.9
Cheese Puffs, Tesco*	1 Bag/17g	99	6.7	580	4.6	52.1	39	0.9

	Measure INFO/WEIGHT	per Measure KCAL	FAT	Nutrition Values per 100g / 100ml KCAL	PROT	CARB	FAT	FIBRE
CRISPS								
Cheese Tasters, M&S*	1 Pack/30g	156	8.7	521	8.2	56.2	29	1
Cheese Tasters, Reduced Fat, M&S*	1 Pack/80g	380	15.9	475	8	65.5	19.9	0.9
Cheese, & Chives, Walkers*	1 Bag/33g	172	10.7	530	6.5	50	33	4.1
Cheese, & Onion, Reduced Fat, Tesco*	1 Pack/25g	116	5.1	463	8.7	57.3	20.4	7.6
Cheeseburger, Classic, Walkers*	1 Multipack/25g	124	6.8	497	5.7	55	27	4.6
Cheesy Wiggles, Asda*	1 Pack/16g	85	4.6	529	7.1	59	29	1.2
Chicken & Thyme, Oven Baked, Walkers*	1 Pack/25g	109	3.4	436	7.1	68	13.6	6.1
Chicken Katsu Curry, Ridge Cut, M&S*	1 Pack/40g	202	11.6	506	7.5	51	28.9	5.7
Chicken Wings, Hot, Strong, Max, Walkers*	1 Bag/30g	160	9.9	532	6.3	51	33	3
Chicken, & Thyme, Oven Roasted, Tesco*	1 Pack/150g	728	40.5	485	6.5	54	27	4.5
Chicken, & Chorizo, Double, Max, Walkers*	1 Pack/140g	683	35	488	7.8	54.9	25	6
Chicken, Chargrilled, Ridged, Snackrite, Aldi*	1 Pack/30g	157	9	524	6.5	54	30	4
Chicken, Roast, Select, Tesco*	1 Bag/25g	134	8.8	536	6.6	48.6	35	4.4
Chicken, Roast, Snack Rite*	1 Bag/25g	132	8.3	526	5.3	51.3	33.3	0
Chickpea Chips, Cheese & Onion, Sainsbury's*	1 Pack/20g	79	1.9	395	11	62.5	9.5	7.5
Chilli, & Lime, Strong, Max, Walkers*	1 Pack/30g	160	9.9	532	6.6	50.9	32.9	3.1
Chip Sticks, Salted, Morrisons*	1/6 Bag/25g	127	7	508	5.2	57	28.2	2.8
Combo Mix, Ready Salted, M&S*	1 Serving/30g	139	6	463	5	63.7	20.1	3.7
Combo Mix, Sour Cream, & Onion, Tesco*	1 Serving/25g	116	4.7	466	4.4	67.9	18.8	3.6
Crinkle Cut, Lower Fat, No Added Salt, Waitrose*	1 Bag/40g	193	10	483	6.5	58	25	3.9
Crinkle Cut, Salt & Vinegar, Coles*	1 Serving/25g	126	7.7	502	0	48.6	30.7	3.6
Crinklys, Baked, Cheese & Onion, Jacob's*	1 Pack/25g	122	5.4	489	8.5	63.4	21.6	2.9
Crinklys, Baked, Chilli Beef, Jacob's*	1 Pack/25g	123	5.6	492	8.3	63.2	22.2	2.6
Crunchy Sticks, Ready Salted, M&S*	1 Pack/75g	398	24.8	530	5.6	52.2	33	3.8
Crunchy Sticks, Ready Salted, Tesco*	1 Serving/25g	119	5.9	475	5.6	60.3	23.5	3
Crunchy Sticks, Salt & Vinegar, Sainsbury's*	1 Bag/25g	118	6.1	474	5.9	58	24.3	2.4
Crunchy Sticks, Salt & Vinegar, Value, Tesco*	1 Bag/22g	112	5.7	509	5	64	25.8	0.8
Duck & Hoisin, Crispy, Walkers*	1 Bag/25g	131	8.2	523	5.8	51.5	32.6	4
Fiery Peri Peri, Max Strong, Walkers*	1 Pack/27g	139	8.4	515	7	51.8	31.1	4.4
Firecracker Ribs, Ridge Cut, TTD, Sainsbury's*	1 Serving/30g	160	10	532	7.4	47.7	33.5	4.8
Flamin' Hot, Fiercely, Max, Walkers*	1 Pack/50g	265	16.4	530	6.5	50.8	32.8	3
Flatbread Chips, Indian Spiced, TTD, Sainsbury's*	1 Serving/30g	135	4.7	449	11.2	61.8	15.5	8.7
Fruit, Apple, Air Dried, 100% Fruit, Spare Snacks*	1 Pack/22g	76	0.1	346	2.3	76.8	0.6	12.2
Fruit, Apple, Air Dried, M&S*	1 Bag/16g	54	0.1	339	1.8	75.9	0.8	10.3
Fruit, Pineapple, Air Dried, M&S*	1 Pack/16g	55	0	341	3.1	76.6	0.1	10.4
Ham, Honey Roast, Hand Cooked, Finest, Tesco*	1 Serving/25g	130	7.3	515	5.1	58.6	28.8	2.5
Ham, Honey Roast, Reduced Fat, M&S*	1 Serving/30g	140	6	467	7.9	61.4	20.1	4.5
Hint of Salt, Natural Sea Salt, Walkers*	1 Pack/25g	126	7	506	6	54.3	28.3	4.7
Honey & Mustard, Mackie's*	1 Pack/30g	150	7.8	499	5.8	60	26	2.7
Hoops, Ready Salted, Snackrite, Aldi*	1 Bag/25g	124	6	494	3.3	65	24	2.6
Hummus Bites, The Foodie Market, Aldi*	1 Bag/20g	94	4.2	468	7.9	59	21	6.1
Jalapeno, & Cheese, Strong, Max, Walkers*	1 Pack/30g	159	9.9	531	6.5	51	33	3.1
Katsu Curry, Yo!, Walkers*	1 Pack/25g	124	6.8	496	6	56	27.2	4.8
Lamb & Mint, Slow Roasted, Sensations, Walkers*	1 Bag/35g	170	9.4	485	6.5	54	27	4.5
Lamb, & Mint, Seabrook*	1 Pack/25g	126	7.2	505	6.3	53.3	28.7	0
Lentil Chips, Himalayan Pink Salt, The Daily Crave*	1 Serving/48g	176	7.7	366	10.7	42.9	16.1	3.6
Lentil Chips, Sea Salt, Proper Crisps*	1 Serving/20g	96	4.2	482	9.7	63.6	20.8	0.7
Lentil Chips, Sour Cream, & Chive, Proper Chips*	1 Pack/20g	93	3.9	466	9.8	63	19.3	1
Lentil Curls, Sour Cream & Chive, Sainsbury's*	1 Pack/20g	95	4.1	476	10.5	61.3	20.3	3.1
Lentil Curls, Sour Cream & Onion, Asda*	1 Pack/20g	98	4.6	490	11	59	23	3.4
Lentil Curls, Sour Cream, & Chive, Tesco*	1 Pack/20g	90	3.1	448	11.3	64.1	15.6	3.3
Lentil Curls, Thai Sweet Chilli, Snaktastic, Lidl*	1 Pack/20g	92	3.6	460	11	61.5	18	3.5
Lentil Waves, Salt & Vinegar, Burts*	1 Pack/20g	92	3.7	462	10.2	62.3	18.3	3.7

	Measure INFO/WEIGHT	per Measure KCAL	FAT	Nutrition Values per 100g / 100ml KCAL	PROT	CARB	FAT	FIBRE
CRISPS								
Marmite, Sunseed, Walkers*	1 Bag/33g	168	9.9	517	7.3	51.1	30.5	4.3
Monster Claws, Flamin' Hot, Snackrite, Aldi*	1 Pack/18g	91	4.7	503	5.9	60	26	1.4
Monster Claws, Flamin' Hot, Snaktastic, Lidl*	1 Pack/18g	92	5	511	6.1	58.3	27.8	0.6
Monster Claws, Pickled Onion, Snackrite, Aldi*	1 Pack/18g	92	4.9	511	6.1	61.1	27.2	2.8
Multi Grain Waves, Sweet Chilli, The Foodie Market, Aldi*	1 Pack/25g	117	5.1	468	8	60	20.4	4.8
Multigrain Waves, Sour Cream & Black Pepper, Tesco*	1 Bag/20g	97	4.6	483	6.4	60.4	23.1	3.9
Multigrain Waves, Sweet Chilli, Tesco *	1 Pack/20g	96	4.6	480	6.5	59.5	23	4
Nacho Cheese, Muchos, Mccoys*	1 Serving/30g	160	9.6	535	6.2	55	32	2.7
Oat, Snackers, Smoked Paprika, GF, Nairn's*	1 Bag/23g	101	4	440	9.7	56.6	17.4	9.3
Onion Rings, Corn Snacks, Average	***1 Bag/25g***	***122***	***6.1***	***486***	***5.8***	***60.9***	***24.2***	***2.7***
Onion, Pickled, Golden Wonder*	1 Bag/25g	131	8.5	524	5.6	49	34	2
Onion, Pickled, Space Raiders, KP Snacks*	1 Bag/13g	64	2.9	495	6.5	65.3	22.8	1
Onion, Pickled, Sunseed, Walkers*	1 Bag/33g	171	10.7	525	6.5	50	33	4
Paprika Mix, Warm & Smoky, Waitrose*	1 Serving/25g	127	7.1	509	4	57.5	28.3	3.9
Paprika, Corn Snacks, Shapers, Boots*	1 Pack/13g	64	3.5	494	8.7	54	27	2.2
Paprika, Hand Cooked, M&S*	1 Pack/40g	210	12.5	524	5.9	52.3	31.3	4.5
Paprika, Max, Walkers*	1 Bag/50g	265	16.3	530	6.5	51.2	32.6	3.1
Parmesan, & Prosciutto, M&S*	1 Pack/40g	206	11.9	516	8.5	50.6	29.8	5.9
Parsnip, Honey Roast, M&S*	1 Serving/50g	275	21.3	550	4.1	30.5	42.6	14.3
Pastrami & Cheese, Crinkle, M&S*	1 Bag/25g	120	5.9	485	6.5	61	24	3.5
Pea Snacks, Snackrite, Aldi*	1 Pack/21g	87	2.7	415	20	49	13	13
Pea Snacks, Sour Cream, & Chive, Passions, Aldi*	1 Bag/21g	89	3	424	18.6	47.6	14.3	13.3
Pea Snacks, Soy, & Balsamic Vinegar, Snaktastic, Lidl*	1 Bag/21g	87	2.9	416	18.6	47.9	13.7	13.5
Peri Peri Chicken, Nandos, Walkers*	1 Pack/25g	124	6.7	496	5.6	56	26.8	4.8
Pickled Onion, Walkers*	1 Std Bag/22g	108	5.5	490	6	60	25	1.7
Pigs in Blankets, Hand Cooked, Christmas, Waitrose*	1 Serving/30g	148	7.8	495	7.3	55.9	26	4
Pigs in Blankets, Irresistible, Co-Op*	¼ Bag/38g	193	11	509	7.6	51	29	5.2
Pigs in Blankets, Walkers*	1 Bag/25g	126	6.7	504	6	56.8	26.8	4.4
Plain, Crinkle Cut, Weight Watchers*	1 Pack/16g	79	3.6	492	8	61.6	22.5	5.5
Pom Bear, Original, Intersnack Ltd*	1 Bag/19g	100	5.3	528	3.2	64	28	2.4
Popchips, Sea Salt & Vinegar	1 Serving/23g	95	3.2	411	5.1	63	14	4
Poppables, BBQ Rib, Walkers*	1 Serving/30g	153	7.8	510	5	63	26	3.7
Popped, Houmous & Lime, Eat Well, M&S*	1 Serving/23g	94	2.2	410	6.1	73.2	9.4	3.9
Popped, Sea Salt, & Apple Cider Vinegar, COU, M&S*	1 Pack/20g	83	2.1	414	6	72.4	10.4	3.5
Popped, Sea Salted, Sainsbury's*	1 Serving/22g	87	1.7	395	6.9	73.2	7.6	3.3
Popped, Smoky BBQ, M&S*	1 Pack/20g	84	2.1	419	6.4	72.6	10.5	4.1
Potato	***1oz/28g***	***148***	***9.6***	***530***	***5.7***	***53.3***	***34.2***	***5.3***
Potato Chips, Cooked, GF, Jumbo Country Chips*	1 Serving/30g	156	9.6	521	6	50.2	32	4.3
Potato Chips, Hand Cooked, Burts*	1 Pack/40g	208	11.5	519	5.1	58.6	28.8	2.5
Potato Loops, Asda*	1 Pack/24g	110	4	458	4.6	70.8	16.7	1.7
Potato Snacks, Original, Snaktastic, Lidl*	1 Serving/50g	266	15	533	4	60	30	3.4
Potato Squares, Ready Salted, Sainsbury's*	1 Bag/50g	192	8	384	6.5	53.8	15.9	7.8
Potato Twirls, Sainsbury's*	1 Serving/50g	218	7.3	435	3	72.8	14.6	3.1
Potato Twists, Salt & Vinegar, Asda*	1/6 Bag/20g	93	3.6	464	4	71	18	2.5
Potato, Low Fat	***1oz/28g***	***128***	***6***	***458***	***6.6***	***63.5***	***21.5***	***5.9***
Potato, Sea Salted, Specially Selected, Aldi*	1 Pack/25g	126	7	504	7.9	53	28	5.2
Prawn Cocktail, Snaktastic, Lidl*	1 Pack/25g	134	8	535	5.9	54	32	3.5
Prawn Cocktail, Spirals, Shapers, Boots*	1 Bag/15g	73	3.8	489	3.3	61	25	3
Prawn Cocktail, Sunseed Oil, Walkers*	1 Bag/33g	171	10.7	525	6.5	50	33	4
Prawn Cocktail, Tayto*	1 Bag/35g	185	12.3	526	7.5	46.6	35	4.5
Prawn Crackers, Tesco*	1 Pack/40g	220	13.3	550	2.2	60.4	33.2	0.6
Prawn Marie Rose, Finest, Tesco*	1 Serving/25g	129	7.7	517	7.4	50.3	30.7	4.7
Prawn, Spirals, Shapers, Boots*	1 Pack/100g	468	22	468	3.1	64	22	2.8

	Measure INFO/WEIGHT	per Measure KCAL	FAT	Nutrition Values per 100g / 100ml KCAL	PROT	CARB	FAT	FIBRE
CRISPS								
Puffs, Chickpea, & Carrot, Tesco*	1 Pack/20g	87	2.5	435	14.3	63.8	12.6	4.4
Puffs, Chickpeas, Salt & Vinegar, Snackrite, Aldi*	1 Serving/30g	132	6	440	11	48	20	15
Ready Salted, Crinkle Cut, Reduced Fat, Tesco*	1 Pack/25g	118	5.4	474	5.6	61.3	21.8	4.9
Ready Salted, Crinkle Cut, Weight Watchers*	1 Bag/16g	77	3.6	481	5.2	62	22.3	5.6
Ready Salted, Sainsbury's*	1 Pack/25g	137	9	550	6.2	48.6	36	3.5
Ready Salted, Stockwell & Co., Tesco*	1 Bag/25g	133	8.2	533	5	52.8	32.7	3.8
Ready Salted, Tesco*	1 Pack/25g	136	8.3	544	5.2	55.6	33.2	2
Ready Salted, Walkers*	1 Bag/21g	91	3.4	434	5	65	16	5
Reggae Reggae, Grove Cut, Levi Roots*	1 Pack/40g	200	11.5	500	5.1	58.6	28.8	2.5
Roast Beef, & Horseradish, Crinkle Cut, Finest, Tesco*	1 Serving/25g	130	7.4	518	7.3	53.3	29.6	4.5
Roast Beef, Walkers*	1 Bag/40g	196	10	490	7	59	25	1.7
Roast Chicken, Walkers*	1 Pack/33g	162	8.8	499	5.7	56	27	4.4
Salt & Pepper, Black, Cracked, Hand Cooked, M&S*	1 Bag/40g	206	11.8	516	7.5	52.2	29.5	6
Salt & Vinegar, Balsamic, Cracker, Jacob's*	1 Serving/25g	118	4.8	470	5.2	67	19.3	2.4
Salt & Vinegar, Balsamic, Delux, Lidl*	1 Pack/25g	121	6.3	484	6	56.8	25.2	4.4
Salt & Vinegar, Balsamic, Handcooked, M&S*	1 Bag/40g	208	12.1	521	6.7	52.8	30.4	4.6
Salt & Vinegar, Balsamic, Kettle Chips*	1 Bag/40g	204	11.2	509	5.7	55.8	28.1	4.9
Salt & Vinegar, Chiplets, M&S*	1 Bag/30g	132	5.7	440	5.7	61.3	18.9	4.7
Salt & Vinegar, Cider Vinegar & Sea Salt, Tyrrells*	1 Pack/40g	192	9.8	481	7.2	60.1	24.6	2.4
Salt & Vinegar, Cider Vinegar, Crinkle Cut, Finest, Tesco*	¼ Pack/38g	186	10	495	6.7	54.6	26.7	4.5
Salt & Black Pepper, Mix, Waitrose*	1 Serving/25g	122	6.1	488	4.4	61.2	24.4	3.2
Salt & Shake, Walkers*	1 Pack/24g	128	7.8	533	6.2	52.2	32.3	4.4
Salt & Vinegar, Average	***1 Bag/25g***	***130***	***8.2***	***519***	***5.5***	***50.3***	***32.9***	***3.4***
Salt & Vinegar, Crinkle Cut, Seabrook*	1 Pack/25g	126	7.2	502	5.9	52.9	28.7	3.9
Salt & Vinegar, Reduced Fat, Crinkle, M&S*	1 Pack/40g	183	7.7	457	6.8	61.9	19.2	4.5
Salt & Vinegar, Squares, Walkers*	1 Bag/28g	122	5	443	6.5	61	18	5.5
Salt & Vinegar, Sunseed Oil, Walkers*	1 Bag/33g	171	10.7	525	6.5	50	33	4
Salt & Vinegar, Thick Ridged, Snackrite, Aldi*	1 Bag/30g	159	9.3	529	5.8	55	31	3.4
Salt Your Own, Excluding Salt, Aldi*	1 Pack/24g	130	8.1	536	6	52.6	33.5	4.5
Salt Your Own, Sainsbury's*	1 Pack/24g	127	7.9	520	5	52.2	32.3	3.7
Salt Your Own, Snackrite, Aldi*	1 Pack/24g	130	8.1	536	6	52.6	33.5	4.5
Salted, Average	***1 Bag/25g***	***127***	***7.4***	***508***	***6.1***	***53.4***	***29.7***	***4***
Salted, Crinkle Cut, Lights, Snackrite, Aldi*	1 Bag/25g	122	5.8	486	7	61	23	3.7
Salted, Reduced Fat, Crinkle, M&S*	1 Pack/40g	188	8.2	471	6.3	62.8	20.6	4.6
Salted, Reduced Fat, Tesco*	1 Pack/25g	114	6.2	456	6.3	52	24.7	5.9
Salted, Sea, Anglesey Sea Salt, Red Sky*	1 Serving/40g	185	8.7	463	6.8	59.8	21.8	5
Salted, Sea, Crinkle Cut, Seabrook *	1 Bag/32g	165	10	517	5.7	53.7	31.1	0
Salted, Sea, Hand Cooked, Specially Selected, Aldi*	¼ Lge Bag/38g	182	9	486	6.2	59	24	4.5
Salted, Sea, Houmous Chips, Eat Real*	1 Serving/28g	126	4.8	449	6.5	68.4	17	4.5
Salted, Sea, Lentil Chips, Eat Real*	1 Serving/28g	133	5.9	478	8	62.1	21	4.5
Salted, Sea, Lightly, Hand Cooked, English, Tyrrells*	1 Pack/25g	125	6.4	501	5.9	49	25.4	5.3
Salted, Sea, Lightly, Potato Chips, Tyrrells*	1 Pack/150g	740	38.1	493	7.7	58.9	25.4	2.6
Salted, Sea, Popchips*	1 Bag/23g	94	3.2	410	5.5	62	14	4.3
Salted, Sea, Potato, Mackies*	1 Pack/40g	200	10.8	499	7.4	55	27	4.5
Salted, Squares, Walkers*	1 Pack/25g	109	4.8	435	6.5	60	19	6
Salted, Sunseed Oil, Walkers*	1 Bag/33g	175	11.1	537	5.9	49.7	34.1	4.2
Sausage, & Tomato, Golden Wonder*	1 Pack/25g	132	7.9	530	6.2	53.8	31.5	3.1
Sausage, & Onion, Mackie's*	1 Serving/30g	148	7.8	492	7.6	55	26	5
Scampi, Smiths, Walkers*	1 Bag/27g	134	7	496	13	52.5	26	0
Sea Salt & Cider Vinegar, Finest, Tesco*	1 Serving/25g	123	6.4	491	6.8	56.3	25.4	5.2
Sea Salt & Malt Vinegar, Baked, M&S*	1 Serving/30g	149	7.9	497	5.4	57.1	26.5	4.2
Sea Salt, Anglesey, Pipers Crisps*	1 Bag/40g	213	12.3	532	5.1	57.2	30.7	3.5
Sea Salt, Original, Terra*	1 Pack/28g	150	9	536	3.6	57.1	32.1	10.7

	Measure INFO/WEIGHT	per Measure KCAL	FAT	Nutrition Values per 100g / 100ml KCAL	PROT	CARB	FAT	FIBRE
CRISPS								
Sea Salted, Furrows, Tyrrells*	1 Pack/50g	262	15.4	524	6.7	52.8	30.9	0
Sea Salted, Morrisons*	1 Serving/50g	257	14.2	514	5.1	57.8	28.3	3.8
Sea Salted. Lightly, Hand Cooked, M&S*	1 Pack/150g	776	44.1	517	5.8	55.2	29.4	4.2
Sheese, & Red Onion, Vegan, Kettle Chips*	1 Serving/30g	154	8.8	514	8	51.7	29.4	5.4
Shells, Prawn Cocktail, Asda*	1 Bag/18g	90	5.3	501	4.6	54.9	29.2	6.2
Smoked Chipotle Chilli, Kent Crisps*	1 Pack/40g	208	11.5	519	5.1	58.6	28.8	2.5
Smoked Paprika, San Nicasio *	½ Pack/75g	428	30	571	6.8	45	40	0
Smoky Bacon Flavour, Average	***1 Bag/25g***	***132***	***8.4***	***527***	***6.2***	***49.7***	***33.7***	***3.2***
Smoky Chilli Chicken, Muchos, McCoys*	1 Serving/30g	152	7.8	507	6.1	60	26	2.9
Snax, Original, Asda*	1 Serving/25g	126	6.5	504	4.5	61	26	4.2
Sour Cream & Onion, Potato Chips, Popchips*	1 Pack/23g	95	3.5	413	28.3	69.6	15.2	4.3
Sour Cream, & Chilli Lentil Curls, M&S*	1 Pack/60g	243	5.2	405	13.6	65.3	8.7	4.3
Sour Cream, & Chive Flavour, Average	***1 Bag/25g***	***127***	***7.7***	***508***	***6.8***	***50.7***	***30.9***	***4.6***
Sour Cream, & Chive, Crinkle, Reduced Fat, M&S*	1 Bag/40g	187	8.1	468	6.7	62.2	20.3	4.6
Sour Cream, & Chives, Quinoa Chips, Eat Real*	1 Pack/30g	165	8.6	550	8	66.4	28.8	2.5
Sour Cream, & Onion, Corn Chips, Popchips*	1 Multipack/17g	72	2.9	422	6.5	65	17	1.9
Sour Cream, & Chive, Hummus Chips, Eat Real*	1 Pack/45g	213	10.4	474	6.7	58	23	5.8
Sour Cream, & Jalapeno, Party Mix, Golden Cross*	1 Serving/25g	116	4.9	464	4.4	68.4	19.6	1.8
Sour Cream, & Mexican Lime, Deluxe, Lidl*	1 Serving/25g	124	5.8	496	6	63.2	23.3	4.5
Sour Cream, & Onion, Stackers, Snackrite, Aldi*	1 Serving/25g	139	9.2	557	3.1	52	37	2.8
Stackers, Salt & Vinegar, Snackrite, Aldi*	½ Pack/83g	401	19.9	483	4.4	62	24	3.5
Steak, & Peppercorn Sauce, Crinkle Cut, Co-Op*	¼ Bag/38g	198	11.8	522	6.6	53	31	3.8
Steak, Flame Grilled, Ridge Cut, McCoys*	1 Bag/47g	250	14.7	526	6.9	53	31	3.9
Steak, Flamed Grilled, Max, Walkers*	1 Pack/50g	266	16.4	533	6.5	51.6	32.8	2.8
Steak, T Bone, Bubble Chips, Roysters*	1 Pack/28g	151	8.9	540	5.5	55	32	2.6
Sticks, Salt & Vinegar, Asda*	1 Serving/25g	126	6.2	504	5.2	63	25	2
Sun Bites, Lightly Sea Salted, Grain Waves, Walkers*	1 Pack/25g	120	5.4	480	7.5	80.7	21.6	6.6
Sunbites, Cheddar & Caramelised Onion, Walkers*	1 Bag/25g	120	5.4	480	7.6	60.8	21.6	6.4
Sundried Tomato, & Garlic, Quinoa Chips, Eat Real*	1 Bag/22g	121	6.4	551	8	66.4	28.9	2.7
Sweet & Salty, Katy's Kettle Corn, Popchips*	1 Serving/28g	128	4	455	6.9	65.9	14.1	5.4
Sweet & Smokin', Hippeas*	1 Pack/22g	90	3.8	411	13.2	51.1	17.4	7.3
Sweet Chilli, & Red Pepper, Potato Chips, Tyrrells*	¼ Pack/37g	180	9.2	481	7.9	59.7	24.5	2.4
Sweet Chilli, & Irish Red Pepper, Keoghs*	1 Bag/50g	263	13.2	526	7.2	49	26.5	5
Sweet Chilli, Average	***1 Bag/25g***	***115***	***5.6***	***461***	***5.1***	***59.9***	***22.6***	***4.6***
Sweet Chilli, Lentil, Curls, Bites, Kettle Chips*	1 Pack/22g	94	2.6	428	13.2	65	11.9	4
Sweet Chilli, Multigrain, Waves, Sainsbury's*	1 Pack/20g	104	5.6	520	6.3	58.6	28	4
Sweet Chilli, Thai, Lentil Waves, Burts*	1 Pack/20g	91	3.3	453	11.7	62.6	16.3	4.9
Sweet Chilli, Thai, Sensations, Walkers*	1 Bag/40g	198	9.9	494	6.9	59	24.7	3.7
Sweet Chilli, Thai, Velvet Crunch, King*	1 Pack/20g	81	1.9	404	1.6	77.5	9.7	2
Sweet Potato Sticks, Sea Salt, Emily Crisps Ltd*	1 Pack/35g	176	9.2	503	3.4	58.6	26.3	9.1
Sweet Potato, Paprika, Oven Baked, with Veg, Walkers*	1 Bag/23g	101	3.4	437	7	66	15	3.9
Sweet Potato, Thai Sweet Chilli, Kettle Chips*	1 Serving/30g	151	7.9	502	7.1	56.5	26.4	4.9
Take it Cheesy, Chickpea Puffs, Organic, Hippeas*	1 Pack/15g	61	2.5	406	14.6	48.8	16.8	8.2
Tangy Salt & Vinegar, KP Snacks*	1 Bag/30g	160	10	532	5	52.6	33.5	2.9
Tangy Toms, Golden Wonder*	1 Pack/81g	411	21	507	5.4	63	25.9	0.5
Thai Bites, Mild, Jacob's*	1 Bag/25g	93	0.8	373	6.9	79	3.3	1
Tomato & Basil, Houmous Chips, Eat Real*	1 Serving/28g	126	4.8	449	6.5	68.4	17	4.5
Tomato & Herbs, Baked Fusions, Snacks, Walkers*	1 Pack/25g	109	3.4	434	6.7	68.3	13.5	6.4
Tomato Ketchup, Golden Wonder*	1 Bag/25g	135	8	521	5.1	54	30.8	3.6
Turkey, & Stuffing, Walkers*	1 Bag/25g	126	6.8	504	6.4	56.4	27.2	4.4
Twirls, Salt & Vinegar, Tesco*	1 Bag/80g	349	14	436	3.9	65.8	17.5	2.4
Unsalted, Seabrook*	1 Bag/30g	163	10.7	544	5.7	47.9	35.8	4.1
Vegetable, Average	***1 Bag/25g***	***118***	***7.4***	***470***	***4.1***	***46.5***	***29.6***	***12.1***

	Measure INFO/WEIGHT	per Measure KCAL	FAT	Nutrition Values per 100g / 100ml KCAL	PROT	CARB	FAT	FIBRE
CRISPS								
Vegetable, Paprika, Punchy, Great Shape, Asda*	1 Pack/23g	99	3	432	3.9	73	13	3.7
Veggie & Kale, Straws, Eat Real*	1 Bag/22g	109	5.6	497	3.1	65.1	25.5	2.8
Veggie Puffs, Pickled Onion, The Foodie Market, Aldi*	1 Pack/21g	87	2.7	415	20	48	13	11
Veggie Puffs, Roast Beef, The Foodie Market, Aldi*	1 Pack/21g	87	2.8	414	21.9	45.7	13.3	11.9
Veggie Straws, The Foodie Market, Aldi*	1 Bag/22g	122	7.7	553	3.2	54	35	3.3
Wasabi, Strong, Max, Walkers*	1 Pack/30g	160	9.9	534	6.3	51.7	32.9	2.9
Wheat Crunchies, Cheese & Onion, KP Snacks*	1 Pack/20g	100	5	498	9.4	57	25	3.6
Wheat Crunchies, Golden Wonder*	1 Pack/35g	172	8.7	491	11.1	55.9	24.8	0
Wheelies, Bacon, Tayto*	1 Pack/20g	98	4.6	492	6.7	63.3	23.1	0
Worcester Sauce, Walkers*	1 Bag/22g	96	3.5	435	5	65	16	5
CRISPY PANCAKE								
Beef Bolognese, Findus*	1 Pancake/65g	104	2.6	160	6.5	25	4	1
Chicken, Bacon & Sweetcorn, Findus*	1 Pancake/63g	101	2.5	160	5.5	26	4	1.1
Minced Beef, As Consumed, Findus*	1 Pancake/115g	178	2.9	155	6.2	26	2.5	1.9
CROISSANT								
All Butter, Bakers Selection, Asda*	1 Croissant/40g	164	8.4	412	6.9	48	21	1.9
All Butter, Finest, Tesco*	1 Croissant/62g	258	14.3	415	7.9	42.9	23.1	1.9
All Butter, Frozen, Sainsbury's*	1 Croissant /44g	169	9	384	8.8	40.1	20.4	2.5
All Butter, Irresistible, Co-Op*	1 Croissant/62g	272	16.1	438	8.6	41	26	2.5
All Butter, Light & Flaky, Specially Selected, Aldi*	1 Croissant/40g	174	10	436	9.2	42	25	1.4
All Butter, M&S*	1 Croissant/40g	179	10.8	447	10.1	40.1	27	1.6
All Butter, Reduced Fat, M&S*	1 Croissant/40g	154	7.1	384	10.9	44.1	17.7	2.2
All Butter, Reduced Fat, Tesco*	1 Croissant/52g	164	5.5	315	7.5	47.4	10.6	1.8
All Butter, Sainsbury's*	1 Croissant/44g	166	7.5	377	9	46.2	17	1.3
All Butter, Tesco*	1 Croissant/44g	168	7.5	383	9	47.2	17	2.6
Almond, Bakery, Tesco*	1 Crossant/84g	342	17.7	407	9.3	43.8	21	2.4
Average	***1 Croissant/50g***	***180***	***10.2***	***360***	***8.3***	***38.3***	***20.3***	***1.6***
Butter, Bakery, Tesco*	1 Croissant/72g	285	13.7	396	9.3	46.1	19	1.6
Butter, Charentes, No.1, Waitrose*	1 Croissant/68g	309	19.3	454	8	40.5	28.4	2.1
Butter, Morrisons*	1 Croissant/44g	196	12.5	446	9.3	38.2	28.4	2
Cheese & Ham, Delice de France*	1 Croissant/91g	225	12.3	247	7	24.4	13.5	2.5
Chocolate Filled, All Butter, Finest, Tesco*	1 Croissant/75g	267	11.3	355	7.4	45.9	15.1	2.8
Chocolate, & Hazelnut, Bakery, Sainsbury's*	1 Croissant/81g	345	19	426	8.6	43.9	23.4	2.7
Flaky Pastry with a Plain Chocolate Filling, Tesco*	1 Croissant/83g	369	20.8	445	8.6	45	25.1	2.6
GF, Free From, Tesco*	1 Croissant/70g	244	11.8	348	3.3	44.5	16.8	2.8
with Cocoa Filling, Max, 7 Days*	1 Croissant/28g	128	7.8	456	6	44	28	0
CROQUETTES								
Cheese, Cheddar, Inspired Cuisine, Aldi*	1 Croquette/42g	129	7.1	306	7.2	24	17	2.5
Potato, Fried in Blended Oil, Average	***1 Croquette/80g***	***171***	***10.5***	***214***	***3.7***	***21.6***	***13.1***	***1.3***
Potato, Frozen, HFC, Tesco*	1 Serving/128g	266	11.7	208	3.3	26.5	9.1	3.2
Serrano Ham & Manchego, World Cafe, Waitrose*	½ Pack/78g	238	14	305	8.4	26.1	18	2.6
CROUTONS								
Black Pepper, & Sea Salt, Oven Baked, Asda*	½ Pack/20g	90	2.6	450	11	69	13	4.8
Cheese, & Shallot, Waitrose*	1 Serving/10g	45	1.4	449	13.1	64.4	14.5	3.4
Fresh, M&S*	1 Serving/10g	53	3.3	530	11.4	50	32.8	3.2
Garlic, Waitrose*	1 Serving/40g	209	12	522	10.8	52.1	30	2.7
Herb, Sainsbury's*	1 Serving/15g	64	1.7	429	13.4	68.2	11.4	2.8
Lightly Sea Salted, Asda*	1 Serving/20g	83	1.9	414	12.9	69.7	9.3	4.3
Mini, Osem*	1 Serving/20g	104	5	522	9.2	65	25	0
Prepacked, Average	***1 Serving/15g***	***74***	***3.6***	***495***	***10.8***	***58.7***	***24***	***2.6***
Sea Salt, & Black Pepper, Belbake, Lidl*	1 Serving/20g	92	3.2	461	11	66	16	4.4
Sea Salt, & Black Pepper, M&S*	½ Pack/43g	210	9.6	488	10.8	58.6	22.4	4.4
Sun Dried Tomato, Sainsbury's*	¼ Pack/15g	75	3.8	497	11.7	55.2	25.5	2.5

	Measure INFO/WEIGHT	per Measure KCAL	FAT	Nutrition Values per 100g / 100ml KCAL	PROT	CARB	FAT	FIBRE
CRUDITES								
Vegetable Sticks, Average	***1 Serving/100g***	***24***	***0.2***	***24***	***0.7***	***4.5***	***0.2***	***1.9***
with Cheese & Chive Dip, Tesco*	1 Pack/115g	132	10.5	115	1.6	5.9	9.1	1.5
with Soured Cream & Chive, Reduced Fat, Dip, Tesco*	1 Pack/53g	30	1.6	56	1.8	5	3	1.9
CRUMBLE								
Almond, & Apricot, Devondale*	1 Cake/80g	314	13.2	392	3.6	57	16.5	9.8
Apple, & Blackberry, M&S*	1 Serving/135g	398	15.1	295	3.5	44.9	11.2	1.6
Apple, & Blackberry, Sainsbury's*	1 Serving/110g	232	6.2	211	3	37.1	5.6	2.1
Apple, & Blackberry, Tesco*	1/6 Pie/90g	286	11.7	318	3	45.8	13	2.8
Apple, & Custard, Asda*	1 Serving/125g	250	8.8	200	2.3	32	7	0
Apple, & Blackberry, Waitrose*	¼ Crumble/125g	296	9.8	236	2.9	37.6	7.8	2.1
Apple, Average	***1 Serving/240g***	***497***	***12***	***207***	***0.9***	***40.5***	***5***	***1.1***
Apple, Flapjack, Finest, Tesco*	¼ Pack/125g	310	13.2	248	5.1	31.2	10.6	3.8
Apple, Golden, Allplants*	1 Serving/100g	242	15	242	3.5	22	15	3.1
Apple, Slices, Frozen, Tesco*	1 Slice/54g	173	8	321	4.9	40.6	14.9	2.8
Apple, with Custard, Green's*	1 Serving/79g	171	5.3	216	1.9	37	6.7	1.2
Apple, with Sultanas, Weight Watchers*	1 Dessert/110g	196	4.3	178	1.4	34.2	3.9	1.3
Berry, Winter, Aldi*	1/6 Crumble/99g	279	9.9	282	3.3	43	10	2.9
Blackcurrant, & Apple, Devondale*	1 Cake/80g	314	13.2	393	3.6	57	16.5	9.8
Fruit	***1 Portion/170g***	***337***	***11.7***	***198***	***2***	***34***	***6.9***	***1.7***
Fruit, Wholemeal	***1oz/28g***	***54***	***2***	***193***	***2.6***	***31.7***	***7.1***	***2.7***
Fruit, with Custard	***1 Serving/270g***	***463***	***17.6***	***171***	***2.4***	***27***	***6.5***	***1.3***
Gooseberry, M&S*	1 Serving/133g	379	14.2	285	3.5	43.3	10.7	1.7
Lemon Meringue, Holly Lane*	1 Tart/50g	213	8.5	426	4.8	63	17	1.8
Rhubarb, Average	***1 Portion/150g***	***330***	***11.1***	***220***	***2.7***	***35.5***	***7.4***	***1.9***
Summer Fruit, Parsley Box*	1 Serving/155g	347	10.2	224	3	35	6.6	6.6
CRUMBLE MIX								
Luxury, Tesco*	¼ Pack/55g	243	9	441	5.7	67.9	16.3	3.2
Topping, Sainsbury's*	1 Serving/47g	188	9.2	401	5.9	50.3	19.6	5.3
CRUMPETS								
Asda*	1 Crumpet/45g	85	0.4	188	6	39	0.9	2.1
Bakers Selection, Asda*	1 Crumpet/50g	106	0.6	211	6.7	42	1.2	2.7
Bunny, Morrisons*	1 Crumpet/57g	107	0.4	187	5.5	38.4	0.7	2.6
Buttermilk, TTD, Sainsbury's*	1 Crumpet/52g	102	0.6	195	6.5	38.5	1.1	2.6
Christmas Tree, Village Bakery, Aldi*	1 Crumpet48g	86	0.3	180	5.5	37	0.7	2.6
Co-Op*	1 Crumpet/40g	70	0.3	175	7	35	0.7	2
Creations, Co-Op*	1 Crumpet/60g	113	0.4	188	5.7	38	0.7	2.5
Essential, Waitrose*	1 Crumpet/52g	94	0.6	182	6.5	35.1	1.1	2.6
Fluffy, Village Bakery, Aldi*	1 Crumpet/57g	117	0.6	206	6.4	42	1	2.4
Golden Sun, Lidl*	1 Crumpet/43g	83	0.7	193	7.8	37.1	1.6	1.6
Ham, Pulled, & Rarebit, M&S*	1 Crumpet/24g	41	0.7	169	9.4	24.7	3	2.7
Jones Village Bakery*	1 Crumpet/55g	95	0.4	172	5.6	34.9	0.7	2
Mcgee's*	1 Crumpet/47g	96	1.1	204	4.8	42.5	2.4	0
Morrisons*	1 Crumpet/40g	90	0.2	225	7.8	47.2	0.5	3.2
Planet Deli*	1 Crumpet/48g	88	0.5	183	6.1	36.6	1	1
Premium, Sainsbury's*	1 Crumpet/50g	96	0.7	191	6.1	38.6	1.4	1.7
Rowan Hill Bakery, Lidl*	1 Crumpet/44g	78	0.5	178	5.5	34.5	1.2	0
Sourdough, Finest, Tesco*	1 Crumpet/55g	100	0.4	181	6	36.5	0.7	2.3
Sourdough, Irresistible, Co-Op*	1 Crumpet /54g	101	0.6	187	6.1	37	1.1	2.2
Sourdough, TTD, Sainsbury's*	1 Crumpet/55g	93	0.3	169	5.6	34.1	0.6	2.4
Sourdough, Waitrose*	1 Crumpet/55g	95	0.4	172	5.6	34.9	0.7	2
Square, Tesco*	1 Crumpet/60g	101	0.5	168	6.3	33.8	0.8	2.7
Tesco*	1 Crumpet/55g	100	0.4	181	6	36.2	0.8	2.3
Toasted, Average	***1 Crumpet/40g***	***80***	***0.4***	***199***	***6.7***	***43.4***	***1***	***2***

	Measure INFO/WEIGHT	per Measure KCAL	FAT	Nutrition Values per 100g / 100ml KCAL	PROT	CARB	FAT	FIBRE
CRUMPETS								
Waitrose*	1 Crumpet/62g	116	0.7	188	6.3	37.9	1.2	2.1
Warburton's*	1 Crumpet/55g	97	0.4	176	6	35.3	0.8	1.9
Wholemeal, Bakers Selection, Asda*	1 Crumpet/50g	94	0.4	189	7.3	36	0.8	3.7
CRUNCHIE								
Blast, Cadbury*	1 Serving/42g	199	8.3	480	4.7	69.6	20.1	0.7
Cadbury*	1 Bar/40g	185	7.5	465	4	69.5	18.9	0.5
Nuggets, Cadbury*	1 Bag/125g	569	20.5	455	3.8	73.1	16.4	0
Treat Size, Cadbury*	1 Bar/17g	79	2.9	463	3	75	17	1.3
CUCUMBER								
Average	***1 Serving/80g***	***8***	***0.1***	***10***	***0.7***	***1.5***	***0.1***	***0.6***
Baby, Pickled, Always Fresh*	1 Serving/30g	14	0.1	47	2	8	0.3	0
Baby, Raw, Tesco*	2 Cucumbers/80g	12	0.5	16	1	1.2	0.6	0.7
Mini, Love Me Tender*	1 Cucumber/33g	6	0.2	19	0.7	3.5	0.5	0.5
CUMIN								
Seeds, Whole, Average	***1 Tsp/2g***	***8***	***0.5***	***375***	***17.8***	***44.2***	***22.7***	***10.5***
CUPCAKES								
Assorted, Sainsbury's*	1 Cake/38g	130	2.3	341	2.2	69.3	6.1	0.4
Birthday, Hostess*	1 Cake/46g	190	8.5	413	1.1	58.7	18.5	0
Carrot, Average	***1 Cake/40g***	***157***	***8.6***	***392***	***3.6***	***45.4***	***21.6***	***0.6***
Celebration, Tesco*	1 Cake/61g	310	17.8	510	2.6	58.5	29.3	1
Chocolate Filled, Free From, Tesco*	1 Cake/52g	238	13.1	459	3.4	53.6	25.3	1.6
Chocolate Fudge, Party Pack, Tesco*	1 Cake/63g	300	17.5	476	4.2	50.7	27.8	3
Chocolate, Average	***1 Cake/40g***	***159***	***6.4***	***398***	***3.5***	***59.9***	***16***	***1.2***
Chocolate, Mini, GF, Free From, Morrisons*	1 Cake/18g	79	3.7	438	4.9	57.3	20.5	2.3
Lemon, Average	***1 Cake/40g***	***184***	***10.1***	***461***	***3***	***55.5***	***25.3***	***1.1***
Lemon, Healthy Option, Average	***1 Cake/40g***	***131***	***1.5***	***328***	***2.7***	***68.9***	***3.7***	***5.2***
Lemon, Mini Fruity Selection, M&S*	1 Cake/23g	105	5.6	458	3.6	55.4	24.6	0.5
Milkshake Flavour, Mini, Co-Op*	1 Cake/22g	23	1.3	106	0	9.5	5.8	0
Raspberry, Mini Fruity Selection, M&S*	1 Cake/23g	104	4.8	453	3.2	62.7	20.9	0.5
Red Velvet, Party Pack, Tesco*	1 Cake/62g	308	17.5	497	2.5	56.8	28.3	2.6
Red Velvet, Tesco*	1 Cake/63g	308	16.6	490	3.1	59.3	26.4	1.2
Sponge Top, Individual, Tesco*	1 Cake/50g	220	10.5	443	3	59.5	21.1	1.3
Strawberry & Cream, Party Pack, Tesco*	1 Cake/65g	316	17.8	486	2.5	56.8	27.3	1.8
Strawberry, Party Selection, Tesco*	1 Cake/46g	229	13.3	496	2	55.8	28.8	2.8
Unicorn, Tesco*	1 Cake/63g	316	17.6	502	3.2	58.6	28	1.1
Vanilla, & Chocolate, Mini, Waitrose*	1 Cake/21g	93	4.8	441	4.1	53.7	22.9	2.2
Vanilla, Mini Fruity Selection, M&S*	1 Cake/23g	106	5.2	463	3.3	61.2	22.7	0.5
Vanilla, Mini, GF, Free From, Morrisons*	1 Cake/18g	29	4.1	162	3.5	60.3	22.8	0.8
Vanilla, Party Platter, Holly Lane, Aldi*	1 Cake/57g	282	16	494	2.6	56	28	2.1
Vanilla, Party Selection, Tesco*	1 Cake/46g	230	13.1	495	2.6	57.2	28.1	1.5
White Chocolate, & Vanilla, Tesco*	1 Cake/76g	390	22.5	513	1.7	59.7	29.6	0.8
CURACAO								
Average	***1 Pub Shot/35ml***	***109***	***0***	***311***	***0***	***28.3***	***0***	***0***
CURLY WURLY								
Cadbury*	1 Bar/26g	118	4.7	453	3.1	70	18	0.7
Squirlies, Cadbury*	1 Squirl/3g	13	0.5	442	3.5	69.2	17.3	0.8
CURRANTS								
Average	***1oz/28g***	***75***	***0.1***	***267***	***2.3***	***67.8***	***0.4***	***1.9***
CURRY								
Aubergine	***1oz/28g***	***33***	***2.8***	***118***	***1.4***	***6.2***	***10.1***	***1.5***
Aubergine, Masala, TTD, Sainsbury's*	½ Pack/115g	135	11.4	117	2.9	4.1	9.9	5.8
Beef Massaman, Thai, Musclefood*	1 Serving/470g	498	17.4	106	8.5	9.8	3.7	1.1
Beef Rendang, COOK!, M&S*	½ Pack/269g	377	10.8	140	21.3	4.2	4	1.1

	Measure INFO/WEIGHT	per Measure KCAL	FAT	Nutrition Values per 100g / 100ml KCAL	PROT	CARB	FAT	FIBRE
CURRY								
Beef, Canned, Tesco*	½ Can/200g	264	15.8	132	9.5	4.3	7.9	2.8
Beef, Sainsbury's*	1 Serving/400g	552	32.8	138	10.7	5.4	8.2	0.9
Beef, Thai, Finest, Tesco*	1 Serving/500g	770	29	154	9	16.5	5.8	1.2
Beef, with Rice, Iceland*,	1 Pack/500g	580	14.5	116	5	16.7	2.9	1.5
Blackeye Bean, Gujerati	***1oz/28g***	***36***	***1.2***	***127***	***7.2***	***16.1***	***4.4***	***2.8***
Butternut & Spinach, Allplants*	1 Serving/376g	425	22.6	113	3.4	9.9	6	2.7
Butternut Squash, & Chickpea, Plant Based, Asda*	1 Pack/388g	400	8.5	103	3.2	17	2.2	1.2
Cabbage	***1oz/28g***	***23***	***1.4***	***82***	***1.9***	***8.1***	***5***	***2.1***
Caribbean Jerk, Rice, & Peas, BOL Foods*	1 Pack/405g	393	11.3	97	3.8	12.3	2.8	3.8
Cauliflower & Potato	***1oz/28g***	***17***	***0.7***	***59***	***3.4***	***6.6***	***2.4***	***1.8***
Cauliflower, Chickpea, & Potato, Vegan, Waitrose*	½ Pack/205g	166	7.4	81	3.2	6.4	3.6	5.2
Chana Saag, Slimming World*	1 Pack/350g	256	4.9	73	4.4	7.3	1.4	6.8
Chettinad, Prawn, King, M&S*	1 Serving/200g	184	7.6	92	8.7	5.1	3.8	1.5
Chick Pea, Whole, Average	***1oz/28g***	***50***	***2.1***	***179***	***9.6***	***21.3***	***7.5***	***4.5***
Chick Pea, Whole, Basic, Average	***1oz/28g***	***30***	***1***	***108***	***6***	***14.2***	***3.6***	***3.3***
Chicken, & Potato, Massaman, Hello Fresh*	1 Serving/607g	704	25.9	116	7.1	12.2	4.3	0
Chicken, & Prawn, Thai Green, Gousto*	1 Serving	347	17.3	347	34	10.7	17.3	6.7
Chicken, & Rice, Calorie Controlled, Tesco*	1 Pack/315g	293	3.8	93	5.4	14.5	1.2	1.6
Chicken, & Rice, Calorie Counted, Asda*	1 Pack/350g	283	3.6	81	4.6	13.1	1	0.9
Chicken, & Rice, Calorie Counted, Asda*	1 Pack/350g	322	4.2	92	5	15	1.2	1
Chicken, & Rice, Dinner, Tesco*	1 Pack/500g	520	12	104	8.2	11.7	2.4	1.3
Chicken, & Rice, Microwaved, Asda*	1 Pack/400g	588	22.2	148	5.5	18	5.6	1.8
Chicken, Butter Masala, Asda*	½ Pack/189g	261	14.4	138	13	4.3	7.6	0.7
Chicken, Butter, & Rice, Taste of India, Tesco*	1 Pack/427g	624	29.9	146	6.4	12.8	7	3.1
Chicken, Butter, Takeaway, Tesco*	½ Pack/175g	224	13.3	128	7.9	6.4	7.6	1.2
Chicken, Chinese with Rice, Ready Meal, Average	***1 Serving/450g***	***490***	***11.5***	***109***	***7.2***	***14.1***	***2.6***	***1.3***
Chicken, Fiery Andhra, Waitrose*	½ Pack/175g	226	11.2	129	13.3	3.7	6.4	1.9
Chicken, Fruity, Meal for One, M&S*	1 Pack/400g	508	15.6	127	6.7	15.6	3.9	1.1
Chicken, Fruity, Mini Meal, M&S*	1 Pack/200g	262	7.4	131	8.2	15.7	3.7	1.1
Chicken, Garlic, Cook*	1 Pack/320g	358	13.7	112	10.7	7.5	4.3	0.5
Chicken, Green Thai, BFY, M&S*	1 Pack/380g	369	6.5	97	7.6	12.4	1.7	1
Chicken, Green Thai, Charlie Bigham's*	½ Pack/300g	342	21	114	8.7	4.8	7	0
Chicken, Green Thai, Cook*	1 Serving/270g	327	16.5	121	11.7	4.4	6.1	0
Chicken, Green, Thai, Jasmine Rice, Sainsbury's*	½ Pack/188g	184	4.7	98	7.9	10.5	2.5	1.3
Chicken, Hot, Can, Tesco*	1 Can/418g	514	26.3	123	9.7	6.9	6.3	0.9
Chicken, Hot, Canned, M&S*	½ Can/200g	246	10.8	123	12.8	4.9	5.4	1.9
Chicken, Kashmiri, Waitrose*	1 Serving/400g	640	36.4	160	14.5	5	9.1	0.6
Chicken, Malaysian, Finest, Tesco*	1 Pack/375g	375	8.3	100	7.4	12.2	2.2	0.8
Chicken, Mild, Canned, Bilash, Aldi*	½ Can/200g	180	7.6	90	9.5	4.5	3.8	0.7
Chicken, Mild, with Fluffy Rice, M&S*	1 Pack/225g	238	5.8	106	6.9	13.3	2.6	0.9
Chicken, Piri Piri, & Cajun Rice, Asda*	1 Pack/380g	410	8.7	108	6.7	14	2.3	2.6
Chicken, Red Thai, BFY, M&S*	1 Pack/380g	399	8.7	105	7.5	13.1	2.3	1
Chicken, Red Thai, Waitrose*	½ Pack/175g	287	19.4	164	9.4	5.8	11.1	2
Chicken, Sweet & Sour, Chinese, Tesco*	1 Pack/507g	684	21.8	135	6.6	16.7	4.3	1.6
Chicken, Thai, Green, & Jasmine Rice, Ready Meal	***1 Serving/450g***	***520***	***17.2***	***116***	***7.7***	***12.6***	***3.8***	***1.1***
Chicken, Thai, Green, No Rice, Average	***1 Serving/200g***	***174***	***7***	***87***	***8.2***	***5***	***3.5***	***1.4***
Chicken, Thai, Red, & Jasmine Rice, Ready Meal	***1 Serving/450g***	***500***	***15.3***	***111***	***7.5***	***12.6***	***3.4***	***1***
Chicken, Thai, Red, & Rice, Ready Meal, Healthy	***1 Serving/400g***	***400***	***7.8***	***100***	***6.4***	***14***	***2***	***1***
Chicken, Thai, Red, & Sticky Rice, Ready Meal	***1 Serving/450g***	***527***	***15.7***	***117***	***6.7***	***14.2***	***3.5***	***1.7***
Chicken, Thai, Red, No Rice, Average	***1 Serving/200g***	***194***	***6.9***	***97***	***7.2***	***9***	***3.4***	***1.4***
Chicken, Tikka, Biryani, Tesco*	1 Pack/365g	599	13.9	164	10.2	20.7	3.8	3.5
Chicken, Weight Watchers*	1 Pack/350g	346	4.6	99	5.2	16.2	1.3	1.1
Chicken, with Rice, Average	***1 Serving/400g***	***465***	***11***	***116***	***5.1***	***17.8***	***2.8***	***0.8***

	Measure INFO/WEIGHT	per Measure KCAL	FAT	Nutrition Values per 100g / 100ml KCAL	PROT	CARB	FAT	FIBRE
CURRY								
Chicken, Yellow Thai Style, HL, Tesco*	1 Pack/450g	504	12.2	112	9.3	12.6	2.7	0.5
Chickpea, & Lentil, Bowl, Spiced, Quorn*	1 Bowl/300g	281	6.6	94	5.3	10.7	2.2	5
Cod, Squid, & King Prawn, Keralan, Waitrose*	½ Pack/185g	211	9.6	114	13.5	3	5.2	0.6
Cod, Yellow Thai, with Lime Rice, Hello Fresh*	1 Serving/569g	597	30.7	105	5.8	8.6	5.4	0.4
Courgette, & Potato	***1oz/28g***	***24***	***1.5***	***86***	***1.9***	***8.7***	***5.2***	***1.2***
Delhi Biryani, Meal Kit, The Spice Tailor*	1 Pack/360g	461	10.4	128	0	22	2.9	1.3
Dupiaza, Lamb, Cook*	1 Pack/300g	468	29.1	156	10.1	6	9.7	0
Fish, & Vegetable, Bangladeshi, Average	***1oz/28g***	***33***	***2.4***	***117***	***9.1***	***1.4***	***8.4***	***0.5***
Fish, Bangladeshi, Average	***1oz/28g***	***35***	***2.2***	***124***	***12.2***	***1.5***	***7.9***	***0.3***
Fish, Red Thai, Waitrose*	1 Pack/500g	275	11	55	5.2	3.7	2.2	1
Fish, Yellow Thai, Asian Fusion, Waitrose*	½ Pack/175g	222	15.8	127	6.8	3.9	9	1.4
Goan, Fiery, Meal Kit, The Spice Tailor*	1 Pack/300g	558	45	186	1.9	9	15	2.6
Goan, Meal Kit, Pataks*	½ Pack/157g	248	18.8	158	2.2	8.3	12	0
Gobi, Sri Lankan, Vegan, Hi Five*	1 Pack/500g	270	15	54	2	6	3	2
Katsu, Chicken, & Rice, G&B, Asda*	1 Pack/370g	388	8.1	105	9.4	11	2.2	1.4
Katsu, Chicken, with Sticky Rice, Asian Fusion, Waitrose*	1 Pack/350g	581	21.7	166	8.3	18.1	6.2	2.1
Katsu, Sweet Potato, Plant Kitchen, M&S*	1 Pack/400g	536	16.8	134	3.2	19.8	4.2	2
Keralan, Butternut Squash, Waitrose*	1 Serving/351g	393	22.1	112	2.8	9.8	6.3	2.6
Laksa, Malaysian, Pot, BOL Foods*	1 Pot/345g	376	10.4	109	3.2	16.1	3	2.4
Lamb, Aromatic, BFY, M&S*	1 Pack/380g	483	7.6	127	9.9	16.3	2	2.3
Madras, Beef, Canned, Sainsbury's*	½ Can/200g	246	13.2	123	11.3	3.9	6.6	2.8
Mushroom, & Pea, Masala, Indian, Sainsbury's*	1 Pack/300g	264	14.7	88	3.3	5.2	4.9	5.1
Mutton, wiith Rice, Island Delight*	1 Pack/400g	548	18.4	137	9	15.6	4.6	0
Panang, Coconut, Thai, BOL Foods*	1 Pack/405g	450	19.4	111	3.2	12.7	4.8	2.1
Peanut, Chickpea, Red Rice, Soulful Food Co*	1 Pot/380g	346	11	91	3.5	15	2.9	4
Pork, & Lentil, with Naan Bread, Hello Fresh*	1 Serving/611g	788	32.9	129	6.8	12.4	5.4	0
Potato & Pea	***1oz/28g***	***26***	***1.1***	***92***	***2.9***	***13***	***3.8***	***2.4***
Prawn, & Mushroom	***1oz/28g***	***47***	***4***	***168***	***7.3***	***2.5***	***14.4***	***1***
Prawn, Coconut & Lime, King, Sainsbury's*	½ Pack/351g	207	8.8	59	3.7	5.4	2.5	1
Prawn, Goan, King, M&S*	1 Pack/400g	680	44.4	170	5.1	11.6	11.1	1.5
Prawn, King, Taste Sri Lanka, M&S*	1 Pack/350g	413	23.4	118	6.3	7.3	6.7	1.6
Prawn, Malay, King, Waitrose*	1 Pack/350g	364	19.2	104	6.6	7.1	5.5	0.9
Prawn, Red Thai, Hello Fresh*	1 Serving/467g	579	23.3	124	5	16	5	0
Prawn, Red Thai, Sainsbury's*	1 Pack/300g	546	39.6	182	6.3	9.4	13.2	1.7
Prawn, Takeaway, Average	***1 Serving/350g***	***410***	***29.8***	***117***	***8.2***	***2.2***	***8.5***	***2***
Prawn, Yellow Thai, Cook*	1 Serving/295g	215	8	73	6.4	5.7	2.7	0.4
Red Kidney Bean, Punjabi	***1oz/28g***	***30***	***1.6***	***106***	***4.7***	***10.1***	***5.6***	***3.8***
Red Thai, Vegetarian, Tesco*	1 Pack/429ml	588	21.9	137	5.4	17.3	5.1	1.6
Rendang, Tempeh, Allplants*	1 Pack/360g	464	24.1	129	3.8	12	6.7	2.6
Roasted Cauliflower, & Paneer, Higgidy*	1 Meal/365g	456	28.8	125	4.4	7.4	7.9	3.7
Salmon, Green, Waitrose*	1 Pack/401g	581	40.5	145	9.1	4.5	10.1	2.7
Sambar, Cauli-Coconut, Sri Lankan, BOL Foods*	1 Pot/345g	304	9.7	88	4.6	7.9	2.8	6.2
Satay, Golden Peanut, Allplants*	1 Serving/377g	611	27.5	162	6.8	15	7.3	3.7
Sweet Potato, & Aubergine, Sri Lankan, Cook*	1 Pack/280g	297	12	106	2.2	15.9	4.3	2.5
Sweet Potato, & Cashew, Plant Kitchen, M&S*	1 Pack/340g	411	10.9	121	4.4	16.7	3.2	3.8
Sweet Potato, & Coconut, Plant Based, Asda*	½ Can/196g	149	8	76	1	8.1	4.1	1.4
Sweet Potato, Katsu, with Rice, Sainsbury's*	1 Pack/377g	550	19.6	146	2.2	21.7	5.2	2
Sweet Potato, Slimfree, Aldi*	1 Pack/500g	250	3	50	2.3	6.5	0.6	4.8
Sweet Potato, What's Cooking, Lidl*	1 Serving/550g	335	7.3	61	2.6	7.9	1.3	3.3
Thai Chicken, Jane Plan*	1 Pack/300g	309	10.2	103	6.6	10.5	3.4	2
Thai Green, & Rice, Co-Op*	1 Pack/380g	429	14.1	113	6.3	13	3.7	0.6
Thai Green, Allplants*	1 Serving/405g	446	23.9	110	4.1	9.1	5.9	2
Thai Green, Creamy, Veg Pot, BOL Foods*	1 Pot/345g	314	8.6	91	2.4	13.8	2.5	2

	Measure INFO/WEIGHT	per Measure KCAL	per Measure FAT	KCAL	PROT	CARB	FAT	FIBRE
				Nutrition Values per 100g / 100ml				
CURRY								
Thai Green, Meal Kit, The Spice Tailor*	½ Pack/137g	200	16.4	146	1.9	7.5	12	1.3
Thai Red, Kit, Asda*	½ Pack/122g	160	13.4	131	1.7	5.1	11	0.9
Thai, Coconut, Veg Pot, Vegan, Bol*	1 Pot/345g	307	8.3	89	1.9	14.1	2.4	1.7
Thai, Red, Coconut, Bol*	1 Serving/345g	297	7.6	86	3	12.4	2.2	2.2
Thai, Yellow, Plant Menu, Aldi*	1 Pack/400g	500	18.8	125	2.6	17	4.7	2.1
Tofu, Red Thai, 1, Waitrose*	½ Pack/175g	345	25.9	197	8.7	6.7	14.8	1.1
Tomato, Lentil, & Chickpea, One Pot, Soulful Food Co*	1 Pot/380g	224	4.6	59	2.6	11	1.2	2.5
Vegetable, & Chickpea, Cook*	1 Serving/330g	224	6.3	68	3.2	7.9	1.9	3.3
Vegetable, Canned, Sainsbury's*	½ Can/200g	200	12.2	100	1.4	9.8	6.1	1.8
Vegetable, Canned, Tesco*	1 Can/400g	308	11.2	77	2	9.7	2.8	2.4
Vegetable, Classic, Jane Plan*	1 Pack/300g	261	7.8	87	2.3	12.8	2.6	1.7
Vegetable, Frozen, Mixed Vegetables, Average	***1oz/28g***	***25***	***1.7***	***88***	***2.5***	***6.9***	***6.1***	***0***
Vegetable, Goan, M&S*	½ Pack/200g	204	12.4	102	1.8	8.9	6.2	1.4
Vegetable, Green Thai, Cook*	1 Pack/280g	314	18.2	112	4.7	8.6	6.5	1.7
Vegetable, in Sweet Sauce, Average	***1 Serving/330g***	***162***	***6.9***	***49***	***1.4***	***6.7***	***2.1***	***1.3***
Vegetable, Indian Meal for One, Tesco*	1 Serving/200g	218	14.4	109	2	9	7.2	1.2
Vegetable, Indian, Sainsbury's*	½ Pack/200g	206	14.6	103	2.5	6.8	7.3	4.6
Vegetable, Indian, Tesco*	1 Serving/225g	257	17.8	114	2.1	8.6	7.9	1.6
Vegetable, Medium, Tesco*	1 Pack/350g	326	21.7	93	2.3	7.1	6.2	1.9
Vegetable, Pakistani, Average	***1oz/28g***	***17***	***0.7***	***60***	***2.2***	***8.7***	***2.6***	***2.2***
Vegetable, Red Thai, with Rice, Tesco*	1 Pack/385g	381	11.5	99	4.4	12.6	3	2.1
Vegetable, Sabzi Tarkari, Patak's*	1 Pack/400g	500	31.2	125	2.5	11.1	7.8	2.2
Vegetable, Takeaway, Average	***1 Serving/330g***	***346***	***24.4***	***105***	***2.5***	***7.6***	***7.4***	***0***
Vegetable, Thai Green, Waitrose*	1 Serving/175g	187	12.9	107	1.3	7.7	7.4	2.3
Vegetable, Tinned, Morrisons*	½ Can/196g	135	3.3	69	2.4	10.2	1.7	1.7
Vegetable, with Rice, Healthy Range, Average	***1 Serving/400g***	***351***	***4.6***	***88***	***2.3***	***16.8***	***1.1***	***1.9***
Vegetable, with Rice, Ready Meal, Average	***1 Serving/400g***	***408***	***12***	***102***	***3.3***	***16.4***	***3***	***0***
Vegetable, with Yoghurt, Average	***1oz/28g***	***17***	***1.1***	***62***	***2.6***	***4.6***	***4.1***	***1.4***
Vegetable, Yellow Thai, Sainsbury's*	1 Pack/400g	624	48.8	156	2.2	9.4	12.2	1.1
Vegetable, Yellow, Cook*	1 Serving/270g	367	25.1	136	2.4	10	9.3	1.6
CURRY LEAVES								
Fresh	***1oz/28g***	***23***	***0.3***	***81***	***6.6***	***11***	***1.1***	***0***
CURRY PASTE								
Balti, Sainsbury's*	¼ Jar/50g	73	4.9	147	3.4	7.6	9.9	6.7
Curry, Katsu, Mild, M&S*	¼ Jar/48g	88	4.2	186	4.8	19.6	8.8	4.7
Green Thai, Average	***1 Tsp/5g***	***6***	***0.4***	***128***	***2.1***	***11.7***	***7.9***	***3.1***
Gulyaskrem Cispos, Le Gusto*	1 Serving/15g	18	1	118	2	9	7	0
Hot Madras, M&S*	¼ Jar/50g	90	5.4	179	2.2	16	10.8	4.4
Jalfrezi, Spice, Pataks*	1/8 Jar/35g	101	8.6	285	3.2	7.8	24.3	7.5
Katsu, M&S*	¼ Pot/48g	76	3.8	161	3	17.6	8.1	2.6
Korma, Asda*	1 Tube/100g	338	23.5	338	5.1	26.6	23.5	1.2
Korma, Asian Home Gourmet*	¼ Sachet/13g	35	2.9	271	3.4	11.1	22.4	0
Korma, Cooks' Ingredients, Waitrose*	1 Serving/50g	76	5	152	3.2	10.6	10	3.4
Madras, Cumin & Chilli, Hot, Patak's*	¼ Jar/70g	202	18.1	289	4.7	7.6	25.9	10.8
Madras, Pot, Patak's*	½ Pot/35g	98	8.1	279	4.4	7	23.1	0
Massaman, Thai, Pot, Blue Dragon*	½ Pot/25g	89	6.8	357	4.9	24	27	9.2
Panang, Sainsbury's*	1 Tbsp/15g	17	0.9	115	2.1	10.4	5.7	6.9
Red, Thai, Average	***1 Tsp/5g***	***7***	***0.5***	***132***	***2.3***	***9.5***	***9.1***	***3***
Rogan Josh, Cooks' Ingredients, Waitrose*	1 Serving/50g	50	3	100	2.6	6.8	6	4.1
Rogan Josh, Easy Paste, Sharwood's*	1 Serving/23g	102	8.9	443	5.2	12.5	38.8	11.5
Rogan Josh, Sainsbury's*	¼ Jar/50g	68	3.7	136	2.7	10.4	7.4	8.7
Rogan Josh, Tomato & Paprika, Patak's*	1 Serving/30g	119	11	397	4.1	12.7	36.7	5.9
Stir Fry, Katsu, Chop*	1 Pot/50g	118	7	235	3.2	24	14	3.4

	Measure INFO/WEIGHT	per Measure KCAL	FAT	Nutrition Values per 100g / 100ml KCAL	PROT	CARB	FAT	FIBRE
CURRY PASTE								
Tikka Masala, Spice, Patak's*	1 Tbsp/15g	40	3.4	270	3	7.8	22.9	6.8
Tikka, Geeta's*	1 Pack/80g	210	15.3	262	1.8	20.7	19.1	2.3
Tikka, M&S*	¼ Jar/50g	110	7.8	219	2.8	13.8	15.5	6.4
Tom Yum, Thai Taste*	1 Tsp/13g	35	2	269	5.4	30.8	15.4	7.7
Yellow Thai, Tesco*	1 Tbsp/15g	15	0.6	100	1.9	13.6	4.1	4.9
Yellow, Thai, Barts*	1 Serving/30g	84	3.8	281	2.7	30.4	12.8	8.3
CURRY POWDER								
Average	***1 Tsp/2g***	***6***	***0.3***	***325***	***12.7***	***41.8***	***13.8***	***0***
CUSTARD								
Banana Flavour, Ambrosia*	1 Sm Pot/135g	139	3.9	103	2.9	16.1	2.9	0
Canned, Essential, Waitrose*	¼ Can/100g	101	3.2	101	2.7	15.3	3.2	0
Chocolate Flavour, Pot, Average	***1 Pot/125g***	***138***	***3.4***	***111***	***3.1***	***18.2***	***2.7***	***0.6***
Devon, Individual Pot, Ambrosia*	1 Pot/125g	120	3.6	96	2.8	14.8	2.9	0.5
Low Fat, Average	***1/3 Pot/141g***	***116***	***1.6***	***82***	***2.9***	***15***	***1.2***	***0***
Powder	***1 Tsp/5g***	***18***	***0***	***354***	***0.6***	***92***	***0.7***	***0.1***
Ready To Serve, Aldi*	¼ Pot/125g	152	7.2	122	2.7	15	5.8	0
Ready to Serve, Average	***1 Serving/50g***	***59***	***2.3***	***118***	***3.3***	***16.1***	***4.6***	***0.2***
Salted Caramel Flavour, Morrisons*	½ Pot/150g	167	4.8	111	2.9	17.4	3.2	0.5
Soya, Vanilla, Dairy Free, Deliciously, Alpro*	1 Tbsp/15g	12	0.3	81	3	13.3	1.8	0.5
Strawberry, Canned, Ambrosia*	1/3 Can/130g	116	3.8	89	2.8	12.9	2.9	0.5
Vanilla Flavour, Pot, Average	***1 Pot/125g***	***128***	***3.5***	***102***	***2.8***	***16.4***	***2.8***	***0***
Vanilla, Oat, Oatly*	¼ Pack/63g	97	6.2	155	1	15	10	0
CUSTARD APPLE								
Cherimoya, Weighed without Skin & Seeds, Average	***1 Serving/312g***	***234***	***2.1***	***75***	***1.6***	***17.7***	***0.7***	***3***
CUTLETS								
Nut, Meat Free, Tesco*	1 Cutlet/82g	198	12.2	241	6.8	15.7	14.9	8.7
Nut, Retail, Fried in Vegetable Oil, Average	***1 Cutlet/90g***	***260***	***20.1***	***289***	***4.8***	***18.7***	***22.3***	***1.7***
Nut, Retail, Grilled, Average	***1 Cutlet/90g***	***191***	***11.7***	***212***	***5.1***	***19.9***	***13***	***1.8***

	Measure INFO/WEIGHT	per Measure KCAL	per Measure FAT	Nutrition Values per 100g / 100ml KCAL	PROT	CARB	FAT	FIBRE
DAB								
Raw	***1oz/28g***	***21***	***0.3***	***74***	***15.7***	***0***	***1.2***	***0***
DAHL								
Bhaji, Allplants*	1 Serving/400g	480	14.4	120	5.3	16	3.6	2.4
Black, Ultimate, Jamie Oliver*	1 Serving/125g	162	6.1	130	6.8	13	4.9	3.9
Cauliflower, Coconut, & Lentil, Plant Kitchen, M&S*	1 Pot/300g	270	9.6	90	4.5	9.2	3.2	3.3
Channa, Jane Plan*	1 Pack/220g	326	18.5	148	3.9	12	8.4	4.4
Chickpea, Canned, Love Your Veg!, Sainsbury's*	½ Can/198g	281	12.5	142	5.8	13.9	6.3	3
Coconut, with Aubergine Pickle, Sri Lankan, Gousto*	1 Serving/343g	652	21.5	190	6.8	23.7	6.3	5
Kale, & Chickpea, Allplants*	1 Serving/420g	508	20.6	121	5.4	12	4.9	3.1
Lentil, & Spinach, Meal Pot, Tideford Organics*	1 Pot/300g	141	5.4	47	2	5.1	1.8	1.2
Lentil, Turmeric, Biona Organic*	1 Serving/175g	135	3.2	77	3.9	9.6	1.8	2.4
Tarka, Indian, Waitrose*	1 Pack/300g	432	21.9	144	6.5	7.2	7.3	11.6
Tarka, Lentil Kit, Classic, Aldi*	½ Pack/200g	238	5	119	4.8	18	2.5	2.7
DAIM								
Mondelez*	1 Bar/28g	148	8.7	530	2.9	59	31	1.2
DAIRYLEA DUNKERS								
with Jumbo Tubes, Kraft*	1 Pack/43g	108	5.1	255	9.1	27	12	0.9
with Ritz Crackers, Dairylea, Kraft*	1 Tub/46g	118	5.5	258	9.6	26	12	2.2
DAMSONS								
Raw, Weighed with Stones, Average	***1oz/28g***	***9***	***0***	***31***	***0.4***	***7.7***	***0***	***1.4***
Raw, Weighed without Stones, Average	***1oz/28g***	***11***	***0***	***38***	***0.5***	***9.6***	***0***	***1.8***
DANDELION & BURDOCK								
Barr*	1 Bottle/250ml	40	0	16	0	4	0	0
Fentiman's*	1 Serving/200ml	94	0	47	0	10.6	0	0
Fermented, Botanical, Fentiman's*	1 Bottle/275ml	130	0	47	0	11.6	0	0
Original, Ben Shaws*	1 Can/440ml	88	0	20	0	4.9	0	0
Sparkling, Diet, Morrisons*	1 Glass/200ml	2	0	1	0	0.3	0	0
DANISH PASTRY								
Apple & Sultana, Tesco*	1 Pastry/72g	293	16.4	407	5.4	45	22.8	1.4
Apple Danish, Bakery, Waitrose*	1 Pastry/123g	400	22.2	325	5.1	35.7	18	2.4
Apple, Fresh Cream, Sainsbury's*	1 Pastry/67g	248	14.6	368	3.1	40.2	21.6	0.4
Average	***1 Pastry/110g***	***411***	***19.4***	***374***	***5.8***	***51.3***	***17.6***	***1.6***
Cherry & Custard, Bar, Tesco*	1 Bar/350g	910	49	260	3.5	29.9	14	7.7
Fruit Bears Claw , Waitrose*	1 Pastry/97g	339	15.8	349	4.6	45	16.3	2
Fruit Filled, Average	***1 Pastry/94g***	***335***	***15.9***	***356***	***5.1***	***47.9***	***17***	***0***
Maple, & Pecan, Plait, Bakery, Sainsbury's*	1 Plait/82g	408	28.1	498	5.5	41.1	34.3	1.4
Maple, & Pecan, Plait, Frozen, Tesco*	1 Pastry/78g	348	22.8	447	5.6	39	29.3	2.7
Mini, Selection, Tesco*	1 Pastry/38g	154	8.4	404	5.7	44.3	22.2	2.2
DATES								
Dried, Average	***1 Date/5g***	***13***	***0***	***266***	***2.8***	***64.1***	***0.4***	***4.1***
Dried, Medjool, Average	***1 Date/20g***	***56***	***0.1***	***279***	***2.2***	***69.3***	***0.3***	***4.3***
Fresh, Raw, Yellow, Average	***1 Date/20g***	***21***	***0***	***107***	***1.3***	***27.1***	***0.1***	***1.5***
Medjool, Stuffed with Walnuts, Tesco*	2 Dates/40g	98	2.3	245	4.4	44	5.7	3.4
Milk Chocolate Covered, Holland & Barrett*	1 Date/17g	65	1.9	384	4.5	66	11.3	2.6
DELI FILLER								
Cheese & Onion, Essential, Waitrose*	1 Pot/170g	692	64.8	407	10.8	4.5	38.1	1.5
Chicken & Bacon, Co-Op*	1 Pack/200g	420	29.6	210	17.6	1	14.8	2.6
Chicken, Bacon, & Sweetcorn, M&S*	1 Serving/30g	65	5	216	10.5	5.7	16.7	0.5
King Prawn & Avocado, M&S*	1 Pack/170g	425	38.8	250	9.5	1.4	22.8	0.5
Prawn & Mayonnaise, M&S*	1 Serving/60g	150	13.8	250	11.3	1	23	0.5
Prawn Cocktail, Eat Well, M&S*	½ Pot/85g	119	7.3	140	9.1	6.4	8.6	0.6
Seafood, & Prawn Cocktail, M&S*	1 Serving/50g	100	7.8	199	5.8	9	15.5	0.5
Tuna, & Sweetcorn, Reduced Fat, M&S*	¼ Pot/55g	86	5.7	157	9.1	6.4	10.3	0

	Measure	per Measure		Nutrition Values per 100g / 100ml				
	INFO/WEIGHT	KCAL	FAT	KCAL	PROT	CARB	FAT	FIBRE
DESSERT								
Apple Crumble, Sainsbury's*	1 Pot/136g	291	10.5	214	3.2	33	7.7	2.7
Banana Split	***1 Serving/175g***	***368***	***25.5***	***210***	***2.2***	***18***	***14.6***	***0.2***
Banoffee, Layered, Sainsbury's*	1 Pot/115g	270	14.7	235	2.2	27.8	12.8	1
Banoffee, Pot, The Coconut Collaborative*	1 Pot/45g	104	9	232	0.7	13	20	1
Banoffee, Sainsbury's*	1 Pot/140g	360	19.1	257	2.7	30.9	13.6	1.3
Billionaire's, Pots, Gastropub, M&S*	1 Pot/80g	293	16.2	366	1.8	43.1	20.3	2
Buche, Aldi*	1 Buche/200g	484	34	242	3	20	17	0.8
Caramel, Pots Of Joy, Dairy Milk, Cadbury*	1 Pot/70g	150	7.3	215	2.5	27.1	10.5	0.1
Caramel, Soya, Creamy, Sweet, Alpro*	1 Pot/125g	106	2.2	85	3.2	13.7	1.8	0.5
Choc Delight, Brooklea, Aldi*	1 Pot/80g	74	1.2	92	4.5	15	1.5	0.6
Chocolate Fix, Belgian, with Mint, Mullerlight, Muller*	1 Pot/100g	97	2.9	97	3.5	14.7	2.9	0
Chocolate, & Orange, Pot, Finest, Tesco*	1 Pot/80g	212	12.3	265	3.9	27	15.4	1.3
Chocolate, & Salted Caramel, Pot, Finest, Tesco*	1 Pot/80g	227	12.6	283	4	31	15.7	1
Chocolate, Brownie, Double, Weight Watchers*	1 Pot/86g	167	3.3	194	5.1	33.7	3.8	2.4
Chocolate, Buttons, Milk, Cadbury*	1 Pot/100g	280	14.9	280	6.2	30.8	14.9	0
Chocolate, Buttons, Twin Pot, Cadbury*	1 Pot/90g	220	11.7	245	4.4	27.5	13	0.6
Chocolate, Creme, King Frais, Lidl*	1 Pot/125g	131	3.6	105	2.6	17	2.9	0
Chocolate, Dark, Soya, Alpro*	1 Pot/125g	118	2.9	94	3	14.7	2.3	1.4
Chocolate, Everyday Value, Tesco*	1 Pot/100g	121	4	121	2.7	18.4	4	0.4
Chocolate, Fix, Mullerlight, Muller*	1 Pot/100g	94	1.9	94	3.2	15.2	1.9	0
Chocolate, Frappe, Skinny, COU, M&S*	1 Pot/100g	116	2.6	116	6.2	16.9	2.6	0.5
Chocolate, Little Choc Pots, The Coconut Collaborative*	1 Pot/45g	103	5.8	228	2.5	24.8	13	1.5
Chocolate, Muffin, Skinny, Low Fat, COU, M&S*	1 Pot/110g	154	3.1	140	5.2	23.5	2.8	0.5
Chocolate, Muffin, Tesco*	1 Serving/104g	354	21.2	340	3.5	35.5	20.4	2.1
Chocolate, Muffin, Waitrose*	1 Serving/110g	138	3	126	5.2	20	2.7	0.4
Chocolate, Pots Of Joy , Dairy Milk, Cadbury*	1 Pot /70g	158	8.2	225	4.2	25.6	11.7	0.1
Chocolate, Salted Caramel, Pot, M&S*	1 Pot/85g	341	25	401	5.2	30.3	29.4	0
Chocolate, Soya, Silky Smooth, Alpro*	1 Pot/125g	104	2.4	83	3	13	1.9	1.1
Chocolate, White Buttons, Pots of Joy, Cadbury*	1 Pot /70g	158	6.6	225	4.8	30.4	9.4	0
Coconut, & Berry, Chia Pot, Allplants*	1 Pot/295g	463	18	157	5	18	6.1	4.7
Coconut, Blueberry, Pot, Plant Kitchen, M&S*	1 Pot/120g	146	10.8	122	0.8	9.4	9	0.1
Coconut, Pot, Plant Kitchen, M&S*	1/3 Pot/117g	146	12.1	125	1.2	6.8	10.3	1
Coconut, Vanilla, Pot, Plant Kitchen, M&S*	1/3 Pot/117g	141	11.7	121	1.2	6.6	10	0.1
Coffee, Italian Style, Free From, Tesco*	1 Pot/90g	210	8.2	233	1.3	36.2	9.1	0.6
Creme Caramel, Sainsbury's*	1 Pot/100g	116	1.6	116	2.6	22.9	1.6	0
Creme, Caramel, Salted, Bonne Maman*	1 Pot/90g	220	13.5	245	1.6	25	15	0.5
Creme, Coffee, Bonne Maman*	1 Pot/90g	178	12.6	198	2.1	15	14	0.5
Creme, Vanilla, Bonne Maman*	1 Pot/90g	190	13.1	211	2.1	17.9	14.6	0
Jaffa Cake, COU, M&S*	1 Serving/120g	138	3.1	115	2.4	20.1	2.6	1
Jaffa Cake, Tesco*	1/6 Pack/100g	162	7.7	162	2.2	20.4	7.7	1.1
Jaffa, COU, M&S*	1 Pot/107g	155	4.9	145	3.4	22.4	4.6	0.5
Jaffa, Skinny, M&S*	1 Pot/107g	167	4	156	2.7	27	3.7	1.7
Key Lime Pie	***1 Serving/125g***	***431***	***25***	***344***	***4.1***	***37.9***	***20***	***1.4***
Limone, Italiamo, Lidl*	1 Serving/75g	191	5	255	2.6	43.4	6.6	0
Mango, & Turmeric, Chia Pot, Allplants*	1 Serving/188g	299	11.3	159	4.8	19	6	3.9
Milky Bar, White Chocolate, Nestle*	1 Pot/70g	105	5.5	150	4.4	18.4	7.9	0
Millionaire's Shortbread, M&S*	1 Dessert/120g	440	27.8	365	3.2	35.5	23.1	1
Mississippi Mud Pie	***1 Serving/125g***	***480***	***32***	***384***	***5.3***	***33.1***	***25.6***	***1.8***
Raspberry, Royale, Essential, Waitrose*	1 Pot/150g	216	10.6	144	1.1	18.9	7.1	0.5
Rolo, Nestle*	1 Pot/70g	170	8.3	243	3.3	30.8	11.9	0.5
Strawberry, & Raspberry, Charlotte, COU, M&S*	1 Pot/110g	153	1.2	139	2.1	29.7	1.1	1.1
Tiramisu	***1 Serving/150g***	***420***	***20.8***	***280***	***4.4***	***34***	***13.9***	***0.8***
Toffee, Cheesecake, Individual, Dessert Menu, Aldi*	1 Dessert/100g	266	12	266	2.5	36	12	0.5

	Measure INFO/WEIGHT	per Measure KCAL	per Measure FAT	Nutrition Values per 100g / 100ml KCAL	PROT	CARB	FAT	FIBRE
DESSERT								
Trifle, Chocolate, Cadbury*	1 Pot /90g	234	13.8	260	4.8	22.5	15.3	0
Vanilla, Soya, Heavenly Velvet, Alpro*	1 Pot/125g	94	2.8	75	3.7	9.5	2.2	1
DHAL								
Black Gram, Average	***1oz/28g***	***21***	***1***	***74***	***4.2***	***7***	***3.4***	***1.7***
Chick Pea	***1oz/28g***	***42***	***1.7***	***149***	***7.4***	***17.7***	***6.1***	***3.8***
Lentil, Red Masoor & Tomato with Butter, Average	***1oz/28g***	***26***	***1.4***	***94***	***4***	***9.7***	***4.9***	***0.9***
Lentil, Red Masoor & Vegetable, Average	***1oz/28g***	***31***	***1.1***	***110***	***5.8***	***14.7***	***3.8***	***1.8***
Lentil, Red Masoor with Vegetable Oil, Average	***1oz/28g***	***48***	***2.2***	***172***	***7.6***	***19.2***	***7.9***	***1.8***
Lentil, Red Masoor, Punjabi, Average	***1oz/28g***	***39***	***1.3***	***139***	***7.2***	***19.2***	***4.6***	***2***
Lentil, Red Masoorl & Mung Bean, Average	***1oz/28g***	***32***	***1.9***	***114***	***4.8***	***9.9***	***6.7***	***1.6***
Mung Bean, Bengali	***1oz/28g***	***20***	***0.9***	***73***	***4.2***	***7.4***	***3.3***	***1.7***
Mung Beans, Dried, Boiled in Unsalted Water	***1oz/28g***	***26***	***0.1***	***92***	***7.8***	***15.3***	***0.4***	***0***
Split Peas, Yellow, Chana, Asda*	1 Serving/275g	300	19.2	109	2.6	9	7	1.8
Tarka, Asda*	½ Pack/150g	216	12	144	6	12	8	6
Tarka, M&S*	1 Serving/250g	235	8.8	94	4.3	9.4	3.5	3.7
Vegetable, Microwaved, Slimming World*	1 Pack/350g	259	2.1	74	5.4	8.3	0.6	7
DHANSAK								
Butternut, Slim Cook, Tesco*	1 Pack/485g	364	3.9	75	3.8	10.5	0.8	5.1
Chicken with Bagara Rice, Waitrose*	1 Pack/450g	549	8.1	122	8.2	18.2	1.8	1.2
Vegetable, Curry, Microwaved, Slimzone, Asda*	1 Portion/459g	225	2.3	49	2.5	7.7	0.5	2.6
Vegetable, Sainsbury's*	1 Serving/200g	148	5.6	74	3.1	8.9	2.8	2.8
DILL								
Dried, Average	***1 Tsp/1g***	***3***	***0***	***253***	***19.9***	***42.2***	***4.4***	***13.6***
Fresh, Average	***1 Tbsp/3g***	***1***	***0***	***25***	***3.7***	***0.9***	***0.8***	***2.5***
DIP								
Aubergine, Eridanous, Lidl*	½ Pack/125g	275	25.5	220	1.2	7.8	20.4	0
Aubergine, Fresh, Waitrose*	1 Serving/85g	159	12.8	187	2.5	10.5	15	1.7
Baba Ganoush, Sabra*	1 Serving/75g	188	17.6	251	3.9	4.4	23.5	0
Babaganoush, Delphi*	1 Serving/30g	51	4.8	169	2.8	2.2	16	2.5
Bean, Mexican, Doritos, Walkers*	1 Tbsp/20g	18	0.7	89	2.7	12.1	3.3	2.4
Beetroot, & Mint, Meadow Fresh, Lidl*	¼ Pack/50g	58	3	116	3.1	10.6	6	3.6
Beetroot, & Mint, The Deli, Aldi*	¼ Pot/50g	66	3.8	131	3.5	10	7.6	4.2
Beetroot, Feta, & Seed, Sainsbury's*	½ Pack/80g	128	8.6	160	5.5	9.1	10.8	2.6
Caramel, Salted, for Mini Doughnuts, Tesco*	1 Dip/3g	11	0.3	386	2.9	68.7	11.1	0
Carrot, & Houmous, Co-Op*	1 Pack/105g	85	4.9	81	2.3	6.3	4.7	2.1
Cheese & Chive, 50% Less Fat, Asda*	1 Pot/125g	261	21.5	209	4.5	9	17.2	0
Cheese & Chive, Asda*	1 Serving/43g	190	19.6	447	4.9	3.4	46	0
Cheese & Chive, Tesco*	¼ Pack/50g	148	13.9	296	3.8	7.5	27.8	0.2
Cheese & Chive, The Deli, Aldi*	1 Serving/31g	107	10.5	345	4.6	5.7	34	0.5
Chilli Cheese, Asda*	1 Serving/50g	131	11	262	8	8	22	1.1
Chilli, M&S*	1 Pot/35g	103	0.1	295	0.4	73.2	0.2	0.4
Cracked Corn, Hella Hot, Wicked Kitchen, Tesco*	1 Serving/30g	27	1.3	90	2	10.2	4.3	1.2
Edamame, & Ginger, Meadow Fresh, Lidl*	¼ Pot/50g	59	3	118	3.3	10.6	5.9	4.6
Endamame & Pea, Waitrose*	¼ Pot/51g	85	5.9	166	6.3	8	11.6	2
Garlic & Herb	***1 Serving/100g***	***584***	***62.4***	***584***	***1.4***	***4.1***	***62.4***	***0.2***
Garlic, & Onion, 30% Less Fat, Asda*	1 Serving/30g	50	3.9	166	3.9	8.2	13	0.5
Garlic, Takeaway Pizza, Goodfella's*	1 Pot/18g	57	5.4	319	0.3	12	30	0
Guacamole, Tex-Mex Multipack Selection, Tesco*	½ Pot/53g	76	6.8	142	1.1	4	12.8	3
Nacho Cheese, Average	***1 Serving/50g***	***175***	***17.2***	***350***	***6.3***	***3.4***	***34.4***	***0.9***
Onion & Garlic, Average	***1 Tbsp/15g***	***62***	***6.4***	***410***	***1.7***	***4.8***	***42.7***	***0.4***
Onion, & Garlic, Reduced Fat, Tesco*	¼ Pot/50g	64	4.8	128	3.7	6.5	9.6	0.6
Onion, Three, Toasted, Wicked Kitchen, Tesco*	½ Pot/85g	269	26.3	317	2.2	7.6	30.9	0.3

	Measure INFO/WEIGHT	per Measure KCAL	FAT	Nutrition Values per 100g / 100ml KCAL	PROT	CARB	FAT	FIBRE
DIP								
Pea & Spinach, Tesco*	¼ Pot/46g	34	1	75	4	7.7	2.1	4.4
Pea, & Mint, The Deli, Aldi*	¼ Pack/50g	52	3	103	3.3	6.4	6.1	4.4
Pea, & Spinach, Tesco*	¼ Pot/46g	61	4	132	3.1	8.6	8.6	3.9
Pea, Yogurt & Mint, Sainsbury's*	¼ Pack/50g	119	10.8	238	3.4	7.5	21.6	2.1
Peanut, Satay Selection, Occasions, Sainsbury's*	1 Serving/2g	4	0.2	186	7.1	13.8	11.4	1.1
Pecorino, Basil & Pine Nut, Fresh, Waitrose*	½ Pot/85g	338	33.7	398	5.1	5.1	39.7	0
Ponzu, for Gyoza, Plant Kitchen, M&S*	1 Pot/22g	12	0	55	2.7	10.4	0.2	0.5
Raita, Tesco*	1 Serving/40g	81	7.8	203	1.6	4.8	19.6	0.3
Red Pepper, Chilli, & Garlic, Morrisons*	¼ Pot/50g	88	7.3	177	2.2	8.8	14.6	0.8
Red Pepper, Meadow Fresh, Lidl*	¼ Pot/50g	59	3	118	3.3	10.6	5.9	4.6
Red Pepper, Sainsbury's*	1 Pot/100g	103	4	103	2.3	14.6	4	0
Red Pepper, The Deli, Aldi*	¼ Pot/50g	60	3	119	3.6	11	6	4
Salsa, Chunky Tomato, Tesco*	1 Pot/170g	68	2.2	40	1.1	5.9	1.3	1.1
Salsa, Chunky, Fresh, Sainsbury's*	1 Serving/100g	51	1.7	51	1.1	7.8	1.7	1.2
Salsa, Hot, Snaktastic, Lidl*	1 Serving/50g	17	0.1	34	1.3	6.1	0.2	1.5
Salsa, Mango, Ginger & Chilli, Spiced, Weight Watchers*	1 Serving/56g	48	0.1	85	1	19.9	0.2	2.6
Salsa, Mild, Asda*	1 Portion/100g	38	0.5	38	1.5	6.7	0.5	0.6
Salsa, Mild, Doritos, Walkers*	1 Tbsp/30g	9	0.1	30	0.8	6	0.3	1.5
Salsa, Mild, Snaktastic, Lidl*	1 Serving/50g	21	0.2	42	1.6	7.7	0.4	0.6
Sour Cream & Chive, Half Fat, Waitrose*	½ Pot/85g	133	9.9	157	5.5	7.6	11.6	0.1
Sour Cream & Chive, Reduced Fat, Tesco*	¼ Pot/50g	80	6.1	159	4.2	7.9	12.2	0.2
Sour Cream & Chive, Average	***1 Tbsp/15g***	***48***	***4.8***	***317***	***3.2***	***4***	***32***	***0.3***
Sour Cream, & Chive, 30% Less Fat, Asda*	¼ Pot/50g	60	4.2	119	3.9	6.9	8.3	0.7
Sour Cream, & Chive, Reduced Fat, M&S*	1 Pack/230g	389	32.7	169	4.7	4.9	14.2	1.5
Sour Cream, & Chive, Reduced Fat, Morrisons*	¼ Pot/50g	70	5.5	139	4	5.8	11	0.1
Soy, Gyoza Selection, Tesco*	1 Pot/30g	30	0.2	100	1.7	21.4	0.7	0.7
Sweetcorn, & Chilli, Tesco*	¼ Pot/46g	53	1.6	115	2.9	17.3	3.4	1.7
Taramasalata, Sainsbury's*	¼ Pot/57g	267	26.6	465	3.3	8.6	46.3	0.5
DOLMADES								
Stffed Vine Leaves, Delphi*	1 Dolmade/30g	36	0.8	119	2.2	21.9	2.5	1.1
Stuffed with Rice, M&S*	1 Leaf/38g	40	1.6	105	2.6	14.2	4.1	1.2
DOPIAZA								
Chicken, Indian, Waitrose*	½ Pack/175g	243	14.5	139	10.2	5	8.3	1.6
Chicken, M&S*	1 Pack/350g	402	21.4	115	11.5	3.7	6.1	2.5
Chicken, Slimming World*	1 Pack/500g	335	6	67	9.1	4.2	1.2	1.6
Mushroom, Retail	***1oz/28g***	***19***	***1.6***	***69***	***1.3***	***3.7***	***5.7***	***1.1***
DORITOS								
Chilli Heatwave, Walkers*	1 Bag/30g	148	7.6	495	6.3	57.3	25.3	6.7
Cool Spice 3ds, Walkers*	1 Bag/24g	108	4.3	450	8	64	18	4.4
Cool, Original, Walkers*	1 Bag/70g	349	17.8	498	5.9	58.1	25.5	5.6
Dippas, Hint of Lime, Walkers*	1 Bag/35g	173	8.8	495	7	60	25	3.5
Dippas, Lightly Salted, Dipping Chips, Walkers*	1 Serving/25g	128	6.8	510	6.5	60	27	3
Lighly Salted, Corn Chips, Doritos*	1 Bag/30g	149	7.1	497	6.9	62.9	23.6	3.3
Sweet Chilli, Walkers*	1 Serving/28g	140	7	500	7.1	64.3	25	3.6
Tangy Cheese, Walkers*	1 Bag/40g	200	10.8	500	7	57	27	3
DOUBLE DECKER								
Cadbury*	1 Bar/54.5g	253	9.3	464	3.7	73	17	1.6
Dinky Deckers, Cadbury*	1 Piece/5g	22	0.8	456	4.2	71	17	1.5
Snack Size, Cadbury*	1 Bar/36g	165	7.4	465	4.8	64.5	20.9	0
DOUGH BALLS								
Garlic, Cooked, Morrisons*	¼ Pack/42g	146	5	349	9.4	50.2	11.9	1.9
with Garlic & Herb Butter, Aldi*	1 Ball/12g	45	2.2	365	7.7	46.7	18.2	1.8
with Garlic Butter Dip, Supermarket, Pizza Express*	4 Balls/46g	130	1	280	10.6	53.1	2.2	2.7

D

	Measure INFO/WEIGHT	per Measure KCAL	FAT	Nutrition Values per 100g / 100ml KCAL	PROT	CARB	FAT	FIBRE
DOUGHNUTS								
Caramel Cream, Baker's Soft, Tesco*	1 Doughnut/61g	200	10.6	328	6.2	35.2	17.4	2.7
Chocolate, Bakery, Tesco*	1 Doughnut/66g	250	12.8	379	6.6	43.5	19.4	2.2
Chocolate, Iced, Ring, Bakery, Sainsbury's*	1 Doughnut/55g	212	10.3	386	6.3	47.4	18.8	1
Custard Filled, Average	***1 Doughnut/75g***	***268***	***14.2***	***358***	***6.2***	***43.3***	***19***	***0***
Glazed, Bakery, Tesco*	1 Doughnut/52g	202	10.1	389	6.5	45.9	19.5	2
Glazed, Ring, Bakery, Sainsbury's*	1 Doughnut/62g	229	12	369	5.5	42.8	19.3	1.1
Iced, Raspberry Filled, Morrisons*	1 Doughnut/65g	245	10.7	378	5.5	51	16.5	1.5
Jam, & Cream, Asda*	1 Doughnut/41g	139	7.4	336	4.9	39	18	0.6
Jam, & Cream, Cream Cake Selection, Tesco*	1 Doughnut/71g	225	10.2	317	6	40.4	14.4	1
Jam, & Fresh Cream, Tesco*	1 Dougnut/71g	223	9.5	314	5.6	41.7	13.4	1.7
Jam, Filled, Average	***1 Doughnut/75g***	***252***	***10.9***	***336***	***5.7***	***48.8***	***14.5***	***0***
Mini, Sainsbury's*	1 Doughnut/14g	53	2.7	379	5.2	47.9	18.9	2.1
Plain, Ring, Average	***1 Doughnut/60g***	***238***	***13***	***397***	***6.1***	***47.2***	***21.7***	***0***
Raspberry Jam, Sainsbury's*	1 Doughnut/58g	203	8.9	350	5.5	46.4	15.3	2.3
Ring, Iced, Average	***1 Doughnut/70g***	***268***	***12.2***	***383***	***4.8***	***55.1***	***17.5***	***0***
Ring, Mini, Bakers Selection, Asda*	1 Doughnut/13g	55	2.8	409	5.2	49	21	1.4
Selection, Bakers Selection, Asda*	1 Doughnut/75g	273	17.9	365	4.5	32	24	1.4
Strawberry, Iced, Ring, Bakery, Tesco*	1 Doughnut/58g	248	14.3	428	5.4	45.3	24.7	1.4
Strawberry, Iced, Ring, Mini, Bakery, Tesco*	1 Doughnut/15g	62	3.1	415	4.9	51.5	20.8	1.3
Sugar, Ring, Bakery, Sainsbury's*	1 Doughnut/51g	222	14	435	5.7	40.7	27.4	2.1
Vanilla, Bakery, Sainsbury's*	1 Doughnut/66g	248	12.9	376	6.1	42.7	19.6	2
White Iced, Ring, Bakery, Sainsbury's*	1 Doughnut/55g	211	10.2	383	7	46.4	18.6	1
Yum Yums, Glazed, Sweet, Waitrose*	1 Doughnut/45g	172	10	382	4	41.6	22.2	2
Yum Yums, M&S*	1 Doughnut/37g	155	8.9	420	4.9	45.7	23.9	1.6
Yum Yums, Sainsbury's*	1 Doughnut/50g	214	12.4	428	4.8	45.8	24.7	1.3
DOVER SOLE								
Fillet, Raw, Average	***1oz/28g***	***25***	***0.5***	***89***	***18.1***	***0***	***1.8***	***0***
DR PEPPER*								
Coca-Cola*	1 Can/330ml	66	0	20	0	4.9	0	0
Zero, Coca-Cola*	1 Can/330ml	2	0	0	0	0	0	0
DRAGON FRUIT								
Raw, Edible Portion, Average	***1 Serving/100g***	***41***	***0.5***	***41***	***0.7***	***9.6***	***0.5***	***3.6***
DRAMBUIE								
39% Volume	***1 Pub Shot/35ml***	***125***	***0***	***358***	***0***	***23***	***0***	***0***
DRESSING								
French, Style, BGTY, Sainsbury's*	1 Tbsp/15ml	11	0.4	76	0.7	12.6	2.5	0.5
Balsamic, & Olive Oil, Sainsbury's*	1 Serving/25ml	104	10.4	415	0.9	9.4	41.8	0.2
Balsamic, & Olive Oil, Tesco*	1 Tbsp/15ml	45	4.2	297	1.1	10.6	27.8	0
Balsamic, BGTY, Sainsbury's*	1 Tbsp/15ml	11	0.1	74	0.5	17.3	0.5	1
Balsamic, Fig Glaze, Tesco*	1 Tbsp/15ml	31	0	208	1.4	47.9	0	0
Balsamic, Low Fat, Tesco*	1 Tbsp/15ml	10	0.2	65	0.2	13.3	1.1	0.9
Balsamic, Sainsbury's*	1 Tbsp/15ml	21	0.8	138	0.5	21.9	5.4	0.5
Balsamic, Sweet, BGTY, Sainsbury's*	1 Tsp/5g	3	0	61	0.5	13.6	0.5	0.5
Balsamic, Vinegar, Asda*	1 Tsp/5ml	7	0.2	146	0.5	27	4	0
Beetroot, & Balsamic, Morrisons*	1 Tbsp/15ml	11	0	73	0.7	16.9	0.2	0.6
Blue Cheese, Hellmann's*	1 Tbsp/15g	69	7.1	459	0.7	6.3	47.2	1.1
Blue Cheese, Salad, Waitrose*	1 Serving/50g	265	25.2	530	2.1	17.3	50.3	4.1
Caesar, Asiago, Briannas*	1 Tbsp/15ml	70	7.5	467	3.3	3.3	50	0
Caesar, Chilled, Reduced Fat, Tesco*	1 Tsp/5ml	13	1.2	252	6.5	3.1	23.7	0.1
Caesar, Classic, Sainsbury's*	1 Tsp/5ml	22	2.3	442	2.7	4.6	45.9	0.5
Caesar, Creamy, Asda*	1 Tbsp/15ml	34	3.3	225	1.5	12	22	1
Caesar, Creamy, M&S*	1 Tbsp/15ml	66	6.5	437	2.6	9.1	43.1	1
Caesar, Fat Free, Average	***1 Tsp/5g***	***4***	***0.2***	***84***	***4.6***	***11***	***4.1***	***0.2***

	Measure INFO/WEIGHT	per Measure KCAL	FAT	Nutrition Values per 100g / 100ml KCAL	PROT	CARB	FAT	FIBRE
DRESSING								
Caesar, Finest, Tesco*	1 Tbsp/15ml	72	7.6	477	1.9	2.8	50.9	0.2
Caesar, Hellmann's*	1 Tsp/6g	30	3.1	499	2.5	4.5	51.7	0.3
Caesar, Low Fat, Average	***1 Tsp/5g***	***4***	***0.1***	***77***	***2.3***	***11.1***	***2.6***	***0.2***
Caesar, Original, Cardini's*	1 Serving/10ml	56	6	555	2.3	1.5	60	0.2
Caesar, Rich & Creamy, Waitrose*	1 Serving/15ml	78	8.3	518	2.2	2.4	55.4	0.8
Caesar, Supermarket, Pizza Express*	1 Serving/20ml	72	7	359	3.3	6.7	35	0.3
Caesar, Tesco*	1 Tbsp/15ml	59	6.1	393	1	4.9	40.9	0.4
Caesar, The Best, Morrisons*	1 Tbsp/15ml	48	4.7	322	3.2	7.1	31.1	0.6
Caesar, Vegan, Sacla*	1 Tbsp/15ml	65	6.9	432	0.3	4.1	46	0
Caesar, Waitrose*	1 Serving/15ml	72	7.6	479	4.5	0.9	50.8	0.2
Caesar, with Smoked Garlic, Hellmann's*	1 Tbsp/15ml	35	3.3	231	2	6.4	22	0
Chilli, & Herb, Morrisons*	1 Tbsp/15ml	21	1.1	140	1.1	17	7.3	0.9
Cucumber, & Mint, M&S*	1 Tbsp/15ml	46	3.9	305	0.7	16.7	26.1	0.1
Drizzle, with Balsamic Vinegar of Modena, Tesco*	1 Tbsp/15ml	27	0	183	0.7	44.4	0	1.1
French, Chilled, Tesco*	1 Tbsp/15ml	63	5.9	421	1.1	15.1	39.6	0
French, Classic, Fresh, M&S*	1 Serving/10ml	52	5.3	515	0.6	8.2	53.1	0.2
French, Classics, M&S*	1 Tbsp/15ml	77	8	516	0.6	8.2	53.1	0.2
French, Fresh, Organic, Sainsbury's*	1 Tbsp/15ml	45	4.6	301	0.4	5.5	31	0.4
French, Fresh, Sainsbury's*	1 Tbsp/15ml	64	6.7	429	0.6	6.6	44.6	0.6
French, LC, Tesco*	1 Tbsp/16g	8	0.3	50	0.8	7.6	1.6	1.1
French, Reduced Fat, M&S*	1 Tbsp/15g	10	0.4	70	0.7	11.5	2.8	0.7
French, Reduced Fat, Tesco*	1 Tbsp/15ml	10	0.2	65	0.5	13	1.3	0
French, Tesco*	1 Serving/25ml	110	11.2	441	0.7	7.2	44.9	0.2
French, Virtually Fat Free, Aldi*	1 Serving/10g	3	0	33	0.9	6.7	0.3	1.1
Garlic & Herb, Tesco*	1 Tbsp/15g	32	3	210	0.9	5.8	20.2	0.8
Glaze, with Balsamic Vinegar Of Modena, Asda*	1 Tbsp/15g	31	0.1	204	1	49	0.5	1
Honey & Mustard, BGTY, Sainsbury's*	1 Tbsp/15g	12	0.2	78	0.5	16.1	1.3	0.5
Honey & Mustard, Finest, Tesco*	1 Serving/25ml	72	5.6	288	1.7	19.6	22.5	0.7
Honey & Mustard, Hellmann's*	1 Serving/15ml	27	0.2	182	0.7	13.7	1.6	0.3
Honey & Mustard, M&S*	1 Tbsp/15ml	47	3.8	313	2.7	16.8	25.5	2.8
Honey & Mustard, Supermarket, Pizza Express*	1 Serving/45ml	197	17.6	437	1.4	18	39	0.9
Honey & Mustard, Tesco*	1 Tbsp/15ml	33	2.3	220	0.8	18.8	15.2	2.5
House, Classic, Salad, Hellmann's*	1 Tbsp/15ml	38	3.9	254	0.5	5.7	26	0
House, Light, Supermarket, Pizza Express*	1 Tbsp/15ml	45	4.5	300	0.7	4.3	30	0.3
House, Supermarket, Pizza Express*	1 Tbsp/15ml	62	6.6	415	0.7	3.3	44	0.3
Lemon, & Black Pepper, Fat Free, Tesco*	1 Tbsp/15ml	11	0	74	0.1	17.8	0.1	0.9
Lemon, & Herb, Counted, Morrisons*	1 Serving/15ml	6	0.3	39	0.5	4.9	1.7	1.2
Light, Salad, Mary Berry*	1 Tbsp/15ml	34	2.8	230	0.8	14	19	0.6
Mary Berry*	1 Serving/15g	77	6.6	513	0.8	28.5	44	0.1
Oil & Lemon	***1 Tbsp/15g***	***97***	***10.6***	***647***	***0.3***	***2.8***	***70.6***	***0***
Ranch, Specially Selected, Aldi*	1 Serving/15ml	32	0.9	216	2.7	37	6.3	0.5
Salad, Balsamic Vinaigrette, Specially Selected, Aldi*	1 Tbsp/15ml	44	3.8	293	3.3	15.3	25.3	3.3
Salad, Balsamic, with Garlic, Spray, Heinz*	1 Spray/1ml	1	0.1	82	0.4	10.3	4.3	0
Salad, Caesar, Inspired Vegan*	1 Tbsp/15ml	51	4.8	340	4	7.7	32.3	0.5
Salad, Lemon, & Thyme, Specially Selected, Aldi*	1 Tbsp/15ml	23	1.2	157	0.5	21	7.9	1.2
Salad, Raspberry Balsamic, Spray, Heinz*	20 Sprays/15ml	23	1.9	156	0.4	9.3	13.1	0
Soy, Chilli, & Ginger, Counted, Morrisons*	1 Tbsp/15ml	8	0	51	0.2	11.8	0.3	0.3
Soy, Chilli, & Ginger, Specially Selected, Aldi*	1 Tbsp/15ml	19	1.2	124	0.5	11	8.3	1.2
Super Nutty, Soy, Wholefood, M&S*	1 Pack/230g	301	11.7	131	5.3	12.8	5.1	6.1
Sweet Chilli, & Coriander, Sainsbury's*	1 Tbsp/15g	38	2.4	255	1.1	26.5	16	0.5
Thousand Island	***1 Tsp/6g***	***19***	***1.8***	***323***	***1.1***	***12.5***	***30.2***	***0.4***
Thousand Island, Reduced Calorie	***1 Tsp/6g***	***12***	***0.9***	***195***	***0.7***	***14.7***	***15.2***	***0***

	Measure INFO/WEIGHT	per Measure KCAL	per Measure FAT	KCAL	PROT	CARB	FAT	FIBRE
				Nutrition Values per 100g / 100ml				
DRIED FRUIT								
Apricots, Soft, Alesto, Lidl*	1 Serving/30g	81	0.1	269	2	61.3	0.3	6.4
Berry, Mix, Diet Chef Ltd*	1 Pack/25g	84	0.2	337	1.4	77.6	0.8	4.8
Fruity Biscuit Shot, Whitworths*	1 Pack/25g	93	2.1	372	2.8	69.2	8.4	4.5
Mixed, Trio, Holland & Barrett*	1 Serving/30g	82	0.2	273	2.3	69.2	0.5	2
Raisin & Chocolate, Shot, Whitworths*	1 Pack/25g	91	2.3	364	4	63.2	9.2	5.6
Summer Berry Burst, Graze*	1 Punnet/26g	80	0.2	306	1.4	69	0.6	7.1
Trail Mix, Kick Start, Wholefoods, Asda*	1 Serving/50g	194	10.2	387	10.9	40	20.4	10.7
Tropical Mix, Alesto, Lidl*	1 Serving/25g	104	4.8	416	3.4	55.9	19	4
DRIED FRUIT MIX								
Average	***1 Tbsp/25g***	***67***	***0.1***	***268***	***2.3***	***68.1***	***0.4***	***2.2***
Berry, Love Life, Waitrose*	1 Serving/30g	89	0.3	296	1.9	70	0.9	3
Continente Puro Prazer*	1 Serving/25g	150	11.2	601	15	32	45	7.8
Garden of England, Graze*	1 Punnet/25g	70	0.2	280	1	71.2	0.7	5.6
Sultanas Raisins & Cranberries, Dunnes*	1 Handful/15g	47	0.1	315	2	80.2	0.9	4.7
DRINK								
Almond, with Caramel Coffee, Free From, Asda*	1 Serving/200ml	72	2.8	36	1	4.5	1.4	0.5
Aloe Vera, Mango, Say Aloe*	1 Bottle/500ml	160	0	32	0	7.9	0	0
Aperitif, Aromatic, Non Alcoholic, AEcorn *	1 Serve/50ml	28	0	55	0.3	8.4	0.1	0
Aperitif, Bitter, Non Alcoholic, AEcorn *	1 Measure/50ml	24	0	47	0.4	8.6	0	0
Aperitif, Bittersweet, Non Alcoholic, Everleaf*	1 Measure/50ml	26	0	51	0	12.6	0	0
Aperitif, Dry, Non Alcoholic, AEcorn*	1 Serve/50ml	18	0	35	2.8	5.6	0.1	0
Appleade, No Added Sugar, Morrisons*	1 Serving/200ml	2	0	1	0	0	0	0
Botanical, Premium, Non Alcoholic, Extra Special, Asda*	1 Shot/25ml	6	0	22	0	5.6	0	0
Chocolate, Plant Protein, Alpro*	1 Serving/200ml	138	5.6	69	5	5.3	2.8	1.3
Chocolate, Sachet, Optifast, Nestle*	1 Sachet/44g	172	4.8	392	36	34	11	6.5
Citrus, & Ginger, Hot Shot, M&S*	1 Shot/100ml	32	0.1	32	0.7	6.9	0.1	0.4
Coconut, Milk Free, Sweetened, Sainsbury's*	1 Serving/100ml	15	0.8	15	0	1.9	0.8	0
Creme Vanille, Optifast, Nestle*	1 Sachet/44g	172	4.8	392	36	34	11	6.5
G&T, Reduced Calorie, Low Alcohol, Tesco*	1 Can/250ml	12	0	5	0	0	0	0
Ginger Zinger, M&S*	1 Bottle/100ml	41	0.1	41	0.2	10.6	0.1	0.1
Grenadine, Le 0%, Teisseire*	1 Serving/20ml	4	0	21	0	1.9	0	0
Hard Seltzer, All Flavours, 5%, Mike's*	1 Can/330ml	99	0	30	0	0.6	0	0
Limone e Menta, Sparkling, Vive, Aldi*	1 Serving/250ml	5	1.2	2	0.5	0.5	0.5	0.5
Malted, Instant, As Sold, Morrisons*	1 Serving/30g	130	2.7	433	8.3	79	9	1.3
Mango & Ginger, Nix And Kix*	1 Can/250ml	50	0.2	20	0.1	5	0.1	0
Oat, Provamel*	1 Serving/200ml	94	2.6	47	0.3	8.1	1.3	0.8
Raspberry, Isotonic, Sports, Tesco*	1 Bottle/500ml	115	0	23	0	5.3	0	0
Seltzer, Hard, Peach & Rose, Sparkl*	1 Bottle/333ml	80	0	24	0	1	0	0
Soda, Mexican Lime, Fever Tree*	1 Bottle/300ml	48	0	16	0	4	0	0
Soda, Pink Guava, Hopt*	1 Bottle/330ml	66	0.3	20	0.1	4.9	0.1	0
Soda, Raspberry & Rose, Fever-Tree*	1 Bottle/500ml	100	0	20	0	4.9	0	0
Soda, Sparkling, Feijoa, Pear, & Elderflower, Mac's*	1 Bottler/330ml	107	0	32	0	8.6	0	0
Soya, Original, Essential, Waitrose*	1 Serving/200ml	82	3.8	41	3.4	2.6	1.9	0
Soya, Unsweetened, Essential, Waitrose*	1 Serving/200ml	70	3.8	35	3.4	0.8	1.9	0.6
Soya, Unsweetened, Organic, Waitrose*	1 Serving/200ml	62	3.8	31	3.3	0.2	1.9	0
Soya, Vanilla, Pingo Doce*	1 Serving/250ml	120	5.2	48	2.9	4.4	2.1	0.4
Turmeric, & Cayenne, Shot, Eat Well, M&S*	1 Bottle/100ml	42	0.1	42	0.3	10	0.1	0.6
Turmeric, Raw, Original, Shot, The Turmeric Co*	1 Shot/60ml	22	0.2	37	0.6	7.9	0.3	0
DRINKING CHOCOLATE								
Cacao A La Taza, Dry Weight, El Canari*	1 Tbsp/15g	51	0.4	340	5.5	72.1	2.9	3.1
Ginger, & Orange, Christmas, Montezuma*	1 Disk/15g	85	6.4	566	8	31	43	11
Made Up with Semi-Skimmed Milk, Average	***1 Mug/227ml***	***129***	***4.3***	***57***	***3.5***	***7***	***1.9***	***0.2***
Made Up with Skimmed Milk, Average	***1 Mug/227ml***	***100***	***1.1***	***44***	***3.5***	***7***	***0.5***	***0***

	Measure INFO/WEIGHT	per Measure KCAL	FAT	Nutrition Values per 100g / 100ml KCAL	PROT	CARB	FAT	FIBRE
DRINKING CHOCOLATE								
Made Up with Whole Milk, Average	***1 Mug/227ml***	***173***	***9.5***	***76***	***3.4***	***6.8***	***4.2***	***0.2***
Mint, Organic, 54%, Montezuma*	1 Disk/15g	82	5.7	547	5	45	38	7
Mochachino, 54%, Montezuma*	1 Disk/15g	79	5.2	526	5	42	35	7
DRIPPING								
Beef	***1oz/28g***	***249***	***27.7***	***891***	***0***	***0***	***99***	***0***
DUCK								
Breast, Meat Only, Cooked, Average	***1oz/28g***	***48***	***2***	***172***	***25.3***	***1.8***	***7***	***0***
Breast, Meat Only, Raw, Average	***1 Serving/160g***	***206***	***6.8***	***128***	***22.6***	***0***	***4.2***	***0.2***
Confit, Bistro, Gressingham*	½ Pack/125g	272	16.2	218	23	1.1	13	0.5
Crispy, Aromatic, Gressingham Foods*	½ Pack/275g	649	22	236	19	12	8	0.8
Leg, Meat & Skin, Average	***1oz/28g***	***80***	***5.6***	***286***	***17.2***	***0.5***	***20***	***0.4***
Raw, Meat, Fat & Skin	***1oz/28g***	***109***	***10.4***	***388***	***13.1***	***0***	***37.3***	***0***
Roasted, Meat Only, Weighed with Fat, Skin & Bone	***1 Serving/100g***	***41***	***2.2***	***41***	***5.3***	***0***	***2.2***	***0***
Roasted, Meat, Fat & Skin	***1oz/28g***	***118***	***10.7***	***423***	***20***	***0***	***38.1***	***0***
Shredded, with Hoisin Sauce, Asda*	1 Pack/191g	387	11.2	203	9	27	5.9	2.3
Vegetarian, Shredded, Hoisin, Frozen, Linda McCartney*	1 Serving/75g	159	6.5	212	24.7	6.7	8.7	4.4
DUCK AROMATIC								
Crispy, Ã,¼, Hoisin Sauce & 6 Pancakes, Tesco*	1/6 Pack/40g	92	3.3	231	13.3	25.3	8.3	1
Crispy, Ã,¼, Hoisin Sauce, Pancakes, M&S*	½ Pack/155g	290	12.1	187	10.5	18.1	7.8	1
Crispy, Ã,½, Duck & Pancakes, M&S*	½ Pack/311g	590	26.7	190	13.9	14	8.6	2.1
Crispy, Ã,½, Hoisin Sauce, & 12 Pancakes, Tesco*	3 Pancakes/106g	263	9.5	248	17.9	23.4	8.9	1
DUCK CANTONESE								
Hoisin, Aldi*	1 Pack/338g	301	1.7	89	2.9	18	0.5	1.1
Style, Roast, Tesco*	1 Pack/300g	375	6.9	125	8.2	17.9	2.3	0.5
DUCK IN								
Chinese Barbecue, Wings, Sainsbury's*	1 Serving/175g	430	25	246	19.4	9.7	14.3	0
Orange Sauce, Breast, Simply, Gressingham Foods*	½ Pack/175g	254	11.9	145	15.9	5.1	6.8	0.4
Orange Sauce, Roast, a L'Orange, M&S*	½ Pack/259g	482	26.9	186	16.2	6.5	10.4	0.8
Plum Sauce, with Egg Fried Rice, Sainsbury's*	1 Pack/379g	576	15.2	152	5	23.2	4	1.4
DUCK PEKING								
Crispy, Aromatic, Sainsbury's*	½ Pack/300g	1236	110.7	412	19.5	0.6	36.9	0.1
DUCK WITH								
Port & Orange Sauce, Legs, Slow Cooked, M&S*	½ Pack/158g	265	16.9	168	14.8	3	10.7	0.5
Pancakes & Hoisin Sauce, M&S*	1 Pack/80g	136	3.2	170	13	19.9	4	0.9
DUMPLINGS								
Average	***1oz/28g***	***58***	***3.3***	***208***	***2.8***	***24.5***	***11.7***	***0.9***
Dim Sum, Assorted Stuffing, Steamed, Restaurant	***1 Serving/100g***	***230***	***8.2***	***230***	***7.9***	***32***	***8.2***	***3***
Dim Sum, Chicken, Steamed, Restaurant	***1 Serving/100g***	***230***	***5.9***	***230***	***7.5***	***37***	***5.9***	***2.1***
Dim Sum, Chinese, Deep Fried, Restaurant	***1 Serving/100g***	***430***	***23***	***430***	***4.9***	***50***	***23***	***1.8***
Dim Sum, From Restaurant, Average	***1 Piece/12g***	***50***	***2.4***	***433***	***28.9***	***31.3***	***20.4***	***0***
Dim Sum, Meat Dumpling, Deep Fried, Restaurant	***1 Serving/100g***	***340***	***16***	***340***	***4.9***	***43***	***16***	***1***
Dim Sum, Pork, Restaurant, Average	***1 Serving/100g***	***270***	***7.3***	***270***	***7.3***	***43***	***7.3***	***1.6***
Dim Sum, Prawn, Steamed, Eat Well, M&S*	1 Dim Sum/20g	28	0.2	138	6.7	25.1	1.1	0.6
Dim Sum, Steamed, Prawn, M&S*	6 Dim Sum/120g	222	3.2	185	1.1	39	2.7	1.5
Dim Sum, Vegetable & Meat, Steamed, Restaurant	***1 Serving/100g***	***240***	***7.9***	***240***	***5.9***	***37***	***7.9***	***2.5***
Dim Sum, Wonton, Deep Fried, Restaurant	***1 Serving/100g***	***430***	***29***	***430***	***9.7***	***32***	***29***	***1.2***
Gyoza, Beef, Korean, Supermarket, Itsu*	1 Gyoza/20g	38	1.6	191	11.3	18	7.8	2.8
Gyoza, Chicken & Vegetable Selection, Sainsbury's*	1 Pack/150g	300	11.1	200	7.2	24	7.4	1.7
Gyoza, Chicken, Sainsbury's*	1 Pack/150g	219	7	146	8.1	17.2	4.7	0
Gyoza, Duck, Aromatic, Supermarket, Itsu*	1 Gyoza/20g	35	0.9	175	4.4	28	4.5	2.1
Gyoza, Legumes, Lidl*	¼ Pack/100g	133	0.9	133	4.9	26	0.9	1.2
Gyoza, Pork, Itsu*	5 Gyoza/100g	185	6.6	185	8.1	22	6.6	2.1
Gyoza, Prawn, Classic, Itsu*	½ Pack/110g	198	5.7	180	5.5	27	5.2	1.9

D

	Measure INFO/WEIGHT	per Measure KCAL	FAT	Nutrition Values per 100g / 100ml KCAL	PROT	CARB	FAT	FIBRE
DUMPLINGS								
Gyoza, Prawn, King, Steamed	5 Gyoza/75g	135	3.9	180	5.5	27	5.2	1.9
Gyoza, Prawn, Thai Tapas*	1 Gyoza/28g	59	2.3	211	6.4	27.8	8.2	1.1
Gyoza, Vegetable, with Ponzu Dip, Ready to Eat, M&S*	1 Pack/68g	87	2.1	128	3.7	20.6	3.1	1.5
Gyozas, Chicken, Microwaved, Iceland*	1 Gyozas/18g	31	0.5	176	8.3	28	2.7	3.3
Hearty, Frozen, As Sold, Aunt Bessies*	1 Dumpling/49g	161	7.3	330	4.7	43	15	1.7
Homestyle, Baked Weight, Frozen, Aunt Bessie's*	1 Dumpling/53g	177	7.9	337	5.4	47	15	3.5
Mix, Cooked as Directed, Aunt Bessie's*	2 Dumpling/53g	126	4.9	238	4.5	33	9.2	2.4
Pork & Garlic Chive, Waitrose*	1 Pack/115g	215	8.1	187	9.4	20.4	7	1.1
Pork, & Beef, Kuljanka*	1 Serving/250g	612	20.8	245	10.4	31.1	8.3	0
Prawn Sui Mai, Selection, M&S*	6 Sui Mai/120g	143	0.8	119	9.4	13.3	0.7	1.5
Prawn, Siu Mai, Chinese, M&S*	1 Dumpling/20g	22	0.3	108	9.4	13.3	1.6	1.5

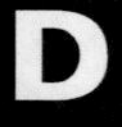

	Measure INFO/WEIGHT	per Measure KCAL	FAT	Nutrition Values per 100g / 100ml KCAL	PROT	CARB	FAT	FIBRE
EASTER EGG								
Aero, Medium, Egg Shell Only, Aero, Nestle*	1 Egg/131g	702	38.9	534	6.2	59.9	29.6	1.6
Buttons, Chocolate Egg Shell Only, Cadbury*	1 Sm Egg/100g	537	31	537	7.3	56	31	2.1
Caramel, Chocolate Egg Shell Only, Cadbury*	1 Lge Egg/343g	1801	102.9	525	7.5	56.8	30	0.7
Chocolate Egg Shell Only, Dairy Milk, Cadbury*	1 Lg Egg/343g	1818	104.6	530	7.6	56.5	30.5	0.7
Chocolate Egg Shell Only, Small, Dairy Milk, Cadbury*	1 Egg/72g	386	22.3	537	7.3	56	31	2.1
Chocolate Orange, Terry's*	1 Egg/196g	1015	52.9	518	8.1	59	27	2.3
Chocolate, Free From, Sainsbury's*	1 Egg/100g	581	35.8	581	3	59.5	35.8	4.5
Chocolate, White, Raspberry, Asda*	½ Pack/100g	566	35	566	5.2	57	35	0.5
Creme Egg, Chocolate Egg Shell Only, Cadbury*	1 Egg/178g	956	55.2	537	7.3	56	31	2.1
Crunchie, Cadbury*	1 Lge Egg/200g	1072	61.9	537	7.3	56	31	2.1
Dairy Milk, Caramel, Egg Shell Only, Cadbury*	1 Egg/176g	945	54.6	537	7.3	56	31	2.1
Ferrero Rocher, Egg Shell Only, Ferrero*	1 Egg/175g	1064	80.2	608	7.3	39.8	45.8	0
Flake, Chocolate Egg Shell Only, Cadbury*	1 Lge Egg/200g	1074	62	537	7.3	56	31	2.1
Freddo Faces, Chocolate Egg Shell Only, Cadbury*	1 Egg/72g	382	22	530	7.6	56.5	30.5	0.7
Kit Kat, Chunky, Nestle*	1 Med Egg/107g	572	31.5	534	6.1	60.4	29.4	1.5
Malteser, Malteaster, Egg Shell Only, Mars*	1 Egg/149g	785	43.2	527	7	59	29	0
Maltesers, Bunny, Egg Shell Only, Mars*	1 Egg/175g	922	50.8	527	7	59	29	0
Maltesers, Truffles, Egg Shell Only, Mars*	1 Egg/175g	922	50.8	527	6.7	59	29	0
Milk Chocolate, Nestle*	½ Egg/42g	205	9.7	489	5	65.2	23.1	0.5
Milky Bar, Nestle*	¼ Egg/18g	97	5.7	543	10.6	53.1	31.7	0
Mini Eggs, Chocolate Egg Shell Only, Cadbury*	¼ Egg/25g	134	7.7	537	7.3	56	31	2.1
Minstrels, Egg Shell Only, Galaxy, Mars*	1 Egg/200g	1056	58	528	7.1	58.9	29	0
Oreo, Cadbury*	1 Egg/31g	175	11.2	563	5	55	36	1.4
Roses, Chocolate Egg Shell Only, Cadbury*	1 Egg/200g	1060	61	530	7.6	56.5	30.5	0.7
Smarties, Nestle*	¼ Egg/31g	160	8.4	524	6	62	27.7	1.4
Twirl, Chocolate Egg Shell Only, Cadbury*	1 Lge Egg/325g	1745	100.8	537	7.3	56	31	2.1
White Chocolate, Thorntons*	1 Egg/360g	1958	109.1	544	5.5	62.2	30.3	2.1
ECLAIR								
Caramel, Asda*	1 Eclair/58g	215	15.1	371	5.6	29	26	0.7
Chocolate, 25% Less Fat, Sainsbury's*	1 Eclair/58g	171	9.3	295	6.8	31.1	16	1.2
Chocolate, Asda*	1 Eclair/33g	144	11	436	6.7	27.3	33.3	4.8
Chocolate, Belgian, & Cream, Essential, Waitrose*	1 Eclair/39g	148	9.5	379	6.2	33	24.4	1.6
Chocolate, Belgian, Fresh Cream, Tesco*	1 Eclair/61g	233	15.4	382	7.3	30.6	25.3	1
Chocolate, Belgian, Sainsbury's*	1 Eclair/34g	127	8.4	374	6.1	30.8	24.8	1.5
Chocolate, Fresh Cream, M&S*	1 Eclair/44g	170	12.2	390	6.3	28.4	27.9	2
Chocolate, Fresh Cream, Sainsbury's*	1 Eclair/35g	130	8.3	372	6.5	32.2	23.8	1.5
Chocolate, Frozen, Free From, Tesco*	1 Eclair/25g	81	4.2	327	4.1	38.9	17	0.8
Chocolate, Frozen, Morrisons*	1 Eclair/31g	116	9.6	374	5	18.8	31	1.3
EEL								
Cooked or Smoked, Dry Heat, Average	***1 Serving/100g***	***236***	***15***	***236***	***23.6***	***0***	***15***	***0***
Jellied, Average	***1oz/28g***	***26***	***1.9***	***93***	***8***	***0***	***6.7***	***0***
Raw, Average	***1oz/28g***	***32***	***2.1***	***113***	***11.1***	***0***	***7.6***	***0***
EGG SUBSTITUTE								
Easy Egg, Vegan, Dry , Orgran*	1 Serving/50g	175	1.6	350	14.9	46.8	3.2	16
Egg Replacer, Free From, Vegan, Free & Easy*	1 Tsp/3g	1	0	30	0.1	8.3	0.1	2.6
Vegan Egg, Follow Your Heart*	1 Serving/10g	40	1.7	401	5	0	17	40
EGGS								
Araucana, Bluebell, Free Range, Finest, Tesco*	1 Egg/50g	66	4.5	131	12.6	0.1	9	0
Blue, Old Cotswold Legbar, Clarence Court*	1 Egg/60g	79	5.4	131	12.4	0	9	0
Duck, Boiled & Salted, Weight with Shell	***1 Egg/75g***	***148***	***11.6***	***198***	***14.6***	***0***	***15.5***	***0***
Duck, Whole, Raw, Weight with Shell	***1 Egg/75g***	***122***	***8.8***	***163***	***14.3***	***0***	***11.8***	***0***
Free Range, Large, Weight with Shell	***1 Egg/68g***	***97***	***6.8***	***143***	***12.6***	***0.8***	***9.9***	***0***
Fried in Veg Oil, Average	***1 Med/60g***	***107***	***8.3***	***179***	***13.6***	***0.7***	***13.9***	***0***

E

	Measure INFO/WEIGHT	per Measure KCAL	FAT	Nutrition Values per 100g / 100ml KCAL	PROT	CARB	FAT	FIBRE
EGGS								
Goose, Whole, Fresh, Raw, Weight with Shell	***1 Egg/144g***	***232***	***16.6***	***161***	***12.1***	***1.2***	***11.5***	***0***
Large, Weight with Shell	***1 Egg/68g***	***97***	***6.8***	***143***	***12.6***	***0.8***	***9.9***	***0***
Medium, Boiled, Weight with Shell	***1 Egg/60g***	***86***	***6***	***143***	***12.6***	***0.8***	***9.9***	***0***
Medium, Weight with Shell	***1 Egg/56g***	***80***	***5.6***	***143***	***12.6***	***0.8***	***9.9***	***0***
Poached, Weight with Shell	***1 Med/58g***	***83***	***5.8***	***143***	***12.6***	***0.8***	***9.9***	***0***
Quail, Whole, Raw, Weight with Shell	***1 Egg/13g***	***20***	***1.4***	***151***	***12.9***	***0.4***	***11.1***	***0***
Savoury, Bites, Mini, Sainsbury's*	1 Bite/12g	34	2.1	285	9.4	21.1	17.9	1.2
Savoury, Bitesize, Tesco*	1 Egg/12g	34	2	287	11.6	21.9	16.7	1.8
Savoury, Mini, Tesco*	1 Egg/20g	55	3.5	274	9.2	20.2	17.4	2.3
Savoury, Vegetarian, Mini, Quorn*	1 Egg/20g	51	2.3	257	15	21	11.5	4.6
Scotch, Retail	***1 Egg/120g***	***301***	***20.5***	***251***	***12***	***13.1***	***17.1***	***0***
Scrambled, Average	***1 Lge Egg/68g***	***97***	***6.8***	***143***	***12.6***	***0.8***	***9.9***	***0***
Very Large, Average, Weight with Shell	***1 Egg/78g***	***112***	***7.8***	***143***	***12.6***	***0.8***	***9.9***	***0***
Whites Only, Raw, Average	***1 Lg Egg/33g***	***17***	***0.1***	***52***	***10.9***	***0.7***	***0.2***	***0***
Yolks, Raw	***1 Yolk/17g***	***55***	***4.5***	***322***	***15.9***	***3.6***	***26.5***	***0***
ELK								
Raw, Meat only	***1 Serving/100g***	***111***	***1.4***	***111***	***23***	***0***	***1.4***	***0***
Roasted, Meat only	***1 Serving/100g***	***146***	***1.9***	***146***	***30.2***	***0***	***1.9***	***0***
ENCHILADAS								
3 Bean, Ready Meal, Average	***1 Pack/400g***	***505***	***16.6***	***126***	***4.4***	***16.9***	***4.2***	***3.2***
Beans, & Rice, Big Bros, Wicked Kitchen, Tesco*	1 Pack/404g	565	15.3	140	4.2	20.5	3.8	3.4
Cheesy, Baked, Meal Kit, Old El Paso*	1 Enchilada/83g	152	2.4	183	5.6	32	2.9	3.2
Chicken, Average	***1 Serving/295g***	***483***	***18.8***	***164***	***11.6***	***16***	***6.4***	***1.7***
Jackfruit, Smoky, with Salsa, Gousto*	1 Serving/420g	483	11.3	115	3	19.2	2.7	1.9
with Cheese & Beef, From Restaurant	***1 Serving/295g***	***496***	***27.1***	***168***	***6.2***	***15.9***	***9.2***	***0***
with Cheese, From Restaurant	***1 Serving/163g***	***319***	***18.8***	***196***	***5.9***	***17.5***	***11.6***	***0***
ENDIVE								
Raw	***1oz/28g***	***2***	***0***	***8***	***1.1***	***0.6***	***0.1***	***1.3***
ENERGY DRINK								
Average	***1 Can/250ml***	***118***	***0***	***47***	***0***	***11.4***	***0***	***0***
BPM Energy*	1 Bottle/500ml	345	0	69	0	14	0	0
Cherry, Lucozade*	1 Bottle/500ml	345	0	69	0	17.1	0	0
Espresso, Vanilla, Monster*	1 Can/250ml	150	5	60	2.2	8.3	2	0
KX, Sugar Free, Diet, Tesco*	1 Can/250ml	5	0	2	0	0	0	0
Mango Loco, Monster*	1 Can/500ml	245	0	49	0	12	0	0
Monster*	1 Can/500ml	240	0	48	0	12	0	0
Natural, Tenzing*	1 Can/250ml	48	0	19	0	4.5	0	0
Origin, Relentless*	1 Can/500ml	110	0	22	0	6.1	0	0
Pacific Punch, Monster*	1 Can/500ml	230	0	46	0	12	0	0
Red Thunder, Diet, Low Calorie, Aldi*	1 Can/250ml	5	0	2	0.1	0	0	0
Relentless, Original, Relentless*	1 Can/500ml	230	0	46	0	10.4	0	0
Sparkling Orange, Dual Energy, Powerade*	1 Bottle/500ml	225	0	45	0	10.5	0	0
Ultra, Zero Calorie, Monster*	1 Can/500ml	10	0	2	0	0.9	0	0
ESCALOPE								
Chicken Style, Vegan, Ocado*	1 Escalope/67g	143	4.5	213	17	19	6.7	4.5
Chicken, Garlic & Herb, with Sourdough, Finest, Tesco*	1 Escalope/153g	343	14.2	224	16.3	18.2	9.3	1.1
Cordon Bleu, de Dinde, Pere Dodu*	1 Escalope/100g	176	7.1	176	14	13	7.1	2.1
Escalope, Average	***1 Escalope/138g***	***341***	***19.3***	***247***	***13.5***	***16.7***	***14***	***0.6***
Escalope, Lemon & Pepper, Average	***1 Escalope/143g***	***371***	***22.6***	***260***	***12.6***	***16.7***	***15.8***	***0.4***
Plant, Vivera*	1 Escalope/100g	188	7.2	188	13	16	7.2	4.7
Vegetarian, Garlic & Mushroom, Creamy, Quorn*	1 Escalope/120g	259	12.3	216	10.4	18.8	10.3	3.7
Vegetarian, Gruyere Cheese, Quorn*	1 Escalope/110g	267	15.4	243	10	18	14	2.6
Vegetarian, Mozzarella & Pesto, Quorn*	1 Escalope/120g	271	15.6	226	10	15	13	4.5

E

	Measure INFO/WEIGHT	per Measure KCAL	FAT	Nutrition Values per 100g / 100ml KCAL	PROT	CARB	FAT	FIBRE
FAGGOTS								
Pork, West Country Sauce, Six Pack, Cooked, Mr Brains*	2 Faggots/218g	190	4.8	87	6	10	2.2	0
FAJITA								
Chicken, Average	***1 Serving/240g***	***357***	***12.8***	***149***	***10.2***	***15***	***5.4***	***2.3***
Kit, Crunchy Nacho, Inspired Cuisine, Aldi*	1 Fajita/63g	207	6	328	7.6	50	9.6	5.8
Kit, Medium, Tesco*	1 Serving/120g	286	6	238	6.4	40.6	5	2.5
Meal Kit, Extra Mild, Old El Paso*	1 Fajita/59g	152	3.6	256	7	42.1	6.1	2.1
Meal Kit, Mild, Tesco*	1 Wrap/59g	144	3.4	247	6.9	40.5	5.8	2.5
Meal Kit, Roasted Tomato, & Pepper, Old El Paso*	1 Fajita/63g	143	2.5	227	6.6	40.1	3.9	2.7
Meal Kit, Sainsbury's*	¼ Pack/118g	280	5.8	237	6.5	40.5	4.9	2.3
Meal Kit, Sizzling, Smoky BBQ, As Sold, Old El Paso*	1 Fajita/63g	141	2.3	224	6.8	40	3.7	1.8
Meal Mix, Asda *	½ Pack/200g	62	1	31	0.9	5.4	0.5	2.1
Medium, Dinner Kit, As Prepared, Inspired Cuisine, Aldi*	1 Fajita/62g	141	2.9	226	6.3	38	4.7	2.7
Mix, Fish, Tesco*	½ Pack/148g	142	3.3	96	13.9	3.9	2.2	2.5
Vegetable	***1 Serving/275g***	***472***	***14.9***	***172***	***4.9***	***25.6***	***5.4***	***1.9***
FALAFEL								
12 pack, Sainsbury's*	1 Falafel/17g	48	2.6	281	6.8	25.2	15.5	6.4
Balls, Meat Free, Meat Free, Tesco*	3 Balls/67g	135	5.3	205	7.1	21.7	8.1	6.3
Beetroot, & Quinoa, Oven Baked, Plant Based, Asda*	3 Falafel/52g	78	1	150	4.2	26	2	6.7
Beetroot, & Feta, World Deli, Waitrose*	1 Falafel/21g	59	3.3	279	7.5	25.1	15.5	4.6
Beetroot, with Red Pepper, & Chilli, Gosh*	4 Falafel/88g	150	6	170	5.4	25.1	6.8	6.4
Chickpea, Cumin, & Coriander, Goodlife*	1 Falafel/19g	39	2	207	7.9	14.1	10.4	12.6
Classic, Vegan, Delphi*	1 Falafel/28g	56	1	200	11.5	31.6	3.7	5.8
Fresh Herb, M&S*	1 Falafel/18g	45	2.2	248	8.3	22.6	12	8.1
Fried in Vegetable Oil, Average	***1 Falafel/25g***	***45***	***2.8***	***179***	***6.4***	***15.6***	***11.2***	***3.4***
Mediterranean, Aldi*	1 Pack/200g	470	24	235	6.4	21	12	7.6
Mezze, Rainbow, Allplants*	1 Serving/360g	457	16.9	127	4.6	15	4.7	3.7
Mini, M&S*	1 Falafel/14g	43	2.5	310	7.9	28.1	18.4	2.6
Moroccan Spiced, Cauldron Foods*	1/3 Pack/60g	143	3.9	239	6	36	6.5	6
Moroccan, Gluten & Milk Free, Free From, Morrisons*	1 Falafel/24g	63	2.4	263	5.8	34	10.1	6.4
Sweet Potato, Bites, Tesco*	¼ Pack/36g	75	2.9	209	6.7	23.4	8	8.7
Sweet Potato, Meat Free, Vegan, Tesco*	3 Falafels/62g	123	6.2	199	4.2	18.1	10	9.6
FANTA								
Grape, Coca-Cola*	1 Can/355ml	170	0	48	0	12.4	0	0
Grape, Zero, Coca-Cola*	1 Can/325ml	13	0	4	0	0.7	0	0
Icy Lemon, Coca-Cola*	1 Can/330ml	112	0	34	0	8.3	0	0
Icy Lemon, Zero, Coca-Cola*	1 Can/330ml	7	0	2	0	0.2	0	0
Lemon, Coca-Cola*	1 Can/330ml	165	0	50	0	12	0	0
Orange, Coca-Cola*	1 Can/330ml	63	0	19	0	4.6	0	0
Orange, Zero, Coca-Cola*	1 Can/330ml	11	0	3	0	0.5	0	0
Pink Grapefruit, Zero Sugar, Coca-Cola*	1 Can/330ml	10	0	3	0	0.3	0	0
Strawberry, Coca-Cola*	1 Can/355ml	160	0	45	0	12.7	0	0
FARFALLE								
Bows, Dry, Average	***1 Serving/75g***	***265***	***1.4***	***353***	***11.4***	***72.6***	***1.9***	***1.9***
FENNEL								
Florence, Boiled in Salted Water	***1oz/28g***	***3***	***0.1***	***11***	***0.9***	***1.5***	***0.2***	***2.3***
Florence, Raw, Unprepared, Average	***1 Bulb/250g***	***24***	***0.4***	***10***	***0.7***	***1.4***	***0.2***	***1.9***
Florence, Steamed	***1 Serving/80g***	***9***	***0.2***	***11***	***9***	***1.5***	***0.2***	***2.3***
FENUGREEK								
Leaves, Raw, Fresh, Average	***10g***	***4***	***0***	***35***	***4.6***	***4.8***	***0.2***	***1.1***
FETTUCCINE								
Chicken, & Parmesan, Italian, Microwaved, Morrisons*	1 Pack/400g	556	15.6	139	9.3	16.2	3.9	1
Edamame & Mung Bean, Explore Asian*	¼ Pack/50g	168	2.1	335	47.2	16.8	4.2	20.6
Konjac, Clean Foods*	½ Pack/100g	6	0.2	6	0.1	0.1	0.2	3.6

F

	Measure INFO/WEIGHT	per Measure KCAL	FAT	Nutrition Values per 100g / 100ml KCAL	PROT	CARB	FAT	FIBRE
FETTUCCINE								
Slim Pasta, Eat Water*	½ Pack/100g	9	0	9	0.2	0	0	4
with Tomato & Mushroom, Easy Cook, Napolina*	1 Pack/120g	461	8.6	384	11.8	67.9	7.2	0
FIG ROLLS								
Asda*	1 Biscuit/19g	71	1.7	372	4.8	68	9	0
Jacob's*	1 Biscuit/17g	66	1.5	386	3.4	72.2	8.6	3
Lyons*	1 Biscuit/19g	71	2.1	374	4.7	62.6	11	3.2
Sainsbury's*	1 Biscuit/19g	67	1.6	360	4.3	64.5	8.7	3.4
FIGS								
Dried, Average	***1 Fig/14g***	***32***	***0.1***	***232***	***3.6***	***53.2***	***1.1***	***8.6***
Dried, with Honey, Intermarche *	4 Figs/30g	80	0.4	268	3.2	57.1	1.2	8.4
Raw, Fresh, Average	***1 Fig/35g***	***16***	***0.1***	***45***	***1.3***	***9.8***	***0.2***	***1.5***
FISH								
3 Fish, Roast, Aldi*	1 Serving/100g	171	10	171	15	5	10	0.7
Ball, Tvi*	4 Balls/60g	61	0.2	101	9.5	15	0.3	0.3
Balls, Fried, Small, Mr Freeds*	1 Ball/19g	35	1.2	188	16.1	16.1	6.6	0
Char, Arctic, Whole, Raw	***1 Serving/100g***	***137***	***6***	***137***	***20.8***	***0***	***6***	***0***
Chargrills, Sun Ripened Tomato, Basil, Birds Eye*	1 Chargrill/163g	127	2.5	75	14	1.4	1.5	0.5
Fillet, Battered Or Breaded, & Fried, From Restaurant	***1 Portion/256g***	***594***	***31.5***	***232***	***14.7***	***17***	***12.3***	***0.5***
Fillet, Breaded, Mini, Cooked, Whitby Seafoods*	1 Fillet/100g	224	9.8	224	11.2	22.2	9.8	1.3
Fillet, Fishless, Battered, Totally Vegan, Quorn*	1 Fillet/97g	202	8.3	209	4.5	27	8.6	2.9
Fillet, Fishless, Breaded, Totally Vegan, Quorn*	1 Fillet/91g	165	2.6	181	4.5	32	2.8	5.2
Fillet, Omega 3, in Bubbly Batter, Chip Shop, Youngs*	1 Fillet/91g	225	13.1	247	10.8	17.9	14.4	1.4
Goujons, Tempura, Fishmonger, Aldi*	½ Pack/100g	222	11	222	10	20	11	0.5
Goujons, Vegetarian, Vivera*	1 Goujon/35g	87	3.5	248	13	25	10	2.7
Grouper	***1 Serving/100g***	***92***	***1***	***92***	***19.4***	***0***	***1***	***0***
Steak, in Creamy Butter Sauce, Youngs*	1 Pouch/121g	104	2.9	86	10.8	5.2	2.4	0.3
Vegan, Fillets, Battered, Fish Free, Plant Chef, Tesco*	1 Fillet/123g	274	8.7	223	13.3	24.7	7.1	3.4
Vegan, Plant, Fillet, Vivera*	1 Fillet/85g	175	7.6	206	14	15	8.9	3.4
White, Breaded, Fillets, Iceland*	1 Fillet/92g	201	8.9	219	12.5	19.9	9.7	1
White, Smoked, Average	***1 Serving/100g***	***108***	***0.9***	***108***	***23.4***	***0***	***0.9***	***0***
FISH & CHIPS								
Cod, Chips, & Peas, Birds Eye*	1 Pack/396g	574	23	145	5	17	5.8	2.4
Feel Good, Gousto*	1 Serving/522g	496	23.5	95	5	10.3	4.5	1.6
Haddock, Breaded, Scottish, M&S*	1 Pack/300g	507	18.6	169	7.5	20.1	6.2	1.2
Mini Meal, 093, Wiltshire Farm Foods*	1 Serving/185g	255	8.3	138	6.9	17.7	4.5	2.8
Takeaway or Fast Food, Average	***1 Serving/469g***	***998***	***115.6***	***213***	***17.7***	***45.7***	***24.6***	***2.6***
with Mushy Peas, Kershaws*	1 Pack/315g	450	18.3	143	6.4	16.4	5.8	1.6
FISH CAKES								
Breaded, Freshly, Fish Counter, Waitrose*	1 Fishcake/124g	188	5.7	152	10.7	16.3	4.6	0.9
Breaded, Oven Baked, Youngs*	1 Fishcake/48g	92	4.4	192	8	18.9	9.1	1.2
Cod, & Parsley, Waitrose*	1 Fishcake/85g	147	6.5	173	9.2	16.9	7.6	1.1
Cod, & Chorizo, Aldi*	1 Fishcake/137g	266	11.5	194	11	18	8.4	1.3
Cod, & Chorizo, Deluxe, Lidl*	1 Fishcake/139g	296	14.6	213	10.2	18.8	10.5	1.2
Cod, & Chorizo, Finest, Tesco*	1 Fishcake/131g	222	9.4	170	11.6	13.8	7.2	1.6
Cod, & Parsley Sauce, The Best, Morrisons*	1 Fishcake/150g	278	13	185	10.2	16.1	8.7	0.7
Cod, & Prawn, Red Thai Style, Extra Special, Asda*	1 Fishcake/140g	227	8.5	162	10	16	6.1	1.4
Cod, Battered, & Crushed Pea, M&S*	1 Fishcake/145g	244	11.3	168	8.9	14.9	7.8	1.1
Cod, Breaded, Frozen, Oven Baked, Iceland*	1 Fishcake/40g	95	4.8	238	8.7	23.1	12.1	1.4
Cod, Breaded, Oven Baked, Youngs*	1 Fishcake/48g	100	4.9	209	8	20.5	10.3	1.4
Cod, Chunky, Breaded, Chilled, Youngs*	1 Fishcake/90g	192	11.5	213	9.5	14.9	12.8	1.2
Cod, Fillet, Free From, Morrisons*	1 Fishcake/131g	252	10.8	193	8.8	20.1	8.3	1.5
Cod, Fillet, GF, Made Without Wheat, M&S*	1 Fishcake/85g	145	6.7	171	8.3	16	7.9	1.4
Cod, Fillet, in Farmhouse Crumb, M&S*	1 Fishcake/85g	142	5.8	167	7.7	18.2	6.8	1.1

	Measure INFO/WEIGHT	per Measure KCAL	FAT	Nutrition Values per 100g / 100ml KCAL	PROT	CARB	FAT	FIBRE
FISH CAKES								
Cod, Fillet, in Golden Farmhouse Crumb, M&S*	1 Fishcake/85g	142	5.8	167	7.7	18.2	6.8	1.1
Cod, HFC, Tesco*	1 Fishcake/48g	86	3.3	181	8.6	20.2	7	1.4
Cod, Homemade, Average	***1 Fishcake/50g***	***120***	***8.3***	***241***	***9.3***	***14.4***	***16.6***	***0.7***
Cod, Katsu, Specially Selected, Aldi*	1 Fishcake/140g	260	12	186	8.7	17	8.6	2
Cod, Melt in the Middle, Specially Selected, Aldi*	1 Fishcake/141g	261	13.7	185	8.1	16	9.7	0.6
Cod, Mornay, Easy to Cook, Waitrose*	1 Fishcake/149g	248	9.4	166	10.6	16.2	6.3	1.4
Cod, Oven Baked, Asda*	1 Fishcake/115g	187	7.2	162	8.5	18	6.2	1.1
Cod, Oven Cooked, Sainsbury's*	1 Fishcake/124g	211	8.3	170	8	19.2	6.7	0.8
Cod, with Lemon & Herb, Tesco*	1 Fishcake/135g	201	5.8	149	10.2	16.5	4.3	1.6
Cod, with Parsley Centre, TTD, Sainsbury's*	1 Fishcake/136g	266	13.4	196	8	18.6	9.9	0.5
Crab, Thai Style, Oven Cooked, TTD, Sainsbury's*	1 Fishcake/141g	296	14.1	210	8.7	20.5	10	1.8
Fried in Blended Oil	***1 Fishcake/50g***	***109***	***6.7***	***218***	***8.6***	***16.8***	***13.4***	***1.2***
Frozen, Average	***1 Fishcake/85g***	***112***	***3.3***	***132***	***8.6***	***16.7***	***3.9***	***0***
Haddock, & Vintage Cheddar, Smoked, Saucy Fish Co*	1 Fishcake/135g	220	7.6	163	9.7	18	5.6	0.9
Haddock, Fillet, Smoked, M&S*	1 Fishcake/145g	245	11.5	169	9.8	15.4	7.9	1
Haddock, Fillet, Smoked, Morrison's*	1 Fishcake/130g	238	9.1	183	11.7	17.7	7	1.6
Haddock, GF, Free From, Sainsbury's*	1 Fishcake/129g	233	10.4	180	10.6	15.8	8	1
Haddock, Melting, Cheddar & Leek, TTD, Sainsbury's*	1 Fishcake/138g	276	13.5	200	9.7	17.8	9.8	0.9
Haddock, Sainsbury's*	1 Fishcake/135g	253	10	188	10.8	18.7	7.4	1.5
Haddock, Smoked, Cheddar, & Leek, TTD, Sainsbury's*	1 Fishcake/138g	276	13.5	200	9.7	17.8	9.8	0.9
Haddock, Smoked, Extra Special, Asda*	1 Fishcake/115g	218	10.9	190	12.8	13.2	9.5	1.3
Haddock, Smoked, Tesco*	1 Fishcake/135g	208	6.2	154	9.9	17.9	4.6	0.7
Haddock, Smoked, with Cheddar Sauce, Asda*	1 Fishcake/142g	302	15.6	213	11	17	11	1.7
Prawn, Cod, Sweet Potato, & Sweet Chilli, Co-Op*	1 Fishcake/135g	255	8.8	189	6.1	26	6.5	1.6
Prawn, Thai Style, Finest, Tesco*	1 Fishcake/135g	196	6.8	145	9.5	14.6	5	1.8
Salmon, & Dill, Waitrose*	1 Fishcake/85g	206	11.9	242	11.5	17.5	14	1.8
Salmon, Fillet, Lochmuir, M&S*	1 Fishcake/85g	180	10.1	212	9	16.5	11.9	1.3
Salmon, Frozen, Oven Baked, Asda*	1 Fishcake/115g	208	8.6	181	11	17	7.5	1.5
Salmon, Homemade, Average	***1 Fishcake/50g***	***136***	***9.8***	***273***	***10.4***	***14.4***	***19.7***	***0.7***
Salmon, Morrisons*	1 Fishcake/90g	241	11.8	268	10.1	27.6	13.1	1.5
Salmon, Rocket, & Watercress, Essential, Waitrose*	1 Fishcake /135g	289	13.9	214	10.5	19	10.3	1.4
Salmon, Scottish, Sainsbury's*	1 Fishcake/130g	240	11.3	184	9.5	16.8	8.7	0.6
Salmon, Spinach & Sicilian Lemon, Finest, Tesco*	1 Fishcake/133g	297	15	223	11.6	17.6	11.3	2.4
Salmon, Sweet Chilli, Aldi*	1 Fishcake/145g	299	12.8	206	8.3	23	8.8	0.9
Salmon,Spinach, & Lemon, Finest, Tesco*	1 Fishcake/133g	297	15	223	11.6	17.6	11.3	2.4
Thai Style Prawn, Chilli & Lemongrass, Aldi*	1 Fishcake/136g	258	11.6	190	7.9	19	8.5	2.8
Tuna, Thai Inspired, Whitby Seafoods*	1 Fishcake/70g	119	4.1	171	9.2	19.6	5.8	2
Vegetarian, Linda McCartney*	1 Fishcake/100g	195	9	195	12.6	13.5	9	4.7
FISH FINGERS								
Breaded, Fishmonger, Aldi*	3 Fingers/86g	168	7.2	195	12	17	8.4	1
Breaded, Frozen, Grilled, Iceland*	4 Fingers/91g	192	8.8	210	13	17.4	9.6	1
Chunky, Cooked, Tesco*	2 Fingers/98g	230	10	235	13.2	21.6	10.2	1.3
Chunky, Extra Large, Captain Birds Eye, Birds Eye*	2 Fingers/120g	247	9.6	206	13	20	8	0.8
Cod, Fried in Blended Oil, Average	***1 Finger/28g***	***67***	***3.9***	***238***	***13.2***	***15.5***	***14.1***	***0.6***
Cod, Frozen, Average	***1 Finger/28g***	***48***	***2.2***	***170***	***11.6***	***14.2***	***7.8***	***0.6***
Cod, Grilled, Average	***1 Finger/28g***	***56***	***2.5***	***200***	***14.3***	***16.6***	***8.9***	***0.7***
Fishless, Squeaky Bean*	1 Finger/27g	68	3	250	13	24	11	3
Free From, Sainsbury's*	1 Finger/30g	56	2.3	188	11.4	18	7.8	0.7
Haddock, Fillet, Chunky, TTD, Sainsbury's*	2 Fingers/113g	244	10.3	216	13.8	19.3	9.1	0.6
Haddock, Fillets, Asda*	1 Finger/30g	62	2.7	205	14	17	9	0
Haddock, in Crispy Batter, Birds Eye*	1 Finger/30g	56	2.3	188	14.3	15.1	7.8	0.7
No Fish, Vegan, Iceland*	2 Fingers/60g	102	2.5	170	13	18	4.1	3.5
Pollock, Omega 3, Birds Eye*	4 Fingers/100g	203	8.2	203	13	19	8.2	0.8

	Measure INFO/WEIGHT	per Measure KCAL	FAT	Nutrition Values per 100g / 100ml KCAL	PROT	CARB	FAT	FIBRE
FISH FINGERS								
Pollock, Sainsbury's*	3 Fingers/85g	160	6.7	188	13	15.9	7.9	0.8
Vegetarian, Fishless, Vegan, Quorn*	1 Finger/20g	37	1.4	187	4.4	24.1	7.1	4.7
FISH IN								
Butter Sauce, Steaks, Ross*	1 Serving/140g	111	4	84	10.6	3.6	3	0.3
Butter Sauce, Steaks, Youngs*	1 Serving/140g	102	2.9	73	9.6	3.7	2.1	0.5
Parsley Sauce, Steaks, Ross*	1 Serving/150g	123	5.6	82	9.1	3.1	3.7	0.1
FIVE SPICE								
Powder, Sharwood's*	1 Tsp/2g	3	0.2	172	12.2	11.6	8.6	23.4
FLAKE								
Dipped, Cadbury*	1 Bar/41g	215	12.5	530	7.6	56.1	30.8	0.8
Luxury, Cadbury*	1 Bar/45g	240	13.6	533	7.3	57.8	30.2	0
Praline, Cadbury*	1 Bar/38g	201	12.9	535	7.7	49.5	34.3	0
FLAN								
Pastry with Fruit	***1oz/28g***	***33***	***1.2***	***118***	***1.4***	***19.3***	***4.4***	***0.7***
Sponge with Fruit	***1oz/28g***	***31***	***0.4***	***112***	***2.8***	***23.3***	***1.5***	***0.6***
FLAN CASE								
Sponge, Average	***1oz/28g***	***90***	***1.5***	***320***	***7***	***62.5***	***5.4***	***0.7***
FLAPJACK								
Lemon Curd, Graze*	1 Punnet/53g	248	12.7	468	6	60	24	6
All Butter, Sainsbury's*	1 Flapjack/35g	156	8	446	5.7	54.5	22.8	2.7
All Butter, Squares, M&S*	1 Flapjack/34g	150	7.2	441	6.2	56.2	21.2	4.4
Apricot & Raisin, Waitrose*	1 Flapjack/38g	143	4.2	376	4.7	64.3	11.1	5.8
Average	***1 Sm/50g***	***242***	***13.3***	***484***	***4.5***	***60.4***	***26.6***	***2.7***
Bites, Sainsbury's*	1 Bite/17g	74	3.4	435	5.3	56	20	4.8
Cacao, Raw, Creative Nature*	1 Bar/38g	136	3.7	359	7.2	64	9.8	11
Chocolate Dipped, M&S*	1 Flapjack/96g	442	21.5	460	6.1	61.3	22.4	3
Chocolate, Belgian, M&S*	1 Bar/80g	372	19.8	465	5.5	52.9	24.7	4.6
Chunky Chocolate, M&S*	1 FlapJack/80g	348	15.1	435	5.8	59.9	18.9	2.2
Cinnamon, Protein, Graze*	1 Punnet/53g	254	13.8	479	16	48	26	7.2
Cranberry, & Orange, Free From, Tesco*	1 Flapjack/30g	131	5.5	440	5.9	60.4	18.5	4.3
Cranberry, Apple & Raisin, LC, Tesco*	1 Flapjack/30g	98	1.7	325	5.7	63.1	5.6	5.7
Free From, Morrisons*	1 Bar/55g	232	7.9	422	4.2	66.9	14.3	4.3
Fruity, M&S*	1 Flapjack/68g	287	11.7	422	5.5	59.3	17.2	4.1
Golden Oaty Fingers, Tesco*	1 Flapjack/34g	142	5.7	420	5.7	59.7	16.8	3.7
Granola, Traybake, Tesco*	1 Serving/46g	202	9.5	440	7.1	54	20.6	5
Honey, & Seed, Protein, Graze*	1 Pack/52g	246	14	473	15.8	42.3	26.9	13.8
Jaffa Cake, Graze*	1 Punnet/53g	242	12.7	457	6	53	24	5
Lemon Drizzle, Graze*	1 Punnet/53g	248	12.7	468	5.9	54	24	5.8
Lemon, Lively, Retail, Graze*	1 Slice/17g	80	4.1	468	5.9	54	24	5.8
Mince Pie, Graze*	1 Punnet/52g	234	10.9	450	4.9	63	21	6.3
Mini, Sainsbury's*	1 Slice/15g	65	2.9	431	5.6	59.3	19	2.7
Oat, Morrisons*	1 Flapjack/50g	228	11	455	5.8	56.3	22.1	3.9
Oats, & Protein, Oatein*	1 Flapjack/40g	161	4.1	402	25	50.6	10.2	3.3
Protein, Cocoa, Vanilla, Graze*	1 Punnet/53g	243	12.7	459	15	44	24	15
Slices, Free From, Tesco*	1 Flapjack/30g	132	5.8	442	6.2	59	19.3	4
Smart, Triple Choc, PhD Nutrition*	1 Bar/60g	226	44.4	376	26	43	74	3.5
Sultana, & Cherry, Bar, Holland & Barrett*	1 Bar/60g	247	10.2	412	6.3	54	17	8.3
Toffee, Finest, Tesco*	1 Flapjack/35g	156	6.7	446	4.9	63.6	19.1	1.3
FLATBREAD								
Brioche, Folded, Deli Kitchen*	1 Flatbread/35g	122	3.4	349	8.3	55.4	9.7	3.1
Cheese, & Tomato, Tesco*	¼ Pack/54g	152	3.8	282	10.3	43.4	7	1.9
Cheese, Three, Thins, Ryvita*	1 Flatbread/7g	29	0.7	420	19.1	60	10.5	4.4
Chicken, & Mango, Stonebaked, Carlos, Aldi*	½ Flatbread/183g	423	17.8	231	9.1	26	9.7	1.6

	Measure INFO/WEIGHT	per Measure KCAL	FAT	Nutrition Values per 100g / 100ml KCAL	PROT	CARB	FAT	FIBRE
FLATBREAD								
Chicken, Chargrilled, COU, M&S*	1 Pack/163g	245	3.1	150	10.8	23	1.9	5.2
Chicken, Harissa, & Roasted Vegetable, M&S*	1 Pack/186g	342	4.8	184	10.7	19.7	2.6	0
Chicken, Mexican, Stonebaked, Finest, Tesco*	1 Pack/155g	280	5.1	180	11.7	25.1	3.3	1.6
Chicken, Moroccan, Shapers, Boots*	1 Pack/164g	289	2.1	176	9.8	30	1.3	2.2
Chicken, Tikka, BGTY, Sainsbury's*	1 Flatbread/186g	292	4.5	157	11.6	20.5	2.4	3.5
Chicken, Tikka, Shapers, Boots*	1 Flatbread/175g	270	4.9	154	11	21	2.8	1.7
Chickpea, & Sesame, Thomas Fudge*	1 Flatbread/11g	48	1.6	439	15	57	15	7
Coronation Chicken, Waitrose*	1 Serving/25g	111	3.6	444	11.2	65.8	14.3	3.5
Crispy, Marmite*	2 Flatbreads/18g	79	2.7	441	20.1	57.4	15.1	0
Feta, COU, M&S*	1 Pack/180g	225	4	125	6.3	20.6	2.2	1.9
Garlic, & Cheese, Co-Op*	1 Serving/66g	194	4.4	294	9.5	39	6.7	1.9
Garlic, & Herb, Oven Baked, Asda*	¼ Pack/61g	185	5.1	302	9.2	46	8.4	2.5
Garlic, Deep Filled, Tesco*	¼ Flatbread/61g	170	4	278	9	44.1	6.5	3.6
Garlic, Mini, Sainsbury's*	½ Flatbread/56g	169	5.1	302	9.3	44.3	9.1	2.5
Garlic, Roasted, & Olive Oil, TTD, Sainsbury's*	¼ Flatbread/53g	168	5.7	319	9.6	44.1	10.8	3.2
Multiseed, Thins, Savour Bakes, Aldi*	1 Flatbread/10g	41	1.2	413	17	56	12	7.7
Olive Oil, Extra Virgin, & Garlic, Waitrose*	¼ Flatbread/41g	146	5.8	357	9	46.9	14.2	2.5
Olive, M&S*	1 Flatbread/25g	113	4.4	453	9.3	61.6	17.4	6.5
Pizza, Meat, Spicy, Asda*	1 Pizza/234g	589	19.9	252	12	31	8.5	2.3
Plain, Thins, Deli Kitchen*	1 Flatbread/35g	103	1.9	295	8.5	51.4	5.3	4.1
Prawn, Tikka, King, Waitrose*	1 Pack/165g	257	3.3	156	9.4	25.1	2	1.5
Roasted Garlic, Waitrose*	¼ Flatbread/61g	181	5.2	297	8.9	44.8	8.6	2.1
Rosemary, & Sea Salt, GF, Nairn's*	1 Flatbread/13g	54	1.8	430	9	63	14.2	7.2
Rosemary, & Sea Salt, Thins, Ryvita*	1 Slice/7g	28	0.4	401	14.8	70.8	5.4	5.2
Salami, Calabrese, Carlos, Aldi*	½ Pizza/181g	490	21.7	271	10	30	12	1.7
Sea Salt, Peters Yard*	1 Flatbread/8g	32	0.8	399	11	72.3	9.4	9.5
White, Folded, Subwich, Deli Kitchen*	1 Flatbread/55g	142	0.6	258	11.2	49.5	1	3
FLAXSEED								
& Goji Berries, Linwoods*	1 Serving/30g	151	11.7	503	20	7.9	39	22
Golden, Ground, P H Foods*	1 Serving/10g	51	4.2	514	18.3	1.6	42.2	27.3
Ground, Organic, Whole Food Earth*	1 Tbsp/15g	80	6.3	534	18.3	1.6	42.2	27.3
Milled, Holland & Barrett*	1 Tbsp/15g	84	5.6	560	20	4.7	37.3	30.6
Milled, Organic, Linwoods*	1 Tsp/5g	25	2	508	22.1	3	40	23.7
FLOUR								
Arrowroot, Average	***1oz/28g***	***100***	***0***	***357***	***0.3***	***88.2***	***0.1***	***3.4***
Bread, White, Strong, Average	***1oz/28g***	***94***	***0.4***	***336***	***11.8***	***68.4***	***1.5***	***3.4***
Bread, Wholemeal, Wessex Mill*	1 Bag/1500g	4635	33	309	15.8	58.2	2.2	12.2
Brown, Chapati, Average	***1 Tbsp/20g***	***67***	***0.2***	***333***	***11.5***	***73.7***	***1.2***	***0***
Brown, Wheat	***1oz/28g***	***90***	***0.5***	***323***	***12.6***	***68.5***	***1.8***	***6.4***
Chick Pea	***1oz/28g***	***88***	***1.5***	***313***	***19.7***	***49.6***	***5.4***	***10.7***
Coconut, Average	***1 Serving/100g***	***344***	***13.6***	***344***	***18.2***	***15.4***	***13.6***	***43.8***
Konjac, Gum, Powder, Special Ingredients*	1 Pinch/2g	4	0	179	0.9	4.1	0	83.5
Oat Fibre, Organic, BuyWholeFoodsOnline*	1 Serving/100g	193	0.3	193	3.3	0.3	0.3	88
Plain, Average	***1oz/28g***	***98***	***0.4***	***349***	***10.3***	***73.8***	***1.5***	***2.2***
Rice	***1 Tsp/5g***	***18***	***0***	***366***	***6.4***	***80.1***	***0.8***	***2***
Soya, Low Fat, Average	***1oz/28g***	***99***	***2***	***352***	***45.3***	***28.2***	***7.2***	***13.5***
Spelt, Average	***1 Serving/57g***	***216***	***1.7***	***381***	***14.3***	***74.5***	***3***	***6.4***
Vital Wheat Gluten, Good Stuff*	1 Serving/100g	403	5	403	81	9	5	1
White, Average	***1oz/28g***	***89***	***0.3***	***319***	***9.8***	***66.8***	***1***	***2.9***
White, Chapati, Average	***1 Tbsp/20g***	***67***	***0.1***	***335***	***9.8***	***77.6***	***0.5***	***0***
White, Self Raising, Average	***1oz/28g***	***94***	***0.4***	***336***	***9.9***	***71.8***	***1.3***	***2.9***
White, Self Raising, Gluten & Wheat Free, Dove's Farm*	1 Serving/100g	344	1	344	5.5	78.1	1	1.4
Wholemeal, Average	***1oz/28g***	***87***	***0.6***	***312***	***12.6***	***61.9***	***2.2***	***9***

	Measure INFO/WEIGHT	per Measure KCAL	FAT	Nutrition Values per 100g / 100ml KCAL	PROT	CARB	FAT	FIBRE
FOOL								
Apricot, Fruit, Tesco*	1 Pot/113g	200	12.7	177	2.6	16.4	11.2	0.3
Apricot, Spanish, The Best, Morrisons*	1 Pot/114g	198	11.6	174	2.7	17.5	10.2	0.5
Fruit, Average	***1 Pot/120g***	***196***	***11.2***	***163***	***1***	***20.2***	***9.3***	***1.2***
Gooseberry, Fruit, Co-Op*	1 Pot/114g	211	11.4	185	3	22	10	1
Gooseberry, Tesco*	1 Pot/112g	225	14.1	200	3	17.8	12.5	0.7
Lemon, Fruit, BGTY, Sainsbury's*	1 Pot/113g	94	3.8	83	3.4	9.7	3.4	0.3
Lemon, Signature, Morrisons*	1 Pot/114g	213	11.8	187	3	20	10.4	0.5
Lemon, Tesco*	1 Pot/114g	213	12	187	2.7	20.3	10.5	0.3
Lemon, Whipped, Sainsbury's*	1 Pot/114g	218	13.9	191	2.9	17.3	12.2	0.5
Raspberry, Fruit, Tesco*	1 Pot/113g	234	12.8	207	2.6	23.6	11.3	0.3
Rhubarb, Fruit, Waitrose*	1 Pot/114g	182	12.9	160	2.7	11.9	11.3	0.3
Strawberry, Fruit, BGTY, Sainsbury's*	1 Pot/120g	100	3.1	83	3.7	11.1	2.6	0.8
Strawberry, Fruit, Co-Op*	1 Pot/114g	188	10.3	165	2	18	9	0.8
FRANKFURTERS								
Average	***1 Sausage/42g***	***123***	***11.2***	***292***	***12***	***1.3***	***26.6***	***0***
Vegetarian, Quorn*	1 Sausage/45g	92	6.3	205	13.5	4.5	14	3.5
Vegetarian, Tivall*	1 Sausage/30g	73	4.8	244	18	7	16	3
FREEKEH								
Dry Weight, Suma*	1 Serving/50g	165	1.4	330	12.6	55.5	2.7	16.5
FRIES								
As Sold, Aunt Bessie's*	1 Serving/100g	150	3.7	150	2.4	26	3.7	1.9
Carrot, & Parsnip, Mash Direct*	½ Pack/150g	231	14	154	1.9	12.8	9.3	5.5
Chips, From Restaurant, Average	***1 Serving/105g***	***294***	***16.3***	***280***	***3.3***	***34***	***15.5***	***2.1***
Classic, Albert Bartlett & Sons Ltd*	1 Serving/150g	279	9.6	186	3.8	27	6.4	3.1
Crinkle, Home, Cooked, McCain*	1 Serving/100g	197	7.7	197	2.4	28	7.7	2.8
Criss Cross, Oven Baked, Iceland*	1 Serving/125g	324	14.1	259	3.5	33.7	11.3	4.4
Curly, Cajun, Weighed Frozen, McCain*	1 Portion/100g	156	8.7	156	1.6	17.7	8.7	1.8
Curly, Lightly Seasoned, McCain*	1 Serving/125g	239	10.8	191	2.3	25.1	8.6	2.4
Curly, Southern Style, Tesco*	1 Serving/50g	95	2.8	189	2.6	29.6	5.6	4.9
Dirty, Cheesy, M&S*	½ Pack/250g	518	30	207	7	16.7	12	2
Dirty, Plant Kitchen, M&S*	1 Pack/400g	564	22.8	141	3	18.4	5.7	1.9
Halloumi, Brew city*	1 Pack/150g	513	36	342	15	15	24	2.2
Halloumi, Iceland*	8 Fries/85g	277	21.7	326	22.5	1.8	25.5	0
Loaded, Tasty, Oven Baked, Aldi*	½ Pack/232g	429	20.6	185	5.5	19	8.9	2.6
Rooster, Frozen Weight, Albert Bartlett & Sons Ltd*	1 Serving/150g	242	7.6	161	2.1	26	5.1	2.1
Seasoned, Frozen, Ovenbaked, Asda*	1/6 Pack/125g	286	10.9	229	3.1	33	8.7	3
Skin On, Bacon Flavour, Oven Baked, Asda*	¼ Pack/77g	144	5.7	186	2.1	26	7.4	2.8
Skin On, Crispy, Four Seasons, Aldi*	1 Serving/100g	198	6.3	198	2.7	31	6.3	2.2
Skin On, Crispy, McCain*	1 Serving/125g	222	7.8	178	2.4	27	6.2	2.6
Skin on, Ovenbaked, Iceland*	1/10 Bag/100g	204	6.9	204	3.3	30.6	6.9	3.2
Skinny, Oven Baked, Tesco*	¼ Pack/125g	151	0.2	121	3.1	25.5	0.2	2.6
Sweet Potato, Co-Op*	¼ Bag/125g	172	6.9	138	1.6	19	5.5	2.9
Sweet Potato, Crispy, McCain*	1 Serving/125g	170	5.7	136	1.6	20.4	4.6	3.5
Sweet Potato, Crispy, Tesco*	½ Pack/150g	320	18.2	213	2.6	21.6	12.1	3.8
Sweet Potato, Lightly Coated, Sainsbury's*	¼ Pack/125g	236	7.5	189	1.3	30.1	6	4.6
Sweet Potato, Oven Baked, Asda*	½ Pack/150g	302	16.5	201	2.6	19	11	4.7
Sweet Potato, Prefried & Frozen, Cooked, Sainsbury's*	1 Serving/125g	297	14.7	237	2.4	28.3	11.7	4.6
Sweet Potato, Ready to Roast, Cooked, Sainsbury's*	½ Pack/116g	201	8.3	174	2.1	23.7	7.2	3.2
Waffle, Potato, Frozen, McCain*	1 Serving/90g	163	6.4	181	2.6	25	7.1	2.5
FRITTATA								
Goats Cheese, & Butternut Squash, Chef Select, Lidl*	1 Pack/130g	189	10.1	145	8.9	9.1	7.8	1.4
Maple Bacon, & Mature Cheddar, Chef Select, Lidl*	½ Pack/65g	97	4.9	149	11.3	8.6	7.5	0
Mushroom, Bacon, & Spinach, Morrisons*	1 Frittata/130g	186	10.3	143	10.8	6.9	7.9	0.6

F

	Measure INFO/WEIGHT	per Measure KCAL	FAT	Nutrition Values per 100g / 100ml KCAL	PROT	CARB	FAT	FIBRE
FRITTATA								
Spinach & Courgette, Meat Free, Tesco*	1 Frittata/120g	199	12.8	166	5.8	10.2	10.7	2.9
Tomato, Pepper & Mozzarella, Morrisons*	1 Frittata/130g	170	7.9	131	9.9	8.7	6.1	0.6
Vegetable, CBY, Asda*	1 Frittata/150g	183	7.8	122	6.2	12.1	5.2	1
FRITTERS								
Black Pudding, Oven Baked, Tony's Chippy*	1 Fritter/85g	234	12.6	275	5.5	28.8	14.8	0
Corn, Plant Chef, Tesco*	2 Fritters/126g	218	10.3	173	3	19.5	8.2	4.7
Courgette, Pea, & Mint, Waitrose*	½ Pack/70g	155	9.7	221	4.9	17.7	13.9	3.4
Courgette, Summer Edition, Sainsbury's*	1 Fritter/27g	45	2.4	168	4.8	15.4	9	2.8
Sweetcorn, Tesco*	1 Fritter/25g	53	2.9	212	5.2	19.9	11.5	4.1
FROMAGE FRAIS								
0% Fat, Isigny Ste Mere*	2 Tbsp/30g	16	0.2	54	8.5	4.7	0.5	0
0% Fat, Vitalinea, Danone*	1 Tbsp/28g	14	0	50	7.4	4.7	0.1	0
Fabby, Loved By Kids, M&S*	1 Pot/43g	45	1.6	105	6.2	12.3	3.7	0
Fat Free, Average	***1 Pot/60g***	***35***	***0.1***	***58***	***7.7***	***6.8***	***0.2***	***0***
High Protein, Tesco*	1 Serving/30g	16	0	54	8.8	4.6	0	0
Kids, Yeo Valley*	1 Serving/90g	111	4.8	123	6.6	12.6	5.3	0
Munch Bunch, Nestle*	1 Pot/42g	44	1.3	105	6.7	12.6	3	0
Plain, Average	***1oz/28g***	***32***	***2***	***113***	***6.8***	***5.7***	***7.1***	***0***
Raspberry, Creamfields*	1 Pot/50g	40	0.4	80	6.9	11.2	0.8	0.2
Raspberry, Savers, Morrisons*	1 Pot/55g	43	1	78	5.5	9.4	1.8	0.4
Raspberry, Value, Tesco*	1 Serving/60g	56	0.8	93	7.2	13.5	1.3	0
Strawberry, Petits Filous, Yoplait*	1 Pot/50g	52	1.4	104	6.7	12.6	2.9	0.2
with Fruit, Average	***1 Avg Pot/90g***	***74***	***2.2***	***83***	***6.1***	***9***	***2.5***	***0.8***
with Fruit, Healthy Range, Average	***1 Avg Pot/90g***	***40***	***0.1***	***45***	***5.8***	***5.1***	***0.2***	***0.3***
FROZEN YOGHURT								
Black Cherry, M&S*	1 Pot/125g	164	1.4	131	3.1	27.1	1.1	0.5
Black Cherry, Split, Co-Op*	1 Scoop/50g	64	1.1	127	4.9	22	2.2	0.5
Cherry Garcia, Low Fat, Ben & Jerry's*	1 Serving/100g	143	2.4	143	3	26	2.4	1
Chocolate, Average	***1 Portion/100g***	***120***	***1.9***	***120***	***4.3***	***22***	***1.9***	***2.1***
Coconut, Pinkberry*	1 Sm Pot/140g	196	0	140	4	30	0	0
Green Tea, Pinkberry*	1 Sm Pot/100g	110	0	110	4	25	0	0
Mango, Pinkberry*	1 Sm Cup/140g	140	0	100	3	23	0	0
Nakedmoo, Yoomoo*	1 Serving/125g	168	2	134	3.3	24.5	1.6	4.1
Natural, Average	***1 Portion/100g***	***101***	***0.8***	***101***	***3.8***	***19.9***	***0.8***	***0.9***
Original, Pinkberry*	1 Sm Pot/140g	140	0	100	3	21	0	0
Strawberry, Average	***1 Portion/100g***	***114***	***2.2***	***114***	***2.6***	***21.2***	***2.2***	***0.5***
Strawberry, Lolly, Yoomoo *	1 Lolly/57g	73	0.8	128	2.8	25.5	1.4	0.5
Tropical, Lolly, Yoomoo *	1 Lolly/57g	74	0.8	130	2.9	26.1	1.4	0.6
Vanilla, Less Than 5% Fat, Tesco*	1 Pot/120g	179	2.9	149	8.1	23.8	2.4	0.7
FRUIT								
Balls, Forest Feast*	1 Pack/100g	434	17.8	434	4.8	61.3	17.8	4.2
Bananas & Berries, Eat Well, M&S*	1 Pack/160g	96	0.3	60	0.9	13.1	0.2	1
Berry Medley, Freshly Prepared, M&S*	1 Pack/180g	90	0.4	50	0.7	10.9	0.2	2.9
Black Forest Fruits, Lidl*	¼ Pack/125g	85	0.8	68	1	10.7	0.6	4.8
Fingers, Melon & Pineapple, Sainsbury's*	1 Pack/240g	74	0.2	31	0.5	6.5	0.1	0.8
Mango, & Watermelon, M&S*	½ Pack/357g	175	1.1	49	0.6	10.3	0.3	1.2
Melon, & Grape, Pot, Co-Op*	1 Pot/130g	48	0.6	37	0.6	7.7	0.5	1.2
Mixed, Fresh, Tesco*	1 Pack/200g	70	0.4	35	0.8	7.4	0.2	1.4
Peach Pieces in Fruit Juice, Tesco*	1 Pot/125g	60	0	48	0.4	11.7	0	1
Peach, Slices, Frozen, Sainsbury's*	1 Serving/80g	30	0	37	1	7.6	0	1.5
Pear, Plum, Figs, & Blackberries, Waitrose*	1 Serving/80g	34	0.2	43	0	9.4	0.2	2.1
Peel, Candied, Average	***1 Serving/30g***	***86***	***0***	***286***	***0.3***	***80.8***	***0***	***5***
Peel, Mixed, Orange & Lemon, Tesco*	1 Serving/25g	75	0.2	301	0.3	70.6	0.9	4.5

	Measure INFO/WEIGHT	per Measure KCAL	FAT	Nutrition Values per 100g / 100ml KCAL	PROT	CARB	FAT	FIBRE
FRUIT								
Red, Mixed, Mercadona*	1 Serving/80g	31	0	39	0.9	5.5	0	0
Summer Berries, M&S*	1 Pack/160g	80	0.3	50	0.7	10	0.2	3
Tropical in Juice, Dole*	1 Pot/113g	59	0	52	0.3	14.2	0	1.8
Tropical, Sun Ripened, Dole*	1 Pack/115g	63	0	55	0.5	12	0	1.2
FRUIT & NUT MIX								
Alesto, Lidl*	1 Serving/30g	150	9.5	500	10.7	39.7	31.7	6.7
Billionaires Shortbread, Graze*	1 Serving/43g	197	10.7	459	8.6	56	25	6.5
Chocolate, & Hazelnut, Shots, Whitworths*	1 Pack/25g	99	3.5	397	5.7	59.9	14	4.2
Chocolate, The Best, Morrisons*	1 Serving/40g	187	10.3	467	7.7	47.7	25.6	7.5
Christmas, Waitrose*	1 Serving/30g	132	6.8	439	9.9	45.9	22.6	6.3
Cranberry, The Best, Morrisons*	1 Serving/40g	192	12.7	481	11.1	34.3	31.8	6.7
Island Mix, Growers Harvest, Tesco*	1 Serving/30g	98	0.2	326	2.1	76.4	0.6	3.4
Pecan, & Berries, with Dark Chocolate, Tesco*	1 Pack/30g	177	13	590	6.7	40.3	43.2	6.8
Pina Colada, Graze*	1 Punnet/32g	141	7.4	441	8.1	54	23	6.2
Selection, Asda*	1 Serving/35g	164	9.8	470	12	42	28	3.7
Trail Mix, Average	***1oz/28g***	***121***	***8***	***432***	***9.1***	***37.2***	***28.5***	***4.3***
Unsalted, Stockwell & Co, Tesco*	1 Serving/25g	120	7.1	478	19.4	33.5	28.3	5.7
Unsalted, Tesco*	1 Serving/25g	112	4.6	449	12.6	58.1	18.5	12.2
Whitworths*	1 Serving/25g	122	7.7	486	18	30.8	30.8	6.9
FRUIT COCKTAIL								
Fresh & Ready, Sainsbury's*	1 Pack/300g	117	0.3	39	0.6	9	0.1	1.2
in Apple Juice, Asda*	1/3 Can/80g	40	0.1	50	0.3	12	0.1	1.6
in Juice, Del Monte*	1 Can/415g	203	0.4	49	0.4	11.2	0.1	0
in Syrup, Morrisons*	½ Can/205g	129	0.2	63	0.3	14.9	0.1	0
in Syrup, Smart Price, Asda*	1 Can/411g	173	0.4	42	0.3	10	0.1	1.6
Tropical, Canned, Asda*	½ Can/200g	120	0	60	0	15	0	1.6
FRUIT COMPOTE								
Apple, & Pear, No Added Sugar, Andros*	1 Tbsp/15g	7	0	46	0.2	9.6	0.3	2.1
Apricot & Prune, Yeo Valley*	1 Pot/225g	207	0.2	92	0.6	22.3	0.1	1.6
Apricot, Bonne Maman*	1 Serving/15g	16	0	108	0.8	25	0.2	1.4
Cherry, Bonne Maman*	1 Serving/15g	17	0	115	1.1	26	0.3	1.9
Peach, Bonne Maman*	1 Serving/15g	16	0	104	0.6	24	0.2	1.7
Rhubarb, Bonne Maman*	1 Serving/15g	15	0	103	0.5	24	0.1	2
Strawberry & Raspberry, M&S*	1 Serving/80g	72	0.1	90	0.7	23.5	0.1	2.3
Summer Berry, Opies*	1 Tbsp/15g	16	0.2	106	0.8	26	1.6	0
FRUIT FLAKES								
Blackcurrant with Yoghurt Coating, Fruit Bowl*	1 Bag/21g	95	4	453	1.3	69	19	3.9
Raspberry with Yoghurt Coating, Fruit Bowl*	1 Serving/21g	95	4	453	1.3	69	19	3.9
Strawberry with Yoghurt Coating, Fruit Bowl*	1 Serving/21g	95	4	453	1.3	69	19	3.9
FRUIT MIX								
Berry Medley, Asda*	1 Pack/220g	121	1.1	55	0.7	12	0.5	1
Black Forest Fruit, Four Seasons, Aldi*	1 Serving/80g	40	0.4	50	0.8	11	0.5	2.1
Date, & Banana, Dried, Asda*	1 Serving/30g	117	4.2	389	2.9	61	14	5.5
Exotic, Frozen, Tesco*	1 Serving/80g	33	0	41	0.6	8.7	0	1.9
in Pineapple Juice, Dole*	1 Pot/100g	54	0	54	0.5	12	0	1
Melon, & Mango, Morrisons*	1 Pot/150g	52	0.2	35	0.6	7.3	0.1	1.2
Pieces, in Juice, Freshona, Lidl*	1 Pot/110g	53	0.1	48	0.3	11.2	0.1	1
Pineapple, Grape, & Apple, Asda*	1 Serving/80g	44	0.4	55	0.5	12	0.5	1.8
Pineapple, Melon, Mango, Tesco*	1 Pack/440g	242	0.9	55	1.1	11.4	0.2	1.3
Pineapple, Watermelon, & Grapes, Asda*	1 Serving/160g	75	0.8	47	0.5	10	0.5	0.9
Plum, & Berries, Eat Well, M&S*	1 Serving/100g	41	0.2	41	0.8	7.8	0.2	2.3
Red, Frozen, Crops*	3 Tbsp/80g	28	0.1	35	1	5.2	0.1	4.6
Sour Mango Tangtastic, Graze*	1 Pack/34g	110	0.2	323	1.3	79.8	0.6	2

	Measure INFO/WEIGHT	per Measure KCAL	FAT	Nutrition Values per 100g / 100ml KCAL	PROT	CARB	FAT	FIBRE
FRUIT MIX								
Summer Fruits, British, Frozen, Waitrose*	1 Pack/300g	111	0.6	37	1.1	6.2	0.2	3.2
Summer Fruits, Frozen, Asda*	1 Serving/100g	28	0	28	0.9	6	0	2.5
Summer Fruits, Frozen, Sainsbury's*	1 Serving/80g	43	0.1	54	0.9	6.9	0.1	2
Watermelon, & Mango, Fingers, Tesco*	½ Pack/136g	64	0.4	47	0.5	9.8	0.3	1.6
Watermelon, Mango, & Blueberries, Tesco*	1 Pack/220g	99	0.7	45	0.6	9.6	0.3	1.1
FRUIT PUREE								
Apple & Peach, Organix*	1 Pot/100g	49	0.3	49	0.6	11	0.3	2.1
Apple, & Mango, Pouch, Tesco*	1 Pouch/70g	40	0.1	57	0	13.5	0.1	1.4
FRUIT SALAD								
Apple, Melon, & Berries, Nutritious, Boots*	1 Pack/257g	118	0.8	46	0.6	9.4	0.3	1.8
Apple, Orange, Pineapple & Grape, Morrisons*	1 Serving/64g	40	0.1	62	0.8	13.1	0.1	2.6
Autumn, Fresh, M&S*	½ Pack/160g	64	0.2	40	0.7	9.4	0.1	2.9
Berry, Seasonal, Asda*	1 Pack/300g	93	0.3	31	0.6	7	0.1	2.1
Canned, in Fruit Juice, Asda*	1/3 Can/136g	60	0.7	44	0.5	10	0.5	0.5
Citrus, Fresh, M&S*	½ Pack/225g	79	0.2	35	0.9	7.7	0.1	1.5
Classic, Fresh, Prepared, Sainsbury's*	1 Pack/320g	157	0.3	49	0.6	10.3	0.1	2
Classic, Waitrose*	1 Pack/330g	162	0.7	49	0.8	10.4	0.2	1.2
Dried, M&S*	½ Pack/125g	269	0.5	215	1.8	51.4	0.4	5.9
Exotic, Fresh, Tesco*	1 Serving/225g	86	0.4	38	0.7	8.4	0.2	1.5
Exotic, Waitrose*	1 Pack/300g	126	0.6	42	0.6	9.5	0.2	1.1
Fresh for You, Tesco*	1 Pack/160g	59	0.3	37	0.6	8.2	0.2	1.1
Fresh, Morrisons*	1 Tub/350g	150	0.4	43	0.7	9.9	0.1	0
Fresh, Tesco*	1 Pack/200g	84	0.4	42	0.7	9.3	0.2	1.5
Freshly Prepared, M&S*	1 Pack/350g	140	0.7	40	0.5	9.3	0.2	1
Frozen, Tesco*	1 Serving/80g	26	0.4	32	0.5	6.1	0.5	1.7
Fruity Cocktail, M&S*	1 Serving/80g	33	0.1	41	0.6	8.5	0.1	1.7
Grapefruit & Orange, Fresh, M&S*	1 Serving/250g	88	0.2	35	0.9	7.4	0.1	1.6
Homemade, Unsweetened, Average	***1 Serving/140g***	***77***	***0.1***	***55***	***0.7***	***13.8***	***0.1***	***1.5***
Juicy Melon, Pineapple & Grapes, Asda*	1 Pot/300g	111	0.3	37	0.5	8.4	0.1	0.9
Kiwi, Pineapple & Grape, Fresh Tastes, Asda*	1 Pack/200g	106	0.6	53	0.6	11	0.3	1.8
Mango, Pineapple & Passion Fruit, Waitrose*	1 Serving/80g	42	0	52	0.8	10.4	0	2.5
Melon & Red Grape, Freshly Prepared, M&S*	1 Pack/450g	158	0.4	35	0.5	8.4	0.1	0.7
Melon & Mango, Shapers, Boots*	1 Pack/80g	29	0.1	36	0.6	7.8	0.1	1.2
Melon, & Grape, Sainsbury's*	1 Pack/159g	59	0.8	37	0.6	7.8	0.5	1.2
Mixed, Average	***1 Bowl/100g***	***42***	***0.2***	***42***	***0.6***	***9.4***	***0.2***	***1.5***
Pineapple, Apple & Strawberries, Tesco*	1 Pack/190g	80	0.2	42	0.4	9.8	0.1	1.4
Pineapple, Melon & Grape, Eat Well, M&S*	1 Pot/130g	53	0.3	41	0.5	8.6	0.2	1.6
Pineapple, Melon, & Mango, Nutritious, Boots*	1 Pack/250g	111	0.5	44	0.6	9.2	0.2	1.6
Pineapple, Strawberry, Grape & Carrot, M&S*	1 Pack/240g	101	1	42	0.6	8.3	0.4	1.4
Plum, Blackberries, & Fig, Tesco*	1 Pot/260g	109	0.5	42	0.8	8.2	0.2	2.5
Rainbow Layers, Tesco*	1 Pack/270g	122	0.5	45	0.5	9.8	0.2	1.1
Rainbow, Fresh, Tesco*	1 Tub/270g	105	0.5	39	0.5	8.8	0.2	0.9
Rainbow, Waitrose*	1 Pack/285g	154	1.4	54	0.7	11.4	0.5	1.5
Seasonal, Fresh, Asda*	1 Pack/125g	55	0.1	44	0.5	10.4	0.1	1.2
Selection, M&S*	½ Pack/275g	140	0.8	51	0.6	10.3	0.3	2.1
Summer, Red, Fresh, M&S*	1 Pack/400g	160	0.8	40	0	10	0.2	1.2
Sunshine, Fresh, M&S*	1 Serving/200g	70	0.2	35	0	8.3	0.1	1.3
Super Fruity, M&S*	1 Pot/150g	88	0.4	59	1	11.6	0.3	3
Tropical Mix, Tesco*	½ Pack/140g	71	0.3	51	0.5	11	0.2	1.5
Tropical, Fresh, Asda*	1 Pack/400g	164	0.8	41	0.7	9	0.2	1.8
Tropical, in Juice, Natures Finest*	1 Pot/125g	61	0.6	49	0	13	0.5	1
Tropical, Tropical Harvest*	1 Serving/100g	52	0	52	0.3	12.8	0	1.4
Virgin Trains*	1 Serving/140g	56	0.1	40	0.4	10	0.1	0.8

	Measure INFO/WEIGHT	per Measure KCAL	FAT	Nutrition Values per 100g / 100ml KCAL	PROT	CARB	FAT	FIBRE
FRUIT SPREAD								
Cherries & Berries, Organic, Meridian Foods*	1 Tbsp/15g	16	0	109	0.5	26	0.3	1.1
Cherry & Berry, Meridian Foods*	1 Serving/10g	14	0.1	138	0.7	33.7	0.6	3.2
Seville Orange, Weight Watchers*	1 Tsp/15g	17	0	111	0.2	27.5	0	0.3
FU YUNG								
Chicken, Chinese Takeaway, Tesco*	1 Pack/350g	315	3.5	90	5.6	14.5	1	0.8
Egg, Average	***1oz/28g***	***67***	***5.8***	***239***	***9.9***	***2.2***	***20.6***	***1.3***
FUDGE								
All Butter, Finest, Tesco*	1 Sweet/10g	43	1.4	429	1.3	73.4	14.5	0
Butter Tablet, Thorntons*	1oz/28g	116	3.1	414	0.9	77.6	11.1	0
Butter, Milk, Thorntons*	1 Sweet/13g	60	2.5	462	3.7	68.5	19.2	0
Cadbury*	1 Bar/25g	118	4	445	2.5	74.5	15	0.5
Chocolate, Average	***1 Sweet/30g***	***132***	***4.1***	***441***	***3.3***	***81.1***	***13.7***	***0***
Chunks for Baking	***1 Serving/100g***	***428***	***12.2***	***428***	***1.7***	***77.2***	***12.2***	***0.6***
Clotted Cream, M&S*	½ Pack/68g	300	9.6	444	0.6	78.2	14.2	0.5
Clotted Cream, Sainsbury's*	1 Sweet/8g	35	0.9	430	1.9	81.5	10.7	0.7
Dairy, Co-Op*	1 Sweet/9g	39	1.2	430	2	76	13	0
Dairy, Morrisons*	3 Sweets/24g	107	3.6	447	1.8	76.1	14.9	0.5
Maple Salt, Specially Selected, Aldi*	3 Pieces/30g	134	4.2	445	0.5	78	14	0.5
Minis, Cadbury*	1 Piece/5g	23	0.9	455	2.6	73	17	0.7
Vanilla, Bar, M&S*	1 Bar/43g	205	10	476	3.7	63	23.3	0.4
Vanilla, Julian Graves*	1 Serving/10g	41	1	407	1	78.9	9.7	0
Vanilla, Thorntons*	1 Bag/100g	465	21.9	465	1.8	65.9	21.9	0
FUSILLI								
Cooked, Average	***1 Serving/210g***	***248***	***1.4***	***118***	***4.2***	***23.8***	***0.6***	***1.2***
Dry, Average	***1 Serving/90g***	***316***	***1.4***	***352***	***12.3***	***72***	***1.6***	***2.2***
Fresh, Cooked, Average	***1 Serving/200g***	***329***	***3.6***	***164***	***6.4***	***30.6***	***1.8***	***1.8***
Fresh, Dry, Average	***1 Serving/75g***	***208***	***2***	***277***	***10.9***	***53.4***	***2.7***	***2.1***
GF, Dry, Average	***1 Serving/60g***	***205***	***0.8***	***341***	***6.8***	***73.7***	***1.3***	***3***
Green Pea, Cooked, Sainsbury's*	1 Serving/170g	291	1.7	171	11	27.5	1	3.8
Red Lentil, Dry, Cook Italian*	1 Serving/80g	283	1.6	354	23	58	2	6
Red Lentil, GF, Dry, Tesco*	1 Serving/70g	296	1.1	423	27.9	70.4	1.6	7.2
Tricolore, Dry, Average	***1 Serving/75g***	***264***	***1.3***	***351***	***12.2***	***71.8***	***1.7***	***2.7***
Whole Wheat, Dry Weight, Average	***1 Serving/90g***	***290***	***2.1***	***322***	***13.1***	***62.3***	***2.3***	***9***
FYBOGEL								
Lemon, Reckitt Benckiser*	1 Serving/4g	4	0	95	2.4	11.3	1.1	64.8
Orange, Reckitt Benckiser*	1 Serving/4g	5	0	106	2.4	12.7	1.1	64.4

F

	Measure INFO/WEIGHT	per Measure KCAL	FAT	Nutrition Values per 100g / 100ml KCAL	PROT	CARB	FAT	FIBRE
GALANGAL								
Raw, Root, Average	***100g***	***71***	***0.6***	***71***	***1.2***	***15.3***	***0.6***	***2.4***
GALAXY								
Cookie Crumble, Mars*	1 Bar/114g	627	37.6	550	6.2	56	33	1.9
Hazelnut, Mars*	1 Piece/6g	37	2.5	582	7.8	49.4	39.2	0
Smooth Caramel, Galaxy, Mars*	1 Serving/25g	124	6.4	498	5.4	60.5	25.7	0
GAMMON								
Breaded, Average	***1oz/28g***	***34***	***0.9***	***120***	***22.5***	***1***	***3***	***0***
Hocks, with Honey & Mustard Sauce, TTD, Sainsbury's*	1 Pack/748g	1114	49.3	149	17.1	4.5	6.6	1.6
Honey & Mustard, Average	***½ Pack/190g***	***294***	***13.5***	***155***	***19.1***	***3.6***	***7.1***	***0.1***
Joint, Boiled, Average	***1 Serving/60g***	***122***	***7.4***	***204***	***23.3***	***0***	***12.3***	***0***
Joint, Honey Glaze, Just Cook, Sainsbury's*	1/3 Pack/123g	242	12.8	197	23.4	2.1	10.4	0
Joint, Raw, Average	***1 Serving/100g***	***138***	***7.5***	***138***	***17.5***	***0***	***7.5***	***0***
Joint, with Honey Glaze, Tesco*	¼ Pack/124g	186	2.6	150	27.4	4.9	2.1	0.6
Shank, with Maple, & Balsamic, Finest, Tesco*	1 Pack/347g	587	15.3	169	25.5	6.6	4.4	0.5
Shanks, with Caramelised Apple Sauce, M&S*	½ Pack/166g	226	6.5	136	14.7	10.5	3.9	0.3
Slow Cooked, British, Thick Sliced, Asda*	1 Slice/33g	40	0.8	121	24	1	2.4	0.7
Steak, with Garden Herb Butter, Co-Op*	½ Pack/150g	207	11	138	17.3	1	7.3	0.4
Steaks, Honey Roast, Average	***1 Steak/100g***	***142***	***5.3***	***142***	***21.5***	***2.3***	***5.3***	***0***
Steaks, Smoked, Average	***1 Steak/110g***	***150***	***5.5***	***137***	***22.7***	***0.1***	***5***	***0.1***
Steaks, Unsmoked, Grilled, Morrisons*	1 Steak/104g	136	2.4	131	26.7	0.5	2.3	0.5
Steaks, with Pineapple & Mango Salsa, Easy, Waitrose*	1 Steak/163g	239	11.6	146	14.1	6.5	7.1	0.5
with Honey & Mustard Glaze, Just Cook, Sainsbury's*	½ Pack/240g	351	6.7	146	23.8	6.1	2.8	0.8
GARAM MASALA								
Dry, Ground, Average	***1 Tbsp/15g***	***57***	***2.3***	***379***	***15.6***	***45.2***	***15.1***	***0***
GARLIC								
Black	***1 Clove/5g***	***13***	***0***	***264***	***13.3***	***53.3***	***0***	***20***
Powder, Average	***1 Tsp/3g***	***7***	***0***	***246***	***18.7***	***42.7***	***1.2***	***9.9***
Raw, Average	***1 Clove/3g***	***3***	***0***	***98***	***7.9***	***16.3***	***0.6***	***2.1***
Wild	***1 Leaf/1g***	***0***	***0***	***23***	***2.8***	***1.7***	***0.6***	***1.9***
GARLIC PUREE								
Average	***1 Tbsp/18g***	***68***	***6***	***380***	***3.5***	***16.9***	***33.6***	***0***
in Vegetable Oil, GIA*	1 Tsp/5g	12	0.9	248	3.6	18.8	17.7	0
GATEAU								
Black Forest, 500g Size, Tesco*	1 Cake/500g	1125	55	225	4	27.1	11	1.8
Black Forest, M&S*	1/8 Cake/77g	207	10.9	269	3.1	31.6	14.1	1.5
Black Forest, Mini, Tesco*	1 Serving/55g	136	5.1	247	5.7	35.3	9.2	1
Caramel, Salted, Dome, Frozen, Tesco*	1 Serving/78g	233	9.9	298	4.2	41.2	12.7	0.9
Caramel, Salted, Profiterole, Tesco*	1 Slice/88g	248	13.6	282	4.3	31	15.5	0.9
Chocolate Layer, M&S*	1 Serving/86g	278	15.7	323	4.2	35.9	18.3	0.9
Chocolate, & Vanilla, Ice Cream, Iceland*	1 Serving/130g	252	12.2	194	3.3	24.1	9.4	0.6
Chocolate, Double, Frozen, Tesco*	1/5 Gateau/70g	115	4.4	255	5.5	34.2	9.8	3.5
Chocolate, Iceland*	1/8 Gateau/75g	201	9.7	268	4.9	31.7	12.9	3
Chocolate, Rich, Tesco*	1 Slice/84g	210	8.6	251	5.1	32.9	10.2	3.4
Chocolate, Swirl, Tesco*	1 Serving/83g	230	13.3	277	3.8	29.3	16	0.2
Strawberry, Co-Op*	1 Serving/77g	222	12.9	288	5.1	29.2	16.7	1
Strawberry, Frozen, Tesco*	1 Serving/75g	144	6.2	192	2.6	26.3	8.3	0.7
Swiss, Cadbury*	1/6 Gateau/60g	228	10.1	380	5.2	52	16.8	0.9
GHEE								
Butter	***1oz/28g***	***251***	***27.9***	***898***	***0***	***0***	***99.8***	***0***
Vegetable	***1oz/28g***	***251***	***27.8***	***895***	***0***	***0***	***99.4***	***0***
GHERKINS								
Pickled, Average	***1 Gherkin/36g***	***4***	***0***	***12***	***0.8***	***2.1***	***0.1***	***1***
Pickled, with Chilli, Bramwells, Aldi*	1 Gherkin/20g	3	0.1	16	0.9	2.6	0.4	1

G

	Measure INFO/WEIGHT	per Measure KCAL	FAT	Nutrition Values per 100g / 100ml KCAL	PROT	CARB	FAT	FIBRE
GIN								
& Diet Tonic, Can, Greenalls*	1 Can/250ml	95	0	38	0	0	0	0
& Tonic, Canned, Ready to Drink, M&S*	1 Can/250ml	175	0.8	70	0.2	5.6	0.3	0.1
& Tonic, Pre-Mixed, Opihr*	1 Bottle/275ml	223	0.6	81	0	8.9	0.2	0
& Tonic, Premixed, Flor De Sevilla, Tanqueray*	1 Bottle/275ml	190	0	69	0	6.6	0	0
37.5% Volume	***1 Pub Shot/35ml***	***72***	***0***	***207***	***0***	***0***	***0***	***0***
40% Volume	***1 Pub Shot/35ml***	***78***	***0***	***224***	***0***	***0***	***0***	***0***
41% Volume	***1 Pub Shot/35ml***	***83***	***0***	***237***	***0***	***0***	***0***	***0***
Average, 43%	***1 Serving/25ml***	***60***	***0***	***241***	***0***	***0***	***0***	***0***
Citrus, Grove 42, Non Alcoholic, Seedlip Ltd*	1 Shot/30ml	0	0	0	0	0	0	0
Clean, Rhubarb, The Clean Liquor Co*	1 Serve/50ml	4	0	8	0	2.6	0	0
Flor De Sevilla, Tanqueray*	1 Single/25ml	64	0	254	0	0	0	0
Gordons & Schweppes Slimline Tonic, Canned, Diageo*	1 Can/250ml	75	0	30	0	0	0	0
Gordons & Schweppes Tonic, Canned, Diageo*	1 Can/250ml	152	0	61	0	6.2	0	0
London, Special Dry, 30%, Gordons*	1 Serve/25ml	52	0	208	0	0	0	0
Mango & Passionfruit, 37.5%, Haysmith's*	1 Serve/25ml	56	0	225	0	0	0	0
Non Alcoholic, Classic, Cedar's*	1 Measure/50ml	2	0	4	0	0	0	0
Peach, & Orange Blossom, 37.5%, Haysmith's*	1 Shot/25ml	57	0	227	0	0	0	0
Pink, & Tonic, Mixed, Can, Gordons*	1 Can/250ml	168	0	67	0	8.7	0	0
Raspberry, Liqueur, Edinburgh Gin Distillery*	1 Serving/25ml	46	0	184	0	18.2	0	0
Rhubarb, & Ginger, Whitley Neill*	1 Shot/25ml	68	0	273	0	0	0	0
Sicilian Lemon, 37.5%, Gordons*	1 Serving/50ml	110	0	221	0	2	0	0
GINGER								
Chunks, Crystallised, Julian Graves*	1 Serving/10g	28	0	283	0.2	70.1	0.2	1.5
Ground, Average	***1 Tsp/2g***	***5***	***0.1***	***258***	***7.4***	***60***	***3.3***	***0***
Minced, Lee Kum Kee*	1 Tsp/10g	1	0	14	0.5	2.9	0.5	0
Root, Raw, Pared, Average	***1 Tsp/2g***	***2***	***0***	***81***	***1.8***	***18***	***0.8***	***2***
Root, Raw, Unprepared, Average	***1 Tsp/2g***	***1***	***0***	***74***	***1.7***	***16.3***	***0.7***	***1.8***
Stem in Sugar Syrup, Sainsbury's*	1 Ball/10g	29	0	292	0.5	71.3	0.5	1.6
Very Lazy, The English Provender Co.*	1 Tsp/5g	3	0	52	0.7	10.9	0.8	0.8
GINGER ALE								
Dry	***1 Glass/250ml***	***38***	***0***	***15***	***0***	***3.9***	***0***	***0***
Orange, Light Spiced, Fever-Tree*	1 Serving/200ml	36	0	18	0	4.3	0	0
GINGER BEER								
Alcoholic, Crabbies*	1 Bottle/500ml	254	0	51	0	7.1	0	0
Classic, Schweppes*	1 Can/330ml	115	0	35	0	8.4	0	0
D & G Old Jamaican*	1 Can/330ml	211	0	64	0	16	0	0
Diet, Crabbies*	1 Bottle/700ml	7	0	1	0	0	0	0
Light, Belvoir Fruit Farms*	1 Serving/200ml	42	0	21	0	4.4	0	0
Light, Waitrose*	1 Glass/250ml	2	0.2	1	0	0	0.1	0.1
No Added Sugar, Canned, Tesco*	1 Can/330ml	3	0.3	1	0	0.1	0.1	0.1
Refreshingly Light, Fever-Tree*	1 Bottle/200ml	38	0	19	0	4.9	0	0
GINGERBREAD								
Average	***1oz/28g***	***106***	***3.5***	***379***	***5.7***	***64.7***	***12.6***	***1.2***
Iced, Sarah The Dinosaur, Waitrose*	1 Biscuit/30g	127	3.3	422	4.5	75.1	11.1	0
Man, Free From, Co-Op*	1 Biscuit/25g	115	3.7	461	4.2	77	15	1.3
Men, GF, Free From, Asda*	1 Biscuit/25g	113	3.5	451	4.3	76	14	1.8
GIRASOLE								
Ricotta, & Spinach, Creamy, Specially Selected, Aldi*	½ Pack/155g	312	15.5	201	7.1	19	10	2.2
Spinach, Buffalo Ricotta, & Pine Nuts, Finest, Tesco*	½ Pack/150g	276	13	184	7.4	16.4	8.7	5.7
GNOCCHI								
Chorizo, Spinach, & Courgette, Hello Fresh*	1 Portion/514g	714	28	139	5	17.3	5.4	0
Cooked, Tesco*	¼ Pack/132g	217	0.4	164	3.5	36.1	0.3	1.7
Fresh, Cooked, Essential, Waitrose*	¼ Pack/134g	242	0.5	181	4.7	39	0.4	1

G

	Measure INFO/WEIGHT	per Measure KCAL	FAT	Nutrition Values per 100g / 100ml KCAL	PROT	CARB	FAT	FIBRE
GNOCCHI								
Fresh, Italian, Chilled, Sainsbury's*	½ Pack/250g	355	1.2	142	2.5	29.9	0.5	4
Italian, Boiled, Asda*	1 Pack/498g	573	2.5	115	1.4	25	0.5	2.2
Italian, Cooked, Morrisons*	1 Serving/250g	385	2.5	154	3.1	32.2	1	1.8
Pan Fried, Rana La Famiglia*	1 Serving/150g	231	1.4	154	2.6	34	0.9	0
Potato, Cooked, Average	***1 Serving/150g***	***200***	***0***	***133***	***0***	***33.2***	***0***	***0***
Pumpkin, Fresh, Dell'ugo*	½ Pack/226g	325	2	144	4.5	28	0.9	3.3
Tomato, & Mozzarella, Italiamo, Lidl*	1 Serving/250g	365	4.8	146	3.5	28	1.9	2.3
Tricolore, Mini, De Marlino*	1 Serving/100g	162	0.5	162	3.6	36	0.5	1.7
Vegetable, Chargrilled, Plant Based, Asda*	1 Pack/384g	338	3.1	88	2.7	17	0.8	1.5
Wholewheat, Cooked, Tesco*	¼ Pack/132g	185	1.1	140	4.7	26.5	0.8	4.3
Wholewheat, Uncooked, Tesco*	¼ Pack/125g	185	1	148	5	27.9	0.8	4.5
GOAT								
Meat, Uncooked	***1 Serving/100g***	***109***	***2.3***	***109***	***20.6***	***0***	***2.3***	***0***
GOJI BERRIES								
Average	***1 Serving/100g***	***287***	***0.7***	***287***	***6.6***	***65.1***	***0.7***	***6.8***
GOOSE								
Meat & Skin, Roasted	***½ Goose/774g***	***2361***	***169.5***	***305***	***25.2***	***0***	***21.9***	***0***
Meat, Raw	***1 Portion/185g***	***298***	***13***	***161***	***23***	***0***	***7***	***0***
Meat, Roasted	***1 Portion/143g***	***340***	***18.1***	***238***	***29***	***0***	***12.7***	***0***
GOOSEBERRIES								
Dessert, Raw, Tops & Tails Removed	***1oz/28g***	***11***	***0.1***	***40***	***0.7***	***9.2***	***0.3***	***2.4***
Stewed with Sugar	***25g***	***14***	***0.1***	***54***	***0.7***	***12.9***	***0.3***	***4.2***
Stewed without Sugar	***25g***	***4***	***0.1***	***16***	***0.9***	***2.5***	***0.3***	***4.4***
GOULASH								
Beef, Average	***1 Serving/300g***	***310***	***9.5***	***103***	***8.1***	***10.4***	***3.2***	***0.9***
Meatball, Beef, with Rice, Hello Fresh*	1 Serving/796g	621	20	78	5.5	8.8	2.5	0
GRAINS								
Gorgeous, Microwave, Sainsbury's*	½ Pack/125g	209	1.6	167	6	30.9	1.3	0
Italian Infused, Pesto-ey, Merchant Gourmet*	1 Pack/250g	452	12.7	181	6.1	25.8	5.1	3.4
Korean Style, Zingy, Merchant Gourmet*	½ Pack/125g	199	3.5	159	6.4	24.8	2.8	4.2
Mediterranean Style, Microwave, Sainsbury's*	½ Pack/125g	222	3.8	178	5.3	29.8	3	5.3
Middle Eastern Style, Golden Sun, Lidl*	½ Pack/125g	220	6.2	176	5.5	24.5	5	5.3
Mixed, Sun Dried Tomato, Merchant Gourmet*	1 Serving/125g	220	3.4	176	6.2	29.5	2.7	4.6
Moroccan Style, M&S*	1 Pack/290g	447	6.4	154	4.7	26.3	2.2	5.1
Piri Piri, Spicy, Merchant Gourmet*	½ Pack/110g	194	4.3	176	4	28.3	3.9	6
Quinoa & Lentils, Persian Style, Merchant Gourmet*	½ Pack/125g	220	3.5	176	6.7	28.6	2.8	4.9
Spanish Style, Worldwide Foods, Aldi*	½ Pouch/125g	231	7.4	185	4.2	27	5.9	4.6
Super, Garlic, & Ginger, Tilda*	½ Pack/110g	165	5.8	150	4.5	19	5.3	4.2
Super, Sweet Potato, Chilli, & Coconut, Tilda*	½ Pouch/110g	161	5.1	146	3.1	22	4.6	2.3
Tomato, & Herb, with Buckwheat, Spelt, & Bulgur, Twistd*	½ Pack/125g	181	3.4	145	4.8	23	2.7	5.2
Wheatberries, & Kale, Sainsbury's*	½ Pack/150g	195	6.8	130	6.6	12	4.5	7.6
Wonder, Mediterranean, Stir & Eat, Quorn*	1 Pot/200g	212	4	106	5.5	14	2	4.9
Wonder, Thai Style, Stir & Eat, Quorn*	1 Pot/200g	252	9.4	126	5.5	14	4.7	3.6
GRAPEFRUIT								
in Juice, Canned, Average	***1/3 Can/179g***	***82***	***0.1***	***46***	***0.5***	***10.6***	***0***	***0.4***
in Syrup, Average	***1oz/28g***	***19***	***0***	***69***	***0.5***	***16.8***	***0.1***	***0.5***
Raw, Flesh Only, Average	***½ Fruit/160g***	***48***	***0.2***	***30***	***0.8***	***6.8***	***0.1***	***1.3***
Raw, Weighed with Skin & Seeds, Average	***1 Lge/340g***	***54***	***0.2***	***16***	***0.3***	***4***	***0***	***0.6***
Ruby Red in Juice, Average	***1 Serving/135g***	***54***	***0.1***	***40***	***0.6***	***9.4***	***0***	***0.5***
GRAPES								
Black, Seedless, Sable, TTD, Sainsbury's*	1 Serving/80g	56	0.4	70	0.5	15.4	0.5	0.7
Candy Floss, Seedless, Raw, Tesco*	1 Serving/80g	58	0.1	73	0.6	17	0.1	0.6
Cotton Candy, 1, Waitrose*	1 Serving/80g	53	0.1	66	0.4	15.4	0.1	0.9

	Measure INFO/WEIGHT	per Measure KCAL	FAT	Nutrition Values per 100g / 100ml KCAL	PROT	CARB	FAT	FIBRE
GRAPES								
Cotton Candy, Black, Seedless, Finest, Tesco*	1 Portion/80g	53	0.1	66	0.4	15.4	0.1	0.7
Green, Average	***1 Grape/5g***	***3***	***0***	***62***	***0.4***	***15.2***	***0.1***	***0.7***
Red & Green Selection, Average	***1 Grape/5g***	***3***	***0***	***62***	***0.4***	***15.2***	***0.1***	***0.8***
Red, Average	***1 Grape/5g***	***3***	***0***	***65***	***0.4***	***15.8***	***0.1***	***0.6***
Sable, 1, Waitrose*	1 Pack/400g	264	0.4	66	0.4	15.4	0.1	0.9
Sable, Finest, Tesco*	1 Serving/80g	53	0.1	66	0.4	15.4	0.1	0.7
Seedless, Red, Average	***1 Grape***	***4***	***0***	***74***	***0.6***	***17***	***0.3***	***0.6***
GRAPPA								
Average	***1 Serving/30ml***	***85***	***0***	***283***	***0***	***6.7***	***0***	***0***
GRATIN								
Aubergine, & Pepper, with Cherry Tomatoes, Higgidy*	1 Pack/390g	320	14.4	82	2.4	7.4	3.7	5
Broccoli, & Cauliflower, Creamy, Iceland*	1 Gratin/112g	204	17.1	182	3.1	7	15.3	1.9
Crab, & Lobster Mac & Cheese, Iceland*	1 Pot/100g	148	7.1	155	7.4	14	7.4	1.5
Dauphinois, Mini, Duc De Coeur, Lidl*	1 Gratin/120g	163	9.7	136	3.2	11.8	8.1	1.4
Haddock, Smoked, Frozen, Tesco*	1 Pot/90g	145	9.2	162	12.4	4.5	10.3	1.1
Ham Hock, Leek, & Potato, The Best, Morrisons*	1 Pack/400g	480	20.4	120	8.3	9.8	5.1	1
Ham, Wiltshire Cured, Specially Selected, Aldi*	1 Pack/400g	616	28	154	7.6	14	7	1.6
Potato, & Spinach, M&S*	1 Serving/225g	259	16	115	2.9	9.1	7.1	1.3
Potato, Cheesy, Oven Baked, Asda*	½ Pack/185g	200	8.1	108	3.8	13	4.4	1.3
Potato, Chef Select, Lidl*	½ Pack/250g	380	22.2	152	2.8	14	8.9	2
Potato, Creamy, M&S*	½ Pack/225g	360	25	160	2.2	11.9	11.1	0.9
Potato, Crispy & Creamy, Oven Baked, Tesco*	½ Pack/218g	233	14	107	2.4	9.4	6.4	1.3
Potato, Dauphinoise, Finest, Tesco*	1 Gratin/107g	210	14.1	196	3.3	15	13.1	2
Potato, Individual, Waitrose*	1 Gratin/120g	230	16.8	192	3.8	11.8	14	1.6
Potato, Oven Cooked, Sainsbury's*	1 Serving/100g	195	12.8	195	2.8	16	12.8	2.4
Potato, Tasty, Aldi*	½ Pack/180g	187	7	104	2.4	14	3.9	2.2
Potato, Waitrose*	½ Pack/207g	275	16.7	133	4.7	9.9	8.1	1.1
Sweet Potato, & Vegetable, Sainsbury's*	1 Gratin/100g	180	14.1	180	2.9	9.1	14.1	2.3
Vegetable, Root, Finest, Tesco*	½ Pack/214g	365	23.9	171	2.4	14	11.2	2
GRAVY								
Beef, Aunt Bessie's*	1 Serving/100g	73	5.3	73	1	5.3	5.3	0.5
Beef, Favourite, Granules, Made Up, Bisto*	1 Serving/50ml	13	0.5	26	0	4.2	1	0
Beef, Free From, Sainsbury's*	½ Pack/151g	47	1.5	31	1.5	4.1	1	0.2
Beef, Fresh, Sainsbury's*	1 Serving/83ml	47	2.7	56	2.4	4.5	3.2	0.6
Beef, Roast, Best in Glass Jar, Made Up, Bisto*	1 Serving/70ml	21	0.3	30	0.3	6.1	0.4	0
Beef, Roast, Traditional, Finest, Tesco*	¼ Pot/125g	68	3	54	2.4	5.5	2.4	0.3
Chicken, & Hint of Sage & Onion, Granules, Oxo*	1 Serving/30g	95	1.8	316	11.1	54.2	6.1	0.7
Chicken, & Turkey, Christmas, TTD, Sainsbury's*	¼ Pot/112g	66	1.7	59	6.9	4.2	1.5	0.5
Chicken, Granules, Dry, Average	***1 Tsp/4g***	***17***	***0.9***	***428***	***4.5***	***49.4***	***23.6***	***1.2***
Chicken, Granules, Made Up, Average	***1 Serving/50ml***	***15***	***0.8***	***30***	***0.4***	***3.6***	***1.5***	***0.1***
Chicken, Roast, Paste, Rich, Bisto*	1 Pack/400ml	140	6	35	0.5	4.9	1.5	0.5
Granules, Instant, Made Up	***1oz/28g***	***10***	***0.7***	***34***	***0.3***	***3***	***2.4***	***0***
Granules, Low Salt, Organic, Made Up, Kallo*	1 Serving/70ml	227	8.5	32	0.3	5.1	1.2	0
Granules, Onion, Dry	1 Tbsp/15g	17	1.1	116	1.9	10.9	7.5	1.9
Granules, Southern Style, As Prepared, Bisto*	1 Serving/50ml	28	1	56	1	8.6	2	1
Lamb, Granules, Dry, Average	***1 Tsp/4g***	***14***	***0.3***	***344***	***10.8***	***56.2***	***8.4***	***2.8***
Onion, Caramelised, Made Up, Bisto*	1 Serving/50ml	14	0.2	29	0.1	6.1	0.4	0.1
Onion, Fresh, Asda*	1/6 Pot/77g	30	1.6	39	1.7	3.3	2.1	0.4
Onion, Granules, Dry Weight, Bisto*	4 Tsp/20g	78	2.9	391	2.4	62.3	14.7	2.3
Onion, Granules, Made Up, Bisto*	1 Serving/50ml	14	0.3	28	0.2	5.6	0.6	0
Onion, Rich, M&S*	½ Pack/150g	60	1.8	40	2	5.9	1.2	0.3
Pork, & Sage, Roast, Classic, Dry, Schwartz*	1 Pack/25g	88	1.4	354	11.8	63.8	5.8	0
Pork, Best, Made Up, Bisto*	1 Serving/50ml	13	0.5	26	1	5.8	1	1

	Measure INFO/WEIGHT	per Measure KCAL	FAT	Nutrition Values per 100g / 100ml KCAL	PROT	CARB	FAT	FIBRE
GRAVY								
Pork, Roast, Best, in Glass Jar, Dry Weight, Bisto*	4 Tsp/20g	67	0.9	333	5.7	66.6	4.7	0.8
Powder, GF, Dry, Allergycare*	1 Tbsp/10g	26	0	260	0.3	63.8	0.4	0
Powder, Made Up, Sainsbury's*	1 Serving/100ml	15	0.1	15	0.4	3.2	0.1	0.1
Reduced Salt, Granules, Chicken, As Prepared, Bisto*	1 Tsp/5g	1	0	28	1	4.4	1	1
Reduced Salt, Granules, Chicken, Dry Weight, Bisto*	1 Tsp/5g	21	0.8	415	2.3	65.5	15.6	1.7
Southern Style, Mayflower, Made Up, Iceland *	1 Serving/50ml	32	1.7	65	0.8	8	3.4	0.3
Turkey, Finest, Tesco*	¼ Pouch/88ml	49	1.4	56	3.9	6.4	1.6	0
Vegan, Plant Kitchen, M&S*	1 Serving/50g	20	0.4	39	1	6.4	0.9	0.4
Vegetable, Granules, Dry Weight, Bisto*	1 Tsp/4g	15	0.5	380	2.1	63	13.3	4.5
Vegetable, Granules, Made Up, Bisto*	1 Serving/50ml	14	0.2	28	0.2	5.6	0.4	0.2
Vegetarian, Granules, Dry Weight, Bisto*	1 Serving/28g	100	3.7	356	2.7	56	13.3	4.5
Vegetarian, Granules, Made Up, Sainsbury's*	1 Serving/50ml	16	1.1	32	0.2	2.8	2.2	0.8
GROUSE								
Meat Only, Roasted	***1oz/28g***	***36***	***0.6***	***128***	***27.6***	***0***	***2***	***0***
GUACAMOLE								
Average	***1 Tbsp/17g***	***33***	***3.3***	***194***	***1.6***	***3.4***	***19.2***	***2.4***
Jalapeno, & Red Pepper, Holy Moly*	1 Serving/30g	38	3.6	126	1.2	1.5	12	4.7
GUAVA								
Canned in Syrup	***1oz/28g***	***17***	***0***	***60***	***0.4***	***15.7***	***0***	***3***
Raw, Flesh Only, Average	***1 Fruit/55g***	***37***	***0.6***	***68***	***3***	***14***	***1***	***5***
GUINEA FOWL								
Boned & Stuffed, Fresh, Fayrefield Foods*	1 Serving/325g	650	39.3	200	19.1	3.3	12.1	0.5
Fresh, Free Range, without Giblets, No.1, Waitrose*	1 Portion/193g	368	16.9	191	27.6	0.5	8.8	0.6
GUMS								
American Hard, Sainsbury's*	1 Sweet/6g	22	0	360	0.1	90	0.1	0
American Hard, Tesco*	1 Serving/200g	646	0	323	0	80.8	0	0
Milk Bottles, Bassett's*	1 Pack/25g	88	0.4	353	6.2	78.3	1.6	0

	Measure INFO/WEIGHT	per Measure KCAL	FAT	Nutrition Values per 100g / 100ml KCAL	PROT	CARB	FAT	FIBRE
HADDOCK								
Fillet, Lightly Dusted, Scottish, Waitrose*	1 Fillet/133g	189	5.5	142	17.3	8.2	4.1	1.4
Fillets, Battered, Average	***1oz/28g***	***64***	***3.4***	***228***	***13.4***	***16.3***	***12.2***	***1.1***
Fillets, in Breadcrumbs, Average	***1 Fillet/125g***	***253***	***12.4***	***203***	***13.5***	***14.9***	***9.9***	***1.2***
Fillets, in White Wine & Onion Sauce, Birds Eye*	1 Fillet/137g	169	7.8	123	16	1.8	5.7	0.5
Fillets, Lightly Dusted, Tesco*	1 Fillet/115g	182	6.7	158	15.3	10.9	5.8	0.6
Fillets, Raw, Average	***1 Fillet/140g***	***111***	***1.2***	***79***	***17.7***	***0.2***	***0.8***	***0***
Fillets, Smoked, Cooked, Average	***1 Pack/300g***	***337***	***7.7***	***112***	***21.9***	***0.4***	***2.6***	***0.1***
Fillets, Smoked, Raw, Average	***1 Pack/227g***	***190***	***1***	***84***	***19.9***	***0.1***	***0.4***	***0.2***
Fillets, Smoked, with Cheese Crumb, Sainsbury's*	1 Fillet/174g	325	23	187	13.6	3.4	13.2	0.5
Flour, Fried in Blended Oil	***1oz/28g***	***39***	***1.1***	***138***	***21.1***	***4.5***	***4.1***	***0.2***
Goujons, Batter, Crispy, M&S*	1 Serving/100g	250	14.1	250	11.7	18.5	14.1	0.8
Mornay, Cheesy, Ready to Cook, Oven Baked, Asda*	½ Pack/140g	133	5	95	14	1.4	3.6	0.5
HAGGIS								
Bon Bons, Simon Howie*	1 Serving/120g	253	10	211	11.3	23	8.3	0
Slices, Uncooked, Malcolm Allan*	1 Slice/56g	178	11.8	318	10.4	21.6	21.1	0
Traditional, Average	***1 Serving/454g***	***1119***	***66.5***	***246***	***12.4***	***17.2***	***14.6***	***1***
Vegetarian, Macsween*	1/3 Pack/151g	412	24.6	273	6	22.9	16.3	6.7
HAKE								
Fillets, in Breadcrumbs, Average	***1oz/28g***	***66***	***3.7***	***234***	***12.9***	***16***	***13.4***	***1***
Goujons, Average	***1 Serving/150g***	***345***	***17.8***	***230***	***12.4***	***18.6***	***11.9***	***1.3***
Raw, Average	***1oz/28g***	***28***	***0.6***	***100***	***20.1***	***0***	***2.2***	***0***
HALIBUT								
Cooked, Dry Heat, Average	***1oz/28g***	***38***	***1.1***	***135***	***24.6***	***0.4***	***4***	***0***
Raw	***1oz/28g***	***28***	***0.5***	***101***	***21.1***	***0***	***1.9***	***0***
HALVA								
Average	***1oz/28g***	***107***	***3.7***	***381***	***1.8***	***68***	***13.2***	***0***
HAM								
Applewood Smoked, Average	***1 Slice/28g***	***31***	***0.8***	***112***	***21.2***	***0.6***	***2.8***	***0.2***
Baked, Average	***1 Slice/74g***	***98***	***3.7***	***133***	***21***	***1***	***5***	***0***
Bavarian, Smoked, Finely Sliced, Asda*	2 Slices/35g	36	0.6	102	21	0.5	1.6	0
Black Forest, Slices, Dulano, Lidl*	1 Slice/11g	26	1.6	240	25	1	15	0.5
Boiled, Average	***1 Pack/113g***	***154***	***6.5***	***136***	***20.6***	***0.6***	***5.8***	***0***
Breaded, Average	***1 Slice/37g***	***57***	***2.3***	***155***	***23.1***	***1.8***	***6.3***	***1.6***
Breaded, Dry Cured, Average	***1 Slice/33g***	***47***	***1.8***	***142***	***22.2***	***1.4***	***5.4***	***0***
Brunswick, Average	***1 Slice/20g***	***32***	***1.8***	***160***	***19.5***	***0.6***	***8.8***	***0***
Cooked, Sliced, Average	***1 Slice/17g***	***18***	***0.5***	***109***	***19***	***1***	***3.2***	***0.1***
Crumbed, Sliced, Average	***1 Slice/28g***	***33***	***0.9***	***117***	***21.5***	***0.9***	***3.1***	***0***
Danish, Average	***1 Slice/11g***	***14***	***0.6***	***125***	***18.4***	***1***	***5.4***	***0***
Dry Cured, Average	***1 Slice/18g***	***26***	***1***	***144***	***22.4***	***1***	***5.6***	***0.2***
Extra Lean, Average	***1 Slice/11g***	***10***	***0.2***	***90***	***18***	***1.4***	***1.4***	***0***
Gammon, Breaded, Average	***1 Serving/25g***	***31***	***0.8***	***122***	***22***	***1.5***	***3.1***	***0***
Gammon, Dry Cured, Sliced, Average	***1 Slice/33g***	***43***	***1.4***	***131***	***22.9***	***0.4***	***4.2***	***0***
Gammon, Honey Roast, Average	***1 Serving/60g***	***81***	***2.8***	***134***	***22.4***	***0.4***	***4.8***	***0***
Gammon, Smoked, Average	***1 Slice/43g***	***59***	***2.1***	***137***	***22.3***	***0.7***	***4.9***	***0.2***
German Black Forest, Average	***½ Pack/35g***	***93***	***6***	***267***	***27.2***	***1.3***	***17***	***0.5***
Heather Honey, Specially Selected, Aldi*	1 Slice/17g	23	0.7	139	22	2.5	4.5	0.6
Hock, Cooked, Shredded, Sainsbury's*	½ Pack55g	100	4.1	182	27.6	0.5	7.5	1
Hock, Mustard Sauce, with Mash, & Peas, Tesco*	1 Pack/450g	387	13	86	7.5	6.8	2.9	1.4
Hock, Pulled, M&S*	1 Pack/100g	165	6.5	165	26.5	0.1	6.5	0.1
Hocks, in Apple Glaze, Simple to Cook, Asda*	1 Serving/270g	358	13	133	18.2	3.6	4.8	0.6
Honey & Mustard, Average	***1oz/28g***	***39***	***1.2***	***140***	***20.8***	***4.6***	***4.3***	***0***
Honey Roast, Average	***1 Slice/20g***	***25***	***0.8***	***123***	***20.3***	***1.6***	***3.8***	***0.1***
Honey Roast, Dry Cured, Average	***1 Slice/33g***	***46***	***1.5***	***140***	***22.7***	***2.3***	***4.4***	***0.2***

	Measure INFO/WEIGHT	per Measure KCAL	FAT	Nutrition Values per 100g / 100ml KCAL	PROT	CARB	FAT	FIBRE
HAM								
Honey Roast, Lean, Average	***1 Serving/25g***	***28***	***0.8***	***111***	***18.2***	***2.7***	***3.1***	***0***
Honey Roast, Wafer Thin, Average	***1 Slice/10g***	***11***	***0.3***	***113***	***17.4***	***3.7***	***3.2***	***0.3***
Jamon, Iberico de Bellota, Hand Carved, 1, Waitrose*	¼ Pack/16g	56	3.9	344	31.5	0.7	23.7	0.9
Joint, Cured, Roasted, Average	***1 Serving/100g***	***138***	***5.2***	***138***	***21.7***	***1***	***5.2***	***0.1***
Joint, Roast, Christmas, Tesco*	1/6 Joint/167g	225	10.8	135	17.9	1.1	6.5	0
Lean, Average	***1 Slice/18g***	***19***	***0.4***	***104***	***19.5***	***1.1***	***2.4***	***0.3***
Oak Smoked, Average	***1 Slice/20g***	***26***	***0.9***	***130***	***21***	***1***	***4.7***	***0.3***
Parma, Average	***1 Slice/10g***	***21***	***1.1***	***213***	***29.3***	***0***	***10.6***	***0***
Parma, Premium, Average	***1 Slice/14g***	***36***	***2.3***	***258***	***27.9***	***0.3***	***16.1***	***0***
Peppered, Average	***1 Slice/12g***	***13***	***0.3***	***110***	***18.5***	***2***	***2.7***	***0***
Prosciutto, Average	***1 Slice/12g***	***27***	***1.5***	***226***	***28.7***	***0***	***12.4***	***0.4***
Pulled, in Mustard Sauce, BFY, M&S*	1 Pack/358g	304	10	85	7.7	6.2	2.8	2.3
Roast, Cooked On The Bone, Finest, Tesco*	1 Slice/25g	32	0.6	130	26.3	0.2	2.6	0.5
Roast, Mini, M&S*	1 Slice/30g	58	3.4	193	21.4	1.2	11.2	0.9
Roast, Thick Cut, M&S*	1 Slice/40g	56	1.9	140	23	1	4.8	1
Roast, Thickly Carved, Extra Special, Asda*	1 Slice/40g	48	0.6	119	25	1	1.5	0.7
Serrano, Average	***1 Slice/20g***	***46***	***2.4***	***230***	***30.5***	***0.4***	***11.8***	***0***
Smoked, Average	***1 Slice/18g***	***21***	***0.7***	***117***	***19.7***	***0.9***	***3.7***	***0***
Smoked, Dry Cured, Average	***1 Slice/28g***	***38***	***1.2***	***137***	***23***	***1.4***	***4.4***	***0.2***
Smoked, Wafer Thin, Average	***1 Serving/40g***	***41***	***1.2***	***102***	***17.7***	***1.2***	***2.9***	***0.2***
Thick Cut, Average	***1 Slice/74g***	***94***	***2.9***	***127***	***22.4***	***0.6***	***3.9***	***0.1***
Tinned, Average	***½ Can/100g***	***136***	***8.8***	***136***	***12.2***	***2***	***8.8***	***0***
Torchon, Aldi*	1 Slice/50g	58	1.4	116	22	1	2.8	0.5
Torchon, French, Sainsbury's*	1 Slice/50g	57	1.5	114	21	0.7	3	0
Torchon, French, Unearthed*	1 Slice/40g	46	1.2	114	21	0.8	3	0
Trimmings, Cooked, Blue Mountain*	1 Serving/180g	200	3.6	111	20	1	2	0
Trimmings, Cooked, Iceland *	1 Serving/30g	31	0.9	103	18.5	0.5	3	0
Vegan, Simply Vamm, Vdeli Slices, Vbites Foods *	3 Slices/33g	70	3.7	212	23.2	4.4	11.3	0.2
Vegetarian, Slices, Deli, Wafer Thin, Deli, Quorn*	1/3 Pack/60g	66	1.3	110	16	6.5	2.2	5.8
Vegetarian, Slices, Quorn*	¼ Pack/25g	30	0.5	122	16	6.5	2.2	5.8
Wafer Thin, Average	***1 Slice/10g***	***10***	***0.3***	***101***	***17.9***	***1.4***	***2.6***	***0.1***
Wiltshire, Average	***1oz/28g***	***41***	***1.7***	***148***	***23.1***	***0***	***6***	***0***
Wiltshire, Breaded, Average	***1oz/28g***	***41***	***1.4***	***145***	***23.9***	***1***	***5***	***0***
HARIBO*								
American Hard Gums, Haribo*	1 Pack/175g	630	3.3	360	0.3	85.5	1.9	0.2
Cola Bottles, Fizzy, Haribo*	1 Pack/175g	595	0.4	340	6.3	78.3	0.2	0.3
Cola Bottles, Haribo*	1 Pack/16g	56	0	348	7.7	78.9	0.2	0.3
Dolly Mixtures, Haribo*	1 Pack/175g	719	8.4	411	1.8	90.2	4.8	0.2
Fantasy Mix, Haribo*	1 Pack/100g	344	0.2	344	6.6	79	0.2	0.3
Gold Bears, Haribo*	1 Pack/100g	343	0.5	343	6.9	77	0.5	0
Happy Cherries, Haribo*	1 Serving/40g	139	0.1	348	7.7	78.9	0.2	0.3
Horror Mix, Haribo*	1 Pack/100g	344	0.2	344	6.6	79	0.2	0.3
Jelly Babies, Haribo*	1 Serving/25g	87	0	348	4.5	82.1	0.2	0.5
Kiddies Super Mix, Haribo*	1 Pack/100g	344	0.2	344	6.6	79	0.2	0.3
Liquorice Favourites, Haribo*	1 Serving/40g	143	1.2	357	2.8	78.8	3	2.3
Maoam Stripes, Haribo*	1 Chew/7g	27	0.4	384	1.2	81.7	6.1	0.3
Milky Mix, Haribo*	1 Pack/175g	607	0.4	347	7.1	79.6	0.2	0.4
Pontefract Cakes, Haribo*	1 Serving/40g	118	0.1	296	5.3	68.2	0.2	0.5
Snakes, Haribo*	1 Snake/8g	28	0	348	7.7	78.9	0.2	0.3
Starmix, Haribo*	1 Pack/100g	344	0.2	344	6.6	79	0.2	0.3
Tangfastics, Haribo*	1 Pack/100g	359	2.3	359	6.3	78.3	2.3	0.5
HARISSA PASTE								
Average	***1 Tsp/5g***	***6***	***0.3***	***123***	***2.9***	***12.9***	***6.7***	***2.8***

	Measure INFO/WEIGHT	per Measure KCAL	per Measure FAT	Nutrition Values per 100g / 100ml KCAL	PROT	CARB	FAT	FIBRE
HARISSA PASTE								
Ruby Rose, Cooks' Ingredients, Waitrose*	1 Tsp/5g	4	0.2	88	1.5	11.3	3.2	4.2
HASH								
Beef, Potato Topped, with Cheddar, TTD, Sainsbury's*	1 Pack/384g	499	18.4	130	9	12.4	4.8	1.1
Beef, Steak, Specially Selected, Aldi*	1 Pack/400g	472	15.6	118	7.4	12	3.9	1.8
Chicken, & Stuffing, Dinner, M&S*	1 Pack/400g	480	18.4	120	8	10.9	4.6	1.3
Corned Beef, Homestyle, Hormel*	1 Can/400g	644	40.7	161	7.2	9.8	10.2	0.8
Corned Beef, in Rich Onion Gravy, Oven Baked, Asda*	1 Pack/374g	438	10.5	117	6.5	16	2.8	1.7
Corned Beef, Waitrose*	1 Pack/385g	516	20.4	134	6.8	13.9	5.3	1.7
Steak, Hash, Extra Special, Asda*	1 Pack/354g	450	11	127	7.5	16	3.1	2.4
HASH BROWNS								
Cauliflower, Strong Roots*	1 Piece/40g	74	4.3	185	1.7	19.4	10.7	1.8
Fries, Oven Baked, Iceland*	1 Serving/150g	375	15	250	3.4	34.7	10	3.5
Golden, Oven Cooked, Aviko*	1 Hashbrown/63g	104	4.4	165	2	22.5	7	2.5
Homestyle, Aunt Bessie's*	2 Pieces/98g	182	9.2	186	1.6	23	9.4	1.9
Iceland*	1 Hashbrown/36g	69	3.2	193	2.2	24.4	9	2.8
Oven Baked, Weighed Frozen, McCain*	1 Piece/40g	60	2.4	150	1.6	21.3	6	2.1
Potatoes, From Restaurant, Average	***1 Portion/150g***	***489***	***32.5***	***326***	***2.6***	***32.1***	***21.6***	***2.7***
Roasted Onion, & Rosemary, Sainsbury's*	1 Hashbrown/52g	96	4.5	185	3	22.3	8.6	3.1
Uncooked, Average	***1 Piece/45g***	***78***	***3.7***	***173***	***2***	***22.5***	***8.3***	***1.9***
HAZELNUTS								
Blanched, Average	***1 Serving/25g***	***164***	***15.9***	***656***	***15.4***	***5.8***	***63.5***	***6.5***
Chopped, Average	***1 Serving/10g***	***67***	***6.4***	***666***	***16.8***	***5.6***	***64***	***6.6***
White Chocolate, & Coconut, Finest, Tesco*	1 Serving/30g	182	13.8	606	9	37	46	4.2
Whole, Average	***10 Whole/10g***	***66***	***6.4***	***655***	***15.4***	***5.8***	***63.5***	***6.5***
HEART								
Lambs, Average	***1 Heart/75g***	***92***	***4.5***	***122***	***16***	***1***	***6***	***0***
Ox, Raw	***1oz/28g***	***23***	***0.8***	***82***	***14.4***	***0***	***2.8***	***0***
Ox, Stewed	***1oz/28g***	***44***	***1.4***	***157***	***27.8***	***0***	***5.1***	***0***
HERRING								
Canned in Tomato Sauce, Average	***1oz/28g***	***57***	***4.3***	***204***	***11.9***	***4.1***	***15.5***	***0.1***
Fillets, Marinated, in Cream Sauce, Lisner*	1 Serving/70g	201	18.8	287	5.4	5.9	26.8	0
Fillets, Raw, Average	***1 Herring/100g***	***139***	***9.4***	***139***	***13.8***	***0***	***9.4***	***0***
Grilled, Average	***1oz/28g***	***51***	***3.1***	***181***	***20.1***	***0***	***11.2***	***0***
Pickled, Average	***1oz/28g***	***42***	***2.9***	***149***	***8.1***	***5.5***	***10.3***	***0***
HONEY								
Acacia Blossom, Sainsbury's*	1 Serving/24g	81	0	339	0.1	84.7	0.1	0.3
Acacia, Tiptree, Wilkin & Sons*	1 Tbsp/15g	43	0	288	0	76	0	0
Clear, with a Hint of Cinnamon, Rowse*	1 Tbsp/15g	49	0.1	329	0.5	81.5	0.5	0.5
Greek, Waitrose*	1 Tsp/6g	18	0	307	0.4	76.4	0	0
Manuka, Mgo 50+, Hiltop*	1 Tsp/5g	17	0	333	0.5	83	0.5	0.5
Manuka, Rowse*	1 Tsp/5g	17	0	348	0	86.9	0.1	0
Pure, Clear, Average	***1 Tbsp/20g***	***63***	***0***	***315***	***0.5***	***78.5***	***0***	***0***
Pure, Set, Average	***1 Tbsp/20g***	***62***	***0***	***312***	***0.4***	***77.6***	***0***	***0***
Raw, British Wildflower, Hilltop*	1 Tsp/5g	17	0	333	0.2	83.1	0.2	0
Scottish Heather, Waitrose*	1 Serving/20g	61	0	307	0.4	76.4	0	0
Spanish Lavender, Hilltop Honey*	1 Tbsp/15g	50	0.1	333	0.5	83	0.5	0.5
Spanish Orange Blossom, Sainsbury's*	1 Tbsp/15g	51	0	339	0.1	84.7	0	0.3
HONEYCOMB								
Chocolate Dipped, M&S*	1 Serving/40g	180	4.6	451	2.6	83.4	11.6	1.1
Natural, Epicure*	1 Serving/100g	290	4.6	290	0.4	74.4	4.6	0
HORLICKS								
Malted Drink, Instant, Dry Weight, Horlicks*	2 Tbsp/30g	108	0.6	359	13.1	74.4	1.9	1.9
Malted Drink, Light, Dry Weight, Horlicks*	1 Serving/32g	116	1.2	364	14.8	72.2	3.8	1.9

H

	Measure INFO/WEIGHT	per Measure KCAL	FAT	Nutrition Values per 100g / 100ml KCAL	PROT	CARB	FAT	FIBRE
HORLICKS								
Powder, Made Up with Semi-Skimmed Milk	***1 Mug/227ml***	***184***	***4.3***	***81***	***4.3***	***12.9***	***1.9***	***0***
Powder, Made Up with Whole Milk	***1 Mug/227ml***	***225***	***8.9***	***99***	***4.2***	***12.7***	***3.9***	***0***
HORSERADISH								
Cream, Strong, Tracklement's*	1 Tsp/5g	15	1.3	299	4.3	7.5	26.5	4.9
Creamed, Sainsbury's*	1 Tsp/10ml	25	1.4	253	2.8	26.9	14.3	2.3
Prepared, Average	***1 Tsp/5g***	***1***	***0***	***28***	***2***	***5***	***0.1***	***2.8***
HOT CHOCOLATE								
Belgian Choc, Options*	1 Sachet/11g	40	0.8	365	8.9	59	7.3	0
Belgian Chocolate, Honeycomb, Options, Ovaltine*	1 Serving/11g	39	0.9	353	8.4	52	8.1	0
Belgian Chocolate, Options, Ovaltine*	1 Serving/11g	40	0.8	365	8.9	59	7.3	0
Cadbury*	1 Serving/12g	44	0.7	370	6.3	73.3	5.9	0
Caramel, Whittards of Chelsea*	1 Serving/20g	71	1.5	355	7.5	64.5	7.5	13
Choc Mint, Highlights, Made Up, Cadbury*	1 Serving/200ml	40	1.4	20	1	2.5	0.7	0.3
Chocolate Au Lait, Options, Ovaltine*	1 Sachet/10g	36	1	355	11.8	54.5	10	7.3
Classic, Hotel Chocolat*	1 Serving/35g	172	2.2	490	4.6	11.7	6.2	1.9
Cocoa, Lidl*	1 Serving/20g	77	1.2	386	6.1	74.1	6.2	0
Dairy Fudge, Highlights, Dry Weight, Cadbury*	1 Serving/11g	38	1.2	347	16	41	11	9.7
Dark, Bournville, Highlights, Made Up, Cadbury*	1 Serving/200ml	35	0.9	18	1.2	2	0.4	0
Dreamy Caramel, Options, Ovaltine*	1 Sachet/11g	39	0.9	354	12.3	48.5	7.8	0
Drink, Organic, Green & Black's*	1 Tsp/5g	20	0.4	396	8.6	67	7.5	12
Fairtrade, Whittards of Chelsea*	4 Tsp/20g	68	0.8	342	7.8	69	3.9	10.9
Frothy, Ultimate, Dry Mix, Galaxy*	1 Serving/25g	97	2	387	4.5	72	8.1	0
Galaxy, Mars*	1 Sachet/25g	97	1.9	386	4.8	71.9	7.7	4.7
Highlights, Instant, Made Up, Cadbury*	1 Cup/200ml	40	1.4	20	1	2.5	0.7	0.3
Instant Break, Cadbury*	1 Sachet/28g	119	3.9	425	10.9	64.2	14	0
Instant, As Prepared, Smart Price, Asda*	1 Serving/227g	109	1.1	48	0.8	10	0.5	0.5
Instant, Highlights, Cadbury*	1 Sachet/22g	80	2.8	364	17.3	44.6	12.7	0
Instant, Powder, As Prepared with Hot Water, Morrisons*	1 Serving/230ml	108	1.1	47	1	9.5	0.5	0.5
Instant, Tesco*	1 Serving/30g	120	2.5	401	7.1	71.6	8.4	5.4
Low Calorie, Dry Weight, As Sold, Average	***1 Sachet/11g***	***41***	***1.2***	***374***	***14.6***	***50***	***10.7***	***11.1***
Maltesers, Malt Drink, Instant, Made Up, Mars*	1 Serving/220ml	104	3	47	0.9	7.7	1.4	0
Milk, Swiss, Powder, Twinings*	1 Serving/20g	78	0.7	389	5	81.3	3.5	0
Milky, 50%, Sachet, Hotel Chocolat*	1 Sachet/35g	199	14.7	568	8.6	33.7	41.9	9.4
Mint Madness, Belgian, Options, Ovaltine*	1 Sachet/11g	38	0.8	348	12.3	49.2	6.9	20
Mint, Highlights, Cadbury*	1 Serving/200ml	40	1.4	20	1	2.5	0.7	0
Mint, Sachet, As Sold, Hotel Chocolat*	1 Sachet/35g	196	14.5	561	7.4	32.9	41.5	11.7
Orange, Supermilk, Sachet, Hotel Chocolat*	1 Sachet/35g	198	15.5	567	9.1	28.6	44.4	10.3
Outrageous Orange, Options, Ovaltine*	1 Serving/11g	38	0.8	348	12.3	49.3	6.9	20
Pods, Galaxy, Mars*	1 Pod/17g	69	1.8	406	5.3	70.6	10.6	0
Salted Caramel, Dry, Specially Selected, Aldi*	1 Serving/20g	75	1.1	373	11	64	5.5	12
Tempting Toffee, Options, Ovaltine*	1 Sachet/11g	43	1	391	13.6	66.4	9.1	0
Wicked White, Options, Ovaltine*	1 Sachet/11g	44	1.1	398	10.5	64.6	10	3.7
Wispa, Hot Frothy, Cadbury*	1 Sachet/27g	107	1.4	395	11	74	5.3	2.9
HOT DOG								
American Style, in Brine, Ye Olde Oak*	1 Hot Dog/45g	111	9.5	247	12.8	1.4	21.1	0
Beef, Campofrio*	1 Hotdog/120g	257	20.4	214	11	3.8	17	0
Bunlimited*	1 Hot Dog/70g	208	18	297	15.7	0.9	25.7	0
Plain, From Restaurant, Average	***1 Hot Dog/98g***	***242***	***14.5***	***247***	***10.6***	***18.4***	***14.8***	***0***
Plant Based, Moving Mountains*	1 Hot Dog/60g	77	5.4	128	7	3	9	3.2
Pork, Red Leicester, & Jalapeno, Finest, Tesco*	1 Hot Dog/86g	244	19.3	284	14.9	5.2	22.5	0.6
Posh Dogs, The Grill, M&S*	1 Hot Dog/100g	264	20.9	264	13.1	5.6	20.9	0.7
Posh Dogs, Vegan, Plant Kitchen, M&S*	1 Hot Dog/80g	174	13.4	218	8.4	4.5	16.7	7.9
Sausage, American Style, Average	***1 Hot Dog/75g***	***180***	***14.3***	***241***	***11.6***	***6.2***	***19***	***0***

H

	Measure INFO/WEIGHT	per Measure KCAL	FAT	Nutrition Values per 100g / 100ml KCAL	PROT	CARB	FAT	FIBRE
HOT DOG								
Sausage, Average	***1 Hot Dog/23g***	***40***	***3***	***175***	***10.8***	***4.3***	***12.8***	***0.3***
Vegetarian, Meat Free, Sainsbury's*	1 Hot Dog/30g	72	5.1	240	17.4	3.8	16.8	2
Vegetarian, Tesco*	1 Hot Dog/30g	66	4.7	222	17.1	1.6	15.8	2.2
HOT POT								
Beef, Classic, 800g, Asda*	1 Serving/400g	400	20.8	100	5.7	7.1	5.2	1.2
Beef, Minced, 3% Fat, Calorie Counted, Asda*	1 Pack/310g	319	7.1	103	4.5	15	2.3	2.2
Beef, Minced, Bisto*	1 Pack/375g	363	13.5	97	4.1	11.3	3.6	1.4
Beef, Minced, Calorie Counted, Oven Baked, Asda*	1 Pack/310g	319	7.1	103	4.5	15	2.3	2.2
Beef, Minced, Classic, Asda*	1 Pack/400g	424	18.4	106	6.8	8.7	4.6	1.1
Beef, Minced, Frozen, Tesco*	1 Pack/360g	377	10.1	105	5.2	11.7	2.8	1.6
Beef, Minced, HFC, Tesco*	1 Pack/362g	347	10	96	5.2	11.7	2.8	1.6
Beef, Minced, Iceland*	1 Pack/500g	500	20	100	2.8	12.1	4	1.8
Beef, Minced, Sainsbury's*	1 Pack/450g	464	22.1	103	5.3	9.5	4.9	2.2
Chicken, Counted, Calorie Controlled, Morrisons*	1 Pack/350g	217	1.8	62	7.3	6.6	0.5	0.9
Chicken, Counted, Morrisons*	1 Pack/350g	196	1.6	56	6.6	6	0.5	0.8
Chicken, Oven Baked, Asda*	1 Pack/368g	364	12.9	99	5.1	11	3.5	1.2
Chicken, Sainsbury's*	1 Pack/400g	340	11	85	5.2	9.8	2.8	1.3
Chicken, Waitrose*	1 Pack/400g	353	13.5	88	4.9	8.9	3.4	1.3
Chicken, Weight Watchers*	1 Pack/320g	296	6.7	93	6.3	11.8	2.1	1.1
Lamb, Chef Select, Lidl*	1 Serving/450g	463	20.8	103	6.1	8.4	4.6	1.6
Lamb, Minced, & Vegetable, COU, M&S*	1 Pack/400g	340	10.8	85	5.7	12.5	2.7	1.8
Lamb, Minced, Classic Kitchen, Tesco*	1 Pack/427g	384	12.8	90	5.6	9.4	3	1.5
Lamb, Minced, Morrison*	1 Pack/400g	376	11.6	94	4.1	11.7	2.9	2.2
Lamb, Onion & Pearl Barley Gravy, BFY, M&S*	1 Pack/375g	304	3	81	7.1	10.7	0.8	1.5
Lamb, Shank, Extra Special, Asda*	1 Pack/450g	508	20.2	113	10.2	7.8	4.5	1.3
Lancashire, M&S*	1 Pack/450g	441	13.5	98	8.4	8.8	3	1.3
Lancashire, Tesco*	½ Pack/225g	205	7	91	6	9.7	3.1	0.5
Lancashire, with Sliced Potatoes, Cooked, Aldi*	1 Pot/450g	460	17	108	7.3	9.3	4	2.7
Sausage, & Vegetable, Vegetarian, Linda McCartney*	1 Pot/400g	516	20.4	129	6.4	15.7	5.1	2.3
Vegetarian, Quorn*	1 Pack/400g	252	8	63	3.3	8	2	1.9
HOUMOUS								
Beetroot, Asda*	1 Serving/30g	57	3.9	191	5.3	11	13	5.6
Beetroot, Roasted, & Mint, Sainsbury's*	¼ Pot/50g	130	10.2	261	5.8	11.5	20.3	4.9
Caramelised Onion, Co-Op*	¼ Pack/43g	106	8.1	249	6.3	11	19	6.3
Caramelised Onion, M&S*	¼ Pot/50g	134	10.4	268	5.8	12.8	20.7	3.8
Caramelised Onion, Meadow Fresh, Lidl*	1 Serving/50g	112	7	224	7.4	14.8	14.1	4.1
Caramelised Onion, Sainsbury's*	1 Serving/30g	68	4.4	225	6.3	15.2	14.5	4.5
Caramelised Onion, Tesco*	¼ Pot/46g	105	7.7	229	5.3	12	16.8	4.1
Chickpea, Smoked, Organic, Daylesford*	1 Serving/50g	91	6.1	182	6.6	7.5	12.2	8.1
Classic, Meadow Fresh, Lidl*	1 Serving/50g	176	15	351	6.6	12	30	3.1
Classic, Sainsburys*	¼ Pot/58g	161	12.8	278	6.7	10.6	22	5.3
Classic, Snappable, Pots, Sainsbury's*	1 Pot/40g	111	8.8	278	6.7	10.6	22	5.3
Classic, So Organic, Sainsbury's*	¼ Pot/50g	146	11.9	292	6.7	10.9	23.8	4
Classic, Triple Selection, The Deli, Aldi*	1 Pot/60g	134	9	224	7.5	10	15	8.9
Extra Virgin Olive Oil, TTD, Sainsbury's*	¼ Pot/43g	133	11.3	310	6.3	10.2	26.2	3.8
Jalapeno, & Red Pepper, Tesco*	¼ Pot/46g	92	5.9	199	6.3	12.3	12.9	3.9
Jalapeno, Mexican, Morrisons*	¼ Pot/50g	162	13.6	325	7.5	9.8	27.3	5.1
Jalapeno, Pepper, Hot & Spicy, Tesco*	¼ Pot/46g	104	6.8	227	8.1	12.8	14.9	4.8
Lemon & Coriander, Sainsbury's*	¼ Tub/50g	146	12.6	291	7	9.1	25.1	6
Lemon & Coriander, M&S*	1 Serving/30g	83	6.6	278	6.7	11.5	21.9	4.1
Lemon & Coriander, Tesco*	¼ Pot/46g	116	8.9	253	6.8	9.9	19.4	5.7
Lemon & Coriander, Waitrose*	¼ Pot/50g	129	9.7	258	6.3	11.8	19.4	5.4
Lentil, Original, Pulse*	1 Serving/30g	70	4.1	232	8.5	15.3	13.8	6.5

H

	Measure INFO/WEIGHT	per Measure KCAL	FAT	Nutrition Values per 100g / 100ml KCAL	PROT	CARB	FAT	FIBRE
HOUMOUS								
Marmite, Marmite*	1 Serving/50g	128	8	257	11	16	16	4.7
Moroccan Inspired, Classic, Co-Op*	¼ Pack/43g	104	7.3	241	6.6	12	17	4.9
Moroccan, Inspired, Finest, Tesco*	¼ Pot/43g	130	10.7	305	5.3	12	25.1	4.7
Moroccan, Sainsbury's*	¼ Pot/50g	114	8.3	229	6	11.1	16.6	5.5
Olive Oil, Extra Virgin, Co-Op*	¼ Pot/42g	135	11.8	321	6.3	7.4	28	7.3
Onion, Caramelised, The Deli, Aldi*	½ Pack/42g	94	5.9	224	7.4	15	14	4.1
Organic, Duchy, Waitrose*	¼ Pot/50g	166	14.2	332	6.8	10.7	28.3	3.5
Organic, M&S*	1 Serving/25g	83	7.4	332	7.2	5.9	29.4	7.3
Pesto, Swirl, M&S*	1 Serving/30g	86	7.2	285	5.7	9.6	24	3.7
Piri Piri, M&S*	¼ Pack/50g	132	10.2	265	6.7	11	20.3	5.5
Red Pepper, & Chilli, 30% Less Fat, Asda*	¼ Pack/50g	77	4	154	5.5	13	7.9	5
Red Pepper, Asda*	1 Serving/30g	68	4.8	225	5.3	12	16	5.1
Red Pepper, Deluxe, Lidl*	1 Serving/30g	90	7	300	6.9	13.3	23.4	4.5
Red Pepper, Meadow Fresh, Lidl*	1 Serving/50g	158	12.9	307	7.1	11	25	5
Red Pepper, Morrisons*	¼ Pot/50g	151	12.4	302	6.8	9.7	24.9	6.1
Red Pepper, Reduced Fat, Tesco*	¼ Pot/46g	81	4.8	176	6.1	12.2	10.5	4.1
Red Pepper, Roasted, M&S*	1 Pack/200g	534	41.8	267	6.1	11.8	20.9	3.8
Red Pepper, Roasted, Reduced Fat, M&S*	¼ Pack/50g	91	5.5	182	5.8	12.7	11	4.5
Red Pepper, Tesco*	1 Serving/25g	56	4.1	223	5.9	11	16.3	4.5
Red Pepper, The Deli, Aldi*	1 Serving/50g	140	10.5	281	7.8	12	21	5.7
Reduced Fat, Average	***1 Tbsp/30g***	***72***	***5***	***241***	***9.2***	***13.3***	***16.8***	***3.6***
Roasted Beetroot, & Mint, Waitrose*	¼ Pot/50g	112	8.1	224	5.9	11.6	16.2	4.1
Roasted Red Pepper, Sainsbury's*	1 Serving/30g	67	4.8	222	5.7	11.6	16.1	4
Smoked, Moorish*	1 Pack/150g	448	36.3	299	7.1	11.5	24.2	3.4
Smoked, Waitrose*	¼ Pot/50g	141	11.2	282	7.2	10.6	22.4	4.5
Sweet Chilli, Co-Op*	¼ Pack/43g	136	10.8	317	5.3	15	25	5.4
Sweet Chilli, Morrisons*	1 Serving/20g	58	4.1	290	7.1	17.5	20.3	4.3
Sweet Chilli, Tesco*	¼ Pot/46g	106	6.8	231	7.1	15	14.7	5.2
White & Green Chickpea, Pesto, Waitrose*	¼ Pot/50g	103	7	206	7.1	11	13.9	4.1
HULA HOOPS								
BBQ Beef, KP Snacks*	1 Bag/24g	120	5.8	500	3.8	65	24	2.2
Beef Puft, KP Snacks*	1 Pack/15g	72	3	478	9	64	20	4
Beef, 55% Less Saturated Fat, KP Snacks*	1 Pack/34g	172	9	505	3.7	61.8	26.4	2.2
Beef, Big Hoops, KP Snacks*	1 Pack/50g	250	12	499	3.8	65	24	2.8
Cheese & Onion 55% Less Saturated Fat, KP Snacks*	1 Bag/34g	175	9.7	515	3.6	61	28.5	1.9
Cheese & Onion, KP Snacks*	1 Pack/24g	120	5.8	502	3.8	66	24	2.5
Original, 55% Less Saturated Fat, KP Snacks*	1 Bag/34g	172	8.8	507	3.3	63	26	2.2
Ready Salted, Puft, KP Snacks*	1 Pack/15g	72	3.2	482	8.3	64	21	4
Salt & Vinegar, 50% Less Saturated Fat, KP Snacks*	1 Pack/25g	128	7	510	3.1	60.9	28.2	1.8
Salt & Vinegar, KP Snacks*	1 Pack/24g	122	5.8	507	3.4	66	24	2.2
Salt & Vinegar, Puft, KP Snacks*	1 Pack/15g	72	3	478	8.1	63	20	3.9
Sweet Chilli, Puft, KP Snacks*	1 Pack/15g	71	3	474	8.1	64	20	4
Tangy Cheese, Flavarings, KP Snacks*	1 Serving/30g	161	10.8	538	5	44	36	8.1

	Measure INFO/WEIGHT	per Measure KCAL	FAT	Nutrition Values per 100g / 100ml KCAL	PROT	CARB	FAT	FIBRE
ICE CREAM								
Baked Alaska, Ben & Jerry's*	1 Serving/100g	260	15	260	4	29	15	0.1
Banana, Pot, Yeo Valley*	1 Pot/100g	171	5.6	171	3.6	26.1	5.6	0.2
Bananas Foster, Haagen-Dazs*	1 Serving/125ml	260	15	208	3.2	22.4	12	0
Banoffee Fudge, Sainsbury's*	1/8 Pot/67g	119	4	178	2.8	28.7	5.9	0.2
Banoffee, Haagen-Dazs*	1 Serving/120ml	274	15.6	228	4	23	13	0
Belgian Chocolate, Haagen-Dazs*	1 Sm Tub/78g	249	16.2	318	4.6	28.4	20.7	0
Belgian Milk Chocolate, Tesco*	1 Lolly/75g	241	15.4	321	3	31.2	20.5	0
Berry Neighbourly, Ben & Jerry's*	1 Scoop/44g	123	7	279	3.5	29	16	0
Birthday Cake, Asda*	1 Scoop/50ml	42	0.8	83	4.1	12	1.7	4.5
Birthday Cake, High Protein, Halo Top*	1 Scoop/50g	30	1	59	4	12	2	2.5
Blondie Brownie, Ben & Jerry's*	1 Scoop/43g	109	6	253	4.2	29	14	0
Blueberries & Cream, Minicup, Haagen-Dazs*	1 Minicup/87g	212	14	244	4.1	20.3	16.1	0.5
Blueberry Crumble, Halo Top*	½ Tub/68g	84	2.3	123	6.8	20	3.4	0
Blueberry, Gelateria, Carte d'Or*	2 Scoops/56g	110	4.1	190	28	31	7	0
Bob Marleys One Love, Ben & Jerry's*	1 Scoop/45g	123	6.3	273	3.2	33	14	0
Bounty, Mini Bar, Mars*	1 Bar/25ml	72	4.8	288	4.5	24.8	19	1
Caffe Latte, The Best, Morrisons*	1/5 Tub/100ml	144	6.6	144	2.9	18	6.6	0.4
Candy Bar, Halo Top*	¼ Tub/118g	90	3.7	76	4.3	14	3.1	2.3
Cappuccino, Tesco*	1 Scoop/54g	121	4.5	224	2.3	34.8	8.3	0.2
Caramel Biscuit & Cream, Minicup, Haagen-Dazs*	1 Minicup/87g	249	16.1	286	4.6	25.5	18.4	0.1
Caramel Chew Chew, Classic Mix, Ben & Jerry's*	1 Minicup/100g	271	15	271	3.6	30	15	0
Caramel Chocolate Crunch, Oppo*	1 Scoop/50g	42	2.2	84	2.5	9.8	4.3	0
Caramel Cookie Fix, Moophoria, Ben & Jerry's*	1 Carton/465ml	576	20.4	124	2.2	17	4.4	0
Caramel Swirl, Gelato, Haagen-Dazs*	1 Mini Tub/72g	139	5.3	193	5.1	23.2	7.4	6.4
Caramel, Chew Chew, Ben & Jerry's*	1 Scoop/45g	122	6.8	270	3.5	28	15	0
Caramel, Diary Milk, Cadbury*	1 Scoop/50ml	93	4.7	186	1.9	23.2	9.4	0.2
Caramella, Sundae, Tesco*	1 Sundae/80g	165	5.5	205	2.2	32.9	6.8	1.9
Caramella, Tesco*	1 Serving/51g	120	5.5	235	2.6	32	10.7	1.1
Cheesecake Brownie, Ben & Jerry's*	1 Serving 100g	260	16	260	4	26	16	0
Cheesecake, Strawberry, Haagen-Dazs*	2 Scoops/86g	226	12.3	262	3.8	29.4	14.3	0.4
Cherry Bakewell, Ripple, Kelly's Of Cornwall*	1 Scoop/50g	112	4.4	223	3.2	32.8	8.7	0.3
Choc Choc Chip, Minicup, Haagen-Dazs*	1 Minicup/87g	245	15.9	281	4.5	24.3	18.2	0.9
Chocolate Chip Cookie Dough, Halo Top*	1 Serving/118g	90	3.1	76	3.9	14	2.6	2.5
Chocolate Chip, Hacendado*	1 Scoop/50g	146	8.5	292	4.6	29	17	2.2
Chocolate Drizzle, Gelato, Mini Cup, Haagen-Dazs*	1 Mini Tub/72g	137	4.9	190	5.9	22.4	6.8	7.5
Chocolate Flavour, Average	***1 Serving/70g***	***149***	***7.9***	***212***	***4.1***	***23.7***	***11.3***	***0.6***
Chocolate Honeycomb, Co-Op*	¼ Pot/81g	186	10.5	230	4	26	13	0.3
Chocolate, Creamy, Breyer's Delights*	1 Serving/100ml	62	1.7	62	3.9	9.3	1.7	0
Chocolate, Dark, Finest, Tesco*	1 Scoop/50g	128	8.2	257	4.8	22.5	16.3	1
Chocolate, Finest, Tesco*	1 Scoop/70g	254	17.7	363	4.4	28.9	25.3	1.1
Chocolate, Fudge, Brownie, Ben & Jerry's*	1 Scoop/42g	102	5.4	245	4.2	29	13	0
Chocolate, Fudge, Brownie, Non-Dairy, Ben & Jerry's*	1 Scoop/40g	88	4.3	222	2.9	26	11	0
Chocolate, Fudge, Oatly*	1 Scoop/50g	118	5.5	235	1.2	32	11	1.4
Chocolate, Gelatelli, Lidl*	1 Portion/50g	126	6.8	251	3.8	27.3	13.6	2.1
Chocolate, Haagen-Dazs*	1 Serving/120ml	269	18	224	4	19	15	0
Chocolate, Heavenly, Non Dairy, Swedish Glace, Wall's*	1 Serving/100g	206	11	206	3.3	23	11	0
Chocolate, Inspiration, Gelateria, Carte d'Or*	1 Serving/100g	210	9	210	3.5	28	9	0
Chocolate, Organic, Green & Black's*	1 Serving/125g	310	17.6	248	5	25.3	14.1	1.1
Chocolate, Plant Kitchen, M&S*	1/5 Tub/62g	119	6.6	192	1.8	19.9	10.6	5.1
Chocolate, Santo Domingo, 1, Waitrose*	1 Serving/66g	220	16.4	333	4.5	22.8	24.8	0.5
Chocolate, Vegan, Jude's*	1 Scoop/50ml	36	1.3	73	0.7	10.9	2.6	0
Chunky Monkey, Non-Dairy, Ben & Jerry's*	1 Scoop/42g	109	5.8	262	2.4	30	14	0
Cinnamon Roll, Tub, Halo Top*	1 Serving/118g	90	3	76	4	15	2.5	2.5

I

	Measure INFO/WEIGHT	per Measure KCAL	FAT	Nutrition Values per 100g / 100ml KCAL	PROT	CARB	FAT	FIBRE
ICE CREAM								
Clotted Cream, Cornish, Kelly's Of Cornwall*	1 Serving/125g	282	18.6	226	2.9	20.1	14.9	0.1
Coconut, Alpro*	1 Serving/100g	167	8.2	167	0.2	16.1	8.2	12.5
Coconut, Toasted, Dairy Free, Halo Top*	1 Scoop/50g	34	1.8	68	2.2	14	3.5	4.2
Coffee, Arabica, Carte d'Or*	1 Scoop/50g	115	4.4	230	3.1	34	8.9	0
Coffee, Carrefour *	1 Scoop/50g	114	4.6	227	3.5	32	9.3	0
Coffee, Colombian, No.1, Waitrose*	1 Sm Pot/81g	197	10.7	243	3.8	27	13.2	0.5
Coffee, Finest, Tesco*	¼ Pot/93g	236	14.9	254	4.9	22.5	16	0
Coffee, Flat White, Jude's*	1 Scoop/50ml	66	3.4	131	3.2	13.4	6.9	0
Coffee, Waitrose*	¼ Tub/125ml	292	16.4	234	3.6	25.4	13.1	0
Cookie Dough, Asda*	1 Scoop/50ml	42	1.4	84	3.8	11	2.8	3.4
Cookie Dough, Ben & Jerry's*	1 Scoop/43g	115	6.4	270	4	30	15	0
Cookie Dough, Tesco*	1 Serving/125g	301	14.2	241	3.3	31	11.4	0.6
Cookies & Cream, Haagen-Dazs*	1 Sm Tub/100ml	226	14.7	226	4	19.5	14.7	0
Cornish Clotted Cream, Soft Scoop, Giannis, Aldi*	1 Scoop/50g	108	6	215	3.6	23	12	0.5
Cornish Clotted, Honeycomb, M&S*	1 Scoop/50g	129	7.8	258	2.5	26.8	15.6	0.2
Creme Egg, Cadbury*	1 Scoop/50ml	100	4	200	2.9	27.5	8	0.2
Dairy, Flavoured	***1oz/28g***	***50***	***2.2***	***179***	***3.5***	***24.7***	***8***	***0***
Double Chocolate, Nestle*	1 Serving/78g	248	14.3	320	4.8	33.7	18.4	0
Double Decker, Cadbury*	1 Scoop/50ml	84	4.8	169	1.6	18.9	9.5	0.5
Dulce De Leche, Minicup, Haagen-Dazs*	1 Minicup/87g	231	13.6	265	4.4	26.7	15.6	0.1
Espresso Caramel, Gelatelli, Lidl*	1 Scoop/50g	38	1	77	4.6	8.6	2	3
Eton Mess, Gelateria, Carte d'Or*	2 Scoops/100g	181	5.8	181	2.2	30	5.8	0
Fig & Orange Blossom Honey, Waitrose*	1 Serving/100g	219	11.8	219	3.9	24.3	11.8	0.4
Gelato, Vanilla	***1 Serving/100g***	***162***	***7.2***	***162***	***2.4***	***22.6***	***7.2***	***0.3***
Gingerbread, Specially Selected, Aldi*	1 Scoop/64g	169	8.3	264	4	33	13	0.6
Half Baked, Ben & Jerry's*	1 Scoop/41g	107	5.3	262	4.1	32	13	0
Hazelnut Chocolate, Alpro*	1 Serving/100g	177	9.4	177	0.8	17.2	9.4	8.6
Home Sweet Honeycomb, Ben & Jerry's*	1 Scoop/43g	114	6.4	266	3.8	30	15	0
Honeycomb & Caramel, Dairy, Sainsbury's*	2 Scoops/76g	180	8	236	3.2	32	10.5	0.6
Lavazza, Carte d'Or*	1 Serving/55g	120	5.4	218	3.5	29	9.9	0
Lemon Meringue Bar, Heston, Waitrose*	1 Serving/60g	108	2.8	181	1.8	32	4.7	1.5
Lemon, Haagen-Dazs*	1 Serving/120ml	144	0.2	120	0.3	29.3	0.2	0
Light Chocolate Ices, Co-Op*	1 Ice/62g	121	8.1	195	2	18	13	0.5
Luscious Mint Choc Chip, Morrisons*	1 Serving/50g	99	5.2	198	2.9	23.1	10.5	0.7
Lychee Cream & Ginger, Haagen-Dazs*	1 Serving/120ml	258	12.7	215	3.6	26.1	10.6	0
Magnum Double Mochaccino, Wall's*	1 Bar/88ml	245	15.9	278	3.3	26	18	0
Magnum, Classic, Tub, Wall's*	1 Scoop/50g	108	7	217	2.4	21	14	0
Magnum, White, Tub, Wall's*	1 Scoop/50g	109	6.5	218	2.5	23	13	0
Maltesers, Mars*	1 Scoop/50g	64	3	128	1.4	17	6	0
Mango & Raspberry, Minicup, Haagen-Dazs*	1 Minicup/87g	211	11.5	243	3.3	27.2	13.3	0.6
Mango, & Raspberry, Haagen-Dazs*	1 Scoop/50g	124	6.7	247	3.4	27.9	13.4	0.6
Mango, Swirl, Passionate, Alpro*	1 Scoop/50g	76	3	153	2.1	16.9	6	10.5
Mince Pie, Farmhouse Dairy, TTD, Sainsbury's*	¼ Pot/100g	272	14.9	272	4.5	29.3	14.9	1.3
Mince Pie, Finest, Tesco*	¼ Pack/188g	476	22.1	254	3.9	33	11.8	1.1
Mini Cups, Giannis, Aldi*	1 Cup/65g	168	10.4	259	4.9	24	16	0
Mint & Chocolate Flavour, Average	***1 Serving/70g***	***129***	***6.3***	***184***	***3***	***22.6***	***9***	***1.2***
Mint, Majestic Luxury, Iceland*	1 Serving/80g	269	14.6	337	3.8	39.3	18.3	1.3
Mint, Specially Selected, Aldi*	1 Scoop/50g	112	6.5	224	6	22	13	0.6
Mint, Viennetta, Wall's*	1 Scoop/50g	125	8	250	2.5	25	16	0
Minter Wonderland, Ben & Jerry's*	1 Scoop/44g	117	7.5	266	4	24	17	0
My Carte D'or, Chocolate, Carte d'Or*	1 Tub/200ml	220	11	110	1.8	12.5	5.5	0.4
Neapolitan, Average	***1 Serving/70g***	***111***	***4.6***	***158***	***3.1***	***21.9***	***6.5***	***0.6***
Neapolitan, Viennetta, Wall's*	1 Scoop/50ml	122	7	245	2.2	27	14	0

I

	Measure INFO/WEIGHT	per Measure KCAL	FAT	Nutrition Values per 100g / 100ml KCAL	PROT	CARB	FAT	FIBRE
ICE CREAM								
Netflix & Chill'd, Ben & Jerry's*	2 Scoops/100g	276	16	276	4.9	28	16	0
Non-Dairy, Reduced Calorie	***1oz/28g***	***33***	***1.7***	***119***	***3.4***	***13.7***	***6***	***0***
Peanut Butter Crunch, Haagen-Dazs*	2 Scoops/100g	343	24.4	343	8.4	21.7	24.4	1.7
Peanut Butter Cup, Ben & Jerry's*	1 Scoop/43g	138	9	320	7	25	21	0
Peanut Butter, & Cookies, Non-Dairy, Ben & Jerry's*	1 Scoop/41g	113	6.5	280	4.3	29	16	0
Peanut Butter, Asda*	1 Scoop/50ml	38	1.1	75	3.7	9.3	2.2	4.6
Phish Food, Ben & Jerry's*	1 Scoop/43g	116	5.2	270	3.5	36	12	0
Pistachio, Haagen-Dazs*	1 Serving/120ml	276	18.8	230	4.4	17.7	15.7	0
Pistachio, Joe Deluccis Gelato*	1 Scoop/70g	148	6.6	211	2.4	28	9.4	0
Poppin' Popcorn, Moophoria, Ben & Jerry's*	2 Scoops/100g	197	7.9	197	3.3	25	7.9	0
Pralines & Cream, Haagen-Dazs*	1 Sm Tub/78g	213	12.9	272	3.9	27.2	16.5	0
Raspberries, Clotted Cream, Waitrose*	1 Tub/500ml	790	39.5	158	2.9	18.9	7.9	0.1
Raspberry Nipple, Oppo*	1 Scoop/50ml	34	1.8	67	2.8	7.4	3.5	0
Raspberry Ripple, & White Chocolate, Gelatelli, Lidl*	1 Tub/450ml	392	14	87	4.5	8.7	3.1	3
Raspberry Ripple, Average	***1 Serving/70g***	***93***	***3.3***	***134***	***1.9***	***20.8***	***4.7***	***0.1***
Raspberry Ripple, Plant Kitchen, M&S*	1/5 Tub/62g	113	6	181	0.8	21.1	9.6	3.4
Really Creamy Chocolate, Asda*	1 Serving/100g	227	11	227	4.1	28	11	0.4
Really Creamy Toffee, Asda*	1 Serving/120ml	146	6	122	1.8	17.5	5	0.1
Red Berries, Solero, Wall's*	1 Lolly/75g	111	2	148	1.4	29	2.7	0
Rocky Road, Sainsbury's*	1/8 Pot/67g	137	4.9	205	3.8	30.9	7.3	1
Rum & Raisin, Haagen-Dazs*	1 Serving/120ml	264	17.6	220	3.4	18.6	14.7	0
Rum & Raisin, TTD, Sainsbury's*	¼ Pot/100g	220	10.4	220	3.8	27.7	10.4	1
Salted Caramel Brownie, Moophoria, Ben & Jerry's*	1 Scoop/50g	93	2.8	186	3.6	28	5.5	0
Salted Caramel, Almond, Alpro*	1 Scoop/50g	90	4.4	181	0.8	18.5	8.8	12.3
Salted Caramel, Carte D'or*	1 Scoop/50g	100	4	200	3	29	8	0
Salted Caramel, Fair Trade, Co-Op*	1/5 Tub/54g	59	1.6	110	6.2	15	2.9	0.6
Salted Caramel, Fairway to Heaven, Ben & Jerry's*	1 Scoop/50ml	110	6.5	221	3.4	23	13	0
Salted Caramel, Goodness, Grahams*	1 Tub/444ml	320	11.1	72	4.5	8	2.5	3
Salted Caramel, High Protein, Gelatelli, Lidl*	1 Scoop/50ml	40	1.2	79	4.5	8	2.5	3
Salted Caramel, High Protein, Morrisons*	1/5 Tub/97ml	57	1.3	59	3.9	7.7	1.3	0.3
Salted Caramel, Low Sugar, Gelatelli, Lidl*	1 Scoop/50g	64	1.6	128	7.1	22.6	3.3	0
Salted Caramel, Minicup, Haagen-Dazs*	1 Minicup/87g	246	15	282	4.1	27.8	17.2	0
Salted Carmael, Good As Gold, Co-Op*	1 Scoop/50g	53	1.2	106	7.1	14	2.3	0.6
Sea Salt Caramel, Dairy Free, Halo Top*	1 Scoop/50g	34	1.2	68	2.2	14	2.5	4
Sicilian Lemon, M&S*	1 Scoop/50g	118	7	237	3.5	24	14	0.3
Sofa So Good , Ben & Jerry's*	1 Scoop/43g	110	5.5	259	4	31	13	0
Soy, Vanilla, Swedish Glace, Wall's*	1 Scoop/50g	87	2.9	174	1	29	5.8	0
Speculoos? Specu-Love, Ben & Jerry's*	1 Scoop/42g	129	8.3	310	3.8	28	20	0
Sticky Toffee Pudding, Co-Op*	1 Scoop/50g	110	5	220	1.9	30	10	0.6
Strawberries & Cream, Minicup, Haagen-Dazs*	1 Minicup/87g	211	13.5	243	3.9	21.8	15.5	0.3
Strawberries & Cream, Haagen-Dazs*	1 Scoop/50g	122	7.8	244	3.9	22.2	15.5	0.3
Strawberry Cheesecake, Ben & Jerry's*	1 Serving 100g	240	14	240	3	27	14	0
Strawberry Cheesecake, Co-Op*	1/6 Pot/86g	163	6	190	3	29	7	0.2
Strawberry Cheesecake, Deluxe, Lidl*	1 Scoop/50ml	70	3.6	139	2.3	16.3	7.1	0
Strawberry Cheesecake, Halo Top*	1 Scoop/50ml	38	1.2	76	3.9	12.5	2.4	0
Strawberry, & Vanilla, Free From, Co-Op*	1 Cone/65g	188	7.8	289	3.5	41.5	12	0.8
Strawberry, Les Classiques, From Multipack, Carte d'Or*	1 Portion/50g	84	3	167	2.8	25	5.9	0
Strawberry, Soft Scoop, Tesco*	1 Serving/46g	78	3.4	170	2.8	23.1	7.4	0.1
Summer Berries & Cream, Minicup, Haagen-Dazs*	1 Minicup/88g	225	14.1	255	3	24.4	16	0.8
Tiramisu, Haagen-Dazs*	1 Serving/120ml	303	19.6	253	3.8	22.7	16.3	0
Toffee & Vanilla, Sainsbury's*	1 Serving/71g	146	6.8	205	3.1	26.7	9.5	0.1
Toffee Fudge, Soft Scoop, Asda*	1 Serving/50g	92	3.5	185	2.6	28	7	0
Toffee Vanilla, HE, Tesco*	1 Serving/73g	106	1.8	145	2.5	28.1	2.5	0.5

	Measure INFO/WEIGHT	per Measure KCAL	FAT	Nutrition Values per 100g / 100ml KCAL	PROT	CARB	FAT	FIBRE
ICE CREAM								
Toffee, & Vanilla, Giannis, Aldi*	1 Scoop/50g	108	5	216	1.7	29	10	0.6
Triple Chocolate, Carte d'Or*	1 Serving/58g	122	5.7	210	3.7	27	9.8	0
Triple Chocolate, Dairy, Morrisons*	1 Serving/100g	233	10.8	233	3.8	30	10.8	0.4
Tutti Frutti, Tesco*	1 Scoop/50g	78	2.4	157	2.3	25.7	4.7	0.6
Vanilla & Caramel, Tesco*	1 Scoop/53g	117	4.4	222	2.4	34.5	8.3	0.1
Vanilla Bean, Jude's*	1 Scoop/50ml	36	1.6	73	2.5	10.4	3.2	0
Vanilla Bean, Light, Deluxe, Lidl*	1 Serving/64g	110	2.5	172	4.7	26.6	3.9	0
Vanilla Caramel Brownie, Minicup, Haagen-Dazs*	1 Minicup/83g	228	13.7	275	4.4	26.9	16.5	0.4
Vanilla Chocolate Brownie, Haagen-Dazs*	1 Pot/78g	217	13.1	278	4.4	27	16.8	0
Vanilla Flavour, Soft Scoop, Sainsbury's*	1 Serving/71g	96	3.9	136	2.9	18.8	5.5	0.2
Vanilla Florentine, Specially Selected, Aldi*	1 Scoop/62g	148	7.4	238	4.4	28	12	0.7
Vanilla, & Chocolate, Viennetta, Wall's*	2 Scoops/100ml	125	7	250	2.5	27	14	0
Vanilla, Alpro*	1 Serving/100g	166	8	166	2.3	16.4	8	9.8
Vanilla, Bean, Halo Top*	1 Serving/118ml	70	2	59	3.9	12	1.7	2.5
Vanilla, Dairy Milk, Cadbury*	1 Serving/120g	259	13.9	216	3.5	26	11.6	0.1
Vanilla, Dairy, Average	**1 Scoop/40g**	**80**	**4.4**	**201**	**3.5**	**23.6**	**11**	**0.7**
Vanilla, High Protein, Asda*	1 Scoop/50g	35	0.9	70	3.9	9.9	1.8	2.7
Vanilla, Les Classiques, From Multipack, Carte d'Or*	1 Portion/50g	86	3.3	172	2.1	26	6.6	0
Vanilla, Low Fat, Average	**1 Scoop/50g**	**59**	**1.7**	**118**	**2.3**	**19.4**	**3.4**	**0.6**
Vanilla, Madagascan, Carte D'or*	1 Scoop/50g	96	3.8	193	2.1	29	7.5	0
Vanilla, Made with Madagascan Vanilla, Sainsbury's*	1 Serving/56g	101	4	181	3	25.6	7.2	0.6
Vanilla, Non-Dairy, Average	**1 Serving/60g**	**107**	**5.2**	**178**	**3.2**	**23.1**	**8.7**	**0**
Vanilla, Pecan, Praline, Oppo*	1 Scoop/50ml	42	2.1	83	2.5	9.8	4.2	2.5
Vanilla, Toffee Crunch, Ben & Jerry's*	1 Tub/407g	1099	65.1	270	4	29	16	0.5
Vanilla, Vanilla Collection, Minicup, Haagen-Dazs*	1 Minicup/87g	217	14.7	249	4.3	19.9	16.9	0
Vanilla, with Almond, Magnum, Pot, Wall's*	1 Scoop/50ml	117	7	234	3.3	22	14	0
Vanilla, with Cherry Sauce, Tesco*	1 Scoop/56g	114	4.1	204	2.1	32.4	7.3	0.2
Viennese Munt, Mini, Aldi*	1 Ice Cream/35g	87	5	249	4.6	25.1	14.3	1.4
White Chocolate, & Raspberry, Giannis, Aldi*	1 Scoop/50g	84	3	169	8.8	18	6.1	3.1
White Chocolate, Minis, Lolly, Multipack, G, Aldi*	1 Lolly/35g	128	8.4	366	3.2	34	24	0.5
ICE CREAM BAR								
Caramel, Biscuits, Gateau, Tesco*	½ Pack/200g	614	33.4	307	5.7	33.3	16.7	0.6
Chocolate Covered	**1 Bar/40g**	**128**	**9.3**	**320**	**5**	**24**	**23.3**	**0**
Chocolate, Dark, & Nordic Berry, Nuii*	1 Bar/66g	235	15.2	356	3.8	33	23	3.3
Cookies, & Mint, Idaho Valley, Nuii*	1 Bar/61g	232	13.4	381	4.3	41	22	0
Crunchie, Cadbury*	1 Bar/60ml	165	9.7	275	3	29.5	16.2	0.5
Dairy Milk, Caramel, Cadbury*	1 Bar/60ml	175	10.3	290	3.6	30.2	17.1	0
Maltesers, Mars*	1 Bar/45ml	113	7	252	2.9	25	15.6	0.7
Sea Salt Caramel, Halo Top*	1 Bar/57g	80	1.5	140	6.7	26	2.6	6.4
Snickers, Mars*	1 Bar/53ml	179	10.4	337	6.5	33.2	19.6	0
Titan, Dairyfine, Aldi*	1 Bar/42g	152	9.2	362	4.1	36	22	0.7
ICE CREAM CONE								
Average	**1 Cone/75g**	**140**	**6.4**	**186**	**3.5**	**25.5**	**8.5**	**0**
Brownie, & Cream, Extreme, Nestle*	1 Cone/71g	207	9.9	292	3.5	38	14	1.5
Chocolate & Nut, Co-Op*	1 Cone/110g	307	17	279	3.9	31	15.5	0.6
Chocolate & Vanilla, Good Choice, Iceland*	1 Cone/110ml	161	7.2	146	2.7	22.9	6.5	0.8
Chocolate Fudge, Gooey, Extreme, Nestle*	1 Cone/73g	218	10.4	299	3.8	37.4	14.3	2.5
Chocolate, Double, Waffle Cone, Co-Op*	1 Cone/135g	209	9	155	2.3	21	6.7	0.9
Chocolate, Mini, Cornetto, Wall's*	1 Cone/36g	110	5.9	300	3.5	34	16	2
Chocolate, Vanilla & Hazelnut, Sainsbury's*	1 Cone/62g	190	10.5	306	4.5	33.9	16.9	0.6
Cookies & Cream, Tesco*	1 Cone/71g	197	7.9	277	3.9	39.8	11.1	1.4
Cornetto, GFY, Asda*	1 Cone/67g	162	6	241	3	37	9	0.1
Cornetto, Soy & GF, Cornetto, Wall's*	1 Cone/60g	179	8.4	299	1.8	40	14	0

	Measure INFO/WEIGHT	per Measure KCAL	FAT	Nutrition Values per 100g / 100ml KCAL	PROT	CARB	FAT	FIBRE
ICE CREAM CONE								
Cornetto, Wall's*	1 Cone/75g	195	9.7	260	3.7	34.5	12.9	0
Cup Cornet, Wafer Cone, Askeys*	1 Cone/4g	13	0.1	376	10.7	77.6	2.5	0
Dairy Milk Buttons, Cadbury*	1 Cone/100ml	204	10.4	204	0	24.6	10.4	0.6
Extreme Raspberry, Cornetto, Nestle*	1 Cone/76g	177	6.2	233	2.4	36.4	8.2	1.5
Flake 99, Cadbury*	1 Cone/125ml	238	12	190	2.6	23.1	9.6	0.5
Mint Choc, Morrisons*	1 Cone/74g	200	8	270	3.3	39.1	10.8	1.8
Mint, & Chocolate, Tesco*	1 Cone/74ml	219	8.8	296	3.5	43.1	11.9	1.6
Mint, Cornetto, Wall's*	1 Cornetto/60g	169	8.4	282	3.4	37	14	0
Peanut Butter, Love, Cornetto, Wall's*	1 Cornetto/75g	245	15	326	3.3	33	20	0
Rainbow, Uni Cone, Co-Op*	1 Cone/135g	198	8.6	147	2	20	6.4	0.7
Salted Butter Caramel, Gelatelli*	1 Cone/76g	216	8.1	284	3.6	43.4	10.6	0
Strawberry & Vanilla, Iceland*	1 Cone/70g	182	7.6	260	3.3	37.5	10.8	0.7
Strawberry & Vanilla, Tesco*	1 Cone/69g	181	7	262	3.3	39	10.1	0.8
Strawberry, Cornetto, Wall's*	1 Cornetto/75g	198	8.2	264	2.1	40	11	0
Strawberry, Swirl Top, Co-Op*	1 Cone/75g	200	8.2	267	3	40	11	0.6
Strawberry, Vegan, No Moo, Iceland*	1 Cone/65g	188	7.8	290	3.6	42	12	0.5
Toffee & Vanilla, Giannis, Aldi*	1 Cone/71g	195	7.1	275	4.5	42	10	0.6
Toffee, & Vanilla, Free From, Tesco*	1 Cone/65g	185	8.9	285	2.1	38	13.7	0.6
Toffee, & Vanilla, Sainsbury's*	1 Cone/72g	176	6.8	244	2.8	37.1	9.4	0.5
Vanilla, & Chocolate, Classico, Cornetto, Wall's*	1 Cornetto/60g	178	9.6	296	3.1	33	16	0
Vanilla, & Chocolate, Ms Molly*	1 Cone/61g	160	7.1	263	3.4	35.9	11.6	0.6
Waffle Cone, Tesco *	1 Cone/12g	49	0.7	411	6.7	81.9	5.6	3.3
ICE CREAM ROLL								
Arctic, Average	***1 Serving/70g***	***140***	***4.6***	***200***	***4.1***	***33.3***	***6.6***	***0***
ICE CREAM SANDWICH								
'Wich, Ben & Jerry's*	1 Pack/117g	398	19.9	340	4	44	17	1
Choc Chip Cookie, Giannis, Aldi*	1 Sandwich/65g	248	12.4	382	5.1	48	19	2.2
Cookies, & Ice Cream, Giannis, Aldi*	1 Sandwich/36g	109	4	303	5.6	45	11	1.7
Freddo, Dairy Milk, Cadbury*	1 Sandwich/34g	98	4	289	4.2	40.8	11.7	2.1
Neapolitan, Gelatelli, Lidl*	1 Sandwich/90ml	134	8	149	1.8	15.1	8.9	0.8
ICE CREAM STICK								
Birthday Cake, Halo Top*	1 Ice Cream/56g	90	3.5	160	6.6	15	6.2	6.4
Biscoff, Lotus*	1 Ice Cream/71g	312	20.6	440	3.4	41	29	0.7
Black Forest, Majestic, Iceland*	1 Ice Cream/63g	210	13.2	333	3.4	30.8	20.9	3.6
Bobble Mania, Giannis, Aldi*	1 Ice Cream/53g	155	8.5	293	2	35	16	0.4
Brunch, Wall's*	1 Ice Cream/90g	170	10.8	189	2.4	18	12	0
Choc Sticks, Free From, Tesco*	1 Ice Cream/70g	234	15.8	335	2.9	28.6	22.6	2.9
Chocolate & Mint, Tesco*	1 Ice Cream/79g	250	15.6	316	3.2	31.3	19.7	0.7
Chocolate, & Almond, Tesco*	1 Ice Cream/77g	268	18	348	4.5	29.2	23.4	1.2
Chocolate, & Caramel, Tesco*	1 Ice Cream/78g	240	14.7	306	3.1	30.5	18.8	0.6
Chocolate, Belgian, Mini, M&S*	1 Ice Cream/35g	113	7	324	3.9	31.9	19.9	0.6
Chocolate, Feast, Wall's*	1 Ice Cream/70g	245	16.1	350	3.6	31	23	0
Chocolate, Milk, Mini, Tesco*	1 Ice Cream/35g	119	7.7	341	3.1	31.9	22.2	0.9
Chocolate, Milk, Sainsbury's*	1 Ice Cream/75g	240	14.8	320	2.9	32.4	19.7	0.7
Chocolate, Mini Milk, Wall's*	1 Ice Cream/23g	32	0.7	138	4.4	22	3.2	0
Chocolate, White, Tesco*	1 Ice Cream/75g	255	17.5	341	3.3	29.4	23.4	0
Cookies, & Cream, Tesco*	1 Ice Cream/73g	238	14.6	326	3.3	33	20	0.7
Crunchie Blast, with Popping Candy, Cadbury*	1 Ice Cream/100g	247	14.9	247	3	24.7	14.9	0.5
Exotic, Solero, Wall's*	1 Ice Cream/68g	98	2.1	144	1.7	27	3.1	0
Kinder*	1 Ice Cream/27g	62	3	229	3.1	30	11	0
Maltesers, Mint, Mars*	1 Ice Cream/100g	235	14.4	235	2.2	24.2	14.4	0
Milk Chocolate, & Chopped Almonds, Minis, Lolly, Aldi*	1 Ice Cream/38g	144	9.5	380	4.5	34	25	1.1
Milk Chocolate, Majestic, Iceland*	1 Ice Cream/83g	267	15.5	320	4.4	33.3	18.6	0.6

I

	Measure INFO/WEIGHT	per Measure KCAL	FAT	Nutrition Values per 100g / 100ml KCAL	PROT	CARB	FAT	FIBRE
ICE CREAM STICK								
Milk Chocolate, Minis, Lolly, Multipack, G, Aldi*	1 Ice Cream/34g	120	7.5	353	3.4	35	22	0.5
Mini Mix, Chocolate Coated, Gelatelli, Lidl*	1 Ice Cream/36g	123	7.8	342	3.9	32	21.8	1.2
Mint Choc, Giannis, Aldi*	1 Ice Cream/58g	87	2.3	150	6.3	21	3.9	5.1
Oreo, Coated, Sandwich, Cadbury*	1 Ice Cream/51g	185	10.2	362	4.8	40	20	1.6
Peanut Butter, Haagen-Dazs*	1 Ice Cream/70g	290	22.1	414	8.4	23.1	31.5	2.3
Peanut Butter, Swirl, Halo Top*	1 Ice Cream/58g	100	5	172	9.1	16	8.6	6.9
Raspberry, Low Calorie, Morrisons*	1 Ice Cream/60g	81	1.6	135	5.1	22.5	2.6	0.5
Raspberry, Luxury, M&S*	1 Ice Cream/67g	211	12.5	315	1.6	34.4	18.7	1.5
Salted Caramel, & Australian Macadamia, Nuii*	1 Ice Cream/68g	246	14.3	361	3.8	38	21	0.8
Salted Caramel, & Glazed Almond, Magnum*	1 Ice Cream/74g	236	15	319	3.4	29.7	20.3	0
Salted Caramel, Chocolate Coated, Oppo*	1 Ice Cream/50g	110	6.4	220	6.6	26	12.8	2
Salted Caramel, Coco Nutters, Coconut Collaborative*	1 Ice Cream/85g	198	11	233	1	21	13	9.9
Salted Caramel, Minis, Jude's*	1 Ice Cream/50ml	94	5.7	189	2.7	18.2	11.4	0
Salted Caramel, No.1, Waitrose*	1 Ice Cream/78g	277	16.4	353	4.2	36.1	20.9	1.6
Salted Caramel, Specially Selected, Aldi*	1 Ice Cream/81g	285	17	353	2.9	37	21	1
Salted Caramel, Tesco*	1 Ice Cream/69g	209	11.6	301	3.2	34.1	16.7	0.6
Spotty Dottie, Sainsbury's*	1 Ice Cream/47g	148	7.8	315	1.8	39.6	16.5	0.5
Stem Ginger with Belgian Chocolate, Waitrose*	1 Ice Cream/110g	255	14.4	232	2.9	25.5	13.1	1.7
Stem Ginger, 1, Waitrose*	1 Ice Cream/79g	287	17.2	364	4.1	37.5	21.8	0.6
Strawberry Cheesecake, Halo Top*	1 Ice Cream/59g	100	4.3	170	6.3	15	7.3	6.1
Strawberry Split, Essential, Waitrose*	1 Ice Cream/73g	80	1.9	110	1.8	19.5	2.6	0.6
Tropical Swirls , Morrisons*	1 Ice Cream/75ml	104	2.8	139	1.8	24.3	3.7	0.6
Vanilla, Chocolate Covered, Swedish Glace, Wall's*	1 Ice Cream/37g	105	6.6	285	1	30	18	0
Vanilla, Dark Coco Nutters, Coconut Collaborative*	1 Ice Cream/69g	134	9.7	194	1	11	14	0
Vanilla, Mini Milk, Wall's*	1 Ice Cream/23g	30	0.7	130	3.9	22	3.1	0
Vanilla, with White Chocolate, Mini, Jude's*	1 Ice Cream/50g	88	5.8	177	2.8	15.1	11.6	0
White Chocolate, Giannis, Aldi*	1 Ice Cream/100g	237	14	237	2.4	24	14	0
ICE LOLLY								
Assorted, Iceland*	1 Lolly/51g	33	0	65	0	16.2	0	0
Baby, Tesco*	1 Lolly/32g	26	0	80	0.1	20	0	0.1
Berry, Mixed, Gelatelli, Lidl*	1 Lolly/73g	104	1.8	143	1.7	27.5	2.5	0
Birthday Cake, Halo Top*	1 Lolly/58g	89	3.4	153	6.4	19	5.8	6.4
Blackcurrant Split, Iceland*	1 Lolly/75g	61	2.4	81	1.1	12	3.2	0.1
Blackcurrant, Dairy Split, Sainsbury's*	1 Lolly/73ml	88	2.6	121	1.8	20.4	3.6	0.1
Blackcurrant, Sainsbury's*	1 Lolly/74g	62	0.4	84	0.5	19.9	0.5	0.6
Bubblegum Swirl, Iceland*	1 Lolly/55g	74	1.4	135	3.1	24.3	2.6	0.6
Bubblegum, Calippo, Wall's*	1 Lolly/106g	90	0.5	85	0.5	21	0.5	0
Bubblegum, Morrisons*	1 Lolly/51g	57	1.2	112	2.4	20.2	2.4	0.4
Bubblegum, Tesco*	1 Lolly/59g	60	1.1	102	1.8	19.2	1.9	0.6
Chai Latte, Waitrose*	1 Lolly/58g	63	1.8	108	0.9	18.8	3.1	0.6
Chocolate Wonderpops, Sainsbury's*	1 Lolly/43g	118	8.3	276	2.6	21.8	19.4	0.7
Chocolate, Plain, Mini, Tesco*	1 Lolly/31g	94	6.6	304	3.1	24.8	21.4	1.2
Cider Refresher, Treats*	1 Lolly/70ml	54	0	77	0	19.2	0	0
Cider, Asda*	1 Lolly/73ml	58	0.4	80	0.5	19	0.5	0.5
Cloudy Apple, Sainsbury's*	1 Lolly/73g	64	0.4	88	0.5	21.5	0.5	0
Coconut, Creamy, Finest, Tesco*	1 Lolly/77g	77	1.6	100	0.4	19.6	2.1	0.6
Coconut, Specially Selected, Aldi*	1 Lolly/73g	68	2	93	0.5	16	2.8	0.5
Cola, Morrisons*	1 Lolly/40g	24	0	59	0.1	14.6	0	0
Dip Dab, Barratt*	1 Lolly/67g	84	0.1	126	0.1	31	0.2	0.1
Drumstick Squashies, Swizzels*	1 Lolly/44g	82	4.1	187	2.7	22.6	9.4	0.5
Exotic Burst, Solo, Iceland*	1 Lolly/75g	100	2.8	134	2.3	22.5	3.7	0.6
Exotic Fruit, Ice Cream, Gelatelli, Lidl*	1 Lolly/110g	148	2.8	135	1.8	25.6	2.5	0
Exotic Fruit, Mini, HL, Tesco*	1 Lolly/31g	41	0.6	131	1	26.4	2	1

	Measure INFO/WEIGHT	per Measure KCAL	FAT	Nutrition Values per 100g / 100ml KCAL	PROT	CARB	FAT	FIBRE
ICE LOLLY								
Fab, Nestle*	1 Lolly/58g	82	2.9	142	0.6	23.1	5.1	0.3
Fab, Strawberry, Mini, Nestle*	1 Lolly/35ml	47	1.6	133	0.5	22.5	4.6	0.3
Forest Fruit, Dairy Free, Giannis, Aldi*	1 Lolly/67g	216	14.1	322	2.5	29	21	2.1
Freeze Pops, Premium, R Whites*	1 Lolly/60g	17	0	29	0	7	0	0
Frozen Yoghurt, Mango, Greek Style, Claudi & Fin*	1 Lolly/26g	29	1.3	112	2.7	12.9	5.2	0.5
Frozen Yoghurt, Mixed Berry, Yoo Moo*	1 Lolly/57g	74	0.8	129	2.8	25.8	1.4	0.5
Frozen Yoghurt, Strawberry, Yoo Moo*	1 Lolly/57g	73	0.8	128	2.8	25.5	1.4	0.5
Frozen Yoghurt, Tropical, Yoo Moo*	1 Lolly/57g	74	0.8	130	2.9	26.1	1.4	0.6
Frozen Yoghurt, with Raspberry Sauce, Guuud, Wall's*	1 Lolly/60g	83	2.1	138	2.7	24	3.5	0
Fruit Blaster, Rowntree's*	1 Lolly/80ml	54	0	67	0.1	15.8	0	0.3
Fruit Ices, Made with Orange Juice, Del Monte*	1 Lolly/75ml	69	0.1	92	1.2	21.5	0.1	0.2
Fruit Juice, Raspberry, Essential, Waitrose*	1 Lolly/38g	32	0.2	84	0.5	19.7	0.5	0.6
Fruit Luxury, Mini, Co-Op*	1 Lolly/45g	58	2.7	130	2	18	6	0.2
Fruit Pastille, Rowntree's*	1 Lolly/65ml	57	0.1	88	0.1	21.1	0.1	0.1
Fruit Spiral, Sainsbury's*	1 Lolly/70g	58	0.4	83	0	20.3	0.5	0
Fruit Split, Waitrose*	1 Lolly/73g	91	2.6	124	2.5	21.7	3.6	0.4
Fruit Splits, Farmfoods*	1 Lolly/49g	48	1.4	98	1.4	16.9	2.8	0
Fruit Stack, Rowntree's*	1 Lolly/70ml	55	0.3	79	0.5	19	0.5	0.5
Fruits of the Forest, Ice Cream, Gelatelli, Lidl*	1 Lolly/110g	145	2.8	132	1.9	24.5	2.5	0
Ice Burst, Aldi*	1 Lolly/60g	67	1.1	112	0.5	24	1.8	0.5
Lemon & Blackcurrant, Twister, Wall's*	1 Lolly/71g	68	0.4	96	0.7	21	0.6	0
Lemon & Lime, Mini, Calippo, Wall's*	1 Lolly/78g	70	0.4	90	0.5	21	0.5	0
Lemon & Lime, Mini, Lemon Core, Twister, Wall's*	1 Lolly/39g	42	0.5	107	0.6	22	1.2	0
Lemon & Lime, Mini, Strawberry Core, Twister, Wall's*	1 Lolly/39g	41	0.5	105	0.6	22	1.2	0
Lemon & Lime, Twister, Wall's*	1 Lolly/71g	76	0.9	107	0.5	22	1.2	0
Lemonade & Cola, Morrisons*	1 Lolly/55ml	36	0	65	0	16.2	0	0
Lemonade Flavour, R White*	1 Lolly/75ml	56	1.1	75	0.5	15.1	1.5	0.1
Love Hearts, Fruit Flavoured, Swizzels*	1 Lolly/65ml	72	0	110	0	25	0	3.4
Mango, & Fresh Mint, Ice Kitchen*	1 Lolly/75g	60	0	80	0.5	18.2	0	1.1
Mango, Max, Wall's*	1 Lolly/75g	74	0.5	98	0.6	21	0.7	0
Mango, Strawberry, Vanilla, 3Ster, Twister, Wall's*	1 Lolly/72g	70	0.5	98	0.6	21	0.7	0
Milk, Blue Parrot Cafe, Sainsbury's*	1 Lolly/30ml	34	1	113	2.7	18	3.3	0.3
Milk, Strawberry, Little, Jude's*	1 Lolly/28g	31	0.7	111	2.4	19.7	2.5	0
Mini Whirlz, Giannis, Aldi*	1 Lolly/40g	46	0.6	114	1	24	1.6	0.5
Mint Chocolate, Tesco*	1 Lolly/47g	160	10.9	342	2.7	30	23.2	1.1
Mixed Fruit, Vimto*	1 Lolly/45ml	39	0.2	87	0.5	20.9	0.5	0.2
No Added Sugar, Tesco*	1 Lolly/32g	26	0	80	0.1	20	0	0.1
Nobbly Bobbly, Nestle*	1 Lolly/70ml	219	11.6	312	2.9	38.1	16.5	0.6
Orange, Average	***1 Lolly/72g***	***66***	***0***	***92***	***0.4***	***22.4***	***0***	***0.1***
Pineapple & Coconut Colada, Waitrose*	1 Lolly/73ml	79	1.5	108	1	21	2.1	0.6
Pineapple, Dairy Split, Sainsbury's*	1 Lolly/72ml	84	2.6	116	1.8	19	3.6	0.1
Pineapple, Real Fruit Juice, Sainsbury's*	1 Lolly/73ml	55	0.1	76	0.1	19	0.1	0.1
Pop Up, CBY, Asda*	1 Lolly/80ml	65	0	81	0	20.1	0	0.3
Rainbow, Iceland*	1 Lolly/65g	54	0.1	83	0.1	20.2	0.2	0.1
Raspberry Smoothie, Del Monte*	1 Lolly/88g	85	0	97	0.3	23	0	1.3
Raspberry, Real Fruit Juice, Sainsbury's*	1 Lolly/72g	62	0.1	86	0.3	21	0.1	0.1
Real Fruit, Dairy Split, Sainsbury's*	1 Lolly/73ml	100	3.1	137	2.1	22.8	4.2	0.1
Refresher, Fruit Flavour, Bassett's*	1 Lolly/45g	56	0.7	125	1.6	26	1.6	0.3
Rocket, Asda*	1 Lolly/60g	44	0.3	73	0.5	17	0.5	0.6
Rocket, Co-Op*	1 Lolly/60g	42	0	70	0	17	0	0
Rocket, Essential, Waitrose*	1 Lolly/58ml	42	0.1	72	0.4	16.8	0.2	0.7
Rocket, Sainsbury's*	1 Lolly/60g	50	0.3	83	0.5	19.9	0.5	0.5
Rocket, Tesco*	1 Lolly/60g	39	0.1	66	0.4	15.2	0.2	0.6

I

	Measure INFO/WEIGHT	per Measure KCAL	FAT	Nutrition Values per 100g / 100ml KCAL	PROT	CARB	FAT	FIBRE
ICE LOLLY								
Rollercoaster, Ice King*	1 Lolly/65g	102	4.2	157	0.5	25	6.4	0.5
Scottish Raspberry, The Best, Morrisons*	1 Lolly/73ml	63	0.1	86	0.5	20.3	0.2	0.6
Seriously Fruity, Mango Sorbet, Waitrose*	1 Lolly/100ml	79	0.3	79	0.8	18.4	0.3	0.5
Solo Smoothies, Iceland*	1 Lolly/44g	53	0.2	121	0.1	29.1	0.5	0
Sorbet, Strawberry, & Watermelon, Asda*	1 Lolly/55ml	39	0.3	71	0.5	17	0.5	0.5
Spiral, Aldi*	1 Lolly/70g	47	0.4	67	0.5	16	0.5	0.5
Spiral, Cherry Cola, Aldi*	1 Lolly/70g	37	0	53	0	12	0	0
Strawberries & Cream, Cadbury*	1 Lolly/100ml	225	11.7	225	2.9	27	11.7	0
Strawberries, & Cream, Ice Kitchen*	1 Lolly/75g	111	5.8	148	0.7	18.4	7.7	0
Strawberry , Rowntrees*	1 Lolly/74ml	62	0.3	84	0.1	19.9	0.4	0.4
Strawberry Split, Average	***1 Lolly/72g***	***78***	***2.3***	***108***	***1.5***	***18.5***	***3.2***	***0.2***
Strawberry Sprinkles, Asda*	1 Lolly/60g	65	0.4	109	0.5	25	0.7	0.5
Strawberry, Blackcurrant & Vanilla, Mini, Twister, Wall's*	1 Lolly/50ml	38	0.3	77	0.7	16	0.7	0
Strawberry, Fruit Split, Iceland*	1 Lolly/73g	77	2.4	105	0.9	17.8	3.3	0.5
Strawberry, Push Up, Rowntree's*	1 Lolly/80ml	55	0.1	69	0.1	15.6	0.1	0.3
Traffic Light, Co-Op*	1 Lolly/52g	55	0.4	105	0.4	25	0.8	0
Tropical, Giannis, Aldi*	1 Lolly/75g	112	3.2	150	1.8	26	4.3	0.6
Tropical, Mmmm, Tesco*	1 Lolly/73g	109	3.1	150	1.2	26.6	4.3	0.4
Twistys, Morrisons*	1 Lolly/70g	51	0.1	73	0.2	17.5	0.2	0
Watermelon, Rowntree's*	1 Lolly/73ml	61	0.3	83	0.1	19	0.4	0.3
Whirlz, Giannis, Aldi*	1 Lolly/50g	49	0.9	98	0	17.4	1.8	0
Yoghurt, & Raspberry, Asda*	1 Lolly/50ml	63	2.1	125	1.4	20	4.2	0
Zoom, Nestle*	1 Lolly/58ml	54	0.4	93	0.9	20.6	0.7	0
IRN BRU								
Diet, Sugar Free, Barr's*	1 Can/330ml	2	0	1	0.5	0	0	0
Original, Barr's*	1 Bottle/500ml	100	0	20	0.5	4.8	0	0

	Measure INFO/WEIGHT	per Measure KCAL	FAT	Nutrition Values per 100g / 100ml KCAL	PROT	CARB	FAT	FIBRE
JACKFRUIT								
Caribbean, Allplants*	1 Serving/410g	549	12.3	134	4.4	20	3	4.6
in Chilli Sauce, Vegan, Waitrose*	1 Pot/350g	259	13	74	2.8	4.7	3.7	5.1
Pulled, Hoisin, Ramen, BOL Foods*	1 Pack/380g	365	8.7	96	2.5	15.4	2.3	1.8
Raw, Average, Flesh Only	***1 Portion/165g***	***155***	***0.5***	***94***	***1.5***	***24.4***	***0.3***	***1.6***
Shredded, in Mexican Sauce, Vegan, Tesco*	1 Pouch/150g	117	4.6	78	2.3	8.9	3.1	2.4
Shredded, in Thai Green Sauce, Vegan, Tesco*	1 Pack/150g	120	8.8	80	1.4	4.6	5.9	1.6
JALFREZI								
Chicken, & Rice, Rice Pot, Sharwood's*	1 Pot/270g	248	1.9	92	3	17.9	0.7	1.1
Chicken, Asda*	½ Pack/191g	201	8	105	12	4.2	4.2	1.9
Chicken, Canned, Morrisons *	½ Can/200g	186	7	93	11.9	1.9	3.5	3
Chicken, Canned, Tesco*	½ Can/200g	190	6.8	95	10.8	4.1	3.4	1.4
Chicken, Hot & Spicy, Sainsbury's*	½ Pack/200g	228	11.4	114	12.8	2.9	5.7	1
Chicken, with Rice, Ready Meal	***1 Serving/450g***	***557***	***18.9***	***124***	***6.9***	***14.5***	***4.2***	***1.5***
Chicken, with Rice, Ready Meal, Healthy Range	***1 Serving/400g***	***363***	***5.7***	***91***	***7.1***	***12.3***	***1.4***	***1.4***
Vegetable, Waitrose*	1 Pack/400g	256	16	64	2.2	4.7	4	3.7
JAM								
Apricot, Average	***1 Tbsp/15g***	***37***	***0***	***248***	***0.2***	***61.6***	***0***	***1.5***
Apricot, Intense, Bonne Maman*	1 Tbsp/15g	25	0	164	0.8	39	0.2	1.6
Black Cherry, Average	***1 Tbsp/15g***	***37***	***0***	***247***	***0.4***	***61.2***	***0.3***	***0.4***
Blackberry, Extra Special, Asda*	1 Tbsp/15g	29	0.1	190	0.9	45	0.7	0
Blackcurrant, Average	***1 Tbsp/15g***	***38***	***0***	***250***	***0.2***	***62.3***	***0***	***1***
Blackcurrant, Reduced Sugar, Average	***1 Tbsp/15g***	***27***	***0***	***178***	***0.4***	***44.4***	***0.2***	***1***
Blueberry, Best, Hartley's*	1 Tsp/15g	37	0	244	0.3	60.6	0.1	0
Chilli, M&S*	1 Tbsp/15g	39	0	262	3	62.4	0.3	4.1
Chilli, Mackays*	1 Tbsp/15g	42	0.3	283	0.9	65.9	1.7	0
Cloudberry, Wild, Scandi Kitchen*	1 Tbsp/15g	25	0.1	169	0.5	42	0.5	3.5
Damson, Extra Fruit, Best, Hartley's*	1 Tbsp/15g	37	0	244	0.2	60.8	0	0
Fig	***1 Tbsp/15g***	***36***	***0***	***242***	***0.5***	***60***	***0***	***0***
Kiwi & Gooseberry, 66% Fruit, Asda*	1 Tbsp/15g	28	0.1	187	0.5	45	0.5	0
Mixed Fruit, Average	***1 Tbsp/15g***	***38***	***0***	***252***	***0.3***	***63.5***	***0***	***0.5***
Peach, & Ginger, Eswatini*	1 Tbsp/15g	38	0	252	0.5	66	0.1	0
Peach, Pure, Summerland Sweets*	1 Tbsp/15g	75	0	500	0	130	0	0
Plum, & Damson, Soft Set, British, M&S*	1 Tbsp/15g	40	0.1	264	0.4	63.7	0.5	1.3
Plum, Tesco*	1 Tbsp/15g	39	0	261	0.2	64.4	0	0.6
Raspberry, & Lychee, Seasonal, Bonne Maman*	1 Tbsp/15g	36	0	241	0.6	58	0.2	2.3
Raspberry, Average	***1 Tbsp/15g***	***36***	***0***	***239***	***0.6***	***58.6***	***0.1***	***0.9***
Raspberry, Intense, Bonne Maman*	1 Tbsp/15g	24	0	162	0.8	37	0.2	4.3
Raspberry, Reduced Sugar, Average	***1 Tbsp/15g***	***24***	***0***	***160***	***0.5***	***39.3***	***0.2***	***0.6***
Raspberry, Seedless, Average	***1 Tbsp/15g***	***39***	***0***	***257***	***0.4***	***63.6***	***0***	***0.3***
Rhubarb & Ginger, Baxters*	1 Tbsp/15g	40	0	264	0.4	65	0.1	0.8
Stem Ginger, Cottage Delight Ltd*	1 Tbsp/15g	49	0	327	0.1	84.7	0.1	0
Strawberry, & Champagne, Fortnum & Mason*	1 Tbsp/15g	40	0	267	0	61	0	0
Strawberry, Average	***1 Tbsp/15g***	***37***	***0***	***243***	***0.3***	***60.2***	***0.1***	***0.7***
Strawberry, Intense, Bonne Maman*	1 Tbsp/15g	24	0	162	0.5	39	0.1	1.6
Strawberry, Reduced Sugar, Average	***1 Tbsp/15g***	***28***	***0***	***187***	***0.4***	***45.8***	***0.3***	***0.2***
Wild Blackberry Jelly, Baxters*	1 Tbsp/15g	32	0	210	0	53	0	1.2
JAMBALAYA								
Cajun Chicken, Cooked, BGTY, Sainsbury's*	1 Pack/389g	389	7.4	100	6.2	12.7	1.9	3.3
Chicken & Prawn, World Cafe, Waitrose*	1 Pack/350g	413	12.2	118	5.3	15.3	3.5	2.3
Chicken, HL, Tesco*	1 Pack/385g	319	5.2	83	7.7	9	1.3	2.1
Ready Meal, Average	***1 Pack/450g***	***569***	***18.2***	***126***	***6.4***	***15.7***	***4***	***1.3***
JELLY								
Apple & Watermelon, Low Calorie, Hartley's*	1 Serving/175g	5	0	3	0	0.3	0	0.3

J

	Measure INFO/WEIGHT	per Measure KCAL	FAT	Nutrition Values per 100g / 100ml KCAL	PROT	CARB	FAT	FIBRE
JELLY								
Apple, & Watermelon, 10 Cal, Hartley's*	1 Pot/175g	7	0.2	4	0.1	0.2	0.1	0
Apple, No Added Sugar, Hartley's*	1 Pot/115g	7	0.3	6	0	1.1	0.3	0
Black Forest Gateau, 10 Cal, Hartley's*	1 Pot/175g	9	0.2	5	0.1	0.2	0.1	0
Blackcurrant & Tahitian Vanilla, M&S*	¼ Pack/143g	77	0.4	54	0.3	12.1	0.3	0.6
Blackcurrant, Low Cal, Pot, Asda*	1 Pot/175g	4	0	2	0	0.5	0	0
Blackcurrant, Made Up, Rowntree's*	¼ Jelly/140ml	100	0.1	71	1.4	16.4	0.1	0
Blackcurrant, Made Up, Sainsbury's*	¼ Jelly/150g	98	0	65	1.2	15.1	0	0
Blackcurrant, Ready to Eat, Pot, Hartleys*	1 Pot/124g	51	0.1	41	0.1	9.5	0.1	0
Blueberry & Blackcurrant, 10 Cal, Hartley's*	1 Pot/175g	4	0.2	2	0.1	0.2	0.1	0.1
Cherry Flavoured, Waitrose*	1 Pot/175g	87	0.5	50	0.3	11.3	0.3	0.2
Cloudy Lemonade, Pot, Hartley's*	1 Pot/183g	11	0.9	6	0.5	0.9	0.5	0
Cranberry & Raspberry, Chivers*	1 Pot/150g	9	0	6	0	0.8	0	0
Cranberry, Tiptree, Wilkin & Sons*	1 Serving/15g	39	0	260	0	65	0	0
Crystals, Strawberry, Made Up, Tesco*	1 Serving/145g	9	0	6	1.3	0.3	0	0
Exotic Fruit, M&S*	1 Pot/175g	140	0.4	80	0.1	18.9	0.2	0.9
Fresh Fruit, M&S*	1 Pot/175g	131	0.2	75	0.2	18.4	0.1	0.3
Fruit Salad, Waitrose*	1 Pot/151g	77	0.8	51	0.5	12	0.5	0.5
Juicy, Naturelly*	1 Pot/120g	38	0.1	32	0.5	7.8	0.1	2.5
Juicy, Strawberry, Hartley's*	1 Pouch/90g	36	0.4	40	0.5	9.6	0.5	0
Lemon & Lime, Ready to Eat, Pot, Hartley's*	1 Pot/125g	51	0.1	41	0.1	9.7	0.1	0
Lemon Cheesecake, 10 Cal, Hartley's*	1Pot/175g	7	0.2	4	0.1	0.1	0.1	0
Lime Flavour, Cubes, Hartley's*	1 Cube/12g	36	0	296	5.1	68.9	0	0
Lime, Made Up, Rowntree's*	¼ Jelly/140ml	100	0.1	71	1.4	16.4	0.1	0
Made Up with Water, Average	***1oz/28g***	***17***	***0***	***61***	***1.2***	***15.1***	***0***	***0***
Mandarin & Pineapple, Sainsbury's*	1 Pot/125g	95	0.1	76	0.2	18.9	0.1	1.2
Mango, Low Cal, Asda*	1 Pot/175g	1	0	1	0	0.3	0	0
Orange, 10 Cal, Hartley's*	1 Pot/175g	4	0.2	2	0.1	0.3	0.1	0
Orange, Sugar Free, Made Up, Hartley's*	1 Serving/145g	9	0.8	6	1.3	0.5	0.5	0
Orange, Sugar Free, Rowntree's*	1 Serving/140ml	8	0	6	1.4	0.1	0	0
Orange, Unprepared, Rowntree's*	1 Square/11g	33	0	296	4.4	69.6	0	0
Orange, with Mandarin Pieces, Tesco*	1 Pot/120g	92	0.1	77	0.1	18.7	0.1	0.5
Pink Lemonade, Waitrose*	1 Pot/150g	81	0.8	54	0.5	12.6	0.5	0.5
Raspberry & Elderflower, Seriously Fruity, Waitrose*	1/6 Pack/103g	71	0.3	69	2.3	13.9	0.3	0.5
Raspberry Flavour, Tesco*	1 Serving/34g	22	0	64	1	15	0	0.1
Raspberry Glitter, Made Up, Hartley's*	1 Serving/150g	94	0	63	0	15.4	0	0
Raspberry, Aldi*	¼ Pack/34g	79	0.2	231	6.6	51	0.5	0
Raspberry, Individual Pot, Waitrose*	1 Pot/175g	94	0.9	54	0.5	12.5	0.5	0.5
Raspberry, M&S*	1 Pot/175g	100	0.5	57	0.4	12.7	0.3	0.7
Redcurrant, Average	***1oz/28g***	***70***	***0***	***250***	***0.2***	***64.4***	***0***	***0***
Strawberry & Raspberry, Sainsbury's*	½ Pot/280g	230	0	82	0.2	20.2	0	1.2
Strawberry Flavour, Sugar Free, Made Up, Rowntree's*	1 Serving/140ml	10	0	7	1.5	0.1	0	0
Strawberry, Glitter, Made Up, Hartley's*	1 Serving/150g	94	0	63	0	15.4	0	0
Strawberry, Sugar Free, Made Up, Hartley's*	1 Serving/145ml	8	0	6	1.1	0.3	0	0
Strawberry, Unprepared, Co-Op*	1 Pack/135g	402	0.1	298	5.5	69.1	0	0
Strawberry, Vegan, Jellipot*	1 Pot/120g	0	0	0	0	0.5	0	0
Strawberry, with Peach, Dole*	1 Pot/123g	92	0.1	75	0.1	18	0.1	0.5
Sugar Free, Dry, Tesco*	1 Pack/13g	36	0	285	55.4	15.6	0	0.2
JELLY BABIES								
Bassett's*	1 Sweet/6g	20	0	335	3.5	79.7	0	0
M&S*	1 Pack/125g	418	0	334	5.2	78	0	0
Mini, Rowntree's*	1 Sm Bag/35g	128	0	366	4.6	86.9	0	0
JELLY BEANS								
Average	***1 Serving/100g***	***365***	***0.1***	***365***	***0.1***	***91.2***	***0.1***	***0.1***

J

	Measure INFO/WEIGHT	per Measure KCAL	FAT	Nutrition Values per 100g / 100ml KCAL	PROT	CARB	FAT	FIBRE
JERKY								
Beef, BBQ Flavour, Kings*	1 Pack/30g	87	1.5	291	36.3	26.3	4.9	1.3
Beef, Honey & Chipotle, Tesco*	1 Pack/40g	123	2.2	307	29.1	34.7	5.4	1.8
Beef, Honey BBQ, Wild West*	1 Pack/100g	288	3.8	288	27.4	35.8	3.8	0.3
Beef, Original, Jack Link's*	1 Pack/25g	65	0.9	260	42	15	3.5	0
Beef, Wagyu, Kings*	1 Pack/25g	94	4.9	374	27	22.5	19.5	0.6
Veggie, Black Bean , Kings*	1 Pack/47g	150	3.3	320	22.5	38.2	7.1	6.8
JUICE								
12 Fruits, Multivitamins, Tropicana*	1 Glass/150ml	70	0	47	0.5	11	0	0.6
Apple & Cranberry, Average	***1 Glass/250ml***	***114***	***0***	***46***	***0.1***	***10.2***	***0***	***0***
Apple & Elderflower, Copella*	1 Glass/250ml	108	0.2	43	0.4	10.2	0.1	0
Apple & Mango, Average	***1 Glass/200ml***	***108***	***0.1***	***54***	***0.3***	***12.6***	***0***	***0.1***
Apple & Orange, Fresh Up*	1 Serving/150ml	63	0	42	0	10.3	0	0
Apple & Raspberry, Average	***1 Serving/150ml***	***67***	***0.1***	***44***	***0.4***	***10.2***	***0***	***0.2***
Apple & Cherry, Sainsbury's*	1 Serving/150ml	72	0	48	0.3	10.8	0	0.8
Apple & Rhubarb, Caxton Vale*	1 Glass/250ml	115	1	46	0.2	9.7	0.4	0
Apple, Cloudy, Pressed, Copella*	1 Glass/100ml	46	0	46	0.2	10.7	0	0.7
Apple, Pineapple, & Grape, Dia*	1 Serving/150ml	75	0	50	0.6	11.8	0	0
Apple, Pure, Average	***1 Glass/250ml***	***116***	***0.1***	***47***	***0.1***	***11.2***	***0***	***0***
Apple, Raspberry, & Rhubarb, Waitrose*	1 Serving/150ml	63	0	42	0.2	10.2	0	0.4
Beetroot, Apple, & Rhubarb, Morrisons*	1 Glass/150ml	68	0.2	45	0.7	9.9	0.1	0.7
Breakfast, Ruby, Tropicana*	1 Glass/200ml	90	0	45	0.8	9.7	0	0.7
Brilliant Beetroot, Cawston Press*	1 Glass/200ml	84	0.2	42	0.9	9.3	0.1	0
Carrot, & Ginger, Natures Choice*	1 Serving/330ml	80	1	24	0.5	3.6	0.3	0.2
Carrot, Average	***1 Glass/200ml***	***48***	***0.2***	***24***	***0.5***	***5.7***	***0.1***	***0***
Cherry, Concentrate, Montmorency, Holland & Barrett*	1 Serving/30ml	102	0	340	3.7	81.7	0	8.7
Citrus Shield, Super Juice, Innocent*	1 Serving/150ml	60	0	40	0	10	0	0
Clementine, 100% Pure Squeezed, Tesco*	1 Serving/150ml	71	0	48	0.4	10.7	0	0.2
Clementine, Morrisons*	1 Serving/100ml	48	0.1	48	0.5	10.9	0.1	0.1
Cranberry, Average	***1 Bottle/250ml***	***139***	***0.2***	***56***	***0.1***	***13.4***	***0.1***	***0.3***
Cranberry, No Added Sugar, Average	***1 Glass/200ml***	***11***	***0.1***	***6***	***0.1***	***0.8***	***0***	***0***
Elderberry, Pressed, Pure, Biona Organic*	1 Serving/200ml	76	0	38	2	7.4	0	0.2
Exotic, No Added Sugar, Morrisons*	1 Glass/150ml	24	0	16	0	3.6	0	0
Fruit, Tropical, Pure Premium, Tropicana*	1 Glass/200ml	98	0	49	0.5	11	0	0.8
Ginger Fix, B Fresh*	1 Bottle/70ml	29	0.2	42	0.7	9.1	0.3	0
Ginger, Boost, Shot, On the Go, Sainsbury's*	1 Shot/100ml	41	0.5	41	0.5	9.9	0.5	0.5
Grape, Purple, Welch's*	1 Serving/200ml	136	0	68	0.1	16.5	0	0
Grape, Red, Average	***1 Glass/250ml***	***155***	***0***	***62***	***0.2***	***15.2***	***0***	***0***
Grape, White, Average	***1 Can/160ml***	***95***	***0.1***	***60***	***0.2***	***14.3***	***0.1***	***0.1***
Grape, White, Sparkling, Non-Alcoholic, M&S*	1 Glass/125ml	90	0.1	72	0.2	17.9	0.1	0
Grapefruit, Pink, Average	***1 Glass/200ml***	***81***	***0.1***	***40***	***0.6***	***9***	***0***	***0.2***
Grapefruit, Pure, Average	***1 Glass/200ml***	***77***	***0.2***	***38***	***0.5***	***8.5***	***0.1***	***0.1***
Lemon, Fresh, Average	***1 Lemon/36ml***	***2***	***0***	***7***	***0.3***	***1.6***	***0***	***0.1***
Lime, Fresh, Average	***1 Tsp/5ml***	***0***	***0***	***9***	***0.4***	***1.6***	***0.1***	***0.1***
Multivitamin, Fruit, Vitafit, Lidl*	1 Carton/250ml	135	0.2	54	0.3	12.5	0.1	0.5
Orange & Pineapple, Average	***1 Glass/120ml***	***56***	***0.6***	***46***	***0.4***	***10.5***	***0.5***	***0.5***
Orange & Grapefruit, Average	***1 Carton/250ml***	***106***	***0.2***	***42***	***0.8***	***9.2***	***0.1***	***0.4***
Orange & Lime, Tropicana*	1 Serving/150ml	69	0	46	1.1	9.4	0	0.6
Orange & Mango, Average	***1 Bottle/375ml***	***176***	***0.4***	***47***	***0.5***	***10.7***	***0.1***	***0.2***
Orange & Passionfruit, Tropicana*	1 Serving/150ml	70	0	47	0.8	10	0	0.7
Orange & Raspberry, Tropicana*	1 Bottle/330ml	139	0	42	0.4	9	0	0.8
Orange, Apple & Mango, Calypso*	1 Carton/200ml	92	0.4	46	0	11	0.2	0.1
Orange, Freshly Squeezed, Average	***1 Serving/150ml***	***50***	***0***	***33***	***0.6***	***8.1***	***0***	***1***
Orange, Pure with Bits, Average	***1 Glass/200ml***	***90***	***0.1***	***45***	***0.6***	***10.2***	***0.1***	***0.1***

J

	Measure INFO/WEIGHT	per Measure KCAL	FAT	Nutrition Values per 100g / 100ml KCAL	PROT	CARB	FAT	FIBRE
JUICE								
Orange, Pure, Smooth, Average	***1 Glass/200ml***	***88***	***0.1***	***44***	***0.7***	***9.8***	***0***	***0.2***
Orange, Sparkling, 55, Britvic*	1 Bottle/275ml	135	0.3	49	0.3	11.3	0.1	0.1
Pear, Granini*	1 Serving/200ml	104	1	52	0.5	12.5	0.5	0
Pineapple, Average	***1 Glass/200ml***	***100***	***0.1***	***50***	***0.3***	***11.7***	***0.1***	***0.2***
Prune, Average	***1 Serving/200ml***	***123***	***0.1***	***61***	***0.6***	***15.3***	***0.1***	***1.8***
Red Fruit, Hacendado*	1 Serving/200ml	64	0.2	32	0.2	5.5	0.1	0.4
Tomato, Average	***1 Glass/200ml***	***40***	***0.1***	***20***	***0.8***	***4***	***0***	***0.4***
Tropical, Farmfoods*	1 Serving/150ml	8	0	5	0	0.9	0	0
Tropical, Jaffa Gold*	1 Serving/200ml	10	1	5	0.5	1	0.5	0.5
Tropical, Pure, Sainsbury's*	1 Glass/200ml	104	0.2	52	0.5	12	0.1	0.1
Vegetable, Original, V8*	1 Glass/150ml	26	0.2	17	0.9	2.8	0.1	0.9
JUICE DRINK								
Aloe Vera, OKF*	1 Bottle/500ml	175	0	35	0	9	0	0
Apple & Raspberry, Sainsbury's*	1 Serving/150ml	84	0.2	56	0.1	13.8	0.1	0.1
Apple & Strawberry, Sainsbury's*	1 Serving/150ml	8	0.1	5	0	1	0	0
Apple & Pomegranate, Sparkling Water, Sainsbury's*	1 Serving/200ml	4	0	2	0	0.3	0	0
Apple & Raspberry, Tesco*	1 Serving/300ml	138	0	46	0.1	11.2	0	0
Apple, & Blackberry, Classic, Fentimans*	1 Glass/200ml	82	0	41	0	10.3	0	0
Apple, & Elderflower, Presse, Sparkling, Finest, Tesco*	1 Serving/150ml	32	0	21	0	5.1	0	0.5
Berries, Mixed, Sparkling, Pressed, Shloer*	1 Can/330ml	66	0	20	0.1	4.6	0	0
Blackcurrant, Extra Light, Ribena*	1 Serving/200ml	8	0	4	0	0.5	0	0
Blood Orange, Sparkling, Aranciata Rossa, San Pellegrino*	1 Can/330ml	73	0	22	0.1	4.9	0	0
Cherry, No Added Sugar, Sainsbury's*	1 Carton/250ml	25	0.1	10	0.2	1.9	0	0
Clarity, Nutriseed*	1 Bottle/250ml	99	0.8	40	0	9.2	0.3	0.5
Cranberry & Raspberry, BGTY, Sainsbury's*	1 Glass/250ml	10	0.2	4	0.1	0.7	0.1	0.1
Cranberry Blend, Ocean Spray*	1 Serving/150ml	89	0	59	0.1	13.9	0	0
Cranberry, & Raspberry, Tesco*	1 Serving/150ml	28	0	19	0	4.4	0	0
Cranberry, Asda*	1 Serving/150ml	30	0	20	0	4.5	0	0
Cranberry, Classic, Ocean Spray*	1 Bottle/500ml	115	0	23	0	5.8	0	0
Cranberry, Light, Classic, Ocean Spray*	1 Glass/200ml	16	0	8	0	1.4	0	0
Cranberry, No Added Sugar, HL, Tesco*	1 Glass/200ml	8	0	4	0	1.1	0	0
Cranberry, Tesco*	1 Serving/150ml	30	0	20	0	4.4	0	0.1
Cranberry, Waitrose*	1 Serving/250ml	145	0	58	0.1	13.9	0	0.1
Elderflower, Wild, & Grape, Sparkling, Shloer*	1 Serving/250ml	75	0	30	0.1	7.2	0	0
Forest Fruits, Asda*	1 Serving/200ml	88	0	44	0.3	10.9	0	0.3
Grape, Apple & Raspberry, Co-Op*	1 Serving/150ml	75	0	50	0.4	12	0	0.1
Grape, Apple & Raspberry, Asda*	1 Glass/200ml	82	1	41	0.5	9.8	0.5	0.5
Grape, Red, Sparkling, Light, Shloer*	1 Serving/250ml	48	0	19	0.1	4.4	0	0
Grape, Red, Sparkling, Shloer*	1 Serving/250ml	52	0	21	0	4.8	0	0
Grape, Rose, Sparkling, Shloer*	1 Serving/200ml	42	0	21	0.1	4.8	0	0
Grape, White, Sparkling, Shloer*	1 Serving/250ml	52	0	21	0.1	4.8	0	0
Grapefruit, & Mint, Spritzed, Shloer*	1 Serving/250ml	45	0	18	0	4	0	0
J20, Apple & Raspberry, Britvic*	1 Bottle/275ml	88	0	32	0.1	7.3	0	0.3
J20, Apple, & Watermelon, Spritz, Britvic*	1 Bottle/275ml	55	0	20	0	4.8	0	0
J20, Orange & Passion Fruit, Britvic*	1 Bottle/275ml	63	0	23	0	4.8	0	0
J20, Pear & Guava, Summer Shine, Britvic*	1 Bottle/275ml	47	0	17	0	3.7	0	0
J2O, Apple & Watermelon, Sparkling, Spritz, Britvic*	1 Serving/250ml	58	0	23	0	5.4	0	0
J2O, Glitterberry, Britvic*	1 Bottle/275ml	77	0	28	0	6.4	0	0
Lemon & Lime, Light, Oasis*	1 Bottle/250ml	6	0	3	0	0.2	0	0
Lemon, Lime, & Apple, Sparkling, Bubbles, Innocent*	1 Can/333ml	90	0	27	0	6.8	0	0
Lemonade, Asda*	1 Glass/200ml	88	0	44	0.1	11	0	0
Lime, Mexican, & Elderflower, Fruit Crush, Freeway*	1 Serving/250ml	8	0.1	3	0	0.4	0	0
Limonata, Organic, San Pellegrino*	1 Bottle/200ml	70	0	35	0	10	0	0

J

	Measure INFO/WEIGHT	per Measure KCAL	FAT	Nutrition Values per 100g / 100ml KCAL	PROT	CARB	FAT	FIBRE
JUICE DRINK								
Mango, & Earl Grey Tea, Rio Doro, Aldi*	1 Bottle/ 330ml	3	0.3	1	0.1	0.3	0.1	0.1
Mango, & Passion Fruit, Tropical, Sparkling, Shloer*	1 Serving/150ml	33	0	22	0.1	5.3	0	0
Mango, No Added Sugar, Morrisons*	1 Serving/150ml	21	0	14	0.1	2.8	0	0.5
Mango, Rubicon*	1 Serving/100ml	54	0.1	54	0.1	13.1	0.1	0
Mango, Sparkling, Rubicon*	1 Can/330ml	172	0	52	0	12.8	0	0
Mixed Berry Crush, Sparkling, CBY, Asda*	1 Glass/250ml	8	0	3	0	0.5	0	0
Mulled Lemonade, Sainsbury's*	1 Serving/150ml	67	0.8	44	0.5	10.8	0.5	0.5
Orange & Lime, Sparkling, Innocent*	1 Can/330ml	93	0	28	0.6	6.5	0	0
Orange & Mango, Spring Water, Sparkling, Rubicon*	1 Bottle/500ml	15	0	3	0	0.5	0	0
Orange, Bitter, Spritzed, Shloer*	1 Serving/250ml	52	0	21	0	4.8	0	0
Orange, Caprisun*	1 Pouch/200ml	89	0	45	0	10.8	0	0
Orange, Mango, & Passionfruit, Morrisons*	1 Serving/200ml	6	0	3	0	0.2	0	0
Orange, Value, Tesco*	1 Glass/250ml	32	0	13	0	3.3	0	0
Orange, Zero, Vive, Aldi*	1 Serving/200ml	2	1	1	0.5	0.5	0.5	0.5
Passion Fruit, Exotic, Rubicon*	1 Serving/200ml	110	0	55	0.1	13.6	0	0
Peach & Apricot, Sparkling, J2O Spritz, Britvic*	1 Serving/250ml	52	0	21	0	4.9	0	0
Peach, & Cherry, Sparkling, Perrier & Juice*	1 Serving/250ml	45	0	18	0	3.9	0	0
Pear & Raspberry, Sparkling, J2O Spritz, Britvic*	1 Serving/250ml	55	0	22	0	5.2	0	0
Pear, Partially Made with Concentrate, Tesco*	1 Glass/200ml	110	0	55	0	12.4	0	0.2
Pink Cranberry Lemonade, Diet, Sparkling, M&S*	1 Bottle/500ml	15	0.5	3	0.1	0.5	0.1	0.1
Pink, Bubbly, Shloer*	1 Serving/125ml	29	0	23	0.1	5.4	0	0
Pomegranate, Rubicon*	1 Can/330ml	108	0	54	0	13.5	0	0
Raspberry, & Apple, Still, Refresh'd, Robinson's*	1 Bottle/500ml	45	0	9	0	2	0	0
Rays & Shine, Innocent*	1 Serving/150ml	56	0	37	0	9.1	0	0
Rhubarb, & Apple, Sparkling, Pressed, Shloer*	1 Can/330ml	63	0	19	0.1	4.4	0	0
Sicilian Lemon & Garden Mint, Presse, Finest, Tesco*	1 Serving/250ml	50	0	20	0	5	0	0
Strawberry, & Lime, Sparkling, Pressed, Shloer*	1 Can/330ml	66	0	20	0.1	4.6	0	0
Summer Fruits, Fresh, Tesco*	1 Glass/250ml	112	0.2	45	0.1	10.8	0.1	0.3
Summer Fruits, Oasis*	1 Bottle/500ml	90	0	18	0	4.2	0	0
Tangerine & Strawberry, Essenza, San Pellegrino*	1 Can/330ml	3	0	1	0	0	0	0
Tropical Fruit, Tesco*	1 Glass/250ml	118	0	47	0	11.4	0	0
Tropical, Be Light, Aldi*	1 Glass/250ml	62	0.2	25	0.2	5.4	0.1	0.2
Tropical, No Added Sugar, Tesco*	1 Carton/250ml	12	0	5	0	1.1	0	0
Virgin Mary, Alcohol Free, M&S*	1 Serving/150ml	30	0.2	20	0.7	4	0.1	0.8
White, Bubbly, Shloer*	1 Serving/125ml	29	0	23	0.1	5.3	0	0

	Measure INFO/WEIGHT	per Measure KCAL	FAT	Nutrition Values per 100g / 100ml KCAL	PROT	CARB	FAT	FIBRE
KALE								
Black, Cavolo Nero, Aldi*	1 Serving/80g	23	0.9	29	2.4	1	1.1	2.8
Curly, Boiled in Salted Water, Average	***1 Serving/60g***	***14***	***0.7***	***24***	***2.4***	***1***	***1.1***	***2.8***
Curly, Raw, Average	***1 Serving/90g***	***25***	***1.2***	***28***	***2.9***	***1.2***	***1.4***	***2.6***
KARELA								
Frozen, Shana*	1 Serving/80g	14	0.1	18	1.4	1.3	0.1	0
KATSU								
Chicken, Pot, Tesco*	1 Pack/132g	187	4.1	141	7.1	20.4	3.1	1.7
Chicken, Red Pepper, & Jasmine Rice, BFY, M&S*	1 Pack/380g	384	8.4	101	9.2	10.5	2.2	1.4
Coconut, Everdine*	1 Serving/450g	585	28.4	130	9.1	7.2	6.3	4.4
Yakisoba, Wasabi Co Ltd*	1 Pack/450g	891	32.8	198	8	24.6	7.3	0
KEBAB								
Beef ,& Pepper, Kofta, Waitrose*	1 Kebab/138g	223	13.9	162	14.8	2.9	10.1	0.6
Beef, BBQ, 5% Fat, Ashfield Farm, Aldi*	1 Kebab/80g	120	2.9	150	21	7.4	3.6	1.2
Beef, BBQ, Sweet & Smoky, Fire Pit, Tesco*	1 Kebab/84g	214	15.1	255	20.7	1.9	18	1.1
Beef, Jalapeno, Ashfield Farm, Aldi*	1 Kebab/48g	125	7.2	261	25	6	15	2.5
Beef, Kofta, Spicy, Oakhurst, Aldi*	1 Kebab/45g	112	6.8	248	20	6.5	15	2.8
Beef, Kofta, Uncooked, Tesco*	1 Kebab/73g	163	12.5	225	14	3.2	17.3	1.2
Chicken, & Chorizo, Fire Pit, Tesco*	1 Kebab/59g	93	3	157	26.4	1.7	5	0.1
Chicken, Breast, Garlic, Lemon, & Herb, Sainsbury's*	2 Kebabs/107g	173	5.7	162	25.8	2.6	5.3	0.5
Chicken, Buttermilk, King, Waitrose*	1/6 Pack/106g	192	9.8	181	24.1	1.6	9.2	0
Chicken, Coronation, Co-Op*	½ Pack/65g	93	1.7	143	28	1.6	2.6	0
Chicken, Indian Spiced, Morrisons*	½ Pack/112g	159	2.7	142	26.7	3.1	2.4	0.5
Chicken, Peri Peri, King, Oakhurst, Aldi*	¼ Pack/177g	301	11	170	24.3	4.3	6.2	1
Chicken, Shawarma, Ashfield Farm, Aldi*	½ Pack/95g	149	3.9	157	17	12	4.1	1.1
Chicken, Shish in Pitta Bread with Salad	***1 Kebab/250g***	***388***	***10.2***	***155***	***13.5***	***17.2***	***4.1***	***1***
Chicken, Shish, Meat Only, Average	***1 Kebab/250g***	***312***	***5.2***	***125***	***25.7***	***0.9***	***2.1***	***0.1***
Chicken, Skewers, Chimichurri, Oakhurst, Aldi*	1 Skewer/83g	135	3.9	163	23	3.9	4.7	1
Chicken, Spanish Style, Good to Go, Waitrose*	1 Pack/80g	148	4.6	185	18.3	13.8	5.7	2.6
Chicken, Sweet Chilli, Birchwood Farm, Lidl*	1 Kebab/80g	110	1.8	138	28.1	1.1	2.2	0
Chicken, Teriyaki, Ashfield Farm, Aldi*	1 Skewer/62g	102	3.7	165	21	6.7	6	0.5
Chicken, Thigh, Sticky Barbecue, M&S*	1 Pack/100g	189	6.8	189	26.3	5.7	6.8	0.1
Courgette, & Feta, Kofta, Vegetarian, Waitrose*	½ Pack/75g	166	7.8	222	5.8	24.2	10.4	4.1
Doner, in Pitta, with Salad, Average	***1 Serving/400g***	***1020***	***64.8***	***255***	***14.2***	***14***	***16.2***	***0.8***
Doner, Meat, & Chips, Heat Me Eat Me*	1 Pack/165g	307	14.9	186	5.4	20	9	2.6
Doner, Meat, Pre Cooked, Frozen, Babek*	1 Serving/100g	300	28	300	14.7	8.1	28	0
Handmade, Seekh, Mumtaz*	½ Pack/94g	201	14.6	214	15.8	2.9	15.5	0
Kofta, Beef, & Cheese, Mini, Oven Baked, Iceland*	2 Koftas/36g	74	3.7	203	18.5	9.1	10.1	1.4
Kofta, Middle Eastern, Slimming World, Iceland*	½ Pack/150g	184	5	123	19.4	3.8	3.3	0.6
Kofta, Seitan, Spiced, Vegan, Waitrose*	3 Koftas/100g	220	11.7	220	17.5	9.3	11.7	3.7
Kofta, Tandoori, Vegan, Waitrose*	1 Kebab/64g	82	2.8	128	5.1	13	4.3	8.5
Koftas, Tex Mex, Vegan, Plant Chef, Tesco*	2 Koftas/64g	125	5.1	196	10.5	18.5	8	4.2
Lamb, & Chicken, Kofta, Tesco*	2 Koftas/38g	97	5.3	255	14.6	16.8	13.9	2
Lamb, Kofta, Citrus Tikka, Sainsbury's*	1 Kebab/84g	199	11.6	235	18.1	9.8	13.7	2.6
Lamb, Kofta, The Butcher's Hook*	1 Kebab/70g	171	13.3	244	13.3	3.5	19	3
Lamb, Mint, Birchwood Farm, Lidl*	1 Kebab/80g	189	10.5	236	23.3	5.8	13.1	1.2
Lamb, Minted, Ashfield Farm, Aldi*	1 Kebab/54g	137	9.2	254	18.5	5.7	17	0
Lamb, Minted, Grilled, Butchers Choice, Asda*	1 Kebab/49g	126	8.8	257	19	3.4	18	2.7
Lamb, Minted, Shish, As prepared, Waitrose*	1 Kebab/57g	123	7.3	217	17.2	7.9	12.9	0.1
Lamb, Shami with a Mint Raita Dip, M&S*	½ Pack/90g	189	12.1	210	12.8	9.7	13.4	3.5
Lamb, Shish, The Grill, M&S*	1 Kebab/74g	168	12.6	227	14.6	3.5	17	0.6
Lamb, with Mint, Tesco*	1 Serving/80g	192	13.4	240	16	5.5	16.7	0.4
Meat, Tasty, Heron*	¼ Pack/125g	364	28.6	291	16.5	4.4	22.9	0.3
Pork, BBQ, Ashfield Farm, Aldi*	1 Kebab/67g	165	9.4	246	23	6.6	14	0.5

	Measure INFO/WEIGHT	per Measure KCAL	FAT	Nutrition Values per 100g / 100ml KCAL	PROT	CARB	FAT	FIBRE
KEBAB								
Pork, BBQ, Sainsbury's*	1 Serving/90g	65	2.2	72	11	1.4	2.4	0.9
Pork, Greek Inspired, Fire Pit, Tesco*	1 Kebab/73g	161	9.4	221	24	1.8	12.9	0.7
Pork, Outdoor Bred, Co-Op*	1 Kebab/100g	174	9.5	174	17	4.5	9.5	0.7
Pork, Sticky Masala, Tesco*	1 Kebab/79g	182	9.4	231	23.4	7.2	11.9	0.6
Salmon, Chilli & Lime, Tesco*	2 Kebabs/78g	187	10.4	240	21.9	8.2	13.3	0
Salmon, Teriyaki, Waitrose *	1 Kebab/50g	90	4.4	181	20.7	4.3	8.8	0.8
Shish, with Onions & Peppers	***1oz/28g***	***59***	***4.5***	***212***	***12.9***	***3.9***	***16.2***	***1.2***
Skewers, Thai BBQ, Moo Ping, Meal Kit, Thai Taste*	½ Pack/85g	139	6.6	163	2.2	2.1	7.8	0
Veggie, Greek, Vivera*	1 Pack/175g	292	15.4	167	14	5.4	8.8	4.4
Veggiebab, Korean Inspired, Plant Menu, Aldi*	1 Veggiebab/55g	78	2.8	141	6.3	15	5	5.2
Veggiebab, Zanzibar Inspired, Plant Menu, Aldi*	1 Veggiebab/55g	76	3.1	138	5.7	15	5.6	7.4
KEDGEREE								
Average	***1oz/28g***	***48***	***2.4***	***171***	***15.9***	***7.8***	***8.7***	***0.1***
Haddock, Smoked, Big Dish, M&S*	1 Pack/450g	585	22.5	130	8.5	13	5	1.9
KETCHUP								
Barbeque, Asda*	1 Tbsp/15g	20	0	136	0.9	33	0	0
BBQ, Heinz*	1 Tbsp/15g	21	0	137	1.3	31.3	0.3	0.3
Chilli, Smoked, Gran Luchito*	1 Tbsp/15g	54	0.1	358	1.8	18.4	0.9	0
Curry, Scharf, Hela*	1 Tbsp/15g	21	0	137	0.8	30.8	0.3	0
Mustard, Sweet, Tracklements*	1 Tbsp/15g	51	2.6	337	8.3	35.3	17.4	4.5
Tomato, Average	***1 Tbsp/15g***	***18***	***0***	***120***	***1.5***	***28.1***	***0.2***	***0.8***
Tomato, GF, Chippa *	1 Tbsp/15g	14	0.1	90	0.9	21.2	0.5	0
Tomato, Reduced Sugar, Average	***1 Tbsp/15g***	***13***	***0.2***	***87***	***2***	***16.9***	***1.2***	***0.9***
KIDNEY								
Lamb, Fried, Average	***1oz/28g***	***53***	***2.9***	***188***	***23.7***	***0***	***10.3***	***0***
Lamb, Raw, Average	***1oz/28g***	***25***	***0.7***	***91***	***17***	***0***	***2.6***	***0***
Ox, Raw	***1oz/28g***	***22***	***0.5***	***77***	***15.1***	***0***	***1.8***	***0***
Pig, Fried	***1oz/28g***	***57***	***2.7***	***202***	***29.2***	***0***	***9.5***	***0***
Pig, Raw	***1oz/28g***	***22***	***0.7***	***77***	***14***	***0***	***2.4***	***0***
Pig, Stewed	***1oz/28g***	***43***	***1.7***	***153***	***24.4***	***0***	***6.1***	***0***
Veal, Raw, Average	***1 Serving/100g***	***99***	***3.1***	***99***	***15.8***	***0.8***	***3.1***	***0***
KIEV								
Chicken, & Garlic, M&S*	1 Kiev/143g	352	23	246	12.8	11.9	16.1	1
Chicken, Cheese & Ham, Morrisons*	1 Kiev/128g	282	16	221	14.3	12	12.5	1.8
Chicken, Cheese, & Ham, Roosters, Aldi*	1 Kiev/112g	266	16.8	238	12	13	15	1.1
Chicken, COU, M&S*	1 Kiev/150g	188	2.7	125	15.8	10.8	1.8	0.5
Chicken, Creamy Peppercorn, Tesco*	1 Kiev/132g	290	17.3	220	13.1	12.1	13.1	0.6
Chicken, Garlic & Parsley Butter, Breaded, Waitrose*	1 Kiev/156g	375	21.3	241	17.5	11.1	13.7	1.4
Chicken, Garlic & Herb Butter, Tesco*	1 Kiev/106g	318	22.3	300	13.6	14	21	0.7
Chicken, Garlic & Herb, Birchwood Farm, Lidl*	1 Kiev/120g	356	26	297	13.1	11.3	21.7	1.9
Chicken, Garlic & Herb, Oven Baked, Asda*	1 Kiev/122g	321	20.7	263	13	14	17	1.9
Chicken, Garlic & Herb, Sainsbury's*	1 Kiev/113g	317	22.8	281	11.5	12.5	20.2	1.2
Chicken, Garlic & Parsley, BGTY, Sainsbury's*	1 Kiev/125g	267	15.5	213	14.7	10.6	12.4	0.5
Chicken, Garlic Butter, HL, Tesco*	1 Kiev/106g	318	22.3	300	13.6	14	21	0.7
Chicken, Garlic, & Herb, Iceland*	1 Kiev/120g	343	24.7	286	13.1	12	20.6	0.2
Chicken, Garlic, Ready to Cook, Co-Op*	1 Kiev/170g	289	13.9	170	18	6	8.2	0.8
Chicken, Garlic, Whole Breast Fillets, Sainsbury's*	1 Kiev/169g	403	23	238	19.8	8.6	13.6	1.2
Chicken, Garlic, Wild, & Cornish Butter, Gastropub, M&S*	1 Kiev/225g	493	32.2	219	17.3	5	14.3	0.6
Chicken, Ham, & Cheese, Tesco*	1 Kiev/143g	307	18.6	215	14.4	9.3	13	1.3
Chicken, Hunters, Tesco*	1 Kiev/122g	285	15.5	234	13.8	15.1	12.7	1.7
Chicken, with Garlic, & Herb, Inspirations, Birds Eye*	1 Kiev/150g	357	19.5	238	16	14	13	0.5
Fish Fillet, Breaded, with Garlic & Herb, Iceland*	1 Kiev/131g	299	20.1	228	9.1	12.8	15.3	1.4
Garlic, Plant Based, The Vegan Factor*	1 Kiev/119g	315	18.8	265	14.3	16	15.8	0.5

	Measure INFO/WEIGHT	per Measure KCAL	per Measure FAT	KCAL	PROT	CARB	FAT	FIBRE
				Nutrition Values per 100g / 100ml				
KIEV								
Mushroom, & Spinach, Oven Baked, Goodlife*	1 Kiev/119g	295	14.8	248	6.9	25.2	12.4	3.7
No Chicken, Mini, Plant Kitchen, M&S*	1 Kiev/30g	79	4.9	264	13.7	13.9	16.4	2.8
No Chicken, Plant Kitchen, M&S*	1 Kiev/140g	340	21.1	243	12.1	13	15.1	3.3
Vegetable, Veggie, M&S*	1 Kiev/155g	267	15.5	172	3.4	15.9	10	2.6
Vegetarian, Mini, Quorn*	1 Kiev/20g	41	2.2	207	14	13	11	6.5
with Garlic Butter, & Parsley, Kiev, Barber Foods*	1 Kiev/140g	243	15.7	243	14.3	10	15.7	0.7
KIMCHI								
Ramyun, Nongshim*	1 Serving/30g	125	3.6	418	7.7	69	12	0
Raw, Vadasz*	1 Serving/50g	8	0.2	15	1.1	1	0.4	1.8
Sliced, Bibigo*	1 Serving/30g	10	0.1	32	1.9	5.4	0.3	0
Spicy, Biona Organic*	1 Serving/50g	12	0.1	24	1.1	3.7	0.2	1.8
Unpasteurised , Kim Kong*	1 Serving/15g	6	0.1	37	2.3	4.4	0.7	2.1
KIPPER								
Baked, Average	***1oz/28g***	***57***	***3.2***	***205***	***25.5***	***0***	***11.4***	***0***
Fillets in Sunflower Oil, John West*	1 Can/140g	321	23.8	229	19	0	17	0
Fillets, Beechwood Smoked, Gold, Ocado*	1 Kipper/110g	268	20.9	244	18	0.5	19	0
Fillets, Raw, Average	***1 Serving/200g***	***384***	***29.1***	***192***	***14.5***	***0***	***14.6***	***0***
Fillets, Scottish, with Butter, Youngs*	1 Pack/170g	350	25.9	226	18.9	0.1	16.7	0
Fillets, Smoked with Butter, Scottish, Boil in Bag, Tesco*	1 Serving/100g	225	17.2	225	17	0	17.2	0
Fillets, Smoked, Scottish, with Butter, Tesco*	1 Fillet/85g	182	13.6	214	16.5	0.9	16	0
Grilled, Average	***1oz/28g***	***71***	***5.4***	***255***	***20.1***	***0***	***19.4***	***0***
Smoked, Average	***1 Serving/150g***	***322***	***23***	***214***	***18.9***	***0***	***15.4***	***0***
Whole, with Bone, Grilled, Average	***1 Serving/100g***	***161***	***12.2***	***161***	***12.7***	***0***	***12.2***	***0***
KIT KAT								
2 Finger, Dark, Nestle*	2 Fingers/21g	107	5.4	510	5.4	62.2	25.5	5.4
2 Finger, Nestle*	2 Fingers/21g	104	5.1	502	6.7	62.7	24.4	2.1
4 Finger, Nestle*	4 Fingers/42g	208	10.2	502	6.7	62.7	24.5	2.1
Chunky, Caramel, Nestle*	1 Bar/48g	259	15.3	539	5.2	58.6	31.8	0
Chunky, Double Caramel, Nestle*	½ Bar/21g	109	5.8	520	6.5	61	27.6	1
Chunky, Nestle*	1 Bar/40g	206	10.2	516	5.4	65.1	25.6	1.7
Chunky, Orange, Nestle*	1 Bar/48g	247	12.5	515	5.8	62	26.1	0
Chunky, Peanut, Nestle*	1 Bar/42g	226	13.2	537	8.4	54.9	31.5	0
Chunky, Salted Caramel, Fudge, Nestle*	1 Bar/42g	222	12.5	529	9.2	55.1	29.7	1.9
Chunky, Snack Size, Nestle*	1 Bar/26g	133	7.1	513	6.6	60.4	27.2	1.1
Cookies & Cream, 2 Finger, Nestle*	1 Bar/21g	106	5.3	507	7.6	60.9	25.4	1.4
Dark, Mint, 2 Finger, Nestle*	1 Bar/21g	105	5.3	502	5.4	60.6	25.3	5.3
Easter Break, Cadburys*	1 Bar/29g	156	9.1	537	6.2	55.6	31.4	2.9
Gold, Nestle*	1 Bar/42g	219	11.6	526	6.2	62.1	27.9	0.8
Kubes, Nestle*	1 Pack/50g	258	13.8	515	5.9	60.9	27.5	1
Lemon Drizzle, Nestle*	1 Bar/21g	105	5.1	505	6.8	63.2	24.5	2.1
Mini, Nestle*	1 Bar/15g	75	3.9	502	7.5	59.4	26	0
Orange, 2 Finger, Nestle*	2 Fingers/21g	107	5.6	507	5.5	61.7	26.5	0
Peanut Butter, Bites, Nestle*	4 Pieces/23g	121	6.5	525	10.8	55.3	28.3	2.1
Ruby, 4 Finger, Kit Kat*	1 Pack/42g	225	13	541	6.5	56.8	31.4	1.4
Senses, Millionaires Shortbread, Nestle*	1 Bar/23g	117	6.1	514	8.1	58.8	26.8	1.5
Senses, Nestle*	1 Bar/31g	165	9.5	531	7.5	56.3	30.7	0
White, Chunky, Nestle*	1 Bar/40g	206	10.6	516	8.1	60.8	26.4	0.5
KIWI FRUIT								
Fresh, Raw, Flesh & Seeds, Average	***1 Kiwi/60g***	***29***	***0.3***	***49***	***1.1***	***10.6***	***0.5***	***1.9***
Weighed with Skin, Average	***1 Kiwi/60g***	***25***	***0.3***	***42***	***0.9***	***9.1***	***0.4***	***1.6***
KOHLRABI								
Boiled in Salted Water	***1oz/28g***	***5***	***0.1***	***18***	***1.2***	***3.1***	***0.2***	***1.9***
Raw	***1oz/28g***	***5***	***0***	***16***	***1.1***	***2.6***	***0.1***	***1.5***

	Measure INFO/WEIGHT	per Measure KCAL	per Measure FAT	Nutrition Values per 100g / 100ml KCAL	PROT	CARB	FAT	FIBRE
KOMBUCHA								
Captain Kombucha*	1 Bottle/333ml	60	0	18	0	4.4	0	0
Cherry Plum, Remedy*	1 Can/250ml	25	1.2	10	0.5	2.2	0.5	0.5
Classic, Kinoko*	1 Can/330ml	86	0.3	26	0.5	4.6	0.1	0.1
Elderflower & Lemon, Naturally Sugar Free, Nexba*	1 Serving/250ml	5	0	2	0	0	0	0
Ginger & Lemon, Organic, Lo Bros Living Drinks*	1 Bottle/330ml	18	1.5	6	0.1	1.1	0.5	0.1
Ginger Beer, Lo Bros Living Drinks*	1 Bottle/330ml	46	1.6	14	0.5	3.4	0.5	0.1
Ginger, & Turmeric, SynerChi*	1 Can/250ml	8	0	3	0.2	0.6	0	0
Ginger, Organic, Equinox*	1 Can/250ml	32	0.2	13	0.1	3.1	0.1	0.5
Leftfield *	1 Bottle/330ml	46	0.3	14	0.1	3.2	0.1	0
No Sugar, Remedy*	1 Can/250ml	25	0.2	10	0.1	2.2	0.1	0.5
Original, Lo Bros Living Drinks*	1 Bottle/330ml	26	0	8	0	2	0	0
Pink Grapefruit, & Guava, Equinox*	1 Bottle/275g	38	0.3	14	0.1	3.3	0.1	0.5
Raspberry Lemonade, No Sugar, Remedy*	1 Can/250ml	8	1.2	3	0.5	1.5	0.5	0.5
Raspberry, & Elderflower, Equinox*	1 Bottle/275g	38	0.3	14	0.1	3.5	0.1	0.5
Raspberry, & Lemon, Lo Bros Living Drinks*	1 Bottle/330ml	30	0	9	0	1.8	0	0
KORMA								
Cashew, & Chickpea, with Black Rice, Mindful Chef*	1 Pack/450g	504	21.2	112	4	11.8	4.7	2.9
Chicken, & Rice, Free From, Tesco*	1 Pack/369g	565	18.8	153	8.3	17.8	5.1	1.5
Chicken, Kashmiri, Sainsbury's*	1 Pack/400g	582	26.6	146	7.6	13.3	6.6	1
Chicken, Rice Pot, As Prepared, Sharwoods*	1 Pot/270g	273	5.9	101	3	17.1	2.2	0.6
Chicken, with Peshwari Coriander Rice, Finest, Tesco*	1 Pack/550g	908	48.4	165	7.5	13.9	8.8	0.9
Chicken, with Rice, Ready Meal	***1 Pack/400g***	***740***	***34.7***	***185***	***8.4***	***18.1***	***8.7***	***1.7***
Mushroom, & Chickpea, Allplants*	1 Serving/390g	499	26.1	128	3.8	12	6.7	3
Vegetable, Takeaway or Restaurant	***1 Serving/300g***	***336***	***13.5***	***112***	***3.4***	***15.4***	***4.5***	***2.6***
Veggie, The Happy Pear*	1 Pack/400g	360	11.6	90	2.2	12	2.9	2.2
KRISPROLLS								
Cracked Wheat, Original, Pagen*	1 Krisproll/13g	48	0.9	380	12	67	7	9
Golden, Swedish Toasts, Pagen*	1 Krisproll/12g	48	1	400	11	69	8.5	5
Organic, Bio, Pagen*	1 Krisproll/12g	46	0.8	380	12	67	7	8
Swedish Toasts, Wholegrain, Pagen*	1 Toast/13g	51	0.8	390	11	67	6.5	8.5
KULFI								
Average	***1oz/28g***	***119***	***11.2***	***424***	***5.4***	***11.8***	***39.9***	***0.6***
KUMQUATS								
Raw	***1 Kumquat/20g***	***9***	***0.1***	***43***	***0.9***	***9.3***	***0.5***	***3.8***
KUNG PO								
Chicken, Sainsbury's*	1 Pack/350g	262	8.8	75	9.2	4	2.5	1
Chicken, Waitrose*	1 Pack/350g	318	3.9	91	8.2	12.1	1.1	1.2

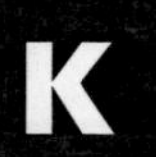

	Measure INFO/WEIGHT	per Measure KCAL	FAT	Nutrition Values per 100g / 100ml KCAL	PROT	CARB	FAT	FIBRE
LAGER								
Alcohol Free, Becks*	1 Serving/275ml	55	0	20	0.7	5	0	0
Alcohol Free, Heineken*	1 Can/330ml	69	0	21	0	4.8	0	0
Amstel, Heineken*	1 Pint/568ml	227	0	40	0.5	3	0	0
Average	***½ Pint/284ml***	***117***	***0***	***41***	***0.3***	***3.1***	***0***	***0***
Becks*	1 Can/275ml	113	0	41	0	3	0	0
Blanc, Kronenbourg*	½ pt/284ml	119	0	42	0	3.3	0	0
Boston, Samuel Adams*	1 Bottle/355ml	160	0	45	0	0	0	0
Bottled, Brahma*	1 Bottle/330ml	125	0	38	0	0	0	0
Budweiser, 66, Anheuser-Busch*	1 Bottle/330ml	102	0	31	0	0	0	0
Budweiser, Light, Anheuser-Busch*	1 Can/440ml	118	0	27	0.3	1.5	0	0
Budweiser, Zero Alcohol, Anheuser-Busch*	1 Can/330ml	46	0	14	0.1	3.3	0	0
Can, Carlsberg*	1 Can/440ml	141	0	32	0	2	0	0
Cinque, Shepherd Neame*	1 Bottle/330ml	129	0.3	39	0.4	2.9	0.1	0
Czech, Low Alcohol, M&S*	1 Bottle/500ml	20	0	4	0	0.4	0	0
Draught, Carling*	1 Pint/568ml	189	0	33	0	1.4	0	0
Export, Carlsberg*	1 Can/440ml	185	0	42	0.4	2.8	0	0.4
Export, Foster's*	1 Pint/568ml	210	0	37	0	2.2	0	0
Foster's*	1 Pint/568ml	193	0	34	0	3.1	0	0
German, Low Alcohol, Sainsbury's*	1 Bottle/330ml	92	0.3	28	0.4	5.9	0.1	0.1
Grolsch*	1 Sm Can/330ml	145	0	44	0	2.2	0	0
Heineken*, 5%, Heineken*	1 Bottle/250ml	110	0	44	0.4	3.4	0	0
Innis & Gunn*	1 Bottle/330ml	132	0	40	0.3	3.5	0	0
Irish, 4%, Rockshore*	1 Can/500ml	160	0	32	0.4	1.9	0	0
Light, 3.5%, Rockshore*	1 Bottle/330ml	73	0	22	0.3	0.6	0	0
Light, Coors*	1 Pint/568ml	170	0	30	0.3	1.5	0	0
Light, Corona*	1 Bottle/330ml	105	0	32	1.5	0	0	0
Low Alcohol	***1 Can/440ml***	***44***	***0***	***10***	***0.2***	***1.5***	***0***	***0***
Perlenbacher, 0% Alcohol, Lidl*	1 Bottle/330ml	69	0	21	0	5.2	0	0
Pils, Holsten*	1 Can/440ml	167	0	38	0.3	2.4	0	0
Pilsner, Efes*	1 Can/500ml	226	0	45	0	7.6	0	0
Pilsner, Premium, Bavaria*	1 Bottle/330ml	142	0	43	0.4	3.5	0	0
Pilsner, Rheinbacher, Aldi*	1 Can/500ml	135	0	27	0	0	0	0
Polish, Tyskie*	1 Can/549ml	236	0	43	0	0	0	0
Premier, Kronenbourg*	½ Pint/284ml	136	0	48	0	0	0	0
Premium	***1 Can/440ml***	***260***	***0***	***59***	***0.3***	***2.4***	***0***	***0***
Premium, French, Biere Speciale, Tesco*	1 Serving/250ml	105	0	42	0.3	3.3	0	0
Premium, Light, Amstel*	1 Can/355ml	95	0	27	0	1.4	0	0
Premium, San Miguel*	1 Bottle/330ml	148	0	45	0.3	3.7	0	0
Shandy, Traditional Style, Asda*	1 Serving/200ml	44	0	22	0	4.6	0	0
Skinny Brands*	1 Bottle/330ml	89	0.3	27	0	0.9	0.1	0
Stella Artois*	1 Can/550ml	220	0	40	0.4	3.1	0	0
Tuborg Green, Carlsberg*	1 Serving/200ml	78	0	39	0.5	2.5	0	0
Vier, Becks*	1 Bottle/275ml	110	0	40	0	3	0	0
LAKSA								
Chicken & Coconut Noodle, Cooked, Tesco*	1 Pack/351g	321	10.6	91	7.1	8.4	3	1.2
Chicken, & Sweet Potato, Irresistible, Co-Op*	½ Pack/300g	156	6.6	52	2.4	5.3	2.2	0.7
Hansells Foods*	1 Pouch/400g	272	21	68	1.7	3.3	5.2	0.4
Prawn, King, & Coconut, G&B, Asda*	1 Pack/367g	268	4.8	73	3.1	11	1.3	1.2
LAMB								
Breast, Lean, Roasted, Average	***1 Serving/100g***	***273***	***18.5***	***273***	***26.7***	***0***	***18.5***	***0***
Chops, Minted, Average	***1 Chop/100g***	***260***	***15.1***	***260***	***25.9***	***5.1***	***15.1***	***0.3***
Cutlets, Neck, Raw, Lean & Fat, Weighed with Bone	***1 Pack 210g***	***359***	***31.7***	***171***	***8.8***	***0***	***15.1***	***0***
Diced, From Supermarket, Healthy Range, Average	***½ Pack/200g***	***277***	***8.9***	***138***	***24.6***	***0.1***	***4.5***	***0***

	Measure INFO/WEIGHT	per Measure KCAL	FAT	Nutrition Values per 100g / 100ml KCAL	PROT	CARB	FAT	FIBRE
LAMB								
Grill Steak, Average	***1oz/28g***	***70***	***4.7***	***250***	***20.2***	***4.4***	***16.9***	***0.4***
Kleftico, Slow Cooked, Waitrose*	¼ Pack/105g	253	18.3	241	20.2	0.8	17.4	0
Lambless, Pieces, Tender, Alt*	½ Pack/160g	248	9.4	155	22	1.9	5.9	3.4
Leg, Joint, Raw, Average	***1 Joint/510g***	***858***	***45.5***	***168***	***20.9***	***1.4***	***8.9***	***0.2***
Leg, Joint, with Mint Sauce, Oven Baked, Iceland*	1/3 Joint/187g	312	13.8	167	21.2	3.5	7.4	0.5
Leg, Roasted, Lean & Fat, Average	***1oz/28g***	***66***	***3.8***	***237***	***28.6***	***0***	***13.6***	***0***
Leg, Roasted, Lean, Average	***1oz/28g***	***58***	***2.7***	***206***	***29.9***	***0***	***9.6***	***0***
Loin, Chop, Grilled, Lean & Fat, Weighed with Bone	***1 Serving/100g***	***193***	***14***	***193***	***16.8***	***0***	***14***	***0***
Loin, Chops, Raw, Lean & Fat, Weighed with Bone	***1 Serving/100g***	***216***	***17.9***	***216***	***13.7***	***0***	***17.9***	***0***
Mince, Average	***1oz/28g***	***58***	***4.2***	***207***	***17.6***	***0.5***	***14.8***	***0***
Mince, Extra Lean, Sainsbury's*	1 Serving/225g	324	11.9	144	24.1	0	5.3	0.1
Mint Gravy, Leg Chops, Tesco*	1 Serving/175g	214	9.8	122	15	3.2	5.6	1.7
Neck Fillet, Lean, Raw	***1 Serving/100g***	***232***	***17.6***	***232***	***18.4***	***0***	***17.6***	***0***
Rack, Raw, Lean & Fat	***1oz/28g***	***79***	***6.7***	***283***	***17.3***	***0***	***23.8***	***0***
Rack, Raw, Lean Only, Weighed with Bone	***1oz/28g***	***21***	***1.1***	***73***	***8.6***	***0***	***4***	***0***
Rack, Roasted, Lean	***1oz/28g***	***63***	***3.6***	***225***	***27.1***	***0***	***13***	***0***
Rack, Roasted, Lean & Fat	***1oz/28g***	***102***	***8.4***	***363***	***23***	***0***	***30.1***	***0***
Shank, in Minted Gravy, Asda*	1 Shank/267g	465	24.6	174	18	4.1	9.2	0.5
Shank, Just Cook, Sainsbury's*	1 Shank/225g	394	18.7	175	22.9	1.8	8.3	0
Shank, Minted, Cooked, Morrisons*	½ Pack/231g	466	16.6	202	29.1	5	7.2	0.2
Shank, with Mint Gravy, Oakhurst, Aldi*	1 Shank/266g	357	11.7	134	22	1.1	4.4	0.5
Shanks, Harissa, Slow Cooked, Waitrose*	1 Shank/222g	492	28.1	222	26.5	0.5	12.7	0.5
Shoulder, Cooked, Lean & Fat	***1oz/28g***	***84***	***6.3***	***301***	***24.4***	***0***	***22.5***	***0***
Shoulder, Fillet, Average	***1oz/28g***	***66***	***5.1***	***235***	***17.6***	***0***	***18.3***	***0***
Shoulder, Raw, Average	***1oz/28g***	***70***	***5.7***	***248***	***16.8***	***0***	***20.2***	***0***
Shoulder, Roasted, Whole, Lean	***1oz/28g***	***61***	***3.4***	***218***	***27.2***	***0***	***12.1***	***0***
Steak, Leg, Raw, Average	***1 Steak/150g***	***169***	***5.5***	***112***	***20***	***0***	***3.6***	***0***
Steak, Minted, Average	***1 Steak/125g***	***212***	***9***	***170***	***22.7***	***3.4***	***7.2***	***0.9***
Steak, Raw, Average	***1 Steak/140g***	***190***	***7.6***	***136***	***21.7***	***0.2***	***5.4***	***0***
Stewing, Raw, Lean & Fat	***1oz/28g***	***57***	***3.5***	***203***	***22.5***	***0***	***12.6***	***0***
Stewing, Stewed, Lean & Fat	***1oz/28g***	***78***	***5.6***	***279***	***24.4***	***0***	***20.1***	***0***
LANGOUSTINE								
Fishmongers, Frozen, Tesco*	½ Pack/229g	262	5.3	114	23	0.1	2.3	0.5
Wholetail, Shelled, Scottish, Bannerman's Seafoods*	½ Bag/170g	129	0.7	76	18	0.1	0.4	0.5
LARD								
Average	***1oz/28g***	***249***	***27.7***	***891***	***0***	***0***	***99***	***0***
LASAGNE								
Al Forno, Aldi*	1 Pack/400g	556	26	139	10	9.3	6.5	1.5
Al Forno, Serves 2, Cook*	½ Pack/370g	585	29.2	158	10	11.1	7.9	1.3
Al Forno, TTD, Sainsbury's*	1 Pack/338g	449	18.6	133	7.6	12.4	5.5	1.6
Beef, & Chunky Vegetable, HL, Tesco*	1 Pack/360g	356	8.9	99	6.5	12	2.5	1.2
Beef, 3% Fat, Oven Cooked, Calorie Counted, Asda*	1 Pack/322g	303	8.7	94	5.9	11	2.7	1.1
Beef, COU, M&S*	1 Pack/365g	358	7.3	98	6.6	12.7	2	1.2
Beef, Counted, Morrisons*	1 Pack/350g	266	5.4	76	6.2	8.8	1.5	1.1
Beef, HFC, Tesco*	1 Pack/400g	420	13.2	105	7.6	10.6	3.3	1.3
Beef, Low Fat, Well & Good, Co-Op*	1 Pack/360g	310	6.5	86	7.1	10	1.8	0.8
Beef, Ready Meal, Average	***1 Serving/400g***	***553***	***24***	***138***	***8.2***	***12.7***	***6***	***1.4***
Butternut Squash, & Lentil, Love Your Veg!, Sainsbury's*	1 Pack/369g	310	10.3	84	3.2	10.3	2.8	2.8
Family, Big Value Pack, Iceland*	¼ Pack/237g	322	14	136	5	15.9	5.9	1.4
for Two, Charlie Bigham's*	½ Pack/345g	545	32.1	158	7	9.5	9.3	0
Mediterranean Vegetable, Jane Plan*	1 Serving/301g	208	18.7	69	0.4	2.8	6.2	0.6
Mushroom Bolognese, Wicked Kitchen, Tesco*	1 Pack/370g	355	12.2	96	2.7	12.8	3.3	2.4
Mushroom, & Spinach, Waitrose*	1 Pack/400g	373	14	93	3.1	12.3	3.5	1.3

	Measure INFO/WEIGHT	per Measure KCAL	FAT	Nutrition Values per 100g / 100ml KCAL	PROT	CARB	FAT	FIBRE
LASAGNE								
My Mamma's, Gino D'Acampo*	1 Pack/525g	735	36.2	140	7.2	12	6.9	0.9
Sheets, Dry, Average	***1 Sheet/20g***	***70***	***0.3***	***349***	***11.9***	***72.1***	***1.5***	***2.9***
Sheets, Wholewheat, Sainsbury's*	1 Serving/63g	216	1.4	346	12.7	64.8	2.3	7.8
Spinach, & Nut Ricotta, Vegan, Allplants*	1 Serving/388g	380	14	98	5	9.9	3.6	2.8
Topped with Cheese Alternative, Plant Kitchen, M&S*	1 Pack/400g	372	7.6	93	5.3	12.3	1.9	2.9
Triple Layered, Plant Chef, Tesco*	1 Serving/415g	532	17.8	128	8.5	12.5	4.3	2.6
Vegetable, Healthy Range, Average	***1 Serving/400g***	***318***	***8.2***	***80***	***3.5***	***11.8***	***2.1***	***1.5***
Vegetable, Mediterranean, Sainsbury's*	1 Pack/392g	337	11	86	3	11.7	2.8	1.1
Vegetable, Ready Meal, Average	***1 Serving/400g***	***408***	***17.6***	***102***	***4.1***	***12.4***	***4.4***	***1***
Vegetarian, Meat Free, Quorn*	½ Pack/250g	251	8.8	109	4.5	13.1	3.8	2.5
Veggie, Roasted, Allplants*	1 Serving/439g	360	13.2	82	4.1	8	3	2.2
LAVERBREAD								
Average	***1oz/28g***	***15***	***1***	***52***	***3.2***	***1.6***	***3.7***	***0***
LEEKS								
Boiled, Average	***1oz/28g***	***6***	***0.2***	***21***	***1.2***	***2.6***	***0.7***	***1.7***
Creamed, Frozen, Waitrose*	1 Serving/225g	115	5.4	51	1.8	5.5	2.4	0
Raw, Unprepared, Average	***1 Leek/166g***	***64***	***1.5***	***39***	***2.8***	***5.1***	***0.9***	***3.9***
LEMON								
Fresh, Raw, Average	***1 Slice/5g***	***1***	***0***	***18***	***0.9***	***2.9***	***0.3***	***2.1***
Peel, Raw, Average	***1 Tbsp/6g***	***3***	***0***	***47***	***1.5***	***16***	***0.3***	***10.6***
Zest, Average	***1 Tsp/2g***	***2***	***0***	***100***	***0***	***25***	***0***	***0***
LEMON CURD								
Average	***1 Tbsp/15g***	***44***	***0.7***	***294***	***0.7***	***62.9***	***4.7***	***0.1***
Luxury, Average	***1 Tsp/7g***	***23***	***0.6***	***326***	***2.8***	***59.7***	***8.4***	***0.1***
Passionfruit, & Lemon, Scarlett & Mustard*	1 Tsp/5g	16	0.5	323	4.2	52.5	10.8	0
LEMON SOLE								
Fillets, Raw, Average	***1 Serving/220g***	***177***	***2.8***	***81***	***17***	***0.2***	***1.3***	***0.3***
Goujons, Average	***1 Serving/150g***	***359***	***18.3***	***239***	***13.9***	***18.5***	***12.2***	***1***
Grilled, Average	***1oz/28g***	***27***	***0.5***	***97***	***20.2***	***0***	***1.7***	***0***
in Breadcrumbs, Average	***1 Fillet/142g***	***322***	***17.4***	***228***	***13.7***	***15.7***	***12.3***	***1***
LEMONADE								
7 Up, Free, Britvic*	1 Bottle/500ml	10	0	2	0	0	0	0
7 Up, Zero, Britvic*	1 Can/330ml	6	0	2	0.1	0.1	0	0
7-Up, Light, Britvic*	1 Can/330ml	4	0	1	0.1	0.2	0	0
Average	***1 Glass/250ml***	***52***	***0.2***	***21***	***0.1***	***5***	***0.1***	***0.1***
Cloudy, Ben Shaws*	½ Bottle/250ml	58	0.2	23	0.1	5.4	0.1	0
Cloudy, Diet, Asda*	1 Serving/200ml	6	1	3	0.5	0.5	0.5	0.5
Cloudy, Diet, Sparkling, M&S*	1 Serving/250ml	8	0.2	3	0.1	0.1	0.1	0.1
Diet, Average	***1 Glass/250ml***	***4***	***0.1***	***2***	***0.1***	***0.2***	***0***	***0***
Diet, Premium, Tesco*	1 Glass/250ml	8	0	3	0	0.4	0	0
Diet, Toppers, Aldi*	1 Glass/100ml	1	0	1	0	0	0	0
Diet, Traditional Style, Tesco*	1 Glass/200ml	6	0	3	0	0.8	0	0
Passion Fruit, Tesco*	1 Can/250ml	10	0	4	0.1	0.4	0	0
Pink, No Added Sugar, Tesco*	1 Glass/250ml	8	0.2	3	0.1	0.3	0.1	0.1
Pink, Zero Calories, Lucozade*	1 Bottle/380ml	8	0	2	0.1	0.1	0	0
Raspberry, & Rose, Tesco*	1 Glass/250ml	5	0.2	2	0.1	0.2	0.1	0.1
Raspberry, Freshly Squeezed, Deluxe, Lidl*	1 Serving/200ml	54	1	27	0.1	5.3	0.5	0.5
Raspberry, R White*	1 Can/330ml	56	0	17	0	3.9	0	0
Schweppes*	1 Can/150ml	27	0	18	0	4.2	0	0
Slimline, Schweppes*	1 Glass/300ml	6	0	2	0	0	0	0
Still, Freshly Squeezed, M&S*	½ Bottle/250ml	100	0.5	40	0.1	9	0.2	0.5
Still, Morrisons*	1 Bottle/330ml	79	0.3	24	0.2	5.6	0.1	0.1

	Measure INFO/WEIGHT	per Measure KCAL	FAT	Nutrition Values per 100g / 100ml KCAL	PROT	CARB	FAT	FIBRE
LEMSIP								
Beechams*	1 Sachet/3g	11	0	387	0	100	0	0
LENTILS								
Black Beluga, Ready to Eat, Merchant Gourmet*	1 Serving/63g	92	0.8	147	10.9	20.5	1.2	5.2
Cakes, Veggie, Beetroot, Kallo*	1 Cake/9g	40	1.1	424	25	51	12	6
French Inspired, Good Grains, Worldwide Foods, Aldi*	½ Pack/125g	149	3	119	7.2	15	2.4	5.2
Good Grains, Aldi*	1 Pack/250g	242	5.2	97	6.6	10	2.1	5
	½ Pouch/125g	252	3	202	11.3	29.7	2.4	8.1
Green & Brown, Dried, Boiled in Salted Water, Average	***1 Tbsp/30g***	***32***	***0.2***	***105***	***8.8***	***16.9***	***0.7***	***3.8***
Green or Brown in Water, Tinned, Average	***½ Can/132g***	***131***	***0.8***	***99***	***8.1***	***15.4***	***0.6***	***3.8***
Green or Brown, Dried, Average	***1 Serving/50g***	***150***	***0.8***	***301***	***22.8***	***49.8***	***1.5***	***9.6***
Lentilles Vertes, Cooked Weight, Tesco*	1 Serving/80g	141	0.5	176	13.4	25	0.6	8.7
Puy, Green, Dry, Average	***1 Serving/100g***	***306***	***1.4***	***306***	***24.7***	***49.5***	***1.4***	***10.3***
Red, Boiled in Unsalted Water, Average	***1oz/28g***	***28***	***0.1***	***102***	***7.6***	***17.5***	***0.4***	***2.6***
Red, Split, Dry, Tesco*	1 Serving/30g	77	0.6	257	19.7	31.3	2	16.3
Wholegrain, & Edamame, COOK!, M&S*	½ Pack/145g	252	7	174	7.8	20.6	4.8	8.7
LETTUCE								
Average, Raw	***½ Cup/28g***	***4***	***0.1***	***13***	***1***	***1.7***	***0.3***	***1.1***
Curly Leaf, Sainsbury's*	1 Serving/80g	11	0.4	14	0.8	1.7	0.5	0
Lamb's, Average	***1 Serving/80g***	***12***	***0.2***	***14***	***1.4***	***1.6***	***0.2***	***1***
Little Gem, Average	***1 Lettuce/90g***	***14***	***0.4***	***15***	***0.8***	***1.8***	***0.5***	***0.7***
Radicchio, Red, Raw, Average	***1 Head/220g***	***29***	***0.2***	***13***	***1.4***	***1.6***	***0.1***	***3***
Red Gem, Tesco*	½ Lettuce/45g	7	0.2	15	0.8	1.7	0.5	0.9
Romaine, Average	***1 Serving/80g***	***12***	***0.4***	***15***	***0.9***	***1.7***	***0.5***	***0.7***
Romaine, Hearts, Average	***1 Serving/80g***	***12***	***0.4***	***16***	***0.9***	***1.7***	***0.6***	***1***
Romaine, Sweet, Average	***1 Serving/80g***	***12***	***0.4***	***16***	***0.9***	***1.6***	***0.6***	***0.8***
Round, Average	***1 Serving/80g***	***10***	***0.2***	***13***	***1.4***	***2.2***	***0.2***	***1.1***
Sweet Gem, TTD, Sainsbury's*	1 Serving/100g	15	0.5	15	0.8	1.7	0.5	0.9
LILT								
Fruit Crush, Coca-Cola*	1 Can/330ml	66	0	20	0	4.6	0	0
Fruit Crush, Zero, Coca-Cola*	1 Can/330ml	12	0	4	0	0.3	0	0
Zero, Coca-Cola*	1 Can/330ml	10	0	3	0	0.3	0	0
LIME								
Peel, Raw	***1 Tbsp/6g***	***3***	***0***	***47***	***1.5***	***16***	***0.3***	***10.6***
Raw, Flesh Only, Average	***1 Lime/71g***	***18***	***0.1***	***25***	***0.6***	***8.8***	***0.2***	***2.4***
Zest, Average	***1 Tsp/2g***	***2***	***0***	***100***	***0***	***25***	***0***	***0***
LINGUINE								
Chicken, with Tomato Pesto, Result Plan*	1 Serving/250g	360	10	144	11.6	14.8	4	1.2
Cooked	***1 Serving/100g***	***133***	***0.7***	***133***	***5.1***	***26.3***	***0.7***	***1.1***
Dry, Average	***1 Serving/100g***	***352***	***2.2***	***352***	***13.1***	***70***	***2.2***	***2.8***
Fresh, Dry, Average	***1 Pack/250g***	***681***	***6.5***	***272***	***12.3***	***51.7***	***2.6***	***4***
Prawn, Calorie Controlled, Tesco*	1 Pack/335g	318	3.7	95	4.8	15.9	1.1	1.1
Prawn, Creamy, Calorie Counted, Asda*	1 Pack/338g	318	7.1	94	4.7	13	2.1	1.2
Prawn, King, & Chilli, Specially Selected, Aldi*	1 Serving/388g	466	13.6	120	5.5	16	3.5	1.4
Prawn, King, Cook*	1 Serving/350g	543	27	155	5.7	13.7	7.7	1.4
Prawn, King, COU, M&S*	1 Meal/360g	400	9	111	5.9	16.4	2.5	0.8
Prawn, King, Fresh Ideas, Morrisons*	1 Pack/390g	343	5.1	88	5.3	12.5	1.3	2.4
Prawn, King, Slimming World*	1 Serving/550g	407	2.2	74	5.3	11.2	0.4	2.3
Prawn, Slim Cook, Tesco*	1 Pack/472g	307	1.4	65	4	11	0.3	1.4
Prawn, with Tomatoes, Chef Select, Lidl*	1 Pack/380g	383	4	101	4.3	17.4	1	2
Salmon, Smoked, Co-Op*	1 Pack/350g	441	16.4	126	5.8	14	4.7	1.8
Seafood, with Prawns, Scallops, Salmon, & Cod, M&S*	1 Pack/368g	379	11.8	103	7.8	10.1	3.2	1.2
Spinach, & Prawn, G&B, Asda*	1 Pack/371g	338	6.7	91	4	14	1.8	1.7

	Measure INFO/WEIGHT	per Measure KCAL	FAT	Nutrition Values per 100g / 100ml KCAL	PROT	CARB	FAT	FIBRE
LINSEEDS								
Average	***1 Tsp/5g***	***23***	***1.7***	***464***	***21.7***	***18.5***	***33.5***	***26.3***
LION BAR								
Milk, Duo, Nestle*	1 Pack/60g	296	13.7	493	5.3	65.7	22.8	1.4
Mini, Nestle*	1 Bar/16g	80	3.6	486	4.6	67.7	21.7	0
Nestle*	1 Bar/52g	248	11.2	478	6.5	64.6	21.6	0
Peanut, Nestle*	1 Bar/40g	195	10	488	8.1	57.1	25	2.3
White, Nestle*	1 Bar/40g	194	8.8	484	5.7	65.2	22.1	0.4
LIQUEURS								
Amaretto, Average	***1 Pub Shot/25ml***	***97***	***0***	***388***	***0***	***60***	***0***	***0***
Chambord*	1 Serving/35ml	79	0	225	0	29.3	0	0
Cointreau, Specialite De France	***1 Serving/37ml***	***80***	***0***	***215***	***0***	***8.5***	***0***	***0***
Cream, Average	***1 Shot/25ml***	***81***	***4***	***325***	***0***	***22.8***	***16.1***	***0***
Grand Marnier*	1 Pub Shot/35ml	94	0	268	0	22.9	0	0
High Strength, Average	***1 Shot/25ml***	***78***	***0***	***314***	***0***	***24.4***	***0***	***0***
Kirsch, Average	***1 Shot/25ml***	***67***	***0***	***267***	***0***	***20***	***0***	***0***
LIQUORICE								
Allsorts, Average	***1 Sm Bag/56g***	***195***	***2.9***	***349***	***3.7***	***76.7***	***5.2***	***2***
Catherine Wheels, Barratt*	1 Wheel/22g	65	0.1	290	3.8	67.2	0.3	0.7
Catherine Wheels, Sainsbury's*	1 Wheel/17g	49	0.1	286	3.8	67.2	0.3	0.7
Filled, Klene*	1 Serving/20g	65	0.1	324	3.6	77	0.4	0
Panda*	1 Bar/32g	109	0.2	340	3.8	78	0.5	0
Raspberry, All Natural, Panda*	1 Bar/32g	98	0.1	307	3.6	72	0.4	0.9
Shapes, Average	***1oz/28g***	***78***	***0.4***	***278***	***5.5***	***65***	***1.4***	***1.9***
Sweet, Sugar Free, Dominion, Aldi*	1/3 Pack/25g	56	0.1	224	0.5	77	0.5	6.3
LIVER								
Calves, Fried	***1oz/28g***	***49***	***2.7***	***176***	***22.3***	***0***	***9.6***	***0***
Calves, Raw	***1oz/28g***	***29***	***1***	***104***	***18.3***	***0***	***3.4***	***0***
Calves, Rose, with Sage Butter, Select Farms, M&S*	½ Pack/94g	150	6.2	160	18.6	6.3	6.6	0.6
Chicken, Cooked, Simmered, Average	***1 Serving/100g***	***167***	***6.5***	***167***	***24.5***	***0.9***	***6.5***	***0***
Chicken, Fried, Average	***1oz/28g***	***47***	***2.5***	***169***	***22.1***	***0***	***8.9***	***0***
Chicken, Raw, Average	***1oz/28g***	***26***	***0.6***	***92***	***17.7***	***0***	***2.3***	***0***
Lamb's, Braised, Average	***1 Serving/100g***	***220***	***8.8***	***220***	***30.6***	***2.5***	***8.8***	***0***
Lamb's, Fried, Average	***1oz/28g***	***66***	***3.6***	***237***	***30.1***	***0***	***12.9***	***0***
Lamb's, Raw, Average	***1 Serving/125g***	***171***	***7.8***	***137***	***20.3***	***0***	***6.2***	***0***
Lambs, & Bacon, Meal for One, M&S*	1 Pack/450g	436	15.3	97	5.7	10.1	3.4	1.5
Ox, Raw	***1oz/28g***	***43***	***2.2***	***155***	***21.1***	***0***	***7.8***	***0***
Pig's, Raw	***1oz/28g***	***32***	***0.9***	***113***	***21.3***	***0***	***3.1***	***0***
Pig's, Stewed	***1 Serving/70g***	***132***	***5.7***	***189***	***25.6***	***3.6***	***8.1***	***0***
Veal, Deluxe, Lidl*	1 Slice/150g	188	5.2	125	19.6	3.8	3.5	0
LIVER & BACON								
& Onions, Cook*	1 Portion/280g	372	21.3	133	11.8	4.3	7.6	0.5
Meal for One, M&S*	1 Pack/452g	430	16.7	95	7	8	3.7	1.2
Mini, Frozen, Waitrose*	1 Pack/250g	277	12	111	5.6	10.6	4.8	1.3
with Fresh Mashed Potato, Waitrose*	1 Pack/400g	416	17.2	104	7.3	9	4.3	1.3
with Mash, Colcannon, Asda*	1 Pack/400g	344	10.4	86	6.6	8.6	2.6	0.8
with Mash, Serves 1, Classic, Sainsbury's*	1 Pack/450g	448	18.7	103	6.4	8.6	4.3	2.5
LIVER SAUSAGE								
Average	***1 Slice/10g***	***22***	***1.5***	***216***	***15.3***	***4.4***	***15.2***	***0.2***
LLAMA								
Steak, Average	***1 Steak/150g***	***158***	***2***	***105***	***23***	***0.2***	***1.3***	***0***
LOBSTER								
Boiled, Average	***1oz/28g***	***29***	***0.4***	***103***	***22.1***	***0***	***1.6***	***0***
Dressed, Canned, John West*	1 Can/43g	45	2.1	105	13	2	5	0

	Measure INFO/WEIGHT	per Measure KCAL	FAT	Nutrition Values per 100g / 100ml KCAL	PROT	CARB	FAT	FIBRE
LOBSTER								
Raw, Average	***1 Serving/100g***	***92***	***1.4***	***92***	***18.7***	***0.3***	***1.4***	***0***
Thermidor, M&S*	1 Serving/140g	287	19.2	205	10.7	9.7	13.7	0
LOGANBERRIES								
Raw	***1oz/28g***	***5***	***0***	***17***	***1.1***	***3.4***	***0***	***2.5***
LOLLIPOPS								
Assorted, Co-Op*	1 Lolly/10g	40	0	400	0	97	0	0
Chupa Chups*	1 Lolly/12g	47	0	388	0	95	0.3	0
Double, Swizzels*	1 Lolly/50g	20	0	41	0	7	0	0
Drumsticks, Swizzels*	1 Lolly/12g	50	0.7	413	0.4	87.9	6.1	0
Refreshers, Bassett's*	1 Lolly/6g	25	0	417	0	108.3	0	0
LOQUATS								
Raw	***1oz/28g***	***5***	***0***	***18***	***0.4***	***4***	***0.1***	***0***
LOZENGES								
Blackcurrant Flavour, Fishermans Friend, Lofthouses*	1 Lozenge/1g	3	0	251	0.1	97.2	1.3	0
Original Extra Strong, Fishermans Friend, Lofthouses*	1 Lozenge/1g	4	0	382	0.3	94.9	0	0.5
Original, Victory V*	1 Lozenge/3g	9	0	350	0	91	0	0
LUCOZADE								
Apple Blast, Lucozade*	1 Serving/200ml	70	0	35	0	8.4	0	0
Energy, Original, GlaxoSmithKline UK Limited*	1 Bottle/380ml	266	0	70	0	17.2	0	0
Orange Energy Drink, GlaxoSmithKline UK Limited*	1 Bottle/500ml	350	0	70	0	17.2	0	0
Orange, Sport Lite, GlaxoSmithKline UK Limited*	1 Serving/500g	50	0	10	0	2	0	0
Orange, Zero, Lucozade*	1 Med Bottle/380ml	15	0	4	0.1	0.5	0	0
Raspberry Sport Body Fuel, GlaxoSmithKline UK Limited*	1 Bottle/500ml	140	0	28	0	6.4	0	0
Zero Calories, Lucozade*	1 Serving/250ml	10	0	4	0.1	0.5	0	0
LUNCHEON MEAT								
Pork, Average	***1oz/28g***	***81***	***6.8***	***288***	***13.3***	***4***	***24.3***	***0***
LYCHEES								
Fresh, Raw, Flesh Only	***1oz/28g***	***16***	***0***	***58***	***0.9***	***14.3***	***0.1***	***0.7***
in Juice, Amoy*	1oz/28g	13	0	46	0.4	10.9	0	0
in Syrup, Average	***1oz/28g***	***19***	***0***	***69***	***0.4***	***17.7***	***0***	***0.4***
Raw, Weighed with Skin & Stone	***1oz/28g***	***6***	***0***	***22***	***0.3***	***5.5***	***0.1***	***0.2***

	Measure INFO/WEIGHT	per Measure KCAL	FAT	Nutrition Values per 100g / 100ml KCAL	PROT	CARB	FAT	FIBRE
M&M'S								
Caramel, Crunchy, Limited Edition, M&M's, Mars*	1 Pack/36g	172	6.6	478	3.7	73.5	18.4	0
Crispy, Mars*	1 Serving/36g	179	8.8	498	4.1	63.9	24.4	2.7
Mars*	1 Pack/45g	218	9.7	485	5	68	21.5	0
Mini, Mars*	1 Pack/36g	176	8.4	489	6.3	63.6	23.2	0
Mix, Mars*	1 Serving/43g	214	10.2	503	7.7	63	24	0
Peanut Butter, Mars*	1 Pack/46g	240	14	520	8.7	56.3	30.3	2.2
Peanut, M&M's, Mars*	1 Serving/45g	230	11.6	516	10	58	26	0
Salted Caramel, M&M's, Mars*	1 Serving/36g	172	6.5	474	4.4	71	18	0
MACADAMIA NUTS								
Plain, Average	***1 Pack/100g***	***750***	***77.6***	***750***	***7.9***	***4.8***	***77.6***	***5.3***
Roasted, Salted, Average	***6 Nuts/10g***	***75***	***7.8***	***748***	***7.9***	***4.8***	***77.6***	***5.3***
MACARONI								
Dry, Average	***1oz/28g***	***99***	***0.5***	***354***	***11.9***	***73.5***	***1.7***	***2.6***
GF, Dry, Free From, Morrisons*	1 Serving/75g	258	0.8	344	5.6	77.1	1.1	1.9
MACARONI CHEESE								
& Mushroom, Vegan, Waitrose*	1 Pack/260g	320	13.5	123	4	14.1	5.2	2.1
Bites, Mac N Cheese, Crispy, M&S*	½ Pack/100g	255	13.8	255	7.9	23.9	13.8	1.6
Butternut Cauli, Plant Chef, Tesco*	1 Pack/450g	518	11.2	115	3.6	18.6	2.5	1.8
Canned	***1oz/28g***	***39***	***1.8***	***138***	***4.5***	***16.4***	***6.5***	***0.4***
Cheddar, Vintage, TTD, Sainsbury's*	1 Pack/366g	571	25.6	156	6.9	15.9	7	0.9
Chilled, HFC, Tesco*	1 Pack/400g	540	16.4	135	5.6	18	4.1	1.9
Mac & Greens, Vegan, Allplants*	1 Serving/410g	570	23.4	139	6.8	13	5.7	3.2
Mini, Serves 1, Sainsbury's*	1 Pack/250g	342	13.8	137	6.4	14.5	5.5	2.2
Ready Meal, Average	***1 Serving/400g***	***580***	***25.5***	***145***	***6***	***15.8***	***6.4***	***1***
Rice, GF, Amy's Kitchen*	1 Pack/257g	416	18.2	162	6.3	18	7.1	0.4
Triple, Finest, Tesco*	1 Pack/400g	645	22.2	174	7.3	22	6	1.4
Vintage Cheddar, Irresistible, Co-Op*	1 Pack/350g	718	33.6	205	9.6	19	9.6	1.3
with Bacon, Microwaved, Iceland*	1 Pack/344g	499	17.6	145	5.8	18.5	5.1	1.2
with Ham, & Cauliflower, Cook*	1 Pack/300g	306	9.6	102	6.5	12.7	3.2	1.7
with Pancetta, Crispy, Deluxe, Lidl*	½ Pack/368g	769	38.3	209	8.9	19.2	10.4	1.7
MACARONS								
Brioche Pasquier*	1 Macaron/10g	46	2.4	456	9.8	50.3	23.5	0
Luxembourgerli, Sprungli*	1 Piece/13g	48	2.5	369	7.7	47.7	19.2	0
MACAROONS								
Coconut, Mini, Sainsbury's*	1 Macaroon/22g	100	5.3	445	3.9	51.6	23.4	6.3
Coconut, Tesco*	1 Macaroon/33g	143	6.3	432	4.5	58	19	5.5
French, Average	***1 Serving/60g***	***225***	***11***	***375***	***6.7***	***46.7***	***18.3***	***3.3***
MACKEREL								
Atlantic, Raw, Average	***1 Fillet/75g***	***154***	***10.4***	***205***	***18.6***	***0***	***13.9***	***0***
Fillets, Honey Smoked, Sainsbury's*	1 Pack/280g	1016	80.9	363	20.5	5.1	28.9	0.5
Fillets, in Brine, Average	***1 Can/88g***	***206***	***15.3***	***234***	***19.4***	***0***	***17.4***	***0***
Fillets, in Mustard Sauce, Average	***1 Can/125g***	***274***	***19.4***	***219***	***14.1***	***5.4***	***15.5***	***0***
Fillets, in Olive Oil, Average	***1 Serving/50g***	***149***	***12.2***	***298***	***18.5***	***1***	***24.4***	***0***
Fillets, in Spicy Tomato Sauce, Average	***1oz/28g***	***56***	***3.9***	***199***	***14.3***	***3.8***	***14***	***0***
Fillets, in Sunflower Oil, Average	***1 Can/94g***	***262***	***20.6***	***279***	***20.2***	***0.2***	***21.9***	***0.2***
Fillets, in Tomato Sauce, Average	***1 Can/125g***	***251***	***18.3***	***200***	***14.3***	***2.7***	***14.7***	***0***
Fillets, Smoked, Average	***1 Fillet/75g***	***251***	***21.1***	***334***	***19.7***	***0.5***	***28.2***	***0.3***
Fillets, Smoked, Skinless, Average	***1 Fillet/65g***	***215***	***17***	***330***	***20.9***	***2.8***	***26.1***	***0.4***
Fillets, Smoked, Sweet Chilli, Market St, Morrisons*	½ Pack/93g	295	21.6	317	19.6	6.4	23.2	2.1
Fried in Blended Oil	***1oz/28g***	***76***	***5.5***	***272***	***24***	***0***	***19.5***	***0***
Grilled	***1oz/28g***	***67***	***4.8***	***239***	***20.8***	***0***	***17.3***	***0***
King, Raw	***1 Fillet/198g***	***208***	***4***	***105***	***20.3***	***0***	***2***	***0***
Raw with Skin, Weighed with Bone, Average	***1oz/28g***	***64***	***4.7***	***227***	***18.9***	***0***	***16.8***	***0***

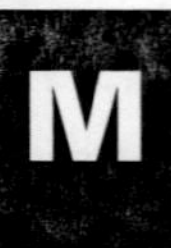

	Measure INFO/WEIGHT	per Measure KCAL	per Measure FAT	Nutrition Values per 100g / 100ml KCAL	PROT	CARB	FAT	FIBRE
MACKEREL								
Smoked, Peppered, Average	***1oz/28g***	***87***	***7***	***310***	***20.4***	***0.3***	***25.2***	***0.2***
Strips, Smoked, Sweetcure, Tesco*	1 Serving/100g	327	24.6	327	21.5	4.8	24.6	0
MADRAS								
Beef, Canned, Cooked, Morrisons*	1 Can/401g	570	33.3	142	11.7	4.7	8.3	1
Beef, Tesco*	1 Pack/460g	616	37.7	134	10.6	4.5	8.2	1.2
Chicken, M&S*	1 Pack/400g	492	25.2	123	12.7	2.7	6.3	2.2
Chicken, M&S*	1 Pack/400g	472	23.2	118	12.9	2.5	5.8	1.9
Chicken, Sainsbury's*	1 Pack/400g	532	29.6	133	11	4.5	7.4	1.9
Chicken, Taste of India, Tesco*	½ Pack/215g	275	14.2	128	10.2	5.7	6.6	2.7
Chicken, Waitrose*	1 Pack/400g	672	42	168	14.6	3.7	10.5	1.8
MAGNUM								
Almond, Mini, Wall's*	1 Mini/55g	155	9.4	281	3.9	27	17	0
Almond, Vegan, Wall's*	1 Magnum/90g	248	16.2	276	2.2	26	18	0
Almond, Wall's*	1 Magnum/73g	243	14.6	332	4.8	32	20	0
Caramel, Double, Mini, Wall's*	1 Mini/50g	174	10	348	3.2	37	20	0
Caramel, Double, Wall's*	1 Magnum/73g	246	14.6	338	3.2	36	20	0
Chocolate, Double, Mini, Wall's*	1 Mini/50g	182	11.5	365	4	33	23	0
Chocolate, Double, Wall's*	1 Magnum/69g	248	15.9	359	4.1	33	23	0
Classic, Mini, Wall's*	1 Mini/50g	168	11	336	3.7	31	22	0
Classic, Vegan, Wall's*	1 Magnum/90g	234	14.3	261	1.3	27	16	0
Classic, Wall's*	1 Magnum/79g	244	15	309	3.6	29	19	1.2
Dark, Mini, Wall's*	1 Mini/50g	165	11	329	3.8	29	22	0
Double Coconut, Wall's*	1 Magnum/88g	239	14.1	272	3.2	27	16	0
Espresso, Black, Mini, Wall's*	1 Mini/50g	159	10.5	317	3.7	29	21	0
Espresso, Black, Wall's*	1 Magnum/82g	237	15.6	289	3.4	27	19	0
Honeycomb, & Almond, Wall's*	1 Magnum/73g	243	15	333	4.5	32.9	20.6	0
Honeycomb, Wall's*	1 Magnum/78g	240	13.2	308	3.6	35	17	0
Mint, Mini, Wall's*	1 Mini/50g	165	10.5	330	4.2	30	21	0
Mint, Wall's*	1 Magnum/78g	244	14	313	3.1	33	18	0
Peanut Butter, Double, Wall's*	1 Magnum/73g	245	15.3	336	4.2	32	21	0
Pistachio, Wall's*	1 Magnum/75g	250	15.8	333	4.2	30	21	0
Raspberry, Pink, Mini, Wall's*	1 Mini/50g	166	11.5	332	2.9	31	23	0
Raspberry, Pink, Wall's*	1 Magnum/73g	239	15.3	328	2.9	30	21	0
Ruby Collection, Wall's*	1 Magnum/78g	237	13	304	4.6	34.7	16.7	0
Ruby, Mini, Wall's*	1 Magnum/43g	136	7.7	317	5	34	18	0
Strawberry, & White, Wall's*	1 Magnum/88g	250	13.2	284	3	34	15	0
White Chocolate, & Cookies, Wall's*	1 Magnum/90g	285	16.2	317	4	34	18	0
White, Mini, Wall's*	1 Mini/55g	137	8.3	248	2.8	26	15	0
White, Wall's*	1 Magnum/79g	239	14.2	303	3.5	33	18	0
MAKHANI								
Chicken, Co-Op*	1 Pack/380g	467	16.3	123	8.7	12	4.3	1.5
Chicken, Morrisons*	½ Pack/175g	301	18.6	172	9.8	8.4	10.6	2
Chicken, Sainsbury's*	½ Pack/199g	313	21.3	157	12.2	2.9	10.7	2.5
Chicken, Tikka, Waitrose*	1 Pack/400g	560	30.4	140	14	3.8	7.6	2.1
MALTESERS								
MaltEaster, Chocolate Bunny, Mars*	1 Bunny/29g	157	9	541	7.1	57	31	0
Mini Bunnies, Mars*	1 Bunny/12g	64	3.6	534	8	53.5	30.2	0
Teasers, Mars*	1 Teaser/9g	48	2.8	538	7.3	57.2	30.8	0
Truffles, Mars*	1 Truffle/9g	51	3.2	565	6.7	53	36	0
MANDARIN ORANGES								
in Juice, Average	***1oz/28g***	***11***	***0***	***39***	***0.7***	***9***	***0***	***0.5***
in Light Syrup, Average	***1 Can/298g***	***201***	***0.1***	***68***	***0.6***	***16***	***0***	***0.1***
Weighed with Peel, Average	***1 Sm/50g***	***14***	***0***	***27***	***0.7***	***6.2***	***0.1***	***0.9***

	Measure INFO/WEIGHT	per Measure KCAL	FAT	Nutrition Values per 100g / 100ml KCAL	PROT	CARB	FAT	FIBRE
MANGE TOUT								
Boiled in Salted Water	***1oz/28g***	***7***	***0***	***26***	***3.2***	***3.3***	***0.1***	***2.2***
Raw, Average	***1 Serving/80g***	***25***	***0.2***	***31***	***3.5***	***4***	***0.2***	***1.1***
Stir-Fried in Blended Oil	***1oz/28g***	***20***	***1.3***	***71***	***3.8***	***3.5***	***4.8***	***2.4***
MANGO								
& Strawberry, Waitrose*	1 Pack/225g	119	1.1	53	0.7	11	0.5	2
Chunks, Co-op*	1 Serving/80g	50	0.4	63	0.7	14	0.5	1.8
Chunks, Fresh, Asda*	1 Serving/80g	56	0.4	70	0.8	15	0.5	1.6
Dried, Average	***1 Serving/50g***	***174***	***0.5***	***347***	***1.4***	***83.1***	***1***	***4.9***
in Syrup, Average	***1oz/28g***	***22***	***0***	***80***	***0.3***	***20.5***	***0***	***0.9***
Ripe, Raw, Weighed with Skin & Stone, Average	***1 Mango/225g***	***60***	***0.2***	***27***	***0.3***	***6.5***	***0.1***	***1.2***
Ripe, Raw, without Peel & Stone, Flesh Only, Average	***1 Mango/207g***	***118***	***0.4***	***57***	***0.7***	***14.1***	***0.2***	***2.6***
Slices, Canned, in Juice, Drained, Tesco*	½ Can/105g	58	0.3	55	1.2	11.6	0.3	0.7
Slices, Canned, in Juice, Tesco*	¼ Can/106g	41	0.1	39	0.4	8.6	0.1	0.8
Slices, Canned, in Light Syrup, M&S*	½ Can/125g	86	0	69	0.5	16.7	0	0.6
MARINADE								
Barbeque, Sticky, Sainsbury's*	¼ Jar/77g	112	2.8	145	0.8	26.7	3.6	1
Peri Peri, Hot, Nando's*	1 Serving/20g	9	0.6	43	0.9	2.4	2.8	0
Peri Peri, Lemon & Herb, Nando's*	1 Serving/20g	13	0.7	63	0.5	5.9	3.6	0
Peri Peri, Mango & Lime, Nando's*	1 Serving/20g	32	1.2	159	0.7	26.9	5.9	0
Peri Peri, Medium, Nando's*	1 Serving/20g	16	0.8	82	1.4	8.1	4.2	0
Peri-Peri, Coat & Cook, Hot , Nando's*	1 Sachet/120g	113	7.9	94	1.9	4.9	6.6	0
Peri-Peri, Coat & Cook, Lemon & Herb, Nando's*	1 Sachet/120g	86	5.8	72	0.5	5.6	4.8	0
Sweet Chilli, Lime, Lemongrass, The Grill, M&S*	1 Bottle/250g	602	11.2	241	0.4	48.3	4.5	3
Tandoori, Oven Bake, Pataks*	½ Pack/60g	65	4.1	109	3	7.9	6.8	0
Tandoori, Spice, Patak's*	1 Tbsp/15g	15	0.4	99	3.5	10.1	2.7	5.9
MARJORAM								
Dried	***1 Tsp/1g***	***2***	***0***	***271***	***12.7***	***42.5***	***7***	***0***
MARMALADE								
Lemon & Lime, Average	***1 Tbsp/20g***	***53***	***0***	***267***	***0.2***	***66.4***	***0.1***	***0.4***
Lemon with Shred, Average	***1 Tbsp/15g***	***37***	***0***	***248***	***0.2***	***61.6***	***0***	***0.6***
Lime with Shred, Average	***1 Tbsp/15g***	***39***	***0***	***261***	***0.2***	***65***	***0.1***	***0.4***
Mandarin, Tangy, Bonne Maman*	1 Tbsp/15g	36	0	239	0.3	59	0.1	0.8
Olde English, Thick Cut, Hartley's*	1 Tbsp/15g	39	0	261	0.3	64.6	0.1	0
Onion, Red, Stokes*	1 Tbsp/15g	37	0	244	1.2	57.2	0.1	1.3
Orange & Ginger, Average	***1 Tbsp/15g***	***40***	***0***	***264***	***0.2***	***65.7***	***0.1***	***0.3***
Orange & Tangerine, Tiptree, Wilkin & Sons*	1 Tbsp/15g	40	0	268	0	67	0	0
Orange with Shred, Average	***1 Tbsp/15g***	***39***	***0***	***263***	***0.2***	***65.2***	***0***	***0.3***
Orange, Med Cut, Tiptree, Wilkin & Sons*	1 Tbsp/15g	41	0	273	0	67	0	0
Orange, Reduced Sugar, Asda*	1 Tbsp/15g	28	0.2	186	0.5	42	1	2
Orange, Reduced Sugar, Average	***1 Tbsp/15g***	***26***	***0***	***170***	***0.4***	***42***	***0.1***	***0.6***
Orange, Seville, Dark, Specially Selected, Aldi*	1 Tbsp/15g	41	0.1	271	0.5	66	0.6	0.5
Orange, Shredless, Average	***1 Tbsp/15g***	***39***	***0***	***261***	***0.2***	***65***	***0***	***0.1***
Orange, Sweet, Bonne Maman*	1 Tbsp/15g	36	0	241	0.3	59	0.1	1.2
Tangy, Fine Cut, Grandessa, Aldi*	1 Tbsp/15g	44	0.1	293	0.7	70	0.9	0.9
Thick Cut, Maribel*	1 Tbsp/15g	36	0	240	0.2	58.3	0.1	1.5
MARMITE*								
Yeast Extract, Marmite*	1 Tsp/9g	23	0	260	34	30	0.5	3.5
MARROW								
Boiled, Average	***1oz/28g***	***3***	***0.1***	***9***	***0.4***	***1.6***	***0.2***	***0.6***
Raw	***1oz/28g***	***2***	***0***	***6***	***0.3***	***1.2***	***0.1***	***0.3***
MARS								
Bar, Duo, Mars*	1 Pack/79g	355	13.3	450	4.3	69.3	16.9	0
Bar, from Multipack, Mars*	1 Bar/39.4g	177	6.6	448	4.4	69.3	16.7	0

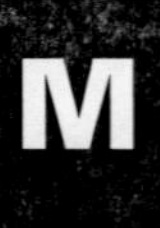

	Measure INFO/WEIGHT	per Measure KCAL	FAT	Nutrition Values per 100g / 100ml KCAL	PROT	CARB	FAT	FIBRE
MARS								
Bar, Funsize, Mars*	1 Bar/18g	80	2.8	443	3.9	70.7	15.7	0
Bar, Protein, Mars*	1 Bar/57g	200	4.6	351	33	39	8.1	0
Bar, Snacksize, Mars*	1 Bar/34g	151	5.7	448	4.3	69	17	0
Bar, Standard, Single, Mars*	1 Bar/51g	228	8.5	448	4.4	69.3	16.7	0
MARSHMALLOWS								
Average	***1 Mallow/5g***	***16***	***0***	***327***	***3.9***	***83.1***	***0***	***0***
Chocolate Mallows, Cadbury*	1 Mallow/13g	56	2.2	435	4.7	64.7	17.4	0.8
Fat Free, Tesco*	1 Mallow/7g	24	0	339	3.4	80.8	0.2	0.5
No Added Sugar, Sainsbury's*	1 Mallow/2g	5	0	206	3.3	77	0.1	0
Pink & White, Co-Op*	1 Mallow/7g	24	0	340	3	82	0	0
Pink & White, Waitrose*	1 Mallow/8g	26	0	327	3.8	77.4	0.1	0.5
Raspberry & Cream, Sainsbury's*	1 Mallow/7g	23	0	330	4.1	78.5	0	0.5
Soft Mallow Pieces, Mr Mallo*	1 Pack/80g	273	0	341	4.2	81	0	0
MARZIPAN								
Chocolate, M&S*	1 Marzipan/10g	47	2.2	470	7.6	58.3	22.1	3.8
Eggs, in Dark Chocolate, Favorina, Lidl*	1 Egg/20g	91	4	454	6.1	62.2	19.9	4.9
Fruits, Almond, M&S*	1 Sweet/12g	52	2	432	5.6	63.4	16.3	4.6
Plain, Average	***1oz/28g***	***115***	***4***	***412***	***5.8***	***67.5***	***14.2***	***1.7***
MASALA								
Beef, Coconut, Indian, Waitrose*	½ Pack/150g	232	15.6	155	10.2	4	10.4	2
Chaat, Chicken Chops, Waitrose*	1 Chop/91g	225	14.3	248	24.9	1.5	15.8	0
Fish, Meal Kit, Aldi*	½ Pack/168g	260	15.3	155	10	6.7	9.1	2.5
Prawn Mango, Waitrose*	½ Pack/175g	175	11.2	100	5.8	4.3	6.4	1.3
Vegetable, Indian, Sainsburys*	1 Pack/300g	273	17.7	91	2.2	5.5	5.9	3.7
MASH								
Carrot, & Swede, Frozen, Microwaved, Iceland*	1 Serving/80g	23	0.4	29	1.1	3.6	0.5	2.7
Carrot, Swede, & Potato, Waitrose*	½ Pack/200g	126	4.6	63	1	8.1	2.3	3
Pea, & Mint, M&S*	1 Serving/151g	134	5.6	89	4.6	6.8	3.7	5.1
Potato, Colcannon, M&S*	½ Pack/200g	210	11.8	105	1.5	10.5	5.9	1.9
Sweet Potato, Frozen, Sainsbury's*	1 Serving/149g	133	3.1	89	1.4	15	2.1	2.2
MAYONNAISE								
Average	***1 Tsp/5g***	***35***	***3.8***	***690***	***0.9***	***1.6***	***75.5***	***0***
Avocado Oil, Vegan, Hunter & Gather*	1 Tsp/5g	27	3	545	2.6	0.7	59.8	0.2
Extra Light, Average	***1 Tbsp/33g***	***34***	***2***	***102***	***0.7***	***10.5***	***6.2***	***0.8***
Garlic, Retail, Average	***1 Tsp/11g***	***44***	***4.4***	***403***	***1.2***	***8.6***	***40.3***	***0***
Reduced Calorie, Average	***1 Tsp/6g***	***18***	***1.7***	***301***	***0.7***	***8.9***	***29***	***0.1***
Vegan, Hellmann's*	1 Serving/15g	98	10.8	654	0.5	3.9	72	0
Vegan, Lowy*	1 Tsp/5g	29	3.1	582	0.2	5.5	62	0.2
Veganaise, Sriracha, Follow Your Heart*	1 Tbsp/15g	75	7.8	503	1.8	7.5	52	0
Vegenaise, Organic, Follow Your Heart*	1 Tbsp/15g	93	10	622	0.8	3.6	67	0
with a Spark of Chilli, Hellmann's*	1 Tbsp/15ml	41	4	276	0.8	7.5	27	0.3
with Dijon Mustard, Hellmann's*	1 Tbsp/15ml	32	3	210	2.9	5.1	19.7	0
MEAL REPLACEMENT								
Breakfast Shake, Chocolate, Be Fast*	1 Bottle/250ml	200	3.8	80	3.3	12	1.5	2.5
Diet, Chocolate & Raspberry , The Protein Works*	1 Meal/60g	200	3.3	333	40	27	5.5	9.3
Drink, Berry, Ready To Drink, Huel*	1 Bottle/500ml	400	18.5	80	4	6.8	3.7	1
Lemon, Bar, Exante Diet*	1 Bar/59g	220	6	373	30.5	37.7	10.1	6.3
Pasta, Green Pesto Flavoured, The 1;1 Diet*	1 Sachet/54g	202	3.3	374	24.1	53.7	6.1	4.6
Pie, Cottage, Country, New You Plan*	1 Pack/49g	176	4	359	33.3	32.1	8.2	11.7
Pizza Mix, Exante Diet*	1 Pack/57g	205	5.3	360	29.8	35.1	9.3	7.7
Porridge, Cinnamon, Pot, Exante Diet*	1 Pot/60g	214	4.7	357	29.3	33	7.8	15
Porridge, Mixed Berry, CWP*	1 Pack/54g	200	2.6	370	23.1	56.1	4.9	4.4
Ready to Drink, Chocolate, Huel*	1 Bottle/500ml	400	19	80	4	6.5	3.8	1.6

	Measure INFO/WEIGHT	per Measure KCAL	FAT	Nutrition Values per 100g / 100ml KCAL	PROT	CARB	FAT	FIBRE
MEAL REPLACEMENT								
Ready to Drink, Vanilla, Huel*	1 Bottle/500ml	400	18.5	80	4	6.8	3.7	1.2
Shake, Breakfast, Nutribuddy*	1 Single/30g	125	3.3	417	13.3	60	11	136.7
Shake, Caffe Latte, Made Up, Shake That Weight*	1 Sachet/250ml	131	3	52	5	5	1.2	0.7
Shake, Caramel Shake, Exante Diet*	1 Shake/50g	201	6.5	402	36	30	13	7.1
Shake, Chocolate, Mediterranean Style, Fast 800*	1 Serving/50g	198	9.8	397	46.1	9.8	19.6	14.7
Shake, Coconut Latte, Exante Diet*	1 Pack/53g	205	6.4	386	32	33	12	6.5
Shake, Coffee Flavour, Huel*	1 Serving/100g	400	13	400	30	37	13	7.7
Shake, Complete Protein, Nutribuddy *	1 Shake/40g	166	5	415	24	45	12.5	13.5
Shake, Complete Protein, Strawberry, Bulk Powders*	2 Scoops/60g	220	4.8	367	67.2	6.5	8	1
Shake, Cookies & Cream, Slim Fast*	1 Bottle/325ml	205	5.2	63	4.6	6.6	1.6	1.5
Shake, Daily Balance, Nuut*	1 Pack/53g	197	4.3	372	37.9	27.7	8.1	8.3
Shake, Keto, Nuut*	1 Pack/42g	206	12.3	490	30.5	23.6	29.3	3.1
Shake, Latte, Smooth, Great Shape, Asda*	1 Bottle/330ml	208	6.9	63	5.5	4.8	2.1	1.6
Shake, Lemon Cheesecake, Exante*	1 Serving/51g	201	6.6	394	33.5	34.7	13	8.2
Shake, Paleo, Nuut*	1 Sachet/55g	207	4.9	376	42.7	23.1	8.9	7.6
Shake, Powder, Strip Fast 5000*	1 Scoop/39g	135	1.4	347	55	24	3.5	4
Shake, Salted Caramel, Exante Diet*	1 Pack/52g	203	6.5	390	32.7	32.7	12.5	6.7
Shake, Strawberry, Delight, Great Shape, Asda*	1 Serving/330ml	198	6.3	60	5.1	5.1	1.9	1.2
Shake, Strawberry, Fast 800*	1 Glass/50ml	199	8.1	398	44.6	9.9	16.2	13.9
Shake, Vanilla, Fast 800*	1 Glass/50ml	199	8.1	398	44.6	9.9	16.2	13.9
Shake, Vanilla, Fast800*	1 Serving/50g	196	9.5	392	44	12.6	19	13.1
Shake, Vanilla, Herbalife*	2 Scoops/25g	90	1	360	36	52	4	12
Shake, Vanilla, Ready to Drink, Advantage, Atkins*	1 Carton/330ml	175	8.9	53	6.2	0.6	2.7	0.9
Shake, Vanilla, Shake That Weight*	1 Sachet/35ml	19	0.5	54	4.5	5.4	1.4	1
Shake, Vanillla, Smooth, Great Shape, Asda*	1 Bottle/330ml	198	6.3	60	5.1	5.1	1.9	1.2
Soup, Chicken, Noodle, Curry, Diet Now*	1 Pack/55g	201	5.1	366	30.7	36.4	9.3	6.9
Ultra Slim, Ready to Drink, Strawberry, Tesco*	1 Carton/330ml	231	3	70	4.2	10.5	0.9	1.5
Ultra Slim, Ready to Drink, Vanilla, Tesco*	1 Carton/330ml	224	3	68	4.2	10.5	0.9	1.5
MEAT LOAF								
Beef & Pork, Co-Op*	¼ Loaf/114g	314	25.1	275	13	7	22	1
Iceland*	1 Serving/150g	332	23.6	221	10.8	9.3	15.7	0.9
Turkey & Bacon, Tesco*	1 Serving/225g	400	22.3	178	14.7	7.4	9.9	1.1
MEATBALLS								
Al Forno, Charlie Bigham's*	½ Pack/324g	532	32.4	164	7	11.5	10	1.1
Beef & Pork, in Rustic Tomato Sauce, Cook*	1 Pack/300g	375	21	125	9.5	6.9	7	1.8
Beef, & Pork, Italian Style, Extra Special, Asda*	½ Pack/170g	466	26	274	29.4	3.5	15.3	0.6
Beef, 10% Fat, Mini, Oven Cooked, Sainsbury's*	4 Meatballs/61g	103	4.7	169	22.9	2	7.7	0.5
Beef, 10% Fat, Oven Cooked, Sainsbury's*	3 Meatballs/87g	148	67	170	22.9	20	77	0.5
Beef, Aberdeen Angus, 12 Pack, Waitrose*	1 Meatball/36g	93	7.1	259	18	2.3	19.8	0.1
Beef, As Sold, Tesco*	1 Meatball/28g	78	6.2	277	16.6	2.3	22.3	0.9
Beef, Ashfield Farm, Aldi*	1 Meatball/20g	45	2.7	232	23	3.9	14	0.5
Beef, Carrot, & Onion, Tesco*	4 Meatballs/94g	179	10.4	190	16.8	4.8	11.1	1.7
Beef, Co-Op*	½ Pack/175g	388	28	222	17	2.7	16	0
Beef, Farm Foods*	1 Meatball/33g	90	6.8	273	18.9	1.8	20.7	0
Beef, Frozen, Iceland*	¼ Pack/150g	364	24.3	243	17.7	5.2	16.2	1.7
Beef, in Onion & Ale Gravy, Classic Kitchen, Tesco*	½ Pack/224g	331	17.6	148	10.5	8.5	7.9	0.5
Beef, in Tomato Sauce, with Parmigiano, Sainsbury's*	½ Pack/217g	467	33	215	13.8	5.5	15.2	0.5
Beef, Irish, Platinum Prime, Aldi*	1 Meatball/20g	30	0.7	150	24.6	4.4	3.6	0.9
Beef, Italian Style, As Consumed, Morrisons*	3 Meatballs/104g	235	14.7	226	19.7	4.5	14.1	0.9
Beef, Lean, Oven Baked, Iceland*	1 Meatballs/19g	28	1.1	150	20.7	3.7	5.7	0.5
Beef, M&S*	6 Meatballs/150g	363	25.5	242	18.3	3.5	17	0.7
Beef, Mini, Oven Cooked, Finest, Tesco*	5 Meatballs/72g	149	8.2	207	21.8	4	11.4	0.8
Beef, Reduced Fat, Tesco*	4 Meatballs/93g	166	6.7	178	21.6	6.2	7.2	0.8

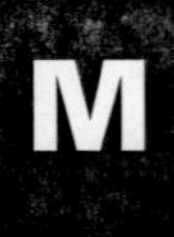

	Measure INFO/WEIGHT	per Measure KCAL	FAT	Nutrition Values per 100g / 100ml KCAL	PROT	CARB	FAT	FIBRE
MEATBALLS								
Beef, Sainsbury's*	1 Meatball/24g	59	4	251	19.6	4.8	16.9	0.5
Beef, Skinny, Mini, 24, M&S*	½ Pack/120g	132	2.9	110	17.9	4.3	2.4	0.5
Chicken, in Barbecue Sauce, Fray Bentos*	½ Can/190g	232	11.8	122	4.3	14.3	6.2	0.8
Chicken, in Tomato Sauce, Average	***1 Can/392g***	***580***	***32.9***	***148***	***7.7***	***10.4***	***8.4***	***0***
Chicken, Mediterranean Inspired, Tesco*	3 Meatballs/64g	120	3.9	188	21.9	11.3	6.1	0.2
Chicken, Spanish Style, Ready to Cook, Asda*	½ Pack/179g	179	6.4	100	8.6	7.4	3.6	1.9
Lamb, Daylesford*	1/3 Pack/112g	203	13.7	181	17.6	0.2	12.2	0
Meat Free, Oven Baked, Plant Based, Asda*	6 Meatballs/118g	176	11.3	149	5.9	5.7	9.6	8
Meat Free, Plant Pioneers, Sainsbury's*	½ Pack/190g	304	12.5	160	15.2	6.7	6.6	6.7
Meat Free, Vegan, Pan Fried, Plant Chef, Tesco*	3 Balls/78g	160	7.1	205	14.2	15	9.1	3.3
Meat-less, Shallow Fried, V Taste, Morrisons*	3 Balls/60g	85	2.5	141	7.8	16.2	4.2	3.7
Plant Based, Moving Mountains*	½ Pack/150g	394	29.4	263	11.7	6.8	19.6	6.5
Pork, & Beef, Swedish Style, Tesco*	1 Meatball/14g	34	2.5	245	14.3	6.5	17.7	2
Pork, & Sage, with Onion Gravy, Gousto*	1 Serving/305g	564	21.7	185	10.5	20.4	7.1	2
Pork, al Forno, Deluxe, Lidl*	½ Pack/400g	620	28	155	7.7	14.3	7	2
Pork, Duchy Originals, Waitrose*	5 Meatballs/68g	184	12.6	270	21.7	4	18.6	0
Pork, Italian, Al Forno, Sainsbury's*	1 Pack/450g	644	23.8	143	6.1	17.6	5.3	1.4
Reduced Fat, Aldi*	3 Meatballs/90g	188	8.6	209	23	6.8	9.5	1.3
Russian, Large, Aida Food*	1 Meatball/50g	116	9	232	17	1.5	18	0
Swedish, Meat Free, Green Cuisine, Birds Eye*	1 Serving/81g	190	12.1	236	16	6.8	15	4.9
Tomato, Spicy, Vegetarian, The Deli, Aldi*	3 Balls/63g	126	5.7	200	5.5	20	9.1	7.5
Turkey, 5% Fat, British, Tesco*	4 Meatballs/95g	126	2.7	132	22.7	2.9	2.8	2.4
Turkey, with Seasoning, Sainsbury's*	3 Meatballs/79g	168	8.5	213	22.8	6	10.8	0.5
Vegan, Gro, Co-Op*	5 Balls/95g	144	7.4	152	14	3	7.8	6.2
Vegan, No Bull, Iceland*	4 Balls/41g	78	3.6	190	13	12	8.8	5.8
Vegetarian, Vivera*	½ Pack/100g	169	7.3	169	17	7.4	7.3	3.3
Vegetarian, Super Greens Balls, as Sold, Heck*	1 Ball/28g	43	0.5	153	6.5	30.3	1.8	5.4
Vegetarian, Swedish Style, Quorn*	½ Bag/150g	195	6.9	130	13.2	7.4	4.6	3
Vegetarian, Swedish, Frozen, Quorn*	¼ Pack/75g	98	3.5	130	13.2	7.4	4.6	3
Vegetarian, Tomato & Basil, Linda McCartney*	5 Meatballs/91g	199	12.2	219	12.8	9	13.4	5.7
MELBA TOAST								
Average	***1 Serving/3g***	***13***	***0.2***	***396***	***12***	***76***	***4.9***	***4.6***
MELON								
Cantaloupe, Flesh Only, Average	***½ Melon/255g***	***87***	***0.5***	***34***	***0.8***	***8.2***	***0.2***	***0.9***
Cantaloupe, Weighed with Rind, Average	***1 Wedge/100g***	***18***	***0.2***	***18***	***0.4***	***4.2***	***0.2***	***0.4***
Galia	***1 Serving/240g***	***60***	***0.1***	***25***	***0.8***	***5.8***	***0***	***0.2***
Honeydew, Raw, Flesh Only, Average	***1oz/28g***	***8***	***0***	***30***	***0.7***	***7***	***0.1***	***0.5***
Medley, Pre Packed, Average	***1 Pack/240g***	***66***	***0.3***	***27***	***0.6***	***6***	***0.1***	***0.5***
MELON & GRAPES								
Fresh, Tesco*	1 Pack/300g	105	0.3	35	0.6	7.2	0.1	1.2
Iceland*	½ Pot/80g	34	0.1	43	0.6	10.5	0.1	0
Meadow Fresh, Lidl*	1 Pack/200g	84	0.4	42	0.8	8.9	0.2	0.5
MERINGUE								
Average	***1 Meringue/8g***	***30***	***0***	***379***	***5.3***	***95.4***	***0***	***0***
Coffee Fresh Cream, Asda*	1 Meringue/28g	109	4.7	396	3.8	57	17	0.3
Cream, Fresh, Sainsbury's*	1 Meringue/35g	142	5.1	407	3.5	65.4	14.6	0.5
Nests, Average	***1 Nest/16g***	***63***	***0***	***397***	***4.8***	***93.3***	***0.1***	***0.1***
Shells, Mini, TTD, Sainsbury's*	1 Shell/5g	19	0	386	4.8	91.2	0.5	0.5
Shells, Mini, Waitrose*	1 Shell/5g	19	0	386	4.8	91.2	0.2	0
Toffee Cream, Tesco*	1 Meringue/30g	114	5	380	4.2	52.9	16.5	0
MIDGET GEMS								
M&S*	1 Bag/113g	367	0.1	325	6.3	75.1	0.1	0
Smart Price, Asda*	1 Pack/178g	586	0.2	329	6	76	0.1	0

	Measure INFO/WEIGHT	per Measure KCAL	FAT	Nutrition Values per 100g / 100ml KCAL	PROT	CARB	FAT	FIBRE
MILK								
Almond, Dark Chocolate, Alpro*	1 Serving/200ml	94	2.6	47	0.8	7.6	1.3	0.8
Almond, Original, Alpro*	1 Serving/200ml	48	2.2	24	0.5	3	1.1	0.2
Almond, Original, Fresh, Alpro*	1 Serving/200ml	48	2.2	24	0.5	3	1.1	0.2
Almond, Original, Roasted, Alpro*	1 Serving/100ml	22	1.1	22	0.4	2.4	1.1	0.4
Almond, Sweetened, UHT, Tesco*	1 Serving/200ml	50	2.4	25	0.7	2.8	1.2	0
Almond, Unsweetened, Actileaf, Aldi*	1 Serving/200ml	40	3	20	0.5	1.3	1.5	0.5
Almond, Unsweetened, Breeze, Blue Diamond*	1 Serving/250ml	32	2.8	13	0.5	0.2	1.1	0.3
Almond, Unsweetened, Morrisons*	1 Serving/100ml	18	1.5	18	0.8	0.1	1.5	0.4
Almond, Unsweetened, Organic, Alpro*	1 Serving/200ml	30	2.4	15	0.5	0	1.2	0.2
Almond, Unsweetened, Roasted, Alpro*	1 Serving/200ml	26	2.2	13	0.4	0	1.1	0.4
Almond, Unsweetened, Sainsbury's*	1 Serving/200ml	36	2.6	18	0.5	1.1	1.3	0
Almond, Unsweetened, Tesco*	1 Serving/100ml	18	1.1	18	0.4	1.3	1.1	0.4
Almond, Unsweetened, UHT, Morrisons*	1 Serving/100ml	14	1	14	0.6	0.6	1	0
Almond, Unsweetened, Unroasted, Alpro*	1 Serving/200ml	26	2.6	13	0.5	0	1.3	0.2
Chocolate, Flavoured, Morrisons*	1 Serving/330ml	236	6.2	72	3.5	9.8	1.9	0.6
Coconut, & Almond, Fresh, Alpro*	1 Serving/200ml	48	2.6	24	0.3	2.6	1.3	0
Coconut, Asia Specialities, Aldi*	1 Serving/100ml	176	18	176	1.5	2.2	18	0.5
Coconut, Average	***1 Can/400ml***	***698***	***69.7***	***174***	***1.4***	***2.9***	***17.4***	***2.9***
Coconut, Canned, Sainsbury's*	1 Can/400ml	764	72.8	191	0.9	5.7	18.2	0.5
Coconut, Canned, Tesco*	¼ Can/100ml	151	15	151	0.9	3.2	15	0
Coconut, Half Fat, Waitrose*	½ Can/135ml	92	8.1	68	0.7	2.7	6	0
Coconut, Light, Tesco*	1 Can/400ml	244	24	61	0.4	1.3	6	0
Coconut, Lighter, Sainsbury's*	¼ Can/100ml	75	6.5	75	0.9	2.9	6.5	0.5
Coconut, Reduced Fat, Average	***1 Serving/100g***	***104***	***10***	***104***	***1***	***2.4***	***10***	***0.4***
Coconut, Sweetened, Sainsbury's*	1 Serving/250ml	45	2.5	18	0.5	2.2	1	0.5
Coconut, Unsweetened, UHT, Alpro*	1 Serving/200ml	28	2.4	14	0.1	0.4	1.2	0
Condensed, Semi Skimmed, Sweetened	***1oz/28g***	***75***	***0.1***	***267***	***10***	***60***	***0.2***	***0***
Condensed, Skimmed, Unsweetened, Average	***1oz/28g***	***30***	***1.1***	***108***	***7.5***	***10.5***	***4***	***0***
Condensed, Whole, Sweetened, Average	***1oz/28g***	***93***	***2.8***	***333***	***8.5***	***55.5***	***10.1***	***0***
Dried, Skimmed, Average	***1oz/28g***	***99***	***0.3***	***355***	***35.4***	***52.3***	***0.9***	***0***
Dried, Whole, Average	***1oz/28g***	***137***	***7.4***	***490***	***26.3***	***39.4***	***26.3***	***0***
Evaporated, Average	***1 Serving/85g***	***136***	***7.6***	***160***	***8.2***	***11.6***	***9***	***0***
Evaporated, Reduced Fat, Average	***1oz/28g***	***33***	***1.5***	***118***	***7.4***	***10.5***	***5.2***	***0***
Goat's, Semi Skimmed, St Helen's Farm*	1 Serving/200ml	88	3.2	44	3	4.3	1.6	0
Goats, Pasteurised	***1 fl oz/30ml***	***18***	***1***	***60***	***3.1***	***4.4***	***3.5***	***0***
Gold Top, Original, Graham's*	1 Tbsp/15ml	12	0.8	80	3.7	4.7	5	0
Kefir, Bibi's Homemade*	1 Glass/210g	128	7.4	61	3.3	4.3	3.5	0
Oat, Cacao, Alpro*	1 Serving/200ml	88	3.4	44	0.5	6.2	1.7	0.7
Plant Based, for Tea, Alpro*	1 Serving/30ml	18	1.3	60	2.1	2	4.3	1.6
Rice, Organic, Provamel*	1 Serving/250ml	122	3.8	49	0.1	9.5	1.5	0
Semi Skimmed, Average	***1fl oz/30ml***	***15***	***0.5***	***49***	***3.4***	***5***	***1.7***	***0***
Semi Skimmed, Lactose Free, Asda*	1 Serving/200ml	96	3.2	48	3.6	4.9	1.6	0.5
Semi Skimmed, Long Life, Average	***1fl oz/30ml***	***15***	***0.5***	***49***	***3.4***	***5***	***1.7***	***0***
Skimmed, Average	***1 Pint/568ml***	***194***	***0.5***	***34***	***3.3***	***5***	***0.1***	***0***
Skimmed, Lactofree, Arla*	1 Serving/200ml	62	1	31	3.7	2.8	0.5	0
Skimmed, Proactiv, Actively Lowers Cholesterol, Flora*	1 Serving/100ml	35	0.3	35	3.2	4.8	0.3	0
Skimmed, Uht, Average	***1fl oz/30ml***	***10***	***0***	***34***	***3.4***	***5***	***0.1***	***0***
Soya, Chocolate, UHT, Alpro*	1 Serving/200ml	122	3.6	61	3.1	7.8	1.8	0.9
Soya, Flavoured, Average	***1 Glass/250ml***	***100***	***4.2***	***40***	***2.8***	***3.6***	***1.7***	***0***
Soya, No Added Sugar, Unsweetened, Average	***1 Serving/250ml***	***85***	***4.8***	***34***	***3.3***	***0.9***	***1.9***	***0.4***
Soya, Strawberry, Alpro*	1 Serving/200ml	124	3.6	62	3.3	7.6	1.8	0.5
Soya, Sweetened, Actileaf, Aldi*	1 Serving/200ml	98	5.2	49	3.5	2.6	2.6	0.5
Soya, Sweetened, Average	***1 Glass/200ml***	***94***	***4.2***	***47***	***3.4***	***3.7***	***2.1***	***0.4***

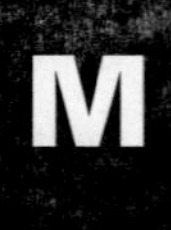

	Measure INFO/WEIGHT	per Measure KCAL	per Measure FAT	KCAL	PROT	CARB	FAT	FIBRE
				Nutrition Values per 100g / 100ml				
MILK								
Soya, Sweetened, Calcium Enriched, Average	***1 Glass/200ml***	***91***	***3.9***	***46***	***3.4***	***3.7***	***2***	***0.3***
Soya, Vanilla, Alpro*	1 Serving/200ml	108	3.4	54	3	6.5	1.7	0.5
Soya, Wholebean, Unsweetened, Alpro*	1 Serving/200ml	66	3.6	33	3.3	0	1.8	0.6
Soya, Wholebean, Unsweetened, Organic, Alpro*	1 Serving/200ml	66	3.6	33	3.3	0	1.8	0.6
Whole, Average	***1 Serving/200ml***	***134***	***7.8***	***67***	***3.3***	***4.7***	***3.9***	***0***
Whole, Lactose Free, Lactofree, Arla*	1 Serving/200ml	114	7	57	3.4	2.8	3.5	0
MILK DRINK								
Almond, Sweetened, Plant Kitchen, M&S*	1 Serving/200ml	58	4	29	1	1.5	2	0.6
Almond, Unsweetened, Plant Kitchen, M&S*	1 Serving/200ml	58	2.4	29	0.5	3.5	1.2	1
Banana, Breakfast, Fuel 10K*	1 Carton/330g	218	4.6	66	6.1	6.7	1.4	1
Breakfast, Chocolate, Protein, Fuel 10K*	1 Carton/330ml	208	3.3	63	6.1	6.9	1	1
Chocolate Coconut, Free From, Tesco*	1 Serving/250ml	125	5.4	49	0.4	6.8	2.1	0.7
Coconut, Plant Kitchen, M&S*	1 Serving/200ml	58	3.8	29	0.2	2.2	1.9	1
Kefir, Natur, Nestle*	1 Glass/250ml	98	3.8	39	3	3.3	1.5	0
Kefir, Natural, Goodness, Graham's The Family Dairy *	½ Bottle/250ml	145	7.5	58	3.4	4.4	3	0
Kefir, Organic, Bio-tiful Dairy*	1 Serving/250g	145	7.5	58	3.2	4.6	3	0
Kefir, Pomegranate, & Blueberry, Light & Free, Danone*	1 Bottle/265ml	69	1.1	26	2.9	4.4	0.4	0
Kvarg, Pro+, Raspberry & Vanilla, Lindahls, Nestle*	1 Serving/250ml	144	1.8	55	8.7	3.4	0.7	0
Original, Mars*	1 Serving/330g	284	6.9	86	3.1	13.7	2.1	0
Strawberry Flavoured, Goodness for Kids, Tesco*	1 Bottle/330ml	248	5.6	75	4	9.9	1.7	0.4
Strawberry, Flavoured, Asda*	1 Bottle/330ml	211	3.6	64	3.6	10	1.1	0.5
Vanilla, Breakfast, Protein, Fuel 10K*	1 Carton/330ml	218	4.6	66	6.1	6.7	1.4	1
MILK SHAKE								
Banana Flavour, Frijj*	1 Bottle/500ml	325	4.5	65	3.7	10.5	0.9	0
Banana, Mix, As Prepared, Morrisons*	1 Serving/216ml	158	3.5	73	3.4	11.3	1.6	0
Banana, Yazoo, Campina*	1 Bottle/200ml	120	2.4	60	3.1	9.6	1.2	0
Chocolate Flavoured, Fresh, Thick, Frijj*	1 Bottle/500ml	350	5	70	3.5	11.7	1	0
Chocolate, Asda*	1 Serving/250ml	198	9.2	79	4.4	7	3.7	0.4
Chocolate, Belgian, M&S*	1 Bottle/300ml	360	14.4	120	4.2	14.6	4.8	0.7
Chocolate, Dry, Cadbury*	1 Serving/14g	54	0.9	387	7.7	64	6.3	21
Chocolate, Fudge, Cowbelle, Aldi*	1 Serving/100ml	74	1.3	74	4.5	11	1.3	0.5
Chocolate, M&M's, Mars*	1 Serving/50g	196	8.3	392	42.6	9	16.6	15.8
Chocolate, Protein, Ufit*	1 Bottle/310ml	170	3.1	55	7.1	3.6	1	1.2
Powder, Made Up with Semi-Skimmed Milk	***1 Serving/250ml***	***172***	***4***	***69***	***3.2***	***11.3***	***1.6***	***0***
Powder, Made Up with Whole Milk	***1 Serving/250ml***	***218***	***9.2***	***87***	***3.1***	***11.1***	***3.7***	***0***
Protein, Supplement, USN*	1 Bottle/310ml	145	0.3	47	8.1	3.4	0.1	0
Strawberry Flavour, Thick, Low Fat, Frijj*	1 Bottle/250ml	155	2	62	3.4	10.1	0.8	0
Strawberry, British, M&S*	1 Bottle/300ml	270	10.2	90	4	10.8	3.4	0.1
Thick, Milky Way, Mars*	1 Bottle/440ml	282	4.8	64	3.4	10	1.1	0.7
White Chocolate, & Vanilla, M&S*	1 Bottle/300ml	315	12.9	105	3.8	12.4	4.3	0.6
MILKY BAR								
Buttons, Nestle*	1 Pack/14g	78	4.6	543	10.6	53.1	31.7	0
Crunchies, Nestle*	1 Pack/30g	168	10.4	560	7	54.9	34.7	0
Egg, White Chocolate, Nestle*	1 Egg/65g	353	20.6	543	10.6	53.1	31.7	0
Funsize, Mars*	1 Bar/17g	75	2.7	449	3.8	71.8	16.3	0.6
Mini Eggs, Nestle*	1 Pack/90g	443	18.5	492	7	69.4	20.6	0
Munchies, Nestle*	1 Serving/70g	392	24.3	560	7	54.9	34.7	0.1
Nestle*	1 Sm Bar/13g	68	4	547	7.3	58.4	31.7	0
MILKY WAY								
Fun Size, Mars*	1 Bar/17g	75	2.7	447	3.8	71.6	16.2	0
Mars*	1 Bar/22g	96	3.3	446	3.9	72.4	15.5	0.6
MINCEMEAT								
Average	***1oz/28g***	***77***	***1.2***	***274***	***0.6***	***62.1***	***4.3***	***1.3***

	Measure INFO/WEIGHT	per Measure KCAL	per Measure FAT	KCAL	PROT	CARB	FAT	FIBRE
				Nutrition Values per 100g / 100ml				
MINSTRELS								
Galaxy, Mars*	1 Serving/39g	196	8.6	498	5.2	69.1	21.9	0
MINT								
Dried, Average	***1 Tsp/5g***	***14***	***0.2***	***279***	***24.8***	***34.6***	***4.6***	***0***
Fresh, Average	***2 Tbsp/3.2g***	***1***	***0***	***43***	***3.8***	***5.3***	***0.7***	***0***
MINTS								
Butter Mintoes, M&S*	1 Sweet/9g	35	0.6	391	0	84	6.8	0
Butter Mintoes, Tesco*	1 Sweet/7g	30	0.5	431	0.1	91.1	7.3	0.5
Butter, Dominion, Aldi*	2 Sweets/14g	23	0.4	167	0.5	35	3.1	0.5
Clear, Co-Op*	1 Sweet/6g	24	0	395	0	98	0	0
Creams, Bassett's*	1 Sweet/11g	40	0	365	0	91.8	0	0
Curiously Strong, M&S*	1 Sweet/1g	4	0	390	0.4	97.5	0	0
Everton, Co-Op*	1 Sweet/6g	25	0.2	410	0.6	92	4	0
Extra Strong, Peppermint, Trebor*	1 Mint/2g	10	0	395	0.3	98.5	0	0
Glacier, Fox's*	1 Sweet/5g	19	0	386	0	96.4	0	0
Humbugs, Co-Op*	1 Sweet/8g	34	0.6	425	0.6	89.9	7	0
Humbugs, M&S*	1 Sweet/9g	37	0.4	407	0.6	91.1	4.4	0
Humbugs, Tesco*	1 Sweet/9g	37	0.2	409	0.3	95.9	2.6	0.5
Humbugs, Thorntons*	1 Sweet/9g	31	0.4	340	1	87.8	4.4	0
Imperials, Co-Op*	1 Sweet/3g	12	0	395	0.3	98	0.2	0
Imperials, M&S*	1 Sweet/3g	12	0	391	0	97.8	0	0
Imperials, Sainsbury's*	1 Sweet/3g	10	0	374	0	92.1	0	0
Imperials, Tesco*	1 Sweet/3g	12	0	397	0.6	98.7	0	0
Mint Assortment, M&S*	1 Sweet/7g	26	0.5	375	0.4	78.2	6.9	0
Peppermints, Strong, Altoids*	1 Sweet/1g	3	0	385	0.5	96	0	0
Soft, Trebor*	1 Pack/48g	182	0	380	0	94.9	0	0
Softmints, Peppermint, Trebor*	1 Pack/48g	170	0	355	0	88.9	0	0
Softmints, Spearmint, Trebor*	1 Pack/45g	170	0	375	0	94.3	0	0
Thins, Chocolate, Waitrose*	1 Thin/5g	27	1.3	509	4.2	69.6	23.8	0.2
MIRIN								
Mikawa, Organic, Clearspring*	1 Tbsp/15ml	24	0.1	163	0.5	39	0.4	0
Rice Wine, Sweetened, Average	***1 Tbsp/15ml***	***35***	***0***	***231***	***0.2***	***41.6***	***0***	***0***
MISO								
Average	***1oz/28g***	***57***	***1.7***	***203***	***13.3***	***23.5***	***6.2***	***0***
Paste, Mellow Yellow, Yutaka*	1 Serving/17g	26	0.8	156	9.7	19	4.8	4.5
Paste, Sainsbury's*	¼ Jar/25g	22	0.6	89	4.6	9.7	2.5	4.4
White, Sweet, Organic, Clearspring*	1 Tbsp/15g	26	0.6	171	7.7	26	4	0.6
MIXED HERBS								
Average	***1 Tsp/5g***	***13***	***0.4***	***260***	***13***	***37.5***	***8.5***	***6.7***
MOLASSES								
Average	***1 Tsp/5g***	***13***	***0***	***266***	***0***	***68.8***	***0.1***	***0***
MONKEY NUTS								
without Shell, Average	***1oz/28g***	***158***	***13.4***	***565***	***25.6***	***8.2***	***48***	***6.3***
MONKFISH								
Grilled	***1oz/28g***	***27***	***0.2***	***96***	***22.7***	***0***	***0.6***	***0***
Raw, Average	***1 Serving/150g***	***114***	***2.2***	***76***	***14***	***0***	***1.5***	***0***
MOUSSAKA								
Allplants*	1 Serving/420g	365	7.1	87	4.1	12	1.7	2.6
Beef, & Lamb, Waitrose*	1 Pack/323g	387	19.4	120	6.2	9.5	6	1.5
Beef, BGTY, Sainsbury's*	1 Pack/400g	300	10.4	75	6.1	6.8	2.6	1.2
Charlie Bigham's*	½ Pack/328g	425	27.8	130	6.1	6.9	8.5	0
for One, Charlie Bigham's*	1 Serving/340g	442	29.2	130	6	6.9	8.6	0
for Two, Charlie Bigham's*	1 Serving/327g	425	27.8	130	6.1	6.9	8.5	0
Lamb, BGTY, Sainsbury's*	1 Pack/400g	296	10.4	74	5	6.1	2.6	3

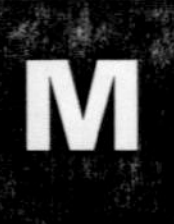

	Measure INFO/WEIGHT	per Measure KCAL	per Measure FAT	Nutrition Values per 100g / 100ml KCAL	PROT	CARB	FAT	FIBRE
MOUSSAKA								
Lamb, Cook*	1 Serving/380g	593	30.8	156	8.3	11.9	8.1	1.3
Lamb, Finest, Tesco*	½ Pack/334g	513	36.5	154	6.4	6.6	10.9	1.5
Lamb, Gastropub, M&S*	1 Pack/409g	528	31.5	129	6.2	7.5	7.7	2.2
Lamb, Greek, Melty, Gousto*	1 Serving/472g	595	28.8	126	7.6	10.3	6.1	2.1
Lamb, Oven Baked, Luxury, Iceland*	1 Pack/424g	903	58.9	213	9.8	11.3	13.9	1.7
Lamb, Serves 2, TTD, Sainsbury's*	½ Pack/400g	546	33.7	141	7.2	8	8.7	1.2
Lidl*	1 Pack/380g	627	34.2	165	6.1	12.1	9	0.5
Vegetable, COU, M&S*	1 Pack/400g	280	10.8	70	2.7	9.1	2.7	2.4
Vegetarian, Quorn*	1 Pack/400g	364	16.4	91	3.6	9.8	4.1	1.2
Voussaka, Vegan, Waitrose*	1 Pack/365g	401	20.8	110	3.6	9.9	5.7	2.4
MOUSSE								
Aero Chocolate, Nestle*	1 Pot/58g	101	3	174	4.8	27.3	5.1	1.1
Apricot, Lite, Onken*	1 Pot/150g	156	2.2	104	4.6	18	1.5	0.3
Banoffee, COU, M&S*	1 Pot/70g	102	1.5	145	2.9	28.8	2.1	1.5
Birthday Cake, Halo Top*	1 Pot/100g	153	7.2	153	6.5	13.6	7.2	3.1
Blackcurrant, Bonne Maman*	1 Pot/70g	116	5.3	166	2.6	20.8	7.6	2
Blackcurrant, Onken*	1 Pot/150g	210	10.2	140	5.2	14.6	6.8	0
Cappuccino, Essential, Waitrose*	1 Pot/100g	279	16.7	279	4.2	27.7	16.7	0.5
Caramel, Meringue, Cadbury*	1 Pot/65g	181	6.7	277	4.6	42.4	10.3	1
Cherry, & Kirsch, Finest, Tesco*	1 Pot/100g	195	11.6	195	2.7	19.6	11.6	0.5
Chocolate	***1 Pot/60g***	***83***	***3.2***	***139***	***4***	***19.9***	***5.4***	***0***
Chocolate, & Hazelnut, Onken*	1 Pot/125g	171	7.5	137	3.3	17.8	6	0
Chocolate, & Mint, COU, M&S*	1 Pot/70g	84	1.8	120	6.2	18.7	2.5	1
Chocolate, & Orange, COU, M&S*	1 Pot/70g	77	1.8	110	5.9	16	2.6	0.9
Chocolate, Bubbly, Aero, Nestle*	1 Pot/58g	93	3	159	5	23.1	5.1	0
Chocolate, Low Fat, Danette, Danone*	1 Pot/60g	73	1.1	121	5.1	20.8	1.9	1.5
Chocolate, Minty, Bubbly, Dessert, Aero, Nestle*	1 Pot/58g	108	5.9	186	4.6	18.9	10.2	0.3
Chocolate, Plain, Low Fat, Nestle*	1 Pot/120g	71	0.9	59	2.4	10.4	0.8	0
Chocolate, Pot, Halo Top*	1 Pot/100g	143	4.3	143	5.7	18.2	4.3	5.4
Chocolate, Pot, Plant Kitchen, M&S*	1 Pot/90g	288	19.4	320	3.5	26.5	21.6	2.8
Chocolate, Wispa, Cadbury*	1 Pot/45g	88	3.6	195	6	25.6	8	1.7
Chocolate, with Vanilla Layer, Cadbury*	1 Pot/100g	162	6.1	162	4.8	21.9	6.1	0
Lemon, COU, M&S*	1 Pot/70g	91	1.8	130	3.1	23.7	2.5	0.6
Lemon, Dessert, Sainsbury's*	1 Pot/63g	114	5.9	182	3.6	20.7	9.4	0.6
Lemon, Freaks Of Nature*	1 Pot/70g	136	4.8	195	1.2	31.8	6.9	0.5
Lemon, Low Fat, Morrisons*	1 Pot/63g	99	5.8	158	3.7	15.4	9.3	0.3
Lemon, Sicillian, Deluxe, Lidl*	1 Pot/100g	210	12.4	210	2.6	22	12.4	0.5
Lemon, Ski, Nestle*	1 Pot/60g	77	2.8	128	3.8	17.8	4.6	0
Lemon, Tesco*	1 Pot/60g	91	4.9	152	3.8	15.4	8.2	0.4
Raspberry, Ripple, Value, Tesco*	1 Pot/47g	70	2.9	149	2.1	21.3	6.1	0.1
Rhubarb, Bonne Maman*	1 Pot/70g	120	5.3	171	2.4	22.8	7.6	1
Rolo, Nestle*	1 Pot/50g	80	3	158	4.7	21.6	5.9	0
Strawberry, Asda*	1 Pot/64g	107	5.8	167	3.5	18	9	0.2
Strawberry, COU, M&S*	1 Pot/70g	90	1.3	128	4.5	23.2	1.8	0.3
Strawberry, Iceland*	1 Pot/100g	158	8.5	158	2.8	16.9	8.5	0.5
Strawberry, Layered, Co-Op*	1 Pot/100g	120	3	120	3	19	3	0.2
Strawberry, Light, Muller*	1 Pot/150g	147	0.6	98	4.3	19.4	0.4	0
Strawberry, Ski, Nestle*	1 Pot/60g	73	2.9	121	3.9	15.4	4.9	0
Strawberry, Tesco*	1 Pot/60g	97	4.6	162	2.7	20.2	7.7	0.5
Summer Fruits, Light, Muller*	1 Pot/149g	143	0.6	96	4.3	18.7	0.4	0
Toffee, M&S*	1 Pot/90g	180	7.2	200	4.5	27.6	8	0.6
White Chocolate, Finest, Tesco*	1 Pot/92g	436	34.5	474	3.9	30.2	37.5	0

MUFFIN	Measure INFO/WEIGHT	per Measure KCAL	FAT	Nutrition Values per 100g / 100ml KCAL	PROT	CARB	FAT	FIBRE
All Butter, M&S*	1 Muffin/65g	175	4.7	270	10.3	40.8	7.3	2.1
Ancient Grain, Rankin Selection*	1 Muffin/70g	212	3.6	303	10.7	49.4	5.2	7.8
Bacon, & Cheddar Cheese, Mini, M&S*	1 Muffin/20g	52	3	260	11.1	19.5	14.8	2.4
Blueberry, American Style, Aldi*	1 Muffin/85g	344	17.3	405	4.3	51.2	20.3	0
Blueberry, American Style, Sainsbury's*	1 Muffin/72g	256	13.1	355	5.1	42.7	18.2	1.9
Blueberry, Asda*	1 Muffin/77g	273	13.1	353	5	45	17	1.3
Blueberry, Bakery, Tesco*	1 Muffin/82g	307	13.1	374	4.3	52.2	16	1.9
Blueberry, Big, Asda*	1 Muffin/105g	342	11.2	326	7.5	49.8	10.7	2.3
Blueberry, Breakfast, Weetabix*	1 Muffin/92g	249	7.3	270	6	42.1	7.9	3.4
Blueberry, GF, Genius*	1 Muffin/95g	352	16.2	370	3.6	51	17.1	1.6
Blueberry, M&S*	1 Muffin/75g	255	12.6	340	4.9	41.9	16.8	1.3
Blueberry, McVitie's*	1 Muffin/80g	328	18.6	405	4.7	47.9	23	1.3
Blueberry, Mini, Tesco*	1 Muffin/28g	104	5.4	370	5.6	43.5	19.3	1.2
Blueberry, PB, Waitrose*	1 Muffin/100g	225	2.2	225	4.6	46.5	2.2	1.8
Blueberry, Rowan Hill Bakery, Lidl*	1 Muffin/72g	283	11.7	393	4.8	55.5	16.2	3.2
Blueberry, Waitrose*	1 Muffin/65g	239	9.2	367	4.7	55.2	14.2	1.7
Brown, Bottom, Rowan Hill Bakery, Lidl*	1 Muffin/65g	160	1.6	246	9.6	44.1	2.4	5
Brown, Oven Bottom, G H Sheldon*	1 Muffin/63g	155	1.5	246	9.5	44	2.4	4.9
Caramel, Cadbury*	1 Muffin/116g	535	30.3	461	5.9	50.8	26.1	0
Caramel, Salted, Filled, Tesco*	1 Muffin/82g	320	15.5	390	4.7	49.5	18.9	1.6
Caramel, Salted, TTD, Sainsbury's*	1 Muffin/113g	447	22	396	4.8	49.6	19.5	1.5
Cheddar, & Spinach, Mini, Higgidy*	1 Muffin/22g	62	3.5	280	12.6	21.7	15.7	1.9
Cheese, Cheddar, & Roasted Onion, M&S*	1 Pack/121g	370	25.4	306	11	17	21	2.4
Cheese, TTD, Sainsbury's*	1 Muffin/69g	200	6	290	11.5	40.2	8.7	2.4
Chocolate Chip, BGTY, Sainsbury's*	1 Muffin/75g	282	12.3	376	5.2	51.8	16.4	1.6
Chocolate Chip, Double, Co-Op*	1 Muffin/60g	246	12.6	410	6	49	21	3
Chocolate Chip, Double, Mini, Asda*	1 Muffin/19g	76	3.7	400	7.4	48.5	19.6	2.7
Chocolate Chip, Double, Tesco*	1 Muffin/100g	360	17.9	360	6.1	44.9	17.9	5.4
Chocolate Chip, Mini, Asda*	1 Muffin/22g	77	2.9	349	7	51	13	2.1
Chocolate Chip, Mini, BGTY, Sainsbury's*	1 Muffin/30g	130	6.7	434	5.5	52.1	22.5	0.8
Chocolate Chip, Mini, Essential, Waitrose*	1 Muffin/27g	108	5.1	399	5.9	49.8	19	2.5
Chocolate Chip, Mini, Tesco*	1 Muffin/25g	108	5.6	436	5	52.5	22.5	1.6
Chocolate Chip, Plain, Tesco*	1 Muffin/72g	270	12.7	375	5	48.1	17.6	1.4
Chocolate Chunk, Morrisons*	1 Muffin/100g	442	23.5	442	5	51.5	23.5	2.2
Chocolate, Double, Mini, M&S*	1 Muffin/32g	133	6.9	416	5.4	49.8	21.7	1.1
Cinnamon, & Sultana, Morrisons*	1 Muffin/74g	199	1.1	269	7.6	54.7	1.5	3.1
Date, Love Yourself Diet*	1 Muffin/70g	133	3	190	4.3	35.7	4.3	0
English, Egg, Cheese, & Sausage, From Restaurant	***1 Muffin/165g***	***487***	***30.9***	***295***	***13.1***	***18.8***	***18.7***	***0***
English, Kingsmill*	1 Muffin/75g	167	1.4	222	9.7	40.4	1.8	2.6
English, Mild Red Cheddar Cheese, Extra Special, Asda*	1 Muffin/70g	201	4.7	288	11	45	6.7	2.7
English, Tesco*	1 Muffin/72g	158	1.1	219	8.4	41.7	1.5	2.7
English, White, Butter, Waitrose*	1 Muffin/62g	166	2.2	266	10	47.7	3.5	1.9
Halloween, Asda*	1 Muffin/84g	346	16.8	412	4.8	53	20	1.3
Lancashire, Oven Bottom, Sheldons*	1 Muffin/65g	166	1.6	255	9.8	47.2	2.5	1.9
Lemon & Poppy Seed, Waitrose*	1 Muffin/121g	460	23.1	380	4.3	46.8	19.1	1.8
Lemon Curd, Patisserie, TTD, Sainsbury's*	1 Muffin/108g	418	20.9	386	5.4	47.1	19.3	1.4
Lemon Curd, Sicilian, Finest, Tesco*	1 Muffin/110g	402	17.5	366	5.1	49.9	15.9	1.4
Mini, Tesco*	1 Muffin/28g	120	6.3	428	6.4	50	22.6	1.2
Muesli, Breakfast, Love Life, Waitrose*	1 Muffin/68g	216	6.2	318	9.1	50	9.1	3.4
Multiseed, Butter, TTD, Sainsbury's*	1 Muffin/70g	208	6.2	297	10.9	40.8	8.9	5.2
Oat, Banana & Chocolate, Fuel 10K*	1 Muffin/60g	218	3.2	364	20.3	55	5.4	6.9
Oat, Double Chocolate, Fuel 10K*	1 Muffin/60g	172	4.6	286	18.7	32.2	7.6	7
Oat, Toffee Apple, Fuel 10K*	1 Muffin/60g	206	3.4	344	19.2	46.7	5.7	15

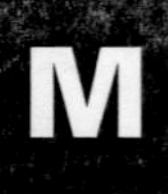

	Measure INFO/WEIGHT	per Measure KCAL	per Measure FAT	Nutrition Values per 100g / 100ml KCAL	PROT	CARB	FAT	FIBRE
MUFFIN								
Oven Bottom, Aldi*	1 Muffin/68g	173	1	255	10	50.4	1.5	2.2
Oven Bottom, Asda*	1 Muffin/65g	175	1.8	269	9	51	2.7	2.1
Oven Bottom, Warburton's*	1 Muffin/63g	173	2.7	274	10.4	49.4	4.3	2.3
Plain, Co-Op*	1 Muffin/60g	135	1.1	225	11.2	41.3	1.9	2.4
Plain, English, Asda*	1 Muffin/66g	158	1.5	241	9.3	45	2.3	2.4
Plain, Prepared From Recipe, Average	***1 Muffin/57g***	***169***	***6.5***	***296***	***6.9***	***41.4***	***11.4***	***2.7***
Plain, with Chocolate Chips, Mini, Holly Lane, Aldi*	1 Muffin/25g	112	6	448	6.2	52	24	2
Raspberry, Cream, Sainsbury's*	1 Muffin/90g	314	19.8	349	3.9	33.8	22	1.3
Sausage, Breakfast, All Day, Rustlers*	1 Muffin/155g	386	13.8	249	11.8	29	8.9	0
Sourdough, Toasting, Specially Selected, Aldi*	1 Muffin/68g	158	1.3	232	9.5	43	1.9	3.2
Toasting, Village Bakery, Aldi*	1 Muffin/68g	158	1.1	232	9.3	43	1.6	3.4
Toasting, Warburton's*	1 Muffin/64g	138	1	216	8.9	41.4	1.6	2.9
Vanilla, & Choc Chip, GFY, Asda*	1 Muffin/59g	152	1.3	260	7	53	2.2	1.6
White Chocolate, & Strawberry Filled, Tesco*	1 Muffin/103g	415	20.3	405	5.2	51.3	19.8	1.3
White Chocolate, Chunk Lemon, Mini, M&S*	1 Muffin/26g	106	5	409	5.7	52.4	19.3	1.2
White, M&S*	1 Muffin/60g	135	1.1	225	11.2	43.7	1.9	2.9
White, Soft, Hovis*	1 Muffin/60g	145	1.7	241	8.9	44	2.8	2.4
White, Tesco*	1 Muffin/72g	173	2.3	240	11.3	41.6	3.2	2.8
Wholemeal, Sainsbury's*	1 Muffin/65g	146	1.5	225	11.1	37.1	2.3	5.5
Wholemeal, Tesco*	1 Muffin/65g	130	1.3	200	12.6	32.9	2	5.7
with Caramel Centre, Dairy Milk, Cadbury*	1 Muffin/80g	313	14	391	4.2	53.6	17.5	1
MULBERRIES								
Raw	***1oz/28g***	***10***	***0***	***36***	***1.3***	***8.1***	***0***	***0***
MULLET								
Grey, Grilled	***1oz/28g***	***42***	***1.5***	***150***	***25.7***	***0***	***5.2***	***0***
Red, Grilled	***1oz/28g***	***34***	***1.2***	***121***	***20.4***	***0***	***4.4***	***0***
MUNCHIES								
Original, Tube, Nestle*	1 Pack/55g	266	12.3	487	5.4	64.6	22.5	1.4
MUSHROOMS								
BBQ, with Sticky Rice, Asian Inspired, Vegan, Waitrose*	1 Pack/370g	451	11.1	122	2.5	20.6	3	1.3
Breaded, Average	***3 Mushroom/51g***	***77***	***2.9***	***152***	***4.3***	***20.8***	***5.7***	***0.6***
Breaded, Garlic, Average	***3 Mushroom/50g***	***92***	***4.9***	***183***	***5.2***	***18.7***	***9.7***	***1.7***
Button, Raw, Average	***1 Serving/50g***	***7***	***0.2***	***15***	***2.3***	***0.5***	***0.4***	***1.2***
Chestnut, Average	***1 Med/5g***	***1***	***0***	***13***	***1.8***	***0.4***	***0.5***	***0.6***
Chinese, Dried, Raw	***1oz/28g***	***80***	***0.5***	***284***	***10***	***59.9***	***1.8***	***0***
Closed Cup, Average	***1 Handful/30g***	***4***	***0.2***	***14***	***1.8***	***0.4***	***0.5***	***1.1***
Common, Boiled in Salted Water, Average	***1oz/28g***	***3***	***0.1***	***11***	***1.8***	***0.4***	***0.3***	***1.1***
Common, Fried, Average	***1oz/28g***	***44***	***4.5***	***157***	***2.4***	***0.3***	***16.2***	***1.5***
Common, Raw, Average	***1 Serving/80g***	***18***	***0.3***	***22***	***3.1***	***3.3***	***0.3***	***1***
Creamed, Average	***1oz/28g***	***23***	***1.5***	***82***	***1.3***	***6.8***	***5.5***	***0.5***
Dried	***1oz/28g***	***45***	***1.7***	***159***	***21.8***	***4.8***	***6***	***13.3***
Enoki, Average	***1 Serving/80g***	***34***	***0***	***42***	***3***	***7***	***0***	***3***
Flat, Large, Average	***1 Mushroom/52g***	***10***	***0.3***	***20***	***3.3***	***0.5***	***0.5***	***0.7***
Garlic, & Cream Cheese, Oaklands, Lidl*	1 Mushroom/94g	98	4.6	104	4.2	10	4.9	1.5
Garlic, Average	***½ Pack/150g***	***159***	***14***	***106***	***2.1***	***3.7***	***9.3***	***1.7***
Mixed, Frozen, Freshona, Lidl*	1 Serving/150g	74	1.5	49	5.3	3.9	1	1.8
Oaklands, Lidl*	1 Pack/650g	46	1.3	7	1	0.3	0.2	0.7
Oyster, Average	***1 Serving/80g***	***10***	***0.2***	***13***	***1.4***	***1.4***	***0.2***	***1.1***
Porcini, Dried, Cooks & Co*	1 Pack/40g	177	2.4	442	30	51	6	32
Porcini, Wild, Dried, Merchant Gourmet*	1 Pack/50g	154	1.1	307	29.6	34.1	2.2	16.5
Portobello, Raw, Average	***1 Mushroom/50g***	***7***	***0.2***	***14***	***1.8***	***0.4***	***0.5***	***1.1***
Portobello, with Chorizo, & Cheddar, The Best, Morrisons*	½ Pack/79g	100	5.8	126	8.7	5.1	7.4	2.1
Shiitake, Cooked	***1oz/28g***	***15***	***0.1***	***55***	***1.6***	***12.3***	***0.2***	***0***

	Measure INFO/WEIGHT	per Measure KCAL	FAT	Nutrition Values per 100g / 100ml KCAL	PROT	CARB	FAT	FIBRE
MUSHROOMS								
Shiitake, Dried, Raw	**1oz/28g**	**83**	**0.3**	**296**	**9.6**	**63.9**	**1**	**0**
Shreds, BBQ, & Greens, Chinese, Wicked Kitchen, Tesco*	1 Serving/356g	467	11.1	131	4.4	19.8	3.1	3
Sliced, Average	**1oz/28g**	**3**	**0.1**	**12**	**1.8**	**0.4**	**0.3**	**1.1**
Steak, No Bull, Iceland*	1 Steak/80g	109	7.2	136	4.1	6.8	9	6.3
Straw, Canned, Drained	**1oz/28g**	**4**	**0.1**	**15**	**2.1**	**1.2**	**0.2**	**0**
Stuffed, Cheese, & Garlic, Mini, Nature's Pick, Aldi*	1 Pack/210g	275	14.7	131	5.5	10	7	2.3
Stuffed, Fire Pit, Tesco*	1 Mushroom/85g	90	4.6	106	6.1	7.5	5.4	1.7
Stuffed, Garlic, & Cheese, Co-Op*	½ Pack/100g	93	4.1	93	3.6	9.8	4.1	1.3
Stuffed, Garlic, Cream Cheese, Herb, Breadcrumbs, Aldi*	½ Pack/92g	105	4.7	114	5.1	11	5.1	2.5
Stuffed, with Chorizo, & Spinach, Asda*	½ Pack/80g	90	5	112	8	4.7	6.3	2.3
Woodland, No.1, Waitrose*	½ Pack/100g	33	0.5	33	2.8	3.3	0.5	2.8
MUSSELS								
Boiled, Flesh Only, Average	**1 Mussel/2g**	**2**	**0.1**	**104**	**16.7**	**3.5**	**2.7**	**0**
Boiled, Weighed in Shell, Average	**1 Mussel/7g**	**2**	**0.1**	**28**	**4.5**	**0.9**	**0.7**	**0**
Pickled, Drained, Average	**1oz/28g**	**32**	**0.6**	**112**	**20**	**1.5**	**2.2**	**0**
Raw, Weighed in Shell, Average	**1oz/28g**	**7**	**0.2**	**23**	**3.4**	**1**	**0.7**	**0**
Ready to Eat, Tesco*	½ Pack/75g	62	1.2	83	14.3	2.8	1.6	0.1
Scottish, Rope Grown, M&S*	1 Serving/150g	140	6.6	93	7.5	5.7	4.4	0.5
with Garlic, & Parsley, Lidl*	1 Pack/125g	381	35	305	8.2	4.6	28	0
MUSSELS IN								
Garlic Butter Sauce, Average	**½ Pack/225g**	**179**	**11.5**	**80**	**6.4**	**2**	**5.1**	**0.2**
Oil, Smoked, Canned, Drained, John West*	1 Can/60g	117	7.3	196	19.9	1.6	12.2	0
Scottish, in Garlic Butter, Waitrose*	½ Pack/120g	108	7.4	90	6.7	1.6	6.2	0.6
Scottish, in White Wine & Cream, Waitrose*	½ Pack/129g	110	4.3	85	6.6	6.8	3.3	0.6
Seasoned White Wine Sauce, Bantry Bay*	1 Serving/450g	270	9	60	6.3	4.1	2	0.1
Tomato Sauce, Cooked, Italiamo, Lidl*	1 Pack/350g	438	34.3	125	7.3	1.9	9.8	0
White Wine Sauce, Sainsbury's*	½ Pack/250g	215	10.2	86	6.4	5.6	4.1	0.7
White Wine, & Garlic Sauce, TTD, Sainsbury's*	1 Dish/101g	179	12.9	177	10	5.2	12.8	0.6
MUSTARD								
American, Average	**1 Tsp/5g**	**5**	**0.2**	**102**	**4.4**	**10.5**	**5**	**2.5**
Coarse Grain, Average	**1 Tsp/5g**	**7**	**0.4**	**141**	**7.7**	**8.4**	**8.3**	**5.9**
Dijon, Average	**1 Tsp/5g**	**8**	**0.6**	**163**	**7.4**	**7.7**	**11.3**	**1.1**
English, Average	**1 Tsp/5g**	**9**	**0.4**	**173**	**6.8**	**19.2**	**7.6**	**1.2**
French, Average	**1 Tsp/5g**	**5**	**0.3**	**106**	**5.4**	**8.1**	**5.6**	**1.8**
German Style, Sainsbury's*	1 Serving/10g	9	0.6	92	5.5	2.8	6.5	0
Honey, Colman's*	1 Tsp/6g	12	0.5	208	7.4	24	8.2	0
Horseradish, Sainsbury's*	1 Tsp/5g	6	0.4	128	5.8	8.3	7.1	3.9
Powder, Average	**1 Tsp/3g**	**15**	**0.9**	**452**	**28.9**	**20.7**	**28.7**	**0**
Smooth, Average	**1 Tsp/8g**	**11**	**0.7**	**139**	**7.1**	**9.7**	**8.2**	**0**
Whole Grain, Average	**1 Tsp/8g**	**11**	**0.8**	**140**	**8.2**	**4.2**	**10.2**	**4.9**
Yellow, New York Deli Style, with Honey, Heinz*	1 Serving/10g	15	0.5	154	5.1	20	4.8	0
MUSTARD CRESS								
Raw	**1oz/28g**	**4**	**0.2**	**13**	**1.6**	**0.4**	**0.6**	**1.1**

N

	Measure INFO/WEIGHT	per Measure KCAL	FAT	Nutrition Values per 100g / 100ml KCAL	PROT	CARB	FAT	FIBRE
NACHOS								
Beef, Chilli, Asda*	1 Serving/200g	208	10	104	10	4.7	5	0.8
Chilli Con, Co-Op*	1 Pack/380g	448	8.4	118	3.9	19	2.2	2.8
Chilli Con, Vegan, Gro, Co-Op*	1 Pack/380g	448	8.4	118	3.9	19	2.2	2.8
Chilli, Sainsbury's*	½ Pack/250g	695	32.2	278	10.9	29.5	12.9	1.3
Kit, Old El Paso*	½ Pack/260g	598	26	230	4	31	10	0
Meal Kit, As Prepared, Sainsbury's*	1 Serving/83g	183	7.1	221	3	31.6	8.5	2.9
with Cheese, From Restaurant, Average	***1 Nacho/16g***	***49***	***2.7***	***306***	***8***	***32.2***	***16.8***	***0***
NASI GORENG								
Asian, Stir Fried, Waitrose*	1 Pack/391g	501	12.1	128	7.7	16.5	3.1	1.8
Indonesian, Asda*	1 Pack/360g	778	22.7	216	7.4	32.3	6.3	1.3
Slimming World*	1 Pack/550g	495	3.3	90	6.8	13.5	0.6	1.6
Vitasia, Lidl*	1 Bowl/250g	438	11	175	7.3	25.8	4.4	1.1
NECTARINES								
Fresh, Raw, Weighed with Stone, Average	***1 Med/140g***	***50***	***0.1***	***36***	***1.2***	***8***	***0.1***	***1.1***
NESQUIK								
Chocolate Flavour, Powder, Dry Weight, Nesquik, Nestle*	1 Serving/15g	56	0.5	372	3	82.9	3.1	6.5
Strawberry Flavour, Powder, Dry Weight, Nesquik, Nestle*	1 Serving/15g	59	0	393	0	98.1	0	0
NETTLES								
Raw, Average	1 Serving/80g	34	0.1	42	2.7	7	0.1	6.9
NIK NAKS								
Cream 'n' Cheesy, KP Snacks*	1 Bag/34g	196	13	575	5.2	52.7	38.1	0.2
Nice 'n' Spicy, KP Snacks*	1 Bag/30g	171	11.5	571	4.6	51.6	38.4	1.6
Rib 'n' Saucy, Golden Wonder*	1 Bag/25g	143	9.4	571	4.5	53.7	37.6	0.5
Scampi 'n' Lemon, KP Snacks*	1 Bag/25g	143	9.4	573	4.9	53.1	37.5	0.1
NOODLES								
Bacon, Dry Supernoodles, Weight, Batchelors*	1 Pack/100g	526	23.6	526	9.4	69.2	23.6	1.6
Beef, BBQ, Instant, Cooked, Aldi*	1 Serving/324g	515	19.4	159	3.7	21.9	6	1.1
Beef, BBQ, Made Up, Supernoodles, Batchelors*	½ Pack/150g	250	11.1	167	3.2	21.3	7.4	1
Beef, Chilli, Ramen, M&S*	1 Pack/484g	532	17.4	110	8.1	11.9	3.6	0.8
Beef, Korean Style, Slimming World*	1 Pack/550g	468	3.3	85	7.5	11.8	0.6	1.4
Beef, Oriental, GFY, Asda*	1 Pack/400g	372	6.8	93	7.4	12.1	1.7	1.7
Beef, Sukiyaki, Cup, Made Up, Nissin*	1 Cup/350g	315	12.2	90	2.2	12.1	3.5	0
Beef, Udon, Shanghai, M&S*	1 Pack/350g	452	14.3	129	7.2	15.1	4.1	1.6
Chicken, & Coconut & Lime, Fuller Longer, M&S*	1 Pack/390g	448	17.6	115	8.7	10	4.5	1.6
Chicken, & Noodle, Sweet Chilli, Tesco*	1 Pot/240g	323	4.3	134	6.4	22.5	1.8	1.3
Chicken, & Red Thai, Easy Steam, Tesco*	1 Serving/400g	556	28.4	139	10.3	8.6	7.1	1.1
Chicken, & Sweetcorn, Snack Pot, Morrisons*	1 Pot/247g	249	1.5	101	4.1	19.8	0.6	1.6
Chicken, & Mushroom, Snack, Made Up, Aldi*	1 Serving/299g	341	7.8	114	18.7	0.5	2.6	2
Chicken, & Prawn, Chinese, Tesco*	½ Pack/298g	307	7.2	103	2.3	16.2	2.4	3.5
Chicken, Aromatic, Weight Watchers*	1 Pack/400g	400	6	100	8.1	12.5	1.5	2.4
Chicken, Chinese, Asda*	1 Pot/302g	305	4.2	101	6	16	1.4	0.8
Chicken, Chinese, Fresh Ideas, Morrisons*	1 Pack/389g	354	7	91	6.3	11.6	1.8	1.8
Chicken, Curry Flavour, Instant, Sainsbury's*	1 Pack/85g	167	6.2	196	4.6	27.9	7.3	0.8
Chicken, Firecracker, Made Up, Naked Noodle*	1 Pot/338g	301	2	89	2.7	17.5	0.6	1.3
Chicken, Flavour, Instant, Made Up, Tesco*	½ Pack/168g	285	10.6	170	4.1	23.7	6.3	1.5
Chicken, Flavour, Instant, Sainsbury's*	1 Pack/335g	549	21.4	164	4.4	22.3	6.4	1.3
Chicken, Hoisin, Box, Co-Op*	1 Pack/243g	265	5.8	109	8.5	12	2.4	1.7
Chicken, Instant, Cooked, Aldi*	½ Pack/150g	248	10.6	165	3.3	21	7.1	1.3
Chicken, Instant, Made Up, HFC, Tesco*	1 Pack/176g	220	7.7	125	3.4	16.4	4.4	3.2
Chicken, Instant, Mama*	1 Pack/350g	238	10.2	68	1.2	9.2	2.9	0
Chicken, Made Up, Supernoodles, Batchelors*	1 Serving/150g	264	11.8	176	3.1	23	7.9	0.4
Chicken, Oriental Style, Instant, Cooked, Koka*	1 Pack/485g	393	16.5	81	1.9	10.4	3.4	0.5
Chicken, Oriental, Slim Choice, Sainsbury's*	1 Pack/490g	333	5.4	68	6.8	6.9	1.1	1.9

	Measure INFO/WEIGHT	per Measure KCAL	FAT	Nutrition Values per 100g / 100ml KCAL	PROT	CARB	FAT	FIBRE
NOODLES								
Chicken, Pad Thai, Waitrose*	1 Pack/400g	588	24	147	6.6	15.5	6	2.6
Chicken, Peri Peri, Super Noodles, Batchelors*	1 Pack/290g	440	18.8	152	3.1	19.5	6.5	1.3
Chicken, Pot, Made Up, Super Noodles, Batchelors*	1 Pot/265g	353	14.9	133	2.5	17.7	5.6	0.9
Chicken, Satay, Fresh Ideas, Morrisons*	1 Pack/400g	468	11.2	117	8.9	13	2.8	2.2
Chicken, Snack Stop, Made Up, Mug Shot*	1 Pack/233g	175	1.2	75	2.3	14	0.5	1.2
Chicken, Soy, Ginger, Slimming World, Iceland*	1 Pack/550g	478	3.8	87	8.1	11.2	0.7	2
Chicken, Spicy, & King Prawn, Bowl, Tesco*	1 Pack/355g	353	2.2	100	7.1	15.2	0.6	2.3
Chicken, Teriyaki, Instant, Nissin*	1 Cup/350g	304	12.6	87	2	11.3	3.6	0
Chow Mein, Made Up, Supernoodles, Batchelors*	½ Pack/150g	262	11.8	175	3	23	7.9	0.4
Chow Mein, Sainsbury's*	1 Pack/125g	136	2.2	109	3.9	19.2	1.8	0.8
Chow Mein, Snack in a Pot, LC, Tesco*	1 Pot/235g	235	1.2	100	3.7	19.4	0.5	1.8
Curry, Instant, Sainsbury's*	1 Pack/335g	412	15.4	123	2.6	17.8	4.6	0.1
Curry, Instant, Vitasia, Lidl*	1 Pack/108g	124	5.3	115	2.5	15.3	4.9	0
Curry, Lost the Pot, Pot Noodle*	1 Pack/92g	132	5.4	144	3.1	19	5.9	0.9
Curry, Mild, Dry Weight, Supernoodles, Batchelors*	½ Pack/50g	260	11.7	520	9.4	67.8	23.4	1.4
Curry, Mild, Made Up, Supernoodles, Batchelors*	1 Serving/100g	157	6.7	157	3.2	20.9	6.7	1
Curry, Singapore, Made Up, Naked Noodle Snack Pot*	1 Pot/329g	270	2	82	2.9	15.7	0.6	0.9
Duck, Shredded, Hoisin, G&B, Asda*	1 Pack/367g	396	6.2	108	5.8	17	1.7	1.8
Egg, Boiled	***1oz/28g***	***17***	***0.1***	***62***	***2.2***	***13***	***0.5***	***0.6***
Egg, Coconut, & Lemongrass, Waitrose*	½ Pack/121g	176	6.2	145	3.6	19.9	5.1	2.7
Egg, Dry, Average	***1 Block/63g***	***218***	***1.2***	***348***	***12.1***	***70.1***	***1.9***	***2.6***
Egg, Fine Thread, Dry, M&S*	1 Serving/63g	220	0.6	350	14.3	71.6	0.9	5.1
Egg, Fine, Blue Dragon*	1 Serving/100g	356	1.7	356	13.8	70	1.7	3.4
Egg, Fine, Dry Weight, Sharwood's*	1 Block/63g	216	1.3	346	12	70	2.1	2.5
Egg, Fine, Fresh, M&S*	1 Pack/275g	330	6.1	120	4.4	20.7	2.2	1.5
Egg, Fine, Morrisons*	¼ Pack/184g	232	0.9	126	4.6	24.8	0.5	1.9
Egg, Fine, Sainsbury's*	1 Nest/150g	256	2.7	171	6	31.8	1.8	1.8
Egg, Fine, Waitrose*	¼ Pack/63g	221	1.6	353	15	67.3	2.6	3.8
Egg, Medium, Asda*	1 Serving/83g	125	0.7	150	4.8	31	0.8	1.3
Egg, Medium, Co-Op*	¼ Pack/144g	168	0.9	117	4.5	23	0.6	1.4
Egg, Medium, Cooked, Sharwood's*	1 Serving/145g	199	1	137	4.7	27.5	0.7	1
Egg, Medium, Dry Weight, Blue Dragon*	1 Nest/50g	186	0.8	372	11.8	77.6	1.6	2.5
Egg, Medium, Dry, Sharwood's*	1 Serving/57g	198	1	348	12	70	1.7	2.5
Egg, Medium, Morrisons*	1 Serving/167g	184	1	110	3.7	22.1	0.6	0.9
Egg, Medium, Sainsbury's*	1 Serving/63g	236	1.2	375	12.5	76.4	1.9	1.3
Egg, Medium, VItasia*	1 Serving/88g	160	1.1	182	6.3	35	1.3	2.4
Egg, Nature's Pick, Aldi*	½ Pack/205g	406	10	198	6.8	30	4.9	3.2
Egg, Raw, Medium, Waitrose*	¼ Pack/63g	221	1.6	353	15	67.3	2.6	3.8
Egg, Tossed in Sesame Oil, Asda*	½ Pack/150g	174	10.5	116	2.3	11	7	0.6
Fried, Average	***1oz/28g***	***43***	***3.2***	***153***	***1.9***	***11.3***	***11.5***	***0.5***
Glass, Dry Weight	***1 Serving/100g***	***351***	***0.1***	***351***	***0.1***	***86.1***	***0.1***	***0.5***
Instant, MR.Noodles *	1 Pack/86g	380	12	442	11.6	67.4	14	2.3
Instant, Spicy Goreng, Hot Heads, Maggie*	1 Pack/119g	547	23.8	460	20	62	20	0
Konjac, Diet, Active Foods, Bulk Powders*	1 Pack/200g	12	1	6	0.5	3.5	0.5	3
Konjac, Raw, Asian Cuisine, Clean Foods*	1 Serving/100g	6	0	6	1	0	0	3.6
Medium, Quick Cook, Sainsbury's*	½ Pack/150g	227	1.5	151	5.4	29	1	2.2
Medium, Ready to Stir Fry, Tesco*	1 Serving/150g	221	2.6	147	5.5	26.3	1.7	2.6
Medium, Soft, Ready to Wok, Asia Specialities, Aldi*	1 Serving/150g	232	0.9	155	6.6	30	0.6	1.6
Mi Goreng, Fried, Instant, Indo Mie*	1 Pack/80g	400	19.4	500	9.6	59.7	24.2	2.3
Nest, Medium, Cooked, Waitrose*	1 Nest/63g	88	0.3	139	5	28.6	0.5	0.6
Pad Kaprao, Thai Taste*	½ Pack/110g	261	5.2	237	6.3	42	4.7	1.4
Pad Thai, Allplants*	1 Serving/387g	507	18.6	131	4.9	16	4.8	2.5
Pad Thai, Chicken, Scratch*	1 Pack/380g	273	6.1	72	7.4	7.9	1.6	1.3

N

	Measure INFO/WEIGHT	per Measure KCAL	FAT	Nutrition Values per 100g / 100ml KCAL	PROT	CARB	FAT	FIBRE
NOODLES								
Pad Thai, Chicken, Waitrose*	½ Pack/100g	170	7.2	170	6.5	18.4	7.2	2.5
Pad Thai, GF, Amy's Kitchen*	1 Pack/268g	407	8.8	152	4.1	26	3.3	1.1
Pad Thai, Ribbon, Ready to Wok, Sharwood's*	1 Serving/150g	206	1.7	137	5	26.3	1.1	1
Pad Thai, Rice, M&S*	½ Pack/137g	246	4	179	3.7	33.4	2.9	2.3
Pea, with Garlic Dressing, High Protein, M&S*	½ Pack/211g	323	5.9	153	8.5	22.4	2.8	2
Plain, Boiled	***1oz/28g***	***17***	***0.1***	***62***	***2.4***	***13***	***0.4***	***0.7***
Plain, Dry	***1oz/28g***	***109***	***1.7***	***388***	***11.7***	***76.1***	***6.2***	***2.9***
Pork, Spicy BBQ, Snack Pot, Tesco*	1 Pot/263g	276	4.5	105	4	17.7	1.7	1.4
Pork, Tonkotsu, Cup, Made Up, Nissin*	1 Cup/350g	322	13.3	92	2.6	11.3	3.8	0
Prawn, Chilli, King, Finest, Tesco*	1 Pack/400g	340	8	85	4	11.9	2	0.9
Prawn, King, Laksa, Slimming World*	1 Pack/550g	346	3.8	63	4.5	8.8	0.7	1.5
Prawn, King, Singapore, Free From, Tesco*	1 Pack/338g	352	11.8	104	3.8	13.8	3.5	1.2
Prawn, Laksa, Diet Chef Ltd*	1 Pack/270g	173	5.4	64	3.1	8.1	2	0.8
Prawn, Tiger, Stir Fry, Tesco*	1 Pack/400g	596	14.8	149	6	23	3.7	2.7
Protein, Stir Fried, Morrisons*	1/3 Pack/95g	141	2.2	148	7.5	24.4	2.3	1.7
Ramen, Morrisons*	1/3 Pack/83g	289	0.7	348	11.1	72.7	0.8	2.8
Ramen, Noodle Kit, Made Up, Blue Dragon*	1 Serving/549g	280	5.5	51	2	8.1	1	0.6
Ribbon, Soft, Sharwood's*	1 Portion/150g	225	1.8	150	5.7	25.7	1.2	6.6
Rice, Cooked	***1 Cup/176g***	***192***	***0.4***	***109***	***0.9***	***24.9***	***0.2***	***1***
Rice, Dry, Blue Dragon*	1 Serving/30g	113	0	376	7	84	0	0
Rice, Gueyteow, Thai Taste*	1 Serving/50g	172	0.6	344	6.7	76.8	1.1	1.4
Rice, Satay, Pot, As Prepared, Itsu*	1 Pot/314g	229	3.5	73	1.7	14	1.1	0.7
Rice, Singapore, Market St, Morrisons*	¼ Pack/90g	192	6.2	214	3.5	33.4	6.9	1.9
Rice, Singapore, Tesco*	½ Pack/150g	316	3.6	211	3.8	43.1	2.4	0.9
Rice, Stir Fry, Tesco*	½ Pack/190g	304	10.8	160	2	24.8	5.7	1
Rice, Sweet Chilli, Ilumi*	1 Pot/375g	292	1.1	78	1.6	17	0.3	0.5
Rice, Vermicelli, Mama*	1 Serving/45g	166	0.4	370	7	81	1	0
Singapore, BGTY, Sainsbury's*	1 Pack/369g	317	10	86	7.2	8.2	2.7	2.1
Singapore, Cook*	1 Serving/275g	289	5.8	105	5.7	16.6	2.1	1.6
Singapore, Sainsbury's*	1 Pack/450g	540	18	120	6.4	13.3	4	2.7
Singapore, Style, Asda*	1 Pack/400g	688	32	172	7	18	8	1
Singapore, Style, Sainsbury's*	½ Pack/150g	320	10.8	214	3.2	33.2	7.2	1.3
Singapore, with Chicken, G&B, Asda*	1 Pack/365g	383	5.5	105	5.4	17	1.5	1
Singapore, with Chicken, Pork, Egg, & Prawns, M&S*	1 Pack/400g	520	20.4	130	6	14.5	5.1	1.2
Soba, Clearspring*	1 Serving/75g	263	2	351	16	64	2.7	3.5
Soba, with Yakisoba Sauce, Instant, Made Up, Nissin*	1 Pot/180g	394	17.6	219	5.3	26.1	9.8	0
Straight to Wok, Medium, Amoy*	1 Pack/150g	240	2.2	160	5.8	31.7	1.5	0
Straight to Wok, Rice, Amoy*	1 Pack/150g	174	0.2	116	1.6	27.4	0.1	0
Straight to Wok, Singapore, Amoy*	1 Serving/150g	206	3.3	137	6.4	21.6	2.2	2.8
Straight to Wok, Thread, Fine, Amoy*	1 Pack/150g	237	3.9	158	5	28.7	2.6	0
Straight to Wok, Udon, Amoy*	1 Pack/150g	212	2	141	4.4	28.8	1.3	0
Sweet & Sour, Asian, Veggie Bowl, Birds Eye*	1 Meal/380g	323	6.8	85	3.5	12.8	1.8	1.7
Sweet & Sour, Cup Shotz, Aldi*	1 Pack/63g	67	0.4	107	2.7	22	0.6	1
Sweet Chilli, Thai, Made Up, Aldi*	1 Pot/338g	301	1.7	89	2.9	18	0.5	1
Teriyaki, Plant Chef, Tesco*	1 Pack/350g	336	8.8	96	1.9	15.2	2.5	2.6
Thai, Style, Sainsbury's*	1 Pack/340g	381	7.8	112	3.3	19.4	2.3	0.7
Thai, Style, Snack, Cupshotz, Aldi*	1 Pack/55g	215	2.8	391	11.4	71.4	5.1	6.9
Udon, Aubergine, Sticky Miso, Sainsbury's*	1 Pack/400g	448	11.2	112	2.6	18.2	2.8	1.7
Udon, Cooked, Just Cook, Sainsbury's*	½ Pack/129g	213	3.6	165	5.1	28.9	2.8	2.3
Udon, Japanese, Sainsbury's*	1 Serving/150g	210	2.7	140	3.9	27.1	1.8	1.2
Udon, Organic, Japanese, Dry Weight, Clearspring*	¼ Pack/50g	177	1	354	14	66	2.1	4.5
Udon, Style, Thick, Ready to Wok, Sharwood's*	1 Pack/150g	233	0.6	155	5.4	32.5	0.4	2.1
Udon, Teriyaki, Allplants*	1 Serving/365g	420	14.6	115	3.8	15	4	2.3

	Measure INFO/WEIGHT	per Measure KCAL	per Measure FAT	Nutrition Values per 100g / 100ml KCAL	PROT	CARB	FAT	FIBRE
NOODLES								
Udon, Yasai Yaki, Allplants*	½ Pack/380g	494	24.3	130	4.4	12	6.4	2.1
Wheat, High Protein, Tesco*	1 Pack/300g	459	3.3	153	9.4	25.4	1.1	1.8
Wholewheat, Cooked Weight, Sharwoods*	1 Portion/161g	215	1.5	134	5	24.8	0.9	2.7
Wholewheat, Dry, Sharwoods*	1 Portion/63g	224	1.4	356	13	66.2	2.3	9.2
Wholewheat, Dry, Tesco*	¼ Pack/66g	227	0.9	342	14.2	64.2	1.4	7.7
Wholewheat, Straight to Wok, Asda*	½ Pack/152g	225	1.2	148	4.9	29	0.8	2.8
NOUGAT								
Average	***1 Sm Bar/28g***	***108***	***2.4***	***384***	***4.4***	***77.3***	***8.5***	***0.9***
Raspberry & Orange Hazelnut, Thorntons*	1 Sweet/9g	39	1.8	433	4.8	60	20	2.2
NUT ROAST								
Average	***1 Serving/200g***	***704***	***51.4***	***352***	***13.3***	***18.3***	***25.7***	***4.2***
Butternut, Almond, & Pecan, Plant Kitchen, M&S*	½ Pack/220g	334	14.1	152	5	14.3	6.4	8.5
Cashew, Quinoa, & Carrot, Deluxe, Lidl*	¼ Pack/88g	252	16.5	286	12.5	14.2	18.7	5.5
Cheese, Melting, Sainsbury's*	1 Nut Roast/140g	364	20.6	260	9.2	19.6	14.7	6.4
Four, Waitrose*	1 Serving/163g	386	23.8	237	5.8	18.8	14.6	3.4
Hazelnut, Cashew, & Cranberry, Deluxe, Lidl*	1/3 Pack/117g	345	21.6	295	12	17.5	18.5	5.4
Kale, & Broccoli, Vegetarian, Tesco*	½ Pack/122g	226	12.1	185	5.9	13.7	9.9	8.8
Lentil, Average	***1oz/28g***	***62***	***3.4***	***222***	***10.6***	***18.8***	***12.1***	***3.8***
Lentil, Red Pepper, & Almond, Vegan, Deluxe, Lidl*	1 Roast/175g	352	17.5	201	8.2	15	10	8.5
Nut, & Cranberry, The Best, Morrisons*	1 Pack/400g	976	52.8	244	5.8	23.7	13.2	3.5
Sweet Potato, & Maple Carrot, Loaf, Sainsbury's*	¼ Loaf/100g	202	12.4	202	9.3	9.6	12.4	7.5
Vegan, GF, Clive's*	1 Serving/140g	216	13.7	154	5.1	20.8	9.8	0
Vegan, Good Health, Waitrose*	½ Pack/143g	315	19.7	220	11.3	7.6	13.8	9.9
NUTMEG								
Ground, Average	***1 Tsp/3g***	***16***	***1.1***	***525***	***5.8***	***45.3***	***36.3***	***0***
NUTS								
Caramelised, Salted, Mixed, Specially Selected, Aldi*	1 Serving/30g	179	13.8	597	5.3	38	46	7.1
Cashews & Peanuts, Honey Roasted, Average	***1 Serving/50g***	***290***	***21.4***	***579***	***21.6***	***26.6***	***42.9***	***4.2***
Chilli, & Lime, Protein, The Foodie Market, Aldi*	1 Pack/25g	154	12.5	614	25	12	50	7.4
Mixed	***1 Pack/40g***	***243***	***21.6***	***607***	***22.9***	***7.9***	***54.1***	***6***
Mixed, Almonds, Brazil, Hazel & Walnuts, M&S*	1 Serving/25g	168	16	670	16	4.8	64	5.4
Mixed, Caramelised, Extra Special, Asda*	1 Serving/30g	180	13.5	599	18	29	45	5.2
Mixed, Chopped, Asda*	1 Serving/30g	181	15.3	604	23	10	51	6
Mixed, Roasted, & Salted, Tesco*	1 Serving/25g	160	13.9	641	20.4	10.7	55.6	8
Mixed, Roasted, Salted, Waitrose*	1 Pack/200g	1252	116.8	626	13.7	11.3	58.4	4.4
Mixed, Roasted, Tesco*	1 Pack/55g	335	26.8	609	23.4	15.1	48.8	7.8
Natural, Collection, M&S*	1 Serving/25g	157	13.7	628	14.8	15.6	54.8	7.6
Selection, Roasted, M&S*	1 Pack/150g	903	74.4	602	24.9	9.5	49.6	9.2
Veggie Burst , Aldi*	1 Pack/25g	140	10	562	30	18	40	4.1
Walnuts, Cashews, & Almonds, Lucky*	1 Box/30g	187	16	622	18.1	15.7	53.5	0
NUTS & RAISINS								
Mixed, Average	***1 Serving/30g***	***144***	***10.2***	***481***	***14.1***	***31.5***	***34.1***	***4.5***
Mixed, Grazin', Holland & Barrett*	1 Pack/200g	888	62	444	8.8	34	31	3.4
Peanuts, Mixed, Average	***1 Pack/40g***	***174***	***10.4***	***435***	***15.3***	***37.5***	***26***	***4.4***
Peanuts, Posh, & Ritzy Raisins, Holland & Barrett*	1 Pack/40g	152	6.2	379	8	54.5	15.4	3
Yoghurt Coated, Waitrose*	1 Serving/50g	264	18.4	527	10.9	38.2	36.7	3
NUTS & SEEDS								
Mixed, Jane Plan*	1 Pack/15g	90	7.8	597	19.4	18.5	52.3	4.2
Paprkia, Smoky, Crunch, Tesco*	1 Pack/35g	152	4.8	434	18	54.5	13.7	10.2
Trail Mix, Natural Days*	1 Serving/30g	133	7.2	442	12	42	24	6

	Measure INFO/WEIGHT	per Measure KCAL	FAT	Nutrition Values per 100g / 100ml KCAL	PROT	CARB	FAT	FIBRE
OAT CAKES								
Ancient Grain, Nairn's*	1 Oatcake/8g	37	1.4	444	13.5	55.3	16.8	8.8
Black Pepper, Savour Bakes, Aldi*	1 Oatcake/10g	45	1.8	450	10	57	18	9.5
Cheese, GF, Nairn's*	1 Oatcake/9g	44	2.2	484	16	45.3	25	7
Cheese, Nairn's*	1 Oatcake/8g	39	2.3	471	13.2	43.3	27.2	6.8
Fine Milled, Nairn's*	1 Oatcake/8g	35	1.7	449	10.5	52.6	21.8	8.6
Fruit, & Seed, On the Go, Nairn's*	1 Oatcake/13g	57	2	437	9.6	60.2	15.5	9.2
Herb & Pumpkin Seed, Nairn's*	1 Oatcake/10g	43	2.1	426	12.2	46.8	21.1	13
Highland, Sainsbury's*	1 Oatcake/13g	56	2.2	446	11	57.4	17.6	7
Highland, Walkers*	1 Oatcake/12g	54	2.5	451	10.3	56	20.6	6.7
Northstaffs Oatcake Bakers Ltd*	1 Oatcake/67g	125	2.3	187	5.8	31.2	3.5	3.9
Oatmeal, Rough, Nairn's*	1 Oatcake/11g	45	1.8	431	10.2	58.6	17.3	8
Oatmeal, Rough, Organic, Nairn's*	1 Oatcake/10g	43	1.7	418	10.2	57.7	16.3	7.5
Orkney, Thick, Stockan's*	1 Oatcake/25g	122	4.6	489	9.8	68	18.2	6.8
Orkney, Thin, Stockan's*	1 Oatcake/13g	65	2.9	501	10.4	62.4	22	6
Retail, Average	***1 Oatcake/13g***	***57***	***2.4***	***441***	***10***	***63***	***18.3***	***2***
Rough with Olive Oil, Paterson's*	1 Oatcake/13g	55	2.1	440	11.7	54.7	17	0
Rough, Crumbly, M&S*	1 Oatcake/13g	58	2.6	463	9.8	56.5	20.5	6.4
Rough, Sainsbury's*	1 Oatcake/10g	47	2	454	9.8	55.4	19.2	10
Rough, Scottish, Tesco*	1 Oatcake/10g	45	1.9	435	11.4	55.3	18.4	8
Scottish, Asda*	1 Oatcake/13g	58	2.3	461	11	59	18	9.8
Seeded, Scottish, Rivercote, Lidl*	1 Oatcake/11g	48	2.1	461	11	54.9	19.9	9.1
Seeded, Waitrose*	1 Oatcake/10g	46	2	461	10.8	54.3	20.3	9.3
Super Seeded, GF, Nairn's*	1 Oatcake/9g	44	2.3	491	12.2	48.4	25.3	10.3
Super Seeded, Organic, Nairns*	1 Oatcake/10g	44	1.9	444	13.4	50.2	19	9.2
Traditional, M&S*	1 Oatcake/11g	49	2	445	11	59.3	18.3	6.6
OAT DRINK								
Barista Edition, Oatly*	1 Serving/200ml	118	6	59	1	6.6	3	0.8
Healthy, Enriched, Oatly*	1 Serving/250ml	112	3.8	45	1	6.5	1.5	0.8
Milk, Acti-Leaf, Aldi*	1 Serving/250ml	120	3.8	48	0.5	7.7	1.5	0.7
Milk, Barista Blend, Califia*	1 Serving/200ml	110	6	55	0.7	5.7	3	0.8
Oat Milk, Barista Blend, Califa Farms*	1 Serving/200ml	110	6	55	0.7	5.7	3	0.8
Oat Milk, Barista, Organic, Rude Health*	1 Serving/200ml	116	4.8	58	0.7	7.8	2.4	0.9
Oat Milk, Organic, Healthy, Oatly*	1 Serving/250ml	100	1.2	40	1	6.7	0.5	0.8
Oat Milk, Unsweetened, Just Free, Lidl*	1 Serving/200ml	74	2.4	37	0.4	5.6	1.2	0.9
Oat, Original, Alpro*	1 Serving/200ml	88	3	44	0.3	6.8	1.5	1.4
Oatmilk, Tesco*	1 Serving/200ml	118	6	59	1	7	3	1
Semi Skimmed, Oatly*	1 Serving/100ml	46	1.5	46	1	6.6	1.5	0.8
Skinny, Oatly*	1 Serving/200ml	74	1	37	1	6.6	0.5	0.8
OCTOPUS								
Chunks in Olive Oil, Palacio De Oriente*	1 Tin/111g	148	4	133	21.6	4.5	3.6	0
Raw	***1oz/28g***	***18***	***0.3***	***66***	***14.1***	***0***	***1***	***0***
OIL								
Avocado, Olivado*	1 Tsp/5ml	40	4.4	802	0	0	88	0
Butter Flavour, Spray, Fry Light*	1 Spray/0.2m	1	0.1	516	0	0.3	53.4	0
Chilli, Average	***1 Tsp/5ml***	***41***	***4.6***	***824***	***0***	***0***	***91.5***	***0***
Coconut, Average	***1 Tsp/5ml***	***45***	***5***	***899***	***0***	***0***	***99.9***	***0***
Cod Liver, Average	***1 Capsule/1g***	***9***	***1***	***900***	***0***	***0***	***100***	***0***
Corn, Average	***1 Tsp/5ml***	***43***	***4.8***	***864***	***0***	***0***	***96***	***0***
Evening Primrose, Average	***1 Serving/1g***	***9***	***1***	***900***	***0***	***0***	***100***	***0***
Fish, Average	***1 Serving/1g***	***9***	***1***	***900***	***0***	***0***	***100***	***0***
Flax Seed, Average	***1 Tbsp/15ml***	***124***	***13.9***	***829***	***0***	***0***	***92.6***	***0***
Garlic, Infuse, Fry Light*	1 Spray/0.2ml	1	0.1	507	0	0.4	52.9	0
Grapeseed, Average	***1 Tsp/5ml***	***43***	***4.8***	***866***	***0***	***0***	***96.2***	***0***

	Measure INFO/WEIGHT	per Measure KCAL	FAT	Nutrition Values per 100g / 100ml KCAL	PROT	CARB	FAT	FIBRE
OIL								
Groundnut, Average	***1 Tsp/5ml***	***41***	***4.6***	***824***	***0***	***0***	***91.8***	***0***
Hazelnut, Average	***1 Tsp/5ml***	***45***	***5***	***899***	***0***	***0***	***99.9***	***0***
MCT, Organic, Nutiva *	1 Tbsp/15ml	130	14	867	0	0	93.3	0
MCT, Pure, C8, Ketosource*	1 Tbsp/15ml	135	15	899	0	0	100	0
Mustard, Average	***1 Serving/100g***	***884***	***100***	***884***	***0***	***0***	***100***	***0***
Olive, Average	***1 Tsp/5ml***	***43***	***4.7***	***855***	***0***	***0***	***94.9***	***0***
Olive, Extra Virgin, Average	***1 Tsp/5ml***	***42***	***4.7***	***848***	***0***	***0***	***94.5***	***0***
Olive, Garlic, Average	***1 Tbsp/15ml***	***127***	***14.1***	***848***	***0***	***0***	***94.3***	***0***
Olive, Mild, Average	***1 Tbsp/15ml***	***129***	***14.4***	***862***	***0***	***0***	***95.7***	***0***
Olive, Spray, Average	***10 Sprays/2ml***	***10***	***1.1***	***508***	***0***	***0***	***54.6***	***0***
Palm, Average	***1 Tsp/5ml***	***45***	***5***	***899***	***0***	***0***	***99.9***	***0***
Peanut, Average	***1 Tsp/5ml***	***45***	***5***	***899***	***0***	***0***	***99.9***	***0***
Rapeseed, Average	***1 Tbsp/15ml***	***130***	***14.4***	***864***	***0***	***0***	***96***	***0***
Rapeseed, Spray, Sizzola*	1 Spray/0.2ml	2	0.2	828	0	0	92	0
Red Palm Fruit, & Rapeseed, Carotino*	1 Tbsp/15ml	124	13.8	828	0	0	92	0
Rice Bran, Average	***1 Tbsp/14g***	***120***	***13.6***	***884***	***0***	***0***	***100***	***0***
Sesame, Average	***1 Tsp/5ml***	***45***	***5***	***892***	***0.1***	***0***	***99.9***	***0***
Sunflower, Average	***1 Tsp/5ml***	***43***	***4.8***	***869***	***0***	***0***	***96.6***	***0***
Sunflower, Spray, Flora*	1 Spray/0.2ml	1	0.2	828	0	0	92	0
Sunflower, Spray, Fry Light*	1 Spray/0.2ml	1	0.1	519	0	0.2	53.9	0
Sunflower, Spray, Sainsbury's*	1 Spray/0.2ml	2	0.2	828	0.5	0.5	92	0.5
Truffle, Black, Truffle Hunter *	1 Tsp/5ml	44	4.9	890	0	1.3	98.3	0
Ultimate Blend, Udo's Choice*	1 Capsule/1ml	9	1	900	1.3	0	96.8	0
Vegetable, Average	***1 Tbsp/15ml***	***129***	***14.3***	***858***	***0***	***0***	***95.3***	***0***
Walnut, Average	***1 Tsp/5ml***	***45***	***5***	***899***	***0***	***0***	***99.9***	***0***
OKRA								
Boiled in Unsalted Water, Average	***1 Serving/80g***	***22***	***0.7***	***28***	***2.5***	***2.7***	***0.9***	***3.6***
Raw, Average	***1 Serving/80g***	***18***	***0.6***	***23***	***2.1***	***2.2***	***0.7***	***3***
Stir-Fried in Corn Oil, Average	***1 Serving/80g***	***215***	***20.9***	***269***	***4.3***	***4.4***	***26.1***	***6.3***
OLIVES								
Basil, & Garlic, Ollys Olives*	1 Pack/50g	75	7.3	149	1.3	1.5	14.6	3.1
Black & Green, with Greek Feta Cheese, Tesco*	1 Pot/100g	200	20.1	200	3.4	0.3	20.1	4.6
Black, & Green, with Greek Feta , Tesco*	1 Serving/30g	54	5	179	4.7	1.4	16.6	2.8
Black, Greek Style, Crespo*	10 Olives/45g	140	13.5	311	2.1	4.5	30	7.5
Black, Pitted, Average	***½ Jar/82g***	***135***	***13.3***	***164***	***1***	***3.5***	***16.2***	***3.1***
Black, Stonless, with Olive Oil, & Sea Salt, Fragata*	½ Pack/60g	97	10.2	161	0.5	0	17	4
Conservolia, & Kalamata, Sainsbury's*	1 Serving/30g	50	4.9	167	1.3	3.1	16.2	1.8
Greek, with Feta, Waitrose*	½ Pot/100g	205	19.2	205	4.7	2.1	19.2	0
Green, Chimichurri, Tesco*	1 Serving/30g	46	4.7	155	1.1	1.1	15.6	2.8
Green, Garlic Stuffed, Asda*	1 Olive/3g	6	0.6	174	1.8	3.5	17	0
Green, Lemon & Thyme, Ollys Olives*	1 Pack/50g	70	7.2	141	1.3	1	14.4	3
Green, Pimento Stuffed, with Gouda & Cumin, Unearthed*	1 Serving/30g	65	6	217	6.6	1	20	2.6
Green, Pitted, Average	***1 Olive/3g***	***4***	***0.4***	***130***	***1.1***	***0.9***	***13.3***	***2.5***
Green, Pitted, in Brine, Drained, The Deli, Aldi*	1 Pot/55g	71	7.2	129	0.9	0.5	13	4.6
Green, Pitted, with Chilli Peppers, Crespo*	1 Pack/70g	132	13.2	189	1.1	0.1	18.9	6.9
Green, Pitted, with Chilli, The Deli, Aldi*	1 Pack/50g	120	12	239	1.4	0.5	24	9
Green, Pitted, with Mixed Herbs, Sainsbury's*	1 Serving/15g	27	2.7	178	1.2	0.6	18.1	4
Green, Stuffed with Almonds, Pitted, Waitrose*	1 Serving/50g	90	8.4	180	3.8	3.2	16.9	2.5
Halkidiki, Stuffed with Garlic, Tesco*	¼ Pack/40g	66	6.7	164	1.3	0.3	16.8	3
Kalamata, in Brine, Drained, Finest, Tesco*	1 Serving/30g	79	8.3	264	1.5	1.2	27.7	1.9
Kalamata, Pitted, Gaea*	1 Serving/15g	26	2.8	172	0.9	2.1	18.7	0
Kalamata, Pitted, Greek, Drained, Sainsbury's*	1 Serving/15g	31	3.2	205	1.6	0.5	21.4	3.2
Kalamata, with Garlic, & Chilli, Waitrose*	1 Serving/30g	83	8.6	278	1.6	2.5	28.5	2.3

	Measure INFO/WEIGHT	per Measure KCAL	FAT	Nutrition Values per 100g / 100ml KCAL	PROT	CARB	FAT	FIBRE
OLIVES								
Manzanilla, & Cheddar, M&S*	1 Pack/180g	391	35.6	217	7	1.4	19.8	2.4
Marinated, Mixed, M&S*	1 Serving/20g	33	3	165	1.6	6.5	14.9	3
Marinated, Selection, M&S*	4 Olives/20g	44	4.4	225	1.4	3.9	22.6	2.1
Mixed, Mediterranean, Morrisons*	1 Serving/30g	74	7.7	248	1	1.6	25.8	2.9
Mixed, with Garlic & Chilli, Tesco*	1 Serving/30g	66	6.8	219	1.2	0.3	22.8	4.3
Mixed, with Mature Cheddar, Tesco*	1/5 Pack/44g	77	7.6	174	3	0.7	17.1	2.6
Spanish, Chimichurri, Specially Selected, Aldi*	¼ Pot/35g	56	5.6	159	1.1	1.4	16	3.1
Spanish, Trio, Sainsbury's*	1/5 Pot/60g	90	7.7	150	1.1	5.1	12.8	5.4
Stuffed, with Garlic, Pimento, & Jalepeno, M&S*	1 Serving/30g	52	5.2	172	1.1	1	17.5	2.9
OMELETTE								
Cheese & Mushroom, Apetito*	1 Serving/320g	486	25	152	6.2	14.4	7.8	1.9
Cheese, 2 Egg, Average	***1 Omelette/180g***	***479***	***40.7***	***266***	***15.9***	***0***	***22.6***	***0***
Cheese, Asda*	1 Omelette/87g	244	19.1	281	15	3.8	22	1.4
Cheese, HFC, Tesco*	1 Omelette/95g	214	16.4	226	13.2	4.1	17.3	0.6
Ham & Mushroom, Farmfoods*	1 Omelette/120g	200	16.7	167	8.7	1.8	13.9	0.1
Mushroom & Cheese, Tesco*	1 Omelette/120g	248	21.5	207	9.8	1.6	17.9	0.2
Plain, 2 Egg	***1 Omelette/120g***	***229***	***19.7***	***191***	***10.9***	***0***	***16.4***	***0***
Potato, Spanish, Waitrose*	1 Pack/500g	710	40	142	6.9	9.5	8	0.5
Spanish	***1oz/28g***	***34***	***2.3***	***120***	***5.7***	***6.2***	***8.3***	***1.4***
Spanish, Plain, with Potatoes, Morrisons*	1 Serving/125g	211	12.1	169	5.1	14	9.7	2.5
Spanish, Unearthed*	1 Pack/250g	362	17.8	145	5.2	15	7.1	1.8
ONION POWDER								
Average	***1 Tsp/2g***	***7***	***0***	***341***	***10.4***	***79.1***	***1***	***15.2***
ONION RINGS								
Battered, Free From, Tesco*	3 Rings/63g	190	9.5	303	3.1	37.3	15.2	2.1
Battered, Harvest Basket, Lidl*	1 Serving/91g	190	9.3	209	3.2	25.3	10.2	1.8
Battered, Mini, Frozen, Tesco*	4 Rings/34g	87	3.9	259	4.2	32.8	11.6	3.3
Battered, Oven Baked, Tesco*	1 Serving/50g	110	5	219	3.9	28.4	10	3.5
Battered, Sainsbury's*	1 Ring/12g	32	1.4	265	3.8	34.4	11.6	4.1
Beer Battered, Frozen, Tesco*	3 Rings/75g	213	10	284	4.6	36	13.3	0.8
Beer Battered, M&S*	1 Serving/70g	151	6.5	216	2.7	29.6	9.3	1.4
Beer Battered, Mash Direct*	½ Pack/100g	283	10.3	283	2.6	23.9	10.3	2.7
Breaded & Fried, From Restaurant	***1 Ring/12g***	***40***	***2.2***	***332***	***4.5***	***37.7***	***18.7***	***0***
Cajun, The Pizza Company*	¼ Pack/68g	172	9.4	253	3.4	27.7	13.8	2.5
Oven Crisp Batter, Tesco*	1 Ring/17g	44	1.9	259	4.1	34.4	11.2	2.1
ONIONS								
Baked	***1oz/28g***	***29***	***0.2***	***103***	***3.5***	***22.3***	***0.6***	***3.9***
Boiled in Unsalted Water	***1oz/28g***	***5***	***0***	***17***	***0.6***	***3.7***	***0.1***	***0.7***
Crispy, Top Taste*	1 Serving/10g	59	4.4	590	6	40	44	0
Dried, Raw, Average	***1oz/28g***	***88***	***0.5***	***313***	***10.2***	***68.6***	***1.7***	***12.1***
Flakes, Dried, Average	***1 Tbsp/15g***	***52***	***0.1***	***349***	***9***	***83.3***	***0.5***	***9.2***
Fried, Average	***1oz/28g***	***46***	***3.1***	***164***	***2.3***	***14.1***	***11.2***	***3.1***
Pickled, Average	***1 Onion/15g***	***3***	***0***	***19***	***0.7***	***4.1***	***0.1***	***0.6***
Pickled, Hot & Spicy, Premium, Barry Norman*	1 Serving/50g	32	0.2	65	1	15	0.5	1.6
Raw, Average	***1 Med/180g***	***69***	***0.4***	***38***	***1.2***	***7.9***	***0.2***	***1.3***
Red, Raw, Average	***1 Med/180g***	***66***	***0.4***	***37***	***1.2***	***7.9***	***0.2***	***1.5***
Spring, Raw, Average	***1 Med/15g***	***4***	***0.1***	***24***	***1.9***	***2.9***	***0.5***	***1.4***
ORANGE CURD								
Jaffa, Luxury, Waitrose*	1 Tbsp/15g	54	1.5	357	3	63.5	10.1	0.1
ORANGES								
Blood, Average	***1 Orange/140g***	***82***	***0***	***58***	***0.8***	***13.3***	***0***	***2.5***
Fresh, Weighed with Peel, Average	***1 Med/220g***	***97***	***0.5***	***44***	***0.9***	***10.8***	***0.2***	***3.2***
Fresh, without Peel, Average	***1 Med/154g***	***97***	***0.5***	***63***	***1.3***	***15.5***	***0.3***	***4.5***

	Measure INFO/WEIGHT	per Measure KCAL	FAT	Nutrition Values per 100g / 100ml KCAL	PROT	CARB	FAT	FIBRE
ORANGES								
Peel Only, Raw, Average	***1 Tbsp/6g***	***6***	***0***	***97***	***1.5***	***25***	***0.2***	***10.6***
OREGANO								
Dried	***1 Tsp/1g***	***3***	***0.1***	***306***	***11***	***49.5***	***10.3***	***0***
Fresh	***1 Tsp/1.3g***	***1***	***0***	***66***	***2.2***	***9.7***	***2***	***0***
*OVALTINE**								
Chocolate, Light, Dry Weight, Ovaltine*	1 Serving/20g	75	1.2	376	4.7	74	5.9	0
Chocolate, Light, Sachet, Ovaltine*	1 Sachet/25g	96	1.5	384	7.4	73	5.9	4.7
Hi Malt, Light, Instant Drink, Ovaltine*	1 Sachet/20g	72	1.2	358	9.1	67.1	5.9	2.8
Powder, Made Up with Semi-Skimmed Milk, Ovaltine*	1 Mug/227ml	179	3.9	79	3.9	13	1.7	0
Powder, Made Up with Whole Milk, Ovaltine*	1 Mug/227ml	220	8.6	97	3.8	12.9	3.8	0
OXTAIL								
Raw	***1oz/28g***	***18***	***1.1***	***65***	***7.6***	***0***	***3.8***	***0***
Stewed, Bone Removed	***1oz/28g***	***68***	***3.8***	***243***	***30.5***	***0***	***13.4***	***0***
OYSTERS								
Raw, Shelled, Shucked	***1 Oyster/14g***	***9***	***0.2***	***65***	***10.8***	***2.7***	***1.3***	***0***

	Measure INFO/WEIGHT	per Measure KCAL	FAT	KCAL	PROT	CARB	FAT	FIBRE
				Nutrition Values per 100g / 100ml				
PAELLA								
Bean, & Vegetable, Spanish, Veg Pot, BOL Foods*	1 Pot/345g	321	8.3	93	2.4	14.6	2.4	1.7
Chicken, & Chorizo, Calorie Controlled, Morrisons*	1 Pack/299g	284	5.7	95	7.6	10.8	1.9	2
Chicken, & Prawn, King, BFY, M&S*	1 Pack/390g	429	10.1	110	8.6	12.1	2.6	1.9
Chicken, & Chorizo, Rice Pot, Tesco*	1 Pack/330g	469	10.6	142	5.5	22	3.2	1.4
Chicken, & Chorizo, SlimWell, Aldi*	1 Pack/500g	430	3.5	86	5.7	13	0.7	2.4
Chicken, & Chorizo, Weight Watchers, Heinz*	1 Meal/399g	395	6.8	99	6.8	13	1.7	2.1
Chicken, & Prawn, BGTY, Sainsbury's*	1 Pack/368g	383	8.8	104	8.2	11.4	2.4	1.9
Chicken, & Prawn, Slim Choice, Sainsbury's*	1 Pack/500g	425	3	85	6.2	13.1	0.6	1.3
Chicken, & Prawn, Slim Cook, Tesco*	1 Pack/500g	380	3	76	6.2	10.5	0.6	2.3
Chorizo, Spanish, Twist'd Flavour Co.*	1 Serving/125g	159	4.6	127	4	18	3.7	1.9
Prawn, King, & Chicken, The Best, Morrisons*	½ Pack/399g	519	19.6	130	5.9	14.7	4.9	1.7
Vegetable, Chunky, Love Your Veg!, Sainsbury's*	1 Pack/382g	367	8	96	2.4	16.1	2.1	1.6
PAIN AU CHOCOLAT								
All Butter, Frozen, Sainsbury's*	1 Pain/53g	205	10.4	386	10.7	40.1	19.7	2.7
Almond, The Delicatessen, Tesco*	1 Pain/100g	406	22	406	0	45	22	0
Average	***1 Pastry/60g***	***253***	***13.7***	***422***	***8***	***45.8***	***22.8***	***3.1***
GF, Schar*	1 Pain/65g	225	9.8	346	3.7	46	15	5.8
Mini, Asda*	1 Pastry/23g	96	5.5	420	8	43	24	3.3
PAIN AU RAISIN								
All Butter, M&S*	1 Pain/90g	287	12.9	319	6.6	38.9	14.3	4.1
Bakery, Sainsbury's*	1 Pastry/100g	335	14.5	335	6	44.6	14.5	1.4
Bakery, Tesco*	1 Pastry/107g	351	14.7	328	6.9	43.3	13.7	1.8
Takeaway, Average	***1 Pastry/100g***	***313***	***13.2***	***313***	***5.2***	***43***	***13.2***	***1.3***
Twist, Extra Special, Asda*	1 Pastry/110g	421	20.9	383	7	46	19	2.5
PAK CHOI								
Raw, Average	***1 Leaf/14g***	***2***	***0***	***11***	***1.3***	***1.9***	***0.2***	***0.9***
PAKORA								
Bhaji, Onion, Fried in Vegetable Oil	***1oz/28g***	***76***	***4.1***	***271***	***9.8***	***26.2***	***14.7***	***5.5***
Bhajia, Potato Carrot & Pea, Fried in Vegetable Oil	***1oz/28g***	***100***	***6.3***	***357***	***10.9***	***28.8***	***22.6***	***6.1***
Bhajia, Vegetable, Retail	***1oz/28g***	***66***	***4.1***	***235***	***6.4***	***21.4***	***14.7***	***3.6***
Chicken, Indian, Sainsbury's*	½ Pack/45g	95	3.3	211	27.7	7.8	7.4	1
Chicken, M&S*	½ Pack/50g	96	4	192	25.2	2.2	8.1	4.6
Chicken, Taste of India, Tesco*	1 Pack/150g	345	10.8	230	26.6	13.8	7.2	1.8
PANCAKE								
American Style, Galberts*	1 Pancake/50g	182	11	365	5.2	36.6	22	0.9
Asda*	1 Pancake/23g	59	1.6	254	4.8	43	7	4
Blueberry, Tesco*	1 Pancake/75g	195	3.1	260	4.8	49.5	4.1	2
Buttermilk, Genesis*	1 Serving/100g	219	3.7	219	4.9	41	3.7	1.1
Buttermilk, Giant , Village Bakery, Aldi*	1 Pancake/65g	146	1.8	225	6.7	42	2.8	1.7
Buttermilk, Large, Tesco*	1 Pancake/65g	176	3.9	270	6.7	46.8	6	1.2
Buttermilk, The Best, Morrisons*	1 Pancake/65g	154	3.4	237	6.4	40.6	5.2	1.3
Classic, Sainsbury's*	1 Pancake/62g	146	8	234	5.1	24	12.8	1.2
Golden Syrup, GF, Free From, Morrisons*	1 Pancake/35g	89	0.6	255	4.4	54.6	1.8	1.6
Mini, Scotch, Tesco*	1 Pancake/16g	44	0.9	277	6.7	50	5.6	1.4
Plain, Prepared From Recipe, Average	***1 Pancake/38g***	***86***	***3.7***	***227***	***6.4***	***28.3***	***9.7***	***0***
Raisin & Lemon, Asda*	1 Serving/30g	92	2.4	304	6	52	8	1.4
Raisin & Lemon, Sainsbury's*	1 Pancake/35g	95	1.5	272	6.3	51.8	4.4	2.2
Ready Made, Average	***1 Sm/30g***	***77***	***1.9***	***258***	***6.1***	***44.2***	***6.4***	***1.7***
Savoury, Made with Skimmed Milk, Average	***1 Pancake/77g***	***192***	***11.3***	***249***	***6.4***	***24.1***	***14.7***	***0.8***
Scotch	***1 Pancake/50g***	***146***	***5.8***	***292***	***5.8***	***43.6***	***11.7***	***1.4***
Sweet, Asda*	1 Pancake/60g	161	6	268	4.8	38	10	0.9
Syrup & Sultana, Kingsmill*	1 Pancake/36g	102	1.7	287	5.7	54.7	4.7	1.7
Syrup, Tesco*	1 Pancake/30g	80	2.5	265	4.7	42.1	8.2	1.5

	Measure INFO/WEIGHT	per Measure KCAL	per Measure FAT	Nutrition Values per 100g / 100ml KCAL	PROT	CARB	FAT	FIBRE
PANCAKE								
Vegetable Roll	***1 Roll/85g***	***185***	***10.6***	***218***	***6.6***	***21***	***12.5***	***0***
with Syrup, American Style, Large, Tesco*	1 Pancake/38g	102	1.3	268	5.1	54.2	3.4	0.9
PANCAKE MIX								
Protein, Myprotein*	1 Serving/50g	186	3.2	372	67	11	6.3	0
Protein, Original, Active Foods*	1 Scoop/50g	168	1.2	336	72	13.8	2.3	1.5
Slender, Dry, Protein World*	1 Serving/50g	172	1.5	343	21.4	57.3	3	2.9
PANCETTA								
Air Dried, Sliced, Cooks' Ingredients, Waitrose*	1 Slice/7g	35	3.3	506	16.9	0.8	48.3	0
Average	***½ Pack/65g***	***212***	***18.7***	***326***	***17***	***0.1***	***28.7***	***0***
Smoked, Diced, Tesco*	¼ Pack/33g	96	7.9	291	18.5	0.3	24	0
PANINI								
Cheese, Tesco*	1 Panini/100g	249	9.1	249	10.5	31.3	9.1	3.1
Chicken, Arrabiata, Ginsters*	1 Panini/200g	489	16.8	245	12.8	29.4	8.4	2.4
Ham, & Cheese, Ginsters*	1 Panini/200g	567	25.6	283	13.3	28.7	12.8	1.6
Mozzarella, & Tomato, M&S*	1 Serving/176g	484	28.5	275	11.3	21.3	16.2	2.1
Tuna, & Sweetcorn, Tesco*	1 Serving/250g	559	16.4	224	12	29.3	6.6	1.4
PANNA COTTA								
BGTY, Sainsbury's*	1 Pot/150g	150	2.8	100	2.4	18.2	1.9	1.4
Caramel, Sainsbury's*	1 Serving/120g	319	15.1	266	4	31.8	12.6	0.7
Caramelon, Milbona, Lidl*	1 Pot/90g	152	8.1	169	2.4	19.5	9	0
Raspberry, COU, M&S*	1 Pot/140g	146	3.5	104	2.6	17.5	2.5	0.6
Raspberry, Hotel Chocolat*	1 Serving/30g	162	11.2	541	6	45.6	37.4	0
Sainsbury's*	1 Pot/100g	304	15.7	304	3	41.5	15.7	4
Strawberry, COU, M&S*	1 Pot/145g	145	3.8	100	2.6	15.7	2.6	0.8
PAPAYA								
Dried, Pieces, Nature's Harvest*	1 Serving/50g	178	0	355	0.2	85.4	0	2.6
Raw, Flesh Only, Average	***1 Serving/140g***	***37***	***0.1***	***26***	***0.4***	***6.6***	***0.1***	***1.2***
PAPPARDELLE								
Beef, Deluxe, Lidl*	1 Serving/400g	472	9.6	118	5.7	176	2.4	1.6
Beef, Ragu, Slow Cooked, M&S*	½ Pack/400g	512	22	128	7	12	5.5	1.1
Egg, Dry, Average	***1 Serving/100g***	***364***	***3.7***	***364***	***14.1***	***68.5***	***3.7***	***2.1***
Italian, Fresh, Waitrose *	1/3 Pack/117g	182	1.8	156	5.9	29.1	1.5	1.2
PAPRIKA								
Average	***1 Tsp/2g***	***6***	***0.3***	***289***	***14.8***	***34.9***	***13***	***0***
PARATHA								
Aloo Gobi, Shana*	1 Paratha/100g	224	7	224	5.5	34.8	7	0
Average	***1 Paratha/80g***	***258***	***11.4***	***322***	***8***	***43.2***	***14.3***	***4***
Roti, Plain, Crown Farms*	1 Slice/80g	250	10	312	5	46.2	12.5	1.2
PARCELS								
Chicken, & Bacon, Sainsbury's*	½ Pack/170g	406	28.6	239	21.9	0.1	16.8	0
Chicken, & Bacon, Specially Selected, Aldi*	1 Parcel/190g	572	34.2	301	12	22	18	0.5
Feta, & Spinach, Filo, Sainsbury's*	1 Parcel/27g	83	5.6	307	5.8	23.8	20.7	1.8
Goats Cheese, & Caramelised Onion, Asda*	1 Parcel/22g	71	4.2	325	6.6	30	19	2.3
Mac & Cheese, Bacon Wrapped, Stacks, M&S*	1 Parcel/20g	55	3.6	277	14.5	13.2	17.8	1.1
Salmon, Iceland*	1 Parcel/140g	365	21.1	261	10.3	20.7	15.1	0.6
Salmon, Puff Pastry, Cream Cheese Sauce & Dill, Tesco*	1 Parcel/124g	334	19.4	269	10.7	20.5	15.6	1.8
Vegetable, Katsura, Crispy, M&S*	1 Pack/100g	281	13.7	281	5.6	32.8	13.7	2
PARSLEY								
Dried	***1 Tsp/1g***	***2***	***0.1***	***181***	***15.8***	***14.5***	***7***	***26.9***
Fresh, Average	***1 Tbsp/3.8g***	***1***	***0***	***27***	***2.4***	***2.2***	***1***	***4***
Root, Raw, Average	***1 Avg Root/33g***	***18***	***0.2***	***55***	***2.3***	***12.3***	***0.6***	***4.3***
PARSNIP								
Boiled, Average	***1 Serving/80g***	***53***	***1***	***66***	***1.6***	***12.9***	***1.2***	***4.7***

	Measure INFO/WEIGHT	per Measure KCAL	FAT	Nutrition Values per 100g / 100ml KCAL	PROT	CARB	FAT	FIBRE
PARSNIP								
Honey Glazed, Roast, Baked, Aunt Bessie's*	1 Serving/100g	158	12	158	1.1	8.6	12	5.1
Honey Glazed, Roast, Deluxe, Lidl*	1 Serving/100g	134	5.7	134	1.4	17.2	5.7	4
Honey Roast, Oven Baked, Iceland*	1 Serving/100g	164	7.5	164	2	19.3	7.5	5.4
Honey Roasted, Tesco*	½ Pack/142g	159	5	112	1.2	16.8	3.5	4.2
Raw, Unprepared, Average	***1 Serving/100g***	***62***	***1***	***62***	***1.7***	***11.6***	***1***	***4.3***
Roast, Honey Glazed, Frozen, Aunt Bessie's*	¼ Pack/125g	234	16.2	187	1.4	14	13	4.4
PARTRIDGE								
Breast, Fillets, No.1, Waitrose*	1 Pack/150g	189	3.6	126	25.7	0.1	2.4	0.5
Meat Only, Roasted	***1 Partridge/260g***	***551***	***18.7***	***212***	***36.7***	***0***	***7.2***	***0***
PASSATA								
Fina, Biona Organic*	1 Serving/100ml	34	0.2	34	1.4	5.8	0.2	1.7
Italian, Rustica, TTD, Sainsbury's*	1 Bottle/430g	155	6.9	36	1.1	3.7	1.6	1
Italian, with Onion & Garlic, Classic, Sainsbury's*	¼ Carton/125g	29	0.6	23	1.3	3.6	0.5	1.2
Italian, with Onion, & Garlic, Sainsbury's*	1 Pack/390g	117	2	30	1.9	4.3	0.5	1.5
Tomato, Freshona, Lidl*	1 Carton/500g	170	2.5	34	1.5	4.6	0.5	1.3
Tomato, Napolina*	½ Carton/196g	55	0.4	28	1.7	4.3	0.2	1.1
Tomato, with Garlic & Herb, Italian, Tesco*	½ Carton/250g	55	0.5	22	1.2	2.9	0.2	1.8
PASSION FRUIT								
Raw, Fresh, Average	***1 Fruit/18g***	***7***	***0.1***	***36***	***2.6***	***5.8***	***0.4***	***3.3***
Weighed with Skin, Average	***1 Fruit/30g***	***7***	***0.1***	***22***	***1.6***	***3.5***	***0.2***	***2***
PASTA								
Alphabet Shapes, Dry, Sainsbury's*	1 Serving/70g	223	1	319	10.2	65	1.4	2.8
Arrabiata, Roasted Vegetable, Low Fat, Co-Op*	1 Pack/380g	391	7.6	103	3.3	17	2	1.7
Beefy Bolognese, Pot Pasta, Pot Noodle*	1 Pot/268g	252	5.1	94	3.3	15	1.9	1.6
Butternut Mac, Oven Baked, Plant Based, Asda*	1 Pack/349g	391	5.2	112	3.7	20	1.5	1.8
Cappelletti, Prosciutto, Italian, Sainsbury's*	½ Pack/200g	362	9.4	181	9.6	23.9	4.7	2.2
Casarecce, Cooked Weight, Free From, Sainsbury's*	1 Serving/200g	342	2.6	171	3.7	35.8	1.3	1.1
Cavatoni, Dry, Italiamo, Lidl*	1 Serving/60g	213	1	355	11	73	1.6	2.3
Cheese Feast, Fully Loaded, Sainsbury's*	½ Pack/283g	382	13.3	135	6.2	15.6	4.7	2.7
Cheese, Leek, & Ham, Pasta n Sauce, Batchelors*	½ Pack/184g	235	3.9	128	5	21.9	2.1	0.7
Cheese, Macaroni, Dry, Pasta n Sauce, Batchelors*	1 Pack/108g	402	5.1	372	17.2	65.2	4.7	2.7
Cheese, Three, Melt, Co-Op*	½ Pack/400g	632	21	158	7	20	5.2	1.2
Chicken, & Chorizo, Average	***1 Pack/400g***	***174***	***5.7***	***174***	***10.1***	***20.3***	***5.7***	***1.5***
Chicken, & Mushroom, Made Up, Mug Shot*	1 Serving/260g	221	3.6	85	2.2	15.7	1.4	0.5
Chicken, & Bacon, Italian, Iceland*	1 Pack/400g	492	11.6	123	6.8	16.9	2.9	1
Chicken, & Bacon, Made Up, Pasta n Sauce, Batchelors*	½ Pack/183g	211	2.9	115	4.4	20.6	1.6	0.6
Chicken, & Mushroom, Free From, Tesco*	1 Pack/373g	393	5.6	105	4.4	18.1	1.5	0.9
Chicken, & Tomato, Calorie Controlled, Tesco*	1 Pack/300g	357	1.8	119	7.8	20.1	0.6	1.2
Chicken, Creamy, Microwaved, G&B, Asda*	½ Pack/303g	352	7.9	116	7.5	15	2.6	2.2
Chicken, Peri Peri, No Mayonnaise, Tesco*	1 Pack/300g	363	5.1	121	4.3	21.4	1.7	1.4
Chicken, Pesto, & Tomato, Fresh Ideas, Morrisons*	1 Pack/379g	466	10.2	123	7.1	15.7	2.7	3.9
Chicken, Roast, As Consumed, Mug Shot*	1 Serving/258g	201	2.6	78	2.8	14.2	1	0.5
Chicken, Tomato, & Basil, Tesco*	1 Pack/300g	471	11.1	157	6.7	23.3	3.7	1.6
Conchiglie, Cooked, Cucina, Aldi*	1 Serving/150g	216	0.9	144	5	29	0.6	1.3
Conchiglie, Dry Weight, Cucina, Aldi*	1 Serving/60g	188	0.6	314	11	63	1	2.9
Farfalle, Spinach, Cooked Weight, Tesco*	1 Serving/170g	300	1.2	176	5.8	35.7	0.7	2.2
Fettuccine, Edamame, & Mung Bean, Cooked, Aldi*	¼ Pack/158g	183	4	116	16	3	2.5	8.3
Fusillata Casareccia, Cooked, The Best, Morrisons*	1 Serving/180g	326	1.1	181	7.2	35.8	0.6	2.2
Girasoli, Ricotta, & Spinach, Creamy, Aldi*	½ Pack/155g	312	15.5	201	7.1	19	10	2.2
Green Pea, GF, As Prepared, Love Life, Waitrose*	1 Serving/175g	276	1.6	158	10.5	24.1	0.9	5.5
Green Pea, GF, Dry, Free From, Morrisons*	1 Serving/75g	262	1.1	349	18.5	61.1	1.5	9.1
Ham, & Mushroom, Melt, Italian, Morrisons*	½ Pack/387g	631	21.7	163	7.5	20.3	5.6	0.9
Itailan Style, with Peppers, Morrisons*	1 Pack/550g	902	42.4	164	3.4	19.4	7.7	1.5

P

	Measure	per Measure		Nutrition Values per 100g / 100ml				
	INFO/WEIGHT	KCAL	FAT	KCAL	PROT	CARB	FAT	FIBRE
PASTA								
King Prawn Alfredo, Luxury, Iceland*	1 Pack/437g	620	25.3	142	6	15.7	5.8	1.8
Mac & Greens, Vegan, Waitrose*	1 Pack/380g	437	17.1	115	3.2	13.7	4.5	3.7
Macaroni, Butternut Cauli Mac, Plant Chef, Tesco*	1 Pack/377g	434	9.4	115	3.6	18.6	2.5	1.8
Macaroni, GF, Free From, Morrisons*	1 Serving/50g	86	0.3	172	2.8	38.6	0.6	0.9
Margherite, Basil, & Pinenut, TTD, Sainsbury's*	½ Pack/125g	259	10.9	207	7.8	23.5	8.7	1.5
Meat Feast, Microwaved, Slimming World*	1 Pack/550g	478	7.2	87	7.3	10.9	1.3	1.3
Orzo, Cooked Weight, TTD, Sainsbury's*	1 Serving/200g	318	1.2	159	6.2	31.4	0.6	1.5
Orzo, Cooked, Finest, Tesco*	1 Serving/170g	289	0.8	170	6.8	33.9	0.5	1.2
Orzo, Dry, Average	***1 Serving/100g***	***348***	***1.5***	***348***	***12.4***	***71.9***	***1.5***	***3***
Pesto, with Semi Dried Tomatoes, Tesco*	1 Pack/225g	432	18.2	192	5.6	23.4	8.1	1.7
Pumpkin, & Pine Nut, Stuffed, Fiorelli, Fresh, Waitrose*	½ Pack/125g	225	7.5	180	8	22.3	6	2.3
Ravioli, Crab & Crayfish, Dell'ugo*	½ Pack/125g	229	8.1	183	7.4	23	6.5	1.4
Raviolini, Ricotta, & Spinach, The Fresh Pasta Company*	½ Pack/125g	316	16	253	9.7	23.8	12.8	2
Rotolo, Beef, & Pancetta, Deluxe, Lidl*	½ Pack/376g	703	39.8	187	8.2	13.8	10.6	1.7
Sausage, in Tomato & Basil Sauce, Sainsbury's*	1 Pack/393g	471	14.1	120	4.6	16.5	3.6	1.5
Shapes, Cooked, Smart Price, Asda*	1 Serving/175g	257	1.2	147	4.6	30	0.7	1.7
Shapes, Dry, Smart Price, Asda*	1 Serving/75g	265	1.3	353	11	72	1.7	4.1
Tomato, & Chorizo, Micro Pasta, Asda*	1 Pack/200g	356	7.2	178	6.5	28	3.6	4.7
Triangoli, Wild Porcini Mushroom, & Truffle, Cooked, Aldi*	1 Pack/349g	708	33.1	203	7	21	9.5	2.3
Tuna, & Sweetcorn, Tesco*	½ Pot/150g	253	11.6	169	6.5	17.9	7.7	0.9
Vegetable, Mediterranean, Cooked, BGTY, Sainsbury's*	1 Pack/400g	347	5.5	89	2.8	15.2	1.4	1.9
Wholewheat, Cooked, Tesco*	1 Serving/200g	284	1.8	142	5.7	27.9	0.9	4.5
PASTA BAKE								
Bacon & Leek, Average	***1 Serving/400g***	***633***	***32.3***	***158***	***6.7***	***14.8***	***8.1***	***1.3***
Beef, Bolognese, Meal to Share, M&S*	½ Pack/400g	700	30.8	175	9.3	16.6	7.7	1.2
Bolognese, Weight Watchers*	1 Pack/359g	230	2.5	64	4.3	9.4	0.7	1.3
Cheese, & Tomato, Italiano, Tesco*	1 Bake/300g	354	12.6	118	3.9	16.1	4.2	1
Chicken, & Bacon, Average	***1 Serving/400g***	***627***	***28.7***	***157***	***9***	***13.7***	***7.2***	***1.6***
Chicken, Bacon & Mushroom, Average	***1 Serving/400g***	***632***	***29.2***	***158***	***7.8***	***15.1***	***7.3***	***2.3***
Chicken, Pesto, & Mozzarella, Meal to Share, M&S*	½ Pack/400g	632	24.4	158	8.3	16.7	6.1	1.3
Mac 'n' Greens, Slimming World*	½ Pack/275g	190	1.1	69	3.9	11.5	0.4	1.7
Mac 'n' Greens, Vegan, Slimming World*	1 Pack/550g	473	1.1	86	3.6	16.1	0.2	3
Meat Feast, Average	***1 Serving/400g***	***601***	***21.4***	***150***	***5.8***	***19.2***	***5.4***	***1.4***
Pepperoni, Tesco*	1 Pack/436g	575	16.1	132	6.1	17.8	3.7	1.6
Sausage, Average	***1 Serving/400g***	***591***	***24***	***148***	***5.5***	***17.7***	***6***	***1.9***
	1 Pack/400g	628	20	157	5.5	21	5	2
Tomato, & Mozzarella, Average	***1 Serving/400g***	***500***	***12.4***	***125***	***5.3***	***17.3***	***3.1***	***1.5***
Tomato, & Mascarpone, Iceland*	1 Pack/413g	491	13.6	119	4.1	17.4	3.3	1.6
Tomato, Creamy, Dolmio*	1 Serving/125g	141	9	113	2.3	8.4	7.2	0
Tomato, Inspired Cuisine, Aldi*	1 Pack/600g	774	21	129	7.8	16	3.5	2.3
Tuna, & Sweetcorn, Average	***1 Pack/400g***	***423***	***22.4***	***106***	***5***	***8.6***	***5.6***	***1.9***
Tuna, Aldi*	1 Pack/400g	568	16	142	7.9	18	4	1.1
Tuna, Co-Op*	1 Pack/501g	626	18	125	79	15	3.6	1
Tuna, Italian, Waitrose*	1 Pack/385g	578	20.4	150	8.6	16.5	5.3	0.9
Tuna, M&S*	1 Pack/380g	555	20.5	146	9.2	14.6	5.4	1.1
Vegetable, M&S*	1 Pack/350g	396	13.3	113	4.4	14.5	3.8	1.4
PASTA QUILLS								
Dry, Average	***1 Serving/75g***	***256***	***0.9***	***342***	***12***	***72.3***	***1.2***	***2***
GF, Salute*	1 Serving/75g	269	1.4	359	7.5	78	1.9	0
PASTA SALAD								
BLT, Asda*	1 Pack/301g	406	16.8	135	4.6	16	5.6	1.6
Cheese, Average	***1 Serving/370g***	***782***	***56.8***	***211***	***5.5***	***12.8***	***15.4***	***1.2***
Chicken, & Bacon, Caesar, Asda*	1 Pack/300g	552	30	184	6.9	16	10	1.2

	Measure INFO/WEIGHT	per Measure KCAL	per Measure FAT	Nutrition Values per 100g / 100ml KCAL	PROT	CARB	FAT	FIBRE
PASTA SALAD								
Chicken, & Bacon, Caesar, Tesco*	1 Pack/265g	418	18.3	158	11.5	12.1	6.9	0.7
Chicken, & Bacon, Tesco*	½ Pack/233g	487	28.6	209	6.6	17.6	12.3	0.9
Chicken, Bacon, & Sweetcorn, M&S*	1 Pack/380g	680	33.1	179	8.2	16.1	8.7	1.7
Chicken, Piri Piri, Asda*	1 Pack/320g	333	9	104	6	13	2.8	2
Chicken, Spicy, Asda*	1 Pack/309g	346	7.1	112	5.3	17	2.3	1.2
Chicken, Spicy, On the Go, Sainsbury's*	1 Pot/300g	455	10.8	152	6.4	22.7	3.6	1.5
Chicken, Sweet Chilli, Asda*	1 Pack/225g	259	5.4	115	5.2	17	2.4	2.5
Chicken, Tomato, & Basil, 205g Pot, M&S*	1 Pack/205g	340	14.6	166	8	16.7	7.1	1.4
Chicken, Tomato, & Basil, Tesco*	1 Pack/260g	235	3.9	90	7.7	10.8	1.5	1.1
Feta, & Red Pepper, Bowl, Co-Op*	1 Pack/260g	420	16	162	5.8	19.6	6.2	2.2
Feta, & Slow Roasted Tomato, M&S*	1 Pack/190g	344	13.3	181	6.5	22.3	7	2.5
Goats Cheese, & Mixed Pepper, Sainsbury's*	1 Pack/200g	366	18.8	183	6.4	18.2	9.4	1.5
Ham, & Cheese, Asda*	½ Pack/160g	213	10.7	133	4.9	12	6.7	1.8
Orzo, Specially Selected, Aldi*	1 Pack/210g	328	10.5	156	4	23	5	0.8
Pesto, & Pine Nut, Asda*	1 Serving/125g	306	13.8	245	6.7	29	11	3.7
Pesto, Spicy Chilli, Sainsbury's*	¼ Pot/63g	170	12.3	272	3.8	20.1	19.6	1.6
Prawn Cocktail, Layered, Shapers, Boots*	1 Pot/210g	181	5.2	86	3.6	13	2.5	1.3
Prawn, Co-Op*	1 Pack/281g	323	14.6	115	4.5	12	5.2	1.8
Prawn, Growers Selection, Asda*	1 Pack/380g	365	9.1	96	5.1	13	2.4	1.2
Prawn, Morrison's*	1 Pack/250g	528	35.5	211	3.7	16.5	14.2	1.1
Salmon, Hot Smoked, Boots*	1 Pack/230g	341	16	148	6.1	15.6	7	0.6
Spinach, & Pine Nut, Sainsbury's*	½ Pot/100g	226	11.6	226	6.4	23	11.6	2.2
Tomato, & Basil, Sainsbury's*	1 Serving/83g	121	3.4	145	3.7	22.7	4.1	1.6
Tomato, & Basil, Asda*	1 Pack/550g	605	9.4	110	3.8	19	1.7	1.8
Tomato, & Basil, The Deli, Aldi*	1 Bowl/375g	514	12	137	4.2	22	3.2	1.9
Tuna, & Sweetcorn, HE, Tesco*	1 Pot/200g	230	5.4	115	5.7	17	2.7	1.3
Tuna, & Sweetcorn, Meadow Fresh, Lidl*	½ Pack/190g	272	19	143	17.5	31.2	10	3
Tuna, & Sweetcorn, On the Go, Sainsbury's*	1 Pack/300g	492	17.1	164	5.9	21.6	5.7	1.4
Tuna, Jane Plan*	1 Pack/220g	242	7.7	110	6.9	12	3.5	0.8
Vegetable, Chargrilled, Sainsbury's*	1 Serving/178g	192	4.8	108	2.7	15.9	2.7	4.7
PASTA SAUCE								
Amatriciana, M&S*	1 Jar/340g	425	32.3	125	3.4	6.3	9.5	2.9
Arrabbiata, Finest, Tesco*	½ Pot/175g	214	10.5	122	3.7	13	6	1.1
Arrabbiata, Fresh, Tesco*	½ Pot/175g	84	3.2	48	0.8	6.7	1.8	0.9
Arrabbiata, Waitrose*	1/3 Jar/116g	67	3.7	58	1.3	5.2	3.2	1.7
Arrabiata, Barilla*	1 Serving/100g	47	3	47	1.5	3.5	3	0
Arrabiata, Fresh, Co-Op*	½ Pot/150g	82	4.5	55	1	5	3	1
Arrabiata, GFY, Asda*	1 Serving/350g	133	3.9	38	1.1	6	1.1	0
Artichoke, Sacla*	½ Pot/95g	249	21.8	262	1.9	9.2	23	5.3
Bacon, Smoky, Loyd Grossman*	½ Jar/175g	142	8.4	81	3	6.1	4.8	0.8
Basilico, Healthier Choice, Mr Organic*	1 Jar/350g	528	3.5	151	1.7	5.6	1	1.5
Bolognese, Baresa, Lidl*	¼ Jar/125g	55	0.5	44	1.6	7.6	0.4	1.6
Bolognese, Cucina, Aldi*	1 Serving/100g	37	0.5	37	0.9	7	0.5	0.9
Bolognese, Free From, Tesco*	¼ Jar/125g	63	0.9	51	1.9	8.4	0.7	1.5
Bolognese, Garlic & Onion, Intense, Dolmio*	1 Jar/500g	210	1	42	1.7	7.4	0.2	1.8
Bolognese, Napolina*	½ Jar/175g	89	1.9	51	1.9	6.4	1.1	3.8
Bolognese, Organic, Seeds of Change*	1 Jar/500g	290	6	58	1.3	10.4	1.2	0.8
Bolognese, Original, Sainsbury's*	¼ Jar/136g	90	2.9	66	1.9	9.9	2.1	1.3
Bolognese, Smooth, Hidden Vegetables, Dolmio*	1 Portion/125g	60	1	48	1.4	7.7	0.8	1.9
Bolognese, Specially Selected, Aldi*	1 Jar/340g	187	9.2	55	1.5	5.5	2.7	1.1
Bolognese, Tesco*	1 Serving/100g	41	0.7	41	1.4	6.6	0.7	1.3
Bolognese, Tomato, & Herb, Sainsbury's*	1 Jar/500g	280	7	56	2	7.9	1.4	2
Bolognese, Waitrose*	¼ Jar/125g	79	5.2	63	1.2	4.4	4.2	1.5

	Measure INFO/WEIGHT	per Measure KCAL	FAT	Nutrition Values per 100g / 100ml KCAL	PROT	CARB	FAT	FIBRE
PASTA SAUCE								
Bolognese, with Beef, Tesco*	½ Pack/175g	170	10	97	5.6	4.7	5.7	2.1
Cacciatore, Fresh, Sainsbury's*	½ Pot/150g	152	8.8	101	5.4	8.1	5.9	1.5
Carbonara, Asda*	½ Pot/175g	359	29.8	205	7	6	17	0.1
Carbonara, Co-Op*	½ Pot/150g	270	25.5	180	3	4	17	0.1
Carbonara, Creamy, Dolmio Express, Dolmio*	1 Pack/150g	166	13.2	111	3.3	4.7	8.8	0.1
Carbonara, Creamy, Stir in Sauce, Dolmio*	1 Serving/75g	98	8	130	3.3	5.2	10.6	0.2
Carbonara, Italian, Fresh, Sainsbury's*	½ Pot/176g	209	16.3	119	5.4	3.4	9.3	0.9
Cheese, Four, Sainsbury's*	1 Serving/150g	296	25.5	197	6.6	4.5	17	0.8
Cheese, Three, Co-Op*	1 Pack/300g	405	27	135	6	6	9	0.1
Chunky Vegetable, Co-Op*	¼ Jar/125g	48	0.6	38	1.5	6.9	0.5	0.5
Lasagne, White, Morrisons*	½ Jar/215g	245	20.2	114	2	5.2	9.4	0.5
Lasagne, White, Ragu, Knorr*	1 Jar/475g	755	72.2	159	0.5	5.1	15.2	0.3
Mac & Cheese, Pasta Bake, Sainsbury's*	¼ Jar/118g	176	14.9	149	1.8	6.9	12.6	0.5
Macaroni Cheese, Pasta Bake, Asda*	¼ Jar/118g	147	11.3	125	1.5	8	9.6	0.5
Mediterranean, Fresh, Waitrose*	1 Pot/350g	214	13.6	61	1.4	5	3.9	2.4
Mushroom, & Cream, M&S*	1oz/28g	45	4	160	1.5	6.6	14.3	0.6
Mushroom, Chunky, Cucina, Aldi*	1 Jar/500g	200	2.5	40	1.6	7.4	0.5	1.3
Mushroom, Italian, Sainsbury's*	1 Serving/85g	56	1.8	66	2	9.8	2.1	1.7
Mushroom, Sainsbury's*	1 Serving/100g	66	2.1	66	2	9.8	2.1	1.7
Mushroom, Tesco*	1/6 Jar/120g	48	0.6	40	1.2	6.9	0.5	1.5
Napoletana, M&S*	½ Jar/170g	126	7.8	74	1.9	4.5	4.6	3.7
Napoletana, Sainsbury's*	½ Pot/150g	126	8.4	84	1.9	6.6	5.6	0.9
Puttanesca, Loyd Grossman*	½ Jar/175g	117	6	67	1.4	5.5	3.4	0.7
Spaghetti, Sweet Filipino, Ufc*	1 Serving/61g	40	0	66	0	16.4	0	0
Sun Dried Tomato, Stir In, Baresa, Lidl*	½ Pack/75g	86	6	115	0.9	9.2	8	0.9
Sun-Dried Tomato, Stir In, Cucina, Aldi*	½ Pot/75g	77	5	103	2	8	6.7	1.2
Sweet Pepper, Tesco*	½ Pot/77g	47	1.8	61	1.3	8.2	2.4	0.7
Toamto, & Basil, M&S*	½ Pack/175g	163	11.8	93	1.6	5.9	6.8	1.4
Tomato, & Basil, Dolmio*	1 Serving/170g	95	3.6	56	1.4	7.9	2.1	0
Tomato, & Basil, Loyd Grossman*	½ Jar/175g	107	6	61	1.5	5.8	3.4	0.8
Tomato, & Basil, Morrisons*	½ Jar/140g	76	0.7	54	1.7	10.1	0.5	1.3
Tomato, & Chilli, Pour Over, M&S*	1 Jar/330g	231	12.5	70	1.3	7.6	3.8	1.8
Tomato, & Garlic, Roasted, CBY, Asda*	1 Pot/350g	122	2.1	35	1.5	5	0.6	1.7
Tomato, & Garlic, Roasted, Loyd Grossman*	½ Jar/175g	133	5.6	76	2	9	3.2	1.4
Tomato, & Herb, Sainsbury's*	¼ Jar/125g	70	1.8	56	2	7.9	1.4	2
Tomato, & Mascarpone, Sainsbury's*	½ Pot/150g	137	9.9	91	2.1	5.9	6.6	1.2
Tomato, & Onions, Original, Morrisons*	1 Serving/125g	51	1.4	41	1.4	6.3	1.1	1.2
Tomato, & Parmesan, Seeds of Change*	1 Serving/150g	100	4.4	67	2.5	7.8	2.9	1.1
Tomato, & Ricotta, Italian, Sainsbury's*	1 Pack/390g	238	11.7	61	2.5	6.1	3	1.2
Tomato, & Tuna, Loyd Grossman*	½ Jar/175g	154	7.7	88	4.4	7.5	4.4	0.8
Tomato, & Basil, Chef Select, Lidl*	½ Pack/175g	68	2.3	39	1.2	4.6	1.3	2
Tomato, & Basil, Fresh, Co-Op*	1 Pot/300g	135	4.8	45	1.6	4.5	1.6	3.3
Tomato, & Basil, Inspired Cuisine, Aldi*	½ Pot/175g	96	3.5	55	1.7	7	2	1
Tomato, & Basil, Morrisons*	½ Pot/175g	110	5.1	63	1.8	6.4	2.9	2.1
Tomato, & Basil, No Added Sugar, Dolmio*	1 Jar/350g	182	7	52	1.6	6.1	2	1.6
Tomato, & Basil, Tesco*	1 Serving/175g	89	3.7	51	1.1	6.3	2.1	1.1
Tomato, & Herb, HFC, Tesco*	¼ Jar/110g	36	0.8	33	0.8	5.5	0.7	0.8
Tomato, & Mascarpone, Fresh, Tesco*	½ Pot/175g	161	11.4	92	2.7	5.3	6.5	0.8
Tomato, & Mascarpone, Inspired Cuisine, Aldi*	½ Pack/176g	123	7.6	70	1.8	5.9	4.3	0.7
Tomato, & Pepperoni, Morrisons*	½ Pot/175g	189	13	108	4.2	4.6	7.4	2.9
Tomato, & Sweet Garlic, M&S*	½ Jar/170g	104	5.1	61	1.3	7	3	0.5
Tomato, Bacon, & Mushroom, Asda*	½ Pot/50g	33	1.8	66	2.5	6	3.6	0
Tomato, Lasagne, Cucina, Aldi*	1 Jar/500g	165	2.5	33	1.2	6.3	0.5	0.8

	Measure INFO/WEIGHT	per Measure KCAL	FAT	Nutrition Values per 100g / 100ml KCAL	PROT	CARB	FAT	FIBRE
PASTA SAUCE								
Tomato, Onion, & Garlic, Baresa, Lidl*	1 Jar/500g	240	2.5	48	2.1	7.8	0.5	1.8
Tomato, Smooth, Cucina, Aldi*	1 Jar/500g	275	4.5	55	1.8	7	0.9	1.2
Tomato, with Basil Pesto, Rich, Express, Dolmio*	1 Pack/170g	146	10	86	2	6.2	5.9	0
Vegetable, Chargrilled, Stir-In, Sainsbury's*	½ Pot/75g	67	3.5	89	1.7	8.5	4.7	2.8
Vegetable, Chunky, Tesco*	1 Jar/500g	235	5	47	1.8	6.8	1	1.8
Vegetable, Mediterranean, Tesco*	1 Serving/166g	95	2.8	57	1.4	9	1.7	1.2
Vegetable, Morrisons*	¼ Jar/125g	56	1.1	45	1.4	7	0.9	1.6
Vegetable, Roasted, Sainsbury's*	½ Pot/151g	103	5.9	68	1.6	6.7	3.9	0.4
PASTA SHELLS								
Dry, Average	***1 Serving/75g***	***265***	***1.5***	***353***	***11.1***	***71.8***	***2***	***2***
Egg, Fresh, Average	***1 Serving/125g***	***344***	***3.6***	***275***	***11.5***	***49.8***	***2.8***	***3.4***
PASTA TWISTS								
Dry, Average	***1oz/28g***	***99***	***0.4***	***354***	***12.2***	***71.8***	***1.5***	***2.2***
Wheat & GF, Glutafin*	1 Serving/75g	262	1.5	350	8	75	2	0.1
PASTE								
'Nduja, Cooks' Ingredients, Waitrose*	1 Tbsp/15g	80	7.6	536	15.7	2.4	50.8	3.3
Barbacoa, Tesco*	1 Serving/30g	32	0.8	107	1.9	16.7	2.6	4.5
Beef, Asda*	1 Serving/37g	72	5.2	194	17	0.1	14	0
Beef, Princes*	1 Serving/18g	42	3.1	231	15.2	3.4	17.4	0
Beef, Sainsbury's*	1 Jar/75g	142	9.9	189	16	1.5	13.2	1.4
Chicken, & Ham, Tesco*	1 Serving/19g	44	3.7	231	12.5	1.4	19.5	0
Chicken, Tesco*	1 Serving/12g	30	2.4	248	14.8	2.3	20	0.1
Chilli, Chipotle, M&S*	¼ Jar/24g	36	1.1	151	2.2	22.8	4.4	5.9
Chilli, Sainsbury's*	1 Tsp/6g	5	0.4	82	1	2.9	5.8	7.3
Chipotle, Chilli, Tesco*	1 Tsp/5g	8	0.2	158	2.8	23.3	4.8	5.2
Crab, Sainsbury's*	1 Spread/5g	6	0.2	115	16.5	1.7	4.7	0.5
Ginger, Barts*	1 Tsp/5g	6	0.6	127	0.6	5	11.2	0
Mediterranean, M&S*	¼ Jar/50g	66	1.8	133	2.5	21.4	3.5	2.7
Nasi Goreng, Waitrose*	½ Pack/50g	69	3.6	138	2	15.7	7.3	1.1
Salmon, & Haddock, Sainsbury's*	1 Tbsp/17g	21	0.9	123	14.3	4.4	5.1	1.3
Salmon, Asda*	1 Tbap/15g	30	2.2	198	12	4.2	15	1.4
Salmon, Value, Tesco*	1 Serving/10g	16	1	165	14	4.6	10.1	0.8
Sardine, & Tomato, Princes*	1 Jar/75g	130	8.1	173	13.9	3.4	10.8	3.2
Sardine, & Tomato, Sainsbury's*	1 Mini Pot/35g	60	3.8	170	16.9	1.2	10.8	1.3
Tamarind, M&S*	¼ Jar/30g	38	0	125	0.9	30.1	0.1	0.5
Tuna Mayo, Asda*	1 Pot/75g	137	9	183	16	3.2	12	0.6
Tuna, & Mayonnaise, Tesco*	1 Serving/15g	32	2.3	215	15.8	0.7	15.6	2.2
PASTILLES								
Fruit, 30% Less Sugar, Rowntree's*	1 Sweet/3g	9	0	312	6.5	62	0.1	16.2
Fruit, Average	***1 Tube/33g***	***108***	***0***	***327***	***2.8***	***84.2***	***0***	***0***
Fruit, Rowntree's*	1 Tube/53g	186	0	351	4.4	83.7	0	0
PASTRAMI								
Beef, Average	***1 Serving/40g***	***51***	***1.4***	***128***	***23.1***	***1.1***	***3.6***	***0.2***
Style, Vegan, Slices, Squeaky Bean*	1 Pack/100g	223	6.5	223	31	5.9	6.5	7.9
Turkey, Average	***½ Pack/35g***	***38***	***0.5***	***107***	***21.8***	***1.7***	***1.5***	***0.5***
PASTRY								
Apricot, Danish, Bakery in Store, M&S*	1 Pastry/130g	347	15	267	5.4	34.6	11.5	1.8
Case, From Supermarket, Average	***1 Case/230g***	***1081***	***58.9***	***470***	***5.8***	***55.9***	***25.6***	***1.2***
Cheese, & Spinach, Lattice, Aldi*	1 Serving/138g	406	26.2	294	7	24	19	2.2
Chicken, & Mushroom, Lattice, Tesco*	1 Lattice/110g	222	6	202	8.4	28.8	5.5	2.1
Choux, Cooked, Average	***1oz/28g***	***91***	***5.5***	***325***	***8.5***	***29.8***	***19.8***	***1.2***
Churros, with Chocolate Dip, Plant Kitchen, M&S*	1 Churro/19g	76	4.8	398	4	38.2	25.2	1.2
Cinnamon Swirls, Bake it Fresh, Jus-Rol*	1 Swirl/45g	162	7.1	360	6.2	47.7	15.7	1.6

	Measure INFO/WEIGHT	per Measure KCAL	FAT	Nutrition Values per 100g / 100ml KCAL	PROT	CARB	FAT	FIBRE
PASTRY								
Cinnamon Swirls, Danish Selection, Tesco*	1 Swirl/35g	151	8.8	432	6.4	43.5	25.2	2.8
Cream Horn, Fresh, Asda*	1 Horn/50g	207	12	414	4.9	43	24	2
Crown, Raspberry, Sainsbury's*	1 Pastry/87g	334	18.1	384	5.7	42.3	20.8	2.2
Feta, Herb, & Spinach, Tesco*	2 Pastries/65g	168	8.3	258	7.4	27.2	12.8	2.3
Filo, Average	***1 Sheet/45g***	***137***	***1.2***	***304***	***9***	***61.4***	***2.7***	***0.9***
Flaky, Cooked, Average	***1oz/28g***	***157***	***11.4***	***560***	***5.6***	***45.9***	***40.6***	***1.8***
Horn, Filled with Jam, & Cream, M&S*	1 Horn/54g	218	12.3	404	3.9	45.6	22.8	0.6
Jambons, Fajita Chicken, Golden Bake*	1 Jambon/104g	280	17.7	269	7.3	22	17	1.5
Lattice, Spinach, Leek, & Cheddar, Mae's Kitchen, Aldi*	1 Lattice/138g	406	26.2	294	7	24	19	2.2
Lattice, Vegetarian, Aldi*	1 Lattice/138g	345	20	250	5	22.5	14.5	2.8
Prawn, Roses, Finest, Tesco*	1 Rose/17g	52	3.1	303	10.7	23.4	18.1	1.8
Puff, Block, Tesco*	1 Block/500g	2095	137	419	6.1	35.4	27.4	3.2
Puff, Frozen, Average	***1 Serving/47g***	***188***	***12***	***400***	***5***	***29.2***	***25.6***	***0***
Puff, GF, Jus-Rol*	1 Serving/50g	170	9.8	341	2.5	36.8	19.6	4
Puff, Light, Sheet, Jus-Rol*	1 Serving/50g	166	8.2	332	6.4	38.3	16.5	2.3
Puff, Lighter, Ready Rolled, Tesco*	1 Serving/60g	241	10.9	401	9	48.7	18.1	3.6
Puff, Palmier, Jam, & Cream, Asda*	1 Palmier/92g	432	27.5	472	5.5	44	30	1.8
Puff, Ready Rolled, Finest, Tesco*	1 Pack/320g	1478	103	462	9.2	32.6	32.2	2.3
Quorn, Roll, Ginsters*	1 Roll/100g	299	18.8	299	8.2	21	18.8	6.2
Shortcrust, Cooked, Average	***1oz/28g***	***146***	***9***	***521***	***6.6***	***54.2***	***32.3***	***2.2***
Shortcrust, Raw, Average	***1oz/28g***	***127***	***8.1***	***453***	***5.6***	***44***	***29.1***	***1.3***
Slices, Cream, Cream Cake Selection, Tesco*	1 Slice/65g	249	12.4	383	4	48.3	19	1.2
Steak, & Onion, Lattice, Pastry, Tesco*	1 Serving/167g	374	17.9	223	12	18.9	10.7	1.7
Sweet Heart, All Butter, Brompton House*	1 Pastry/11g	59	3.5	539	5.9	56	32	1.6
Swirl, Sweet, Lidl*	1 Pastry/37g	171	9.2	461	6.8	51	25	2.3
Twists, Chocolate, All Butter, M&S*	1 Twist/71g	280	15.1	394	7.6	41.4	21.3	3.1
Twists, Sea Salt, & Pepper, M&S*	1 Twist/9g	44	2.2	491	10.2	56.3	24.2	3.4
Vanilla Slice, Frozen, Tesco*	1 Slice/38g	136	6	359	4.7	48.9	15.8	1.5
PASTY								
Beef, Iceland*	1 Pasty/130g	324	16.2	249	5.5	26.8	12.5	1.8
Beef, Mini, Asda*	1 Pasty/16g	55	3.3	337	8.1	30	20	2.3
Cauliflower, Curried, Wicked Kitchen, Tesco*	1 Pasty/150g	361	19.5	241	4.1	26.2	13	1.1
Cheese, & Onion, Average	***1 Pasty/150g***	***435***	***27.6***	***290***	***7.3***	***24.5***	***18.4***	***1.4***
Chicken, Tikka, Asda*	1 Pasty/30g	103	6	343	8	31	20	2.3
Cornish, Average	***1 Pasty/160g***	***450***	***27.7***	***281***	***7***	***24.2***	***17.3***	***1.6***
Cornish, Frozen, Baked, Ginsters*	1 Pasty/130g	343	20.4	264	6.6	23.2	15.7	1.9
Cornish, Mini, Sainsbury's*	1 Pasty/70g	280	20.1	400	7.3	28.1	28.7	1.5
Meat Free, Quorn*	1 Pasty/141g	285	10.3	202	5.6	26.6	7.3	3.4
No Beef, Vegan, Mae's Kitchen, Aldi*	1 Pasty/170g	420	25.5	247	5.9	20	15	3
No Bull, Meat Free, Vegan, Oven Baked, Iceland*	1 Pasty/190g	431	22.6	227	5.5	23.3	11.9	2.5
No Cheese, & Onion, Iceland*	1 Pastry/170g	471	31.3	277	4.4	22.4	18.4	2.3
Quorn, Vegan, Ginsters*	1 Pasty/180g	436	23.8	242	6.4	23.1	13.2	2.7
Vegan, Waitrose*	1 Pasty/130g	346	20.3	266	7.7	22.3	15.6	2.6
Vegetable	***1oz/28g***	***77***	***4.2***	***274***	***4.1***	***33.3***	***14.9***	***1.9***
Vegetable, Moroccan, Ginsters*	1 Pasty/180g	409	22.5	227	3.8	23.6	12.5	2.4
Vegetarian, Cornish Style, Quorn*	1 Pasty/150g	320	15	213	6.9	22.5	10	3
PATE								
Ardennes, BGTY, Sainsbury's*	1 Serving/30g	59	4.5	197	12.3	3.2	15	0.5
Ardennes, Coarse, with Smoked Bacon, Tesco*	1 Serving/40g	78	5.8	194	10.7	5.1	14.4	0.8
Ardennes, Reduced Fat, Essential, Waitrose*	¼ Pack/43g	103	7.5	242	14.4	6	17.7	0.5
Ardennes, Tesco*	1 Tbsp/15g	53	5	354	13.3	0.5	33.2	1.2
Ardennes, with Bacon, Tesco*	½ Pack/85g	241	20.6	284	11.4	5.1	24.2	1.1
Brussels, & Garlic, Tesco*	1 Serving/40g	145	13.5	363	8.7	6	33.8	0

P

	Measure INFO/WEIGHT	per Measure KCAL	FAT	Nutrition Values per 100g / 100ml KCAL	PROT	CARB	FAT	FIBRE
PATE								
Brussels, & Garlic, Morrisons*	1 Serving/50g	132	11	263	9.4	6.2	22	1.3
Brussels, 25% Less Fat, Morrisons*	¼ Pack/43g	106	8.8	249	14.2	0.7	20.6	0
Brussels, Co-Op*	1 Serving/15g	51	4.6	340	11	4	31	2
Brussels, M&S*	1 Spread/7g	23	2.1	323	9.9	1.9	30.5	0.5
Brussels, Reduced Fat, Warren & Sons, Lidl*	1 Serving/35g	71	5.2	204	12	5	15	0.7
Brussels, Sainsbury's*	1 Pack/170g	663	64.9	390	10.6	1.1	38.2	0.1
Brussels, Smooth, Eastmans, Tesco*	1/5 Pack/35g	87	9.2	249	9.6	4.6	26.2	0.5
Brussels, Smooth, Spreadable, Sainsbury's*	1 Serving/30g	97	8.7	323	10.7	4.7	29	0
Brussels, with Caramelised Shallots, The Best, Morrisons*	1 Serving/30g	91	7.5	304	8.8	10.7	25	0.5
Brussels, with Mushrooms, Wild, The Best, Morrisons*	1 Serving/30g	92	7.9	308	9.7	7.2	26.3	1.8
Chicken Liver, Smooth, M&S*	¼ Pack/42g	108	9	255	7.8	8	21.2	0.5
Chicken Liver, Smooth, Specially Selected, Aldi*	¼ Pack/43g	126	11.5	296	8.6	4.2	27	0.5
Chicken, Liver, French, Waitrose*	¼ Pack/40g	162	16.1	406	8.8	1.9	40.2	0.5
Chicken, Liver, M&S*	½ Pack/85g	173	13.1	204	11	5	15.4	0.5
Chicken, Liver, Parfait, Specially Selected, Aldi*	1 Portion/85g	278	26.4	327	11	2.1	31	0.6
Chicken, Liver, Parfait, Waitrose*	1 Pack/100g	258	22.9	258	7.5	4.8	22.9	1.1
Chicken, Liver, with Madeira Jelly, Waitrose*	½ Pack/40g	100	8.7	251	6.4	6.8	21.7	1.4
De Campagne, Extra Special, Asda*	1 Pate/55g	163	13.2	296	17	2.5	24	0
De Campagne, M&S*	1 Serving/30g	47	2.7	158	13.6	5.4	8.9	0.9
De Campagne, Sainsbury's*	1 Serving/55g	129	10	235	16.3	1.4	18.2	0
De Campagne, Waitrose*	¼ Pack/40g	145	13.1	362	13.1	3.2	32.7	1.1
Duck, Liver, with Port, TTD, Sainsbury's*	1/5 Pack/30g	71	5.6	238	8.2	8.3	18.8	1.3
Farmhouse, Co-Op*	1 Serving/57g	148	11.9	261	14	4.3	21	0
Farmhouse, with Mushrooms, Sainsbury's*	1 Serving/30g	76	6.8	252	11.3	1.2	22.5	0.5
Garlic, & Herb, Yeast, Tartex*	1 Serving/30g	69	5.4	230	7	10	18	0
Layered, Duck, & Pork, Sainsbury's*	1 Serving/30g	94	8	313	11.3	6.8	26.7	0.5
Mackerel, Smoked	***1oz/28g***	***103***	***9.6***	***368***	***13.4***	***1.3***	***34.4***	***0***
Mackerel, Tesco*	1 Serving/29g	102	9.5	353	14.3	0.5	32.6	0
Mushroom, Coarse, Roasted, M&S*	1 Serving/30g	57	4.8	190	3.4	8	15.9	0.7
Mushroom, Sainsbury's*	½ Pot/58g	85	6.7	147	3.9	5.8	11.6	0
Mushroom, Vegan, Suma*	1 Serving/50g	115	9.1	230	8.3	5.8	18.2	4.8
Mushroom, Wild, Yeast, GranoVita*	1 Serving/50g	106	8.5	213	10	5	17	0
Pork, Hyperu*	1 Serving/28g	104	9.8	372	10	4.3	35	0
Salmon, Smoked, Coarse, M&S*	1 Serving/30g	61	4.4	202	14.4	2.9	14.7	0.6
Salmon, Smoked, Waitrose*	1 Serving/38g	70	4.7	185	16.8	1.3	12.4	0.5
Trout, Smoked, Waitrose*	1 Serving/34g	59	3.7	176	18.3	0.6	11.1	0
Tuna, Coarse, M&S*	½ Pack/57g	136	10.5	239	14.8	3.3	18.5	0.6
Tuna, Tesco*	1 Pack/115g	332	26.7	289	19.8	0.3	23.2	0.2
Tuna, with Butter & Lemon Juice, Sainsbury's*	½ Pot/58g	145	11.5	251	15.5	2.2	19.9	0.6
Vegetable	***1oz/28g***	***48***	***3.8***	***173***	***7.5***	***5.9***	***13.4***	***0***
PATTY								
Lamb, Curried, Island Delight*	1 Patty/140g	451	28	322	6.4	28	20	1.4
Lamb, Jamaican, Port Royal*	1 Patty/130g	352	17.4	271	7.2	30.5	13.4	0
Vegetable, Jamaican, Patty, Island Delight*	1 Patty/140g	423	22.4	302	5.2	35	16	0
Vegetarian, Jamaican, Port Royal*	1 Patty/130g	315	13.8	242	12.5	24.1	10.6	0
PAVLOVA								
Base, Cooks' Ingredients, Waitrose*	1 Serving/17g	62	0	366	4.8	91.2	0.2	0
Maltesers, Mars*	1 Serving/50g	205	8.1	410	3.6	61.7	16.2	0
Raspberry, Individual, M&S*	1 Serving/65g	133	1.6	205	4	41.8	2.4	0.2
Raspberry, M&S*	1 Serving/84g	193	8.1	230	2.3	33.3	9.6	0.3
Raspberry, Tesco*	1 Serving/65g	191	8.4	294	2.7	41.8	12.9	1.1
Sticky Toffee, Sainsbury's*	1 Serving/60g	249	9.8	415	3.7	63.1	16.4	0.9

	Measure INFO/WEIGHT	per Measure KCAL	FAT	Nutrition Values per 100g / 100ml KCAL	PROT	CARB	FAT	FIBRE
PAW-PAW								
Raw, Fresh	***1oz/28g***	***10***	***0***	***36***	***0.5***	***8.8***	***0.1***	***2.2***
Raw, Weighed with Skin & Pips	***1oz/28g***	***6***	***0***	***20***	***0.3***	***5***	***0.1***	***1.3***
PEACH								
Dried, Average	***1 Pack/250g***	***472***	***1.6***	***189***	***2.6***	***45***	***0.6***	***6.9***
in Fruit Juice, Average	***1oz/28g***	***13***	***0***	***47***	***0.5***	***11.2***	***0***	***0.7***
in Light Syrup, Canned, As Sold	***1 Serving/100g***	***66***	***0***	***66***	***0.4***	***15.9***	***0***	***1***
Raw, Stoned, Average	***1oz/28g***	***9***	***0***	***33***	***1***	***7.6***	***0.1***	***1.5***
Raw, Weighed with Stone, Average	***1 Peach/125g***	***39***	***0.1***	***31***	***1***	***7.2***	***0.1***	***1.3***
Slices in Fruit Juice, Average	***1 Serving/100g***	***49***	***0***	***49***	***0.6***	***11.6***	***0***	***0.5***
Slices, Canned, in Water, Drained, Morrisons*	1 Serving/81g	25	0.2	31	0.3	6.4	0.2	1.4
PEANUT BUTTER								
Crunchy, 100% Nuts, Morrisons*	1 Tbsp/15g	91	7.2	606	26.4	12.2	48.3	8.7
Crunchy, Mister Choc, Lidl*	1 Tbsp/15g	92	7.4	614	25.3	12	49	7.2
Crunchy, Natural, No Added Sugar or Salt, Average	***1 Tbsp/15g***	***91***	***7.3***	***606***	***27.6***	***12.2***	***48.4***	***7***
Crunchy, Rich Roast, 100% Nuts, Meridian Foods*	1 Tbsp/15g	93	7.6	622	25	13	51	6.5
Crunchy, Sainsbury's*	1 Tbsp/15g	92	7.4	610	25.4	12.8	49	8.3
Crunchy, Sun Pat*	1 Tbsp/15g	92	7.3	611	24.8	14.5	48.7	7.3
Crunchy, The Foodie Market, Aldi*	1 Tbsp/15g	94	7.5	628	29	12	50	6.5
Dark, Roasted, Crunchy, Whole Earth*	1 Tbsp/15g	89	6.9	594	28.9	10.3	46.3	8.3
Marmite, Crunchy, Marmite*	1 Tbsp/15g	86	6.8	574	28	12	45	7.9
Salted Date, Yumello*	1 Tbsp/15g	84	7.2	558	22.6	19.6	47.7	8.5
Smooth, Average	***1 Tbsp/15g***	***93***	***8.1***	***623***	***22.6***	***13.1***	***53.7***	***5.4***
Smooth, No Added Sugar, Organic, Whole Earth*	1 Tbsp/15g	94	7.7	628	25.6	13.7	51.2	4.9
Smooth, No Added Sugar, Sunpat*	1 Tbsp/15g	92	7.3	610	24.4	14.7	48.8	7.2
Smooth, Reduced Fat, 30%, Morrisons*	1 Tbsp/15g	84	5.6	562	18	36.3	37.2	5
Smooth, Unsalted, Biona Organic*	1 Tbsp/15g	89	7.4	594	25.8	16.1	49.2	8.5
Whole Nut, Crunchy, Average	***1 Tbsp/15g***	***91***	***8***	***606***	***24.9***	***7.7***	***53.1***	***6***
PEANUTS								
Chilli, Average	***½ Pack/50g***	***303***	***25.3***	***605***	***28.2***	***9.3***	***50.6***	***6.8***
Chilli, Spicy, Jumbo, KP Snacks*	1 Serving/30g	183	14.7	609	29	7.5	49	8.5
Chilli, Sweet, Nobby's*	1 Bag/40g	214	13.6	535	15	42	34	3
Chocolate, Milk, Sainsbury's*	1 Pack/180g	1013	65.2	563	15.5	35.5	36.2	7
Crispy, Tesco*	1/8 Bag/25g	144	10	574	16.2	35.5	39.8	4.7
Dry Roasted, Average	***1 Serving/20g***	***117***	***9.8***	***587***	***25.7***	***11.5***	***48.8***	***6.5***
Honey Roasted, Average	***1oz/28g***	***169***	***13.2***	***605***	***26.8***	***23.6***	***47***	***5.5***
in Chilli Oil, Laoganma*	1 Serving/30g	189	15.9	629	7.4	28	53	0
Plain, Average	***10 Whole/10g***	***59***	***5***	***592***	***24.7***	***11***	***50***	***6.3***
Red Skin, BuyWholeFoodsOnline*	1 Serving/30g	169	13.8	563	25.6	12.5	46	0
Roast, Salted, Average	***10 Whole/12g***	***74***	***6.3***	***614***	***27.8***	***7.9***	***52.4***	***4.9***
Roasted, Salted, Jumbo, Tesco*	1 Portion/25g	154	12.5	616	28.9	9.2	49.9	7.2
Salted, Average	***10 Whole/6g***	***37***	***3.1***	***609***	***27***	***8.3***	***52***	***5.4***
Wasabi Coated, Alesto, Lidl*	1 Serving/30g	153	9.4	511	14.1	40.6	31.5	4.5
PEARL BARLEY								
Boiled	***1oz/28g***	***34***	***0.1***	***123***	***2.3***	***28.2***	***0.4***	***3.8***
Cooked, Average	***1 Serving/150g***	***184***	***0.7***	***123***	***2.3***	***28.2***	***0.4***	***3.8***
Raw, Average	***1oz/28g***	***99***	***0.3***	***352***	***9.9***	***77.7***	***1.2***	***15.6***
PEARS								
Abate Fetel, Average	***1 Med/133g***	***48***	***0.1***	***36***	***0.4***	***8.3***	***0.1***	***2.2***
Asian, Nashi, Raw, Average	***1 Lge/209g***	***80***	***0.4***	***38***	***0.5***	***9.7***	***0.2***	***3.3***
Comice, Raw, Weighed with Core	***1 Med/170g***	***56***	***0***	***33***	***0.3***	***8.5***	***0***	***2***
Conference, Average	***1 Lge/209g***	***88***	***0.2***	***42***	***0.3***	***10.1***	***0.1***	***2***
Dried, Average	***1 Pear Half/16g***	***33***	***0.1***	***204***	***1.9***	***48.4***	***0.5***	***9.7***
in Fruit Juice, Average	***1 Serving/225g***	***102***	***0.1***	***45***	***0.3***	***10.9***	***0***	***1.2***

P

	Measure INFO/WEIGHT	per Measure KCAL	FAT	Nutrition Values per 100g / 100ml KCAL	PROT	CARB	FAT	FIBRE
PEARS								
in Syrup, Average	***1oz/28g***	***16***	***0***	***58***	***0.2***	***14.4***	***0.1***	***1.4***
Prickly, Raw, Fresh	***1oz/28g***	***8***	***0.1***	***30***	***0.4***	***7***	***0.2***	***0***
Raw, Weighed with Core, Average	***1 Med/166g***	***58***	***0.2***	***35***	***0.3***	***8.4***	***0.1***	***1.3***
William, Raw, Average	***1 Med/170g***	***58***	***0.2***	***34***	***0.4***	***8.3***	***0.1***	***2.2***
PEAS								
Dried, Boiled in Unsalted Water, Average	***1oz/28g***	***31***	***0.2***	***109***	***6.9***	***19.9***	***0.8***	***5.5***
Dried, Raw, Average	***1oz/28g***	***85***	***0.7***	***303***	***21.6***	***52***	***2.4***	***13***
Edible Podded, Raw	***1 Cup/63g***	***25***	***0.1***	***39***	***2.6***	***7.1***	***0.2***	***2.4***
Frozen, Average	***1 Serving/85g***	***62***	***0.8***	***73***	***6***	***9.7***	***1***	***4.5***
Frozen, Boiled, Average	***1 Serving/75g***	***51***	***0.7***	***68***	***6***	***9.4***	***0.9***	***5.1***
Garden, Canned with Sugar & Salt, Average	***1 Serving/90g***	***59***	***0.6***	***66***	***5.3***	***9.3***	***0.7***	***5.1***
Garden, Canned, No Sugar Or Salt, Average	***1 Can/80g***	***36***	***0.3***	***45***	***4.4***	***6***	***0.4***	***2.8***
Garden, Frozen, Average	***1 Serving/90g***	***66***	***1***	***74***	***6.3***	***9.8***	***1.1***	***3.3***
Garden, Minted, Average	***1 Serving/80g***	***59***	***0.9***	***74***	***6.3***	***9.7***	***1.1***	***5.9***
Marrowfat, Average	***1 Sm Can/160g***	***134***	***0.9***	***84***	***6.1***	***13.7***	***0.6***	***3.7***
Mushy, Average	***1 Can/200g***	***173***	***1***	***86***	***6.2***	***14.4***	***0.5***	***2.2***
Mushy, Canned, British, Sainsbury's*	½ Can/150g	123	0.9	82	4.7	12.8	0.6	3.4
Processed, Canned, Average	***1 Sm Can/220g***	***162***	***1.6***	***74***	***5.6***	***11.3***	***0.7***	***3.4***
Roasted, Chocolate, & Salted Caramel, Brave*	1 Pack/30g	129	5.1	431	16	44	17	16
Roasted, Paprika, & Chilli, Brave*	1 Pack/35g	132	3.8	378	19	41	11	20
Roasted, Sea Salt, & Vinegar, Brave*	1 Pack/35g	134	3.8	383	19	41	11	19
Roasted, Sea Salt, Classic, Brave*	1 Pack/35g	134	3.8	382	20	41	11	20
Roasted, Sour Cream, & Chive, Brave*	1 Pack/35g	132	3.8	377	20	41	11	20
Sea Salt & Balsamic Vinegar, Snacks, Podberry*	1 Pack/20g	67	0.4	334	22.9	44.8	1.9	22.9
Snow	***1 Serving/80g***	***24***	***0.2***	***29***	***3.3***	***3.9***	***0.2***	***2.1***
Sugar Snap, Average	***1 Serving/80g***	***27***	***0.2***	***33***	***3.2***	***4.8***	***0.2***	***1.4***
Wasabi, Average	***1 Serving/28g***	***114***	***3.8***	***406***	***15.2***	***54***	***13.7***	***8.6***
with Leeks & Pancetta, Finest, Tesco*	½ Pack/122g	146	7.4	120	6.3	7.6	6.1	4.6
PEASE PUDDING								
Canned, Re-Heated, Drained	***1oz/28g***	***26***	***0.2***	***93***	***6.8***	***16.1***	***0.6***	***1.8***
PECAN NUTS								
Average	***3 Nuts/6g***	***42***	***4.2***	***692***	***10***	***5.6***	***70.1***	***4.7***
Roasted, Salted, Waitrose *	1 Serving/25g	183	18.2	733	11.2	3.9	72.7	9.1
PENNE								
Arrabbiata, Slimming World, Iceland*	1 Pack/550g	429	2.2	78	3.5	13.8	0.4	2.3
Arrabiata, BGTY, Sainsbury's*	1 Pack/450g	414	7.2	92	2.9	16.5	1.6	1.9
Brown Rice, GF, Pasta, Waitrose*	¼ Pack/125g	250	2.1	200	4.1	41	1.7	1.9
Chickpea, Peaz*	1 Portion/75g	264	4.4	352	26	43	5.8	11
Cooked, Average	***1 Serving/185g***	***244***	***1.3***	***132***	***4.7***	***26.7***	***0.7***	***1.1***
Dry, Average	***1 Serving/100g***	***352***	***1.9***	***352***	***12.4***	***71.3***	***1.9***	***2.7***
Egg, Fresh, Average	***1 Serving/125g***	***352***	***4***	***282***	***11.1***	***52.2***	***3.2***	***2***
Free From, Tesco*	1 Serving/100g	340	2	340	8	72.5	2	2.5
Fresh, Dry, Average	***1 Serving/125g***	***222***	***2.4***	***178***	***7.3***	***32.2***	***1.9***	***1.6***
GF, Cooked, Free From, Morrisons*	1 Serving/170g	287	1	169	3.3	36.7	0.6	1.6
GF, Dry Weight, Free From, Tesco*	1 Serving/75g	266	0.8	355	7	78.4	1	2
Penne, Cooked, Asda*	1 Serving/180g	279	1.1	155	5.3	31	0.6	2.1
Penne, Mozzarella, Morrisons*	1 Pack/400g	568	16.4	142	5.5	20	4.1	1.7
Penne, Spinach, Cooked, Morrisons*	1 Serving/180g	342	1.1	190	6.9	38.1	0.6	2.4
Red Pepper, Roasted, GFY, Asda*	1 Pack/400g	212	2.4	53	1.9	10	0.6	0.8
Rigate, Dry Weight, Average	***1 Serving/90g***	***318***	***1.6***	***353***	***12.3***	***72.1***	***1.8***	***1.8***
Sausage, Tuscan, Spicy Tomato , Meal for One, M&S*	1 Pack/400g	640	36.8	160	4.7	13.9	9.2	1.6
Wholewheat, Asda*	1 Serving/100g	333	2.1	333	12.1	66.3	2.1	6.9

	Measure INFO/WEIGHT	per Measure KCAL	FAT	Nutrition Values per 100g / 100ml KCAL	PROT	CARB	FAT	FIBRE
PEPERAMI*								
Beef, Bars, Peperami*	1 Bar/20g	69	3.4	345	26	22	17	0
Hot, Peperami*	1 Stick/23g	112	9.9	497	22	3.2	44	1.2
Lunchbox Minis, 30% Less Fat, Peperami*	1 Stick/10g	40	3.1	400	26	5.5	31	3
Original, Peperami*	1 Stick/25g	126	11	504	24	2.5	44	0.1
Tender, Peperami*	1 Serving/20g	64	2.2	322	39	16.5	11	0
PEPPER								
Black, Freshly Ground, Average	***1 Tsp/2g***	***5***	***0.1***	***255***	***11***	***64.8***	***3.3***	***26.5***
Cayenne, Ground	***1 Tsp/2g***	***6***	***0.3***	***318***	***12***	***31.7***	***17.3***	***0***
White	***½ Tsp/1g***	***3***	***0***	***296***	***10.4***	***68.6***	***2.1***	***26.2***
PEPPERCORNS								
Black, Schwartz*	1 Tsp/2g	11	0.4	529	13	68.7	22.5	27
Green, Average	***1 Tsp/10g***	***4***	***0.1***	***44***	***1.6***	***5.3***	***0.8***	***4.7***
PEPPERONI								
Asda*	1 Slice/6g	26	2.2	434	26	1.6	36	0
for Pizza, Slices, Tesco*	6 Slices/20g	97	9.2	485	15.6	2.2	45.9	0.1
Sliced, Tesco*	1 Slice/5g	20	1.7	402	20	2.4	34.7	0
Sliced, Waitrose*	1 Slice/2g	8	0.7	425	23.7	0.1	36.6	0
Slices, Pork, Cured, with Chilli & Paprika, Sainsbury's*	1 Pack/42g	155	12.2	368	26	1	29	0.5
PEPPERS								
Chargrilled, The Deli, Aldi*	1 Jar/170g	116	9.5	68	0.7	2.8	5.6	1.7
Cherry Bell, Stuffed, Cream Cheese, Morrisons*	¼ Pack/37g	98	8.3	264	2.4	12.6	22.3	1.6
Cherry, Hot, Stuffed with Ricotta, Waitrose*	1 Pack/135g	185	10.3	137	5.4	10.5	7.6	2.7
Cherry, Stuffed with Ricotta , The Deli, Aldi*	¼ Pack/33g	39	2.1	117	2.7	11	6.5	1.9
Chilli, Dried, Flakes, Average	***1 Tsp/3g***	***13***	***0.4***	***425***	***16***	***56***	***15***	***44***
Chilli, Green, Raw, Unprepared, Average	***1 Med/13g***	***4***	***0***	***29***	***1.5***	***6.9***	***0.1***	***1.1***
Chilli, Red, Raw, Unprepared, Average	***1 Med/45g***	***13***	***0.1***	***29***	***1.5***	***6.9***	***0.1***	***1.1***
Chilli, Red, Very Lazy, The English Provender Co.*	1 Serving/15g	17	0.6	114	4.2	15.3	4	0.5
Green, Boiled in Salted Water	***1oz/28g***	***5***	***0.1***	***18***	***1***	***2.6***	***0.5***	***1.8***
Green, Raw, Unprepared, Average	***1 Med/160g***	***20***	***0.4***	***13***	***0.7***	***2.2***	***0.3***	***1.3***
Jalapeno, Raw	***1 Pepper/14g***	***4***	***0.1***	***28***	***1.2***	***5.4***	***0.6***	***2.6***
Jalapenos, Sliced, in Spirit Vinegar, Drained, Sainsbury's*	¼ Jar/23g	5	0.1	22	0.5	2.5	0.5	3.3
Mixed Bag, From Supermarket, Average	***1oz/28g***	***7***	***0.1***	***25***	***1***	***4.4***	***0.4***	***1.7***
Orange, Sweet, Raw, Average	***1oz/28g***	***8***	***0.1***	***30***	***1.8***	***5***	***0.3***	***1.5***
Red, Boiled in Salted Water	***1oz/28g***	***10***	***0.1***	***34***	***1.1***	***7***	***0.4***	***1.7***
Red, Raw, Unprepared, Average	***½ Med/80g***	***21***	***0.3***	***27***	***0.8***	***5.3***	***0.3***	***1.3***
Red, Roasted, Cypressa*	1 Serving/30g	5	0.2	16	0.8	3.1	0.5	1.4
Stuffed, Cream Cheese, Sweet, Aldi*	1 Serving/60g	92	7.2	154	3.7	6.9	12	2.1
Stuffed, Goats Cheese, Finest, Tesco*	1/3 Jar/61g	91	5.1	149	4.5	12.8	8.4	2.1
Stuffed, with Rice Based Filling, Average	***1oz/28g***	***24***	***0.7***	***85***	***1.5***	***15.4***	***2.4***	***1.3***
Stuffed, with Vegetables, Cheese Topping, Average	***1oz/28g***	***31***	***1.9***	***111***	***3.4***	***9.8***	***6.7***	***1.5***
Yellow, Raw, Unprepared, Average	***1 Med/160g***	***35***	***0.3***	***22***	***1***	***4.4***	***0.2***	***1.4***
PERCH								
Raw, Atlantic	***1oz/28g***	***26***	***0.5***	***94***	***18.6***	***0***	***1.6***	***0***
PESTO								
Bail, Cucina, Aldi*	¼ Jar/48g	217	21.6	452	4.2	6.9	45	1.7
Basil, Bright & Green, Waitrose*	¼ Jar/48g	217	22.5	453	4.5	2.3	46.9	1.6
Basil, Finest, Tesco*	½ Pack/65g	278	27.4	428	7.9	3.6	42.2	0.9
Basil, Fresh, Sainsbury's*	1 Tbsp/15g	60	5.8	403	9.6	3.7	38.6	1.3
Black Olive, Wicked Kitchen, Tesco*	1 Serving/48g	159	14.9	331	2.6	9	31.1	2.5
Green, Average	***1 Tbsp/20g***	***103***	***9.5***	***517***	***20.4***	***2***	***47.5***	***0***
Green, Basil, Free From, Tesco*	¼ Jar/47g	198	18.6	422	3.7	11.6	39.7	1.5
Green, Free From, Asda*	¼ Jar/48g	172	17.1	362	2.9	6	36	1.1
Green, Reduced Fat, Tesco*	¼ Jar /49g	96	9.5	195	2.6	0.7	19.4	3.4

P

	Measure INFO/WEIGHT	per Measure KCAL	per Measure FAT	Nutrition Values per 100g / 100ml KCAL	PROT	CARB	FAT	FIBRE
PESTO								
Pink Beetroot, Wicked Kitchen, Tesco*	¼ Jar/48g	179	16.8	372	4.3	8.6	35	2.8
Pumpkin, Orange, Wicked Kitchen, Tesco*	¼ Jar/48g	158	14.6	330	2.1	10.7	30.5	2.3
Red, Morrisons*	1 Tbsp/15g	47	4.4	311	5.7	6.6	29	5.9
Red, Rosso, Sundried Tomato, Finest, Tesco*	¼ Jar/47g	166	16.1	353	4	5.6	34.3	3.2
Sauce, Alla Genovese, Waitrose*	1 Serving/10g	38	3.8	380	5	3.1	38.2	2.1
Sauce, Green, Lighter, Sainsbury's*	¼ Jar/47g	98	8.8	207	4.1	4.1	18.5	4.1
Sauce, Sun Dried Tomato, Extra Special, Asda*	¼ Jar/48g	159	15.7	334	3.4	4.8	33	2
Spinach, & Ricotta, Tesco*	1 Tbsp/15g	44	4.2	291	3	3.5	28.2	5
Tomato, Sun Dried, Filippo Berio*	1 Tbsp/15g	73	6.3	484	7.3	18	42	0
PETIT POIS								
& Baby Carrots, Canned, Drained, Average	***½ Can/122g***	***58***	***0.8***	***47***	***2.9***	***7***	***0.7***	***3.2***
Canned, Drained, Average	***1 Sm Can/200g***	***125***	***1***	***63***	***4.8***	***8.9***	***0.5***	***2.6***
Fresh, Frozen, Average	***1 Serving/80g***	***51***	***0.8***	***63***	***5.4***	***7.1***	***1***	***4.8***
Leeks, & Pancetta, Extra Special, Asda*	½ Pack/120g	163	11.1	136	5.7	4.6	9.3	5.6
PHEASANT								
Meat Only, Roasted	***1oz/28g***	***62***	***3.4***	***220***	***27.9***	***0***	***12***	***0***
Meat Only, Roasted, Weighed with Bone	***1oz/28g***	***32***	***1.7***	***114***	***14.5***	***0***	***6.2***	***0***
Stuffed, Easy Carve, Finest, Tesco*	1 Serving/200g	540	37.4	270	23.2	2.2	18.7	0.9
PHYSALIS								
Raw, without Husk, Average	***5 Fruits/30g***	***16***	***0.2***	***53***	***1.9***	***11.2***	***0.7***	***0.4***
PICCALILLI								
Haywards*	1 Serving/28g	18	0.2	66	0.6	12	0.7	0.7
Heinz*	1 Serving/10g	10	0.1	99	1	20.5	0.6	0.6
Morrisons*	1 Serving/50g	38	0.4	75	1.6	15	0.7	0.6
Mustard, Asda*	1 Tbsp/15g	11	0.1	73	0.5	16	0.5	1.3
Original, Bartons*	1 Tbsp/15g	7	0.1	48	0.8	10.4	0.4	0
PICKLE								
Banana Habanero , Mr Vikkis*	¼ Jar/55g	122	3.4	222	1.4	42.4	6.1	0
Branston, Original, Crosse & Blackwell*	1 Serving/12g	19	0.1	157	0.5	34	0.7	1.8
Branston, Sm Chunk, Squeezy, Crosse & Blackwell*	1 Serving/15g	19	0	127	0.9	29.8	0.2	1.1
Branston, Smooth, Squeezy, Crosse & Blackwell*	1 Serving/15g	19	0	127	0.9	29.8	0.2	1.1
Brinjal, Patak's*	1 Tsp/16g	61	4	381	2.1	34.5	24.8	0
Cornichons, Freshona, Lidl*	1 Serving/50g	18	0.2	35	1.2	5.5	0.3	0
Cornichons, with Herbs, The Deli, Aldi*	1 Cornichon/6g	2	0	33	1.9	4.3	0.5	2.3
Garlic, Patak's*	1 Tsp/16g	42	3	261	3.6	20	18.5	1.6
Hot Chilli Jam, What A Pickle*	1 Tsp/8g	14	0	178	0.6	44	0.1	1.2
Lime, Hot, Patak's*	1 Tsp/16g	31	3	194	2.2	4	18.7	0.4
Lime, Oily	***1 Serving/39g***	***70***	***6.1***	***178***	***1.9***	***8.3***	***15.5***	***0***
Mild Mustard, Heinz*	1 Tbsp/10g	13	0.1	129	2.2	25.7	1.3	0.9
Mixed, Drained	***1 Serving/100g***	***14***	***0.2***	***14***	***1***	***1.9***	***0.2***	***1***
Red Cabbage, Asda*	1 Serving/50g	16	0	32	1.6	6	0.1	0
Sandwich, Tesco*	1 Tbsp/30g	38	0	126	0.7	29.5	0.1	1.9
Sweet	***1 Tsp/10g***	***14***	***0***	***141***	***0.6***	***36***	***0.1***	***1.2***
Tangy, Sandwich, Heinz*	1 Tsp/10g	13	0	134	0.7	31.4	0.2	0.9
PICNIC								
Cadbury*	1 Bar/38g	182	8.7	479	7.3	60	23	2.5
PIE								
Aloo Gobi, GF, Clive's*	1 Pie/235g	486	29.3	207	3	19.2	12.5	0
Apple, & Blackberry, Co-Op*	1 Serving/138g	338	15.2	245	3	33	11	2
Apple, & Blackberry, Shortcrust, M&S*	1 Serving/142g	469	17.8	330	4.3	50.2	12.5	1.1
Apple, Bramley, Free From, Tesco*	1 Serving/67g	173	7.6	260	0.6	37.5	11.4	2.6
Apple, Bramley, Individual, Mr Kipling*	1 Pie/60g	210	7.9	351	3.4	54	13.2	1.4
Apple, Bramley, Individual, Sainsbury's*	1 Pie/54g	165	5	307	3.6	52.2	9.3	1.3

	Measure INFO/WEIGHT	per Measure KCAL	FAT	Nutrition Values per 100g / 100ml KCAL	PROT	CARB	FAT	FIBRE
PIE								
Apple, Bramley, Individual, Tesco*	1 Pie/60g	221	7.6	362	4	57.5	12.5	1.9
Apple, Commercially Prepared	***1 Slice/125g***	***296***	***13.8***	***237***	***1.9***	***34***	***11***	***1.6***
Apple, GF, Genius *	1 Pie/160g	387	17.8	242	1	38	11.1	3.3
Apple, Pastry Top & Bottom	***1oz/28g***	***74***	***3.7***	***266***	***2.9***	***35.8***	***13.3***	***1.7***
Apple, Prepared From Recipe, Average	***1oz/28g***	***74***	***3.5***	***265***	***2.4***	***37.1***	***12.5***	***0***
Apple, Shortcrust, Made Without Wheat, M&S*	¼ Pie/129g	317	9.9	246	3	40.1	7.7	2.3
Apple, with Custard	***1 Serving/217g***	***353***	***18.8***	***163***	***2.4***	***25.2***	***8.7***	***1.1***
Banoffee, Mini, Waitrose*	1 Pie/26g	115	5.8	444	3.3	57	22.5	1.2
Banoffee, Tesco*	1/6 Pie/83g	217	11.2	261	2.6	31.5	13.5	1.5
Beef, & Onion, Minced, Tesco*	1 Pie/150g	454	28.5	303	5.7	27.4	19	1.7
Beef, & Onion, Pukka Pies Ltd*	1 Serving/231g	529	32.6	229	7.6	17.9	14.1	3
Beef, Mince, Round, Munro The Butchers *	1 Round/523g	1271	51.3	243	13.7	24.4	9.8	1.3
Beef, Minced, Aberdeen Angus, Shortcrust, M&S*	1 Pie/171g	435	26.6	255	9.3	19.3	15.6	3
Caramel, Crumble, Extra Special, Asda*	1 Pie/45g	179	6.7	402	3.4	63	15	2.3
Cauliflower, & Mushroom, Wicked Kitchen, Tesco*	1 Pie/381g	583	32.4	153	3.6	14.2	8.5	2.8
Cheese, & Onion, Oven Baked, Average	***1 Serving/200g***	***654***	***40***	***327***	***8.2***	***30.4***	***20***	***1.2***
Cheese, & Potato	***1oz/28g***	***39***	***2.3***	***139***	***4.8***	***12.6***	***8.1***	***0.7***
Cheese, Veggie, with Scone Pastry, Waitrose*	1 Pie/170g	408	24.5	240	8.2	18.6	14.4	1.5
Cherry, Bakery, Tesco*	1/6 Pie/87g	240	9.7	276	2.6	40.5	11.2	1.3
Cherry, Morello, Sainsbury's*	1/6 Pie/92g	258	10.2	281	2.6	41.7	11.1	2.3
Chicken, & Asparagus, Tesco*	1 Serving/170g	468	28.7	275	8.3	22.4	16.9	0.8
Chicken, & Gravy, Just, Fray Bentos*	½ Pie/215g	267	7.3	124	5.6	17.2	3.4	0.6
Chicken, & Gravy, Roast, Deep Fill, Tesco*	¼ Pie/157g	358	16	228	9.7	23.7	10.2	1.5
Chicken, & Gravy, Shortcrust Pastry, Tesco*	1 Pie/250g	618	34.5	247	6.8	23.9	13.8	1
Chicken, & Ham, Deep Filled, Sainsbury's*	1 Pie/210g	594	37.2	283	8	23	17.7	1
Chicken, & Leek, & Bacon, Deluxe, Lidl*	1/3 Pie/171g	511	30.8	299	11	22	18	2.7
Chicken, & Leek, & Ham, Morrisons*	¼ Pie/137g	393	23.9	286	10.1	21.7	17.4	1
Chicken, & Leek, LC, Tesco*	1 Pie/350g	298	5.6	85	6.6	10.3	1.6	1.3
Chicken, & Leek, M&S*	1oz/28g	70	4.2	250	10.1	18.8	15.1	1.1
Chicken, & Mushroom, Average	***1 Serving/200g***	***540***	***31.7***	***270***	***8***	***23.8***	***15.9***	***1***
Chicken, & Mushroom, Puff Pastry Topped, Waitrose*	1 Pie/200g	558	35.4	279	9.3	19.9	17.7	1.4
Chicken, & Wiltshire Ham, Finest, Tesco*	1 Pie/250g	688	37.2	275	11.6	22.7	14.9	1.1
Chicken, & Bacon, Crestwood, Aldi*	1 Pie/235g	585	34	249	9.4	19.6	14.5	0.9
Chicken, & Bacon, Puff Pastry Lid, Tesco*	1 Pie/131g	300	15.7	229	7.6	22	12	1.4
Chicken, & Bacon, Puff Pastry, Sainsbury's*	1 Pie/200g	464	21.6	232	9.5	23.1	10.8	2
Chicken, & Bacon, Tesco*	1 Pie/131g	295	14.1	225	8.9	22.3	10.8	1.4
Chicken, & Gravy, Chef Select, Lidl*	1/3 Pie/183g	518	30.9	283	10	21.4	16.9	2.6
Chicken, & Gravy, Classic, Waitrose*	1 Pie/200g	552	31.4	276	8.8	24.4	15.7	1.3
Chicken, & Leek, Filo , COU, M&S*	1 Pack/150g	160	2.8	107	10	12.1	1.9	0.8
Chicken, & Mushroom, COU, M&S*	1 Pack/293g	220	4.1	75	7.7	7.2	1.4	1.2
Chicken, & Porcini Mushroom, TTD, Sainsbury's*	1 Pie/250g	538	26.5	215	8.5	20.7	10.6	1.6
Chicken, & Vegetable, Crestwood, Aldi*	1 Pie/140g	350	21	250	8.2	19	15	2.1
Chicken, & Vegetable, Frozen, Tesco*	1 Pie/129g	282	14.4	219	7.2	21.6	11.2	1.4
Chicken, Bacon, Smoked, & Leeks, TTD, Sainsbury's*	1 Pack/378g	491	25.7	130	8.4	8.2	6.8	1.5
Chicken, Creamy, Potato Topped, Gousto*	1 Serving/640g	461	10.2	72	6.1	8.9	1.6	1.4
Chicken, Deep Filled, Puff Pastry, Sainsbury's*	1 Pie/210g	538	31.9	256	10	19.9	15.2	3.1
Chicken, Ham Hock, & Leek, Finest, Tesco*	1 Pie/250g	562	28	225	9.2	21.2	11.2	1.3
Chicken, Individual, Ready Made, Average	***1 Pie/155g***	***392***	***22.3***	***253***	***9.5***	***20.9***	***14.4***	***1.6***
Chicken, Leek, & Smoked Bacon, Gastropub, M&S*	½ Pie/250g	693	46.5	277	13	13.5	18.6	1.7
Chicken, Leek, & Wholegrain Mustard, Deluxe, Lidl*	1/3 Pie/167g	427	22.8	255	8.7	23.3	13.6	2.5
Chicken, Meat Free, Birds Eye*	1 Pie/155g	400	20.2	258	7.3	27	13	1.8
Chicken, Shortcrust Pastry, Individual, M&S*	1 Pie/150g	363	18.6	242	12.4	19.4	12.4	1.6
Chicken, Shortcrust, Oven Baked, Birds Eye*	1 Pie/155g	417	23.1	271	8.4	25	15	1.2

	Measure INFO/WEIGHT	per Measure KCAL	FAT	Nutrition Values per 100g / 100ml KCAL	PROT	CARB	FAT	FIBRE
PIE								
Chicken, with Root Veg Topping, Moreish, M&S*	1 Pack/400g	352	14	88	5.9	7.4	3.5	1.6
Cod, & Haddock, Smoked, COU, M&S*	1 Pack/400g	320	9.6	80	6.1	9	2.4	1.2
Cottage, 1, Waitrose*	1 Pack/400g	580	30.4	145	8.2	10.3	7.6	1.6
Cottage, Calorie Controlled, Love Life, Waitrose*	1 Pack/320g	253	4.5	79	4.5	11.3	1.4	1.6
Cottage, Calorie Controlled, Tesco*	1 Pack/314g	264	6.6	84	4.9	10.6	2.1	1.6
Cottage, Calorie Counted, Asda*	1 Pack/350g	243	4.9	80	4.1	11	1.6	1.9
Cottage, Chilled, 400g, Quorn*	1 Pack/380g	315	8	83	3.4	11	2.1	3
Cottage, Frozen, 400g, Quorn*	1 Pack/400g	396	14	99	4.2	11	3.5	4
Cottage, Lentil, Plant Based, Asda*	1 Pack/400g	300	2	75	3.2	13	0.5	4.1
Cottage, Lentil, with Sweet Potato Mash, Kirstys*	1 Pack/400g	270	2	68	2.6	12.1	0.5	2.1
Cottage, Lentil, with Sweet Potato Mash, Sainsbury's*	1 Pack/382g	283	6.1	74	2.6	10.4	1.6	4
Cottage, Low Fat, Well & Good, Co-Op*	1 Pack/400g	332	10	83	2.8	11	2.5	2.4
Cottage, Meat Free, Morrisons*	1 Pack/337g	239	4.4	71	2.5	10.9	1.3	3
Cottage, Mushroom, Plant Chef, Tesco*	1 Serving/388g	353	10.5	91	3.2	11.6	2.7	4
Cottage, Plant Kitchen, M&S*	1 Pack/400g	436	15.2	109	4.2	13.8	3.8	1.6
Cottage, Retail, Average	***1 Pack/400g***	***399***	***15.7***	***100***	***5.5***	***10.5***	***3.9***	***1.3***
Cottage, Slim Cook, Tesco*	1 Pack/443g	381	9.7	86	9.2	6.3	2.2	2
Cottage, Veggie, Meal for One, M&S*	1 Pack/400g	356	12.8	89	2.4	11.9	3.2	1.7
Cottage, with Ale Gravy, The Best, Morrisons*	1 Pack/391g	481	21.5	123	8.1	9.6	5.5	1.4
Cottage, with Red Wine, & Cheddar Crumb, Sainsbury's*	1 Pack/375g	488	23.3	130	6.8	10.2	6.2	3.3
Cumberland, Classic, Sainsbury's*	1 Pack/353g	438	18.7	124	5.7	12.3	5.3	2
Cumberland, Oven Cooked, Morrisons*	1 Pack/439g	404	14.9	92	6.2	8.5	3.4	1.2
Cumberland, Serves 1, Classic, Sainsbury's*	1 Pack/353g	438	18.7	124	5.7	12.3	5.3	2
Cumberland, Waitrose*	1 Pack/328g	269	10.5	82	3.8	9	3.2	1.1
Fish	***1 Serving/250g***	***262***	***7.5***	***105***	***8***	***12.3***	***3***	***0.7***
Fish, Admirals, Frozen, Oven Baked, Youngs*	1 Pack/250g	290	11	116	4.9	13.7	4.4	1
Fish, Buttery, Gastropub, M&S*	1 Pack/400g	484	24.8	121	7.6	8.3	6.2	1
Fish, HL, Tesco*	1 Pack/384g	311	7.7	81	3.9	11.4	2	0.9
Fish, Serves 1, BGTY, Sainsbury's*	1 Pie/450g	369	8.6	90	6.7	10.2	2.1	1.6
Fish, Serves 1, No.1, Waitrose*	1 Pack/334g	457	26	137	6.4	9.4	7.8	1.7
Fisherman's, Youngs*	1 Pack/340g	377	13.6	111	5.6	12.8	4	0.8
Fishermans, Traditional, Morrison's*	1 Pie/327g	425	19.6	130	5.2	13.4	6	0.8
Fruit, Autumn, M&S*	1 Serving/116g	271	7.2	234	1.9	41.8	6.2	1.7
Fruit, Pastry Top & Bottom	***1oz/28g***	***73***	***3.7***	***260***	***3***	***34***	***13.3***	***1.8***
Fruit, Selection, Mr Kipling*	1 Pie/66g	232	9	350	3.5	53.5	13.6	1.3
Lemon Meringue	***1 Portion/120g***	***383***	***17.3***	***319***	***4.5***	***45.9***	***14.4***	***0.7***
Lentil, & Olive, Greek, Clive's*	1 Pie/235g	477	25.4	203	4.5	20	10.8	0
Meat, & Potato, Hollands*	1 Pie/179g	385	18.4	215	5.5	24	10.3	0
Mince, All Butter, Average	***1 Pie/65g***	***251***	***8.9***	***386***	***4***	***60.2***	***13.8***	***2.4***
Mince, All Butter, Crumble Topped, Finest, Tesco*	1 Mince Pie/44g	185	5.8	420	4.1	69.3	13.2	3.4
Mince, All Butter, Florentine, Extra Special, Asda*	1 Pie/52g	204	8.4	393	4.9	54.7	16.2	4.5
Mince, All Butter, Mini, Average	***1 Pie/20g***	***78***	***2.8***	***389***	***4.3***	***61.6***	***13.8***	***2.8***
Mince, All Butter, Puff Pastry, Average	***1 Pie60g***	***228***	***10.5***	***381***	***4.3***	***51.1***	***17.4***	***2.2***
Mince, Deep Fill, Holly Lane, Aldi*	1 Pie/61g	235	8.5	386	4	59	14	2.7
Mince, Deep Filled, All Butter Pastry, Finest, Tesco*	1 Pie/65g	259	10.8	401	5	56.2	16.7	2.7
Mince, Deep, Morrisons*	1 Pie/65g	243	9.1	371	3.7	57.8	13.9	1.5
Mince, Dusted, Mini, Finest, Tesco*	1 Pie/20g	76	2.4	379	7.3	62.9	12.2	5
Mince, Frangipane, Specially Selected, Aldi*	1 Pie/46g	191	9.2	415	5.7	52	20	2.8
Mince, Free From, Sainsbury's*	1 Pie/58g	226	7.5	393	2.3	64	13	2.5
Mince, Iced Top, Asda*	1 Pie/55g	220	7.7	399	2.8	63	14	4.7
Mince, Individual, Average	***1 Pie/65g***	***260***	***11***	***400***	***4.2***	***56.3***	***17***	***1.6***
Mince, Luxury, Deep Filled, M&S*	1 Pie/65g	234	9	360	4.3	55	13.8	3.8
Mince, Mini, M&S*	1 Pie/28g	105	4	380	4.3	57.8	14.6	4

PIE	Measure INFO/WEIGHT	per Measure KCAL	FAT	Nutrition Values per 100g / 100ml KCAL	PROT	CARB	FAT	FIBRE
Mince, Mini, Specially Selected, Aldi*	1 Pie/29g	111	4.1	382	4	59	14	2.7
Mince, Plant Kitchen, M&S*	1 Pie/62g	243	8.5	390	3.7	61.9	13.6	2.7
Mince, Puff Pastry, Co-Op*	1 Pie/72g	245	11.9	340	5	43.1	16.5	2.6
Mince, Vegan, & GF, Holland & Barrett*	1 Pie/60g	217	7.8	361	2.3	60	13	2.6
Mushroom, & Camembert, Puff Pastry Topped, Tesco*	1 Pie/162g	434	26.2	268	5.6	24	16.2	2.1
Mushroom, Plant Kitchen, M&S*	1 Pie/200g	450	24.6	225	4.2	23.9	12.3	1.1
Parsnip, & Portobello Mushroom, Deluxe, Lidl*	1 Pie/190g	475	26.8	250	3.9	25.6	14.1	2.7
Pork, & Egg, M&S*	¼ Pie/110g	411	31	374	10.9	18.4	28.2	1.5
Pork, & Festive Fruit Stuffing, Morrisons*	1 Pie/28g	94	5.7	336	12.5	24.9	20.3	2
Pork, & Pickle, Mini, Sainsbury's*	1 Pie/50g	177	11.5	354	9.5	26.2	23	2.1
Pork, & Pickle, Snack, Sainsbury's*	1 Pie/65g	246	15.8	379	8.9	29.9	24.4	2.3
Pork, BBQ, Mini, Tesco*	1 Pie/50g	198	13.2	396	10.7	28.2	26.3	1.9
Pork, Bitesize, Tesco*	1 Pie/25g	98	6.5	393	10.8	28.1	26.1	1.5
Pork, Cheese & Pickle, Mini, Tesco*	1 Pie/49g	191	12.8	389	9.2	29.3	26.1	1.2
Pork, Cheese, & Pickle, Mini, Morrisons*	1 Pie/50g	228	14.9	456	9	36.9	29.8	2
Pork, Cheese, & Pickle, Snack, Morrisons*	1 Pie/75g	326	22.1	435	9.8	31.4	29.5	2.4
Pork, Dinky, Melton Mowbray, M&S*	1 Pie/25g	101	6.8	404	13.2	26.1	27	1.7
Pork, Individual	***1 Pie/75g***	***272***	***19.3***	***363***	***10.8***	***23.7***	***25.7***	***0.9***
Pork, Lattice, Large, Market St, Morrisons*	1 Pie/450g	1742	132.8	387	7.9	21.6	29.5	1.8
Pork, Melton Mowbray, Crestwood, Aldi*	1 Pie/50g	211	14.5	422	9.8	28	29	2.1
Pork, Melton Mowbray, Cured, Mini, M&S*	1 Pie/50g	192	12.2	385	9.8	32.6	24.4	1
Pork, Melton Mowbray, Individual, Sainsbury's*	½ Pie/70g	234	15.1	334	11.1	22.8	21.6	1.8
Pork, Melton Mowbray, Mini, Asda*	1 Pie/50g	220	15.5	440	8.9	31	31	0.7
Pork, Melton Mowbray, Mini, M&S*	1 Pie/50g	185	12.1	370	11.6	26.1	24.2	1.6
Pork, Melton Mowbray, Mini, Morrisons*	1 Pie/50g	197	12.5	393	10.9	31.3	24.9	0.9
Pork, Melton Mowbray, Mini, Tesco*	1 Pie/50g	192	12.8	383	10.6	26.9	25.6	1.5
Pork, Melton Mowbray, Mini, TTD, Sainsbury's*	1 Pie/50g	204	14.2	407	10.6	26.5	28.4	1.7
Pork, Mini, Retail, Average	***1 Mini/50g***	***198***	***13.7***	***396***	***10.8***	***26.4***	***27.4***	***2.4***
Pork, Sliced	***1 Slice/100g***	***380***	***29.9***	***380***	***10.2***	***18.7***	***29.9***	***0***
Rhubarb, Lattice, Individual, Baked by Us, Morrisons*	1 Pie/135g	433	19.2	321	3.9	43.4	14.2	2
Rhubarb, Shortcrust Pastry, Bakery, Tesco*	1 Slice/87g	219	9.3	251	3.1	34.8	10.7	1.7
Sausage, & Mash, Tesco*	½ Pack/365g	288	5.1	79	2.3	13.7	1.4	1.2
Scotch, Co-Op*	1 Pie/132g	408	24.9	309	7.3	27.3	18.9	1.5
Shepherd's, Average	***1oz/28g***	***31***	***1.7***	***112***	***6***	***9.3***	***5.9***	***0.7***
Shepherd's, Vegetarian, Average	***1 Serving/400g***	***371***	***14.6***	***93***	***4***	***10.4***	***3.6***	***2.5***
Shepherds, Allplants*	1 Serving/455g	450	6.8	99	4.1	16	1.5	2.8
Spinach, Courgette, & Feta Cheese, Vegetarian, Waitrose*	1 Pie/170g	408	25	240	7.4	18.5	14.7	1.8
Spinach, Feta, & Pine Nut, Higgidy*	1 Pie/265g	684	47.4	258	9.2	15.6	17.9	1.5
Steak, & Ale with Chips & Gravy	***1 Serving/400g***	***825***	***42.2***	***206***	***7.2***	***20.5***	***10.6***	***0.5***
Steak, & Ale, Average	***1 Pie/200g***	***507***	***28.7***	***253***	***9.8***	***21.1***	***14.4***	***1.3***
Steak, & Kidney, Individual	***1 Pie/200g***	***646***	***42.4***	***323***	***9.1***	***25.6***	***21.2***	***0.9***
Steak, & Kidney, Puff Pastry, Sainsbury's*	1 Pie/150g	423	23.6	282	8.2	26.9	15.7	0.9
Steak, & Ale, Puff Pastry, Finest, Tesco*	1 Pie/250g	560	24.2	224	11	22.6	9.7	1.3
Steak, & Ale, Puff Pastry, Serves 3, Sainsbury's*	1 Serving/183g	464	24.9	253	9.5	22.7	13.6	0.9
Steak, & Craft Ale, Tesco*	1 Pie/198g	449	20.6	227	11.4	21.1	10.4	1.2
Steak, & Gravy, Puff Pastry Topped, Oven Baked, Asda*	1 Pie/150g	419	23.9	280	8.3	25	16	1.5
Steak, & Horseradish, Frozen, Deluxe, Lidl*	1 Pie/194g	650	42.5	335	10.9	22.6	21.9	2.1
Steak, & Old Peculiar Ale, Deluxe, Lidl*	1 Serving/167g	426	22.4	255	9.1	23.3	13.4	2.4
Steak, & Red Wine Gravy, Finest, Tesco*	½ Pie/250g	650	32	260	12.3	22.9	12.8	1.6
Steak, & Red Wine, GF, Made Without Wheat, M&S*	1 Pie/180g	522	31.7	290	10.3	21.7	17.6	1.8
Steak, & Red Wine, Shortcrust Topped, Cook*	1 Serving/295g	496	24.2	168	11.6	10.5	8.2	1.2
Steak, & Stilton, TTD, Sainsbury's*	1 Pie/250g	615	31	246	12.1	20.4	12.4	2.2
Steak, Aberdeen Angus, Top Crust, Waitrose*	½ Pie/280g	476	24.1	170	10	13.4	8.6	4.1

P

	Measure INFO/WEIGHT	per Measure KCAL	FAT	Nutrition Values per 100g / 100ml KCAL	PROT	CARB	FAT	FIBRE
PIE								
Steak, British, & Craft Ale, Specially Selected, Aldi*	1 Pie/190g	549	34.2	289	8.3	22	18	1.9
Steak, British, Slow Cooked, Extra Special, Asda*	1/3 Pie/186g	494	26.1	265	13	21	14	1.2
Steak, Puff Pastry, Average	***¼ Pie/100g***	***259***	***14.5***	***259***	***9.4***	***21.8***	***14.5***	***1.9***
Steak, Puff Pastry, Top Crust, M&S*	1 Pie/200g	520	30.8	260	12.7	17	15.4	1.1
Steak, Red Wine, & Mushroom, Higgidy*	1 Pie/250g	601	31.6	240	10.4	21.4	12.6	1.3
Steak, Shortcrust, Average	***¼ Pie/100g***	***253***	***14.1***	***253***	***9.9***	***21.6***	***14.1***	***1.4***
Sweet Potato, & Feta, with Pumpkin Seeds, Higgidy*	1 Pie/270g	756	49.4	280	7.2	22.9	18.3	2.1
Sweet Potato, Feta, & Sunflower Seed, Deluxe, Aldi*	1 Pie/250g	660	42.8	264	6.3	19	17.1	1.6
Vegetable	***1oz/28g***	***42***	***2.1***	***151***	***3***	***18.9***	***7.6***	***1.5***
Vegetable, & Cheese, Asda*	1 Pie/141g	330	16.2	234	5.8	26.9	11.5	1
Vegetable, & Feta, Moroccan, Little, Higgidy*	1 Pie/180g	418	22.5	232	5.1	24.7	12.5	0.6
Vegetable, Indian Spiced, Higgidy*	1 Pie/200g	450	28	225	4.7	21.4	14	2.5
Vegetable, Retail, Average	***1 Serving/200g***	***348***	***19***	***174***	***3.7***	***18.6***	***9.5***	***1.1***
Vegetarian, Chicken Style, & Mushroom, Quorn*	1 Pie/235g	588	33.2	250	5.5	23.7	14.1	3
Vegetarian, Deep Country, Linda McCartney*	1 Pie/166g	413	23.6	249	5.2	24.9	14.2	2.6
Vegetarian, Mince & Potato, Quorn*	1 Pie/200g	388	16	194	6.5	22.5	8	3
Vegetarian, Mushroom & Ale, Linda McCartney*	1 Pie/200g	439	23.5	219	4.1	25	11.7	1.2
Vegetarian, Steak, Meat Free, Quorn*	1 Pie/235g	439	18.8	187	5.6	22	8	2
PIE FILLING								
Apple, Sainsbury's*	1 Serving/75g	67	0.1	89	0.1	22.1	0.1	1
Cherry	***1oz/28g***	***23***	***0***	***82***	***0.4***	***21.5***	***0***	***0.4***
PIGEON								
Meat Only, Roasted, Average	***1 Pigeon/115g***	***215***	***9.1***	***187***	***29***	***0***	***7.9***	***0***
Meat Only, Roasted, Weighed with Bone, Average	***1oz/28g***	***12***	***0.5***	***41***	***6.4***	***0***	***1.7***	***0***
PIKELETS								
Buttermilk, Waitrose*	1 Pikelet/28g	54	0.2	192	7.1	37.7	0.8	2.6
Sainsbury's*	1 Pikelet/24g	55	0.3	230	7.6	45.1	1.4	3.3
Tesco*	1 Pikelet/27g	52	0.3	193	6.6	38.1	1	2.4
PILAF								
Beef, with Tomatoes, & Green Beans, Hello Fresh*	1 Serving/448g	667	20	149	7.6	19.9	4.5	0.2
Bulgur Wheat, Sainsbury's*	1 Pack/381g	347	11.1	91	3.9	12.3	2.9	6.3
Chicken, Co-Op*	1 Pack/550g	891	45.7	162	8.9	12	8.3	1.8
Chicken, Middle Eastern Inspired, Waitrose*	½ Pack/275g	639	28.9	232	13.2	19.9	10.5	2.7
with Tomato, Average	***1oz/28g***	***40***	***0.9***	***144***	***2.5***	***28***	***3.3***	***0.4***
PILCHARDS								
Fillets in Tomato Sauce, Average	***1 Can/120g***	***158***	***7.8***	***132***	***16.2***	***2.2***	***6.5***	***0.1***
Fillets in Virgin Olive Oil, Glenryck*	1 Serving/92g	223	14.4	242	23.3	2	15.7	0
in Hot Chilli Sauce, Glenryck*	1 Tin/155g	219	13.2	141	15.2	1	8.5	1
PIMMS*								
& Lemonade, Premixed, Canned, Pimms*	1 Can/250ml	160	0	64	0	8.4	0	0
25% Volume, Pimms*	1 Serving/50ml	80	0	160	0	5	0	0
PINE NUTS								
Average	***1 Tbsp/8g***	***56***	***5.5***	***695***	***15.7***	***3.9***	***68.6***	***1.9***
PINEAPPLE								
Chunks, Average	***1 Serving/100g***	***66***	***0.1***	***66***	***0.5***	***15.5***	***0.1***	***0.3***
in Juice, Canned, Average	***1 Can/106g***	***57***	***0***	***53***	***0.3***	***12.9***	***0***	***0.6***
Raw, Flesh Only, Average	***1 Med Slice/80g***	***40***	***0.1***	***50***	***0.5***	***13.1***	***0.1***	***1.4***
PISTACHIO NUTS								
Chilli, & Lime, Morrisons*	1 Pack/55g	334	27.6	608	25.6	8.8	50.1	9.5
Raw, Average, without Shells	***1 Serving/20g***	***111***	***8.9***	***557***	***20.6***	***28***	***44.4***	***10.3***
Roasted & Salted, without Shells, Average	***1 Serving/25g***	***152***	***13.6***	***608***	***19.6***	***9.9***	***54.5***	***6.1***
Salted, Roasted, Weighed with Shell	***1 Serving/100g***	***331***	***30.5***	***331***	***9.8***	***4.5***	***30.5***	***3.4***
Salted, Roasted, without Shells	***1 Serving/100g***	***601***	***55.4***	***601***	***17.9***	***8.2***	***55.4***	***6.1***

P

PIZZA	Measure INFO/WEIGHT	per Measure KCAL	per Measure FAT	KCAL	PROT	CARB	FAT	FIBRE
'Nduja, & Burrata, Sourdough Base, No.1, Waitrose*	¼ Pizza/129g	284	10.6	220	8.9	26.5	8.2	2.1
American, Hot, Thin & Crispy, Stonebaked, Aldi*	½ Pizza/149g	357	16.4	240	9.7	25	11	2.8
American, Supermarket, Pizza Express*	½ Pizza/130g	352	14.5	271	11.3	30.5	11.2	1.5
Bacon, & Mushroom, Thin & Crispy, Sainsbury's*	½ Pizza/150g	396	15.9	264	12.9	29.2	10.6	1.7
BBQ Meat Feast, Sourdough, Carlos, Aldi*	1 Slice/45g	127	5.4	282	14	29	12	1.8
BBQ Meat Feast, Stuffed Crust, Carlos, Aldi*	½ Pizza/250g	622	18.8	249	9.9	34	7.5	2.4
Beef, Chilli, Classic Crust, Tex Mex, Tesco*	½ Pizza/260g	655	26.5	252	10.9	27.9	10.2	2.5
Buffalo Chicken, Fully Loaded, Iceland*	¼ Pizza/168g	420	13.4	251	9.5	34	8	2.4
Buffalo Mozzarella, & Tomatoes, Finest, Tesco*	1 Pizza/207g	502	16.7	243	10.5	31.1	8.1	2.3
Cajun Chicken, Stonebaked, Chef Select, Lidl*	½ Pizza/160g	330	8	206	10.8	27.9	5	2.9
Caprino Verde, Specially Selected, Aldi*	½ Pizza/193g	490	21.2	254	9.4	27	11	2.9
Carbonara, Romana, Supermarket, Pizza Express*	½ Pizza/182g	486	17.8	267	12.2	31.2	9.8	2.5
Cauliflower, Spicy, Stonebaked, Plant Menu, Aldi*	½ Pizza/170g	406	13.8	239	6.8	33	8.1	4
Chargrilled Veg, Stone Baked, Tesco*	½ Pizza/162g	337	10.4	208	10.2	26.4	6.4	1.9
Chargrilled Vegetable & Basil Pesto, Sourdough, Asda*	1 Serving/239g	468	15.5	196	8.1	25	6.5	2
Cheese & Tomato, Average	***1 Serving/300g***	***711***	***35.4***	***237***	***9.1***	***25.2***	***11.8***	***1.4***
Cheese & Tomato, Baguette, Tesco*	1 Baguette/125g	275	8.5	220	11	28	6.8	2.8
Cheese & Tomato, Deep Pan, Goodfella's*	¼ Pizza/102g	259	10.8	253	11.5	29.6	10.5	3.7
Cheese & Tomato, Mini, M&S*	1 Pizza/95g	233	5.5	245	10	38.7	5.8	1.6
Cheese & Tomato, Retail, Frozen	***1oz/28g***	***70***	***3***	***250***	***7.5***	***32.9***	***10.7***	***1.4***
Cheese & Tomato, Thin & Crispy, Essential, Waitrose*	½ Pizza/112g	306	10.6	273	14.3	30.7	9.5	3.5
Cheese & Tomato, Thin & Crispy, Sainsbury's*	1 Serving/135g	344	10	255	14.9	32.2	7.4	5
Cheese & Tomato, Thin & Crispy, Waitrose*	1 Pizza/280g	658	28.3	235	12.3	23.6	10.1	2.3
Cheese & Tomato, Thin, HFC, Tesco*	½ Pizza/144g	361	9.6	250	10.9	35.5	6.7	2.3
Cheese & Tomato, Snack, Co-Op*	1 Pizza/259g	738	21.2	285	10	41	8.2	2.8
Cheese & Tomato, Thin & Crispy, M&S*	¼ Pizza/116g	314	12.3	271	12.3	30.7	10.6	1.8
Cheese Feast, Deep Crust, Carlos, Aldi*	1 Pizza/155g	432	14.9	279	9.7	37.3	9.6	2.1
Cheese Feast, Stuffed Crust, Asda*	½ Pizza/204g	521	18.8	255	13	29	9.2	2.2
Cheese Feast, Stuffed Crust, Iceland*	½ Pizza/227g	624	22.9	275	13.4	31.2	10.1	2.8
Cheese Feast, Thin Crust, Chilled, Tesco*	½ Pizza/175g	467	22.4	267	14.7	23.4	12.8	2.5
Cheese Medley, Tiger Crust, Chicago Town*	1 Pizza/298g	992	47.7	333	14	32	16	1.5
Cheese Meltdown, Thin & Crispy, 10", Asda*	1 Pizza/287g	723	28.7	252	12	28	10	1.7
Cheese, & Garlic, Tesco*	½ Pizza/102g	304	11.7	298	9.2	38.1	11.5	2.4
Cheese, & Tomato, Lidl*	1 Pizza/120g	190	5.3	158	10.4	17.9	4.4	2.5
Cheese, & Tomato, Snack, Asda*	1 Pizza/110g	302	9.1	275	10	38	8.3	2.7
Cheese, Four, Deep Dish, Chicago Town*	1 Pizza/148g	433	17.8	292	12	33	12	0
Cheese, Four, Finest, Tesco*	½ Pizza/230g	575	21.2	250	12.1	29.8	9.2	1.3
Cheese, Four, Stonebaked, Thin, Carlos, Aldi*	½ Pizza/176g	498	17.4	283	13	34	9.9	2.8
Cheese, Four, Thin & Crispy, Iceland*	½ Pizza/148g	354	12.6	239	10.7	29.1	8.5	1.6
Cheese, Loaded, Stuffed Crust, Takeaway, Chicago Town*	¼ Pizza/150g	436	17.9	292	12	33	12	0
Cheese, Stuffed Crust, Takeaway, Tesco*	½ Pizza/203g	521	17.7	256	11.5	31.8	8.7	2.5
Cheese, Thick Crust, From Restaurant, Average	***1 Pizza/976g***	***2655***	***107.3***	***272***	***12***	***31.3***	***11***	***1.8***
Cheese, Thin Crust, From Restaurant, Average	***1 Pizza/627g***	***1906***	***98.3***	***304***	***14.2***	***26.5***	***15.7***	***2***
Chicken Tikka, Ultra Thin, Iceland*	½ Pizza/159g	404	15.9	254	11.9	27.6	10	2.7
Chicken, & Chorizo, 12", TTD, Sainsbury's*	½ Pizza/290g	702	20.9	242	12.2	32.1	7.2	2.6
Chicken, & Chorizo, Sourdough, Carlos, Aldi*	½ Pizza/165g	406	14.2	246	12	29	8.6	4.7
Chicken, & Sweetcorn, Stonebaked, Tesco*	1 Serving/177g	354	9.6	200	11.9	26	5.4	2
Chicken, & Vegetable, Stone Baked, GFY, Asda*	½ Pizza/161g	349	3.7	217	13	36	2.3	1.7
Chicken, & Bacon, Stonebaked, Tesco*	½ Pizza/147g	376	14.7	256	13	27.1	10	2.5
Chicken, BBQ, & Bacon, Stuffed Crust, Takeaway, Iceland*	1 Pizza/460g	1219	38.2	265	13.1	32.8	8.3	3.2
Chicken, BBQ, M&S*	½ Pizza/210g	430	11.8	205	11.6	27.5	5.6	1.8
Chicken, BBQ, Stonebaked, Tesco*	½ Pizza/158g	285	9.5	180	10.5	20.9	6	3.9
Chicken, BBQ, Thin & Crispy, Sainsbury's*	½ Pizza/167g	399	12.4	238	11.4	30.4	7.4	2.2

Nutrition Values per 100g / 100ml

P

	Measure INFO/WEIGHT	per Measure KCAL	FAT	Nutrition Values per 100g / 100ml KCAL	PROT	CARB	FAT	FIBRE
PIZZA								
Chicken, Cajun Style, Stonebaked, Tesco*	1 Pizza/561g	1318	55	235	11.9	24.8	9.8	1.4
Chicken, Cajun, Sainsbury's*	½ Pizza/146g	285	2.6	195	12.9	31.8	1.8	2.6
Chicken, Chargrilled, Iceland*	1 Pizza/381g	804	25.5	211	12.3	25.4	6.7	2
Chicken, Chargrilled, Thin & Crispy, Asda*	1 Pizza/373g	780	18.6	209	9	32	5	1.6
Chicken, Club, Deep Dish, Chicago Town*	1 Pizza/155g	404	14.9	261	11	32	9.6	0
Chicken, Garlic, Thin & Crispy, Stonebake, Sainsbury's*	½ Pizza/160g	386	17.3	241	10.7	25.2	10.8	3.5
Chicken, Hot & Spicy, Deep Pan, Tesco*	½ Pizza/222g	423	7.3	191	10.5	30	3.3	2.1
Chicken, Piri Piri, Classic Crust, Takeaway, Tesco*	1 Pizza/550g	1196	38.4	217	10.3	28.3	7	2.4
Chicken, Romano, Goodfella's*	½ Pizza/189g	447	17.6	236	11	26	9.3	0
Chicken, Spicy, Thin & Crispy, Morrisons*	½ Pizza/144g	330	8.8	229	11.4	30.8	6.1	2.7
Chicken, Sweet Chilli, BGTY, Sainsbury's*	½ Pizza/138g	276	2.3	200	13	33.2	1.7	2.1
Chicken, Sweet Chilli, Extra Thin, Morrison's*	½ Pizza/146g	301	7.9	206	10.7	27.9	5.4	1.7
Chilli Salsiccia, Irresistible, Co-Op*	1 Pizza/212g	577	19.7	272	12	34	9.3	1.2
Double Pepperoni, Spicy, Iceland*	½ Pizza/171g	394	14	231	9.4	28.5	8.2	2.8
Double Pepperoni, Thin & Crispy, Stonebaked, Co-Op*	1 Slice/40g	106	4	266	11	31	10	2.5
Double Pepperoni, Tiger Crust, Chicago Town*	½ Pizza/160g	538	27.2	336	13	31	17	1.5
Falafel, Vegan, Stonebaked, Goodfellas *	½ Pizza/182g	397	12.7	218	6.4	30	7	0
Feta, Mascarpone, & Caramelised Onion, M&S*	½ Pizza/240g	612	28.1	255	9.8	26.9	11.7	1.6
Funghi, Ristorante, Dr Oetker*	1 Pizza/365g	847	43.4	232	7.6	22.5	11.9	1.8
Goats Cheese, & Red Onion, Tesco *	½ Pizza/210g	559	24.2	266	10.4	29.1	11.5	1.9
Ham, & Mushroom, Average	***1 Serving/250g***	***533***	***16***	***213***	***10.5***	***28.4***	***6.4***	***2.1***
Ham, & Pineapple, Average	***1 Serving/250g***	***555***	***16.8***	***222***	***11***	***29.2***	***6.7***	***2.1***
Ham, & Pineapple, Stone Bake, M&S*	1 Pizza/345g	690	19.7	200	10.1	28.3	5.7	1.6
Ham, & Pineapple, Thin & Crispy Italian, Morrisons*	1 Pizza/375g	746	22.9	199	10.2	24.9	6.1	0
Ham, & Cheese, Thin & Crispy, Essential, Waitrose*	½ Pizza/72g	170	4.9	237	12.9	29.7	6.8	2.8
Ham, & Mushroom, COU, M&S*	1 Pizza/194g	353	6.6	182	11.9	24.9	3.4	2.2
Ham, & Mushroom, Deep Pan, Oven Baked, Iceland*	1/3 Pizza/100g	245	7.3	245	11.1	32.2	7.3	2.9
Ham, & Pineapple, Stonebaked, Thin & Crispy, Tesco*	¼ Pizza/88g	192	5.9	219	11.5	26.6	6.7	3.2
Ham, & Pineapple, Thin Stonebaked, Asda*	1 Slice/52g	111	3.5	213	11	26	6.7	2.2
Hawaiian, Stonebaked, Cucina, Aldi*	½ Pizza/165g	326	5.6	198	9.5	32	3.4	1.6
Hawaiian, Thin Crust, Tesco*	½ Pizza/192g	365	9.4	190	10.3	25.6	4.9	1.8
Hoisin Pork, The Best, Morrisons*	½ Pizza/211g	499	15.4	236	10.6	30.9	7.3	1.9
Jackfruit, BBQ, Aldi*	½ Pizza/180g	418	13.7	232	6.6	32	7.6	3.9
King Prawn, Garlic & Chilli, No.1, Waitrose*	¼ Pizza/124g	273	9.1	220	10.8	27	7.3	1.6
La Reine, Supermarket, Pizza Express*	½ Pack/145g	320	9.4	221	11.1	28.3	6.5	2.3
Margherita, 12", Finest, Tesco*	½ Pizza/255g	433	9.2	170	8.1	26.4	3.6	2.7
Margherita, Average	***1 Slice/108g***	***239***	***8.6***	***239***	***11***	***30.5***	***8.6***	***1.2***
Margherita, Classic, Supermarket, Pizza Express*	½ Pizza/127g	312	10.8	245	10	31.5	8.5	1.4
Margherita, Classico, Italiano, Tesco*	½ Pizza/191g	414	11.8	217	11.2	29.1	6.2	2.5
Margherita, GF, Free From, Sainsbury's*	½ Pizza/150g	430	18.6	287	8.5	33.3	12.4	3.9
Margherita, GF, Supermarket, Pizza Express*	½ Pizza/134g	341	13	254	9	31.3	9.7	2.6
Margherita, Sourdough, Pizzeria, Crosta & Mollica*	½ Pizza/201g	462	14.7	230	10	30	7.3	2.3
Margherita, Stone Baked, Goodfella's*	1 Slice/36g	95	4.1	263	10.9	31.9	11.4	7.6
Margherita, Stonebaked, 10", Sainsbury's*	½ Pizza/139g	359	11.3	258	12.4	32.2	8.1	3.5
Margherita, Stonebaked, Hand Stretched, Sainsbury's*	½ Pizza/133g	347	11.7	262	12.8	31.5	8.8	2.6
Margherita, Supermarket, Pizza Express*	½ Pizza/127g	312	10.8	245	10	31.5	8.5	1.4
Margherita, The Best, Morrisons*	½ Pizza/216g	569	20.8	263	9.8	32.7	9.6	3.5
Margherita, Thin & Crispy, Stonebaked, Co-Op*	½ Pizza/147g	350	10.6	238	11	31	7.2	2.6
Margherita, Thin Crust, Takeaway, Goodfella's*	½ Pizza/206g	594	26.7	289	13	29	13	0
Margherita, Three Cheezly, Vegan, One Planet*	½ Pizza/214g	445	10.9	208	5.6	35.8	5.1	2.2
Margherita, Vegan, Plant Chef, Tesco*	¼ Pizza/65g	164	5.7	254	6	35.8	8.9	3.5
Margherita, Wood Fired, Irresistible, Co-Op*	1 Slice/70g	181	7	258	9.9	30	10	3.4
Meat Feast, Deep & Loaded, Sainsbury's*	½ Pizza/298g	818	30	275	13.2	32.7	10.1	2.6

P

	Measure INFO/WEIGHT	per Measure KCAL	FAT	Nutrition Values per 100g / 100ml KCAL	PROT	CARB	FAT	FIBRE
PIZZA								
Meat Feast, Deep Pean, Sainsbury's*	½ Pizza/193g	492	16.8	255	11.9	31.2	8.7	2
Meat Feast, Mega, Asda*	½ Pizza/428g	1044	33.8	244	9.5	33.6	7.9	3.2
Meat Feast, Sourdough, Morrisons*	½ Pizza/177g	469	20.5	265	13.7	24.3	11.6	4.1
Meat Feast, Stone Baked Thin, Goodfella's*	1 Pizza/341g	897	34.1	263	13	29	10	2.6
Meat Feast, Thin & Crispy, Asda*	½ Pizza/183g	410	14.6	224	11	27	8	1.4
Meat Feast, Thin Crust, Tesco*	½ Pizza/178g	430	20.2	242	13.6	21.3	11.4	2.3
Meats, Italian, Finest, Tesco*	½ Pizza/217g	449	8.5	207	13.6	29.4	3.9	1.3
Meaty, Mega, Deep Dish, Chicago Town*	1 Pizza/157g	442	18.9	281	11	31	12	0
Mini, Party, Tesco*	1 Pizza/11g	26	1.1	248	11.4	28.6	10.5	1.9
Mozzarella, & Basil, Sourdough, Carlos, Aldi*	¼ Pizza/83g	218	7.8	261	12	31	9.3	2
Mozzarella, & Sunblush Tomato, 12", TTD, Sainsbury's*	½ Pizza/251g	638	17.8	254	12.4	35	7.1	2.6
Mozzarella, Italian, & Basil, Ultra-Thin, Wood Fired, M&S*	1 Pack/173g	420	20.1	243	11.1	22.7	11.6	1.8
Mozzarella, Ristorante, Dr Oetker*	½ Pizza/184g	472	23.9	257	10	25	13	0
Mushroom, & Truffle, Sourdough, No.1, Waitrose*	¼ Pizza/120g	334	16.5	279	9.1	28.7	13.8	2
Mushroom, & Roasted Pepper, Allplants*	1 Pizza/353g	660	22.9	187	1.3	32.7	6.5	3.7
Mushroom, Garlic, Thin Crust, Tesco*	½ Pizza/163g	340	14.6	209	11	21.1	9	3.6
Mushroom, Vegan, Plant Chef, Tesco*	¼ Pizza/73g	180	6.5	246	5.6	34.7	8.9	2.5
New Yorker, Stuffed Crust, Iceland*	1/3 Pizza/176g	445	21.5	253	11	24	12.2	1.6
Pancetta, Mushroom, & Mascarpone, Crosta & Mollica*	½ Pizza/223g	580	26.8	260	11	26	12	1.8
Pepperoni, & Cheese, Asda*	½ Pizza/150g	386	13.5	257	10	34	9	2.7
Pepperoni, & Jalapeno Chill, Asda*	1 Pizza/277g	742	22.2	268	10	39	8	1.8
Pepperoni, Average	***1 Serving/250g***	***671***	***28.4***	***269***	***11.8***	***29.6***	***11.4***	***2.1***
Pepperoni, Deep & Crispy, Iceland*	1 Serving/175g	490	21	280	11.9	31.1	12	1.8
Pepperoni, Double, Deep Pan, Asda*	¼ Pizza/80g	223	8.8	280	12	32	11	2.1
Pepperoni, Double, Deep Pan, Chicago Town*	½ Pizza/199g	575	23.9	289	12	32	12	0
Pepperoni, Double, Iceland*	½ Pizza/154g	471	22.3	306	13	29.8	14.5	1.9
Pepperoni, Double, Thin & Crispy, Sainsbury's*	½ Pizza/174g	470	20	270	11.2	29.5	11.5	1.9
Pepperoni, Flatbread, Asda*	1 Pizza/237g	670	23.7	283	11	35	10	2.7
Pepperoni, Hand Stretched, Stone Baked, Sainsbury's*	1 Pizza/298g	852	31.3	286	13	33.3	10.5	3
Pepperoni, Hot & Spicy, Stuffed Crust, Asda*	1 Pizza/245g	666	30	272	13.9	26.5	12.2	2.4
Pepperoni, Mini, Tesco*	1 Serving/22g	71	3.7	323	11.8	30.5	16.8	2.7
Pepperoni, Reg Crust, From Restaurant, Average	***1 Pizza/959g***	***2445***	***94***	***255***	***14.3***	***28***	***9.8***	***0***
Pepperoni, Salame, Ristorante, Dr Oetker*	½ Pizza/165g	465	23.2	281	10	28	14	0
Pepperoni, Spicy, Meat'zza, M&S*	½ Pizza/155g	431	34.3	278	12	6.7	22.1	1.9
Pepperoni, Stone Baked, Tesco*	½ Pizza/140g	399	17.5	285	12.7	29.1	12.5	2.8
Pepperoni, Stone Baked, Thin Crust, Asda*	1 Pizza/289g	754	34.7	261	12	26	12	1.8
Pepperoni, Stonebaked, Chef Select, Lidl*	¼ Pizza/85g	209	7.4	246	11.1	29.5	8.7	2.4
Pepperoni, Stonebaked, Pizzeria, Waitrose*	1/3 Pizza/121g	390	16.5	323	13.6	35.1	13.7	2.6
Pepperoni, Thin & Crispy, Sainsbury's*	½ Pizza/139g	393	18.3	282	12.5	27.6	13.1	1.8
Pepperoni, Thin & Crispy, Essential, Waitrose*	½ Pizza/133g	380	18	286	12.3	28.8	13.5	1
Pepperoni, Thin & Crispy, HFC, Tesco*	½ Pizza/148g	383	13.2	258	10.6	32.8	8.9	2.4
Pepperoni, Thin, Stone Baked, Goodfella's*	½ Pizza/159g	432	19.1	271	13	27	12	2.2
Peppers, Courgettes, Olives, & Pesto, TTD, Sainsbury's*	¼ Pizza/115g	250	7.4	217	9.4	29	6.4	2.9
Pesto Chicken, Stonebaked, The Best, Morrisons*	¼ Pizza/106g	245	6.8	231	10.4	31.6	6.4	2.8
Philly Cheese Steak, Co-Op*	½ Pizza/241g	599	21.7	249	11	30	9	2.5
Pollo, ad Astra, Supermarket, Pizza Express*	½ Pizza/144g	315	8.7	218	11.3	28.9	6	1.8
Pollo, Primavera, Wood Fired, Ultra Thin, M&S*	1 Pizza/185g	414	15.9	224	10.4	25.3	8.6	1.9
Pollo, Ristorante, As Sold, Dr Oetker*	½ Pizza/183g	408	16.5	223	8.8	25.7	9	1.8
Pork, Pulled, BBQ, Fully Loaded, Takeaway, Sainsbury's*	½ Pizza/262g	691	26.7	264	10.5	31.4	10.2	2.2
Prawn, King, Garlic, Wood Fired, Finest, Tesco*	½ Pizza/222g	471	14.7	212	10.4	26.8	6.6	2.1
Prosciutto Cotto, Mushroom, & Mascarpone, Co-Op*	½ Pizza/227g	513	17	226	11	27	7.5	2.4
Quattro Formaggi, Ristorante, Dr Oetker*	½ Pizza/170g	457	23.8	269	10.8	24.1	14	1.6
Roasted Vegetable, & Houmous, Plant Based, Asda*	½ Pizza/188g	360	7.1	192	5.9	32	3.8	4.1

P

	Measure INFO/WEIGHT	per Measure KCAL	FAT	Nutrition Values per 100g / 100ml KCAL	PROT	CARB	FAT	FIBRE
PIZZA								
Salami, & Ham, Pizzeria, Waitrose*	½ Pizza/205g	443	13.7	216	10.1	28.7	6.7	1.8
Salami, & Pepperoni, Waitrose*	½ Pizza/190g	578	30.8	304	13.4	23.9	16.2	2.1
Salami, Napoli Diavolo, Pizza, Wood Fired, M&S*	½ Pizza/244g	549	24.9	225	10.8	21.7	10.2	1.7
Salami, Ultra Thin Italian, Tesco*	1 Serving/263g	692	25.5	263	12	31.9	9.7	1
Salami, Ventricina, Truly Irresistible, Co-Op*	½ Pizza/230g	577	19.6	251	8.5	34	8.5	2.6
Selection, Slices, M&S*	1 Serving/52g	120	4.1	230	9.4	30.3	7.8	1.9
Sloppy Giuseppe, Supermarket, Pizza Express*	½ Pizza/151g	333	10.9	220	10	28.1	7.2	1.6
Spicy Italian Salami, Sourdough, Specially Selected, Aldi*	½ Pizza/265g	657	24.4	248	10	30	9.2	3.1
Spicy Salami, & Red Chill, Finest, Tesco*	½ Pizza/187g	484	18.5	259	12.4	31.7	9.9	1.4
Spinach & Ricotta, Carlos, Aldi*	½ Pizza/170g	362	14.4	213	9.1	24	8.5	2.6
Spinach, & Ricotta, Classic Italian, Stonebaked, Tesco*	½ Pizza/190g	460	16.3	240	10.3	29	8.5	1.2
Spinach, & Ricotta, Thin & Crispy, Baked, Morrisons*	½ Pizza/158g	317	10.4	201	8.1	25.9	6.6	2.6
Spinach, & Ricotta, Thin Crust, Italian, Tesco*	½ Pizza/190g	365	16.7	192	9.6	18.7	8.8	1.9
Spinach, & Ricotta, Chef Select, Lidl*	½ Pizza/160g	339	10.6	212	9.8	26.6	6.6	3.7
Spinach, & Ricotta, Irresistible, Co-Op*	¼ Pizza/105g	270	11.5	258	9.5	30	11	2.2
Spinach, & Ricotta, Stonebaked, M&S*	½ Pizza/253g	543	17.4	215	8	29.2	6.9	2.1
Sub, Cheese & Tomato, Ovenbaked, Asda*	1 Baguette/122g	277	8.3	227	11	29	6.8	2.7
Sub, Pepperoni Pizza, Ovenbaked, Asda*	1 Baguette/122g	272	9.3	223	11	26	7.6	3.1
Super Spicy, Stonebaked, As Sold, Gino D'Acampo*	1 Pizza/458g	1113	50.4	243	8.8	26	11	2.4
The Vegan Gardener, The White Rabbit Pizza Co.*	1 Pizza/340g	656	23.8	193	1.7	32.8	7	3.9
The Whole Hog, Deep & Loaded, M&S*	½ Pizza/345g	823	33.4	239	12.3	24.9	9.7	1.5
Tomato, Mozzarella, & Pesto, Momenti, Dr Oetker*	1 Pizza/182g	422	14.9	232	8.5	30	8.2	2.3
Truffle, Salsiccia, Truly Irresistible, Co-Op*	½ Pack/97g	296	12.6	305	13	33	13	1.2
Vegan, Alfredo, Lidl*	1 Pizza/390g	573	10.5	147	4.9	24.3	2.7	0
Vegan, Hacendado*	1 Pizza/400g	724	21.2	181	6.4	26	5.3	2.5
Vegan, No Cheese, Houmous Style Sauce, Iceland*	½ Pizza/140g	346	18.2	247	6.1	24	13	4.7
Vegetable, & Peppers, Fire Roasted, Waitrose*	½ Pizza/235g	442	16.7	188	9.8	21.3	7.1	2.7
Vegetable, & Pesto, Chargrilled, Specially Selected, Aldi*	½ Pizza/305g	756	29	248	9.2	30	9.5	2.9
Vegetable, Average	***1 Avg Slice/70g***	***133***	***3.7***	***190***	***8.2***	***27.5***	***5.2***	***2.4***
Vegetable, Balsamic Roast, & Mozzarella, Sainsbury's*	½ Pizza/200g	444	15.6	222	8.5	29.4	7.8	2.4
Vegetable, Chargrilled, Frozen, BGTY, Sainsbury's*	1 Pizza/290g	548	13.3	189	10.2	26.7	4.6	3
Vegetable, Deep Pan, Co-Op*	1 Pizza/425g	829	29.8	195	8	25	7	2
Vegetable, Extra Thin, Morrisons*	1 Serving/176g	385	17.1	219	8.3	22.9	9.7	3.4
Vegetable, Frozen, HL, Tesco*	1 Pizza/400g	604	10.8	151	8.1	23.5	2.7	4.4
Vegetable, GFY, Asda*	¼ Pizza/94g	141	2.7	150	7	24	2.9	3.7
Vegetable, Mediterranean, Stonebaked, Carlos, Aldi*	½ Pizza/173g	323	8.7	187	7.5	26.6	5	2.9
Vegetable, Mediterranean, Thin & Crispy, Tesco*	½ Pizza/179g	350	10.7	195	7.1	27.3	6	2.1
Vegetable, Romano, Goodfella's*	½ Pizza/195g	419	15	215	9	26	7.7	0
Vegetable, Salsa, Spicy, Stonebaked, Vegan, Goodfella's*	½ Pizza/181g	385	11.4	213	5.8	32	6.3	2.9
Vegetable, Thin & Crispy, Iceland*	½ Pizza/150g	345	11	230	9.8	29.9	7.3	2.9
Vegetable, Thin & Crispy, Sainsbury's*	½ Pizza/198g	427	14	216	8.6	28.2	7.1	2.3
Veggie Delight, Classic Crust, Takeaway, Sainsbury's*	1 Serving/132g	283	7.3	214	10.1	29.6	5.5	2.6
Veggie Feast, Thin Crust, Stonebaked, Asda*	½ Pizza/168g	360	13.6	214	7.9	26	8.1	3.1
Veggie Feast, Vegan, Flatbread, Asda*	1 Pizza/219g	486	15.1	222	5.6	33	6.9	3.1
Veggie, Very, Stonebaked, M&S*	½ Pizza/274g	537	15.9	196	7.9	27	5.8	2.1
PIZZA BASE								
Deep Pan, Italian, Sainsbury's*	1 Base/220g	684	11	311	7	59.5	5	1.4
Deep Pan, Napolina*	1 Base/260g	757	7.8	291	7.9	58	3	0.2
Dough, Ready Rolled, Tesco*	1 Base/400g	1248	22.4	312	10	54	5.6	2.9
GF, Schar*	1 Pizza/150g	436	5.2	291	3	60	3.5	4.7
Italian, Classic, Sainsbury's*	1 Base/150g	452	7.2	301	7.6	57	4.8	1.5
Light & Crispy, Napolina*	1 Base/150g	436	4.5	291	7.9	58	3	0.2
Low Carb, Thin & Crispy, Lizza*	1 Base/100g	233	11	233	22	2.4	11	19

	Measure INFO/WEIGHT	per Measure KCAL	FAT	Nutrition Values per 100g / 100ml KCAL	PROT	CARB	FAT	FIBRE
PIZZA BASE								
M&S*	1 Base/150g	418	8.1	279	9.2	47.5	5.4	1.9
Mini, Napolina*	1 Base/75g	218	2.2	291	7.9	58	3	0.2
Original, Dough, Frozen, Northern Dough Co. *	1 Base/220g	451	2.9	205	7.1	39.4	1.3	3.4
Stone Baked, GF, BFree*	½ Pizza/90g	231	2.6	257	3.5	49.2	2.9	10
Thin & Crispy, Sainsbury's*	1 Base/150g	504	7.8	336	9.9	62.3	5.2	4.3
Wholemeal, Multiseed, Dough It Yourself*	1 Base/200g	544	9.4	272	12.4	49.1	4.7	0
with Tomato Sauce, Crosta & Mollica*	½ Pizza/135g	282	4.9	209	6	40.7	3.6	3
PLAICE								
Fillets, in Breadcrumbs, Average	***1 Serving/150g***	***331***	***17.9***	***221***	***12.8***	***15.5***	***11.9***	***0.8***
Fillets, Lightly Dusted, Average	***1 Fillet/113g***	***188***	***9.2***	***166***	***12.9***	***10.4***	***8.2***	***0.6***
Fillets, Raw, Average	***1oz/28g***	***24***	***0.4***	***87***	***18.2***	***0***	***1.5***	***0***
Goujons, Baked	***1oz/28g***	***85***	***5.1***	***304***	***8.8***	***27.7***	***18.3***	***0***
Goujons, Fried in Blended Oil	***1oz/28g***	***119***	***9***	***426***	***8.5***	***27***	***32.3***	***0***
Grilled	***1oz/28g***	***27***	***0.5***	***96***	***20.1***	***0***	***1.7***	***0***
in Batter, Fried in Blended Oil	***1oz/28g***	***72***	***4.7***	***257***	***15.2***	***12***	***16.8***	***0.5***
Steamed	***1oz/28g***	***26***	***0.5***	***93***	***18.9***	***0***	***1.9***	***0***
PLANTAIN								
Boiled in Unsalted Water	***1oz/28g***	***31***	***0.1***	***112***	***0.8***	***28.5***	***0.2***	***1.2***
Raw, Average	***1 Med/179g***	***218***	***0.7***	***122***	***1.3***	***31.9***	***0.4***	***2.3***
Ripe, Fried in Vegetable Oil	***1oz/28g***	***75***	***2.6***	***267***	***1.5***	***47.5***	***9.2***	***2.3***
PLUMS								
Average, Stewed without Sugar	***1oz/28g***	***8***	***0***	***30***	***0.5***	***7.3***	***0.1***	***1.3***
Dried, in Port, Chocolate Covered, Hotel Chocolat*	2 Plums/20g	80	6.4	401	4.5	40	32	9.8
Fresh, Raw, Weighed without Stone, Average	***1 Plum/66g***	***24***	***0.1***	***36***	***0.6***	***8.6***	***0.1***	***1.9***
Weighed with Stone, Average	***1 Plum/90g***	***31***	***0.1***	***34***	***0.5***	***8.1***	***0.1***	***1.8***
Yellow, Waitrose*	1 Plum/50g	20	0	39	0.6	8.8	0.1	1.5
POLLOCK								
Fillet, Breaded, Skinless & Boneless, Savers, Morrisons*	1 Fillet/142g	311	11.5	219	13.1	22.9	8.1	1
Fillets, Breaded, HFC, Tesco*	1 Fillet/128g	269	8.2	210	14.6	22.4	6.4	2.1
White Fish, Fillets, Basics, Sainsbury's*	1 Fillet/74g	62	0.4	84	20.4	0	0.5	0
POLO								
Fruits, Nestle*	1 Tube/37g	142	0	383	0	96	0	0
Mints, Original, Nestle*	1 Sweet/2g	8	0	402	0	98.2	1	0
Spearmint, Nestle*	1 Tube/35g	141	0.4	402	0	98.2	1.1	0
POMEGRANATE								
Raw, Fresh, Flesh Only, Average	***1 Sm Fruit/86g***	***59***	***0.3***	***68***	***1***	***17.2***	***0.3***	***0.6***
Raw, Weighed with Rind & Skin, Average	***1 Sm Fruit/154g***	***59***	***0.3***	***38***	***0.5***	***9.6***	***0.2***	***0***
POMELO								
Fresh, Raw, Weighed with Skin & Seeds	***100 Grams/100g***	***11***	***0.1***	***11***	***0.2***	***2.5***	***0.1***	***0***
Raw, Flesh Only, Average	***1 Fruit/340g***	***129***	***0.1***	***38***	***0.8***	***9.6***	***0***	***1***
POP TARTS								
Chocolate, Kellogg's*	1 Pop Tart/50g	198	8.5	396	5	136	17	2
Cookies 'n' Creme, Kellogg's*	1 Pop Tart/50g	190	5	380	4	70	10	2
Frosted Blueberry, Mini Crisps, Kellogg's*	1 Pop Tart/23g	100	2.5	435	4.4	78.3	10.9	0
Frosted Brown Sugar Cinnamon, Kellogg's*	1 Pop Tart/50g	210	7	420	6	68	14	2
Frosted Chocolate Fudge, Kellogg's*	1 Pop Tart/52g	200	5	385	5.8	71.2	9.6	1.9
Frosted Hot Fudge Sundae, Kellogg's*	1 Pop Tart/48g	190	4.5	396	4.2	70.8	9.4	2.1
Frosted Raspberry, Kellogg's*	1 Pop Tart/52g	200	5	385	3.8	73.1	9.6	1.9
Strawberry Sensation, Kellogg's*	1 Pop Tart/50g	198	5.5	395	4	70	11	2
POPCORN								
Air Popped, Plain, Average	***1 Sm Bag/17g***	***66***	***0.8***	***387***	***12.9***	***77.9***	***4.5***	***14.5***
Butter, Microwave, Act II*	1 Bag/90g	425	16.2	472	9	69	18	9

P

	Measure INFO/WEIGHT	per Measure KCAL	FAT	Nutrition Values per 100g / 100ml KCAL	PROT	CARB	FAT	FIBRE
POPCORN								
Butter, Microwave, Popz*	1 Serving/100g	480	27.5	480	7.5	51.1	27.5	9.2
Butter, Toffee, Belgian Milk Chocolate Coated, M&S*	1 Pack/100g	505	25	505	6.5	60.4	25	4.1
Butter, Toffee, Tesco*	1 Pack/175g	709	13.5	405	2.2	81.7	7.7	4.3
Butterfly, Sweet & Salty, Sainsbury's*	1 Pack/14g	68	3.5	487	8.4	52	24.7	11.6
Caramel, Salted, Bloom's*	1 Bag/28g	135	6.6	483	4.9	60.3	23.4	5.8
Caramel, Salted, Butterkist*	1 Serving/20g	83	1.9	417	3.4	77.7	9.5	3.5
Chocolate, & Pecan, M&S*	1 Pack/27g	130	5.2	480	3.3	72.9	19.3	3.6
Coconut, & Vanilla, The Foodie Market, Aldi*	1 Serving/27g	130	6.2	483	9.2	57	23	8.2
Cookie, Tesco*	1 Serving/25g	113	3.3	452	3.3	79	13.2	1.8
Corn Triangles, Popped, Sweet & Salty, M&S*	1/3 Pack/23g	98	2.3	427	6.4	76.3	10	3.1
Cotton Candy, American Style, Epic*	1 Pot/150g	766	41.7	511	6.1	59.7	27.8	7
Kernels, Wholegrain, Kelkin*	1 Bowl/40g	142	1.4	354	10.2	71	3.4	10.5
Maple, Shapers, Boots*	1 Bag/20g	94	3.6	469	12	59	18	10
Original, Cracker Jack*	1 Pack/35g	148	3	424	5.6	81.9	8.5	5.6
Peanut Butter, & Almond, Propercorn*	1 Serving/25g	115	5	460	12.9	50.2	20.2	12.9
Peanut Butter, The Foodie Market, Aldi*	1 Pack/27g	133	6.5	493	12	53	24	8.3
Peanut, & Almond, Smooth, Propercorn*	1 Serving/25g	120	5.9	481	11.9	49.4	23.5	12.2
Plain, Oil Popped, Average	***1 Bag/74g***	***439***	***31.7***	***593***	***6.2***	***48.7***	***42.8***	***0***
Popping Corn, Average	***1 Serving/30g***	***112***	***1.3***	***375***	***10.9***	***73.1***	***4.3***	***12.7***
Salt & Vinegar, Snack-A-Jacks, Quaker*	1 Sm Pack/13g	47	1.3	360	12	55	9.9	14
Salted Caramel, Propercorn*	1 Serving/20g	97	4.6	484	4.7	61.8	22.9	5.9
Salted, Blockbuster*	1 Bowl/25g	99	2.9	397	10.6	62.2	11.7	8.6
Salted, Cineworld, Munchbox*	1 Serving/55g	235	9.1	427	9.6	52.7	16.6	14.4
Salted, Crunch Corn, Propercorn*	1 Serving/30g	140	7.9	468	5	52.1	26.4	12.2
Salted, Diet Chef Ltd*	1 Pack/23g	107	3.8	465	10.5	68.6	16.6	14
Salted, Light, Microwave, Act II*	1 Pack/85g	336	6.5	395	10.6	71	7.6	15.8
Salted, Lightly, Popping Corn, Graze*	1 Punnet/28g	127	7	454	8	44	25	13
Salted, Lightly, Sea, Propercorn*	1 Bag/10g	44	1.7	436	8.6	56.7	16.9	11
Salted, Lightly, The Foodie Market, Aldi*	1 Pack/27g	127	5.7	471	11	56	21	7.6
Salted, Microwave, Popz*	1 Serving/20g	101	6	504	7	51.5	30	9.2
Salted, Microwave, Propercorn*	1 Pack/20g	84	3.8	418	8.5	47.4	19.1	11.4
Salted, Microwave, Snaktastic, Lidl*	1 Pack/100g	483	23	483	10.7	53	23	10.8
Salted, Microwave, Sunsnacks*	1 Pack/100g	498	22.9	498	10.7	51.3	22.9	10.8
Salted, Sea Salt, Skinny, Topcorn, Metcalfe's Food Co*	1 Pack/23g	108	5.6	471	6.6	63.7	24.4	15.2
Salted, Variety Pack, Tesco*	1 Bag/11g	57	3.4	522	7.6	48.3	31.3	8.5
Salted, Variety, Asda*	1 Bag/11g	54	2.8	489	8.3	52	25	510
San Carlo*	1 Serving/20g	97	5	485	9.5	50	25	11
Sour Cream & Black Pepper, Propercorn*	1 Bag/20g	88	3.7	440	10.8	50.1	18.3	15.9
Sweet & Salty, Microwave, Butterkist*	1 Pack/70g	298	14.1	425	8.2	48.5	20.2	8.4
Sweet & Salt, Metcalfe's Food Co*	1 Pack/100g	481	23.8	481	8.1	53.4	23.8	10.3
Sweet & Salted, Snackrite, Aldi*	1 Serving/30g	141	6	471	7.1	62	20	7.5
Sweet & Salty, Bloom's*	1 Portion/28g	138	7	492	4	58.6	25	8.5
Sweet & Salty, M&S*	1 Bag/15g	73	3.7	488	7.7	55.4	24.4	7.8
Sweet & Salty, Propercorn*	1 Bag/14g	63	2.5	451	5.4	63.2	18	10.8
Sweet & Salty, Tesco*	¼ Bag/27g	132	6.3	488	6.3	60	23.4	6.1
Sweet, & Salted, Snaktastic, Lidl*	1 Serving/25g	122	5.8	486	7.7	59	23	6.3
Sweet, & Salted, The Foodie Market, Aldi*	1 Bag/27g	120	4.2	444	9.3	63	15.6	7.4
Sweet, Asda*	1 Bag/13g	63	2.9	483	5.3	62	22	7.7
Sweet, Butterkist, Butterkist*	1 Pack/120g	612	29.8	510	2.8	68.5	24.8	5.6
Sweet, Cinema Style, Basics, Sainsbury's*	1 Handful/20g	90	4.4	450	5.9	57.5	21.8	11.1
Sweet, Cinema Style, Butterkist*	1 Bag/85g	447	22	526	5.2	65.2	25.9	5.8
Sweet, Coconut & Vanilla, Propercorn*	1 Bag/25g	122	5.5	486	6	61.6	22.1	7.7
Sweet, Deli, Passions, Aldi*	1 Bag/27g	121	4.2	448	7	74.8	15.6	10.7

	Measure INFO/WEIGHT	per Measure KCAL	FAT	Nutrition Values per 100g / 100ml KCAL	PROT	CARB	FAT	FIBRE
POPCORN								
Sweet, Microwave, Butterkist*	1 Pack/70g	316	15.4	452	7	53	22	7.2
Sweet, Propercorn*	1 Pack/20g	93	3.7	464	5.8	65.5	18.5	6.3
Toffee, Butterkist*	1 Sm Bag/50g	212	4.7	424	3.1	80.1	9.4	3.2
Toffee, Sainsbury's*	1 Serving/50g	208	6.4	415	1.8	73.8	12.7	3.3
Toffee, Snack Pack, Butterkist*	1 Bag/25g	106	2.4	424	3.1	80.1	9.4	3.2
Toffee, Snaktastic, Lidl*	1 Serving/25g	106	2.1	424	2.4	82.8	8.4	2.8
POPPADOMS								
Balti, Mini, Vitasia, Lidl*	½ Bag/30g	153	9.5	510	18.4	34.3	31.6	7.4
Fried in Vegetable Oil, Takeaway, Average	***1 Poppadom/13g***	***65***	***5***	***501***	***11.5***	***28.3***	***38.8***	***5.8***
Garlic & Coriander, Ready to Eat, Sharwood's*	1 Poppadom/9g	39	1.9	438	18.4	43	21.4	6.5
Indian, Asda*	1 Pack/45g	232	15.7	516	14.5	36.2	34.8	7.8
Mango Chutney Flavour, Mini, M&S*	1 Poppadom/25g	130	8.3	518	13.1	39.9	33	4.5
Mini, Sainsbury's*	½ Pack/50g	249	16.2	498	14.9	36.9	32.3	7.6
Plain, Asda*	1 Poppadom/9g	44	2.5	484	18	40	28	0
Plain, Bilash, Aldi*	1 Poppadom/8g	36	1.8	448	20	38	22	9.7
Plain, Cook to Eat, Sharwood's*	1 Poppadom/12g	32	0.1	273	21.9	45.7	1	10.1
Plain, Indian to Go, Sainsbury's*	1 Poppadom/8g	34	1.5	405	18.4	43.4	17.5	9
Plain, Low Fat, Sharwood's*	1 Poppadom/12g	35	0.1	295	20.7	46.5	0.9	9
Plain, Mini, Cook to Eat, Sharwood's*	1 Poppadom/4g	11	0	273	21.9	45.7	0.3	10.1
Plain, Ready to Eat, Average	***2 Poppadom/16g***	***68***	***2.8***	***427***	***19.8***	***46.6***	***17.3***	***6.6***
Plain, Ready to Eat, Sharwood's*	1 Poppadom/8g	37	1.8	461	19.4	46.3	22	5.6
Plain, Taste of India, Lidl*	1 Poppadom/8g	36	1.6	449	19.5	40	20.4	12.8
Plain, Taste of India, Tesco*	1 Poppadom/8g	36	1.6	449	19.5	40	20.4	13.8
Plain, Tesco*	1 Poppadom/9g	41	2	439	17.8	44.4	21.1	4.6
Plain, Waitrose*	1 Poppadom/9g	37	1.7	408	21	39.3	18.6	9.1
Spicy, Cook to Eat, Sharwood's*	1 Poppadom/12g	30	0.1	257	20.2	43	0.5	13
Spicy, COU, M&S*	1 Pack/26g	84	0.6	325	23.5	51.9	2.4	8.1
POPPETS*								
Chocolate Raisins, Poppets*	1 Pack/35g	140	4.7	401	4.9	65.4	13.3	0
Toffee, Milk Chocolate, Poppets*	1 Box/100g	491	23	491	5.3	68	23	0
PORK								
& Stuffing, Sliced, Asda*	1 Slice/53g	79	2.7	148	23	2.2	5.1	0.7
Belly Slices, Maple, Oven Baked, Asda*	½ Pack/141g	501	36.6	356	27	3.8	26	1
Belly, Fresh, Raw, Weighed with Skin, Average	***1 Serving/100g***	***518***	***53***	***518***	***9.3***	***0***	***53***	***0***
Belly, Roasted, Lean & Fat	***1oz/28g***	***82***	***6***	***293***	***25.1***	***0***	***21.4***	***0***
Belly, Slices, Woodside Farms, Tesco*	1 Slice/125g	382	33.5	306	15.9	0.1	26.8	0.3
Chop, British, Grilled, Sainsbury's*	1 Chop/121g	409	31	338	25.3	1.3	25.6	0.8
Chops, Thick Cut, Hampshire Bred, The Best, Morrisons*	1 Chop/350g	945	76	270	18.6	0	21.7	0
Diced, Lean, Average	***1oz/28g***	***31***	***0.5***	***109***	***22***	***0***	***1.8***	***0***
Escalope, Average	***1 Escalope/75g***	***108***	***1.7***	***144***	***31***	***0***	***2.2***	***0***
Escalope, Lean, Healthy Range, Average	***1 Escalope/75g***	***80***	***1.5***	***106***	***22***	***0***	***2***	***0***
Frikadellen, Patties, Dulano, Lidl*	1 Patty/100g	287	22	287	13.9	8	22	0.5
Ham, Hock, Raw, Weighed with Bone, Fat & Skin	***100g***	***124***	***5***	***124***	***18.4***	***0***	***5***	***0***
Joint with Crackling, Ready to Roast, Average	***1 Joint/567g***	***1283***	***80.1***	***226***	***24.2***	***0.8***	***14.1***	***0***
Joint, Ready to Roast, Average	***½ Joint/254g***	***375***	***18***	***148***	***19.2***	***2.3***	***7.1***	***0.2***
Kabanos, Smoked, Dried, Polish, Krakus*	1 Serving/30g	169	14.1	563	28	7	47	0
Kebabs, Maple BBQ, Sticky, Co-Op*	1 Kebab/100g	174	9.5	174	17	4.5	9.5	0.7
Leg, Joint, Healthy Range, Average	***1 Serving/200g***	***206***	***4.4***	***103***	***20***	***0.6***	***2.2***	***0***
Loin, Applewood Smoked, Asda*	1 Slice/15g	18	0.5	122	21.8	0.5	3.6	0
Loin, Chop, Raw, Lean & Fat, Boneless	***1 Avg Chop/185g***	***287***	***12.8***	***155***	***21.6***	***0***	***6.9***	***0***
Loin, Chop, Raw, Lean Only, Boneless	***1 Avg Chop/155g***	***197***	***5.3***	***127***	***22.4***	***0***	***3.4***	***0***
Loin, Chops, Boneless, Grilled, Average	***1oz/28g***	***83***	***4.1***	***298***	***27***	***0***	***14.6***	***0***
Loin, Chops, Grilled, Lean	***1oz/28g***	***52***	***1.8***	***184***	***31.6***	***0***	***6.4***	***0***

P

	Measure INFO/WEIGHT	per Measure KCAL	FAT	Nutrition Values per 100g / 100ml KCAL	PROT	CARB	FAT	FIBRE
PORK								
Loin, Chops, Raw, Lean & Fat, Weighed with Bone	***1 Chop/130g***	***248***	***19.9***	***191***	***13.2***	***0***	***15.3***	***0***
Loin, Joint, Roast, Lean	***1oz/28g***	***51***	***1.9***	***182***	***30.1***	***0***	***6.8***	***0***
Loin, Joint, Roasted, Lean & Fat	***1oz/28g***	***71***	***4.3***	***253***	***26.3***	***0***	***15.3***	***0***
Loin, Peppered, Roast, Aldi*	1 Slice/20g	26	0.9	132	21	2	4.6	0.5
Loin, Steak, Cajun, Smoky, Cooked, Tesco*	½ Pack/151g	340	22.8	225	19.1	2.7	15.1	1.1
Loin, Steak, Fried, Lean	***1oz/28g***	***53***	***2***	***191***	***31.5***	***0***	***7.2***	***0***
Loin, Steak, Fried, Lean & Fat	***1oz/28g***	***77***	***5.2***	***276***	***27.5***	***0***	***18.4***	***0***
Loin, Steak, Lean, Raw, Average	***1 Serving/175g***	***345***	***19.6***	***197***	***22.7***	***0***	***11.2***	***0.4***
Loin, Steak, Pepper Crusted, M&S*	½ Pack/150g	189	6	126	22.5	1	4	1
Loin, Steaks, Beechwood Smoked, Sainsbury's*	2 Steaks/123g	216	5.2	176	30.7	3.6	4.2	0.6
Loin, Steaks, Maple BBQ, Fire Pit, Tesco*	1 Steak/76g	210	13.3	277	23.4	5	17.6	2
Loin, Steaks, Memphis BBQ, Ashfield Farm, Aldi*	½ Pack/220g	598	35.2	272	28	4.5	16	0.5
Loin, Steaks, Smokey BBQ, Birchwood Farm, Lidl*	1 Steak/89g	190	11.5	213	19.7	4	12.9	1
Loin, Steaks, Sweet Chilli, Grilled, Asda*	1 Loin/110g	267	13.2	243	28	6.2	12	1
Loin, with Beans,& Apple Gravy, Tesco*	1 Pack/372g	294	7.1	79	7.4	7.3	1.9	1.5
Loin, with Rind, Uncooked, Average	***1 Serving/100g***	***246***	***18.8***	***246***	***19.3***	***0***	***18.8***	***0***
Lorne, Slices, Plum Tree Farm*	1 Slice/60g	34	2.4	56	2.5	2.8	4	0.1
Luncheon, Meat, Slices, Morrisons*	1 Slice/13g	28	2.3	216	12.6	2.3	17.4	0.1
Medallions, Average	***1 Medallion/125g***	***140***	***2.6***	***112***	***22.6***	***0***	***2***	***0***
Mince, Lean, Healthy Range, Average	***1 Pack/400g***	***504***	***20.2***	***126***	***19.8***	***0.4***	***5***	***0.3***
Mince, Raw	***1oz/28g***	***46***	***2.7***	***164***	***19.2***	***0***	***9.7***	***0***
Mince, Stewed	***1oz/28g***	***53***	***2.9***	***191***	***24.4***	***0***	***10.4***	***0***
Patties, Breakfast, Frozen, Oakhurst, Aldi*	1 Pattie/45g	132	9.4	293	25	1.6	21	0.5
Pibil, Slow Cooked, Mexican, Waitrose*	½ Pack/184g	374	23.7	203	21.2	0.5	12.9	0.5
Pulled, Slow Cooked, M&S*	½ Pack/85g	143	4.8	168	17.6	11.5	5.7	0.2
Pulled, Vegetarian, Linda McCartney*	1 Pack/300g	567	25.8	189	19.5	6.2	8.6	0
Raw, Lean, Average	***1oz/28g***	***42***	***1.2***	***151***	***28.6***	***0***	***4.1***	***0***
Rissole, Low Fat, Oh So Lean*	1 Rissole/50g	89	1.2	178	16.6	10.4	2.3	0
Roast, Lean Only, Average	***1oz/28g***	***34***	***0.9***	***121***	***22.7***	***0.3***	***3.3***	***0***
Roast, Slices, Average	***1 Slice/30g***	***40***	***1.4***	***134***	***22.7***	***0.4***	***4.5***	***0***
Saltimbocca, Cook with, M&S*	½ Pack/143g	207	9.6	145	19.6	1.5	6.7	0.1
Saucisson Sec, Slices, Tesco*	3 Slices/15g	53	4.1	355	26	0.6	27.4	1.1
Schnitzel, XXL, Farmfoods*	1 Schnitzel/250g	530	25	212	16	14	10	0
Shoulder, Boneless, Average	***1 Piece/430g***	***127***	***3.4***	***127***	***22.5***	***0***	***3.4***	***0***
Shoulder, Steaks, British, Sainsbury's*	1 Steak/113g	305	19.5	270	27.2	0.9	17.3	0.8
Shoulder, Steaks, Raw, The Butchers Market, Iceland*	1 Steak/160g	298	19.8	186	18.5	0	12.4	0
Shoulder, Whole, Lean & Fat, Raw, Average	***100g***	***236***	***18***	***236***	***17.2***	***0***	***18***	***0***
Shoulder, Whole, Lean Only, Roasted	***1 Serving/150g***	***345***	***20.3***	***230***	***25.3***	***0***	***13.5***	***0***
Steak, Lean & Fat, Average	***1oz/28g***	***61***	***3.8***	***219***	***23.8***	***0***	***13.7***	***0.1***
Steak, Lean, Stewed	***1oz/28g***	***49***	***1.3***	***176***	***33.6***	***0***	***4.6***	***0***
Steak, Loin, BBQ Chinese, Tesco*	1 Steak/81g	219	14.4	270	21.9	5.3	17.7	1.1
Stir Fry Strips, Lean, Healthy Range, Average	***¼ Pack/113g***	***118***	***2.3***	***104***	***21.3***	***0***	***2***	***0***
Tenderloin, Lean, Boneless, Raw, Average	***1 Serving/100g***	***109***	***2.2***	***109***	***21***	***0***	***2.2***	***0***
Thai Style, Rice Bowl, Hello Fresh*	1 Serving/373g	720	26.1	193	9	22	7	0
PORK CRACKLING								
BBQ, Low & Sow, The Snaffling Pig Co.*	1 Bag/14g	87	6.6	621	43.9	0.5	47.5	0
PORK DINNER								
Roast, 103, Oakhouse Foods Ltd*	1 Dinner/400g	376	14.8	94	6.7	8.3	3.7	1.4
Roast, Birds Eye*	1 Pack/340g	410	12	121	7.6	14.7	3.5	1.6
PORK IN								
Gravy, Baby Potatoes, Carrots, & Savoy Cabbage, M&S*	1 Pack395g	288	9.9	73	6.2	5.7	2.5	1.6
Mustard & Cream, Chops	***1oz/28g***	***73***	***6***	***261***	***14.5***	***2.4***	***21.6***	***0.3***

	Measure INFO/WEIGHT	per Measure KCAL	FAT	Nutrition Values per 100g / 100ml KCAL	PROT	CARB	FAT	FIBRE
PORK SCRATCHINGS								
Crispy Strips, Mr Porky*	1 Bag/20g	102	5.7	508	62.4	0.6	28.4	0
Crunch, Mr Porky*	1 Pack/25g	129	6.9	515	65.7	0.6	27.7	0
Crunch, Traditional Black Country*	1 Bag/25g	138	8.9	554	57.8	0.4	35.7	0
Hand Cooked, Mr Porky*	½ Pack/33g	212	17.1	653	44.3	0.4	52.7	0
Jays*	1 Serving/60g	369	27.7	615	49.7	0.2	46.2	0
KP Snacks*	1 Pack/20g	125	9.6	624	47.3	0.5	48.1	0.5
Pn, Proteinium*	1 Bag/30g	156	7.9	520	69.7	0.1	26.2	0
Puffs, Original Salted, The Curators*	1 Serving/22g	118	6.1	536	71.1	0.1	27.8	0.7
Puffs, Spicy BBQ, The Curators*	1 Pack/25g	128	7.1	513	60.3	10	28.4	1
PORT								
Average	***1 Serving/50ml***	***78***	***0***	***157***	***0.1***	***12***	***0***	***0***
White, Average	***1 Glass/125ml***	***182***	***0***	***146***	***0.1***	***11***	***0***	***0***
POT NOODLE*								
Beef & Tomato, King, Made Up, Pot Noodle*	1 Pot/420g	543	19.8	129	3.3	18.5	4.7	1.1
Beef & Tomato, Made Up, Pot Noodle*	1 Pot/320g	426	14.7	133	3.4	19.4	4.6	1.3
Bombay Bad Boy, King, Made Up , Pot Noodle*	1 Pot/420g	542	19.7	129	3.3	18.5	4.7	1.1
Bombay Bad Boy, Made Up, Pot Noodle*	1 Pot/320g	415	15.3	130	3.3	18.4	4.8	1.1
Chicken & Mushroom, King, Made Up, Pot Noodle*	1 Pot/420g	545	19.3	130	3.3	18.8	4.6	1
Chicken & Mushroom, Made Up, Pot Noodle*	1 Pot/305g	430	18	141	3	19	5.9	1
Chilli Beef, Made Up, Pot Noodle*	1 Pot/305g	384	14.6	126	3	17.7	4.8	0.8
Chow Mein Chinese, Made Up, Pot Noodle*	1 Pot/320g	416	14.7	130	3.2	19	4.6	1.3
Curry, Original, King, Made Up, Pot Noodle*	1 Pot/420g	507	18.1	121	2.6	17.9	4.3	1
Curry, Original, Made Up, Pot Noodle*	1 Pot/320g	431	15	135	3.1	20	4.7	1.2
Curry, Spicy, Made Up, Pot Noodle*	1 Pot/300g	393	14.4	131	2.9	19.1	4.8	1.1
Jerk Chicken Flavour, Made Up, Pot Noodle*	1 Pot/303g	433	17.9	143	3.2	18	5.9	1
Piri Piri Chicken, Made Up, Pot Noodle*	1 Pot/307g	430	15.4	140	3	20	5	0
Sweet & Sour, Made Up, Pot Noodle*	1 Pot/305g	436	17.1	143	2.6	20	5.6	1.2
POTATO BOMBAY								
Average	***½ Pack/150g***	***176***	***10.2***	***117***	***2***	***13.7***	***6.8***	***1.2***
POTATO CAKES								
Average	***1 Cake/70g***	***127***	***1.2***	***180***	***3.8***	***37.5***	***1.7***	***2.4***
Fried, Average	***1oz/28g***	***66***	***2.5***	***237***	***4.9***	***35***	***9***	***0.8***
POTATO SALAD								
& Egg, with Mayonnaise, Tesco*	½ Tub/150g	115	8.5	77	2.9	3.1	5.7	1.2
& Yoghurt, Meadow Fresh, Lidl*	1 Portion/50g	72	4	144	1.8	15.4	8	1.8
Baby, Finest, Tesco*	¼ Pack/69g	143	11.8	206	1.4	11.3	17	0.7
Charlotte, Extra Special, Asda*	1/3 Pack/92g	119	7.9	130	1.3	11	8.6	2.3
Charlotte, TTD, Sainsbury's*	½ Pack/150g	212	14.1	141	2	11	9.4	2
From Restaurant, Average	***1/3 Cup/95g***	***108***	***5.7***	***114***	***1.5***	***13.5***	***6***	***0***
Reduced Calorie, Pre Packed	***1oz/28g***	***27***	***1.1***	***97***	***1.3***	***14.8***	***4.1***	***0.8***
Vegan, Sainsbury's*	¼ Pot/75g	139	10.4	185	1.7	12.2	13.9	2.1
with Mayonnaise, Retail	***1oz/28g***	***80***	***7.4***	***287***	***1.5***	***11.4***	***26.5***	***0.8***
POTATO SKINS								
Cheese & Bacon, Loaded, Asda*	½ Pack/125g	275	15	220	13	15	12	3.3
Cheese, & Bacon, Sainsbury's*	1 Skin/97g	154	6.6	159	6.9	16.2	6.8	2.9
Cheese, & Chive, Mini, Co-Op*	1 Skin/28g	48	2.3	172	7.1	15	8.2	3.8
Cheese, & Chive, Oven Baked, Asda*	1 Pack/245g	392	15.7	160	5.9	18	6.4	3
with Sour Cream	***1 Serving/275g***	***541***	***34.6***	***197***	***7.2***	***13.8***	***12.6***	***2.2***
POTATO WAFFLES								
Frozen, Cooked	***1oz/28g***	***56***	***2.3***	***200***	***3.2***	***30.3***	***8.2***	***2.3***
Potato, & Carrot, Mini, Oven Baked, Asda*	1 Serving/60g	124	3.8	205	3.2	32	6.3	3.3
Sweet Potato, Birds Eye*	1 Waffle/59g	150	9.4	255	2.2	24	16	2.9

P

	Measure INFO/WEIGHT	per Measure KCAL	FAT	Nutrition Values per 100g / 100ml KCAL	PROT	CARB	FAT	FIBRE
POTATO WEDGES								
Aldi*	1 Serving/100g	150	6.8	150	2.1	20.2	6.8	0
Crispy, M&S*	1 Serving/200g	340	14.2	170	1.3	25.3	7.1	1.7
Fiery & Filthy, Wicked Kitchen, Tesco*	½ Pack/219g	285	7.2	130	2.1	21.5	3.3	3.1
Frozen, Average	***1 Serving/120g***	***145***	***4.1***	***121***	***2***	***20.5***	***3.4***	***2.2***
Garlic, & Rosemary, Frozen, Jumbo frozen*	1/3 Pack/200g	276	8.8	138	2.5	21	4.4	2.3
Harvest Basket, Lidl*	1 Serving/175g	215	6	123	2.2	20	3.4	2.6
Loaded, Mexican Beef, with Spring Onion, Hello Fresh*	1 Serving/757g	742	31	98	6.2	8.8	4.1	2
Maris Piper, Aldi*	1 Serving/100g	189	7.8	189	2.3	26	7.8	2.6
Southern Fried, Oven Baked, Iceland*	1 Serving/100g	190	6.2	190	2.9	28.4	6.2	4.3
Spicy, Asda*	1 Serving/100g	145	5.7	145	1.8	21.8	5.7	2.1
Spicy, Oven Cooked, Green Isle*	1 Serving/150g	339	15	226	3.4	28	10	3.4
Sweet Potato, Spiced, Allplants*	1 Serving/130g	240	8.3	185	2.4	28	6.4	3.4
with Sour Cream Dip, Waitrose *	½ Pack/201g	273	8.2	136	2.8	20.2	4.1	3.7
POTATOES								
Alphabites, Captain Birds Eye, Birds Eye*	9 Bites/56g	75	3	134	2	19.5	5.3	1.4
Anya, Raw, TTD, Sainsbury's*	1 Serving/100g	75	0.3	75	1.5	17.8	0.3	1.1
Apache, Albert Bartlett & Sons Ltd*	1 Serving/175g	278	17.3	159	2.4	14	9.9	6.5
Baby, Herby, Microwave, Nature's Pick, Aldi*	½ Pack/193g	171	3.5	89	2.2	15	1.8	2.2
Baby, Raw, Linroyale*	1 Serving/100g	65	0.3	65	1.4	14.1	0.3	0
Baby, Salad, Boiled with Skins, Garden Of Elveden*	1 Serving/100g	64	0.1	64	1.8	14.9	0.1	13.8
Baby, with Herbs & Butter, Morrisons*	1 Serving/100g	94	2.3	94	1.9	14.6	2.3	1.9
Baby, with Herbs, & Butter, Sainsbury's*	½ Pack/193g	145	3.5	75	2.8	11.1	1.8	1.9
Baked, & Cheese, Waitrose*	½ Pack/220g	281	8.6	128	3.7	18.1	3.9	2.6
Baked, Chilli Con Carne, COU, M&S*	1 Pack/300g	270	6.3	90	6	11.1	2.1	1.2
Baked, Flesh & Skin, Average	***1 Med/200g***	***218***	***0.2***	***109***	***2.3***	***25.2***	***0.1***	***2.4***
Baked, Flesh Only, Weighed with Skin, Average	***1oz/28g***	***20***	***0***	***72***	***1.5***	***16.6***	***0.1***	***1.2***
Baked, in Microwave, Flesh & Skin, Average	***1oz/28g***	***29***	***0***	***105***	***2.4***	***24.1***	***0.1***	***2.3***
Baked, in Microwave, Flesh Only, Average	***1oz/28g***	***28***	***0***	***100***	***2.1***	***23.3***	***0.1***	***1.6***
Baked, in Microwave, Skin Only, Average	***1oz/28g***	***37***	***0***	***132***	***4.4***	***29.6***	***0.1***	***5.5***
Baked, Mature Cheddar Cheese, M&S*	½ Pack/206g	225	6.6	109	3.6	16.9	3.2	1
Baked, Skin Only, Average	***1oz/28g***	***55***	***0***	***198***	***4.3***	***46.1***	***0.1***	***7.9***
Baked, Tuna & Sweetcorn, Average	***1 Serving/300g***	***273***	***6.8***	***91***	***5***	***12.6***	***2.2***	***0.9***
Baked, with Cheese & Butter, Tesco*	1 Potato/214g	212	4.2	99	3	16.4	2	1.9
Baking, Raw, Average	***1 Med/250g***	***198***	***0.2***	***79***	***2.1***	***18***	***0.1***	***1.6***
Boiled with Skin	***1 Potato/125g***	***98***	***0.1***	***78***	***2.9***	***17.2***	***0.1***	***3.3***
Boiled, Average	***1 Serving/120g***	***86***	***0.1***	***72***	***1.8***	***17***	***0.1***	***1.2***
Bombay, for Two, Sainsbury's*	½ Pack/144g	155	9	108	1.8	9.8	6.3	2.2
Bombay, Tasty Bite*	½ Pack/143g	122	4.9	85	2.9	10.4	3.4	2.7
Boulangere, M&S*	½ Pack/225g	180	2	80	2.8	15.9	0.9	0.9
Charlotte, Average	***1 Serving/184g***	***139***	***0.5***	***76***	***1.6***	***17.4***	***0.2***	***3.3***
Crispy, Slices, Co-Op*	½ Pack/150g	435	27	290	2.5	28	18	3.1
Dauphinoise, Average	***1 Serving/200g***	***335***	***23.9***	***168***	***2.2***	***12.8***	***12***	***1.5***
Desiree, Average	***1 Serving/200g***	***152***	***0.4***	***76***	***2.2***	***16.4***	***0.2***	***0.6***
Fritters, Crispy, Oven Baked, Birds Eye*	1 Fritter/20g	29	1.6	145	2	16.3	8	1.2
Hasselback, Average	***1 Serving/175g***	***182***	***1.6***	***104***	***1.9***	***22***	***0.9***	***2.9***
Jersey Royal, Canned, Average	***1 Can/186g***	***116***	***0.2***	***62***	***1.4***	***14***	***0.1***	***1.2***
Jersey Royal, New, Raw, Average	***1oz/28g***	***21***	***0.1***	***75***	***1.6***	***17.2***	***0.2***	***1.5***
Lattices, Golden, Oven Baked, Asda*	1/6 Pack/91g	180	7.3	198	3	26	8	5.1
Lattices, Tesco*	¼ Pack/103g	221	8.4	215	3	29.8	8.2	5.2
Maris Piper, Raw, Average	***1 Serving/200g***	***151***	***0.4***	***75***	***2***	***16.5***	***0.2***	***1.4***
Mash, Buttery, Creamy, Finest, Tesco*	½ Pack/215g	219	9.5	102	2	13	4.4	1.3
Mash, Creamy, Maris Piper, Extra Special, Asda*	½ Pack/200g	202	10	101	1.3	12	5	2.3
Mash, Creamy, Morrisons*	½ Pack/243g	386	24.3	159	2.1	14.2	10	1.6

	Measure INFO/WEIGHT	per Measure KCAL	FAT	Nutrition Values per 100g / 100ml KCAL	PROT	CARB	FAT	FIBRE
POTATOES								
Mashed, Cheddar Cheese, Idahoan*	1 Pack/109g	88	2.4	81	1.8	12.9	2.2	0
Mashed, Cubes, Fluffy & Buttery, Frozen, Aunt Bessie's*	15 Cubes/123g	127	5.1	103	1.9	14	4.1	0.9
Mashed, From Restaurant, Average	***1/3 Cup/80g***	***66***	***1***	***83***	***2.3***	***16.1***	***1.2***	***0***
Mashed, From Supermarket, Healthy Range, Average	***1 Serving/200g***	***160***	***3.1***	***80***	***1.8***	***14.6***	***1.6***	***1.3***
Mashed, Home Prepared with Whole Milk	***1 Cup/210g***	***162***	***1.2***	***77***	***1.9***	***17.6***	***0.6***	***2***
Mashed, Jersey Butter & Black Pepper, TTD, Sainsbury's*	½ Pack/225g	243	13.7	108	1.4	11.2	6.1	1.5
Mashed, Made Up with Water, Average	***1 Serving/180g***	***118***	***0.3***	***66***	***1.7***	***14.5***	***0.2***	***1.3***
Mashed, with Cream & Butter, Ultimate, M&S*	½ Pack/225g	268	13.7	119	2.5	12.8	6.1	1.2
New, & Vegetables, M&S*	1 Pot/170g	76	3.2	45	1.1	4.8	1.9	1.9
New, Average	***1 Serving/100g***	***75***	***0.3***	***75***	***1.5***	***17.8***	***0.3***	***1.1***
New, Baby, Average	***1 Serving/180g***	***135***	***0.5***	***75***	***1.7***	***17***	***0.3***	***1.6***
New, Baby, Canned, Average	***1 Can/120g***	***69***	***0.2***	***58***	***1.4***	***12.9***	***0.2***	***1.4***
New, Easy Steam with Herbs & Butter, Tesco*	1 Serving/125g	94	3.5	75	1.8	9.6	2.8	1.7
New, with Herb Dressing, Morrisons*	½ Pack/146g	114	1.6	78	1.7	14.3	1.1	1.9
Pan Fried, Aldi*	1 Serving/250g	182	2	73	2.7	13.7	0.8	0
Raw, Peeled, Flesh Only	***1 Serving/100g***	***75***	***0.2***	***75***	***2***	***17.3***	***0.2***	***1.4***
Red, Flesh Only, Average	***1 Serving/300g***	***218***	***0.4***	***72***	***2***	***16.4***	***0.2***	***1.2***
Roast, Dry, No Oil, No fat	***1 Serving/100g***	***79***	***0.1***	***79***	***2.7***	***18***	***0.1***	***1.6***
Roast, Frozen, Average	***1 Potato/70g***	***105***	***3.5***	***149***	***2.6***	***23.5***	***5***	***1.4***
Roast, Garlic & Rosemary, Miniature, Tesco*	¼ Pack/125g	85	0.9	68	1.8	12.5	0.7	2.3
Roast, Goose Fat, Oven Baked, Luxury, Iceland*	1 Serving/100g	215	7.7	215	3	31.5	7.7	3.5
Roast, in Lard, Average	***1oz/28g***	***42***	***1.3***	***149***	***2.9***	***25.9***	***4.5***	***1.8***
Roast, in Oil, Average	***1oz/28g***	***42***	***1.3***	***149***	***2.9***	***25.9***	***4.5***	***1.8***
Roast, New, Rosemary, Ainsley Harriott*	1 Serving/150g	133	4	89	2	16	2.7	1.3
Roast, with Goose Fat, TTD, Sainsbury's*	½ Pack/185g	216	4.4	117	2.7	21.1	2.4	3
Roasting, Average	***1 Serving/150g***	***202***	***5.2***	***135***	***2.5***	***23.4***	***3.5***	***1.6***
Scallops, Battered, Deep Fried, Average	***1 Scallop/67g***	***216***	***14.5***	***323***	***5.4***	***27.3***	***21.6***	***0***
Smiles, Weighed Baked, McCain*	1 Serving/100g	193	7.7	193	2.4	27.3	7.7	2.8
Smiles, Weighed Frozen, McCain*	½ Pack/228g	406	16.2	178	2.1	24.9	7.1	2.8
Smiley Stars, Golden, Oven Baked, Asda*	1 Serving/122g	192	6.5	157	2.4	24	5.3	1.5
White, Raw, Flesh & Skin	***1 Lge/369g***	***284***	***0.3***	***77***	***2***	***17.5***	***0.1***	***2.2***
White, Raw, Weighed with Skin, Flesh Only, Average	***1 Med/213g***	***153***	***0.3***	***72***	***1.9***	***16.1***	***0.2***	***1.2***
POUSSIN								
Meat & Skin, Raw, Average	***1oz/28g***	***57***	***3.9***	***202***	***19.1***	***0***	***13.9***	***0***
Spatchcock, British, Waitrose*	½ Poussin/225g	364	20.2	162	19	1.2	9	0
POWERADE								
Berry & Tropical Fruit, Coca-Cola*	1 Bottle/500ml	90	0	18	0	4.1	0	0
Isotonic, Sports Drink, Coca-Cola*	1 Bottle/500ml	120	0	24	0	5.6	0	0
PRAWN COCKTAIL								
Asda*	1 Pot/170g	371	30.6	218	8.9	3.9	18	0
BGTY, Sainsbury's*	½ Pot/85g	119	7.9	140	9.1	4.7	9.3	0.5
Delicious, Boots*	1 Pack/250g	285	6.5	114	5.5	17	2.6	1.2
Fishmonger, Aldi*	1 Pot/170g	266	18.8	156	8.1	6	11	0.6
International Seafood Co, Morrisons*	½ Pot/90g	316	30.6	351	8.3	3	34	0
King, Extra Special, Asda*	1 Pack/204g	474	22.5	232	8.9	23	11	1.8
LC, Tesco*	1 Pot/140g	210	16	150	7.5	4.3	11.4	1.3
Lobster & Prawn, Posh, Christmas, M&S*	1 Cocktail/90g	244	21.6	271	11.2	2.4	24	0.3
Reduced Fat, 30%, Tesco*	½ Pot/85g	122	8	143	10.6	3.6	9.4	0.6
PRAWN COCKTAIL								
Reduced Fat, Good Health, Waitrose*	½ Pot/100g	208	16.5	208	10.9	3.6	16.5	0.5
Reduced Fat, M&S*	1 Pack/200g	296	20	148	9.9	4.5	10	0.5
PRAWN CRACKERS								
Asda*	1 Serving/25g	134	8.8	535	2	53	35	0

P

	Measure INFO/WEIGHT	per Measure KCAL	FAT	Nutrition Values per 100g / 100ml KCAL	PROT	CARB	FAT	FIBRE
PRAWN CRACKERS								
M&S*	1 Bag/50g	262	15.6	525	2.8	57.4	31.3	0.8
Meal for Two, Meal Box, Tesco*	½ Pack/23g	127	8	554	2	57.3	35	1.1
Ready to Eat, Sharwood's*	1 Bag/60g	316	18.5	527	0.5	62	30.8	1.2
Sainsbury's*	1 Serving/25g	134	7.8	534	2.1	60.8	31.3	0.6
Snackrite, Aldi*	1 Pack/25g	136	8	546	2.6	61	32	1.1
Snaktastic, Lidl*	1 Serving/15g	80	4.6	533	2.1	61.2	31	0.5
Sweet Chilli, Thai Dragon, Aldi*	1 Serving/20g	95	4	475	1.6	71	20	0
Thai Sriracha, Three Tigers*	1 Bag/60g	319	18.2	531	1.8	61.9	30.4	1.4
PRAWN TOAST								
from Chinese Selection, Ken Hom, Tesco*	1 Toast/14g	50	3.8	364	11	17.1	27.4	2.6
Mini, Oriental Selection, Party, Iceland*	1 Toast/15g	52	3.6	345	10.5	22	23.9	2.1
Oriental Snack Selection, Sainsbury's*	1 Toast/20g	57	2.5	283	9.4	31.7	12.3	3.8
Oven Baked, Asda*	1 Toast/24g	89	6.5	372	9	22	27	2.2
Oven Cooked, Sainsbury's*	½ Pack/59g	237	17.7	401	11.8	19.7	30	2.7
Sesame Prawn, Toasted Triangles, M&S*	1 Pack/220g	616	39.6	280	12.4	17.3	18	2
Stars, Asian Prawn Selection, Let's Party, Aldi*	1 Star/14g	47	2.9	334	9.5	25	21	5.4
PRAWNS								
Al Ajillo, Aguinamar*	1 Pack/105g	239	21	228	12	0	20	0
Batter Crisp, Lyons*	1 Pack/160g	350	20.3	219	8	18.2	12.7	1.1
Boiled	***1 Prawn/3g***	***3***	***0***	***99***	***22.6***	***0***	***0.9***	***0***
Breaded, Coconut, Oven Baked, Sainsbury's*	½ Pack/84g	214	10.7	255	12.3	22.3	12.7	1.4
Cooked & Peeled, Average	***1oz/28g***	***21***	***0.2***	***77***	***17.6***	***0.2***	***0.6***	***0***
Cooked, Canadian, Frozen, Finest, Tesco*	1 Pack/226g	156	2.7	69	14.2	0.1	1.2	0.5
Gratinee, At Home, Cote*	1 Serving/220g	251	14.7	114	5.3	4	6.7	0.8
Hot & Spicy, Average	***1 Serving/170g***	***461***	***26.9***	***271***	***9.4***	***22.8***	***15.8***	***2.2***
Icelandic, Raw, Average	***1oz/28g***	***30***	***0.4***	***106***	***22.7***	***0***	***1.6***	***0***
Jumbo, Tempura, Oven Baked, Iceland*	1 Prawn/11g	40	2.5	362	12.6	26.6	22.7	0.8
King, Basil Pesto Marinated, M&S*	½ Pack/70g	103	6.4	147	15.8	0.3	9.1	0.1
King, Breaded	***1 Prawn/13g***	***33***	***1.8***	***260***	***15.1***	***17.8***	***14***	***1.2***
King, Chilli, & Coriander, Tesco*	1 Pack/75g	68	1.8	91	17.1	0.1	2.4	0.1
King, Cooked, Organic, M&S*	½ Pack/75g	61	0.8	81	17.9	0.4	1	0.4
King, Crispy, Wrapped, Finest, Tesco*	1 Prawn/19g	64	3.7	335	10.7	28.6	19.6	0.9
King, Fisherman, seaside favourites *	½ Pack/70g	42	0.2	60	14.6	0.2	0.3	0.5
King, Frozen, Cooked, Co-Op*	½ Pack/90g	59	0.4	66	16	0.5	0.5	0.5
King, Garlic Butter, Sainsbury's*	½ Pack/80g	95	4.3	119	17.4	0.5	5.4	0.5
King, in Sweet Chilli Sauce, Oven Baked, Iceland*	1 Serving/120g	88	0.2	73	13.4	4	0.2	0.7
King, in Tomato, & Garlic Sauce, Iceland*	½ Pack/116g	128	8	110	10.2	1.2	6.9	1
King, Jumbo, Cooked & Peeled, Finest, Tesco*	½ Pack/75g	60	0.4	80	18.4	0.4	0.5	0.1
King, Jumbo, Frozen, Artic Royal*	1 Serving/100g	36	0.1	36	7.8	1.2	0.1	0
King, Large, Finest Catch*	1 Serving/100g	61	0.4	61	14.2	0	0.4	0
King, Large, Peeled, Raw, Tesco*	½ Pack/82g	51	0.4	62	14.3	0.1	0.5	0.1
King, Lemon & Garlic, Finest, Tesco*	½ Pack/75g	70	2	94	16.2	1.1	2.6	0.6
King, Organic, Raw, Duchy, Waitrose*	½ Pack/83g	91	1.7	110	22.2	0.3	2.1	0.5
King, Peeled, & Cooked, Fisherman*	½ Pack/70g	42	0.2	60	14.6	0.2	0.3	0.5
King, Raw, Average	***1 Bag/200g***	***145***	***1.9***	***72***	***15.8***	***0.2***	***1***	***0.1***
King, Raw, Frozen, As Prepared, Essential, Waitrose*	½ Pack/62g	80	2	129	24.5	0.5	3.3	0.5
King, Selection, Cone, Deluxe, Lidl*	1 Cone/19g	56	2.9	296	10.5	27.8	15.3	2.3
King, Selection, Lollipop, Deluxe, Lidl*	1 Lollipop/19g	53	2.9	281	9.2	24.5	15.5	3.4
King, Semi-Dried Tomatoes, & Basil, M&S*	1 Pack/145g	270	20	186	11.2	4	13.8	0.5
King, Shell On, As Sold, Iceland*	1 Pack/225g	173	1.6	77	17.6	0	0.7	0
King, Sweet & Sour, Tesco*	½ Pack/193g	147	0.8	76	12.3	5.2	0.4	1.3
King, Tails, Sea Spray, Iceland*	½ Pack/85g	95	0.8	112	7.6	18.1	0.9	0.6
King, Tandoori, Average	***1 Prawn/59g***	***33***	***0.6***	***55***	***5.7***	***5.9***	***1.1***	***0.7***

	Measure INFO/WEIGHT	per Measure KCAL	FAT	Nutrition Values per 100g / 100ml KCAL	PROT	CARB	FAT	FIBRE
PRAWNS								
King, Thai Chilli, Oven Cooked, Specially Selected, Aldi*	½ Pack/86g	55	0.7	64	14	0.5	0.8	0.5
King, Whole, Shell On, Raw, Iceland*	1 Serving/113g	87	0.8	77	17.6	0	0.7	0
North Atlantic, Peeled, Cooked, Average	***1oz/28g***	***22***	***0.3***	***80***	***17.5***	***0***	***1.1***	***0***
North Atlantic, Raw, Average	***1oz/28g***	***17***	***0.1***	***62***	***14.4***	***0***	***0.4***	***0***
Piri Piri, with Peppers, M&S*	½ Pack/115g	102	1.7	89	13.5	5	1.5	0.8
Poke, Bowl, M&S*	1 Pack/298g	364	5.1	122	4.5	21.6	1.7	1.3
Sesame, Rainbow Layer Pot, M&S*	1 Pot/270g	324	14.6	120	6.3	9.2	5.4	4.6
Tempura, with Sweet Chilli, M&S*	1 Serving/100g	221	10.8	221	9.9	20.5	10.8	1.2
Tiger, Black, Extra Large, M&S*	1 Serving/100g	98	0.2	98	22.4	1.7	0.2	0.1
Tiger, Black, Whole, Raw, The Best, Morrisons*	1/3 Pack/116g	89	0.8	77	17.6	0	0.7	0
Tiger, Cooked & Peeled, Average	***1 Pack/180g***	***151***	***2***	***84***	***18.4***	***0.1***	***1.1***	***0***
Tiger, Jumbo, Average	***1 Serving/50g***	***39***	***0.2***	***78***	***18.2***	***0.3***	***0.5***	***0***
Tiger, Raw, Average	***1 Prawn/30g***	***19***	***0.2***	***64***	***14.2***	***0***	***0.7***	***0***
Tiger, Tempura, M&S*	1 Prawn/18g	49	3.1	274	8.8	20.1	17.3	1.2
PRAWNS CHILLI								
Crispy, with Sweet Chilli Dipping Sauce, M&S*	1 Pack/240g	490	20.2	204	8.2	23.6	8.4	0.6
King, Chilli & Coriander Marinated, Just Add, M&S*	1 Pack/80g	82	2.1	102	19	0.1	2.6	0
King, with a Sweet Chilli Sauce, Succulent, Birds Eye*	1 Serving/140g	251	17.2	179	10.5	6.5	12.3	0.1
Skewers, Sweet Chilli, King, BBQ Favourites, Asda*	1 Skewer/48g	48	0.5	100	16.6	5.4	1.1	1
PRAWNS WITH								
Chilli, Coriander & Lime, King, Waitrose*	1 Pack/140g	143	3.2	102	19.9	0.5	2.3	0.6
Chorizo, & Lentils, Cook*	1 Pot/315g	246	5.4	78	5.7	8.2	1.7	0
Ginger & Spring Onion, Sainsbury's*	1 Pack/300g	198	9.3	66	4.7	4.7	3.1	0.3
King, with a Creamy Cocktail Sauce, M&S*	1 Pack/120g	278	23.3	232	12.6	1.3	19.4	1.1
King, with Garlic Butter, M&S*	1 Serving/100g	165	9	165	12.5	9.1	9	0.5
Orzo, Harissa, Hello Fresh*	1 Serving/358g	584	14.3	163	9	23	4	0
PRESERVE								
Bramble, Seedless, Mackays*	1 Tbsp/15g	40	0	269	0.3	66.8	0.1	0
Ginger Shred, Robertsons*	1 Tbsp/15g	40	0	267	0.1	66	0	0
Ginger, Asda*	1 Tbsp/15g	39	0.1	261	0.5	63	0.5	1.7
Ginger, Stem, Curd, Woolliss & Son Ltd*	1 Tbsp/15g	51	1.3	343	2.6	65	8.4	0
Red Currant Jelly, Tiptree, Wilkin & Sons*	1 Tbsp/15g	40	0	264	0	66	0	0
Rhubarb & Ginger, Mackays Ltd*	1 Tbsp/15g	40	0	269	0.3	66.7	0	0
The Ruby Red, Prebiotic, Leon Restaurants*	1 Tbsp/15g	19	0.1	124	0.9	27.1	0.5	2.7
Three Berry, Scottish, Mackays*	1 Tbsp/15g	41	0	272	0.4	67.6	0	0
PRETZELS								
Bavarian, Bakery Instore, Lidl*	1 Pretzel/85g	251	5	295	9.4	50.6	5.9	0
Bites, Rock Salt, Indie Bay Snacks *	1 Pack/26g	99	1.1	381	13.1	71.2	4.2	3.1
Bites, Spelt, Easy Cheesy, Indie Bay*	1 Pack/26g	99	1.2	380	12.9	70.1	4.6	3.1
Jumbo, Tesco*	1 Serving/50g	194	3.4	388	9.7	71.9	6.8	5.4
Mini, M&S*	1 Pack/45g	194	6	430	10.4	66.6	13.4	4.9
Peanut Butter, Kirkland Signature, Costco*	1 Pretzel/3g	16	0.7	464	15	49	22	5
Pieces, Jalapeno, Snyders*	1 Pack/125g	590	23.3	472	7.1	67.4	18.6	3.2
Plain, Bakery, Tesco*	1 Pretzel/108g	316	5.8	293	9.5	50.3	5.4	2.7
Salted Caramel, Tesco*	1 Serving/25g	104	1.9	416	9.8	75.2	7.6	3.6
Salted, Average	***1 Serving/30g***	***114***	***0.8***	***380***	***10.3***	***79.8***	***2.6***	***3***
Salted, Mini, M&S*	1 Pack/25g	96	0.5	382	10.9	78	2.1	3.9
Soft, Cinnamon Sugar, Auntie Anne's*	1 Pretzel/112g	380	1	339	7.1	75	0.9	1.8
Soft, Salted, Original, Auntie Anne's*	1 Pretzel/112g	310	1	277	7.1	58	0.9	1.8
Sour Cream & Onion, M&S*	1 Serving/30g	136	4.4	455	11	70.9	14.5	0.7
Sour Cream & Chive, Christmas Trees, Snackrite, Aldi*	1 Serving/25g	106	2.2	422	10	74	8.9	3
Sour Cream & Chive, Penn State Pretzels*	1 Serving/25g	111	3.2	443	8.9	71.8	12.9	2
Sticks, Salted, Co-Op*	1 Serving/15g	60	0.6	397	11	77	4.3	3.6

	Measure INFO/WEIGHT	per Measure KCAL	FAT	Nutrition Values per 100g / 100ml KCAL	PROT	CARB	FAT	FIBRE
PRETZELS								
Superseeds, Crunchy, Indie Bay*	1 Pack/26g	106	2.9	408	18.7	54.7	11.3	6.4
Turkey, Emmental, & Avocado, Finest, Tesco*	1 Pretzel/192g	487	21.9	254	13.1	23.9	11.4	1.6
Wheat, GF, Trufree*	1 Bag/60g	282	12	470	0.5	72	20	0.7
PRINGLES*								
Barbecue, Pringles*	1 Serving/50g	266	18	533	4.9	48	36	5.1
BBQ Spare Rib, Rice Infusions, Pringles*	1 Pack/23g	108	5.3	469	5.1	60	23	2.6
Cheese & Onion, Pringles*	1 Serving/25g	132	8.5	528	4.1	50	34	3.4
Hot & Spicy, Pringles*	1 Serving/25g	132	8.5	530	4.6	49	34	3.7
Light, Original, Pringles*	1 Serving/25g	121	6.2	484	4.3	59	25	3.6
Light, Sour Cream & Onion, Pringles*	1 Serving/25g	122	6.2	487	4.7	57	25	3.6
Margarita Pizza, Classic Takeaways, Pringles*	1 Serving/25g	134	8	538	3.9	53	32	2.6
Minis, Original, Pringles*	1 Pack/23g	118	6.9	514	5.1	55	30	3.7
Minis, Sour Cream & Onion, Pringles*	1 Pack/23g	118	6.7	511	5.2	56	29	3.5
Original, Pringles*	1 Serving/25g	130	8.5	522	3.8	51	34	2.6
Paprika, Pringles*	1 Serving/25g	132	8.5	529	4.9	49	34	6.5
Peking Duck with Hoisin Sauce, Rice Fusions, Pringles*	1 Serving/30g	146	8.1	485	4.4	55	27	2.5
Prawn Cocktail, Pringles*	1 Serving/25g	130	8	518	4.1	53	32	2.5
Salt & Vinegar, Pringles*	1 Serving/25g	128	8	512	3.9	52	32	2.4
Sour Cream & Onion, Pringles*	1 Serving/30g	154	9.6	515	4.2	51	32	2.9
Texas BBQ Sauce, Pringles*	1 Serving/25g	132	8.5	527	4.2	50	34	3.5
PROFITEROLES								
12 Chocolate, Waitrose*	3 Profiteroles/65g	284	21.4	437	6	28.7	33	0.4
Asda*	1 Serving/64g	218	17.2	343	5	20	27	0
Black Forest, Tesco*	1 Profiterole/19g	71	4.3	374	4.9	37.4	22.6	0.7
Chocolate Orange, Tesco*	1 Profiterole/17g	67	4.5	393	5.2	32.8	26.5	1.2
Chocolate, 8 Pack, Co-Op*	¼ Pack/112g	330	17.9	295	6	31	16	2
Chocolate, Sainsbury's*	1/6 Pot/95g	192	8.5	202	5.4	25.1	8.9	0.8
Chocolate, Stack, Sainsbury's*	¼ Pack/76g	311	19.5	409	5.3	39.3	25.6	2
Chocolate, Tesco*	4 Profiteroles/59g	202	16.1	343	5.2	18.5	27.4	1
Choux & Chocolate Sauce, Tesco*	1 Serving/77g	295	22	386	5.1	26.9	28.7	0.5
Classic French, Sainsbury's*	1 Serving/90g	284	15.5	316	6.6	33.7	17.2	0.1
Filled with Cream, Stack, Fresh, M&S*	1 Serving/75g	303	22.8	404	5.6	26.3	30.4	1.5
Hazelnut, Praline , Partytime, Lidl*	3 Profiteroles/54g	228	15.9	422	5.4	32.8	29.4	2.2
in a Pot, Waitrose*	1 Pot/80g	207	11.3	259	6.3	25.6	14.1	2.9
Savoury with Cheese & Chive, CBY, Asda*	¼ Pack/15g	95	7.7	634	9.1	32.1	51.3	3.5
Waitrose*	4 Profiteroles/75g	269	17.9	359	4.8	31.1	23.9	0.7
PROSECCO								
12%, Average	***1 Sm/125ml***	***112***	***0***	***89***	***0***	***1.4***	***0***	***0***
Extra Dry , M&S*	1 Glass/125ml	85	0	68	0	0	0	0
PRUNES								
Dried, Average	***1 Prune/7g***	***11***	***0***	***158***	***2.5***	***36.4***	***0.4***	***5.8***
in Apple Juice, Average	***1 Serving/90g***	***76***	***0.1***	***84***	***0.8***	***19.8***	***0.1***	***1.4***
in Fruit Juice, Average	***1oz/28g***	***24***	***0***	***86***	***0.9***	***20.9***	***0.2***	***2.9***
in Syrup, Average	***1oz/28g***	***25***	***0***	***89***	***0.9***	***21.5***	***0.2***	***2.6***
Stewed with Sugar	***1oz/28g***	***29***	***0.1***	***103***	***1.3***	***25.5***	***0.2***	***3.1***
Stewed without Sugar	***1oz/28g***	***23***	***0.1***	***81***	***1.4***	***19.5***	***0.3***	***3.3***
PUDDING								
Banoffee, Sticky, Allplants*	1 Serving/85g	246	12.8	289	3	35	15	1.9
Beef, & Onion, Minced, Hollands*	1 Pudding/165g	353	19	214	6.5	20.6	11.5	0
Black Forest, Brilliant, Graze*	1 Punnet/37g	97	3.3	262	4	40	9	2
Bread, Retail Average	***1 Slice/120g***	***301***	***8***	***251***	***8.4***	***41.8***	***6.7***	***0.5***
Cherry Bakewell, Freaks Of Nature*	1 Pudding/100g	322	16.4	322	4.6	36.9	16.4	2.6
Chocolate Brownie, Classic, Co-Op*	¼ Pack/100g	429	25	429	6.1	44	25	2.4

	Measure INFO/WEIGHT	per Measure KCAL	FAT	Nutrition Values per 100g / 100ml KCAL	PROT	CARB	FAT	FIBRE
PUDDING								
Chocolate, Brownie, Waitrose*	1 Serving/98g	391	24.8	399	4.5	37.7	25.3	1
Chocolate, Colombian, Pot, Pots & Co*	1 Pot/65g	196	12.3	301	4.2	27.8	18.9	0
Chocolate, Fudge, Hot, Freaks Of Nature*	1 Pudding/100g	279	10.5	279	2.7	42.5	10.5	1.9
Chocolate, Ganache, Mini Pot, Gu*	1 Pot/45g	199	16.6	442	3.3	26.4	36.8	2.3
Chocolate, M&S*	¼ Pudding/76g	265	12	350	4.1	48	15.8	2.1
Chocolate, Melt in The Middle, Frozen, Waitrose*	1 Pudding/90g	310	14.4	344	6.7	41.4	16	3.5
Chocolate, Melt in The Middle, Mini, Tesco*	1 Pudding/20g	85	5.9	427	7.5	30.2	29.5	5.5
Chocolate, Melting Middle, Hot, Puds, Gu*	1 Pud/100g	409	26.9	409	6	36	26.9	2.7
Chocolate, Melting Middle, M&S*	1 Pudding/155g	510	27.8	330	5.8	36.2	18	3.1
Chocolate, No Moo, Iceland*	1 Pudding/80g	298	18.4	372	5.6	35	23	0.8
Chocolate, Steamed, Aunty's*	1 Pudding/95g	298	5.9	314	4.2	52.8	6.2	2
Eve's, Average	***1oz/28g***	***67***	***3.7***	***241***	***3.5***	***28.9***	***13.1***	***1.4***
Eves, with Apple Compote, Sainsbury's*	1 Pot/110g	256	9	235	3.2	36.2	8.3	1.2
Fondant, Chocolate Peanut, Allplants*	1 Serving/92g	363	23	395	8.3	32	25	2.9
Golden Syrup, Steamed, Aunty's*	1 Pudding/100g	293	4.1	293	3.3	57.3	4.1	0.8
Jam, Roly Poly, Sainsbury's*	¼ Pack/81g	291	11.5	359	4.4	53.3	14.2	0.5
Liegeois, Zott*	1 Pot/175g	163	4.2	93	1.2	16.4	2.4	0
Pease, Canned, Forsight*	1/3 Can/138g	134	1	97	6	15.9	0.7	1.7
Pease, Durham Foods *	1/3 Pack/70g	66	0.4	95	5.9	16.8	0.5	1.6
Queen of Puddings	***1oz/28g***	***60***	***2.2***	***213***	***4.8***	***33.1***	***7.8***	***0.2***
Roly Poly, Jam, Aunt Bessie's*	1 Serving/75g	278	9	370	3.6	62	12	1.4
Souffle, Hot Chocolate, Gu*	1 Pot/65g	298	23.5	458	6	24.1	36.2	2.5
Sponge, Spotted Dick, Asda*	1 Pudding/95g	401	21.9	422	4.4	489	23	1.7
Steak & Kidney, Meaty Puds, Fray Bentos*	1 Pack/400g	856	44	214	6.6	22.7	11	0.8
Sticky Toffee, Co-Op*	¼ Pudding/100g	355	20	355	3	40	20	0.7
Sticky Toffee, Deluxe, Lidl*	½ Pudding/225g	806	36	358	2.5	50	16	2.1
Sticky Toffee, Donald Russell*	1 Pudding/140g	511	22.4	365	2.7	54	16	0.3
Sticky Toffee, Extra Special, Asda*	¼ Pudding/100g	378	18	378	1.9	52	18	1.8
Sticky Toffee, Gro, Co-Op*	1 Pudding/95g	252	6.7	265	0.9	48	7.1	3
Sticky Toffee, Gu*	1 Pudding/85g	277	14.5	326	2.3	40.5	17.1	1.4
Sticky Toffee, Irresistible, Co-Op*	1 Serving/100g	335	14	335	2.1	48	14	3.7
Sticky Toffee, Plant Kitchen, M&S*	¼ Pack/119g	381	8.9	321	3.4	58.5	7.5	2.9
Sticky Toffee, Puree, Wiltshire Farm Foods*	1 Pack/155g	277	17	179	1.4	19	11	0
Sticky Toffee, Steamed, Aunty's*	1 Pudding/95g	279	4.6	294	3.4	55.6	4.8	1
Sticky Toffee, Tesco*	1 Serving/110g	287	14.7	261	3.3	31.8	13.4	0.7
Strawberry, Jelly Pud, with Devon Custard, Ambrosia*	1 Pot/150g	129	1.2	86	0.7	19.4	0.8	0
Suet, Average	***1oz/28g***	***94***	***5.1***	***335***	***4.4***	***40.5***	***18.3***	***0.9***
Summer Fruits, Eat Well, M&S*	1 Pudding/135g	128	0.7	95	1.7	20.8	0.5	3
Summer, Layered, Individual, Waitrose*	1 Pudding/150g	150	0.8	100	2.1	21	0.5	1.5
Summer, Layered, Waitrose*	¼ Pudding/101g	95	0.5	94	2.1	19.3	0.5	2
Syrup, M&S*	1 Serving/105g	370	10.5	352	3.9	61.7	10	0.8
Torte, Cheeky Little Chocolate, Gu*	1 Pud/50g	211	14.6	422	5.7	31.6	29.1	1.8
PUMPKIN								
Boiled in Salted Water	***1oz/28g***	***4***	***0.1***	***13***	***0.6***	***2.1***	***0.3***	***1.1***
Potimarron, Raw, Average	***1 Serving/80g***	***21***	***0.1***	***26***	***1***	***6.5***	***0.1***	***1.9***
Puree, Baking Buddy*	1 Serving/53g	22	0	42	1.7	6.7	0	2.5

P

	Measure INFO/WEIGHT	per Measure KCAL	per Measure FAT	KCAL	PROT	CARB	FAT	FIBRE
				Nutrition Values per 100g / 100ml				
QUAVERS								
Cheese, Walkers*	1 Bag/20g	107	6	534	2.7	62.5	30.1	1.1
Prawn Cocktail, Walkers*	1 Bag/16g	88	5.1	537	2.1	62	31	1.2
QUESADILLA								
Beef, Mexican, Aldi*	1 Quesadilla/150g	345	17.1	230	14.8	16.8	11.4	0
Chicken, from Restaurant, Average	***1 Serving/300g***	***867***	***46.7***	***289***	***15.6***	***22.2***	***15.6***	***1.7***
Meal Kit, Mexican, Asda *	¼ Pack/119g	281	4.3	236	6.9	44	3.6	1.1
Meal Kit, Toasted Cheese, Old El Paso*	1 Quesadilla/63g	135	2.1	215	6.6	38.4	3.4	2.2
QUICHE								
Asparagus, & Mushroom, Tesco*	½ Quiche/200g	474	32.8	237	5.1	17.2	16.4	1.2
Asparagus, & Vegetable, Herby Summer, Higgidy*	1 Quiche/400g	848	50	212	5.9	18.9	12.5	2.7
Bacon, & Cheese, Sainsbury's*	¼ Quiche/100g	237	15	237	7	18.6	15	0.7
Bacon, & Leek, From Our Deli, As Consumed, Morrisons*	1 Quiche/160g	435	28	272	7.8	20	17.5	1.6
Bacon, & Leek, Morrisons*	1 Quiche/400g	1224	87.6	306	8.3	18.4	21.9	0.8
Bacon, Cheese, & Tomato, Asda*	1/3 Pack/133g	345	22.6	259	6.5	20	17	0.7
Bacon, Cherry Wood Smoked, Specially Selected, Aldi*	¼ Quiche/100g	287	19	287	8.9	18	19	1.6
Bacon, Leek & Mushroom, M&S*	¼ Quiche/100g	245	16.4	245	6.9	17.2	16.4	1.3
Bacon, Smoked, & Mature Cheddar, Higgidy*	1/6 Quiche/67g	176	11.7	262	9.5	17.4	17.4	1.1
Balsamic Onion, & Cheddar, Mature, Aldi*	¼ Quiche/100g	298	18	298	8.4	24	18	2
Balsamic Onion, & Mature Cheddar, Deluxe, Lidl*	1 Quiche/420g	1428	91.1	340	9.6	26	21.7	1.1
Balsamic Onion, Sweet, Higgidy*	¼ Quiche/100g	292	18.5	292	9.2	22.6	18.5	1.3
Brie, & Bacon, Waitrose*	¼ Quiche/100g	271	17.4	271	8.9	19.1	17.4	1.1
Brie, & Winter Spiced Chutney, Higgidy*	¼ Quiche/100g	246	15.5	246	7.4	19.7	15.5	1.4
Broccoli, & Cheddar, Crustless, Oven Baked, Asda*	1 Quiche/150g	296	18	197	7.4	14	12	1.9
Broccoli, & Cheddar, Family, Oven Baked, Asda*	1/3 Quiche/133g	325	20	244	6.5	21	15	1.5
Broccoli, Cheese, & Tomato, M&S*	1/3 Quiche/133g	293	18.2	220	6.2	17	13.7	1.7
Broccoli, Spinach, & Ricotta, Waitrose*	¼ Quiche/100g	223	14.6	223	8.2	13.8	14.6	1.7
Broccoli, Tesco*	1 Serving/100g	249	17.2	249	6	17.6	17.2	1.4
Broccoli, Tomato, & Cheese, Crestwood, Aldi*	¼ Quiche/100g	212	12	212	5.9	19	12	1.8
Broccoli, Tomato, & Cheese, Sainsbury's*	¼ Quiche/100g	214	12.7	214	5.6	18.5	12.7	2
Butternut, Kale, & Chilli, Crustless, Tesco*	1 Quiche/160g	345	22.8	216	8.7	12.3	14.3	1.7
Cauliflower, Cheese, Higgidy*	½ Quiche/200g	540	37.2	270	9	17.4	18.6	1.5
Cheddar, & Bacon, Crustless, Crestwood, Aldi*	¼ Quiche/85g	242	16	285	12.9	15.3	18.8	0.6
Cheddar, & Onion, Tesco*	¼ Quiche/100g	260	16.5	260	9.6	17.9	16.5	0.8
Cheddar, Somerset, & Tomato, Jon Thorners*	½ Quiche/200g	436	24	218	8.2	14	12	0
Cheddar, Vintage, & Broccoli, Jon Thorners*	1/3 Quiche/200g	556	34	278	12	16	17	0
Cheddar, Vintage, & Maple Bacon, Irresistible, Co-Op*	¼ Quiche/100g	268	18	268	8.7	18	18	1.3
Cheese, & Bacon, Crustless, Tesco*	¼ Quiche/85g	196	13.4	230	9.8	11.8	15.7	1.5
Cheese, & Broccoli, Morrisons*	1/3 Quiche/134g	338	22.4	253	7.1	18.4	16.8	1.7
Cheese, & Egg	***1oz/28g***	***88***	***6.2***	***314***	***12.5***	***17.3***	***22.2***	***0.6***
Cheese, & Leek, & Chive, Sainsbury's*	1/3 Quiche/125g	292	20.2	234	7.1	14.9	16.2	1.3
Cheese, & Onion, Caramelised Onion, Finest, Tesco*	¼ Quiche/100g	300	18.6	300	9.4	22.4	18.6	1.7
Cheese, & Onion, Crustless, Deli, Morrisons*	1 Quiche/388g	1005	68.3	259	9.7	14.9	17.6	1
Cheese, & Onion, Crustless, Weight Watchers*	1 Quiche/160g	267	12.3	167	11.3	11.1	7.7	4.3
Cheese, & Onion, Mature Cheddar, Crustless, Higgidy*	¼ Quiche/95g	254	16.9	267	7.4	18.7	17.8	1
Cheese, & Onion, Reduced Fat, Eat Smart, Morrisons*	1 Quiche/400g	824	36.8	206	7.7	16.9	9.2	0.7
Cheese, & Onion, Retail, Average	***¼ Quiche/100g***	***262***	***17.8***	***262***	***8.4***	***17.1***	***17.8***	***1.3***
Cheese, & Tomato, Retail, Average	***¼ Quiche/100g***	***268***	***17.1***	***268***	***8***	***20.2***	***17.1***	***1.1***
Cheese, & Bacon, Crustless, Ovenbaked, Iceland*	¼ Quiche/85g	178	11.8	209	9.5	11.4	13.9	0.5
Cheese, & Bacon, Eastmans, Tesco*	¼ Quiche/100g	256	15.8	256	8.4	19.5	15.8	0.9
Cheese, & Onion, Crustless, Tesco*	¼ Quiche/85g	211	14.4	249	10.8	12.8	16.9	1.2
Cheese, & Pickle, Asda *	¼ Quiche/100g	255	14	255	7.9	23	14	0.9
Cheese, Pickle, & Tomato, Waitrose*	1 Quiche/400g	976	58.8	244	7.4	20	14.7	10
Cherry Tomato, & Mozzarella, Crustless, Booths*	¼ Quiche/85g	155	9	182	7.8	13.5	10.6	0.9

Q

	Measure INFO/WEIGHT	per Measure KCAL	FAT	Nutrition Values per 100g / 100ml KCAL	PROT	CARB	FAT	FIBRE
QUICHE								
Goats Cheese, & Red Pepper, Morrisons*	1 Quiche/160g	450	29.9	281	7	20.7	18.7	1.1
Lorraine, Crustless, Asda*	1 Quiche/160g	259	12.6	162	9.3	13.5	7.9	1.1
Lorraine, Crustless, Individual, 150g, Sainsbury's*	1 Quiche/150g	369	23.7	246	10.6	15	15.8	0.7
Lorraine, Crustless, Individual, Asda*	1 Quiche/150g	353	21	235	10	17	14	0.6
Lorraine, Crustless, LC, Tesco*	1 Pack/160g	280	13.4	175	12.6	11.8	8.4	2.5
Lorraine, Crustless, You Count, Love Life, Waitrose*	1 Quiche/160g	295	15.4	185	8.9	15.2	9.6	0.9
Lorraine, Retail, Average	***¼ Quiche/100g***	***280***	***19.5***	***280***	***9***	***16.8***	***19.5***	***2***
Lorraine, Smoked Bacon & Cheese, M&S*	¼ Quiche/100g	270	18.4	270	9.7	16.4	18.4	1.6
Mediterranean Style, Vegetable, Individual, Waitrose*	1 Quiche/155g	364	22.2	235	7.6	18.5	14.3	1.1
Mediterranean Vegetable, Waitrose *	1 Serving/100g	236	15.3	236	7.2	16.6	15.3	1.5
Mushroom	***1oz/28g***	***80***	***5.5***	***284***	***10***	***18.3***	***19.5***	***0.9***
Pea, Higgidy*	1 Serving/65g	161	10.3	248	8.5	18.4	15.8	1.7
Pea, Minted, & Bacon, Waitrose*	¼ Quiche/100g	253	14.9	253	8	21.1	14.9	1.4
Red Pepper, & Greek Feta, The Best, Morrisons*	¼ Quiche/100g	273	17.6	273	7.2	20.8	17.6	1.2
Salmon, & Spinach, Sainsbury's*	1/3 Quiche/125g	318	21.9	254	8.2	15.9	17.5	1
Salmon, & Spinach, Smoked, Little, Higgidy*	1 Quiche/155g	448	31.5	289	8.6	17.5	20.3	0.9
Salmon, & Spinach, with Cheddar Crumb, Higgidy*	¼ Quiche/100g	267	18	267	10	16.9	18	1.3
Salmon, & Broccoli, Jon Thorners*	¼ Quiche/100g	289	16.6	289	12.8	16.9	16.6	0
Scotch Egg, Tesco*	1 Quiche/180g	494	31	274	10.7	18.7	17.2	1.2
Spanish, 501, Oakhouse Foods Ltd*	1 Serving/117g	252	14.6	216	7.7	18.2	12.5	0.8
Spinach, & Red Pepper, Goats Cheese, Waitrose*	1 Serving/100g	218	14.3	218	6.5	15.8	14.3	2.6
Spinach, & Ricotta, Tesco*	¼ Quiche/100g	237	14.9	237	5.8	19.9	14.9	1
Spinach, & Roast Red Pepper, Little, Higgidy*	1 Quiche/155g	397	27.3	256	9.1	15.2	17.6	1.2
Spinach, & Feta, Home Chef*	1 Quiche/200g	466	29	233	8.6	16.2	14.5	0
Spinach, Edamame, & Kale, Crustless, Tesco*	1 Quiche/160g	350	22.2	219	8.7	13.9	13.8	2.2
Spinach, Feta, & Roasted Red Pepper, Higgidy*	½ Quiche/200g	526	35.8	263	8.8	17.4	17.9	1.8
Spinach, Feta, & Roasted Tomato, Higgidy*	1 Quiche/155g	435	29.3	281	10.2	20	18.9	1.8
Swiss Gruyere, & Cheddar, Best Ever, M&S*	¼ Quiche/100g	274	18.2	274	13	13	18.2	1.2
Tomato, & Goats Cheese, Shortcrust, Waitrose*	¼ Quiche/100g	271	18.3	271	5.9	20.1	18.3	1
Tomato, Mozzarella, & Pesto, Crustless, Morrisons*	¼ Quiche/85g	201	13.9	237	8.2	13.6	16.4	1.1
Tomato, Roasted, & Pesto, Higgidy*	¼ Quiche/100g	281	19.7	281	7.9	20	19.7	1.8
Vegetable, & Sundried Tomato, Tesco*	¼ Quiche/100g	211	12.9	211	6.7	16.4	12.9	1.3
Vegetable, Mediterranean Style, Classic, Sainsbury's*	1 Quiche/400g	868	50.4	217	6.2	19.8	12.6	2.2
QUINCE								
Average	***1 Avg fruit/209g***	***37***	***0.1***	***18***	***0.2***	***4.3***	***0.1***	***1.3***
QUINOA								
Bean, Zesty, Steam Bag, Microwaved, Iceland*	1 Bag/125g	174	7.4	139	6.1	13.6	5.9	3.5
Bio, Mix, Dry Weight, Provida*	1 Serving/45g	159	2.7	353	14	57	6	7
Cajun, Good Grains, Worldwide Foods, Aldi*	½ Pack/110g	185	3.5	168	7.7	24	3.2	6.4
Dry Weight, Average	***1 Serving/70g***	***258***	***4.2***	***368***	***14.1***	***64.2***	***6.1***	***7***
Mediterranean, Aldi*	1 Pack/125g	179	5.1	143	4.1	20.8	4.1	3.2
Puffed, Organic, As Sold, BuyWholeFoodsOnline*	1 Serving/50g	178	0.5	355	7	77	1	3
Red	***1 Serving/100g***	***358***	***6***	***358***	***12.9***	***62.2***	***6***	***9.7***
Red & White, Microwaveable, Good Grains, Aldi*	½ Pouch/125g	239	4.6	191	6	32	3.7	2.7
White, Red, & Black, Cooked, Sainsbury's*	1 Serving/120g	176	3.2	147	5.2	23.3	2.7	4.2

	Measure INFO/WEIGHT	per Measure KCAL	FAT	Nutrition Values per 100g / 100ml KCAL	PROT	CARB	FAT	FIBRE
RABBIT								
Meat Only, Raw	***1oz/28g***	***38***	***1.5***	***137***	***21.9***	***0***	***5.5***	***0***
Meat Only, Raw, Weighed with Bone	***1 Serving/200g***	***164***	***6.6***	***82***	***13.1***	***0***	***3.3***	***0***
Meat Only, Stewed	***1oz/28g***	***32***	***0.9***	***114***	***21.2***	***0***	***3.2***	***0***
Meat Only, Stewed, Weighed with Bone	***1oz/28g***	***11***	***0.3***	***41***	***7.6***	***0***	***1.1***	***0***
RADISH								
Black, Raw, Average	***1 Lge/9g***	***1***	***0***	***16***	***1***	***3***	***0***	***2***
Red, Unprepared, Average	***1 Radish/8g***	***1***	***0***	***11***	***0.6***	***1.7***	***0.2***	***0.8***
White, Mooli, Raw	***1oz/28g***	***4***	***0***	***13***	***0.7***	***2.5***	***0.1***	***0***
RAISINS								
& Sultanas, Jumbo, M&S*	1 Serving/80g	212	0.4	265	2.4	62.4	0.5	2.6
& Sultanas, The Fruit Factory*	1 Box/14g	43	0.1	305	3	72.3	0.5	4
Chocolate, Milk, Mister Choc, Lidl*	1 Serving/40g	172	5.9	431	4.2	69.2	14.8	2.1
Flame, Tesco*	1 Serving/30g	86	0	288	3.7	66	0	4.2
Lime Infused, Tangy, Nak'd*	1 Pack/25g	68	0	272	2.1	69.3	0	0
Milk Chocolate, Belgian, M&S*	½ Pack/63g	274	9.6	438	4.6	68.9	15.3	2.9
Raspberry, Chocolate, Super Nature*	1 Pack/40g	201	11.2	502	3	59	28	0
Ruby Chocolate, Holland & Barrett*	1 Serving/30g	134	6.6	448	4.6	60	22	1.2
Seedless, Average	***1 Serving/75g***	***215***	***0.4***	***287***	***2.2***	***68.5***	***0.5***	***3.2***
Three, Mix, Asda*	1 Serving/30g	88	0.2	293	2.1	69	0.5	2
Yoghurt Coated, Fruit Bowl*	1 Pack/25g	114	4.8	455	2	67	19	3
Yoghurt Coated, Snack Bag, Asda*	1 Pack/25g	106	4	422	2.4	67	16	1
Yoghurt, Cranberry Foods Ltd*	1 Pack/50g	222	9.8	445	2.6	66.4	19.5	1.4
RAITA								
Plain, Average	***1oz/28g***	***16***	***0.6***	***57***	***4.2***	***5.8***	***2.2***	***0***
RASPBERRIES								
Fresh, Raw, Average	***1 Serving/80g***	***20***	***0.2***	***25***	***1.3***	***4.7***	***0.3***	***4.5***
Frozen, Average	***1 Serving/100g***	***27***	***0.3***	***27***	***1.3***	***4.7***	***0.3***	***4.5***
in Juice, Canned, Morrisons*	½ Can/150g	81	0.3	54	0.4	12	0.2	1.4
RATATOUILLE								
Average	***1oz/28g***	***23***	***2***	***82***	***1.3***	***3.8***	***7***	***1.8***
Canned, Freshona, Lidl*	¼ Can/188g	66	2.3	35	0.9	4.5	1.2	1.2
Les Legumes Cuisines, Frozen, Picard*	1 Serving/250g	115	5.7	46	1.3	4.1	2.3	1.8
Provencale, Canned, Cassegrain*	½ Can/188g	156	9.6	83	1.5	5.9	5.1	3.9
Tuscan Bean, Allplants*	1 Serving/453g	403	12.7	89	4.3	10	2.8	2.7
RAVIOLI								
Asparagus, & Mozzarella, Dell'ugo*	½ Pack/125g	220	5.4	176	6.8	26.3	4.3	2.8
Asparagus, Waitrose*	1 Serving/150g	303	9	202	10.5	26.4	6	2
Beef	***1 Serving/300g***	***501***	***13.7***	***167***	***6.4***	***25***	***4.6***	***1.4***
Beef, & Red Wine, Italiano, Tesco*	½ Pack/200g	424	13	212	7.3	30	6.5	2.3
Beef, Canned, Bramwells, Aldi*	½ Can/200g	146	2.6	73	2	13	1.3	0.7
Beef, in Tomato Sauce, Heinz*	½ Can/200g	147	3.2	74	2.5	12	1.6	0.8
Butternut Squash, & Marjoram , M&S*	½ Pack/125g	336	15.5	269	8.9	29.2	12.4	2.5
Cheese, & Spinach, G&B, Asda*	1 Pack/368g	302	8.5	82	3.3	11	2.3	1.9
Cheese, & Tomato, Canned, Sainsbury's*	½ Can/200g	170	2	85	3.5	15	1	0.9
Chicken, & Bacon, Cucina, Aldi*	1 Pack/250g	455	14	182	6.9	24.7	5.6	2.7
Crab, & Crayfish, Dell'ugo*	½ Pack/125g	266	10.4	213	12.6	21.5	8.3	0.7
Gorgonzola, & Walnut, M&S*	½ Pack/125g	345	15.8	276	10.6	29.2	12.6	1.5
Lasagne, M&S*	½ Pack/125g	335	16.1	268	11.2	25.8	12.9	1.9
Lemon, Mozzarella, & Sage Butter, Pasta Evangelists*	½ Pack/114g	332	20.9	291	15.4	16.9	18.3	0
Parmesan, M&S*	½ Pack/125g	331	13.9	265	10.2	30.2	11.1	1.5
Porcini Mushroom, Soli*	½ Pack/125g	276	11.6	221	8.6	26	9.3	0
Pork, Fennel, & Chilli, Cooked, Waitrose*	½ Pack/125g	228	7.2	182	8.6	22.9	5.8	1.8
Spinach, & Ricotta, Waitrose*	1 Serving/125g	309	9	247	10.5	35	7.2	1.9

R

	Measure INFO/WEIGHT	per Measure KCAL	FAT	Nutrition Values per 100g / 100ml KCAL	PROT	CARB	FAT	FIBRE
RAVIOLI								
Spinach, & Ricotta, Deluxe, Lidl*	1 Pack/400g	419	12.2	105	3.8	14.6	3	2
Spinach, & Ricotta, Meal for One, M&S*	1 Serving/375g	555	22.1	148	5.1	17.6	5.9	1.8
Spinach, Vegan, Cooked, Waitrose*	½ Pack/159g	249	4.9	157	4.5	26.7	3.1	2.1
Tomato, & Pancetta, Boiled, Tesco*	½ Pack/225g	394	9.7	175	7.5	25.2	4.3	3
REDCURRANTS								
Raw, Average	***1oz/28g***	***6***	***0***	***20***	***1.1***	***4.3***	***0***	***3.3***
Raw, Stalks Removed	***1 Serving/100g***	***21***	***0***	***21***	***1.1***	***4.4***	***0***	***0***
RELISH								
Barbeque, Sainsbury's*	1 Serving/50g	50	1	100	1	19.3	2.1	1.1
Chilli, Slowly Reduced, Irresistible, Co-Op*	1 Tbsp/15g	30	0.1	202	0.6	48	0.6	1.4
Cucumber, & Dill, with Green Pepper, Baxters*	1 Jar/220g	266	0.4	121	0.6	28.6	0.2	0.9
Onion, Red, Caramelised, Burger, Branston*	1 Squeeze/15g	23	0.2	151	0.8	32	1.4	1.4
Onion, Red, Caramelised, Tesco*	1 Serving/10g	28	0	280	0.6	69.1	0.1	0.7
Onion, Sainsbury's*	1 Serving/15g	23	0.1	151	0.9	36	0.4	0.7
Pickle, Deli, New York, French's*	1 Tbsp/15g	14	0	92	1	21.1	0.1	1.6
Red Pepper, & Sweetcorn, Burger, Aldi*	1 Tbsp/15g	16	0.1	105	1.2	23	0.6	1.3
Sweetcorn, American Style, Maryland, Tesco*	1 Serving/15g	15	0	101	1.1	23.9	0.1	0.9
Tomato, Spicy, Bick's*	1 Serving/28g	28	0.1	99	1.3	23.2	0.2	0
REVELS								
Mars*	1 Pack/35g	169	7.4	483	5.2	67.6	21	0
RHUBARB								
Chunks, Frozen, Picard*	1 Serving/80g	11	0.4	14	1	1.4	0.5	2.3
In Juice, Canned, Drained, Average	***1 Serving/100g***	***46***	***0***	***46***	***0.5***	***10.8***	***0***	***0.8***
Raw, Average	***1 Serving/80g***	***17***	***0.2***	***21***	***0.9***	***4.5***	***0.2***	***1.8***
Stewed with Sugar, Average	***1oz/28g***	***32***	***0***	***116***	***0.4***	***31.2***	***0***	***2***
RIBENA*								
Blackcurrant Juice Drink, Ready Made, Ribena*	1 Carton/200ml	82	0	41	0	10.6	0	0
Blackcurrant, Diluted with Water, Ribena*	1 Serving/100ml	46	0	46	0	11.4	0	0
Blackcurrant, Original, Undiluted, Ribena*	1 Serving/50ml	108	0	216	0	53	0	0
Blackcurrant, Really Light, No Added Sugar, Ribena*	1 Carton/250ml	8	0	3	0	0.8	0	0
Light, Ribena*	1 Carton/288ml	26	0	9	0.1	2.1	0	0
Pineapple & Passion Fruit, Juice Drink, Ribena*	½ Bottle/250ml	103	0	41	0	9.9	0	0
Strawberry Juice Drink, Ribena*	1 Carton/288ml	12	0	4	0	0.5	0	0
RIBS								
Peking, Taste of China, Tesco*	½ Pack/104g	222	12.4	214	16.4	10.1	12	0
Pork, Barbecue, Meat Only, Cooked, Average	***1 Serving/130g***	***360***	***23.4***	***275***	***21.4***	***7.2***	***17.9***	***0.3***
Pork, Chinese Style, Average	***1 Serving/300g***	***736***	***44.7***	***245***	***17.9***	***10***	***14.9***	***0.7***
Pork, Chops, Raw, Lean & Fat, Weighed with Bone	***1 Chop/130g***	***241***	***16.1***	***186***	***18.5***	***0***	***12.4***	***0***
Pork, Full Rack, Sainsbury's*	1 Serving/225g	567	38.7	252	18	6.5	17.2	0.9
Pork, Rack, Slow Cooked, Sweet BBQ, Morrisons*	½ Pack/158g	442	26.4	280	21	11.1	16.7	0.7
Pork, Salt & Chilli, Tesco*	½ Pack/99g	316	23.3	319	24.8	1.6	23.5	1
Pork, Smokey BBQ, Slow Cooked, Sainsbury's*	½ Pack/165g	455	25.6	276	24.8	8.7	15.5	1
Pork, Smoky BBQ, Rack, Tex Mex, Tesco*	½ Pack/158g	337	21.1	213	17.6	5.6	13.3	0.2
Pork, Spare, BBQ, Cooked, Iceland*	½ Pack/150g	290	16.8	193	16.5	6.2	11.2	1.1
Spare, Barbecue, Chinese Style, Farmfoods*	1 Pack/400g	464	25.2	116	9.3	5.6	6.3	0.1
Spare, Cantonese, Mini, Sainsbury's*	1 Rib/38g	97	5	259	17.2	17.3	13.4	1
Spare, Chinese Style, Summer Eating, Asda*	1 Serving/116g	334	18.6	288	32	4.1	16	0.8
Spare, Sweet, Sticky, Mini, M&S*	½ Pack/75g	215	12.9	286	22.7	9.8	17.2	0.8
Veggie, BBQ, Sweet n Smoky, Ribz, Plant Power*	1 Serving/150g	244	8.8	163	10.4	14.9	5.9	3.2
RICE								
Arborio, Dry, Average	***1 Serving/80g***	***279***	***0.6***	***348***	***7.1***	***78.3***	***0.8***	***0.8***
Basmati, & Wild, Cooked, Sainsbury's*	½ Pack/125g	150	0.8	120	3.1	25.7	0.6	1.3
Basmati, & Wild, Dry Weight, Tilda*	1 Serving/70g	244	0.3	349	9.4	77	0.5	1

R

	Measure INFO/WEIGHT	per Measure KCAL	FAT	Nutrition Values per 100g / 100ml KCAL	PROT	CARB	FAT	FIBRE
RICE								
Basmati, Boil in the Bag, Dry, Average	***1 Serving/50g***	***176***	***0.4***	***352***	***8.4***	***77.8***	***0.8***	***0.4***
Basmati, Brown, Dry, Average	***1 Serving/50g***	***177***	***1.5***	***353***	***9.5***	***71.8***	***3***	***2.2***
Basmati, Cooked, Average	***1 Serving/140g***	***190***	***3.9***	***136***	***2.4***	***25.6***	***2.8***	***0.8***
Basmati, Dry Weight, Average	***1 Serving/60g***	***212***	***0.6***	***353***	***8.1***	***77.9***	***1***	***0.6***
Basmati, Indian, Dry, Average	***1 Serving/75g***	***260***	***0.7***	***346***	***8.4***	***76.1***	***0.9***	***0.1***
Basmati, Lemon & Herb, Steamed, Tilda*	1 Serving/125g	172	2.8	137	2.6	26.1	2.2	1.2
Basmati, Mexican, Spicy, Tilda*	½ Pack/125g	152	3.1	122	2.4	21.6	2.5	1.8
Basmati, Microwave, Cooked, Average	***1 Serving/125g***	***182***	***2.3***	***146***	***2.7***	***30***	***1.8***	***0***
Basmati, Peri Peri, Tilda*	1 Pack/250g	325	6.2	130	2.5	23.5	2.5	1.8
Basmati, White, Dry, Average	***1 Serving/75g***	***262***	***0.4***	***349***	***8.1***	***77.1***	***0.6***	***2.2***
Basmati, Wholegrain & Wild, Pouch, Tilda*	½ Pack/125g	160	2.6	128	3	23.4	2.1	1.7
Basmati, Wholegrain, Cooked, Tilda*	1 Portion/180g	203	1.6	113	3.3	23	0.9	3.2
Beef, Super Rice, As Prepared, Batchelors*	½ Pack/116g	159	1.2	137	3.8	27.3	1	1.7
Black, Dry Weight, Holland & Barrett*	1 Serving/60g	208	1.9	346	9.8	67.6	3.1	3.9
Brown, Basmati, Microwave Pouch, Sainsbury's*	1 Pouch/250g	340	3	136	3.2	27.6	1.2	0.9
Brown, Basmati, Wholegrain, Classic, GF, Tilda*	½ Pack/125g	161	2.6	129	2.8	23.3	2.1	3
Brown, Cooked, Average	***1 Serving/140g***	***173***	***1.5***	***123***	***2.6***	***26.6***	***1.1***	***0.9***
Brown, Dry, Average	***1 Serving/75g***	***266***	***2.3***	***355***	***7.5***	***76.2***	***3***	***1.4***
Brown, Long Grain, Dry, Average	***1 Serving/50g***	***182***	***1.4***	***364***	***7.6***	***76.8***	***2.8***	***2***
Brown, Long Grain, Microwave Pouch, Sainsbury's*	½ Pack/125g	214	2.5	171	3.3	32.2	2	5.3
Brown, Short Grain, Dry, Average	***1 Serving/50g***	***176***	***1.4***	***351***	***6.8***	***77.6***	***2.8***	***1***
Brown, Spelt, & Quinoa, Dry Weight, Lassie*	¼ Pack/69g	245	1.9	355	11.1	68.9	2.8	5
Brown, Whole Grain, Cooked, Average	***1 Serving/170g***	***223***	***1.9***	***132***	***2.6***	***27.8***	***1.1***	***1.2***
Brown, Whole Grain, Dry, Average	***1 Serving/40g***	***138***	***1.2***	***344***	***7.4***	***71.6***	***2.9***	***3***
Cauliflower, Frozen, Tesco*	1 Sachet/150g	36	0.3	24	1.8	2.1	0.2	3.2
Cauliflower, Microwaved, G&B, Asda*	½ Pack/200g	68	1.8	34	2.9	2.1	0.9	2.7
Chicken, & Sweetcorn, Microwave, Sainsbury's*	½ Pack/125g	204	2.6	163	3.9	31.2	2.1	1.9
Chinese Style, Express, Uncle Ben's*	1 Pack/250g	392	5.5	157	3.4	30.9	2.2	0.4
Coconut, Chilli, & Lemongrass, Worldwide Foods, Aldi*	½ Pack/125g	218	5.7	174	2.8	29	4.6	2
Coconut, Lime, & Coriander, Waitrose*	½ Pack/125g	200	3.1	160	3.1	30.8	2.5	1.4
Coconut, Worldwide Foods, Aldi*	1 Serving/125g	210	5.2	168	3.5	28	4.2	1.2
Egg Fried, Average	***1 Serving/300g***	***624***	***31.8***	***208***	***4.2***	***25.7***	***10.6***	***0.4***
Egg Fried, Wholegrain, Pouch, Uncle Ben's*	½ Pouch/125g	194	4.5	155	4.3	25	3.6	1.8
Egg Fried, with Peas, M&S*	½ Pack/150g	328	14.2	219	4.1	28.5	9.5	1.4
Fried, Chicken, Takeaway, Iceland*	1 Pack/336g	631	18.1	188	7.5	26.5	5.4	1.5
Garlic, Roasted, Express Rice, Uncle Ben's*	½ Pack/125g	190	2.6	152	3.2	30	2.1	0.9
Golden Veg, Micro, Asda*	½ Pack/125g	195	1.9	156	3.5	31.2	1.5	2.3
Golden Vegetable, Savoury Rice, Batchelors*	½ Pack/116g	157	0.8	135	3.9	27.5	0.7	1.6
Golden Vegetable, Savoury, Sainsbury's*	½ Pack/147g	189	0.9	129	2.9	27.1	0.6	2
Golden Vegetable, Special, Worldwide Foods, Aldi*	½ Pack/125g	181	2.1	145	3.7	27	1.7	3
Golden, Savoury, Steam Bags, Iceland*	1 Bag/149g	179	3.1	120	3.1	21.4	2.1	1.6
Golden, Steamed, Sainsbury's*	1 Bag/189g	210	2.1	111	3	21	1.1	2.3
Golden, Super Rice, Cooked, Batchelors*	1 Serving/116g	157	0.8	135	4	27.4	0.7	1.7
Jasmine, Microwave, Tesco*	½ Pouch/125g	206	1.6	165	3.3	34.4	1.3	1
Jasmine, Thai, Microwave, Morrisons*	½ Pack/125g	222	2	178	3.1	37.3	1.6	0.8
Lemon, & Thyme, Uncle Ben's*	½ Pouch/125g	192	2.8	154	3.3	30	2.2	1
Long Grain, & Wild, Dry, Average	***1 Serving/75g***	***254***	***1.5***	***338***	***7.6***	***72.6***	***2***	***1.7***
Long Grain, & Wild, Microwave, M&S*	1 Pack/130g	212	1.2	163	3.9	34	0.9	1.5
Long Grain, & Wild, Microwave, Morrisons*	½ Pack/110g	182	1.4	166	3.7	34.4	1.3	0.9
Long Grain, & Wild, Microwave, Uncle Ben's*	½ Pack/125g	188	1.6	150	3.2	30.9	1.3	0.9
Long Grain, American, Cooked, Average	***1 Serving/160g***	***229***	***2.8***	***143***	***3***	***28.8***	***1.8***	***0.2***
Long Grain, American, Dry, Average	***1 Serving/50g***	***175***	***0.5***	***350***	***7.2***	***77.8***	***1.1***	***0.6***
Long Grain, Dry, Average	***1 Serving/50g***	***169***	***0.5***	***337***	***7.4***	***75.5***	***1***	***1.7***

	Measure INFO/WEIGHT	per Measure KCAL	FAT	Nutrition Values per 100g / 100ml KCAL	PROT	CARB	FAT	FIBRE
RICE								
Long Grain, Microwavable, Cooked, Average	***1 Serving/150g***	***180***	***0.9***	***120***	***2.7***	***25.8***	***0.6***	***0.7***
Mexican Inspired, Micro, Tesco*	1 Bag/142g	184	2	130	3.2	25.5	1.4	1.1
Mexican Style, Microwave, Lidl*	½ Pack/125g	235	3.5	188	3	37	2.8	1.3
Mexican Style, Special, Worldwide Foods, Aldi*	½ Pack/181g	262	3.3	145	3.1	28	1.8	2.9
Mexican, M&S*	1 Serving/250g	368	5.5	147	3.3	27.5	2.2	2.2
Mushroom, M&S*	1 Pack/300g	417	15	139	3	19.6	5	1.6
Mushroom, Pilau, Indian, Sainsbury's*	1 Serving/100g	119	2.4	119	3	21.3	2.4	1.9
Mushroom, Roasted, Taste of India, Tesco*	½ Pack/135g	177	3.5	131	3.2	23	2.6	1.6
Onion Bhaji, Uncle Ben's*	½ Pack/125g	200	2.9	160	3.3	31	2.3	1.4
Paella, Spanish, Dry, Tesco*	1 Serving/75g	262	0.4	349	6.3	78.9	0.6	1.5
Pilau, Cooked, Average	***1 Serving/200g***	***349***	***8.8***	***174***	***3.5***	***30.3***	***4.4***	***0.8***
Pilau, Dry, Average	***1oz/28g***	***101***	***0.7***	***362***	***8.4***	***78.2***	***2.4***	***3.4***
Pilau, Microwave, Sainsbury's*	½ Pouch/125g	202	1.4	161	3.3	33.6	1.1	1.9
Pudding, Dry Weight, Average	***1 Serving/100g***	***356***	***1.1***	***356***	***6.9***	***82***	***1.1***	***0.4***
Rainbow, Vegan, Nature's Pick, Aldi*	1 Serving/80g	23	0.4	29	1.6	3.9	0.5	2.4
Red, Dry, Ingredients, Tesco*	1 Serving/60g	209	1.8	349	8.2	69.8	3	5
Risotto, Dry, Average	***1 Serving/50g***	***174***	***0.6***	***348***	***7.8***	***76.2***	***1.3***	***2.4***
Saffron, Cooked, Average	***1 Serving/150g***	***208***	***4.7***	***139***	***2.6***	***25.3***	***3.2***	***0.5***
Singapore, Stir Fry, Waitrose*	½ Pack/140g	158	4.5	113	1.9	17.5	3.2	3.3
Special Fried, Chinese Takeaway, Iceland*	1 Pack/350g	630	17.5	180	5.5	28.2	5	1.2
Special Fried, Chinese, Tesco*	1 Serving/300g	618	33.3	206	6.5	19.9	11.1	0.8
Special Fried, M&S*	½ Pack/150g	300	12.3	200	6.7	24.2	8.2	1.2
Spicy Mexican, Microwave, Uncle Ben's*	½ Pouch/125g	199	3.8	159	3.8	28	3	1.5
Spinach, & Carrot, Pilau, Waitrose*	1 Pack/350g	466	8.4	133	3.1	24.8	2.4	1.2
Thai, Black, Sainsbury's*	1 Serving/180g	205	2	114	3.7	20.4	1.1	3.8
Thai, Cooked, Average	***1 Serving/100g***	***136***	***1.8***	***136***	***2.5***	***27.4***	***1.8***	***0.3***
Thai, Dry, Average	***1 Serving/50g***	***174***	***0.2***	***348***	***7.1***	***78.9***	***0.4***	***0.9***
Thai, Fragrant, Dry, Average	***1 Serving/75g***	***272***	***0.5***	***363***	***7.2***	***82***	***0.7***	***0.3***
Thai, Glutinous, Sticky, White, Dry, Raw	***1 Serving/100g***	***370***	***0.6***	***370***	***6.8***	***81.7***	***0.6***	***2.8***
Tomato, & Basil, Morrisons*	½ Pack/110g	176	2.8	160	4	29.3	2.5	1.8
Tomato, & Basil, Tilda*	½ Pack/125g	154	3.1	123	2.1	22.4	2.5	1.1
Vegetable, Golden, Freshly Frozen, Asda*	1 Sachet/200g	238	2.6	119	3.2	23.6	1.3	1.3
Vegetable, Mediterranean, SteamFresh, Birds Eye*	1 Bag/190g	218	4.9	115	2.4	20	2.6	1.2
White, Cooked, Average	***1 Serving/140g***	***182***	***1.1***	***130***	***2.6***	***28.7***	***0.8***	***0.2***
White, Cooked, Frozen, Average	***1 Serving/150g***	***168***	***0.8***	***112***	***2.9***	***23.8***	***0.6***	***1.2***
White, Fried	***1oz/28g***	***37***	***0.9***	***131***	***2.2***	***25***	***3.2***	***0.6***
White, Long Grain, Dry Weight, Average	***1 Serving/50g***	***181***	***1***	***362***	***7.1***	***79.1***	***1.9***	***0.4***
White, Microwave, Cooked, Average	***½ Pack/125g***	***185***	***2.4***	***148***	***3.3***	***29.4***	***1.9***	***1.4***
White, Steam & Serve, Frozen, Steamed, Morrisons*	1 Sachet/200g	280	0.8	140	2.8	31.1	0.4	0.5
Whole Grain, Dry, Average	***1 Serving/50g***	***171***	***1.2***	***342***	***8.2***	***72***	***2.3***	***4***
Whole Grain, Microwave, Waitrose*	1 Serving/125g	188	2.6	150	3.3	26.9	2.1	5.3
Whole Grains, 5, Microwave, Golden Sun, Lidl*	½ Pack/110g	170	3.2	155	4.1	26.4	2.9	3.5
Wholegrain, & 5 Grains, Microwave, Sainsbury's*	½ Pack/125g	222	1.5	178	4.4	35.4	1.2	3.8
Wholegrain, & Freekeh, Sainsbury's*	½ Pack/125g	206	3.2	165	4.4	29.2	2.6	3.6
Wholegrain, & Quinoa, Sainsbury's*	½ Pack/125g	204	2.1	163	3.8	31.6	1.7	3.2
Wholegrain, & Wild, Sainsbury's*	½ Pack/125g	197	2	157	3.4	30.8	1.6	3.1
Wholegrain, Basmati, & Wild, Microwave, Tilda*	½ Pack/125g	169	3.3	135	3.1	23.3	2.6	3
Wholegrain, Classic, Worldwide Foods, Aldi*	½ Pack/125g	205	2.6	164	4.1	31	2.1	2.6
Wholegrain, Cooked, Uncle Ben's*	1 Serving/150g	252	1.7	168	3.9	35	1.1	1.6
Wholegrain, Duchy, Waitrose*	1 Serving/75g	106	0.7	142	3.6	29.2	0.9	1.5
Wholegrain, Micro Rice, Asda*	1 Pack/250g	412	5	165	3.9	31	2	3.4
Wholegrain, Microwave, Uncle Ben's*	½ Pack/125g	205	3.1	164	3.7	31	2.5	1.9
Wholegrain, Wild, & Red, Worldwide Foods, Aldi*	½ Pack/125g	218	3.4	174	4.5	31	2.7	4.4

	Measure INFO/WEIGHT	per Measure KCAL	FAT	Nutrition Values per 100g / 100ml KCAL	PROT	CARB	FAT	FIBRE
RICE								
Wild, Cooked, Average	***1 Cup/164g***	***166***	***0.6***	***101***	***4***	***21.3***	***0.3***	***1.8***
with Mixed Vegetables, White & Wild, Steam Bag, Tesco*	1 Bag/150g	168	1.8	112	2.6	21.7	1.2	1.9
With Red Kidney Beans, Average	***1oz/28g***	***49***	***1***	***175***	***5.6***	***32.4***	***3.5***	***2.5***
Yellow Lentil, Slim Rice, Eat Water*	1 Serving/249g	244	5.5	98	4.4	15.2	2.2	2.4
RICE CAKES								
& Corn, Salt & Vinegar, Sainsbury's*	1 Rice Cake/9g	34	0.3	375	7.3	77	3.5	3.3
Asda*	1 Rice Cake/8g	31	0.2	386	8.7	81.1	3	2.8
Bar, Kelkin*	1 Bar/20g	95	3.6	474	5.8	71	18	2.2
Caramel, Flavour, Kallo*	1 Rice Cake/10g	38	0.5	383	6.2	78.9	4.8	3.9
Caramel, Free From, Tesco*	1 Rice Cake/11g	41	0.3	373	5.9	80.9	2.5	1.8
Caramel, Jumbo, Snack-A-Jacks*	1 Rice Cake/13g	51	0.3	390	5.5	87	2.1	1.4
Caramel, Jumbo, Tesco*	1 Rice Cake/10g	34	0.3	340	7	74	3	5
Cheese, & Onion, Snack, Snack-A-Jacks*	1 Bag/30g	120	2.2	400	6.7	77	7.5	1.5
Chocolate Coated, Mini, Snack-A-Jacks*	1 Pack/14g	69	3.4	493	6.4	62.9	24.3	2.9
Chocolate Covered, Thin, Kallo*	1 Rice Cake/11g	54	2.5	495	7.8	63	23	3.5
Chocolate Orange, Tesco*	1 Rice Cake/18g	85	3.6	472	5.1	65.4	20	5.1
Chocolate, Chip, Jumbo, Snack-A-Jacks*	1 Rice Cake/15g	62	1	410	6	81	7	1.7
Chocolate, Dark, Organic, Kallo*	1 Rice Cake/12g	57	2.9	471	6.8	57.2	24.1	7.4
Chocolate, Milk, Kallo*	1 Rice Cake/17g	83	3.7	486	7	65	22	0
Chocolate, Milk, Mini, Sainsbury's*	1 Pack/30g	138	5	459	7.8	67.9	16.8	2.9
Chocolate, Milk, Minis, Kids, Kallo*	1 Pack/14g	69	3.3	496	6.6	62.6	23.8	0
Chocolate, Milk, Sainsbury's*	1 Pack/38g	178	7	469	7.7	66.2	18.5	3.2
Corn, Salt & Vinegar, Co-Op*	1 Rice Cake/9g	33	0.5	367	8.9	75.6	5.6	5.6
Dark Chocolate, Minis, Kallo*	1 Pack/21g	102	4.8	486	6.2	61	23	5.2
Dark Chocolate, Morrisons*	1 Rice Cake/17g	80	3.3	473	6.5	65.1	19.5	4.5
Idly, Average	***1 Idly/40g***	***59***	***0.4***	***149***	***4.1***	***30.8***	***1***	***1.3***
Low Fat, BGTY, Sainsbury's*	1 Rice Cake/7g	29	0.2	388	8.1	81.5	2.4	3.9
Milk Chocolate, & Salted Caramel, The Best, Morrisons*	1 Rice Cake/17g	85	3.6	487	5.9	67.4	20.9	2.6
Multigrain, Harvest Morn, Aldi*	1 Rice Cake/8g	30	0.2	374	11	72	2.3	11
Multigrain, High Protein, M&S*	1 Rice Cake/8g	31	0.2	387	21.8	67.4	2.8	2.3
Multigrain, Ryvita*	3 Rice Cakes/11g	43	0.5	384	9.1	76.2	4.7	5.3
Pea, & Lentil, Protein, Sainsbury's*	1 Rice Cake/8g	31	0.2	370	21.6	60.6	2.5	9.3
Pear, & Berries, Tesco*	1 Rice Cake/2g	7	0	372	7.3	84	0.6	0.7
Salt & Vinegar, Asda*	1 Rice Cake/8g	30	0.2	353	9.1	72	2.6	3.4
Salt & Vinegar, Morrisons*	1 Rice Cake/9g	30	0.2	335	6.7	69.2	2.6	3.8
Salt & Vinegar, Tesco*	1 Rice Cake/12g	47	0.7	392	6.3	78	5.7	1.8
Salt, & Vinegar, Jumbo, Snack-A-Jacks*	1 Rice Cake/10g	41	0.6	391	7.4	75.4	5.7	1.6
Salt, & Vinegar, Jumbo, Tesco*	1 Rice Cake/9g	31	0.2	347	8.4	72.7	2.5	6
Salt, & Vinegar, Wholegrain, Tesco*	1 Rice Cake/9g	28	0.2	314	8.4	61.9	2.6	6
Salted Caramel, M&S*	1 Rice Cake/19g	90	3.7	474	6.8	66.8	19.5	2.6
Salted, Lightly, Thick Slice, Low Fat, Kallo*	1 Rice Cake/8g	28	0.2	372	8	78.7	2.8	5.1
Salted, Sea, Harvest Morn, Aldi*	1 Rice Cake/7g	27	0.2	379	8.7	78	2.2	5.1
Salted, Slightly, Organic, Thin Slice, Kallo*	1 Rice Cake/5g	17	0.1	372	8	78.7	2.8	5.1
Salted, Slightly, Thick Slice, Organic, Kallo*	1 Rice Cake/8g	28	0.2	372	8	78.7	2.8	5.1
Sesame, No Added Salt, Thick Sliced, Organic, Kallo*	1 Rice Cake/10g	37	0.3	373	8	78	3.2	5.4
Sesame, Toasted, Ryvita*	1 Pack/11g	43	0.5	391	8.4	78.4	4.9	3.5
Sour Cream, & Black Pepper, M&S*	1 Rice Cake/9g	39	1	432	7.1	75.8	10.8	1.6
Sour Cream, & Chive, Snack, The Foodie Market, Aldi*	1 Pack/23g	101	1.9	437	7.5	82	8.4	1.2
Sweet Chilli, Harvest Morn, Aldi*	1 Rice Cake/10g	47	1.7	452	7.2	67	16	4.4
Thai Chilli, Snaktastic, Lidl*	1 Serving/25	137	8.1	549	3.4	60.4	32.5	0
Thin Slice, No Added Salt, Organic, Kallo*	1 Rice Cake/5g	19	0.1	372	8	78.7	2.8	5.1
RICE PUDDING								
& Jam, Fat Free, Aunt Bessie's*	¼ Pack/131g	136	0.3	104	2.4	23	0.2	0.6

	Measure INFO/WEIGHT	per Measure KCAL	FAT	Nutrition Values per 100g / 100ml KCAL	PROT	CARB	FAT	FIBRE
RICE PUDDING								
50% Less Fat, Asda*	½ Can/212g	180	1.7	85	3.3	16.2	0.8	0.2
830, Wiltshire Farm Foods*	1 Serving/160g	181	4.8	113	2.9	18	3	0
Apple, Ambrosia*	1 Pot/150g	125	2.3	104	2.7	18.8	1.9	0.5
Apple, Brooklea, Aldi*	1 Pot/180g	200	3.2	111	2.9	21	1.8	0.5
Canned, Average	***1oz/28g***	***25***	***0.7***	***89***	***3.4***	***14***	***2.5***	***0.2***
Canned, Light, Salco, Lidl*	1 Can/400g	316	2.8	79	2.8	15.1	0.7	0.5
Clotted Cream, Morrisons*	1 Pudding/145g	265	17.3	183	3.1	15.5	11.9	0.7
Clotted Cream, Waitrose*	1 Pot/150g	286	18	191	3.1	17.3	12	0.7
Creamed, Canned, Ambrosia*	1 Can/425g	382	8.1	90	3.1	15.2	1.9	0
Creamed, Pot, Ambrosia*	1 Pot/150g	156	3.8	104	3.3	17	2.5	0.1
Creamed, Value, Tesco*	1 Can/425g	348	3.4	82	3.2	15.5	0.8	0
Creamed, with British Milk, Canned, Simply, M&S*	½ Can/200g	230	9.8	115	3.2	13.9	4.9	1.2
Creamy, Tesco*	1 Pudding/172g	249	12.4	145	2.6	17	7.2	1
Light, Ambrosia*	1 Pot/150g	120	0.9	80	3.3	15.3	0.6	0.5
Light, Tesco*	½ Can/200g	152	1.6	76	2.8	14.4	0.8	0.1
Low Fat, Devon, Creamed, Ambrosia*	½ Can/213g	193	2.8	91	3.2	16.5	1.3	0
Low Fat, Muller Rice, Muller*	1 Serving/180g	182	4.7	101	3.4	16.1	2.6	0
Pot, Ambrosia*	1 Pot/125g	126	3.1	101	3.3	16.3	2.5	0
Raspberry, Low Fat, Muller Rice, Muller*	1 Pot/180g	189	4	105	3	18.4	2.2	0
Raspberry, Mullerice, Muller*	1 Pot/190g	201	4.4	106	3.2	18.2	2.3	0.5
Riz Au Lait, Bonne Maman*	1 Pot/100g	149	5.3	149	3.3	22	5.3	0.1
Stockwell & Co., Tesco*	½ Can/200g	162	1.6	81	3.1	15.3	0.8	0
Strawberry, Muller*	1 Pot/180g	191	4	106	3	18.6	2.2	0
Vanilla Custard, Mullerrice, Muller*	1 Pot/200g	230	5	115	3.4	19.8	2.5	0.3
RICE WINE								
Sake, Average	***1 Tbsp/15ml***	***20***	***0***	***134***	***0.5***	***5***	***0***	***0***
RIGATONI								
Dried, Specially Selected, Aldi*	1 Serving/75g	263	1	351	14	70	1.4	3.1
Dry, Average	***1 Serving/80g***	***272***	***1.2***	***340***	***11.4***	***68.4***	***1.5***	***2.7***
Mezzi, Dry Weight, TTD, Sainsbury's*	1 Serving/100g	318	1.2	318	12.4	62.8	1.2	3
RISOTTO								
aux Asperges, Vertes, Frozen, Picard*	½ Pack/250g	308	11	123	3.1	17	4.4	0.6
Balls, Green Vegetable, & Mozzarella, Sainsbury's*	1 Ball/50g	126	6.4	252	6.8	26	12.7	3
Butternut Squash, Fresh Ideas, M Kitchen, Morrisons*	1 Pot/350g	371	11.9	106	1.8	16.8	3.4	0.7
Butternut Squash, Kale, & Spelt, Tesco*	1 Pack/361g	347	8.7	96	3.4	14.1	2.4	2.4
Cherry Tomato, & Basil, Napolina*	1 Serving/320g	285	10.6	89	1.8	12.4	3.3	0
Chicken	***1 Serving/380g***	***494***	***17.4***	***130***	***7.2***	***15.2***	***4.6***	***1.3***
Chicken, & Lemon, Weight Watchers*	1 Pack/320g	353	6.3	107	6.3	15.8	1.9	0.7
Chicken, & Mushroom, for Two, Charlie Bigham's*	1 Serving/350g	556	26.2	159	7.2	15.8	7.5	0
Chicken, & Asparagus, COU, M&S*	1 Pack/360g	320	4.3	89	7.7	11.7	1.2	0.5
Chicken, & Chorizo, Super, Bachelors *	½ Pack/130g	178	2	137	4.2	26.4	1.5	0.7
Chicken, & Mushroom, BFY, M&S*	1 Pack/380g	407	10.3	107	8.8	11.4	2.7	0.9
Chicken, & Mushroom, Chef Select, Lidl*	1 Pack/333g	330	9	99	6.6	11.5	2.7	1
Chicken, & Mushroom, Extra Special, Asda*	1 Pack/400g	532	16	133	5.8	18	4	0.7
Chicken, & Mushroom, Italian Inspired, Asda*	1 Pack/373g	403	10.8	108	6.6	14	2.9	0.5
Chicken, & Mushroom, Meal for One, M&S*	1 Pack/400g	468	13.2	117	8.1	13.3	3.3	0.8
Chicken, & Mushroom, Portobello, Finest, Tesco*	1 Pack/372g	454	12.3	122	8	14.2	3.3	1.2
Courgette, & Pea, Vegan, Waitrose*	½ Pack/187g	172	6.2	92	3.2	11	3.3	2.7
Green Bean, Asparagus & Pecorino, Finest, Tesco*	1 Pack/400g	460	15.6	115	4.4	15	3.9	1.5
Haddock, Smoked, Finest, Tesco*	1 Pack/396g	412	8.7	104	5.6	15.1	2.2	1
Mediterranean Inspired, Calorie Controlled, Tesco*	1 Pack/350g	294	0.5	84	3.9	16.8	0.1	1.2
Mushroom, Calorie Counted, Tesco*	1 Pack/365g	339	8.4	93	3.4	14	2.3	1.4
Mushroom, Creamy, Co-Op*	1 Pack/401g	497	20	124	4.2	15	5	0.6

R

	Measure INFO/WEIGHT	per Measure KCAL	FAT	Nutrition Values per 100g / 100ml KCAL	PROT	CARB	FAT	FIBRE
RISOTTO								
Mushroom, HL, Tesco*	1 Pack/366g	339	8.3	93	3.4	14	2.3	1.4
Mushroom, Plant Based, Asda*	1 Pack/400g	448	15.6	112	2.2	16	3.9	1.8
Mushroom, Risotto, Cook*	1 Serving/340g	530	23.5	156	4.2	19.7	6.9	0
Mushroom, Three, Allplants*	1 Serving/378g	507	19.3	134	4.2	17	5.1	1.9
Prawn, COU, M&S*	1 Pack/350g	378	7.7	108	4.3	17.3	2.2	0.8
Prawn, Pea & Mint, King, M&S*	½ Pack/300g	405	18.6	135	3.8	15.9	6.2	0.9
Pumpkin, & Feta, Woolworths*	1 Serve/350g	430	18.2	123	3.2	15.1	5.2	0
Red Pepper, & Italian Cheese, Roasted, M&S*	1 Pack/400g	500	13.2	125	2.9	20.4	3.3	1
Roasted Pumpkin, Pre-Mix, Belladotti*	1 Serving/58g	209	1.6	361	7.4	72.3	2.7	0
Seafood, Youngs*	1 Pack/350g	424	13	121	4.5	17.4	3.7	0.1
Squash, Orzo, Sumptuous, Orzotto, Jamie Oliver*	½ Pack/125g	169	3.9	135	5	19	3.1	5.6
Tomato, with Crispy Aubergine, Gousto*	1 Serving/404g	461	8.5	114	3.8	20.6	2.1	1.7
Vegetable, Average	***1oz/28g***	***41***	***1.8***	***147***	***4.2***	***19.2***	***6.5***	***2.2***
Vegetable, Brown Rice, Average	***1oz/28g***	***40***	***1.8***	***143***	***4.1***	***18.6***	***6.4***	***2.4***
Vert, Serves 1, At Home, Cote*	1 Pack/374g	606	32.9	162	4.1	15.9	8.8	1.5
with Mushroom, & Garlic, Cucina, Aldi*	1 Serving/200g	214	3	107	2.6	20	1.5	1
ROCK SALMON								
Raw, Flesh Only, Average	***1oz/28g***	***43***	***2.7***	***154***	***16.6***	***0***	***9.7***	***0***
ROCKET								
Fresh, Raw, Average	***1 Serving/80g***	***12***	***0.4***	***16***	***0.8***	***1.7***	***0.5***	***1.2***
ROE								
Cod, Average	***1 Can/100g***	***96***	***2.8***	***96***	***17.1***	***0.5***	***2.8***	***0***
Cod, Hard, Coated in Batter, Fried	***1oz/28g***	***53***	***3.3***	***189***	***12.4***	***8.9***	***11.8***	***0.2***
Cod, Hard, Fried in Blended Oil	***1oz/28g***	***57***	***3.3***	***202***	***20.9***	***3***	***11.9***	***0.1***
Herring, Soft, Fried in Blended Oil	***1oz/28g***	***74***	***4.4***	***265***	***26.3***	***4.7***	***15.8***	***0.2***
Herring, Soft, Raw	***1oz/28g***	***22***	***0.1***	***78***	***18.2***	***0.5***	***0.4***	***0***
ROGAN JOSH								
Chicken, & Pilau Rice, Morrisons*	1 Pack/419g	528	13.8	126	7.4	15.2	3.3	2.9
Chicken, Breast, Chunks, Hot, Sainsbury's*	½ Pack/114g	143	2	126	23.6	3.9	1.8	1
Chicken, Munch*	1 Pack/197g	292	4.1	148	10.4	20.7	2.1	0
Chicken, with Pilau Rice, Farmfoods*	1 Pack/325g	354	6.8	109	5.3	17.1	2.1	0.4
Chickpea, & Kale, Tideford Organics*	1 Pot/300g	180	6.9	60	2.5	6.2	2.3	1.8
Lamb, Indian, Takeaway, CBY, Asda*	½ Pack/200g	218	12	109	8	5.1	6	1.4
Lamb, Sainsbury's*	1 Pack/400g	660	44.4	165	11.3	4.9	11.1	1.9
Lamb, Takeaway, Tesco*	½ Pack/192g	228	14	119	6.3	5.7	7.3	2.5
Prawn, COU, M&S*	1 Pack/400g	360	2.4	90	4.9	16.2	0.6	0.8
ROLL								
Bacon, Breakfast, Co-Op*	1 Roll/134g	355	11.7	265	17	29	8.7	1.8
Beef, & Roast Onion Mayo, Soft White, M&S*	1 Pack/215g	522	17.6	243	11.5	30	8.2	1.5
Cheddar, & Onion Chutney, Veggie, Higgidy*	1 Roll/27g	93	5.5	345	8.6	33.3	20.4	1.6
Cheese & Onion, Oven Baked, Asda*	1 Roll/60g	174	9.6	290	6.6	29	16	2.7
Cheese, & Onion, Co-Op*	1 Roll/66g	195	11.9	295	7	26	18	2
Cheese, & Onion, Iceland*	1 Roll/67g	222	13.6	332	7.5	29.6	20.4	1.5
Cheese, & Onion, M&S*	1 Roll/25g	80	5.1	320	9.6	24.7	20.5	1.3
Cheese, & Onion, Tesco*	1 Roll/67g	203	12.1	305	7.3	28	18.1	1.9
Cheese, & Pickle, Sainsbury's*	1 Roll/136g	359	13.6	264	10.6	35.1	10	0
Cheese, & Bacon, Snack, Sainsbury's*	1 Roll/30g	95	5.3	318	9.9	28.5	17.8	2.4
Cheese, & Onion, Mini, Sainsbury's*	1 Roll/10g	29	1.5	292	6.9	30.6	15.4	1.9
Cheese, & Onion, Sainsbury's*	1 Roll/66g	190	9.8	288	6.9	30.6	14.8	2.5
Chicken, & Mayonnaise, Roast, Big, Sainsbury's*	1 Pack/185g	479	27.4	259	9.6	21.8	14.8	0
Chicken, Deep Fried, Shazans*	3 Rolls/138g	298	3.9	216	12.7	37.5	2.8	4.8
Cornish, in Pastry, Pork Farms*	1 Roll/75g	226	15.1	301	6.6	24.5	20.1	0
Egg Mayo, & Cress, Fullfillers*	1 Roll/125g	266	11.8	213	10	25.7	9.4	0

R

	Measure INFO/WEIGHT	per Measure KCAL	FAT	Nutrition Values per 100g / 100ml KCAL	PROT	CARB	FAT	FIBRE
ROLL								
Egg Mayonnaise, & Cress, Sub, Delicious, Boots*	1 Pack/205g	399	14.1	195	10	23	6.9	2.4
Egg, & Cress, HL, Tesco*	1 Pack/175g	322	6.8	184	9.6	27.7	3.9	1.2
Feta, & Red Pepper, Specially Selected, Aldi*	1 Roll/27g	103	6.7	387	8.9	31	25	3.3
Feta, & Red Pepper,, Veggie, Higgidy*	1 Roll/27g	97	6	360	9.3	32.3	22.3	2
Ham, & Salad, BGTY, Sainsbury's*	1 Roll/178g	292	3.4	164	10.8	25.9	1.9	0
Ham, & Salad, J D Gross, Lidl*	1 Roll/154g	293	9.2	190	7.7	29.1	6	1.9
Ham, & Tomato, Taste!*	1 Serving/112g	211	4.8	188	10.4	27	4.3	0
Ham, Darwins Deli*	1 Serving/125g	298	7.5	238	11	37.4	6	0
Mushroom, Miso, Vegan, Higgidy*	1 Roll/27g	92	5.1	345	7.1	37.3	19	3.9
Ploughman's, Large, Ginsters*	1 Pack/140g	473	33.5	338	10.2	20.5	23.9	1.8
Pork, Stuffing, & Apple Sauce, Roast, Boots*	1 Roll/218g	602	26.2	276	10	32	12	1.8
Salmon, Oak Smoked, M&S*	1 Roll/55g	139	6.2	252	14.6	23.1	11.3	1.2
Sausage, Lincolnshire, COU, M&S*	1 Roll/175g	280	4.7	160	10	23.2	2.7	2.6
Tuna Mayo, & Cucumber, Taste!*	1 Serving/111g	274	12.5	247	9	27.3	11.3	0
Tuna Mayonnaise, with Cucumber, Yummies*	1 Serving/132g	340	18.6	257	10.4	22.5	14	0
Tuna, & Sweetcorn, with Mayonnaise, Shell*	1 Pack/180g	536	26.3	298	13.1	28.6	14.6	0
Tuna, Cheese Melt, Boots*	1 Roll/199g	612	35.8	308	13	23	18	1.2
Turkey, Salad, Northern Bites*	1 Roll/231g	323	8.3	140	8.6	19.6	3.6	3
Vegetable Samosa, & Mango Chutney, Vegan, Higgidy*	1 Roll/27g	86	4.7	318	4.9	36	17.4	2.7
ROLO								
Little, Nestle*	1 Pack/40g	196	9.4	491	4	65.5	23.5	0.5
Nestle*	1 Sweet/5g	24	1	478	4.4	68.2	20.4	1.1
ROOT BEER								
Average	***1 Can/330ml***	***135***	***0***	***41***	***0***	***10.6***	***0***	***0***
ROSEMARY								
Dried	***1 Tsp/1g***	***3***	***0.2***	***331***	***4.9***	***46.4***	***15.2***	***0***
Fresh	***1 Tsp/0.7g***	***1***	***0***	***99***	***1.4***	***13.5***	***4.4***	***0***
ROSTI								
Baskets, Vegetable Jalfrezi, Aldi*	1 Rosti/279g	472	20.4	169	3.2	21	7.3	2.2
Cheese, & Onion, Tesco*	1 Rosti/92g	202	10.9	220	5.1	21.6	11.9	3.2
Maris Piper & Onion, M&S*	1 Rosti/35g	77	4.2	219	1.9	24.7	12	2.4
Potato & Root Vegetable, COU, M&S*	1 Rosti/100g	85	2.7	85	1.6	13.3	2.7	1.5
Potato Cakes, Baby, M&S*	1 Rosti/23g	40	1.5	175	3.5	25.1	6.7	1.6
Potato, McCain*	1 Rosti/95g	161	8.6	169	2.2	19.6	9.1	0
Sweet Potato, Tesco*	½ Pack/91g	258	16	283	2.7	26.2	17.6	4.4
ROULADE								
Black Forest, Finest, Tesco*	1/8 Roulade/74g	206	6.5	280	3.2	46.4	8.8	1
Chocolate, Dark, & Valencian Orange, Extra Special, Asda*	1/8 Roulade/53g	174	6.4	329	2.9	50	12	2.6
Chocolate, Finest, Tesco*	1 Serving/80g	222	4.5	277	3.4	53.2	5.6	2.3
Chocolate, Sainsbury's*	1 Serving/72g	264	15.7	367	5.7	36.9	21.8	1.8
Kir Royale, Boozy, Deluxe, Lidl*	1 Slice/73g	215	4.3	294	2.6	57.2	5.9	1
Peach, M&S*	1 Slice/47g	126	5.9	268	4.3	33.7	12.6	1.1
Raspberry, Finest, Tesco*	1/6 Roulade/75g	220	9.2	295	2.7	41.5	12.4	2.7
Turkey, with Pork, Leek, & Bacon Stuffing, M&S*	½ Pack/250g	382	14.5	153	20.6	4.4	5.8	0.3
RUM								
37.5% Volume	***1 Pub Shot/35ml***	***72***	***0***	***207***	***0***	***0***	***0***	***0***
40% Volume	***1 Pub Shot/35ml***	***78***	***0***	***222***	***0***	***0***	***0***	***0***
Captain Morgans & Cola, Premixed, Canned, Diageo*	1 Can/250ml	180	0	72	0	9.1	0	0
Malibu, 21% Volume, Pernod Ricard*	1 Pub shot/25ml	50	0	200	0	29	0	0
Spiced Gold, 28%, Captain Morgan*	1 Shot/25ml	50	0	201	0	1.3	0	0
Spiced, Original, 35%, Captain Morgan*	1 Shot/25ml	48	0	193	0	0.4	0	0
White	***1 Pub Shot/35ml***	***72***	***0***	***207***	***0***	***0***	***0***	***0***

R

	Measure INFO/WEIGHT	per Measure KCAL	FAT	Nutrition Values per 100g / 100ml KCAL	PROT	CARB	FAT	FIBRE
RUSKS								
Reduced Sugar, Farleys *	1 Rusk/17g	70	1.5	409	7.9	73.8	8.5	2.8
Wheat, Crispy, Elite*	1 Rusk/10g	38	0.7	396	13.7	68.9	6.8	3.1

R

	Measure INFO/WEIGHT	per Measure KCAL	FAT	Nutrition Values per 100g / 100ml KCAL	PROT	CARB	FAT	FIBRE
SAAG								
Aloo, M&S*	½ Pack/125g	121	7.1	97	1.6	8.7	5.7	2.1
Chicken, Microwaved, Slimming World, Iceland*	1 Pack/500g	395	8	79	11.5	3.9	1.6	1.6
Chicken, Slim Choice, Sainsbury's*	1 Pack/476g	352	5.7	74	11.9	3.7	1.2	0.8
Chicken, SlimWell, Aldi*	1 Pack/480g	331	7.2	69	11	2.1	1.5	1.8
Chicken, with Gunpowder Potatoes, Tesco*	1 Pack/348g	369	15	106	6.7	8.3	4.3	3.9
Paneer, Sainsbury's*	1 Pack/300g	441	32.7	147	7.1	3.9	10.9	2.5
SAFFRON								
Average	***1 Tsp/1g***	***2***	***0***	***310***	***11.4***	***61.5***	***5.9***	***0***
SAGE								
Dried, Ground	***1 Tsp/1g***	***3***	***0.1***	***315***	***10.6***	***42.7***	***12.7***	***0***
Fresh	***1oz/28g***	***33***	***1.3***	***119***	***3.9***	***15.6***	***4.6***	***0***
SALAD								
3 Bean, with Mint Vinaigrette, M&S*	1 Pack/250g	285	4.5	114	6.5	14.8	1.8	6.1
Agretti, Raw, Average	***1 Serving/80g***	***14***	***0***	***17***	***1.8***	***2.2***	***0***	***2.3***
Asian Inspired, Sainsbury's*	½ Pack/113g	98	6.8	87	1.9	4.9	6	3.2
Avocado, & Egg, Nourish Bowl, M&S*	1 Pack/285g	333	15.4	117	6.3	6.6	5.4	8.3
Avocado, & Feta, & Rice, Good to Go, Waitrose*	1 Pack/240g	350	13.4	146	3.4	18.4	5.6	4.1
Avocado, & Feta, Gourmet To Go, M&S*	1 Pack/320g	512	32	160	5.4	12.1	10	3.1
Avocado, & Feta, Side, Waitrose*	1 Pack/201g	285	17.5	142	4.4	10.3	8.7	2.6
Baby Leaf, & Beetroot, Bistro, M&S*	1 Pack/165g	41	0	25	2	3.6	0	2
Baby Leaf, & Rocket, Florette*	1 Serving/25g	5	0.1	20	2.1	0.9	0.5	2
Baby Leaf, Aldi*	1 Serving/50g	11	0	22	3.5	1	0.1	1.5
Baby Leaf, Italian Style, M&S*	1 Bag/65g	14	0.3	22	1.3	2.3	0.5	1.3
Baby Leaf, Mix, Nature's Pick, Aldi*	½ Bag/55g	15	0.3	27	2.4	2.5	0.5	1.8
Baby Leaf, Peppery, Nature's Pick, Aldi*	1 Serving/75g	26	0.4	34	1.9	4.6	0.5	2.1
Baby Leaf, Seasonal, Morrisons*	½ Pack/50g	10	0.3	21	1.4	1.6	0.6	1.8
Bean, 3, Sainsbury's*	1 Tub/270g	281	6.2	104	7.1	13.6	2.3	5.9
Bean, Four, Sainsbury's*	½ Pot/125g	121	3.2	107	6.6	11.5	2.8	4.8
Bean, Mixed, Canned, in Vinaigrette, Sainsbury's*	½ Can/133g	144	1.1	108	6	16.7	0.8	5.1
Bean, Three, with Mint Vinaigrette, M&S*	1 Pack/250g	250	6	100	5.9	8.2	2.4	11.1
Beetroot, & Feta, Veggie Pot, Eat Well, M&S*	1 Pot/140g	182	10.5	130	4.4	8.9	7.5	4.7
Beetroot, & Lettuce, Asda*	1 Serving/30g	5	0	16	1.4	2.7	0	2.5
Beetroot, & Carrot, Baby Leaf, Morrisons*	½ Pack/60g	17	0.2	29	1.8	4	0.3	1.5
Beetroot, & Goats Cheese, Sainsbury's*	½ Pack/68g	72	4.9	106	5.1	4.5	7.2	1.2
Beetroot, & Tomato, Santini, M&S*	½ Pack/110g	58	1.8	53	1.3	7.8	1.6	1.1
Beetroot, Aldi*	1/3 Pot/100g	35	0.5	35	0.8	6.1	0.5	2.1
Beetroot, Carrot, & Roasted Lentil, M&S*	1 Pack/230g	109	4.7	47	1.4	4.7	2	2.2
Beetroot, Goats Cheese, & Rocket, Tesco*	1 Pack/120g	72	3.4	60	2.7	5.3	2.8	1.4
Beetroot, Lambs Lettuce, & Red Chard, Bistro, Lidl*	1 Serving/80g	20	0.2	25	1.8	2.9	0.2	2.3
Beetroot, Lidl*	1 Serving/50g	30	0.4	59	1	11	0.8	2.1
Beetroot, Morrisons*	1 Tsp/10g	4	0	42	1.2	7	0.4	2.7
Beetroot, Rocket, & Feta, M&S*	1 Pack/140g	182	10.5	130	4.4	8.9	7.5	2.7
Beetroot, Tesco*	1 Tub/305g	143	2.7	47	1	7.7	0.9	2.2
Bistro, Asda*	1 Serving/180g	29	0	16	1.4	2.7	0	2.5
Bowl, Essential, Waitrose*	1 Pack/330g	92	1.6	28	1.3	3.6	0.5	1.8
Broccoli, & Peanut, Finest, Tesco*	½ Pack/105g	196	9.2	187	6.9	18.4	8.8	3.3
Burrito, BBQ, Bowl, Allplants*	½ Pack/380g	543	12.2	143	4.2	21	3.2	5.3
Butterhead, & Spinach, Waitrose*	½ Pack/70g	15	0.4	22	1.7	1.5	0.6	1.7
Caesar	***1 Serving/200g***	***352***	***27.8***	***176***	***4.8***	***8.1***	***13.9***	***0.7***
Caesar, Chicken, Shapers, Boots*	1 Pack/200g	205	5.8	102	8.2	10	2.9	1
Caesar, Kit, Tesco*	1 Pack/262g	404	31.7	154	3.4	7.3	12.1	1.2
Caesar, Kit, Waitrose*	1 Bag/250g	436	36.1	174	4.4	6.1	14.4	1.3
Caesar, with Dressing, Croutons & Parmesan, M&S*	1 Serving/115g	190	15.5	165	4.3	6.4	13.5	1.4

S

	Measure INFO/WEIGHT	per Measure KCAL	FAT	Nutrition Values per 100g / 100ml KCAL	PROT	CARB	FAT	FIBRE
SALAD								
Cheese, & Onion, Market St, Morrisons*	1 Pack/260g	330	19.8	127	4.6	9.3	7.6	1.6
Chicken, Caesar, Chargrilled, Eat & Go, Aldi*	1 Pack/175g	294	16.4	168	12	8.9	9.4	1.2
Chicken, Chargrilled, High Protein, M&S*	1 Pack/270g	243	10	90	7.6	5	3.7	3.1
Chicken, Harissa, & Grain, Eat & Go, Aldi*	1 Pack/242g	358	13.3	148	9.2	14	5.5	2.3
Chicken, Katsu, & Sticky Rice, M&S*	1 Pack/270g	367	11.3	136	6.4	17.7	4.2	0.8
Chicken, Noodle, Sweet Chilli, Eat & Go, Aldi*	1 Serving/332g	345	4	104	6.4	16	1.2	1.4
Chicken, Nourish Bowl, On the Go, Sainsbury's*	1 Pack/282g	415	23.1	147	8.4	8	8.2	4.1
Chicken, Piri Piri, Rice, & Bean, Waitrose*	1 Pack/176g	155	4	88	7.1	8.8	2.3	1.7
Chicken, Spiced, & Mango, Asda*	1 Pack/225g	133	4	59	4.4	5.1	1.8	2.3
Chickpea, & Bean, Dahl, Waitrose*	½ Pack/95g	145	5.1	153	5.6	17.3	5.4	6.4
Classic, Asda*	1 Pack/185g	43	1.5	23	1	2.4	0.8	1.1
Coleslaw, Deli Style, Waitrose*	½ Pack/110g	99	8.1	90	1.1	4.5	7.4	1
Corn, Smokey Charred, Waitrose*	½ Pack/113g	108	2.6	96	2.7	15	2.3	2.4
Cous Cous, & Vegetable, Roasted, Waitrose*	1 Pack/220g	396	13.4	180	5.1	26.1	6.1	1.2
Cous Cous, Beetroot, & Feta, Asda*	1 Pack/275g	272	10.4	99	4	12	3.8	1.3
Crayfish, & Mango, Sainsbury's*	1 Pack/310g	329	6.5	106	4.1	17	2.1	1.2
Crisp, Mixed, Morrisons*	1 Pack/230g	39	0.7	17	1	2.8	0.3	0
Crisp, Mixed, Tesco*	1 Pack/200g	40	0.6	20	1.1	3.2	0.3	2
Crunchy, & Crisp, Asda*	1 Pack/250g	55	1.5	22	0.8	3.3	0.6	1.4
Crunchy, Side, Florette*	1 Serving/80g	25	0.4	31	1.1	4	0.5	3.1
Deli, with New Potatoes, & Mustard Mayonnaise, M&S*	1 Pack/295g	298	18.6	101	6.4	3.5	6.3	2.4
Duck, & Herb, Crispy, M&S*	½ Pack/140g	378	25.6	270	20.7	3.7	18.3	1.4
Edamame, & Petit Pois, Finest, Tesco*	½ Pack/100g	108	4.3	108	6	9.3	4.3	3.9
Edamame, & Black Rice, Plant Kitchen, M&S*	1 Pack/295g	395	16.2	134	5.6	12.8	5.5	5.3
Edamame, & Feta, High Protein, M&S*	1 Pack/215g	209	9	97	7.5	5.1	4.2	4.3
Edamame, & Sprouting Pea, Finest, Tesco*	1 Serving/100g	136	5.7	136	7.6	11.4	5.7	4.4
Edamame, Asda*	½ Pack/110g	90	3.3	82	5.9	4.8	3	5.9
Egg, & Ham, with Salad Cream Dressing, M&S*	1 Pack/240g	149	7.2	62	4.9	3.2	3	1.2
Egg, & Spinach, Baby, Waitrose*	1 Pack/215g	167	13.5	78	3.5	1.8	6.3	1
Egg, & Avocado, Free Range, M&S*	1 Pack/225g	268	14.4	119	6.9	7.4	6.4	2.3
Egg, & Avocado, Grains, Waitrose*	1 Pack/260g	351	16.1	135	5.3	13.1	6.2	2.9
Egg, & Spinach, High Protein, M&S*	1 Pot/105g	130	8.1	124	11.9	1.7	7.7	0.5
Egg, Free Range, & Bacon, Side, Eat Well, M&S*	1 Pack/205g	242	16.2	118	9.8	1.6	7.9	0.6
English Garden, Tesco*	1 Serving/180g	22	0.4	12	0.7	1.8	0.2	0.7
Falafel, Bulgur Wheat & Houmous, Eat Well, M&S*	1 Pack/300g	375	15.3	125	4.1	13.2	5.1	4.8
Feta, & Sunblushed Tomato, M&S*	1 Serving/190g	361	21.1	190	5.5	17.2	11.1	2.1
Freekeh, Feta, & Roast Grape, Gousto*	1 Serving/229g	509	20.6	222	10.3	21.8	9	6.5
Goats Cheese, & Lentil, M&S*	1 Pack/215g	316	10.3	147	6.9	17.4	4.8	3.3
Grain, Mixed, Courgette, & Pea, Waitrose *	½ Pack/150g	242	6.8	161	4.8	23.8	4.5	2.9
Grain, Mixed, Deluxe, Lidl*	1 Pack/215g	275	9.2	128	4.1	15.3	4.3	5.8
Grain, Triple, Tesco*	1 Pack/225g	212	1.4	94	3.7	17.2	0.6	2.7
Greek	***1oz/28g***	***36***	***3.5***	***130***	***2.7***	***1.9***	***12.5***	***0.8***
Greek Style, with Feta, M&S*	1 Pack/270g	348	17.8	129	4.3	12.5	6.6	1.7
Greek, M&S*	1 Pack/200g	228	19.6	114	3.6	2.2	9.8	1.5
Greek, Style, Bowl, M&S*	1 Bowl/223g	212	18.3	95	2.5	2.4	8.2	0.7
Greek, Style, Feta, Tip & Mix, M&S*	1 Pack/195g	214	18.3	110	4	2.5	9.4	1.6
Green Bean, Aldi*	½ Pack/80g	62	2.7	77	4.6	5	3.4	3.9
Green, Average	***1oz/28g***	***4***	***0.1***	***13***	***0.8***	***1.8***	***0.3***	***0.9***
Green, Complete, Sainsbury's*	1/3 Pack/55g	92	6.7	168	4.2	10.3	12.2	1.4
Green, Mixed, Average	***1 Serving/100g***	***12***	***0.3***	***12***	***0.7***	***1.8***	***0.3***	***1***
Green, Side, M&S*	1 Serving/200g	30	0.4	15	0.9	2.5	0.2	0
Greens, Oriental Inspired, Tesco*	1 Serving/90g	47	2.2	52	2.3	4.4	2.4	2
Ham Hock, & Piccalilli, Waitrose*	1 Pack/240g	257	7.4	107	4.7	14	3.1	2.3

S

	Measure INFO/WEIGHT	per Measure KCAL	FAT	Nutrition Values per 100g / 100ml KCAL	PROT	CARB	FAT	FIBRE
SALAD								
Ham Hock, Ploughmans, Waitrose*	1 Pack/185g	170	8.1	92	7.1	5.4	4.4	0.9
Ham, & Egg, Free Range, G&B, Asda*	1 Pack/250g	150	6.2	60	5.3	3.1	2.5	1.9
Hipster, Wicked Kitchen, Tesco*	½ Pack/100g	146	7.9	146	2.8	14	7.9	3.8
House, Side, Tesco*	1 Pack/120g	24	0.4	20	1.2	2.4	0.3	1.4
Italian, Meadow Fresh, Lidl*	1 Serving/80g	19	0.2	24	2	2.2	0.3	2.2
Italian, Strong & Peppery, Sainsbury's*	1 Serving/80g	18	0.4	22	2.5	1	0.5	1.8
Italian, Tomato, Balsamic, & Italian Cheese, Sainsbury's*	½ Pack/80g	56	3.6	70	3.3	3.6	4.5	0.8
Italian, with Pesto Dressing, Tesco*	½ Pack/128g	205	14.9	160	6.8	6.1	11.6	1.9
Italiana, Freshcoolis*	1 Bag/100g	25	0.1	25	1.6	3.4	0.1	1.8
Lambs Lettuce, Sainsbury's*	1 Serving/80g	12	0.4	15	1.7	0.6	0.5	0.7
Large, Bowl, Sainsbury's*	1/6 Pack/52g	12	0.2	23	0.9	4.3	0.3	1.1
Leaves, Meadow Fresh, Lidl*	1 Serving/80g	25	0.2	31	2.4	3.4	0.3	2.3
Leaves, Mixed, Little Leaves*	½ Bag/63g	12	0.3	19	2.5	1.2	0.5	1.8
Lettuce, Lambs, & Pea Shoot, Good Health, Waitrose*	1 Bag/100g	21	0.5	21	1.9	1.3	0.5	1.7
Mediterranean Style, Bowl, with Dressing, Sainsbury's*	1 Pack/155g	67	1.9	43	1.1	6	1.2	1.8
Mediterranean, Style, Asda*	½ Pack/135g	22	0	16	1	3	0	0
Mixed Grains, Chipotle, Tesco*	1 Pack/250g	348	4.5	139	5	22.4	1.8	6.5
Mixed Leaf, Medley, Waitrose*	1 Serving/25g	4	0.1	15	0.8	1.7	0.5	1.4
Mixed Leaf, Tesco*	1 Serving/20g	3	0.1	14	0.9	1.6	0.4	0.9
Mixed Leaf, Tomato & Olive, Tesco*	1 Serving/170g	150	13.3	88	1	3.4	7.8	2
Mixed Leaf, with Beetroot, Earthy, Waitrose*	1 Bag/140g	34	0.6	24	1.5	3.6	0.4	2.1
Mixed Leaves, Carrot, Tomatoes, & Cucumber, Co-Op*	½ Pack/80g	22	0.6	27	1	3.7	0.7	0.9
Mixed Rice, Tesco*	1 Pack/215g	198	0.9	92	2.3	18.9	0.4	1.7
Mixed, Bowl, Waitrose*	¼ Pack/64g	9	0.3	14	0.8	1.6	0.5	1.4
Mixed, Medley, Bowl, Waitrose*	¼ Pack/60g	9	0.3	15	0.9	1.7	0.5	1
Mixed, Sweet & Crispy, Tesco*	1 Serving/200g	48	0.6	24	1	4.2	0.3	2
New Potato, Tuna, & Egg, M&S*	1 Pack/340g	255	12.9	75	3.8	6.7	3.8	0.7
Noodle, Chicken, Hoisin, Well & Good, Co-Op*	1 Pack/244g	288	7.8	118	8.3	13	3.2	1.2
Noodle, Coconutty, Meal for One, M&S*	1 Pack/300g	366	14.4	122	2.9	15.7	4.8	2
Noodle, Prawn, Sesame, M&S*	1 Pack/220g	242	8.1	110	5.6	12.9	3.7	1.5
Octopus, Drained, Medusa*	1 Serving/100g	163	11	163	15	1.6	11	0
Pasta, Mediterranean Orzo, Love Life, Waitrose*	1 Pack/220g	299	10.8	136	3.9	19	4.9	3.2
Pea Shoot, Mild, Asda*	1 Serving/80g	20	0.4	25	2.5	2.4	0.5	2.1
Pea Shoots, Purple Radish, & Garlic Chives, Morrisons*	½ Pack/35g	15	0.4	42	4.4	2.5	1.2	1.6
Potato, Baby, & Free Range Egg, Asda*	1 Pack/270g	159	7.6	59	1.9	5.9	2.8	1.2
Prawn, & Avocado, M&S*	1 Serving/240g	254	16.3	106	3	2	6.8	3.1
Prawn, Cocktail, Tesco*	1 Pack/300g	360	18	120	5.7	10.9	6	0.8
Prawn, King, & Asian Slaw, Aldi*	1 Pack/230g	244	8	106	3.9	14	3.5	0.9
Prawn, Layer, Eat Well, M&S*	1 Pack/220g	205	8.2	93	4.1	10.5	3.7	0.6
Prawn, Layered, Co-Op*	1 Pack/300g	375	18	125	4	14	6	2
Prawn, Layered, M&S*	1 Pack/400g	396	17.2	99	4.1	10.4	4.3	1.1
Protein Power Bowl, Allplants*	1 Serving/421g	530	21.5	126	6.3	12	5.1	3.4
Quinoa, & Kale, Supergreen, Asda*	½ Pot/135g	232	10	172	6.4	16	7.4	8.9
Quinoa, & Supergreen, Eat Well, M&S*	1 Pack/180g	180	10.4	100	4.3	5	5.8	5.3
Quinoa, Tomato, Red Pepper, & Mango, Lidl*	1 Pot/210g	191	4.2	91	2.6	14.1	2	2.5
Rainbow, Feta, & Beetroot, Layered, M&S*	1 Pack/265g	339	18	128	4.2	10.3	6.8	4.3
Rainbow, Morrisons*	½ Bowl/72g	20	0.1	27	1.4	3.7	0.2	2.5
Rainbow, Nature's Pick, Aldi*	½ Pack/75g	21	0.4	28	1.1	3.9	0.5	1.5
Rainbow, Side, Waitrose*	1 Pack/120g	30	0.6	25	1.4	3.2	0.5	2
Ranch, Kit, Morrisons*	¼ Pack/73g	107	7.1	147	4.7	9.2	9.7	1.8
Ribbon, Asda*	1 Pack/115g	33	0.6	29	1.6	4.3	0.5	0.5
Rice, Hoisin, M&S*	1 Pack/200g	312	8.6	156	3.1	25.4	4.3	1.6

S

	Measure INFO/WEIGHT	per Measure KCAL	FAT	Nutrition Values per 100g / 100ml KCAL	PROT	CARB	FAT	FIBRE
SALAD								
Rocket, & Parmesan, Wild, Italian, Sainsbury's*	1 Serving/50g	88	7.4	177	7.5	3.4	14.8	0.5
Root Vegetable, & Grains, Co-Op*	½ Pack/150g	148	4.5	99	3.3	13.3	3	3.1
Salmon, Lime, & Miso, with Sticky Rice, M&S*	1 Pack/285g	396	13.4	139	5.3	18.2	4.7	1.4
Salmon, Moroccan Style, Light Lunch, John West*	1 Pack/220g	299	11.7	136	11.7	8.8	5.3	3.4
Salmon, Oak Smoked, Aldi*	1 Pack/129g	254	5.8	197	5	8.6	4.5	1.3
Side, Garden, with Cherry Tomatoes, Waitrose*	1 Pack/170g	25	0.7	15	0.8	2	0.4	1.3
Side, Simple, with Dressing, Tesco*	½ Pack/83g	69	5.4	83	1.2	4.2	6.5	1.6
Side, Sweet & Crisp, Tesco*	1 Pack/128g	65	2.4	51	3.7	3.9	1.9	1.6
Simple, Bowl, Sainsbury's*	1 Bowl/130g	26	0.6	20	1.2	3	0.5	1.2
Simple, Bowl, Tesco*	1 Bowl/135g	32	0.4	24	1.3	2.9	0.3	2.1
Simple, with Sour Cream, & Chive, Tesco*	1 Pack/165g	139	10.9	84	1.2	4.2	6.6	1.5
Spinach, & Pine Nut, Deluxe, Lidl*	1 Serving/50g	135	7.7	270	6.8	25.3	15.4	1.5
Sweet & Crispy, M&S*	1 Serving/140g	49	1.4	35	1.7	4.7	1	1.6
Sweet & Crisp, Asda*	1 Serving/80g	26	0.4	32	1.5	4.4	0.5	2.3
Sweet & Crispy, Bowl, Sainsbury's*	½ Pack/110g	118	11.2	107	1	2	10.2	1.8
Sweet & Crunchy, Bowl, Sainsbury's*	¼ Pack/85g	42	0.6	49	1.6	8.2	0.7	2
Sweet & Crunchy, Side, Eat Well, M&S*	1 Pack/145g	48	0.9	33	1.5	4.3	0.6	2.3
Sweet Leaf, Fully Prepared, Fresh, Sainsbury's*	¼ Pack/75g	12	0.1	16	0.8	3	0.1	2.1
Sweet Pepper, Market St, Morrisons*	1 Pack/140g	41	0.4	29	0.9	4.5	0.3	2.2
Sweet Potato, & Red Pepper, Deli, M&S*	1 Serving/250g	113	5.6	45	0.8	5.6	2.2	0.9
Sweet Potato, Skinny, M&S*	1 Serving/70g	69	2.9	99	2	12	4.2	2.6
Sweet, & Crunchy, Co-Op*	1 Pack/160g	43	1.1	27	1	3.7	0.7	0.9
Tabbouleh, & Dill Carrot, Pickled, Waitrose*	1 Pack/299g	266	11.4	89	3	8.7	3.8	3.8
Tabbouleh, Aldi*	1 Serving/70g	42	1	60	0	1.1	1.4	0
Tomato, & Onion	***1oz/28g***	***20***	***1.7***	***72***	***0.8***	***4***	***6.1***	***1***
Tomato, Cherry, Tesco*	1 Pack/210g	136	9.4	65	0.9	4.2	4.5	1.1
Tuna, & Potato, Beautifully Balanced, Tesco*	1 Pack/258g	124	1.8	48	5.7	3.6	0.7	2.1
Tuna, & Potato, Tesco*	1 Pack/180g	99	0.9	55	5.5	6.4	0.5	1.4
Tuna, Bowl, Fresh, Asda*	1 Serving/160g	184	11.2	115	8	5	7	0
Tuna, French Style, Light Lunch, John West*	1 Pack/220g	218	6.2	99	7.5	9.8	2.8	2.5
Tuna, Italian Style, Light Lunch, John West*	1 Pack/220g	205	5.7	93	7.3	9.8	2.6	0.5
Tuna, Mediterranean Inspired, Tesco*	1 Pack/220g	200	2	91	8.5	10.5	0.9	3.4
Tuna, Mediterranean Style, Light Lunch, John West*	1 Pack/220g	211	4.2	96	8.5	10	1.9	2.4
Tuna, Mediterranean Style, Nixe, Lidl*	1 Pack/220g	254	5.5	116	10	12	2.5	2.8
Tuna, Mexican Style, Nixe, Lidl*	1 Pack/220g	277	9	126	10.6	11.5	4.1	0.5
Tuna, Nicoise, Tesco*	1 Pack/240g	392	29	163	6.2	6.8	12.1	1.2
Tuna, White, & Egg, Co-Op*	1 Serving/240g	242	13	101	11.8	0.5	5.4	0
Tuna, with Lime, & Black Pepper Dressing, John West*	1 Pack/230g	239	6.9	104	8.5	9.4	3	2.5
Tuna, with Rice, Nixe, Lidl*	1 Pack/220g	308	14.3	140	8.9	11.3	6.5	0.5
Tuna, with Spicy Tomato Sauce, Jane Plan*	1 Pack/220g	224	7	102	7	10	3.2	2.8
Vegetable, Mixed, without Dressing, From Restaurant	***1 ½ Cups/207g***	***33***	***0.1***	***16***	***1.2***	***3.2***	***0.1***	***2.1***
Vitality Mix, Superfood, Florette*	½ Bag/60g	14	0	23	1.8	1.7	0	2.3
Waldorf, Average	***1 Serving/100g***	***193***	***17.7***	***193***	***1.4***	***7.5***	***17.7***	***1.3***
Watercress, Spinach & Rocket, Prepared , Tesco*	½ Pack/40g	10	0.3	26	2.5	1.1	0.8	2
Watercress, Spinach & Rocket, Waitrose*	1 Bag/145g	30	1.2	21	2.2	1.2	0.8	1.5
Wheatberries, Lentils, & Green Vegetables, Waitrose*	½ Pack/150g	218	7	145	5.9	16.5	4.7	6.4
Wholefood, Super Nutty, M&S*	1 Pack/285g	430	20.5	151	7.1	11.4	7.2	6.3
Wholefood, Super, Creamy Lemon & Mint Dressing, M&S*	1 Pack/290g	374	12.2	129	8.8	10.6	4.2	6.6
SALAD CREAM								
30% Less Fat, Bramwells, Aldi*	1 Tbsp/15g	29	2.2	193	1	15	15	0.5
70% Less Fat, Heinz*	1 Tbsp/15g	18	1.1	120	1.8	11.2	7.1	0.5
Average	***1 Tbsp/15g***	***50***	***4.2***	***335***	***1.7***	***18.6***	***27.8***	***0.1***
Free From, Tesco*	1 Tbsp/15g	35	2.6	232	0.3	18.8	17.2	0.5

S

	Measure INFO/WEIGHT	per Measure KCAL	FAT	Nutrition Values per 100g / 100ml KCAL	PROT	CARB	FAT	FIBRE
SALAD CREAM								
Light, Batts*	1 Tbsp/15g	30	2.3	200	0.7	14.7	15.3	3.3
Original, Heinz*	1 Tbsp/15g	45	3.6	303	1.3	20.3	23.7	0
Reduced Calorie, Average	***1 Tbsp/15g***	***19***	***1.2***	***130***	***1***	***12.9***	***7.9***	***0.2***
Vegan, GranoVita*	1 Tbsp/15g	37	3.4	247	0.9	9.9	22.6	0
SALAMI								
Average	***1 Slice/5g***	***18***	***1.3***	***360***	***28.4***	***1.8***	***26.2***	***0***
Beechwood Smoked, German, Waitrose*	2 Slices/17g	51	4	302	21.7	0.4	23.5	0.9
Brunswick, German, Wafer Thin, M&S*	3 Slices/25g	80	6.5	322	21	0.7	26	0.7
Calabrian, Salsiccia, Piccante, No.1, Waitrose*	1 Serving/30g	117	8.8	390	30.3	0.5	29.5	0.7
Danish, Average	***1 Serving/17g***	***89***	***8.8***	***524***	***13.2***	***1.3***	***51.7***	***0***
German, Average	***1 Serving/60g***	***200***	***16.4***	***333***	***20.3***	***1.6***	***27.3***	***0.1***
German, Peppered, Average	***3 Slices/25g***	***86***	***6.8***	***342***	***22.2***	***2.5***	***27.1***	***0.2***
German, Smoky & Savoury , Asda*	3 Slices/18g	69	5.9	383	20	1.3	33	1
German, Smoky Selection, Iceland*	1 Slice/4g	13	1	330	24.6	1	25.6	1
Milano, Antipasto Selection, The Deli, Aldi*	1 Slice/5g	19	1.6	389	24	1	32	1.1
Milano, Average	***1 Serving/70g***	***278***	***22.6***	***397***	***25.9***	***0.9***	***32.2***	***0***
Milano, Smoked Prosciutto & Salmon Platter, Tesco*	1 Slice/8g	29	2.3	363	26	0.5	28.5	0
Napoli, Antipasto Selection, The Deli, Aldi*	1 Slice/5g	19	1.6	388	25	1.5	31	1
Napoli, Average	***1 Slice/5g***	***17***	***1.3***	***342***	***27.1***	***0.8***	***25.5***	***0***
Napoli, Salami & Cheese Selection, The Deli, Aldi*	3 Slices/13g	48	3.9	369	24	0	30	0.9
Napoli, Smoked Prosciutto & Salami Platter, Tesco*	1 Slice/8g	27	2.1	343	25.5	0.5	26.5	0
Pork, Cured, Sliced, Continental Selection, Tesco*	1 Slice/4g	14	1.1	363	26	0.5	28.5	0
Smoked, Dulano, Lidl*	1 Slice/23g	82	6.9	356	20.2	1	30	0
Ventricina, Morrisons*	1 Slice/6g	21	1.7	350	24	0.6	28	0
SALMON								
Chestnut Smoked, Scottish, No.1, Waitrose*	½ Pack/50g	88	4.6	176	22.8	0.6	9.1	0.5
Cooked, Prepacked, Average	***1 Fillet/93g***	***180***	***11.1***	***194***	***21.8***	***0***	***11.9***	***0***
Cooked, with Broccoli, & Green Beans, Tesco*	1 Pack/371g	289	7.8	78	6.9	7.2	2.1	1.3
Fillet, Hot Smoked, Honey Roast, Market St, Morrisons*	1 Fillet/90g	273	18.9	303	24.3	4	21	0.3
Fillet, Market St, Morrisons*	1 Fillet/97g	230	15.7	237	22.2	0.5	16.2	0.3
Fillet, Sockeye, Wild Caught, Finest, Tesco*	1 Fillet/106g	176	7.8	166	24.3	0.1	7.4	0.7
Fillets, Boneless, Fishmonger, Aldi*	1 Fillet/120g	199	9.1	166	22	1.6	7.6	0.6
Fillets, Boneless, Scottish, Oven Cooked, Waitrose*	1 Fillet/93g	166	8.8	178	23.4	0	9.4	0
Fillets, Boneless, Scottish, Raw, Waitrose*	1 Fillet/130g	180	9.5	138	18.2	0	7.3	0
Fillets, Boneless, Skin-On, Fresh, Cooked, Average	***1 Sm Fillet/120g***	***265***	***17.1***	***221***	***23.2***	***0.2***	***14.2***	***0.1***
Fillets, Honey Roast, Sainsbury's*	1 Fillet/90g	203	12.1	226	23	3.4	13.4	0
Fillets, Hot Smoked, Sweet Chilli, Waitrose*	1 Fillet/72g	178	9.9	247	26.2	4.5	13.8	0.5
Fillets, in Teriyaki Marinade, Good Health, Waitrose*	1 Fillet/91g	176	9.2	193	23	2.1	10.1	0.9
Fillets, Lighthouse Bay, Lidl*	1 Fillet/115g	245	16	213	21.6	0.1	13.9	0.5
Fillets, Lightly Smoked, Scottish, Waitrose*	1 Serving/175g	382	26.6	218	18.7	1.3	15.2	0.6
Fillets, Pink, Boneless, Wild, Iceland*	1 Serving/100g	179	10.1	179	22.1	0	10.1	0
Fillets, Poached , Sainsbury's*	1 Fillet/90g	218	15.4	242	20.9	0.9	17.1	0.5
Fillets, Poached, M&S*	1 Fillet/98g	164	7.9	167	23.3	0.1	8.1	0.1
Fillets, Raw, Average	***1 Sm Fillet/120g***	***227***	***14***	***189***	***20.9***	***0.1***	***11.7***	***0.1***
Fillets, Raw, Skin-On, Average	***1 Avg Fillet/120g***	***214***	***13.9***	***179***	***18.3***	***0.2***	***11.6***	***0.2***
Fillets, Red Thai Marinade, Infused, Fishmonger, Aldi*	1 Fillet/110g	189	12.1	172	17	1.4	11	0.5
Fillets, Scottish, Deluxe, Lidl*	1 Fillet/120g	256	16.7	213	21.6	0.1	13.9	0.5
Fillets, Scottish, Specially Selected, Aldi*	1 Fillet/120g	176	7.7	147	22	0	6.4	0
Fillets, Skin On, TTD, Sainsbury's*	1 Fillet/126g	249	14.3	197	23.5	0.2	11.3	0
Fillets, Sweet Chilli, Hot Smoked, Ready to Eat, Tesco*	1 Fillet/90g	211	12.4	234	22.7	4.6	13.8	0.4
Fillets, Traditionally Smoked, Finest, Tesco*	1 Fillet/113g	226	13.3	200	23.4	0	11.8	0
Fillets, Wild Alaskan, Keta, Sainsbury's*	1 Fillet/115g	178	6.4	155	25.9	0.2	5.6	0.3
Fillets, with Miso, & Maple Glaze, Waitrose*	½ Pack/112g	233	14.8	208	17.2	4.8	13.2	0.5

S

	Measure INFO/WEIGHT	per Measure KCAL	FAT	Nutrition Values per 100g / 100ml KCAL	PROT	CARB	FAT	FIBRE
SALMON								
Flakes, Honey Roast, Average	***1oz/28g***	***56***	***3***	***198***	***24***	***1.9***	***10.7***	***0.2***
Flakes, Honey Roast, Kiln Smoked, M&S*	1 Pack/120g	265	14.6	221	24.6	3.1	12.2	0.6
Flakes, Sweet Chilli, M&S*	½ Pack/70g	143	4.6	204	24.5	11.7	6.6	0.6
Goujons, Average	***1 Pack/150g***	***321***	***16.4***	***214***	***16.4***	***12.4***	***11***	***1.1***
Gravadlax Marinated, Fishmonger, Aldi*	1 Pack/149g	286	16.4	192	19	4.6	11	0.5
Gravadlax, Cured with Salt, Sugar & Herbs	***1 Serving/100g***	***119***	***3.3***	***119***	***18.3***	***3.1***	***3.3***	***0.4***
Grilled	***1oz/28g***	***60***	***3.7***	***215***	***24.2***	***0***	***13.1***	***0***
Hot Smoked, Average	***1 Serving/62g***	***103***	***4.4***	***166***	***24***	***0.9***	***7.2***	***0.1***
Hot Smoked, Scottish, Slices, Waitrose*	½ Pack/75g	149	8.5	199	24.2	0	11.3	0
Kiln Smoked, Honey Roast, Slices, M&S*	½ Pack/63g	138	7.6	221	24.6	3.1	12.2	0.6
Mild Oak Smoked, Average	***1 Slice/25g***	***46***	***2.5***	***182***	***22.6***	***0.1***	***10.2***	***0***
Oak Smoked, Scottish, Sliced, Specially Selected, Aldi*	½ Pack/50g	93	4.2	186	25	3.1	8.3	0
Oak Smoked, Speybay, M&S*	1 Pack/100g	158	6.5	158	22	2.4	6.5	0.7
Pink in Brine, Average	***1 Sm Can/105g***	***129***	***5.5***	***122***	***18.8***	***0***	***5.3***	***0***
Pink, Canned, Average	***1 Serving/125g***	***162***	***7.2***	***130***	***19.5***	***0.1***	***5.8***	***0.1***
Poached, Average	***1 Serving/90g***	***176***	***10.5***	***195***	***22.5***	***0.2***	***11.7***	***0.3***
Red in Brine, Average	***1oz/28g***	***42***	***2.2***	***149***	***19.7***	***0***	***7.8***	***0***
Red, Average	***½ Can/90g***	***141***	***7.4***	***156***	***20.4***	***0.1***	***8.2***	***0.1***
Ribbons, Oak Smoked, M&S*	1 Serving/100g	207	9.7	207	27.9	1.9	9.7	0.6
Skewers, Chilli, Lime, & Soy, Morrisons*	1 Skewer/101g	228	14.7	226	18.8	4.6	14.6	0.3
Smoked, Average	***1 Serving/70g***	***126***	***7***	***179***	***21.9***	***0.5***	***10***	***0.1***
Smoked, Lightly, Lemon & Herb, Tesco*	¼ Pack/128g	334	23	261	22.1	2	18	1.2
Smoked, Scottish, Mild & Delicate, Extra Special, Asda*	½ Pack/60g	120	7.2	200	22	0.5	12	0.5
Smoked, Scottish, Mild & Delicate, Sliced, M&S*	½ Pack/50g	90	4.6	181	22.9	1.2	9.3	0.6
Smoked, Scottish, Slices, Finest, Tesco*	½ Pack/60g	110	5.8	184	22.7	1.4	9.6	0.5
Smoked, Slices, Fishmonger, Aldi*	½ Pack/100g	158	7.9	158	21	0.5	7.9	0.5
Smoked, Trimmings, Asda*	1 Serving/60g	119	7.8	198	19	0.5	13	0
Smoked, Trimmings, Average	***1 Serving/55g***	***101***	***5.7***	***184***	***22.8***	***0.2***	***10.3***	***0***
Smoked, Wild Alaskan, Red Sockeye, Slices, M&S*	1 Slice/25g	28	0.2	113	24.2	1.6	1	0.6
Steaks	***1 Serving/100g***	***180***	***11***	***180***	***20.2***	***0***	***11***	***0***
Steamed	***1oz/28g***	***55***	***3.6***	***197***	***20.1***	***0***	***13***	***0***
Teriyaki, Specially Selected, Aldi*	1 Pack/85g	213	11.9	251	18	13	14	0.5
with New Potatoes, Broccoli, Green Beans, BFY, M&S*	1 Pack/385g	358	18.9	93	7	4.4	4.9	1.8
SALMON EN CROUTE								
Frozen, Tesco*	1 Serving/166g	365	18.4	220	10.1	19.1	11.1	1.1
Retail, Average	***1oz/28g***	***81***	***5.3***	***288***	***11.8***	***18***	***19.1***	***0***
SALSA								
Beetroot, Love Beets*	1 Serving/80g	75	0.2	94	1.2	20	0.3	2.9
Chipotle, Smokey, M&S*	¼ Pack/51g	37	0.4	73	1.8	13.2	0.8	3
Chunky, Sainsbury's*	½ Pot/84g	43	1.4	51	1.1	7.8	1.7	1.2
Classic, Medium, Shake & Squeeze, Asda*	1 Tbsp/15g	4	0.1	30	1	4.7	0.5	1.2
Cool, Sainsbury's*	¼ Pot/58g	30	1.2	52	1.4	6.3	2.1	1.1
Mild, Original, Old El Paso*	1 Sachet/144g	60	0.7	42	1.6	9	0.5	0
Original from Dinner Kit, Old El Paso*	1 Jar/226g	71	0.7	32	1.2	6	0.3	0
Red, Medium, M&S*	¼ Jar/49g	34	1.5	69	1.4	8.3	3	1.8
Spicy Mango & Lime, Morrisons*	½ Pot/85g	62	0.3	73	1	15.9	0.4	1.3
Spicy Red Pepper, Fresh, Waitrose*	½ Pot/85g	27	0.8	32	1.9	4.1	0.9	1.6
Tomato, Chunky, Tesco*	1 Pot/170g	68	2.2	40	1.1	5.9	1.3	1.1
Tomato, Cool, Asda*	1 Pot/215g	84	1.1	39	1.4	6.4	0.5	1.5
Tomato, Onion, Coriander & Chilli, Fresh, Waitrose*	1 Tub/170g	110	5.3	65	1.3	8	3.1	1.2
Tomato, Sun Ripened, Tesco*	1 Serving/40g	46	1.7	115	5	14.2	4.2	4.6
SALT								
Alternative, Reduced Sodium, Losalt*	½ Tsp/1g	0	0	0	0	0	0	0

S

	Measure INFO/WEIGHT	per Measure KCAL	FAT	Nutrition Values per 100g / 100ml KCAL	PROT	CARB	FAT	FIBRE
SALT								
Himalayan Pink, Coarse, Perrin's Fine Foods*	1 Pinch/0.1g	0	0	0	0	0	0	0
Kosher, Average	***1 Tsp/5g***	***0***	***0***	***0***	***0***	***0***	***0***	***0***
Rock, Average	***¼ Tsp/1g***	***0***	***0***	***0***	***0***	***0***	***0***	***0***
Table, Average	***1 Tsp/5g***	***0***	***0***	***0***	***0***	***0***	***0***	***0***
SAMBUCA								
Average	***1 Pub Shot/35ml***	***122***	***0***	***348***	***0***	***37.2***	***0***	***0***
SAMOSAS								
Chicken, Indian, Waitrose*	1 Samosa/50g	124	7.2	248	7.8	21	14.4	1.8
Chicken, Premier*	1 Slice/110g	272	14.3	247	5.9	25.7	13	0
Chicken, Tikka, Indian, Sainsbury's*	1 Samosa/55g	131	5.5	237	9.4	25	10	4.6
Indian Style Selection, Co-Op*	1 Samosa/21g	50	2.7	240	5	27	13	3
Lamb, Premier*	1 Slice/110g	260	11.8	236	6	28	10.7	0
Meat, Takeaway, Average	***1 Samosa/110g***	***299***	***19***	***272***	***11.4***	***18.9***	***17.3***	***2.4***
Punjabi, Cofresh*	1 Samosa/50g	81	5	162	2	16	10	3
Vegetable, Aldi*	1 Samosa/50g	138	8.6	276	4.2	23.6	17.3	4.2
Vegetable, Average	***1 Samosa/110g***	***258***	***12.8***	***235***	***4.8***	***26.9***	***11.6***	***2.5***
Vegetable, Indian Snack Selection, 12, Sainsbury's*	2 Samosas/45g	114	5.5	253	4.9	28.5	12.3	4.1
Vegetable, Indian Starter Selection, M&S*	1 Samosa/21g	53	2.5	254	5.3	29.3	12.1	3.3
Vegetable, Indian, 4 Pack, Sainsbury's*	1 Samosa/47g	115	5.9	246	4.7	26.3	12.6	4.4
Vegetable, Large, Individual, Sainsbury's*	1 Samosa/110g	254	16.5	231	3.3	20.7	15	2.1
Vegetable, Large, Tesco*	1 Samosa/98g	214	8.9	219	5.3	27.6	9.1	2.8
Vegetable, Mini, Asda*	1 Samosa/23g	52	2	233	6	32	9	2.6
Vegetable, Mini, Indian Snack Selection, Tesco*	1 Samosa/32g	76	4.2	238	4.7	25.5	13	3.3
SANDWICH								
All Day Breakfast, Tesco Classic*	1 Pack/374g	636	29.9	170	8	14.5	8	3
Bacon, & Egg, Co-Op*	1 Pack/188g	536	32	285	13	20	17	2
Bacon, & Egg, Sainsbury's*	1 Pack/160g	384	17.8	240	13	22	11.1	1.8
Bacon, & Egg, Tesco*	1 Pack/213g	494	19.6	232	14.8	21.6	9.2	1.8
Bacon, On the Go, Sainsbury's*	1 Pack/163g	454	17.9	279	13.2	30.9	11	1.6
Beef, & Horseradish, Sainsbury's*	1 Pack/187g	391	12.5	209	12.5	23.8	6.7	1.5
Beef, & Pate, M&S*	1 Pack/188g	310	7.3	165	11.2	21.6	3.9	2.4
Beef, & Horseradish, Tesco*	1 Pack/175g	364	9.6	208	13.2	25.7	5.5	1.6
Beef, Med Rare, & Stilton, Finest, Tesco*	1 Pack/201g	461	15.3	229	13.5	25.8	7.6	1.9
Beef, Roast, & Onion, Sub Roll, M&S*	1 Pack/205g	435	12.5	212	12.6	25.1	6.1	2.9
BLT, Asda*	1 Pack/172g	325	11.9	189	9.9	21.8	6.9	4.6
BLT, Classic, Waitrose*	1 Pack/181g	347	13	192	9.1	21.5	7.2	2.2
BLT, Made Without Wheat, M&S*	1 Pack/206g	476	25.1	231	7.2	21.2	12.2	4
BLT, on Malted Brown Bread, Tesco*	1 Pack/185g	454	21.7	245	10.9	22.9	11.7	2.4
Brie, & Cranberry, Morrisons*	1 Pack/178g	438	20.3	246	10.4	24.4	11.4	2.2
Brie, & Grape, Finest, Tesco*	1 Pack/209g	527	31.6	252	8.5	20.6	15.1	1.5
Brie, & Bacon, with Chilli Relish, Waitrose*	1 Pack/219g	525	27.1	240	11.6	19.4	12.4	2.1
Brie, & Cranberry, on Malted Brown, Tesco*	1 Pack/159g	387	17.6	244	8.9	25.9	11.1	2.3
Cheddar, & Ham, M&S*	1 Pack/165g	396	18.6	240	15.1	20	11.3	1.7
Cheddar, & Tomato, Red, Tesco*	1 Pack/165g	474	23.8	287	9.2	29.2	14.4	1.9
Cheddar, Cheese, Farmhouse, & Celery, M&S*	1 Pack/200g	482	25.4	241	11.1	19.4	12.7	2.1
Cheese, & Ham, & Pickle, HL, Tesco*	1 Pack/201g	312	4.2	155	13.1	21	2.1	1.7
Cheese, & Ham, & Pickle, Tesco*	1 Pack/215g	497	24.7	231	11.7	20.3	11.5	1.8
Cheese, & Ham, Smoked, Co-Op*	1 Pack/167g	334	8.4	200	15	24	5	2
Cheese, & Onion, Tesco*	1 Pack/172g	505	28.3	294	10.2	24.5	16.5	3.3
Cheese, & Pickle, Tesco*	1 Pack/140g	400	19.3	286	12.7	27.8	13.8	1.4
Cheese, & Salad, COU, M&S*	1 Pack/188g	244	3	130	12.1	17	1.6	2.4
Cheese, & Tomato, Asda*	1 Pack/154g	388	19.7	252	11	23.2	12.8	3.7
Cheese, & Tomato, Co-Op*	1 Pack/155g	365	18.5	235	10.6	21.8	11.9	1.9

S

	Measure INFO/WEIGHT	per Measure KCAL	per Measure FAT	Nutrition Values per 100g / 100ml KCAL	PROT	CARB	FAT	FIBRE
SANDWICH								
Cheese, & Tomato, Organic, M&S*	1 Pack/165g	559	35.3	339	11.8	24.8	21.4	1.9
Cheese, & Onion, Soft Oatmeal Bread, M&S*	1 Pack/170g	497	30.1	292	10.3	21.9	17.7	2.1
Cheese, & Pickle, On Malted Bread, Waitrose*	1 Pack/148g	433	21	293	12.3	27.6	14.2	2.7
Cheese, & Red Onion, Co-Op*	1 Pack/150g	411	21	274	11	24	14	2.7
Cheese, Cheddar, on White, Asda*	1 Pack/147g	418	20.5	285	13	27	14	1.6
Cheese, Simply, Boots*	1 Pack/138g	375	13.9	272	13.8	30.4	10.1	2.2
Chicken Mayo, on Malted Bread, Asda*	1 Pack/165g	362	10.6	219	13	26	6.4	1.8
Chicken Salad, Tesco*	1 Pack/226g	369	8.6	163	12.6	18.5	3.8	2.4
Chicken, & Avocado, Black Pepper Mayo, Waitrose*	1 Pack/213g	392	12.4	184	9.8	21.8	5.8	2.5
Chicken, & Avocado, Roast, on Soft Malted Bread, M&S*	1 Pack/200g	412	14.2	206	11.2	23	7.1	2.7
Chicken, & Avocado, Roast, Tesco*	1 Pack/173g	360	13.3	208	12.1	21.4	7.7	2.4
Chicken, & Bacon, & Avocado, M&S*	1 Pack/242g	508	28.3	210	10.7	15.8	11.7	3.2
Chicken, & Bacon, COU, M&S*	1 Pack/179g	250	3.6	140	13.5	15.8	2	3.8
Chicken, & Bacon, Deep Filled, Co-Op*	1 Pack/166g	556	33.2	335	16	23	20	3
Chicken, & Bacon, Tesco*	1 Pack/195g	486	24.2	249	14.3	20	12.4	2.7
Chicken, & Chorizo, with Red Pepper Sauce, Tesco*	1 Pack/186g	394	13.2	212	13	23.1	7.1	1.8
Chicken, & Salad, Aldi*	1 Pack/195g	338	4.5	173	11.5	23.8	2.3	2
Chicken, & Salad, Roast, Waitrose*	1 Pack/217g	482	24.1	222	9.4	21.1	11.1	2
Chicken, & Salad, Sainsbury's*	1 Pack/247g	461	12.6	187	11.8	22.6	5.1	1.6
Chicken, & Stuffing, Co-Op*	1 Pack/208g	420	13	202	13.5	22.6	6.2	2.4
Chicken, & Stuffing, Waitrose*	1 Pack/183g	450	18.8	246	12.8	25.6	10.3	1.5
Chicken, & Sweetcorn, British, Eat Well, M&S*	1 Pack/194g	340	10.5	175	11.4	19.6	5.4	3.1
Chicken, & Sweetcorn, Malted Bread, Sainsbury's*	1 Pack/193g	370	9.8	192	12.3	22.9	5.1	2.6
Chicken, & Sweetcorn, Tesco*	1 Pack/174g	355	11	204	10.8	24.6	6.3	3
Chicken, & Sweetcorn, with Seasoned Mayo, Aldi*	1 Pack/160g	327	7.3	204	14.4	25.6	4.6	2.4
Chicken, & Avocado, Limited Edition, Co-Op*	1 Pack/192g	362	11.9	188	10	21	6.2	2.9
Chicken, & Bacon, Caesar, Triple, Morrisons*	1 Pack/279g	713	32.3	256	12.2	25	11.6	1.2
Chicken, & Bacon, with Mayonnaise, Tesco*	1 Pack/160g	355	13.9	222	13.6	21.4	8.7	1.9
Chicken, & Mayo, Deli Club, Tesco*	1 Pack/183g	384	10.8	210	15.5	22.8	5.9	2.1
Chicken, & Stuffin', Vegan, Gro, Co-Op*	1 Pack/194g	466	16.5	240	11	28	8.5	3.6
Chicken, & Stuffing, Asda*	1 Pack/190g	393	10.3	207	13	25	5.4	1.9
Chicken, Bacon, & Lettuce, Tesco*	1 Pack/173g	420	19.2	243	14.8	19.4	11.1	3.2
Chicken, Bacon, & Mayo, Tesco*	1 Pack/160g	355	13.9	222	13.6	21.4	8.7	1.9
Chicken, Club, The, Tesco*	1 Pack/246g	613	29.8	249	12.9	21.1	12.1	2.1
Chicken, Coronation, M&S*	1 Pack/210g	420	20.4	200	11.2	20.2	9.7	3.1
Chicken, Roast, & Bacon, M&S*	1 Pack/219g	473	17.9	216	14.5	20	8.2	2.1
Chicken, Roast, & Mayo, Essential, Waitrose*	1 Pack/150g	329	10.5	219	12.6	25.5	7	1.8
Chicken, Roast, Mozzarella, & Pesto, Tesco*	1 Pack/231g	468	18.4	203	11.8	20	8	1.8
Chicken, Salad, Lighter, On the Go, Sainsbury's*	1 Pack/201g	321	5	160	12.3	21.2	2.5	1.7
Chicken, Tikka, & Mango Chutney, Tesco*	1 Pack/201g	352	4.8	175	11.6	25.4	2.4	2.6
Chicken, Tikka, COU, M&S*	1 Pack/185g	268	3.3	145	12.1	20.5	1.8	3.2
Chicken, Triple, On the Go, Sainsbury's*	1 Pack/275g	637	22.2	232	13	23.4	8.1	1.9
Chickpea, Smashin', Wicked Kitchen, Tesco*	1 Pack/220g	480	17.1	218	7	28.7	7.8	2.9
Club, New York Style, Sainsbury's*	1 Pack/212g	608	33.5	287	13.3	22.8	15.8	2.7
Crayfish, & Rocket, Finest, Tesco*	1 Pack/178g	365	10.5	205	9.8	27.5	5.9	2.1
Egg & Cress, on Malted Bread, Tesco*	1 Pack/178g	352	11.4	198	9.3	24.8	6.4	2.2
Egg Mayo, Free Range, Asda*	1 Pack/178g	311	10.1	175	9.3	21.5	5.7	2.1
Egg Mayonnaise, & Cress, Co-Op*	1 Pack/159g	405	24	255	8.8	20.8	15.1	1.9
Egg Mayonnaise, & Cress, Go Simple, Asda*	1 Pack/169g	370	18.6	219	10	20	11	1.7
Egg Mayonnaise, & Cress, HL, Tesco*	1 Pack/149g	271	7.7	182	9	23.5	5.2	2.6
Egg Mayonnaise, Double, Tesco*	1 Pack/189g	412	19.3	218	10.3	20.4	10.2	1.5
Egg, & Avocado, & Chilli Chutney, M&S*	1 Pack/209g	368	15.1	176	7.7	18.3	7.2	3.5
Egg, & Bacon, Handmade, Tesco*	1 Pack/217g	489	20.4	225	13.4	20.8	9.4	2

S

	Measure INFO/WEIGHT	per Measure KCAL	FAT	Nutrition Values per 100g / 100ml KCAL	PROT	CARB	FAT	FIBRE
SANDWICH								
Egg, & Cress, BGTY, Sainsbury's*	1 Pack/145g	268	7.5	185	9.1	25.4	5.2	2.7
Egg, & Cress, Co-Op*	1 Pack/159g	398	23.8	250	9	21	15	2
Egg, & Cress, COU, M&S*	1 Pack/192g	240	5.2	125	9.8	15.5	2.7	2.8
Egg, & Cress, Free Range, M&S*	1 Pack/192g	307	9	160	10.7	17.8	4.7	3
Egg, & Cress, Free Range, Sainsbury's*	1 Pack/185g	359	13	194	9.8	21.8	7	2.3
Egg, & Ham, Deli Club, Tesco*	1 Pack/220g	433	15.4	197	11.4	20.5	7	2.7
Egg, & Salad, on Softgrain Bread, HL, Tesco*	1 Pack/197g	290	4.7	147	7	23.6	2.4	1.7
Egg, & Tomato & Salad Cream, M&S*	1 Pack/214g	402	14.8	188	7.8	22.6	6.9	2
Egg, & Watercress, Bloomer, Freshly Prepared, M&S*	1 Pack/221g	465	26.1	210	10.2	15.3	11.8	3
Egg, & Watercress, GF Seeded Bread, Eat Well, M&S*	1 Pack/192g	382	16.9	199	8	20.6	8.8	2.9
Egg, & Cress, on Oatmeal Bread, Asda*	1 Pack/162g	323	11.3	200	9.7	23	7	2.1
Egg, & Salad Cream, with Tomatoes, Waitrose*	1 Pack/190g	357	12.5	188	7.2	23.8	6.6	2.3
Egg, & Watercress, Eat Well, M&S*	1 Pack/190g	355	10.8	187	9.8	22.9	5.7	2.4
Egg, & Watercress, GF, Good to Go, Waitrose*	1 Pack/174g	376	22.8	216	7.9	15	13.1	3.2
Ham Salad, on Malted Bread, BGTY, Sainsbury's*	1 Pack/175g	262	4.2	150	9.1	21.8	2.4	2.2
Ham, & Cheese, & Pickle, Average	***1 Pack/220g***	***524***	***25.1***	***238***	***12.2***	***21.6***	***11.4***	***2.5***
Ham, & Cheese, Honey Roast, Oatmeal Bread, M&S*	1 Pack/181g	436	19.7	241	14	20.6	10.9	2
Ham, & Coleslaw, Smoked, Malted Brown Bread, M&S*	1 Pack/175g	388	16.3	222	9.2	24.2	9.3	2.5
Ham, & Egg, Honey Roast, Tesco*	1 Pack/192g	355	9.8	185	12.8	20.6	5.1	2.5
Ham, & Mustard Mayo, Smoked, Oatmeal Bread, M&S*	1 Pack/150g	282	6.4	188	13.2	23.2	4.3	2
Ham, & Mustard, Tesco*	1 Pack/147g	437	27.9	297	10.6	20.8	19	1.2
Ham, & Salad, On the Go, Sainsbury's*	1 Pack/174g	244	3	140	10.1	20	1.7	2
Ham, & Soft Cheese, Tesco*	1 Pack/164g	333	12.1	203	11.6	22.5	7.4	2.2
Ham, & Cheese, Morrisons*	1 Pack/183g	273	4.6	149	12.5	19.2	2.5	4.1
New Delhi Inspired, Wicked Kitchen, Tesco*	1 Pack/192g	297	2.9	155	6.5	25.5	1.5	6.9
New Yorker, TTD, On the Go, Sainsbury's*	1 Pack/248g	486	17.6	196	10.2	21.8	7.1	2.1
No Turkey Feast, Plant Kitchen, M&S*	1 Pack/179g	354	8.9	198	8.6	27.6	5	4.1
Pastrami, Black Pepper, New York Deli, Deluxe, Lidl*	1 Pack/204g	384	14.3	188	12.4	18	7	1.9
Pastrami, New York Deli, Finest, Tesco*	1 Pack/231g	500	22.7	216	11.9	18.7	9.8	2.9
Ploughman's, Cheese, Cheddar, Deep Fill, Asda*	1 Pack/229g	471	22.9	206	9	20	10	4.3
Ploughmans, Cheddar, Tesco*	1 Pack/186g	418	18.6	225	9	23.4	10	2.8
Ploughmans, Red Leicester, No Mayo, Sainsbury's*	1 Pack/200g	438	17	219	9.4	25.1	8.5	2.4
Prawn Cocktail, Free From, Waitrose*	1 Pack/158g	336	17.2	213	6.6	20.8	10.9	2.6
Prawn Mayo, Egg & Cress, CLT, Triple, Waitrose*	1 Pack/262g	557	22.8	213	9.8	22.7	8.7	2.1
Prawn Mayo, on Oatmeal Bread, On the Go, Sainsbury's*	1 Pack/176g	329	8.8	187	10.6	23.9	5	1.9
Prawn Mayonnaise, Morrisons*	1 Pack/157g	234	3.9	149	9	22.7	2.5	3
Prawn Mayonnaise, on Oatmeal Bread, Tesco*	1 Pack/181g	338	10.1	187	10.2	22.9	5.6	2.1
Prawn Mayonnaise, Soft Malted Brown Bread, M&S*	1 Pack/197g	347	8.9	176	11.6	21.1	4.5	2.3
Prawn, & Salmon, Smoked, M&S*	1 Pack/445g	1135	63.6	255	11.7	19.3	14.3	1.4
Prawn, King, Sainsbury's*	1 Pack/204g	424	16.3	208	11.6	22.3	8	0
Prawn, Marie Rose, Waitrose*	1 Pack/164g	226	5.6	138	8.8	18	3.4	1.9
Roast Chicken, & Salad, on Malted Brown, M&S*	1 Pack/237g	363	6.4	153	11.5	19.1	2.7	2.9
Salmon, & Cucumber, M&S*	1 Pack/168g	329	13.9	196	11	19.5	8.3	2.6
Salmon, & Cucumber, Red, Tesco*	1 Pack/144g	284	9.2	197	11.1	23.8	6.4	1.9
Salmon, & Soft Cheese, Smoked, Waitrose*	1 Pack/180g	416	18	231	11.5	22.6	10	2.2
Salmon, & Cream Cheese, Smoked, Sainsbury*	1 Pack/168g	408	17.5	243	11.7	24.5	10.4	2.2
Salmon, & Cucumber, Good to Go, Waitrose*	1 Pack/185g	316	9.2	171	12.1	18	5	2.8
Salmon, Smoked, Moray Firth, & Egg, Co-Op*	1 Pack/230g	493	22.1	214	12	19	9.6	1.5
Sausage, Bacon, & Egg, Triple, Tesco*	1 Pack/265g	591	21.5	223	10.9	25.2	8.1	2.6
Seafood, Medley, M&S*	1 Pack/227g	468	28.1	206	7.2	16.3	12.4	3.5
Smoked Ham, & Cheddar, Tesco*	1 Pack/168g	414	18.1	247	14.8	21.7	10.8	1.7
Steak	***1 Serving/204g***	***459***	***14.1***	***225***	***14.9***	***25.5***	***6.9***	***0***
Steak, & Peppercorn Sauce, M&S*	1 Pack/190g	378	12.2	199	11.4	23.2	6.4	1.6

S

	Measure INFO/WEIGHT	per Measure KCAL	FAT	Nutrition Values per 100g / 100ml KCAL	PROT	CARB	FAT	FIBRE
SANDWICH								
Sub, Tuna, & Salad, From Restaurant, Average	***1 Serving/256g***	***584***	***28***	***228***	***11.6***	***21.6***	***10.9***	***0***
Tastes of Christmas, Selection, M&S*	1 Pack/205g	484	21.5	236	12.3	22	10.5	1.9
Tofu, Fiery, & Slaw, Wicked Kitchen, Tesco*	1 Pack/236g	425	11.6	180	6.5	26.4	4.9	2.3
Tuna & Cucumber, on Oatmeal Bread, Waitrose*	1 Pack/199g	304	4.8	153	11.8	20.1	2.4	2.1
Tuna Mayo, Essential, Waitrose*	1 Pack/133g	283	7.4	213	13.3	25.9	5.6	2.9
Tuna Mayonnaise, & Cucumber, Finest, Tesco*	1 Pack/183g	387	15	211	10.6	22.5	8.2	2.2
Tuna Mayonnaise, Sainsbury's*	1 Pack/150g	314	9.9	209	11.4	24.5	6.6	2.8
Tuna, & Cucumber, BGTY, Sainsbury's*	1 Pack/178g	268	3.2	151	11.3	22.3	1.8	3.1
Tuna, & Cucumber, COU, M&S*	1 Pack/204g	294	5.1	144	9.1	20.6	2.5	1.5
Tuna, & Cucumber, NUME, Morrisons*	1 Pack/151g	255	3.5	169	12	23.7	2.3	2.5
Tuna, & Cucumber, On the Go, Sainsbury's*	1 Pack/196g	284	5.5	145	9.6	19.4	2.8	2.1
Tuna, & Sweetcorn, Loved by Us, Co-Op*	1 Pack/200g	380	9.2	190	11.7	24.1	4.6	2.4
Tuna, & Sweetcorn, Malted Bread, Asda*	1 Pack/202g	365	10.7	181	11	21	5.3	2.5
Tuna, & Sweetcorn, on Malted Bread, Sainsbury's*	1 Pack/200g	362	9.2	181	11.9	21.8	4.6	2.4
Tuna, & Cucumber, Calorie Controlled, Tesco*	1 Pack/180g	268	3.1	149	10.5	22	1.7	1.8
Tuna, & Sweetcorn, BGTY, Sainsbury's*	1 Pack/187g	309	5.1	165	10.8	24.7	2.7	2.8
Tuna, & Sweetcorn, on Malted Bread, Co-Op*	1 Pack/185g	337	8.5	182	12	22	4.6	2.6
Tuna, & Sweetcorn, on Malted Bread, Tesco*	1 Pack/178g	329	9.8	185	9.7	22.8	5.5	2.6
Tuna, & Sweetcorn, on Malted Brown, M&S*	1 Pack/208g	379	11.9	182	10.7	20.8	5.7	2.3
Tuna, Crunch, HL, Tesco*	1 Pack/180g	261	4.3	145	11	19.9	2.4	0.5
Tuna, Crunch, Tesco*	1 Pack/165g	341	8.6	207	8.7	30.3	5.2	1.9
Tuna, Skip Jack, & Cucumber , Morrisons*	1 Pack/170g	271	3.6	159	10.9	23.2	2.1	2.2
Turkey Feast, GF, M&S*	1 Pack/242g	520	19.8	215	11.9	21.7	8.2	3.2
Turkey, & Cranberry, COU, M&S*	1 Pack/180g	279	3.1	155	12.1	22.8	1.7	2.9
Turkey, & Pastrami, HL, Tesco*	1 Pack/185g	286	4.8	155	9.6	22.1	2.6	2.6
Turkey, & Trimmings, Christmas, Tesco*	1 Pack/209g	476	16.5	228	12.5	25.5	7.9	2.3
Turkey, & Trimmings, Light Choices, HL, Tesco*	1 Pack/154g	256	4.3	166	10.1	24.1	2.8	2.2
Turkey, Mango, & Houmous, Aldi*	1 Pack/165g	291	8.1	176	9.1	22.4	4.9	3.9
SANDWICH FILLER								
Cheese & Spring Onion, M&S*	1 Serving/56g	199	18.8	355	8.5	5	33.6	0.2
Cheese & Onion, Reduced Fat, Supermarket, Average	***1 Serving/100g***	***227***	***18.1***	***227***	***11.8***	***4.4***	***18.1***	***1.7***
Cheese & Onion, Supermarket, Average	***1 Serving/100g***	***405***	***38.6***	***405***	***10.2***	***4.1***	***38.6***	***1.3***
Cheese, & Onion, Double Cheese, Tesco*	1 Serving/50g	102	7.4	205	12.9	4.5	14.9	0.6
Cheese, Three, & Onion, 35% Less Fat, Asda*	1/5 Pack/50g	120	9.5	240	12	5.3	19	0.5
Chicken & Bacon with Sweetcorn, Sainsbury's*	1 Serving/60g	123	9.4	205	12	4	15.7	0.9
Chicken, Coronation, Deli, M&S*	1 Serving/50g	107	7.4	214	11.4	8.8	14.7	0.6
Chicken, Coronation, Deli, Meadow Fresh, Lidl*	1 Serving/30g	78	5.7	261	12	9.8	19	1.2
Chicken, Coronation, Tesco*	1 Serving/50g	108	7.1	217	12.1	10	14.2	0.7
Chicken, Sweetcorn & Bacon, Tesco*	1 Serving/50g	167	14.8	334	12.3	4.3	29.7	1.6
Coronation Chicken, Sainsbury's*	¼ Tub/60g	183	14.8	305	12.1	8.9	24.6	1.2
Egg & Bacon, Fresh, Tesco*	1 Serving/45g	112	9	248	12.7	4.2	20.1	0.6
Egg Mayonnaise, BGTY, Sainsbury's*	1 Serving/63g	71	4.1	113	10.2	3.4	6.5	0.1
Egg Mayonnaise, Country Fresh, Aldi*	¼ Pack/50g	106	8.9	211	9.8	2.9	17.8	0
Egg Mayonnaise, Tesco*	1 Serving/50g	100	7.8	199	10.9	3.5	15.6	0.5
Prawn Marie Rose, Sainsbury's*	1 Serving/60g	121	10.6	201	8.1	2.5	17.6	0.9
Prawn Mayonnaise, Deli, Asda*	1 Serving/50g	170	16.5	339	9	1.6	33	0.4
Seafood Cocktail, Asda*	1 Serving/50g	104	8.5	207	4.8	9	17	0.5
Seafood Cocktail, Sainsbury's*	1 Serving/55g	99	6.9	180	5.9	10.6	12.6	0.5
Smoked Salmon & Soft Cheese, M&S*	1 Pack/170g	450	40.6	265	11.1	4.9	23.9	0
Tuna & Sweetcorn, Reduced Fat, Supermarket	***1 Serving/100g***	***119***	***5.4***	***119***	***11.5***	***5.8***	***5.4***	***1.2***
Tuna & Sweetcorn, Tesco*	1 Serving/54g	127	9.8	235	8.6	8.1	18.1	0.6
Tuna Crunch, Morrisons*	1 Serving/35g	65	4.7	187	10.8	5.7	13.3	0.5
Tuna Mayonnaise, BGTY, Sainsbury's*	1 Serving/100g	114	3.4	114	17.6	3.5	3.4	0.1

S

	Measure INFO/WEIGHT	per Measure KCAL	FAT	Nutrition Values per 100g / 100ml KCAL	PROT	CARB	FAT	FIBRE
SANDWICH SPREAD								
Heinz*	1 Tbsp/10ml	22	1.3	220	1	24	13	1
Light, Heinz*	1 Tbsp/10g	16	0.9	161	1.1	18.2	9.2	0.9
SARDINES								
Canned, in Tomato Sauce, Asda*	1 Can/107g	128	3.8	120	20	1.2	3.6	0.8
Canned, in Tomato Sauce, Essential, Waitrose*	1 Serving/120g	239	16.5	200	17.9	1.2	13.8	0
Canned, in Tomato Sauce, Nixe, Lidl*	1 Can/120g	229	14.4	191	19	1.6	12	0.5
Fillets, with Lemon & Herb Dressing, Morrisons*	1 Can/100g	109	4.9	109	14.3	1.5	4.9	1
Grilled	***1oz/28g***	***55***	***2.9***	***195***	***25.3***	***0***	***10.4***	***0***
in Brine, Canned, Drained	***1oz/28g***	***38***	***2.1***	***136***	***17***	***0***	***7.6***	***0***
in Oil, Canned, Drained	***1oz/28g***	***51***	***3.2***	***180***	***19.1***	***0***	***11.6***	***0***
in Spring Water, Portuguese, Sainsbury's*	1 Can/90g	176	10.5	195	21.3	1.2	11.6	0.5
in Tomato Sauce, Canned	***1oz/28g***	***45***	***2.8***	***162***	***17***	***1.4***	***9.9***	***0***
North Atlantic, with Chilli, Lime & Coriander, Finest, Tesco*	1 Can/105g	302	24.6	288	18.7	0.6	23.4	0.1
Raw, Whole with Head	***1oz/28g***	***22***	***1.2***	***78***	***9.7***	***0***	***4.3***	***0***
SATAY								
Chicken with Peanut Sauce, Waitrose*	1 Pack/250g	492	27	197	18.9	6	10.8	0.5
Chicken, 12 Mini, Taste Original*	1 Stick/10g	21	1.3	217	19.9	3.1	13.6	1.2
Chicken, Indonesian, Mini, Sainsbury's*	1 Stick/10g	17	0.7	171	23	4	7	0.7
Chicken, Sticks, Asda*	1 Stick/20g	43	2.8	216	18	4.5	14	0
Chicken, with Peanut Dip, Sainsbury's*	1 Pack/90g	171	10	190	15.4	6.3	11.1	1.5
Satay, Spicy, with Noodles, G&B, Asda*	1 Pack/365g	336	9.1	92	6.5	10	2.5	1.3
Spicy Chicken & Noodles, Microwaved, Asda*	1 Portion/380g	361	10.3	95	6.4	10	2.7	1.4
SATSUMAS								
Fresh, Raw, Flesh Only, Average	***1 Sm/56g***	***21***	***0***	***37***	***0.9***	***8.6***	***0.1***	***1.3***
Weighed with Peel, Average	***1 Sm/60g***	***16***	***0***	***26***	***0.6***	***6.1***	***0.1***	***0.6***
SAUCE								
Aioli, Garlic, Leon*	1 Jar/245g	1333	137.7	544	0.8	8.3	56.2	0.7
Apple, Bramley, Sainsbury's*	1 Tsp/15g	17	0	111	0.2	27.2	0.1	1.8
Apple, Everyday Value, Tesco*	1 Tbsp/15g	15	0	105	0.1	24.8	0.1	0.5
Arrabiata, Italian, Tesco*	½ Pot/175g	74	0.9	42	1.1	7.9	0.5	1
Arrabiata, M&S*	½ Jar/170g	85	6.3	50	1.8	2	3.7	0.7
Bacon & Tomato, Smoked, Stir in, Dolmio*	½ Tub/75g	74	4.2	98	4.6	7.2	5.6	1.3
Balti, Cooking, Asda*	¼ Jar/125g	64	1.9	51	0.9	7.8	1.5	1.1
Balti, Loyd Grossman*	½ Jar/175g	180	11.7	103	1.3	8.4	6.7	1.7
Barbecue, Sweet, Heinz*	1 Tbsp/15g	27	0	181	0.9	44	0.2	0
Barbeque, Cook in, Homepride*	1 Can/500g	375	7.5	75	0.7	14.6	1.5	0.6
BBQ, Bold Spicy Texas, Bulls-Eye*	1 Serving/20g	27	0	135	1.1	31	0	0
BBQ, Jerk, Reggae Reggae, Levi Roots*	1 Jar/310g	375	0.3	121	1.1	28.8	0.1	0.5
BBQ, Reduced Sugar, & Salt, Tesco*	1 Tbsp/15g	11	0.1	71	0.4	15.9	0.5	0.6
BBQ, Roasted Onion, Heinz*	1 Tbsp/15ml	25	0	169	1.3	37	0.2	0
BBQ, Smoky, Asda*	1 Tbsp/15g	14	0.1	93	1.3	21	0.5	1.2
BBQ, Smoky, Sugar Free, Blend Bros*	1 Serving/15ml	4	0	30	0.7	5.3	0.2	2.2
BBQ, Sticky, Spread & Bake, Heinz*	¼ Jar/78g	131	0.5	168	1	39.6	0.6	1.2
Bearnaise, Sainsbury's*	1 Tbsp/15g	59	6.2	393	0.6	5	41	0
Bechamel, M&S*	1 Jar/425g	480	34.8	113	2.1	7	8.2	1.6
Bechamel, Plant Kitchen, M&S*	1 Jar/410g	377	32.4	92	0.7	3.9	7.9	1.1
Bhuna, Cooking, Sharwood's*	¼ Jar/105g	83	4.9	79	1.1	7.1	4.7	1.9
Biryani, Aromatic, Stir Fry, Just Cook, Sainsbury's*	½ Pack/88ml	75	3.3	86	2.3	9	3.8	2.8
Biryani, Med & Aromati, Oven Bake, Patak's*	½ Jar/175g	140	9.3	80	1.1	6.1	5.3	0
Biryani, Reduced Fat, Waitrose*	1 Serving/115g	55	1.8	48	1.8	5.7	1.6	1.9
Black Bean, & Red Pepper, Sharwood's*	½ Jar/213g	132	3	62	1.9	10.5	1.4	1.2
Black Bean, Canton, Stir Fry, Blue Dragon*	½ Pack/60g	53	1.2	88	2.8	14.8	2	1.5
Black Bean, Cooking, Tesco*	¼ Jar/124g	56	0.7	45	0.2	9.4	0.6	0.5

S

	Measure INFO/WEIGHT	per Measure KCAL	FAT	Nutrition Values per 100g / 100ml KCAL	PROT	CARB	FAT	FIBRE
SAUCE								
Black Bean, M&S*	½ Jar/140g	130	3.8	93	2.9	14.1	2.7	0.5
Black Bean, Stir Fry, Amoy*	½ Pack/60g	58	1.9	96	2.3	14.1	3.2	0.9
Black Bean, Stir Fry, Asda*	1 Pouch/120g	125	2.8	104	1.6	19	2.3	0.7
Black Bean, Stir Fry, Sharwood's*	1 Jar/195g	127	0.6	65	2.3	12.9	0.3	0
Black Bean, Stir Fry, Taste of China, Lidl*	½ Sachet/60g	64	0.9	107	1.4	21.8	1.5	0.5
Bolognese, Dolmio*	1 Serving/100g	33	0.2	33	1.5	6.3	0.2	1.3
Bolognese, Morrisons*	1/5 Jar/145g	52	1	36	1.2	5.6	0.7	1.2
Bolognese, No Added Sugar, Dolmio*	½ Jar/175g	67	1.1	38	1.3	6.2	0.6	1.3
Bolognese, No Added Sugar, Tesco*	¼ Jar/125g	43	0.9	34	1.3	5.4	0.7	0.6
Bolognese, Smart Price, Asda*	¼ Jar/110g	44	1	40	0.1	7.6	0.9	0.5
Bolognese, Vegan, Sacla*	1 Jar/350g	259	13.3	74	3.2	6.2	3.8	1.1
Bouillabaisse, M&S*	½ Pouch/100g	132	11.8	132	1.8	4.3	11.8	0.7
Bread, Made with Semi-Skimmed Milk	***1 Serving/45g***	***42***	***1.4***	***93***	***4.3***	***12.8***	***3.1***	***0.3***
Brown, Bottled	***1 Tsp/6g***	***6***	***0***	***99***	***1.1***	***25.2***	***0***	***0.7***
Brown, Bramwells, Aldi*	1 Tbsp/15g	17	0.1	115	0.5	27	0.5	1
Brown, Original, HP*	1 Tbsp/15g	18	0	122	0.9	28.3	0.1	0.4
Brown, Reduced Salt & Sugar, HP*	1 Tbsp/15g	13	0	87	0.7	20	0.1	0.3
Brown, Reduced Sugar & Salt, Tesco*	1 Tbsp/15g	13	0.1	88	0.7	17.1	0.5	0.8
Brown, Stockwell & Co., Tesco*	1 Tbsp/15g	12	0.1	82	0.3	17.2	0.5	0.5
Burger, Heinz*	1 Tbsp/15g	56	5.3	372	0.9	12	35.5	0
Burger, Hellmann's*	1 Tbsp/15g	36	3.2	240	1.1	12	21	0
Burger, Tesco*	1 Tbsp/15ml	29	2.5	193	1	9.4	16.6	0.8
Butter Chicken, Lidl*	1 Jar/350g	438	29.1	125	1.8	10	8.3	1.4
Butter Chicken, Patak's*	½ Jar/225g	279	20.2	124	1.2	9.1	9	0
Butter Chicken, Tesco*	¼ Jar/125g	134	10.4	107	0.8	6.9	8.3	0.8
Caesar, Dressing, Florette*	1 Tbsp/15g	45	4.6	302	1.4	2.8	31	0.3
Caramel, Salted, Finest, Tesco*	¼ Pot/65g	266	8.5	409	3.2	69	13.1	1.2
Carbonara, Pot, Tesco*	½ Pot/175g	194	13.8	111	4.8	4.8	7.9	0.6
Casserole, Sausage, Morrisons*	¼ Jar/125g	51	0.1	41	0.8	9	0.1	0.2
Ch**se, Vegan, Sacla*	1 Jar/350g	374	33.9	107	0.7	4.3	9.7	0
Cheese, Four, Finest, Tesco*	½ Pot/175g	231	17.8	132	4.1	5.8	10.2	0.1
Cheese, Four, for Pasta, Waitrose*	1 Pot/350g	546	41	156	6.7	5.8	11.7	0.1
Cheese, Four, M&S*	1 Pot/350g	466	32.9	133	7.2	4.8	9.4	0.1
Cheese, Fresh, Waitrose*	1 Pot/350g	458	34.3	131	5.1	5.7	9.8	0
Cheese, Made with Semi-Skimmed Milk	***1 Serving/60g***	***107***	***7.6***	***179***	***8.1***	***9.1***	***12.6***	***0.2***
Cheese, Made with Whole Milk	***1 Serving/60g***	***118***	***8.8***	***197***	***8***	***9***	***14.6***	***0.2***
Chilli & Garlic, Blue Dragon*	1 Serving/30ml	26	0.1	85	1.1	19.7	0.2	0
Chilli Con Carne, Homepride*	½ Jar/250g	145	1.2	58	1.6	11.1	0.5	1.6
Chilli Con Carne, Hot, Asda*	1 Jar/500g	285	3	57	1.9	11	0.6	0.9
Chilli Con Carne, Hot, Uncle Ben's*	1 Jar/500g	295	3	59	2.3	10.9	0.6	1.7
Chilli, Con Carne, Mexican, Co-Op*	¼ Jar/128g	82	0.8	64	2.6	10	0.6	3.2
Chilli, Cooking, Medium, Fiesta, Aldi*	¼ Jar/125g	60	0.6	48	2.3	7.3	0.5	2.7
Chilli, Extra Hot, Maggi*	1 Tbsp/15g	16	0	107	0.7	25.3	0	1.4
Chilli, Hot, Cooking, Asda*	¼ Jar/125g	71	0.7	57	1.9	11	0.6	0.9
Chilli, Hot, Mexican, Morrisons*	¼ Jar/125g	72	0.6	58	2.2	11.2	0.5	2
Chilli, Hunan Smoky, Cooking, Sharwoods*	1 Pack/230g	168	1.2	73	1.2	15.5	0.5	1.3
Chilli, Mild, Tesco*	1 Jar/550g	302	1.6	55	2.3	10	0.3	3.4
Chilli, Tesco*	1 Tsp/5ml	4	0.2	90	1.3	14	3.2	1.1
Chilli, Tomato Based, Bottled, Average	***1 Tbsp/15g***	***16***	***0***	***104***	***2.5***	***19.8***	***0.3***	***5.9***
Chinese, Stir Fry, Ashfield Farm, Aldi*	½ Pack/87g	80	2.5	92	1.4	15	2.9	0.8
Chocolate, Dessert, M&S*	1 Dtsp/11g	35	1	330	2.1	59.3	9.4	1.9
Chow Mein, Stir Fry, Asda*	½ Pack/85g	101	6.3	119	0.8	12	7.4	0.6
Chow Mein, Stir Fry, Asia Specialities, Aldi*	½ Pack/60g	56	0.4	94	0.5	21	0.6	0.5

S

	Measure INFO/WEIGHT	per Measure KCAL	FAT	Nutrition Values per 100g / 100ml KCAL	PROT	CARB	FAT	FIBRE
SAUCE								
Chow Mein, Stir Fry, Blue Dragon*	1 Sachet/120g	127	1.3	106	0.9	23	1.1	0.4
Chow Mein, Stir Fry, Straight to Wok, Amoy*	1 Pack/120g	172	7	143	0.9	21.9	5.8	0.5
Coconut, & Lemon Grass, Tesco*	½ Pack/90g	74	5.3	82	1.3	5.4	5.9	1.2
Country French, Chicken Tonight, Knorr*	¼ Jar/125g	96	7.4	77	0.5	5	5.9	0.6
Cranberry Jelly, Morrisons*	1 Tsp/12g	23	0	189	0.2	47	0	0.1
Cranberry, Sainsbury's*	1 Tsp/15g	26	0.1	170	0.5	41.5	0.5	0.5
Cranberry, Tesco*	1 Tsp/15g	23	0	156	0.1	38.8	0	0.9
Creamy, Vegan, Waitrose*	½ Pot/175g	159	10.8	91	1.6	7	6.2	2.3
Curry, Asda*	1 Tbsp/15g	62	2.1	414	13	59	14	1.3
Curry, Basics, Sainsbury's*	¼ Jar/110g	70	2.8	64	0.7	9.7	2.5	0.9
Curry, Chinese Style, Tesco*	¼ Jar/125g	59	0.5	47	0.4	10.3	0.4	0.5
Curry, Chip Shop, Knorr*	1 Sachet/150ml	146	6.9	97	1.7	12.4	4.6	0.7
Curry, Chip Shop, Prepared, CBY, Asda*	1 Serving/62ml	50	3	80	0.5	8.6	4.8	0.2
Curry, Cook in, Homepride*	½ Can/250g	170	6.2	68	0.8	10.5	2.5	0.7
Curry, Green Thai, Finest, Tesco*	1 Serving/350g	420	37.1	120	1.4	4.8	10.6	0.7
Curry, Medium, Uncle Ben's*	1 Jar/500g	330	10	66	0.9	10.9	2	0
Curry, Mild & Creamy, Cooking, Asda*	¼ Jar/125g	114	5.9	91	1	11	4.7	0.8
Curry, Red Thai, Finest, Tesco*	1 Jar/350g	388	31.5	111	1.3	6.2	9	0.9
Curry, Thai Coconut, Uncle Ben's*	1 Serving/125g	128	6	102	1.4	13.2	4.8	0
Dessert, Strawberry, & Phizzecco, Waitrose*	1 Serving/15g	28	0.1	187	0.7	44.2	0.6	0.8
Dhansak, Sharwood's*	1 Jar/445g	668	34.7	150	4.7	15.2	7.8	1.4
Dill & Lemon, Delicate for Fish, Schwartz*	1 Pack/300g	387	34.2	129	1.1	5.6	11.4	0.5
Dopiaza, Punjabi Style, Cooking, Extra Special, Asda*	1/3 Jar/112g	94	3.8	84	1.8	11	3.4	1.5
Fajita, Asda*	¼ Jar/125g	79	5.4	63	1	5	4.3	1
Fish Pie, As Sold, Schwartz*	1 Serving/75g	85	6.8	113	0.8	6.9	9	0.5
for Meatballs, Cucina, Aldi*	¼ Jar/125g	39	0.6	31	1.1	5.7	0.5	1
Garlic & Chive, Table & Dip, Heinz*	1 Serving/10ml	32	3	323	1	12.1	29.9	0.2
Garlic, & Herb, Asda*	1 Serving/10g	38	4	384	1.6	3.1	40	4.4
Garlic, Creamy, Sainsbury's*	1 Tbsp/15g	44	4.3	296	0.5	7.6	29	1.5
Garlic, Heinz*	1 Tbsp/15g	60	5.4	398	2.2	15	36	0.3
Garlic, Peri Peri, Medium, Nando's*	1 Serving/20g	10	0.6	49	0.8	4.2	3	0.8
Garlic, Turkish Style, Heinz*	1 Tbsp/15g	56	5.2	371	1.9	11	35	0
Hoisin, & Garlic, Blue Dragon*	1 Serving/60g	80	1.6	133	1.2	26.1	2.6	0
Hoisin, & Plum, Stir Fry, HL, Tesco*	1 Serving/250g	148	3.2	59	2.1	9.7	1.3	1.3
Hoisin, & Plum, Deliciously Versatile, M&S*	½ Bottle/75g	112	1.1	149	2.7	29.3	1.5	2.4
Hoisin, & Spring Onion, Stir Fry, Sharwood's*	½ Jar/98g	103	1.6	105	1.7	20.5	1.6	0.9
Hoisin, Dipping, Sharwood's*	1 Tbsp/15g	25	0.2	165	1.5	36.2	1.3	1.4
Hoisin, Rich & Fruity, Tesco*	1 Serving/29g	48	0.4	166	1.7	36.4	1.3	0.8
Hoisin, Sharwood's*	1 Tbsp/15g	32	0	211	2.7	49.5	0.3	0.1
Hoisin, Slimming World*	1 Pot/350g	130	1.4	37	1.8	5.9	0.4	1.4
Hoisin, Stir Fry, Amoy*	½ Pouch/60g	66	1.4	110	2.1	20.3	2.3	0.1
Hoisin, Stir Fry, Asda*	½ Pack/63g	54	0.4	86	0.6	18	0.6	3.1
Hoisin, Stir Fry, Tesco *	½ Pouch/60g	55	0.9	92	0.6	18.9	1.5	0.4
Hollandaise, Cook with, M&S*	1 Serving/50g	136	13.9	271	0.7	4.3	27.8	0.4
Hollandaise, Finest, Tesco*	1 Serving/98g	473	44.5	485	1.4	17.2	45.6	0.3
Hollandaise, Fresh, Average	***1 Pack/150g***	***342***	***32.4***	***228***	***2.4***	***6.1***	***21.6***	***0***
Hollandaise, Fresh, pouch, Sainsbury's*	1 Tbsp/15g	39	3.9	259	1.7	5	25.7	0.5
Hollandaise, Style, Inspired Vegan*	1 Tsp/5g	27	2.8	531	1.7	6.9	55.1	0.2
Honey & Mustard, Chicken Tonight, Knorr*	¼ Jar/125g	132	6.6	106	1	12.6	5.3	1.8
Honey Mustard, Bunlimited*	1 Tbsp/15g	30	2.4	201	0.7	13.8	15.7	0
Horseradish, & Mustard, Hella, Wicked Kitchen, Tesco*	1 Tbsp/15ml	16	0.7	105	3.8	10.9	4.5	2.9
Horseradish, Colman's*	1 Tbsp/15ml	17	0.9	112	1.9	9.8	6.2	2.6
Horseradish, Creamed, M&S*	1 Tsp/5g	16	1.5	325	2.4	12.1	29.3	2.5

S

	Measure INFO/WEIGHT	per Measure KCAL	FAT	Nutrition Values per 100g / 100ml KCAL	PROT	CARB	FAT	FIBRE
SAUCE								
Horseradish, Creamed, Waitrose*	1 Tbsp/16g	30	1.6	185	2.4	19.6	9.9	2.3
Horseradish, Creamy, Sainsbury's*	1 Tsp/5g	11	0.6	223	2.8	28.9	11.8	1.6
Horseradish, Hot, Morrisons*	1 Serving/20g	31	1.5	157	2.2	19.1	7.7	1.7
Horseradish, Hot, Tesco*	1 Tsp/5g	12	0.8	233	1.8	17.4	16.9	2.1
Hot, Pineapple, Barnfathers*	1 Serving/10ml	4	0	43	0.6	7.8	0	0
Jalfrezi, Average	***1 Sm Jar/350g***	***326***	***23.7***	***93***	***1.3***	***6.7***	***6.8***	***1.6***
Kashmiri, Creamy, Sharwood's*	½ Pouch/125g	151	10.6	121	1.2	9.1	8.5	1.6
Katsu Curry, Blue Dragon*	1 Serving/100g	240	2	240	1	54	2	1
Katsu, Curry, Sainsbury's*	½ Jar/170g	138	7.1	81	1.7	8.5	4.2	1
Katsu, Spice & Simmer, Taste of Japan, Asda*	1/3 Jar/115g	142	9.1	123	1.3	11	7.9	1
Kicap Manis, Malay Taste*	1 Tbsp/15ml	36	0.1	237	1.3	55.9	0.9	0
Korma, 2 Step, Sainsbury's*	½ Jar/180g	216	13.3	120	1.6	10.5	7.4	2.6
Korma, 30% Less Fat, Sharwoods*	¼ Jar/105g	101	6.2	96	1.1	9.2	5.9	0.9
Korma, Coconut & Cream, Mild, in Glass Jar, Patak's*	½ Jar/225g	326	25	145	1.2	9.4	11.1	0
Korma, Cooking Sauce, Waitrose*	1 Jar/350g	696	51.8	199	3.4	12.2	14.8	1.8
Korma, Cooking, Asda*	¼ Jar/122g	131	7.8	107	1.5	10	6.4	1.1
Korma, Cooking, Free From, Tesco*	1 Jar/500g	405	21.5	81	0.8	9.3	4.3	1
Korma, Curry, Uncle Ben's*	1 Jar/500g	630	42	126	1.4	11.1	8.4	0
Korma, Deluxe, Lidl*	1 Jar/350g	640	40.2	183	2.7	16.4	11.5	1.5
Korma, Mild Curry, BFY, Morrisons*	¼ Jar/118g	150	7.2	127	1.3	16.8	6.1	1.5
Korma, Milk, Morrisons*	¼ Jar/112g	172	13.5	153	1.7	8.4	12	2.3
Korma, Tesco*	¼ Jar/125g	192	14.6	154	2.4	9.9	11.7	1.3
Lasagne, White, Baresa, Lidl*	1 Jar/470g	794	71.9	169	0.6	7	15.3	0.5
Lasagne, White, Sainsbury's*	¼ Jar/119g	130	11.4	109	0.8	4.5	9.6	0.5
Lemon Chicken, Uncle Ben's*	1 Jar/450g	315	1.4	70	0.3	16.2	0.3	0.3
Madras, Aldi*	1 Serving/113g	68	2.3	60	1.5	9	2	0
Madras, Cooking, Sharwood's*	1 Tsp/2g	2	0.1	86	1.5	6.9	5.8	1.3
Madras, Hot, Patak's*	¼ Jar/113g	92	5.4	82	1.5	7	4.8	0
Makhani, Butter, M&S*	½ Jar/170g	291	22.6	171	1.9	10	13.3	1.9
Marie Rose, The Best, Morrisons*	1 Tbsp/15g	64	5.8	428	2	18.2	38.5	0.1
Mint Jelly, Tesco*	1 Tbsp/15g	34	0	224	0.3	55.2	0.1	0.7
Mint, Asda*	1 Tbsp/15g	13	0.1	88	0.9	19	0.6	2
Mint, Bramwells, Aldi*	1 Serving/30g	28	0.2	93	0.5	21	0.5	0
Mint, British, Finest, Tesco*	1 Tbsp/15g	12	0	77	0.9	17.3	0.2	1.2
Mint, Reduced Sugar, Tesco*	1 Tbsp/15g	12	0.1	81	1.8	16.2	0.5	2.1
Mint, Sainsbury's*	1 Dtsp/10g	13	0	126	2.5	28.7	0.1	4
Mint, Value, Tesco*	1 Serving/10g	4	0	41	1.1	9	0.1	1.8
Mushroom, Creamy, Asda*	¼ Jar/121g	126	9.8	104	0.8	6.7	8.1	0.5
Mushroom, Creamy, Chicken Tonight, Knorr*	¼ Jar/125g	100	7.4	80	0.8	5.7	5.9	0.6
Olive, & Tomato, Asda*	1 Jar/340g	374	28.9	110	1.6	5.7	8.5	2
Oyster & Spring Onion, Stir Fry, Blue Dragon*	1 Sachet/120g	134	0	112	1.5	26.3	0	0
Oyster, Blue Dragon*	1 Tsp/5ml	6	0	121	3.4	26.9	0	0
Pad Thai, M&S*	1 Sachet/125g	120	1	96	2.8	18.5	0.8	1.3
Pad Thai, Stir Fry, Morrisons*	1 Pack/120g	142	5.2	118	2.2	17.4	4.3	0.4
Parsley, Fishmongers, Morrisons*	½ Pack/90g	112	8.9	124	2.1	6.2	9.9	0.9
Parsley, Fresh, Microwaved, Sainsbury's*	1/3 Pot/100g	78	5.4	78	1.7	5.3	5.4	0.5
Parsley, Tesco*	½ Pack/89g	85	5.1	95	2.8	8.1	5.7	1.1
Pasta Bake, Tomato & Herb, Homepride*	¼ Jar/121g	126	8.8	104	1.8	7.2	7.3	1
Pasta Bake, Tuna, Homepride*	½ Jar/250g	208	13	83	1.4	7.6	5.2	0.9
Peanut Satay, Stir Fry, Amoy*	1 Pack/120g	217	11.9	181	5.2	16.9	9.9	2.5
Peanut, Sainsbury's*	1 Sachet/70g	185	9.2	264	1.9	34.7	13.1	1.6
Pecorino, & Black Pepper, Finest, Tesco*	½ Tub/175g	166	11.6	95	4.3	4.2	6.6	0.6
Pepper, As Prepared, Colman's*	1 Portion/75ml	89	4.7	119	4.7	11	6.3	0

	Measure INFO/WEIGHT	per Measure KCAL	FAT	Nutrition Values per 100g / 100ml KCAL	PROT	CARB	FAT	FIBRE
SAUCE								
Pepper, Creamy, As Sold, Schwartz*	1 Serving/85g	71	5.8	83	1.3	4	6.8	0.5
Peppercorn, Morrisons*	¼ Pack/51g	49	3.8	97	1	5.9	7.6	0.7
Peppercorn, Waitrose*	1 Serving/60g	64	4.7	107	4.1	4.5	7.9	0.5
Peppercorn, with a Dash of Brandy, M&S*	½ Pouch/100g	100	7.9	100	1.5	5.4	7.9	0.5
Peri Peri, Hot, Bramwells, Aldi*	1 Tbsp/15g	29	2.4	193	0.6	10	16	1.8
Perinaise, Hot, Squeezy Bottle, Nando's*	1 Tbsp/15ml	49	4.4	327	0.5	14	29	0
Perinaise, Mild, Squeezy Bottle, Nando's*	1 Serving/15g	46	4.2	309	0.3	13	28	0
Perinaise, Vegan, Squeezy Bottle, Nando's*	1 Tbsp/15g	46	4.1	307	0.8	13.4	27.5	0
Pesto, Green, Baresa, Lidl*	1 Tbsp/15g	55	5.4	364	4.1	4.8	35.9	2.6
Pesto, Red, Italian Inspirations, Co-Op*	1 Tbsp/15g	45	4	298	4.7	8.1	27	2.5
Pesto, with Basil, Buitoni*	1 Serving/62g	290	27	467	11.3	8.1	43.5	0
Plum, & Hoisin, Rich & Vibrant, Waitrose*	½ Pack/70g	99	0.4	141	1.6	32.1	0.5	1.1
Plum, & Hoisin, Stir Fry, Morrisons*	½ Pack/90g	103	0.1	114	0.6	27.6	0.1	0.1
Plum, Dipping, M&S*	1 Tbsp/15g	34	0	228	0.1	56.2	0.2	0.3
Plum, Sticky, Stir Fry, Blue Dragon*	1 Serving/60g	145	0.2	242	0.1	35.6	0.3	0
Pomodoro, TTD, Sainsbury's*	½ Pot/175g	152	10.7	87	1.8	5.3	6.1	1.8
Prawn Cocktail, Morrisons*	1 Portion/15ml	81	8.5	540	1.4	5.5	56.9	1.1
Ranch, American, Morrisons*	1 Tbsp/15g	72	7.2	479	2.4	9.8	47.7	0.2
Raspberry, Dessert, M&S*	1 Serving/20g	24	0.1	120	0.5	28.7	0.3	2.6
Raspberry, Tangy, Dessert, Specially Selected, Aldi*	1 Tbsp/15g	33	0.1	218	0.5	54	0.5	0.5
Red Hot, Buffalo Wings, Bramwells, Aldi*	1 Tbsp/15g	8	0.4	53	1.5	4.6	2.6	2.5
Red Hot, Wings, Buffalo, Franks*	1 Tbsp/15g	4	0.2	30	0.8	2	1.5	2.5
Red Pepper, & Chilli, M&S*	½ Pack/75g	63	3.6	84	1.6	7.7	4.8	1.9
Red Pepper, M&S*	1 Pot/180g	270	17.3	150	0.8	14.3	9.6	1.7
Red Pepper, Roasted, & Chorizo, Waitrose*	1 Serving/50g	125	11.2	250	3.2	7	22.5	3.1
Redcurrant, Colman's*	1 Tsp/12g	44	0	368	0.7	90	0	0
Rogan Josh, Deluxe, Lidl*	1/3 Jar/116g	122	7.3	105	2.3	8.8	6.3	1.9
Rogan Josh, Low Fat, Tesco*	¼ Jar/125g	38	0.6	31	0.9	4.9	0.5	1.4
Rogan Josh, Medium, Sharwood's*	½ Jar/210g	151	7.6	72	1.4	8.6	3.6	0.5
Rogan Josh, Patak's*	¼ Jar/173g	112	5	65	1.2	8	2.9	0
Rogan Josh, Sizzle, Spice, Patak's*	1 Jar/360g	310	14.8	86	1.2	10	4.1	0
Rogan Josh, Spice & Simmer, Asda*	1/3 Jar/120g	101	5.6	84	1.3	8.3	4.7	1.5
Saag Masala, 2 Step Cooking, Sainsbury's*	½ Jar/178g	141	6.4	79	2.1	7.8	3.6	3.3
Saag Masala, Cooking, Specially Selected, Aldi*	1/3 Jar/120g	90	4.6	75	1.6	7.4	3.8	2.6
Salted Caramel, Dipping, Waitrose*	1 Tsp/5g	21	1.2	425	2.4	46.4	24.5	4.4
Satay, Dipping, Inspired Cuisine, Aldi*	1 Tbsp/15g	28	1.6	188	5	17	11	1.5
Satay, Stir Fry, Tesco*	1 Pack/120g	144	7.4	120	3.3	11.6	6.2	1.9
Satay, Tesco*	1 Jar/180g	265	14	147	4.7	10.9	7.8	7.1
Saucy, Heinz*	1 Serving/10g	43	4.1	432	0.9	14.7	40.8	0
Sausage Casserole, Cook in, Homepride*	½ Jar/250g	92	0.5	37	0.7	8	0.2	0.6
Seafood, Average	***1 Tsp/5g***	***20***	***1.9***	***410***	***1.4***	***15.4***	***38***	***0.2***
Seafood, Colman's*	1 Tbsp/15g	44	3.4	296	0.9	21.5	22.9	0.4
Seafood, Ocean Spray*	¼ Jar/52g	180	16.6	346	1.5	17.7	32	0.5
Shepherds Pie, Homepride*	¼ Pie/122g	50	0.6	41	1.3	7.6	0.5	1.2
Soy & Ginger, Sticky, Sainsbury's*	¼ Jar/38g	54	0.8	143	1.7	29	2.2	0.5
Soy, & Garlic, Stir Fry, Fresh Tastes, Asda*	1 Pack/180g	175	6.7	97	1.7	14.1	3.7	0.5
Soy, & Chilli, M&S*	½ Pack/75g	70	0.1	93	0.9	21.9	0.1	0.5
Soy, & Garlic, Stir Fry, Asda*	½ Pack/85g	89	3	105	0.9	17	3.5	0.5
Soy, Average	***1 Tsp/5ml***	***3***	***0***	***64***	***8.7***	***8.3***	***0***	***0***
Soy, Dark, Average	***1 Tsp/5g***	***4***	***0***	***84***	***4***	***16.7***	***0.1***	***0.2***
Soy, Dark, Blue Dragon*	1 Serving/10ml	10	0	97	1.1	23	0.5	0
Soy, Dark, Premium, Lee Kum Kee*	1 Tbsp/15ml	22	0.1	148	6.1	31	0.5	0
Soy, Dark, Sainsbury's*	1 Tsp/5ml	6	0	123	0.8	29.2	0.5	1.2

S

	Measure INFO/WEIGHT	per Measure KCAL	FAT	Nutrition Values per 100g / 100ml KCAL	PROT	CARB	FAT	FIBRE
SAUCE								
Soy, Light, Amoy*	1 Tsp/5ml	3	0	52	2.5	10.5	0	0
Soy, Light, Premium, Lee Kum Kee*	1 Tbsp/15ml	14	0.1	92	7.7	14	0.5	0
Soy, Light, Sainsbury's*	1 Tsp/5ml	4	0	71	1.8	15.3	0.5	1.1
Soy, Reduced Salt, Amoy*	1 Tsp/5ml	3	0	56	4	10	0	0
Soy, Sushi & Sashimi, Kikkoman*	1 Tbsp/15ml	12	0	82	8.2	8.8	0	0
Spanish Chicken, Batts, Lidl*	½ Jar/250g	122	4.8	49	1.3	5.9	1.9	1.4
Spanish Chicken, Chicken Tonight, Knorr*	¼ Jar/125g	68	2	55	1.6	7.3	1.6	2.3
Spanish Style Chicken, Cooking, Lidl*	¼ Jar/125g	66	1.4	53	1.8	8.1	1.1	1.7
Spare Rib, Lee Kum Kee*	2 Tbsp/38g	80	1	211	2.6	39.5	2.6	2.6
Sriracha, Hot & Fiery, Sainsbury's*	1 Tsp/5g	3	0	69	0.8	13.6	0.9	1.6
Sriracha, M&S*	1 Tsp/5g	6	0	125	1.4	25.4	1	4.2
Sriracha, Thai Style, Oh So Delish, Aldi*	1 Pack/26g	109	3.4	420	11	60	13	9.3
Stir Fry, Firecracker, Spicy, Blue Dragon*	½ Sachet/60g	86	1.9	144	0.5	29	3.1	0
Stir Fry, Katsu Curry, M&S*	½ Pouch/75g	82	3.9	109	1.2	13.1	5.2	2.3
Stir Fry, Katsu, Aromatic, Blue Dragon*	1 Serving/60g	62	2.7	104	1	15	4.5	0
Stir Fry, Pad Thai, Passage To India *	¼ Pack/50g	55	0.2	110	1.1	25.1	0.3	0
Stir Fry, Sichuan Style, Hot & Spicy, Lee Kum Kee*	1 Jar/360g	457	19.1	127	3.6	13	5.3	0
Stir Fry, Sweet Chilli, Morrisons*	½ Pouch/60g	84	0.2	140	0.3	34	0.3	0.6
Stir Fry, Szechuan, Tomato, Blue Dragon*	1 Sachet/120g	143	3.2	119	1	22.4	2.7	0
Stir Fry, Vegetarian, Lee Kum Kee*	1 Serving/40g	53	0.2	133	1.3	32	0.5	0
Stroganoff, Cooking Sauce, Lloyd Grossman*	½ Pack/165g	203	14.8	123	1.6	8.6	9	0.7
Stroganoff, Cooking, Loyd Grossman*	½ Pack/165g	203	14.8	123	1.6	8.6	9	0.7
Stroganoff, Creamy, M&S*	1 Pouch/200g	190	15.2	95	0.6	4.6	7.6	1.8
Sun-Dried Tomato, & Basil, Stir in, M&S*	½ Pot/75g	106	9.2	141	1.4	3.9	12.3	4.7
Sweet & Sour, Cook In, Glass Jar, Homepride*	1 Jar/500g	335	0.5	67	0.3	16.2	0.1	0.5
Sweet & Sour, Spicy, Sharwood's*	1 Serving/138g	142	0.7	103	0.7	23.8	0.5	0.4
Sweet & Sour, Spicy, Uncle Ben's*	1 Jar/400g	364	0.4	91	0.6	22.1	0.1	0
Sweet & Sour, Take-Away	***1oz/28g***	***44***	***1***	***157***	***0.2***	***32.8***	***3.4***	***0***
Sweet & Sour, 30% Less Sugar, Sharwood's*	¼ Jar/104g	70	0.8	67	0.5	14.3	0.8	0.5
Sweet & Sour, Cooking, Asda*	1 Jar/500g	350	2.5	70	0.5	17	0.5	0.5
Sweet & Sour, Cooking, HL, Tesco*	½ Jar/250g	98	1	39	0.2	8.3	0.4	0.6
Sweet & Sour, Cooking, Tesco*	¼ Jar/127g	98	0.1	77	0.5	18.4	0.1	0.4
Sweet & Sour, Extra Pineapple, Uncle Ben's*	½ Jar/225g	164	0.4	73	0.3	16.9	0.2	0.8
Sweet & Sour, HFC, Tesco*	¼ Jar/110g	65	0.4	59	0.4	13	0.4	0.8
Sweet & Sour, Light, Uncle Ben's*	¼ Jar/125g	71	0.1	57	0.4	12.6	0.1	0.9
Sweet & Sour, M&S*	½ Jar/145g	144	1	99	1.1	22	0.7	0.5
Sweet & Sour, No Added Sugar, Uncle Ben's*	1 Jar/440g	123	0.4	28	0.4	5.5	0.1	0.8
Sweet & Sour, Sharwoods*	¼ Jar/105g	110	0.5	105	0.5	24.3	0.5	0.5
Sweet & Sour, Stir Fry, Pouch, Average	***1 Pouch/120g***	***148***	***2.3***	***124***	***0.8***	***25.7***	***1.9***	***1***
Sweet & Sour, Stir Fry, Sachet, Blue Dragon*	1 Sachet/120g	157	0.1	132	0.2	32.7	0.1	0.3
Sweet Chilli & Garlic, Stir Fry & Dipping, Tesco*	½ Jar/95ml	78	0	82	0.3	20.1	0	0.1
Sweet Chilli, Aromatic & Sweet, Waitrose*	½ Pouch/70g	58	0.4	83	0.9	18.1	0.5	1
Sweet Chilli, Dipping, M&S*	1 Tbsp/15g	34	0.1	225	0.9	53.2	0.7	0.6
Sweet Chilli, Dipping, Morrisons*	1 fl oz/30ml	64	0.6	212	0.4	47.3	2.1	1
Sweet Chilli, Dipping, Taste of Asia, Lidl*	1 Tbsp/15g	30	0	203	0.5	49.3	0.2	1.1
Sweet Chilli, Heinz*	1 Serving/25g	38	0.1	150	0.3	36.5	0.4	6.4
Sweet Chilli, Hot, Squeezy, Blue Dragon*	1 Serving/10ml	18	0.1	184	0.5	43.6	0.6	1.3
Sweet Chilli, M&S*	½ Pack/75g	72	0.3	96	0.8	21.9	0.4	0.8
Sweet Chilli, Stir Fry, Additions, Tesco*	1 Serving/50g	106	3.8	211	0.3	35.2	7.6	0.6
Sweet Chilli, Stir Fry, Tesco*	½ Pack/90g	100	1.4	111	0.4	23.8	1.5	0.6
Sweet Chilli, Szuchuan Inspired, Tesco*	¼ Jar/126g	106	0.5	84	0.4	19.2	0.4	1
Sweet Chilli, Thai, Blue Dragon*	1 Serving/15g	28	0.1	188	0.5	45.5	0.6	0
Sweet Curry, Eazy Squirt, Heinz*	1 Serving/10ml	12	0	124	0.7	29	0.3	0.5

	Measure INFO/WEIGHT	per Measure KCAL	FAT	Nutrition Values per 100g / 100ml KCAL	PROT	CARB	FAT	FIBRE
SAUCE								
Sweet Pepper, Stir in, Dolmio*	½ Pot/75g	77	4.6	103	1.4	9.6	6.2	1.6
Sweet Thai Chilli, Flavour Burst, Uncle Ben's*	1 Serving/75g	83	0.4	110	0.5	27	0.5	0.5
Szechuan Style, Stir Fry, Fresh Ideas, Tesco*	1 Sachet/50g	114	4.8	228	1.9	33.4	9.7	0.1
Szechuan, Spicy Tomato, Stir Fry, Blue Dragon*	½ Sachet/60g	59	1.8	98	1.3	15.8	3	0.9
Tamarind & Lime, Stir Fry, Sainsbury's*	1 Serving/75g	88	5.6	117	1.1	11.4	7.4	0.8
Tartare	***1oz/28g***	***84***	***6.9***	***299***	***1.3***	***17.9***	***24.6***	***0***
Tartare, Asda*	1 Tbsp/15g	48	5	323	1.1	5.6	33	1
Tartare, Batts, Lidl*	1 Tsp/5g	18	1.6	369	0.7	19.1	32.1	0.5
Tartare, Classic, Co-Op*	1 Tbsp/15g	52	4.6	349	1.1	16	31	0.4
Tartare, Colman's*	1 Tbsp/15g	45	3.7	290	1.5	17	24	0.6
Tartare, Finest, Tesco*	1 Tbsp/15g	47	4.7	312	1.3	5.7	31.1	2.1
Tartare, Maille*	1 Tsp/5g	29	3	574	1	7.1	61	0.5
Tartare, Mild & Creamy, Heinz*	1 Tbsp/15g	47	4.2	312	0.9	13.4	28.3	0.1
Tartare, Sainsbury's*	1 Tbsp/15ml	42	3.6	281	1.4	15.4	23.7	0.5
Tartare, Tesco*	1 Tbsp/15g	47	3.9	312	0.7	18.7	25.8	1.1
Teriyaki, Asda*	1 Serving/98g	99	0.1	101	2.1	23	0.1	0
Teriyaki, Deliciously Versatile, M&S*	1 Tbsp/15g	19	0.2	127	2.6	25.7	1.3	0
Teriyaki, Lee Kum Kee*	1 Serving/15g	27	0	178	2.2	42.4	0	0.5
Teriyaki, Rich & Savoury, Waitrose*	1 Serving/70g	122	0.4	174	0.5	42.6	0.5	0.5
Teriyaki, Sainsbury's*	1 Tbsp/15ml	31	0.1	209	1.6	49.2	0.5	1.8
Teriyaki, Sticky, Sainsbury's*	¼ Bottle/71g	81	0.4	113	1.1	26.3	0.5	1
Teriyaki, Stir Fry, Blue Dragon*	1 Pack/120g	131	0.2	109	0.9	25.9	0.2	0
Teriyaki, Stir Fry, Tesco*	½ Pack/90g	101	0.7	112	1.8	24.2	0.8	0.6
Teriyaki, Tesco*	1 Tsp/5ml	8	0	161	4	36	0.1	0
Thai Green Style, M&S*	½ Pack/75g	76	4.6	101	1.5	9.4	6.2	1
Thai Sweet Chilli, No Added Sugar, Blue Dragon*	1 Serving/25g	14	0.1	58	0.5	14	0.5	0
Tikka Masala, Cooking, HL, Tesco*	¼ Jar/125g	78	3.1	62	0.4	9	2.5	0.7
Tikka Masala, Cooking, Sainsbury's*	¼ Jar/125g	131	7.6	105	1.5	10.1	6.1	1.6
Tikka Masala, Cooking, Specially Selected, Aldi*	1/3 Jar/120g	113	6.5	94	1.4	6.9	5.4	2.2
Tikka Masala, Cooking, Tesco*	1 Jar/500g	430	21	86	1.2	10.5	4.2	0.9
Tikka Masala, Deluxe, Lidl*	1/3 Jar/116g	126	7.2	109	2.7	10	6.2	1.3
Tikka Masala, GFY, Asda*	½ Jar/250g	190	8	76	2.9	9	3.2	0.5
Tikka Masala, Low Fat, Tesco*	¼ Jar/125g	60	2.5	48	0.5	6.7	2	0.7
Tikka Masala, M&S*	½ Jar/170g	309	26.9	182	1.8	7.2	15.8	2
Tikka Masala, Medium, Cooking, Sharwood's*	1/3 Jar/140g	150	9.7	107	1.3	9.7	6.9	0.5
Tikka Masala, Mild, Low Fat, Morrisons*	¼ Jar/112g	73	2.5	65	1.3	9.3	2.2	1.4
Tikka Masala, Ready Made, Average	***1 Sm Jar/350g***	***422***	***28.8***	***121***	***2***	***9.6***	***8.2***	***1.2***
Tikka Masala, Sizzle & Spice, Pataks*	½ Jar/180g	220	13.7	122	1.5	11	7.6	0
Tikka, Low Fat, Cooking, Calorie Counted, Asda*	1 Jar/500g	255	10	51	0.9	7	2	0.8
Toffee, GFY, Asda*	1 Serving/5g	15	0.1	306	2.2	68	2.8	0
Tomato & Cheese, Pasta Bake, Dolmio*	¼ Jar/125g	70	1.5	56	2.1	9.1	1.2	1.2
Tomato & Marscapone, Finest, Tesco*	1 Serving/350g	270	17.5	77	2.7	5.4	5	0.8
Tomato & Mushroom, Pasta, Cucina, Aldi*	¼ Jar/125g	59	0.6	47	2	8.2	0.5	1.4
Tomato & Basil Sauce, Fresh, Tesco*	1 Pot/500g	245	9	49	1.5	6.8	1.8	0.8
Tomato & Basil, for Meatballs, Dolmio*	¼ Jar/125g	48	0.2	38	1.5	6.9	0.2	1.3
Tomato & Basil, Italian, Fresh, Asda*	½ Tub/175g	107	5.7	60	1.5	6.1	3.2	0.6
Tomato & Basil, Italian, Sainsbury's*	½ Pot/175g	88	3	50	1.9	6.2	1.7	1
Tomato, & Bacon, Pasta Bake, Aldi*	¼ Jar/123g	107	6.8	87	1.5	7.4	5.5	0.9
Tomato, & Basil, Rich & Herby, M&S*	½ Pot/175g	124	6.1	71	1.8	7.4	3.5	1.5
Tomato, & Chorizo, Stir in, Morrisons*	½ Pot/78g	68	4.1	87	2.4	7.3	5.2	0.5
Tomato, & Garlic, Stir In, Morrisons *	½ Pot/78g	62	3.2	80	1.9	7.9	4.1	1.7
Tomato, & Mascarpone, Vegan, Waitrose*	½ Pot/50g	49	3.4	98	1.9	7.3	6.7	0.5
Tomato, & Red Pepper, Extra Special, Asda*	½ Pot/175g	96	2.3	55	1.3	8.6	1.3	1.6

S

	Measure INFO/WEIGHT	per Measure KCAL	FAT	Nutrition Values per 100g / 100ml KCAL	PROT	CARB	FAT	FIBRE
SAUCE								
Tomato, Heinz*	1 Tbsp/17g	18	0	103	0.9	24.1	0.1	0.7
Tomato, Pomodorini, Finest, Tesco*	½ Pot/125g	79	3.9	63	1.2	5.8	3.1	3.7
Vindaloo, Hot, Patak's*	1 Jar/540g	518	34.6	96	1.5	6.4	6.4	0
Watercress, & Stilton, Creamy for Fish, Schwartz*	1 Pack/300g	141	12.3	47	0.6	2	4.1	0.7
Watercress, Creamy, Schwartz*	1 Serving/75g	49	3.3	65	0.5	5.5	4.4	0.5
Watercress, Sainsbury's*	1 Serving/100g	87	6.4	87	2.8	4.2	6.4	0.5
White Wine, & Cream, Cook in, Classic, Homepride*	¼ Can/125g	101	5.1	81	1	8	4.1	0.4
White, Savoury, Made with Semi-Skimmed Milk	***1oz/28g***	***36***	***2.2***	***128***	***4.2***	***11.1***	***7.8***	***0.2***
White, Savoury, Made with Whole Milk	***1oz/28g***	***42***	***2.9***	***150***	***4.1***	***10.9***	***10.3***	***0.2***
White, Vegan, Sacla*	1 Jar/350g	382	31.8	109	0.7	6.1	9.1	0
Worcestershire, Average	***1 Tsp/5g***	***3***	***0***	***65***	***1.4***	***15.5***	***0.1***	***0***
Yuzu, & Soy, Waitrose*	½ Pack/60g	68	0.3	113	1.9	25.1	0.5	0.9
SAUCE MIX								
Beef Bourguignon, Colman's*	1 Pack/40g	136	0.8	340	7	72	2	3
Beef Stroganoff, Colman's*	1 Pack/40g	140	3.6	350	11.6	56.1	8.9	2.7
Bolognese, As Prepared, Morrisons*	¼ Pack/283g	280	4	99	7.5	13.3	1.4	1.4
Bread, As Sold, M&S*	¼ Pack/18g	64	1.2	368	11.4	62.4	6.9	5.5
Bread, Made Up, Colman's*	1 Serving/75ml	70	1.5	95	5	14	2	0.6
Cheddar Cheese, Colman's *	1 Serving/75g	79	2.7	105	6.1	12	3.6	0.5
Cheddar Cheese, Colman's*	1 Pack/40g	164	6	410	19	51	15	2
Cheddar Cheese, Dry Mix, Schwartz*	1 Pack/40g	144	3	361	18.4	55.1	7.4	2.3
Cheese Flavour, Dairy Free, Free & Easy*	4 Teasp/15g	4	0.1	26	0.6	4.9	0.4	0.3
Cheese, Made Up with Skimmed Milk	***1 Serving/60g***	***47***	***1.4***	***78***	***5.4***	***9.5***	***2.3***	***0***
Chicken Chasseur, Schwartz*	1 Pack/40g	126	1.8	316	9.6	59.1	4.6	6.8
Chilli Con Carne, Asda*	1 Sachet/50g	157	0.8	314	7	68	1.6	2.5
Chilli Con Carne, Recipe Mix, Schwartz*	1 Pack/41g	133	1.5	324	8.2	60.8	3.6	0
Chip Shop Curry, Dry Weight, Bisto*	1 Dtsp/9g	38	1.6	427	3.4	63.5	17.7	1.3
Dauphinoise Potato Bake, Schwartz*	1 Pack/40g	161	10.5	402	6.8	34.7	26.3	15.8
Four Cheese, Colman's*	1 Pack/35g	127	3.9	362	17.1	48.4	11.1	1.8
Hollandaise, Colman's*	1 Pack/28g	104	3.1	372	6.4	61.6	11.1	1.8
Hollandaise, Made Up, Schwartz*	1 Serving/79g	58	2	73	3.9	8.7	2.5	0
Lemon Butter for Fish, Schwartz*	1 Pack/38g	136	3	357	6.1	65.3	8	5.8
Mushroom, Wild, Schwartz*	½ Sachet/15g	55	1.2	368	10.5	61.5	8.1	2.8
Paprika For Chicken, So Juicy, Maggi*	1 Pack/34g	91	1.4	267	8.8	45.5	4	7.1
Parsley & Chive for Fish, Schwartz*	1 Pack/38g	150	4.3	394	9.4	61.8	11.4	3.5
Parsley, Creamy, Made Up, Schwartz*	1 Serving/79g	59	2	75	4.2	8.7	2.5	0.3
Parsley, Elmwood, Co-Op*	1 Pack/21g	15	0.5	72	3.7	9.1	2.2	0.5
Parsley, Made Up, Bisto*	1 Serving/50ml	43	2.5	86	1	9.6	5	1
Peppercorn, Made Up with Water, CBY, Asda*	1 Serving/63ml	52	3.9	84	0.7	5.4	6.2	1.7
Peppercorn, Mild, Creamy, Schwartz*	1 Pack/25g	88	2.2	352	13.8	55	8.6	5
Peri-Peri, Medium, Nando's*	1 Serving/20g	9	0.7	45	0.7	1.1	3.4	0
Sausage Casserole, Schwartz*	1 Pack/35g	116	0.8	330	10	63.2	2.2	8.8
Savoury Mince, Schwartz*	1 Pack/35g	108	0.7	310	14.6	58.3	2	1.8
Shepherd's Pie, Schwartz*	1 Pack/38g	118	0.9	311	8.2	60.3	2.3	11.1
Spaghetti Bolognese, Colman's*	1 Pack/40g	120	0.4	300	8.9	64.1	0.9	5.2
Spaghetti Bolognese, Schwartz*	1 Pack/40g	114	0.6	285	9.2	59	1.6	7
Spaghetti Carbonara, Schwartz*	1 Pack/32g	135	6.4	421	10.4	49.4	20.1	7.2
Stroganoff, Beef, Schwartz*	1 Pack/35g	125	3.6	358	15.6	50.8	10.3	4.4
Stroganoff, Mushroom, Schwartz*	1 Pack/35g	121	3.1	345	10.9	52.4	8.9	5.9
White, Dry Weight, Bisto*	1 Dtsp/9g	45	2.5	496	3.2	57.4	28.2	0.4
White, Dry Weight, Sainsbury's*	1 Pack/25g	90	1.7	358	15.4	57.7	6.8	22
White, Made Up with Semi-Skimmed Milk	***1oz/28g***	***20***	***0.7***	***73***	***4***	***9.6***	***2.4***	***0***
White, Made Up with Skimmed Milk	***1oz/28g***	***17***	***0.3***	***59***	***4***	***9.6***	***0.9***	***0***

S

	Measure INFO/WEIGHT	per Measure KCAL	FAT	Nutrition Values per 100g / 100ml KCAL	PROT	CARB	FAT	FIBRE
SAUCE MIX								
White, Savoury, Colman's*	1 Pack/25g	105	3.8	420	9	63	15	2
SAUERKRAUT								
Average	***1oz/28g***	***3***	***0***	***11***	***1.1***	***1.6***	***0***	***0.9***
Tumeric, & Cumin, Slaw, Hurly Burly *	1 Serving/30g	10	0.1	32	1.5	4.7	0.2	2.8
SAUSAGE								
Beef, Average	***1 Sausage/60g***	***151***	***11.1***	***252***	***14.5***	***7***	***18.5***	***0.6***
Best Of British, Quorn*	1 Sausage/56g	115	5.8	206	15	10.4	10.4	5.4
Bockwurst, Average	***1 Sausage/45g***	***114***	***10.4***	***253***	***10.8***	***0.8***	***23***	***0***
Bratwurst, German, Morrisons*	1 Sausage/90g	279	25.5	310	12.7	0.8	28.3	0.5
Chicken, British, Tesco*	1 Sausage/57g	99	4.4	175	17.2	8.4	7.8	1.1
Chicken, Grilled, Brannans, Aldi*	1 Sausage/40g	84	5.6	210	14	7.3	14	0.7
Chicken, Italia, Grilled, Heck*	1 Sausage/34g	49	0.9	145	28.5	2.4	2.6	0
Chipolata, Average	***1 Chipolata/28g***	***81***	***6.5***	***291***	***12.1***	***8.7***	***23.1***	***0.7***
Chipolata, Chicken, Italian, Grilled, Heck*	2 Chipolatas/59g	76	2.3	129	21.5	1.6	3.9	0
Chipolata, Chicken, Paprika, Heck*	2 Chipolatas/60g	78	2	130	22	2.4	3.4	0
Chipolata, Chicken, Simply, Grilled, Heck*	2 Chipolatas/58g	77	2.3	133	22.2	1.8	3.9	0
Chipolata, Chicken, Tomato, & Basil, M&S*	2 Chipolatas/68g	116	7.1	170	14.2	3.7	10.4	2.4
Chipolata, Cumberland, Grilled, Morrisons*	1 Chipolata/27g	67	4.6	250	19.9	3.6	17.1	1
Chipolata, Pork, Black Pepper & Nutmeg, Waitrose*	1 Chipolata/22g	50	2.4	229	20	12.7	10.9	0.5
Chipolata, Pork, Chorizo, Specially Selected, Aldi*	2 Chipolatas/59g	182	14.8	308	14	5.6	25	1
Chipolata, Pork, Tomato, & Mozzarella, Morrisons*	1 Chipolata/26g	69	4.6	265	21.5	4.6	17.7	1.2
Chipolata, Pork, with Rosemary, & Thyme, Waitrose*	2 Chipolatas/46g	137	9.9	297	24.6	0.5	21.5	1
Chipolata, Premium, Average	***1 Chipolata/80g***	***187***	***13.8***	***234***	***14.8***	***4.7***	***17.3***	***1.2***
Chipolatas, Chicken, TTD, Sainsbury's*	2 Chipolata/49g	75	3.6	154	16.8	4.9	7.3	1
Chorizo Style, Bangrs, Grilled, Wicked Kitchen, Tesco*	2 Sausages/99g	152	4	154	11.5	15.2	4	5.8
Chorizo Style, Extra Special, Asda*	1 Sausage/57g	156	12.5	273	16	4	22	1.8
Chorizo, Average	***1 Serving/80g***	***250***	***19.4***	***313***	***21.1***	***2.6***	***24.2***	***0.2***
Chorizo, Lean, Average	***1 Sausage/67g***	***131***	***9.2***	***195***	***15.7***	***2.3***	***13.7***	***0.8***
Cocktail, Average	***1 Sausage/7g***	***23***	***1.9***	***323***	***12.1***	***8.6***	***26.7***	***0.9***
Cocktail, Veggie, Gosh!*	1 Serving/40g	96	5.1	241	6.4	21	12.9	7.2
Cumberland, Average	***1 Sausage/57g***	***167***	***13***	***293***	***13.8***	***8.6***	***22.8***	***0.8***
Cumberland, Cauldron Foods*	1 Sausage/46g	75	4	163	14	6.5	8.6	2
Cumberland, Meat Free, Quorn*	1 Sausage/47g	105	4.7	222	17.9	12.5	9.9	5.9
French, Garlic, Slices, Deli Special, Iceland*	1 Pack/90g	187	14	208	16.4	0.7	15.5	0
Garlic, Average	***1 Slice/11g***	***25***	***2***	***227***	***15.7***	***0.8***	***18.2***	***0***
Honey, & Mustard, Dinky, M&S*	1 Sausage/15g	42	3.1	277	15.1	8.2	20.2	1.1
Irish, Average	***1 Sausage/40g***	***119***	***8.3***	***298***	***10.7***	***17.2***	***20.7***	***0.7***
Lincolnshire, Average	***1 Sausage/42g***	***122***	***9.1***	***291***	***14.6***	***9.2***	***21.8***	***0.6***
Lincolnshire, Vegetarian, Grilled, Linda McCartney*	1 Sausage/50g	104	5.8	209	13.6	10.2	11.5	5
Lorne, Average	***1 Sausage/25g***	***78***	***5.8***	***312***	***10.8***	***16***	***23.1***	***0.6***
Meat Free, Green Cuisine, Birds Eye*	1 Sausage/60g	126	7.2	210	16	6.4	12	6
Meat Free, High Protein, Pan Fried, Heck*	2 Sausages/79g	77	1.1	97	6.6	11	1.4	7.2
Meat Free, Richmond*	2 Sausage/79g	115	4.3	145	8.8	14	5.4	3.6
Meat Free, Succulent, Green Cuisine, Birds Eye*	2 Sausages/100g	210	12	210	16	6.4	12	6
Meat Free, The Meatless Farm Co*	1 Sausage/50g	117	8	234	14.4	6.8	15.9	3.2
Merguez	***1 Merguez/55g***	***165***	***14.3***	***300***	***16***	***0.6***	***26***	***0***
Mushroom, & Leek, Bangers, Vegan, Waitrose*	2 Sausages/86g	95	2.1	111	6.8	13.3	2.4	4.4
Non-Meaty, Mighty, Oven Baked, Goodlife*	1 Sausage/39g	57	1.6	147	11.7	13.6	4	5.1
Patties, Breakfast, Iceland*	1 Pattie/48g	125	8.8	261	20.2	3.5	18.3	1
Pigs in Blankets , M&S*	1 Sausage/24g	72	6	300	15.3	3.6	24.9	0.1
Pigs In Blankets, Cooked, Sainsbury's*	1 Roll/15g	42	2.8	280	3.1	11.2	18.5	1
Pigs in Blankets, Morrisons*	2 Pigs/30g	84	5.9	279	22.4	3.2	19.6	0
Pigs In Blankets, Oven Baked, Iceland*	1 Pig/18g	42	2.5	236	20	6.7	13.8	2.3

S

	Measure	per Measure		Nutrition Values per 100g / 100ml				
	INFO/WEIGHT	KCAL	FAT	KCAL	PROT	CARB	FAT	FIBRE
SAUSAGE								
Pigs In Blankets, TTD, Sainsbury's*	2 Pigs/42g	77	4.9	183	16.9	1.9	11.7	1.2
Plant Based, Vegan, Moving Mountains*	1 Sausage/56g	140	7.6	250	14	6.7	13.6	5.6
Plant-Based, Brat, Original, Beyond Meat*	1 Sausage/76g	190	12	250	21	6.6	15.8	4
Polish Kabanos, Sainsbury's*	1 Sausage/25g	92	7.6	366	23	0.1	30.4	0.1
Pork & Beef, Average	***1 Sausage/45g***	***133***	***10.2***	***295***	***8.7***	***13.6***	***22.7***	***0.5***
Pork & Herb, Average	***1 Sausage/75g***	***231***	***19.5***	***308***	***13.2***	***5.4***	***26***	***0.4***
Pork & Tomato, Grilled, Average	***1 Sausage/47g***	***127***	***9.7***	***273***	***13.9***	***7.5***	***20.8***	***0.4***
Pork & Apple, Average	***1 Sausage/57g***	***146***	***10.7***	***256***	***14.5***	***7.5***	***18.8***	***1.9***
Pork, & Caramelised Onion, Grilled, Finest, Tesco*	2 Sausages/94g	291	22.8	309	13.5	9	24.2	0.7
Pork, & N'duja, Whorl, Waitrose*	1 Whorl/80g	224	17.5	280	15.5	4.2	21.9	2.1
Pork, Average	***1 Sausage/45g***	***139***	***11.2***	***309***	***11.9***	***9.8***	***25***	***0.8***
Pork, Battered, Thick, Average	***1oz/28g***	***126***	***10.2***	***448***	***17.3***	***21.7***	***36.3***	***2***
Pork, Chorizo, Mini, Sainsbury's*	2 Sausages/36g	166	14.4	458	19.7	4.5	39.8	1.6
Pork, Cocktail, Asda*	1 Sausage/10g	29	2.1	289	11	13	21	2.3
Pork, Extra Lean, Average	***1 Sausage/54g***	***84***	***3.7***	***155***	***17.3***	***6.1***	***6.8***	***0.8***
Pork, Firecracker, Grilled, TTD, Sainsbury's*	2 Sausages/106g	342	28.2	323	175	31	26.6	10
Pork, Frozen, Fried	***1oz/28g***	***88***	***6.9***	***316***	***13.8***	***10***	***24.8***	***0***
Pork, Frozen, Grilled	***1oz/28g***	***81***	***5.9***	***289***	***14.8***	***10.5***	***21.2***	***0***
Pork, Garlic & Herb, Average	***1 Sausage/76g***	***203***	***16.5***	***268***	***12***	***6***	***21.8***	***1.2***
Pork, GF, Finest, Tesco*	2 Sausages/102g	320	26.5	314	18.5	1.5	26	0.5
Pork, Italian Style, M&S*	1 Sausage/67g	149	11.9	222	13.1	1.7	17.8	1.2
Pork, Link, Simon Howie*	2 Sausages/42g	90	6	214	12.9	8.9	14.3	1.5
Pork, Premium, Average	***1 Sausage/74g***	***191***	***13.6***	***258***	***14.9***	***8.3***	***18.4***	***1***
Pork, Reduced Fat, Chilled, Grilled	***1 Sausage/45g***	***104***	***6.2***	***230***	***16.2***	***10.8***	***13.8***	***1.5***
Pork, Reduced Fat, Healthy Range, Average	***1 Sausage/57g***	***86***	***3.4***	***151***	***15.6***	***9***	***6***	***0.9***
Pork, Silesian, Dulano, Lidl*	1 Sausage/83g	198	14.9	239	16	3	18	0.5
Pork, Skinless, Average	***1oz/28g***	***81***	***6.6***	***291***	***11.7***	***8.2***	***23.6***	***0.6***
Pork, Square, Squig*	1 Square/85g	226	17	266	11.8	9.6	20	0
Pork, Thick, Average	***1 Sausage/39g***	***115***	***8.7***	***296***	***13.3***	***10***	***22.4***	***1***
Premium, Chilled, Fried	***1oz/28g***	***77***	***5.8***	***275***	***15.8***	***6.7***	***20.7***	***0***
Premium, Chilled, Grilled	***1oz/28g***	***82***	***6.3***	***292***	***16.8***	***6.3***	***22.4***	***0***
Red Pepper, & Butternut Squash, The Deli, Aldi*	1 Sausage/42g	50	0.6	118	4.8	18	1.4	6.8
Saveloy, Unbattered, Takeaway, Average	***1 Saveloy/65g***	***192***	***14.5***	***296***	***13.8***	***10.8***	***22.3***	***0.8***
Shroomdog, Cumberland, Plant Pioneers, Sainsbury's*	2 Sausages/88g	128	4	145	7.6	16.1	4.6	4.6
Shroomdogs, Chorizo, Plant Pioneers, Sainsbury's*	2 Sausages/66g	104	4.4	158	6	16	6.6	5.3
Smoked Pork, Reduced Fat, Mattessons*	1 Serving/50g	120	10	240	16	0	20	0
Smoked, Average	***1 Sausage/174g***	***588***	***52.2***	***338***	***13***	***4***	***30***	***0***
Soy, Little Willies, The Vegetarian Butcher*	3 Willies/80g	121	7	151	14.6	5.4	8.7	0.8
Tofu, Sizzlers, Tofoo Co.*	2 Sizzlers/125g	260	14.6	208	11.2	13.1	11.7	2.8
Toulouse, with Cannellini Bean Stew, Hello Fresh*	1 Serving/666g	553	15.1	83	4.8	10.5	2.3	0
Turkey & Chicken, Average	***1 Sausage/57g***	***126***	***8.2***	***222***	***14.4***	***8.2***	***14.6***	***1.8***
Turkey, Average	***1 Sausage/57g***	***90***	***4.6***	***157***	***15.7***	***6.3***	***8***	***0***
Turkey, Caramelised Red Onion, Sainsbury's*	2 Sausages/104g	165	6.5	158	18.3	6.9	6.2	0.5
Turkey, Low Fat, Mallons*	1 Sausage/39g	43	1.1	110	19	1.6	2.8	1.2
Vegan, Bangers, Herby, Grilled, Plant Chef, Tesco*	2 Sausages/91g	156	7.7	171	16.9	4	8.5	5.6
Vegan, Breakfast, Grilled, Heck*	2 Sausages/77g	112	6	146	5.5	8.1	7.8	10.3
Vegan, Cumberland Style, Bangers, Plant Chef, Tesco*	2 Sausages/103g	175	7.7	170	8.6	15.6	7.5	3
Vegan, Naked Glory*	2 Sausages/73g	111	4.1	152	9.9	14	5.6	3.9
Vegan, Smoked, Like Meat*	1 Sausage/25g	54	3	218	13	11	12	4.9
Vegetarian, Bangers, Quorn*	1 Sausage/50g	58	2.4	116	11.7	6.6	4.8	3
Vegetarian, Chorizo Puppies, Plant Kitchen, M&S*	2 Sausages/90g	164	10.9	182	6.7	7.5	12.1	7.9
Vegetarian, Chorizo, & Red Pepper, Linda McCartney*	2 Sausages/90g	142	5.8	158	14.1	8.1	6.4	6.2
Vegetarian, Cocktail, Quorn*	1 Sausage/15g	31	1.7	206	12.4	11.6	11.3	4.3

	Measure INFO/WEIGHT	per Measure KCAL	FAT	Nutrition Values per 100g / 100ml KCAL	PROT	CARB	FAT	FIBRE
SAUSAGE								
Vegetarian, Outrageously Succulent, Linda McCartney*	2 Sausages/84g	129	5.2	153	18.6	2.3	6.2	6.6
Vegetarian, Quorn*	1 Sausage/40g	79	4.5	198	11.2	10.6	11.1	5.5
Venison & Pork, Waitrose*	1 Sausage/64g	93	4	146	16.5	5.3	6.3	1.1
Wiejska, Polish, Sainsbury's*	1/8 Pack/50g	78	4.5	157	18.7	0.4	9	0.5
Wild Boar	***1 Sausage/85g***	***220***	***17***	***259***	***16.5***	***1.2***	***20***	***0***
SAUSAGE & MASH								
2 British Pork & Rich Onion Gravy, M&S*	1 Pack/400g	340	6.8	85	5.7	12.2	1.7	1.3
Bangers, Microwaved, Iceland*	1 Pack/500g	455	16.5	91	3	11.4	3.3	1.8
Bangers, Vegan, Plant Chef, Tesco*	1 Serving/397g	429	12.7	108	4	14.6	3.2	2.5
Classic Kitchen, Tesco*	1 Pack/450g	510	23.2	113	4	12	5.1	1.3
Cumberland, Finest, Tesco*	1 Pack/387g	712	46.8	184	7.5	10.2	12.1	1.6
Cumberland, Good Choice, Iceland*	1 Pack/460g	580	27.1	126	5.3	12.2	5.9	1.8
Frozen, HFC, Tesco*	1 Pack/380g	371	8.4	98	3.3	15.5	2.2	1.4
in Rich Onion Gravy, Tesco*	1 Serving/400g	392	12	98	3.6	13.5	3	1
Inspired Cuisine, Aldi*	1 Pack/435g	491	22.6	113	4.8	11	5.2	1.4
LC, Tesco*	1 Pack/400g	360	8.8	90	4.4	11.8	2.2	1.4
Shroomdogs, Plant Pioneers, Sainsbury's*	1 Pack/384g	353	8.1	92	3	14.1	2.1	1.9
with Onion Gravy, Bangers, British Classic, Sainsbury's*	1 Pack/450g	562	30.6	125	4.8	9.9	6.8	2.6
SAUSAGE MEAT								
Pork, Average	***1oz/28g***	***96***	***8.2***	***344***	***9.9***	***10.2***	***29.4***	***0.6***
Pork, British, Sainsbury's*	1 Serving/60g	143	9	239	14	12	15	0.5
Pork, with Black Pepper, & Nutmeg, Waitrose*	1/6 Pack/56g	137	10	245	15.9	4.8	17.8	0.8
SAUSAGE ROLL								
Artisan, Mini, Donald Russell*	1 Roll/58g	176	12.4	303	11.8	14.7	21.3	2.6
Bacon, & Cheddar, Smoked, M&S*	1 Roll/45g	167	10.7	372	13.8	24.9	23.8	1.4
Bacon, & Cheddar, Smoked, Vintage, Finest, Tesco*	1 Roll/47g	199	15.1	423	12.6	20.2	32.1	1.3
Best Ever, M&S*	1 Roll/80g	235	14.9	294	11.1	19.5	18.6	2.2
Cheese, & Bacon, Tesco*	1 Roll/60g	181	10.7	301	9.1	25.4	17.8	1.7
Chicken Style, Vegan, Fry's*	1 Roll/80g	274	16	342	10.6	31	20	4.1
Cocktail, Average	***1 Roll/15g***	***57***	***3.7***	***378***	***8.9***	***29.4***	***24.9***	***1.9***
Dinky, Hand Crafted, M&S*	1 Roll/15g	55	3.6	369	11.5	25.5	24.1	2.2
Eastmans, Tesco*	1 Roll/60g	179	9.6	299	7.5	30	16	2.6
Jumbo, Iceland*	1 Roll/117g	302	14.7	258	10.1	24.6	12.6	2.9
Jumbo, Sainsbury's*	1 Roll/145g	456	26.3	314	9.5	27.2	18.1	2.3
Kingsize, Pork Farms*	½ Roll/50g	241	15.9	483	10.5	39.9	31.8	0
Linda McCartney*	1 Roll/51g	145	8.2	287	10.9	22.7	16.2	3.8
Meat Free, Mini, Frys*	1 Roll/22g	73	3.7	325	12	31	16.3	3.3
Meat Free, No Porkies, Oven Baked, Iceland*	1 Roll/90g	271	15.6	301	9.3	25.1	17.3	4.2
Mini, Greggs, Iceland*	1 Roll/26g	72	4.4	277	7.8	23	17	0
Mini, Linda McCartney*	1 Roll/14g	41	2.2	293	11.3	23.7	15.8	5.2
Mini, M&S*	1 Roll/30g	112	8.2	373	9.5	21.7	27.2	1.6
Mini, Waitrose*	1 Roll/35g	124	9.2	353	13	16.1	26.3	1
No Pork, Vegan, Plant Menu, Aldi*	1 Roll/60g	169	7.8	281	7.1	33	13	4.1
No Sausage, Vegan, Mini, Plant Pioneers, Sainsbury's*	1 Roll/30g	84	4	279	6.3	31	13.4	4.6
Pork, & Cranberry, Higgidy*	1 Roll/26g	106	6.4	402	8.3	39.1	24.1	2
Pork, Allcroft's*	2 Rolls/100g	331	19.4	331	9.8	28.2	19.4	2
Pork, Bowyers*	1 Roll /45g	147	8.4	326	7	31.7	18.6	2.4
Pork, Cocktail, Asda*	2 Rolls/29g	86	4.3	298	8.3	31	15	2.3
Pork, Cocktail, Mini, M&S*	1 Roll/42g	152	9.9	361	11.1	25.5	23.5	1.6
Pork, Finest, Tesco*	1 Roll/47g	174	11.5	371	12.2	24.9	24.4	1.5
Pork, Mini, Tesco*	1 Roll/10g	37	2.2	374	10.2	32.6	22.1	1.9
Pork, Morrisons*	1 Roll/70g	195	9	278	9.6	31.2	12.8	1.5
Pork, TTD, Sainsbury's*	1 Roll/65g	242	16.8	372	11.5	22.9	25.8	1.1

S

	Measure INFO/WEIGHT	per Measure KCAL	FAT	Nutrition Values per 100g / 100ml KCAL	PROT	CARB	FAT	FIBRE
SAUSAGE ROLL								
Puff Pastry	***1 Roll/60g***	***230***	***16.6***	***383***	***9.9***	***25.4***	***27.6***	***1***
TTD, Sainsbury's*	1 Roll/27g	103	7	383	12.3	23.9	26.1	1.4
Vegan, Mae's Kitchen, Aldi*	1 Roll/90g	284	17.1	316	8.2	27	19	3.9
Vegan, No Pork, Plant Kitchen, M&S*	1 Roll/60g	180	10.9	300	9.7	22.8	18.2	3.7
Vegetarian, Chilled, Quorn*	1 Roll/70g	181	8.8	259	10.1	24.5	12.5	3.9
Vegetarian, Chilled, Single Pack, Quorn*	1 Roll/130g	292	12.1	225	12.3	21.2	9.3	3.8
SCALLOPS								
& Prawns, King, in Creamy Lobster Sauce, Sainsbury's*	1 Dish/112g	204	14.4	182	12.3	4	12.9	0.5
Coquilles St Jacques, M&S*	1 Serving/150g	177	9.2	118	6.5	8.9	6.1	0.9
Raw, Bay or Sea with Roe, Average	***1 Scallop/15g***	***13***	***0.1***	***88***	***16.8***	***2.4***	***0.8***	***0***
Steamed, Average	***1oz/28g***	***33***	***0.4***	***118***	***23.2***	***3.4***	***1.4***	***0***
SCAMPI								
& Chips, with Peas	***1 Serving/490g***	***822***	***43.6***	***168***	***10.1***	***11.3***	***8.9***	***1.2***
Bites, Breaded, Oven Baked, Whitby Seafoods*	1 Serving/100g	225	9.7	225	9.7	24	9.7	1.4
Bites, Everyday, Value, Tesco*	½ Pack/125g	262	10	210	9.4	23.4	8	1.2
Bites, Vegetarian, Linda McCartney*	½ Pack/125g	279	11.5	223	14.7	18.3	9.2	3.7
Breaded, Baked, Average	***½ Pack/255g***	***565***	***27.4***	***222***	***10.7***	***20.5***	***10.7***	***1***
Breaded, Co-Op*	1 Pack/200g	428	18.4	214	8.2	24	9.2	0.9
Breaded, Free From, Tesco*	½ Pack/101g	192	7.2	190	15.6	15.1	7.1	1.6
Breaded, Fried in Oil, Average	***1 Serving/100g***	***237***	***13.6***	***237***	***9.4***	***20.5***	***13.6***	***0***
Popcorn, Bites, Oven Bites, Youngs*	½ Pack/91g	218	11.8	240	7.8	22.1	13	1.6
White Tail, Aldi*	½ Pack/125g	256	9.6	205	10	23	7.7	2.4
Wholetail, Breaded, Fresh, Waitrose*	1 Serving/81g	176	7.9	217	13.6	17.9	9.7	1.7
Wholetail, Breaded, Ocean Sea, Lidl*	1 Serving/100g	214	9.6	214	9.2	22	9.6	1.6
Wholetail, Deluxe, Lidl*	½ Pack/101g	262	12.1	259	12.5	23.9	12	2.9
Wholetail, in Breadcrumb Coating, Morrisons*	½ Pack/113g	244	8.7	216	11	24.5	7.7	2.5
Wholetail, Jumbo, Chilled, Whitby Seafoods*	½ Pack/100g	201	7	201	9.6	24.2	7	1.4
Wholetail, Jumbo, Gastro, Youngs*	½ Pack/115g	238	9.5	207	11.3	21.1	8.3	1.3
SCONE								
All Butter, & Cherry, Finest, Tesco*	1 Scone/70g	245	7.2	349	7.1	56	10.3	1.9
All Butter, Finest, Tesco*	1 Scone/70g	258	10.5	369	7.5	50.1	15	1.8
All Butter, Sultana, TTD, Sainsbury's*	1 Scone/70g	241	7	344	7.7	54	10	3.7
All Butter, Tesco*	1 Scone/60g	222	7.6	371	6.4	56.7	12.7	2
All Butter, Waitrose*	1 Scone/75g	237	7.3	316	8.7	47.2	9.7	2.5
Buttermilk, M&S*	1 Scone/70g	258	10.8	368	7.4	49.1	15.4	1.9
Cheddar, Cheese, Farmhouse, TTD, Sainsbury's*	1 Scone/70g	235	9.7	335	12	39.4	13.8	2.8
Cheese & Black Pepper, Mini, M&S*	1 Scone/18g	67	3.3	370	10.2	41.1	18.3	1.7
Cheese, Average	***1 Scone/40g***	***145***	***7.1***	***363***	***10.1***	***43.2***	***17.8***	***1.6***
Cherry, M&S*	1 Scone/60g	202	7.3	337	6.9	49.7	12.2	1.9
Clotted Cream, Cornish, TTD, Sainsbury's*	1 Scone/70g	269	12.7	384	8.4	46.6	18.2	2.1
Cream, Mini, Co-Op*	1 Scone/24g	86	4.1	360	6.8	44	17	1.1
Devon, M&S*	1 Scone/59g	225	9.6	380	7.1	50.8	16.2	1.5
Fresh Cream with Strawberry Jam, Tesco*	1 Scone/88g	299	12.9	340	6.3	44.7	14.7	1.8
Fruit, Average	***1 Scone/40g***	***126***	***3.9***	***316***	***7.3***	***52.9***	***9.8***	***0***
Plain, All Butter, Sainsbury's*	1 Scone/58g	213	7.4	366	8.1	54.1	12.7	1.6
Plain, Average	***1 Scone/40g***	***145***	***5.8***	***362***	***7.2***	***53.8***	***14.6***	***1.9***
Potato, Average	***1 Scone/40g***	***118***	***5.7***	***296***	***5.1***	***39.1***	***14.3***	***1.6***
Red Berry, Mixed, Finest, Tesco*	1 Scone/110g	344	9.5	313	7.8	50.1	8.6	1.9
Specially Selected, Aldi*	1 Scone/65g	226	6.2	347	8.9	55	9.5	2.5
Strawberry, Fresh Cream, BGTY, Sainsbury's*	1 Scone/50g	154	5.6	309	5.1	47	11.2	1.1
Sultana, All Butter, Aldi*	1 Scone/75g	254	5.4	339	7.5	60	7.2	2.2
Sultana, All Butter, Tesco*	1 Scone/60g	216	6.5	360	4.6	59.1	10.9	3.5
Sultana, All Butter, The Best, Morrisons*	1 Scone/67g	222	6.4	332	7.4	52.5	9.5	3.5

	Measure INFO/WEIGHT	per Measure KCAL	FAT	Nutrition Values per 100g / 100ml KCAL	PROT	CARB	FAT	FIBRE
SCONE								
Sultana, Finest, Tesco*	1 Scone/70g	238	7.6	340	8.9	50.9	10.9	2.1
Sultana, H.W. Nevill's*	1 Scone/41g	136	3.1	334	6.8	58.6	7.5	2.3
Sultana, M&S*	1 Scone/66g	231	8.2	350	6.5	53	12.5	2
Sultana, Tesco*	1 Scone/90g	304	6.8	338	7.2	59.5	7.6	1.6
Sultana, Value, Tesco*	1 Scone/40g	134	4	335	6.5	53.8	10.1	2.7
Tattie, Scottish, Tesco*	1 Scone/33g	89	1.2	269	5.6	53.3	3.7	2.2
Wholemeal	***1 Scone/40g***	***130***	***5.8***	***326***	***8.7***	***43.1***	***14.4***	***5.2***
Wholemeal, Fruit	***1 Scone/40g***	***130***	***5.1***	***324***	***8.1***	***47.2***	***12.8***	***4.9***
SEA BASS								
Butterflied, Fishmonger, Aldi*	1 Pack/180g	284	13.1	158	23	0.5	7.3	0.5
Cooked, Dry Heat, Average	***1 Fillet/100g***	***124***	***2.6***	***124***	***23.6***	***0***	***2.6***	***0***
Fillet, Lemon & Pepper, Tesco*	½ Pack/82g	180	12.4	220	19.4	1	15.1	1.7
Fillets, Caramelised Ginger & Lime Butter, Sainsbury's*	1 Fillet/115g	258	18.1	224	19.9	0.5	15.7	0.5
Fillets, Large, Frozen, Iceland*	1 Fillet/140g	235	13.7	168	20	0	9.8	0
Fillets, Lemon & Herb, Market St, Morrisons*	½ Pack/90g	197	12.2	219	23.3	0.5	13.6	0.6
Fillets, with Butter, Cooked, Tesco*	1 Fillet/86g	189	13	220	19.4	1	15.1	1.7
Fillets, With Rocket Pesto Butter, Waitrose*	½ Pack/95g	220	15.4	232	20.1	1.2	16.2	0.5
Raw, Fillet, Average	***1 Fillet/95g***	***108***	***3.4***	***113***	***20.3***	***0***	***3.5***	***0.1***
SEA BREAM								
Butterflied, Pan Fried, Sainsbury's*	1 Fillet/116g	252	13.9	217	25	1.6	12	0.6
Fillet, Cooked, Dry Heat, Average	***1 Serving/100g***	***124***	***3***	***124***	***24***	***0***	***3***	***0***
Fillets, Raw, Average	***1oz/28g***	***27***	***0.8***	***96***	***17.5***	***0***	***2.9***	***0***
Fillets, with Rocket Pesto Butter, Waitrose*	1 Fillet/87g	220	15.4	253	22.7	0.5	17.7	0.5
SEAFOOD								
& Prawn Cocktail, Deli Filler, Waitrose*	½ Tub/100g	199	15.5	199	5.8	9	15.5	0.5
Cocktail, Average	***1oz/28g***	***24***	***0.4***	***87***	***15.6***	***2.9***	***1.5***	***0***
Mix, Cooked, Iceland*	1 Pack/500g	440	7	88	15.1	3.8	1.4	0.1
Selection, Fresh, Tesco*	1 Pack/234g	187	2.3	80	17.7	0.1	1	0
Selection, Ready to Eat, Asda*	1 Pack/240g	230	5.8	96	12	6.5	2.4	0.5
Selection, Sainsbury's*	½ Pack/100g	75	1	75	15.2	1.3	1	0.5
Shells, Waitrose*	1 Shell/60g	86	4.7	143	16.2	1.6	7.9	0
SEAFOOD STICKS								
Average	***1 Stick/15g***	***16***	***0***	***106***	***8***	***18.4***	***0.2***	***0.2***
SEASONING MIX								
Butter Chicken, as Sold, Maggi*	1 Pack/46g	172	4	373	6	65.5	8.8	4
Chicken Casserole, Newgate, Lidl*	½ Pack/19g	58	0.4	305	7.5	61.9	1.9	5.3
Chicken, Lemon & Herb, Tray Bake, Schwartz*	1 Serving/110g	352	3.1	320	7.7	60.9	2.8	10.1
Chicken, Provencal Herb, Tray Bake, Schwartz*	1 Pack/30g	89	0.6	296	9.3	55.3	2	9.9
Chinese Marinade, Flava it*	1 Serving/8g	28	0.1	349	1.4	83.7	0.8	1.1
Cottage Pie, GF, Schwartz*	1 Pack/30g	91	0.6	302	10.2	59	1.9	0
Cumin, & Chipotle, Fajita Mix, Capsicana*	1 Bag/28g	82	2.3	294	10.5	51.3	8.2	0
Dukkah, Cooks' Ingredients, Waitrose*	1 Serving/5g	19	0.8	388	18.3	30.7	17	19.6
Fajita, Original, Mild, Latin American Kitchen, Santa Maria*	¼ Sachet/7g	20	0.4	283	8.6	46	5	11
Fajita, Schwartz*	1 Serving/5g	14	0.2	278	7.5	55	4.2	0
Fajitas, Smoky BBQ, Old El Paso*	1 Pack/35g	110	0.5	313	6.3	67.2	1.3	3.5
Fish Pie, Colman's*	1 Pack/20g	65	0.3	326	9.8	64	1.4	3.6
Garlic, Papyrus Sheets, SoTender, Maggi*	1 Sheet/6g	25	1.9	438	6.3	24.4	32.5	11.4
Italian Herb, Schwartz*	1 Tsp/1g	3	0	338	11	64.5	4	0
Italian Herbs, Papyrus Sheets, SoTender, Maggi*	1 Sheet/6g	26	2	440	7.3	22.1	34.1	7.7
Jamaican Jerk Chicken, Recipe, Schwartz*	1 Pack/27g	75	0.8	276	9.8	69.8	3	17.2
Katsu, Street Food, Schwartz*	1 Pack/15g	44	0.6	294	10.9	49.9	3.8	0
Lamb Hot Pot, Colman's*	¼ Pack/10g	32	0.2	320	12	61	1.5	4
Lasagne, Schwartz*	1 Pack/35g	116	0.4	330	6.9	71	1.2	3.6

S

	Measure INFO/WEIGHT	per Measure KCAL	FAT	Nutrition Values per 100g / 100ml KCAL	PROT	CARB	FAT	FIBRE
SEASONING MIX								
Lemon & Herb, for Chicken, Cook in Bag, Average	***1 Bag/34g***	***121***	***1.9***	***356***	***10.8***	***63.7***	***5.5***	***4.1***
Lemon, & Pepper, Maggi*	1 Pack/80g	250	1.6	313	8.3	62.5	2	7.6
Mediterranean Chicken, Season & Shake, Colman's*	1 Pack/33g	99	0.7	300	10.3	56.8	2.1	5.9
Mediterranean, for Chicken, Cook in Bag, Average	***1 Bag/33g***	***99***	***0.7***	***302***	***10.6***	***56.6***	***2***	***7***
Mexican Chicken, As Sold, So Juicy, Maggi*	1 Pack/40g	123	1.7	308	7.4	57.2	4.2	6
Paprika, for Chicken, Cook in Bag, Average	***1 Bag/34g***	***96***	***1.3***	***283***	***12.3***	***45.8***	***4***	***8.1***
PIri Piri, Smoky & Aromatic, Maggi*	1 Pack/27g	87	1.4	324	6.9	58	5	9.7
Potato Wedges, Garlic & Herb, Schwartz*	1 Pack/38g	106	1.9	278	11.4	47.1	4.9	11.7
Roast Chicken, Garlic & Herb, Schwartz*	1 Tsp/3g	8	0.2	280	11.5	40.1	6.2	8.6
Satay, Globo*	1 Serving/25g	103	2.4	413	9.3	70	9.8	4
Shepherds Pie, Colman's*	1 Pack/50g	158	0.8	315	12	60	1.6	5.4
Smoked Paprika Chicken, As Sold, Schwartz*	1 Pack/28g	87	1.6	309	10.3	44.4	5.7	0
Spaghetti Bolognese, Bramwells, Aldi*	1 Sachet/44g	132	2	300	10.9	57.3	4.6	7.3
Sweet Chilli, for Chicken, Bake in Bag, Colman's*	1 Pack/45g	162	0.9	360	1.5	82	2	2
Taco, Old El Paso*	¼ Pack/9g	30	0.4	334	5.5	69	4	0
Takeaway, Classic Flavour, Spice Bag, McDonnell's*	1 Tbsp/15g	29	1	192	18.2	9.1	7	0
SEAWEED								
Crispy, Average	***1oz/28g***	***182***	***17.3***	***651***	***7.5***	***15.6***	***61.9***	***7***
Laverbread, Selwyn's*	1 Serving/10g	3	0	28	3.3	1.3	0.4	0
Nori, Dried, Raw	***1oz/28g***	***38***	***0.4***	***136***	***30.7***	***0***	***1.5***	***44.4***
Seaveg, Crispies, Clearspring*	1 Pack/4g	18	1.2	462	30	0.1	31	31
Wakame, Dried, Raw	***1oz/28g***	***20***	***0.7***	***71***	***12.4***	***0***	***2.4***	***47.1***
SEED MIX								
3, Toasted, Tesco*	1 Serving/25g	141	11.5	562	26	1.4	45.9	19.8
Chia & Flaxseed, Sprinkles, Tesco*	1 Serving/26g	135	9.2	518	24.2	15.9	35.3	20.2
Choccy Ginger, Munchy Seeds*	1 Pack/25g	120	7.8	481	9.1	44	31	3.4
Four, Whitworths*	1 Serving/25g	141	11.8	565	26.8	1.4	47.2	14.5
Omega, Morrisons*	¼ Pack/25g	138	11.4	554	20.9	15	45.6	6.4
Omega, Munchy Seeds*	1 Bag/30g	184	14.9	613	28.4	13.1	49.7	2.2
Pumpkin, & Sunflower, Holland & Barrett*	1 Serving/30g	171	13.8	570	22	17	46	5.6
Salad Topper, Lite, Natursource*	¼ Cup/28g	157	10.4	561	17	37	37	6
Seven, Tamari Mix, Munchy Seeds*	1 Serving/30g	172	14.4	575	22	18	48	8
Super Seeds, Salad Topper, Good4U*	1 Serving/25g	144	11.2	575	30	7	45	10
The Foodie Market, Aldi*	1 Serving/30g	172	13.8	575	23	12	46	8.7
Warm Cinnamon, Munchy Seeds*	1 Pack/25g	129	9	516	16	34	36	6.3
SEEDS								
Chia, Bio, Chia Direct*	1 Tbsp/15g	69	4.7	460	21.2	3.8	31.4	33.7
Chia, Black, The Chia Co*	1 Tbsp/15g	67	5.2	447	20	45	35	37
Chia, Clever, Holland & Barrett*	1 Tbsp/15g	74	4.6	490	18	6	31	38
Chia, Milled, Mix, Natural Selection*	1 Tbsp/15g	80	6.3	530	24	5.4	42	19
Chia, Organic, BuyWholeFoodsOnline*	1 Tsp/5g	22	1.6	436	20	2	31	37.9
Chia, Organic, Sevenhills Wholefoods*	1 Tbsp/15g	66	4.3	437	22.1	6.7	28.8	31.3
Chia, Sainsbury's*	1 Tbsp/15g	62	3.8	414	21.8	8.6	25	33.6
Chia, Tesco*	1 Tbsp/15g	64	4.3	428	22.3	2.6	28.8	34.7
Chia, White, The Chia Co*	1 Tbsp/15g	67	4.7	447	20.7	4.7	31.3	37.3
Chironji, Raw, Average	***1 Serving/10g***	***7***	***0.6***	***66***	***1.9***	***1.2***	***5.9***	***0.4***
Fiery, Graze*	1 Pack/34g	173	14.8	510	21.8	17.3	43.5	7.9
Flaxseed, Sunflower & Pumpkin, Milled, Linwoods*	1 Scoop/10g	54	4.9	542	22.7	2.4	49.1	16.2
Hemp, Hulled, Ceres Organic*	1 Tsp/5g	30	2.6	600	32.1	0.9	51.7	0
Hemp, Shelled, Linwoods*	2 Tbsps/30g	178	14.8	593	35.1	7.6	49.5	5.9
Milled, with Flax, & Chia, Tesco*	1 Tbsp/15g	85	6.7	567	26.4	6.4	44.8	16.4
Mixed, Wholesome, Love Life, Waitrose*	1 Serving/30g	166	13.6	554	21.3	15.5	45.2	8
Mixed, with Salted Caramel, Whitworths*	1 Serving/25g	148	11.9	591	26.8	10.7	47.6	6.4

S

	Measure INFO/WEIGHT	per Measure KCAL	FAT	Nutrition Values per 100g / 100ml KCAL	PROT	CARB	FAT	FIBRE
SEEDS								
Mustard, Average	***1 Tsp/3.3g***	***15***	***0.9***	***469***	***34.9***	***34.9***	***28.8***	***14.7***
Nigella, Average	***1 Tsp/5g***	***20***	***1.7***	***392***	***21.3***	***1.9***	***33.3***	***8.4***
Phool Makhana, Raw, Average	***1 Serving/10g***	***35***	***0***	***350***	***9.7***	***77***	***0.1***	***7.6***
Poppy, Average	***1 Tbsp/9g***	***47***	***3.9***	***533***	***18***	***23.7***	***44.7***	***10***
Pumpkin, & Sunflower, Toasted, Sainsbury's*	1 Serving/10g	64	5.6	643	28	1.9	56	9.8
Pumpkin, Average	***1 Tbsp/10g***	***57***	***4.6***	***568***	***27.9***	***13***	***45.9***	***3.8***
Sesame, Average	***1 Tsp/2g***	***12***	***1.1***	***610***	***22.3***	***3.6***	***56.4***	***7.8***
Sesame, Black, Sainsbury's*	1 Tsp/5g	30	2.6	593	21.4	1.8	52.6	13.6
Sesame, Snappy, Holland & Barrett*	1 Pack/300g	1794	174	598	18	0.9	58	7.9
Sesame, White, M&S*	1 Tsp/5g	31	2.9	615	18.3	0.9	58	8.3
Sunflower, Average	***1 Tbsp/10g***	***59***	***4.9***	***585***	***23.4***	***15***	***48.7***	***5.7***
SEMOLINA								
Average	***1oz/28g***	***98***	***0.5***	***348***	***11***	***75.2***	***1.8***	***2.1***
Pudding, Creamed, Ambrosia*	1 Can/425g	344	7.2	81	3.3	13.1	1.7	0.2
Pudding, Creamed, Co-Op*	1 Can/425g	382	8.5	90	4	15	2	0
SHALLOTS								
Pickled in Hot & Spicy Vinegar, Tesco*	1 Onion/18g	14	0	77	1	18	0.1	1.9
Pickled, Drained, Garners*	1 Shallot/15g	15	0.1	97	1	21.6	0.5	2.5
Raw, Average	***1 Serving/80g***	***16***	***0.2***	***20***	***1.5***	***3.3***	***0.2***	***1.4***
SHANDY								
Bitter, Original, Ben Shaws*	1 Can/330ml	89	0	27	0	6	0	0
Canned, Morrisons*	1 Can/330ml	36	0	11	0	1.8	0	0
Homemade, Average	***1 Pint/568ml***	***148***	***0***	***26***	***0.2***	***2.9***	***0***	***0***
Lager, 0.9%, Bavaria*	1 Can/330ml	76	0	23	0.1	5	0	0
Lemonade, Traditional Style, Tesco*	1 Can/330ml	63	0	19	0	4.7	0	0
Panache, Carrefour*	1 Bottle/250ml	68	0	27	0.5	6.3	0	0
SHARON FRUIT								
Average	***1oz/28g***	***19***	***0***	***68***	***0.7***	***17.3***	***0***	***1.5***
SHERRY								
Dry, Average	***1 Glass/120ml***	***139***	***0***	***116***	***0.2***	***1.4***	***0***	***0***
Medium	***1 Serving/50ml***	***58***	***0***	***116***	***0.1***	***5.9***	***0***	***0***
Sweet	***1 Serving/50ml***	***68***	***0***	***136***	***0.3***	***6.9***	***0***	***0***
SHORTBREAD								
All Butter, Deans*	1 Biscuit/15g	77	3.8	511	4.9	65.7	25.4	1.2
All Butter, Deluxe, Lidl*	1 Biscuit/20g	103	5.3	517	4.3	64.9	26.5	1
All Butter, Finger, Highland, TTD, Sainsbury's*	1 Biscuit/20g	103	5.5	515	4.6	61.8	27.4	1.2
All Butter, Fingers, Highland, Sainsbury's*	2 Biscuits/40g	208	11.5	521	4.8	59.4	28.8	2.7
All Butter, Giant, Fingers, Higland, Sainsbury's*	1 Biscuit/35g	182	10.1	520	4.8	59.4	28.8	1.8
All Butter, Petticoat Tails, Co-Op*	1 Biscuit/13g	68	3.8	520	5	60	29	2
All Butter, Round, Luxury, M&S*	1 Biscuit/20g	105	5.8	525	6.2	60	29	2
All Butter, Selection, Waitrose*	1 Biscuit/18g	95	11	527	5.3	58.3	61.1	3
All Butter, Trufree*	1 Biscuit/11g	58	3.1	524	2	66	28	0.9
All Butter, with Toffee, Scottish, M&S*	1 Biscuit/6g	32	1.7	515	5.7	61.9	26.9	1.2
Average	***1oz/28g***	***139***	***7.3***	***498***	***5.9***	***63.9***	***26.1***	***1.9***
Belgian Chocolate Chunk, Asda*	1 Biscuit/20g	106	6.2	531	7	56	31	1.8
Choc Chip, Fair Trade, Co-Op*	1 Biscuit/19g	100	6	526	5.3	57.9	31.6	2.6
Chocolate Chip, Jacob's*	1 Biscuit/17g	87	4.7	513	5.2	61.2	27.5	1.8
Chocolate, Belgian, Chunky, TTD, Sainsbury's*	1 Piece/70g	353	19	505	5.5	58.8	27.2	1.4
Chocolate, Triple, Finest, Tesco*	1 Square/63g	325	18.5	516	5.8	56.3	29.4	1.5
Clotted Cream, Finest, Tesco*	1 Biscuit/20g	109	6.4	543	5.2	58	32.2	1.7
Demerara, Rounds, TTD, Sainsbury's*	1 Biscuit/22g	113	5.9	508	5.1	62.2	26.5	1.8
Fingers, Asda*	1 Finger/18g	93	5.1	519	5.8	60.3	28.3	18
Fingers, Clotted Cream, Paterson's*	1 Finger/15g	76	3.8	507	6.4	62.4	25.3	0

S

	Measure INFO/WEIGHT	per Measure KCAL	FAT	Nutrition Values per 100g / 100ml KCAL	PROT	CARB	FAT	FIBRE
SHORTBREAD								
Fingers, Highland Speciality*	1 Finger/10g	49	2.3	488	5.9	66.1	23	0
Fingers, Scottish, Finest, Tesco*	1 Finger/21g	104	5	498	5.1	65.5	23.9	2
Lavender, Waitrose*	1 Biscuit/53g	282	14.8	532	5.5	63.5	28	2
Millionaire, Salted Caramel, M&S*	1 Slice/55g	261	12.5	475	4	63	22.7	1.2
Millionaire, Squares, Free From, Asda*	1 Square/30g	153	8.4	510	2.9	60	28	1.7
Mini Bites, Co-Op*	1 Biscuit/10g	53	3	530	7	59	30	2
Mini, Bites, Tesco*	1 Bite/12g	63	3.5	528	7.2	58.1	29.3	1.3
Oatflake, Sinclair Of Rhynie*	1 Biscuit/23g	112	6.6	486	4.6	53.6	28.8	2.2
Pecan All Butter, Sainsbury's*	1 Biscuit/18g	99	6.5	548	5.3	49.9	36.3	2.5
Petticoat Tails, All Butter, Highland, Sainsbury's*	1 Biscuit/12g	65	3.6	521	6.3	58	28.8	2.2
Pure Butter, GF, Walkers*	1 Biscuit/16g	83	4.4	518	3.6	63.5	27.4	1.3
Pure Butter, Scottie, Mini, Walkers*	1 Scottie/3g	15	0.8	509	5.8	63.3	25.3	2.3
Rings, Handbaked, Border*	1 Biscuit/17g	86	4.9	520	6.2	61.2	29.5	0
Rose Petal, & Chinese Tea, 1, Waitrose*	1 Biscuit/10g	53	2.9	527	5.8	59.6	29	2.1
Rounds, All Butter, Toffee & Pecan, M&S*	1 Biscuit/20g	111	7	553	4.7	54.1	34.9	2
Salted Caramel, Scottish, Morrisons*	1 Biscuit/20g	106	6.1	530	5.5	57.5	30.5	2
Stem Ginger, All Butter, Duchy, Waitrose*	1 Biscuit/13g	65	3.2	502	5	63.4	25	1.7
Wheat & GF, Free From Range, Tesco*	1 Shortbread/18g	93	4.9	521	5.4	61.7	27.6	1.9
SHORTCAKE								
Caramel, Baked in the Tray, Tesco*	1 Slice/49g	247	13.2	504	3.4	61.6	26.9	1.1
Caramel, Mini, Thorntons*	1 Piece/14g	69	4.1	491	5	50.6	29.5	0
Caramel, Slice, Holly Lane, Aldi*	1 Slice/50g	252	14	503	5.4	57	28	1.7
Caramel, Slices, Sainsbury's*	1 Slice/33g	162	8.4	491	5.3	59.6	25.5	1.3
Squares, Caramel, Tesco*	1 Slice/25g	127	7.7	506	6.3	54.3	30.7	2.4
SHRIMP								
Boiled, Average	***1 Serving/60g***	***70***	***1.4***	***117***	***23.8***	***0***	***2.4***	***0***
Frozen, Average	***1oz/28g***	***20***	***0.2***	***73***	***16.5***	***0***	***0.8***	***0***
in Tomato Sauce, Arbi*	1 Pack/300g	504	41.1	168	10	0.9	13.7	0.5
Panko Breaded, Kirkland Signature, Costco*	1 Shrimp/26g	62	3.4	240	12.7	17	13.2	1.1
Shredded, Jeeny's*	1 Pack/30g	81	0.3	269	30.1	35.2	0.9	0
SKATE								
Grilled	***1oz/28g***	***22***	***0.1***	***79***	***18.9***	***0***	***0.5***	***0***
in Batter, Fried in Blended Oil	***1oz/28g***	***47***	***2.8***	***168***	***14.7***	***4.9***	***10.1***	***0.2***
Raw, Edible Portion	***1oz/28g***	***18***	***0.1***	***64***	***15.1***	***0***	***0.4***	***0***
SKIPS								
Cheesy, KP Snacks*	1 Bag/17g	89	5	524	6.2	58.5	29.5	1
Prawn Cocktail, KP Snacks*	1 Bag/17g	92	5.4	543	4.7	57	32	2.4
SKITTLES								
Giants, Skittles*	1/3 Pack/47g	191	2	406	0	91.4	4.2	0
Mars*	1 Pack/55g	223	2.4	406	0	90.6	4.4	0
Sweet Heat, Mars*	¼ Pack/49g	196	2.1	399	0	89.8	4.2	0
SLICES								
Bacon & Cheese, Pastry, Tesco*	1 Slice/165g	480	32	291	7.4	21.7	19.4	1
Bean, Cheesy, Pastry, Sainsbury's*	1 Slice/180g	524	28.3	291	7.5	25.9	15.7	3.4
Beef, Minced Steak & Onion, Tesco*	1 Slice/150g	424	27.2	283	8.7	21.3	18.1	1.6
Cheese & Onion, Pastry, Tesco*	1 Slice/150g	502	37	335	8	20.1	24.7	1.4
Chicken & Mushroom, Tesco*	1 Slice/165g	457	28.9	277	9.2	20.6	17.5	0.9
Chicken & Bacon, Wall's*	1 Slice/225g	576	33.5	256	10.5	19.9	14.9	0
Chicken & Mushroom, Ginsters*	1 Slice/180g	439	26.8	244	8.3	19.1	14.9	1.8
Chicken & Mushroom, Sainsbury's*	1 Slice/164g	427	26.5	259	7.3	21.3	16.1	1
Chicken Fajita, Puff Pastry, Sainsbury's*	1 Slice/165g	404	17.6	245	9.2	27	10.7	2
Chicken, & Bacon, Asda*	1 Slice/156g	416	21.9	266	10	24	14	1.4
Chicken, & Mushroom, Iceland*	1 Slice/130g	322	16.6	248	7	25.4	12.8	1.6

	Measure INFO/WEIGHT	per Measure KCAL	FAT	Nutrition Values per 100g / 100ml KCAL	PROT	CARB	FAT	FIBRE
SLICES								
Custard, Pastry, Tesco*	1 Slice/94g	266	10.7	283	3.2	41.6	11.3	0.9
Fresh Cream, Tesco*	1 Slice/75g	311	21	414	3.5	37.4	27.9	1
Minced Steak & Onion, Sainsbury's*	1 Slice/165g	475	29.9	288	15.2	16	18.1	2.5
Steak, Large, Ginsters*	1 Slice/204g	516	30.6	253	10.9	17.9	15	0
Steak, Peppered, Ginsters*	1 Slice/180g	457	27	254	8.4	21.3	15	1.6
Steak, Puff Pastry, Sainsbury's*	1 Slice/150g	328	11.7	219	8.4	27.7	7.8	2.3
Steak, Puff Pastry, Tesco*	1 Slice/150g	387	22	258	8.5	22.1	14.7	1.6
Vanilla, Baked by Us, Morrisons*	1 Slice/103g	290	12.4	282	3	40	12	0.9
Yoghurt, Crownfield, Lidl*	2 Slices/37g	160	5	433	6.2	70.6	13.4	2.4
SLIM FAST*								
Bars, Chocolate Caramel Treat, Snack, Slim Fast*	1 Bar/26g	95	2.6	360	3.5	63	10	1.5
Bars, Chocolate, Nutty, Nougat, Snack, Slim Fast*	1 Bar/25g	95	3	380	4	63	12	1.5
Bars, Heavenly Chocolate Delight, Snack, Slim Fast*	1 Bar/24g	95	3.2	390	5	58	13	7
Bars, Heavenly Chocolate, Crunch Snack, Slim Fast*	1 Bar/24g	95	3.2	390	5	58	13	7
Bars, Nutty Salted Caramel, Meal, Slim Fast*	1 Bar/60g	218	6.8	364	25.4	26.9	11.3	18.7
Bars, Summer Berry, Meal, Slim Fast*	1 Bar/60g	210	5	350	23.3	51.7	8.3	5.8
Chunky Chocolate, Shake, Ready to Drink, Slimfast*	1 Shake/325ml	204	5.2	63	4.6	6.6	1.6	1.5
Crackers, Cheddar Flavour Bites, Snack Bag, Slim Fast*	1 Pack/22g	92	2	417	9.6	72.8	9.2	2.5
Milk Shake, Blissful Banana, Powder, Dry, Slim Fast*	2 Scoops/37g	131	2.4	359	13.4	60.2	6.7	11
Milk Shake, Chunky Chocolate, Powder, Dry, Slim Fast*	2 Scoops/37g	132	2.7	363	13.9	59	7.5	10.9
Milk Shake, Simply Vanilla, Powder, Dry, Slim Fast*	2 Scoops/37g	131	2.4	360	13.4	60.9	6.5	11
Milk Shake, Summer Strawberry, Powder, Dry, Slim Fast*	2 Scoops/37g	139	2.4	380	13.5	60.1	6.6	11.1
Milk Shake,Caramel Temptation, Powder, Dry, Slim Fast*	1 Serving/37g	139	2.2	380	14	62	6	11
Noodles, Chicken Tikka Masala, Box, Slim Fast*	1 Box/250g	81	2.2	33	2.3	2.7	0.9	2.5
Noodles, Spicy Thai, Slim Fast*	1 Box/240g	70	3.1	29	0.9	2.4	1.3	2.4
Pretzels, Sour Cream & Chive, Snack Bag, Slim Fast*	1 Pack/23g	99	2.2	432	9.7	74.9	9.5	4.1
Tortillas, Barbecue Flavour, Snack Bag, Slim Fast*	1 Bag/22g	96	2.6	435	6.5	73.9	11.8	3.6
SMARTIES								
Mini Eggs, Nestle*	5 Eggs/17g	85	3.5	499	3.9	73.5	20.4	2.8
Mini, Treat Size, Smarties, Nestle*	1 Carton/14g	68	2.8	471	5	68.1	19.6	1
Nestle*	1 Tube/40g	188	7.1	469	3.9	72.5	17.7	2.4
SMOOTHIE								
Almond, & Banana, Allplants*	1 Serving/140g	302	14.1	216	6.5	24.2	10.1	4.4
Almond, & Berry, Allplants*	1 Serving/140g	186	6.2	133	6.5	18	4.4	3.4
Berry Set Go, Innocent*	1 Bottle/330ml	142	0	43	0	11	0	0
Berry, & Beetroot, Sachet, M&S*	1 Sachet/110g	65	0.2	59	1.2	12.1	0.2	2.2
Berry, & Mango, Allplants*	1 Serving/140g	106	1.5	76	1.2	16	1.1	2.8
Berry, Dry Weight, Lighter Life*	1 Scoop/20g	71	1.2	354	17	48	5.8	20
Blackberries & Blueberries, Innocent*	1 Bottle/250ml	120	0.2	48	0.5	12	0.1	2.1
Blackcurrant, & Blueberry, Asda*	1 Serving/250ml	125	1.2	50	0.5	12	0.5	0.6
Blue Spark, Super Smoothie, Innocent*	1 Serving/150ml	81	0	54	0.3	12	0	1
Bolt from the Blue, Innocent*	1 Serving/150ml	62	0	41	0	10	0	0
Breakfast Oats, Mindful Chef*	1 Pack/140g	158	2.8	113	2.5	19.1	2	3
Cacao, & Black Cherry, Super Smoothie, Innocent*	1 Serving/248ml	154	0	62	0.8	14	0	0.9
Carrot, Mango, & Turmeric, Plant Kitchen, M&S*	1 Bottle/250ml	165	2.2	66	0.7	13.5	0.9	0.4
Cherries, & Strawberries,, Just For Kids, Innocent*	1 Carton/180ml	92	0	51	0.4	11	0	1.3
Cucumber, Avocado, & Lime, M&S*	1 Bottle/250ml	148	3.5	59	0.4	10.4	1.4	1.4
Green, Lean, Mindful Chef*	1 Pack/140g	78	0.8	56	1.3	10	0.6	2.5
Kefir, Cacao, Bio-tiful Dairy*	1 Bottle/250ml	162	6.8	65	3.1	6.8	2.7	0
Kefir, Raspberry, Bio-tiful Dairy*	1 Bottle/250ml	162	6.8	65	3	7.2	2.7	0
Kiwi, & Cucumber, Lean, Naked Juice Co*	1 Bottle/350ml	98	0	28	0.2	6.9	0	0
Magnificent Mango, Innocent*	1 Bottle/250ml	136	0	54	0.4	12	0	1.4
Mango, & Greens, Allplants*	1 Serving/140g	102	1.1	73	1.8	15	0.8	2.7

S

	Measure INFO/WEIGHT	per Measure KCAL	FAT	Nutrition Values per 100g / 100ml KCAL	PROT	CARB	FAT	FIBRE
SMOOTHIE								
Mango, Avocado, Pear, & Matcha, Super, M&S*	1 Glass/150ml	117	0.9	78	0.7	15	0.6	0.5
Mango, Pineapple, & Passion Fruit, Eat Well, M&S*	1 Bottle/250g	170	1.2	68	0.5	14.9	0.5	0.9
Mangoes & Passion Fruits, Pure Fruit, Innocent*	1 Bottle/250ml	135	0	54	0.4	12	0	1.4
Mixed Berry, CBY, Asda*	1 Glass/250ml	143	0	57	0.6	12.6	0	1.6
Orange, Banana, Mango, Morning Boost, Tropicana*	1 Serving/250ml	125	0	50	0.1	9.2	0	2.3
Orange, Mango, & Passionfruit, On the Go, Sainsbury's*	1 Serving/150g	84	0.8	56	0.5	12.8	0.5	0.7
Oranges, Mangoes & Pineapples For Kids, Innocent*	1 Carton/180ml	94	0.2	52	0.7	11.7	0.1	0.9
Peaches & Passionfruit, for Kids, Innocent*	1 Carton/180ml	95	0	53	0.6	14.7	0	0.9
Pear, Kiwi, Kale, & Fennel, Waitrose*	1 Serving/150ml	64	0	43	0.5	9.8	0	0.9
Pineapple, Apple, & Carrot, Innocent*	1 Carton/180ml	94	0	52	0.6	12	0	0.3
Pineapple, Banana & Coconut, CBY, Asda*	1 Glass/250ml	178	2.8	71	0.7	13.6	1.1	1
Pineapples, Bananas & Coconuts, Innocent*	1 Bottle/250ml	172	2.8	69	0.7	13.6	1.1	1
Pomegranates, Blueberries & Acai, Special, Innocent*	1 Serving/250ml	170	0.5	68	0.6	15.6	0.2	0.8
Protein Superfood, Mango & Banana, PhD Nutrition*	1 Serving/130g	175	7.7	135	15.4	4.2	5.9	1.4
Raspberry & Blueberry, Plus, Tesco*	1 Serving/100ml	59	0.3	59	2.6	11.6	0.3	0.5
Revitalise, The Juice Company, Aldi*	1 Serving/150ml	75	0.5	50	0.4	12	0.3	0.5
Strawberries & Bananas, Pure Fruit, Innocent*	1 Bottle/250ml	132	0.2	53	0.7	13.1	0.1	1.3
Strawberry & Banana, Tesco*	1 Bottle/250ml	112	0.5	45	0.6	10.1	0.2	0.8
Strawberry, & Banana, Ready Made, Asda*	1 Glass/150ml	90	0	60	0.7	13	0	1.8
Summer Sunrise, Mindful Chef*	1 Pack/140g	78	0.3	56	0.9	11.6	0.2	1.8
Super Berry, M&S*	1 Bottle/150g	94	0.8	63	1	13.1	0.5	1
Super, Power, M&S*	1 Bottle/250ml	388	2.8	155	2.2	10.5	1.1	0.7
Super, Protect, M&S*	1 Bottle/250ml	190	7	76	0.8	11.4	2.8	0.8
Vanilla Bean, M&S*	1 Bottle/500ml	450	13	90	3.3	13.9	2.6	0
Vitamin Bundle, Innocent*	1 Bottle/300ml	135	0	45	0	11	0	0.5
Watermelon, & Raspberry, Lean, Naked Juice Co*	1 Bottle/360ml	97	0	27	0.2	6.6	0	0
SMOOTHIE MIX								
Banana, Kale & Mango, As Sold, Iceland*	1 Sachet/150g	90	0.4	60	1.1	12.2	0.3	2.3
Beautiful Berries, My Goodness, Sainsbury's*	1 Serving/80g	39	0.4	49	1	8.9	0.5	3.7
Berry, Banana, Frozen, Sainsbury's*	1 Serving/80g	43	0.4	54	0.8	10.3	0.5	3.1
Berry, Frozen, Love Life, Waitrose*	1 Serving/80g	31	0	39	1.1	7.2	0	2.9
Carrot Kick, Sainsbury's*	1 Serving/80ml	39	0.4	49	0.7	10	0.5	2.1
Detox Zing, Love Smoothies*	1 Bag/120g	68	0.4	57	1.1	11.3	0.3	2.2
Detox, Pack'd*	1 Pouch/140g	69	0.7	49	2.3	11	0.5	2.2
Energy, Pack'd*	1 Pouch/140g	85	0.8	61	1.4	14	0.6	3.3
Gorgeous Greens, Asda*	1 Serving/80g	34	0.4	43	1.2	7.8	0.5	1.2
Grape Escape, Love Smoothies*	1 Serving/120ml	74	0.4	62	0.7	13	0.3	2.3
Green, Four Seasons, Aldi*	1 Serving/100g	47	0.6	47	1.6	8.1	0.6	1.6
Greens, Glowing, My Goodness, Sainsbury's*	1 Serving/80g	47	2.1	59	2.1	5.5	2.6	2.6
Mango, & Pineapple, Totally Tropical, Asda*	1 Serving/80g	44	0.4	55	0.6	12	0.5	2.1
Melange Vert, Lidl*	1 Sachet/150g	60	0.3	40	0.5	8.1	0.2	0
Orange, Lidl*	1 Pack/148g	61	0.3	41	2	8.1	0.2	0
Strawberry & Banana, Frozen, Love Life, Waitrose*	1 Serving/80g	37	0.3	46	0.7	8.2	0.4	3.4
Strawberry, & Banana, Frozen, Iceland*	1 Serving/80g	51	0.2	64	0.9	13.2	0.3	2.6
Strawberry, Blueberry, & Banana, Lidl*	1 Pack/150g	82	0.6	55	1	9.9	0.4	2.6
Summer Fruits, & Banana, Frozen, Asda*	1 Serving/80g	41	0.4	51	1	10	0.5	1.4
Tropical, Frozen, Love Life, Waitrose*	1 Serving/80g	45	0.2	57	0.7	11.8	0.3	1.9
Tropical, Lidl*	1 Serving/75g	39	0.2	52	0.5	11.4	0.2	0.8
Very Berry, Sainsbury's*	1 Serving/80g	39	0.4	49	0.9	9.2	0.5	3.1
Vitality, Pack'D*	1 Pouch/140g	97	1.4	69	1.1	13	1	1.8
Yellow Frozen, Morrisons*	1 Portion/80g	41	0.2	51	0.5	10.9	0.2	1.9
SNACKS								
Amaretti, & Almond, Chocolate Curiosities, Graze*	1 Punnet/32g	171	12.2	535	17	33	38	9.4

	Measure INFO/WEIGHT	per Measure KCAL	FAT	Nutrition Values per 100g / 100ml KCAL	PROT	CARB	FAT	FIBRE
SNACKS								
Apple, Grape, Pineapple, & Cheese, Waitrose*	½ Pack/110g	152	8.8	138	6.1	9.9	8	1.2
Balls, Cotton Candy , Herr's*	1 Serving/28g	160	10	571	3.6	53.6	35.7	3.6
BBq Chilli Crunch, Co-Op*	1 Serving/30g	156	9.3	520	12	45	31	4.9
Bean, Crunch, Chilli, Graze*	1 Punnet/30g	135	5.7	451	17	48	19	9.2
Boondi, Regal Snacks*	1 Serving/15g	81	5.4	542	8.2	44.4	36.3	0
Box, Smokehouse BBQ, Crunch, Graze*	1 Pack/31g	137	4.6	441	9.9	60	15	7.3
Cheese Savouries, Morrisons*	1 Serving/25g	130	7.5	520	11.3	49.2	30	3.8
Cheese Savouries, Tesco*	1 Serving/25g	133	7.8	531	11.3	50	31.3	2.1
Chickpea Mix, Crunchy, Salt & Vinegar, Co-Op*	1 Pack/30g	127	6.6	422	16	37	22	17
Chili & Lime, Nutty Protein Power, Punchy, Graze*	1 Punnet/41g	245	19.7	597	22	21	48	8.3
Choccy Wonders, Almond, & Coconut, Graze*	1 Punnet/36g	189	14.8	524	12	21	41	20
Choccy Wonders, Banana & Peanut, Graze*	1 Punnet/37g	186	12.6	503	13	29	34	17
Choccy Wonders, Pretzel & Hazelnut, Graze*	1 Punnet/31g	160	10.8	516	13	32	35	16
Chocolate, Dark, Cherry, & Pecan Mix, Co-Op*	1 Serving/30g	131	6.9	438	4.4	51	23	4.5
Chorizo, Cheddar, & Toasts, Bodega*	1 Pack/64g	240	14.5	375	21.4	20.7	22.7	0
Classic, Aperitivo, Mix, Aldi*	1 Serving/25g	125	6.5	500	16	49	26	0
Cocoa Paradise , Graze*	1 Punnet/28g	140	8.7	501	4.8	50	31	6.8
CocoTop, Organic, Tiana*	1 Tub/50g	292	20.6	583	6.9	46.2	41.3	25.5
Corn, Giant, Sweet Red Pepper, Sainsbury's*	1 Pack/35g	160	5.6	457	5.7	70	16	5.4
Corn, Original, Mister Corn*	1 Serving/30g	145	6.3	482	7.6	63	21	5.5
Crunch, Sea Salted, Lightly, Graze*	1 Serving/31g	128	4	413	16	53	13	11
Dexter the Dog, Morrisons*	1 Bag/15g	78	4.3	522	2.8	61.6	29	2
Dip Dip Hooray, Graze*	1 Serving/25g	134	8.5	535	18	33	34	9.1
Grilled Cheese Crunch, Graze*	1 Punnet/27g	150	10.5	555	18	35	39	7.4
Honey, Sesame, Chinese Style, Graze*	1 Punnet/30g	46	2.7	153	7.9	8.6	9	3.1
Hot Pepper Kick, M&S*	1 Pack/110g	557	29	506	15.4	48.8	26.4	6
Lion, Lightly Salted, Sainsbury's*	1 Pack/15g	78	4.4	522	2.8	61.6	29	2
Macaron, Coconut, White Chocolate, Graze*	1 Punnet/29g	162	11.6	557	9.8	43	40	5.4
Mini C's, Cheese, GF, Schar*	1 Serving/30g	137	5.1	457	7.3	67	17	3.5
Mix, Sweet & Salty, Reese's*	½ Pack/28g	139	7.6	496	12.4	54.7	27.1	0
Mumbai Street Mix, Sensations, Walkers*	1 Serving/30g	167	11	556	14.3	40.8	36.5	3.7
Nut Mix, Acti-Snack*	1 Pack/40g	250	21.4	625	22.7	17.9	53.4	8.8
Nutty Protein Mix, Snacking Essentials*	1 Serving/25g	150	12.4	600	22.6	12.9	49.5	6
Pea Snaps, Sweet Chilli, & Lemon, Yushoi*	1 Pack/21g	90	3.2	429	17.1	48.1	15.2	12.9
Peanut Butter, Protein, Power, Graze*	1 Punnet/27g	136	8.1	503	22	33	30	6.2
Poppy Seed, & Onion, Bagel Crunch, Graze*	1 Punnet/37g	207	14.1	560	18	35	38	4.1
Pretzel, & Peanut, Chocolate Curiosities, Graze*	1 Pack/36g	177	9.4	492	17	44	26	9
Pretzel, Sweet Mustard, Graze*	1 Punnet/25g	129	7.2	517	14	48	29	4.1
Protein Mix, Bare Nature*	1 Serving/30g	156	9.7	519	32.6	19.9	32.4	8.9
Protein Mix, Veggie, Sainsbury's*	¼ Pack/30g	142	7.9	473	29.2	22.1	26.3	15.5
Protein Power, Veggie, Alesto, Lidl*	1 Serving/28g	134	7.3	479	30.3	25.5	26	10.7
Rice, Sushi Mix, Mitsuba*	1 Serving/30g	124	2.3	412	9	75.5	7.7	2.1
Salt & Pepper, Combo Mix, Sainsbury's*	1 Serving/30g	143	6.4	476	4.3	65.5	21.2	3.1
Salt & Vinegar, Crunch, Graze*	1 Punnet/28g	124	4.8	444	16	51	17	12
Slightly Salted, Baked Pea Sticks, Yushoi *	1 Pack/21g	88	3.2	419	19.4	43.1	15.4	15.5
Smoky Barbecue, Crunch, Retail, Graze*	1 Pack/31g	137	5	443	11	57	16	7.9
Sour Cream & Onion, Lentil Curls, Passions Deli, Aldi*	1 Pack/20g	91	3.4	454	11	63	17	3.6
Soy & Balsamic Vinegar, Baked Pea Sticks, Yushoi *	1 Serving/21g	88	2.9	417	18.6	47.9	13.7	13.5
Super, Rosemary & Sea Salt, The Food Doctor*	1 Serving/30g	174	15.3	580	20.6	17.2	51.1	8.2
Sweet & Salty, Veggie Protein Power, Graze*	1 Punnet/30g	162	10.2	539	25	30	34	8.2
Sweet Chilli, Crunch, Graze*	1 Punnet/31g	139	5.3	448	15	55	17	9.9
Sweet Chilli, with Lemon, Baked Pea Sticks, Yushoi *	1 Pack/21g	90	3.2	428	17.4	48.1	15.3	13.1
Sweet Memphis BBQ, Veggie Protein Power, Graze*	1 Pack/38g	193	10.3	509	17	44	27	5.3

S

	Measure INFO/WEIGHT	per Measure KCAL	FAT	Nutrition Values per 100g / 100ml KCAL	PROT	CARB	FAT	FIBRE
SNACKS								
Teddy Faces, Snackrite, Aldi*	1 Bag/19g	96	5.1	505	3.4	61	27	2.7
Texan Style BBQ Crunch, Lidl*	1 Pack/31g	130	3.2	419	8.9	69	10.4	7
Thai Sriracha Mix, Natural Selection*	1 Pack/26g	109	3.4	420	11	60	13	9.3
Thai Sweet Chilli, Weight Watchers*	1 Bag/22g	87	2	395	34.6	38.6	9.1	10.9
Triple Berry Fusion, Graze*	1 Punnet/36g	122	0.3	340	2.2	82	0.9	4.5
Veggie Caesar, Graze*	1 Punnet/24g	115	4.6	478	17	52	19	9.4
SNAILS								
in Garlic Butter, Average	***6 Snails/50g***	***219***	***20.8***	***438***	***9.7***	***8***	***41.5***	***1***
Raw, Average	***1 Snail/5g***	***4***	***0.1***	***90***	***16.1***	***2***	***1.4***	***0***
SNAPPER								
Red, Fried in Blended Oil	***1oz/28g***	***35***	***0.9***	***126***	***24.5***	***0***	***3.1***	***0***
Red, Weighed with Bone, Raw	***1oz/28g***	***12***	***0.2***	***42***	***9.2***	***0***	***0.6***	***0***
SNICKERS								
Crispy, Mars*	1 Serving/20g	97	4.6	483	7.1	61	23	0
Mars*	1 Single/48g	245	13.4	510	9.5	54.3	27.9	1.3
Peanut Butter, Crunchy, Snickers*	1 Bar/26g	130	7	500	11.5	57.7	26.9	3.8
Protein, Mars*	1 Bar/51g	199	7.1	391	35.6	36.1	13.9	0
White, Mars*	1 Bar/49g	241	11.8	491	9	59	24	0
SOLE								
Dover, on the Bone, Pan Fried, Sainsbury's*	1 Fillet/200g	190	2.2	95	19.4	1.5	1.1	0.5
Fillet, Yellowfin, Lightly Dusted, Northern Catch, Aldi*	1 Fillet/114g	171	4.6	150	20	7.6	4	2.5
Fillets, Lemon & Pepper, Co-Op*	1 Fillet/113g	232	13.6	205	11	13	12	0.8
Fillets, Lightly Dusted, Salt, & Black Pepper, Co-Op*	1 Fillet/113g	220	12.4	195	12	11	11	1
Goujons, Lemon & Pepper, Premium, Foxwood*	1 Pack/500g	1055	50.5	211	15.5	14.3	10.1	0.8
Yellow Fin, Fillets, Lemon & Parsley, Tasty Catch, Aldi*	1 Fillet/115g	193	8.3	168	15	10	7.2	1
Yellow, Fillet, Lightly Dusted, As Consumed, Morrisons*	1 Fillet/124g	218	8.5	176	14	13.9	6.9	1
Yellowfin, Fillets, Ocean Trader, Lidl*	1 Fillet/106g	153	6.1	144	14.5	8.1	5.8	0.5
Yellowfin, Lightly Dusted, Garlic & Herb Crumb, Aldi*	1 Fillet/113g	177	6.8	157	16	9.7	6	0.7
SOPOCKA								
Sliced, Cured, Pork Loin	***1 Serving/100g***	***101***	***2.9***	***101***	***17.8***	***0.8***	***2.9***	***0***
SORBET								
Blackcurrant, Yorvale Ltd*	1 Serving/100g	120	0.2	120	0	28.8	0.2	0
Damson, Mary's farmhouse*	1 Scoop/50g	42	0	85	0.3	21	0	0
Exotic Fruit, Sainsbury's*	1 Serving/75g	90	1.5	120	1.2	24.1	2	0
Granita, al Limone, Grom*	2 Scoops/100g	116	0.5	116	0.5	28.5	0.5	0
Jamaican Me Crazy, Ben & Jerry's*	1 Serving/100g	130	0	130	0.2	32	0	0.4
Lemon	***1 Scoop/60g***	***79***	***0***	***131***	***0.9***	***34.2***	***0***	***0***
Mandarin Orange, Yorvale Ltd*	1 Serving/100g	125	0.2	125	0.1	30.5	0.2	0
Mango, Tesco*	1 Scoop/50g	57	0.4	113	0.5	25.6	0.8	0.8
Mango, Waitrose*	1 Pot/100g	90	0	90	0.1	22.1	0	0.6
Orange, Del Monte*	1 Sorbet/500g	625	0.5	125	0.2	32.1	0.1	0
Passion Fruit, Yorvale Ltd*	1 Serving/100g	109	0.2	109	0.1	26.6	0.2	0
Raspberry & Blackberry, Fat Free, M&S*	1 Sorbet/125g	140	0	112	0.4	27.5	0	0.6
Raspberry, Gelatelli, Lidl*	1 Serving/50g	62	0.2	124	0.2	29.1	0.3	1.2
Raspberry, Haagen-Dazs*	½ Cup/105g	120	0	114	0	28.6	0	1.9
Raspberry, Sainsbury's*	1 Scoop/50ml	54	0.2	109	0.5	25	0.5	0.5
Raspberry, Tesco*	1 Scoop/64g	73	0.3	114	0.2	26.8	0.5	0.5
SOUFFLE								
Cheese	***1oz/28g***	***71***	***5.4***	***253***	***11.4***	***9.3***	***19.2***	***0.3***
Cheese, Mini, Waitrose*	1 Souffle/14g	32	2.4	232	16	2.9	17.4	2.4
Lemon, Finest, Tesco*	1 Pot/80g	270	20.5	338	2.9	24.1	25.6	0.2
Ricotta & Spinach, M&S*	1 Serving/120g	186	13.3	155	8	6.2	11.1	2.1
Strawberry, M&S*	1 Serving/95g	171	10.1	180	1.6	19.5	10.6	0.9

S

	Measure INFO/WEIGHT	per Measure KCAL	FAT	Nutrition Values per 100g / 100ml KCAL	PROT	CARB	FAT	FIBRE
SOUP								
Almond, Deluxe, Lidl*	1 Serving/280g	409	40	146	1.4	2.1	14.3	1.4
Asparagus, Chef's Selection, Knorr*	1 Serving/250ml	76	3	30	0.7	4.4	1.2	0.2
Asparagus, Cream of, Canned, M&S*	½ Can/200g	108	7.2	54	0.9	4.3	3.6	0.2
Asparagus, in a Cup, Made Up, Sainsbury's*	1 Sachet/224ml	139	4.9	62	1.3	8.8	2.2	0.7
Asparagus, with Croutons, Aldi*	1 Sachet/229ml	96	3.7	42	0.5	6.5	1.6	0.5
Bacon, & Bean, Smoked, Diet Chef Ltd*	1 Pack/300g	162	3.3	54	2.8	8.2	1.1	2.1
Bacon, & Bean, Three, Smoked, Chunky, Baxters*	1 Can/400g	232	4.8	58	2.9	8.8	1.2	1.8
Bacon, & Lentil, CBY, Asda*	½ Pot/300g	177	4.2	59	3.8	7.2	1.4	1.2
Bacon, Smoked, & Kale, Sainsbury's*	1 Pot/600g	366	21	61	1.4	5.7	3.5	0.8
Bean, & Vegetable, Three, LC, Tesco*	½ Can/200g	110	0.6	55	2.6	9.7	0.3	1.9
Bean, & Veg, Stew, Mighty, Big Soup, Heinz*	1 Can/500g	355	4.5	71	3	11.8	0.9	3
Bean, & Vegetable, Chunky, Sainsbury's*	1 Can/400g	268	4	67	3.5	9.3	1	3.6
Bean, Butter, & Chorizo, Meal, Sainsbury's*	1 Pot/400g	257	9.6	64	3.9	5.6	2.4	2.3
Bean, Chilli, Mexican, Tesco*	1 Carton/600g	270	6.6	45	2.2	6.4	1.1	1.9
Bean, Hearty, Italian Inspired, Love Life, Waitrose*	½ Pot/300g	151	6.6	50	1.5	5.2	2.2	1.8
Bean, Italian Style, Tesco*	1 Can/300g	153	3.6	51	2.8	7.3	1.2	1.1
Bean, Mexican, Fresh, Morrisons*	½ Pot/300g	171	3.9	57	2.1	8.3	1.3	1.9
Bean, Tuscan, Chunky, Love Life, Waitrose*	½ Can/200g	101	1	50	2.6	7.6	0.5	2.3
Bean, Tuscan, Slimming World, Iceland*	½ Pot/250g	100	0.5	40	2.6	5.1	0.2	3.7
Bean, Tuscan, Tesco*	1 Can/400g	212	2.8	53	2.8	7.7	0.7	2.4
Beef, & Mushroom, Big Soup, Heinz*	1 Can/515g	216	2.6	42	2.3	7	0.5	0.7
Beef, & Tomato, Cup a Soup, Made Up, Batchelors*	1 Serving/252g	83	1.6	33	0.6	6.3	0.6	0.4
Beef, & Vegetable, Big Soup, Heinz*	1 Can/400g	212	4	53	3.5	7.5	1	0.9
Beef, & Vegetables, Chunky, Newgate, Lidl*	1 Tin/400g	232	3.2	58	3.6	8.2	0.8	1.8
Beef, Broth, Big Soup, Heinz*	1 Can/400g	184	2.8	46	2.5	7	0.7	0.9
Beef, Broth, Classic, Heinz*	1 Can/400g	180	2	45	1.9	7.6	0.5	0.8
Beef, Chilli, Chunky, Asda*	1 Can/400g	212	4	53	4.2	5.7	1	2.4
Beef, Fiery, Pho, Vietnamese, Naked Soup*	1 Pack/300g	108	2.1	36	0.9	6.5	0.7	0
Beetroot, Carrot, & Apple, Waitrose*	1 Pot/350g	105	3.2	30	0.7	4.2	0.9	1.1
Beetroot, Curly Kale, with Quinoa, Tideford Organics*	½ Pack/300g	87	2.1	29	0.8	4.2	0.7	1.1
Black Bean, Mexican, Extra Special, Asda*	½ Pot/263g	194	10.8	74	2.3	7	4.1	1.7
Bone Broth, Beef, Grass Fed, Organic, Borough Broth Co.*	1 Sachet/324g	81	1.6	25	4.3	0.7	0.5	0.5
Bone Broth, Mushroom, & Barley, Super Good, Baxters*	1 Can/400g	168	6.4	42	1.4	5.2	1.6	0.8
Bread, with Fruit Mix, Estonia, Tartu Mill*	1 Serving/50g	162	0.4	323	4.7	70.6	0.9	6.7
Broccoli, & Stilton, Canned, Sainsbury's*	½ Can/200g	84	4	42	1.5	4.2	2	0.6
Broccoli, & Stilton, Classics, Fresh, Tesco*	½ Pot/300g	156	10.8	52	2.4	1.8	3.6	1.5
Broccoli, & Stilton, Cup Soup, Ainsley Harriott*	1 Sachet/230g	99	2.1	43	0.9	7.8	0.9	0.2
Broccoli, & Stilton, Fresh, Sainsbury's*	½ Pot/300ml	141	9.9	47	2.7	1.8	3.3	1.5
Broccoli, & Spinach, Souper, M&S*	½ Pot/300g	102	3.9	34	2.1	2.7	1.3	1.6
Broccoli, & Stilton, Canned, Tesco*	½ Can/200g	100	5	50	1.8	4.9	2.5	0.5
Broccoli, Pea, & Basil, Soupologie*	½ Pot/300g	124	6.2	41	2.4	2.7	2.1	1.4
Broccoli, Salmon & Watercress, Stay Full, Baxters*	1 Can/400g	244	8.8	61	3.3	5.8	2.2	2.4
Butternut Squash, & Bacon, Smoked, Aldi*	½ Can/200g	122	8	61	1.8	4.2	4	0.5
Butternut Squash, & Chilli, Sainsbury's*	½ Pot/300g	112	7.2	37	0.7	3.1	2.4	0.2
Butternut Squash, & Tarragon, Waitrose*	½ Pot/300g	123	6.6	41	0.8	4.5	2.2	1
Butternut Squash, & Chickpea, Spiced, Heinz*	½ Can/200g	69	1	35	1.1	6.3	0.5	1.2
Butternut Squash, & Lentil Dhansak, Plant Based, Baxters*	1 Can/380g	171	1.5	45	2.4	7.2	0.4	1.5
Butternut Squash, Fresh, Waitrose*	½ Pot/300g	153	8.7	51	0.5	5.8	2.9	0.8
Butternut Squash, M&S*	1 Serving/400g	132	3.2	33	0.6	5.3	0.8	1
Butternut Squash, New England, Skinnylicious, Glorious!*	½ Pot/300g	87	2.1	29	0.5	4.5	0.7	1.4
Butternut Squash, Soupreme, Aldi*	½ Pot/300g	60	3.3	20	0.5	1.5	1.1	1.5
Butternut Squash, Tesco*	½ Pot/300g	82	4.3	27	0.4	2.5	1.4	1.5
Butternut, & Sage, Crosse & Blackwell*	1 Can/400g	215	12.4	54	0.5	5.8	3.1	0.4

	Measure INFO/WEIGHT	per Measure KCAL	FAT	Nutrition Values per 100g / 100ml KCAL	PROT	CARB	FAT	FIBRE
SOUP								
Butternut, Spiced, New Covent Garden Food Co*	½ Pack/280g	95	4.8	34	0.8	3.3	1.7	1.1
Carrot, & Butter Bean, Vegetarian, Baxters*	1 Can/400g	232	7.6	58	1.7	7.2	1.9	2.1
Carrot, & Coriander, Average	***1 Can/400g***	***167***	***8.6***	***42***	***0.6***	***4.8***	***2.2***	***1***
Carrot, & Coriander, Fresh, New Covent Garden Food Co*	½ Carton/280g	123	5.3	44	0.8	5.2	1.9	1.2
Carrot, & Coriander, Fresh, Tesco*	½ Pot/300g	99	4.8	33	0.6	2.9	1.6	2.2
Carrot, & Ginger, Fresh, Sainsbury's*	1 Pot/600g	150	5.4	25	0.4	3.9	0.9	1
Carrot, & Lentil, Weight Watchers*	1 Can/295g	87	0.3	29	1.3	5.5	0.1	0.7
Carrot, & Coriander, Vegetarian, Baxters*	1 Can/400g	214	12.3	54	0.5	5.4	3.1	1
Carrot, & Lentil, Farmers Market, Heinz*	1 Serving/200g	84	0.3	42	1.7	7.8	0.2	0.9
Carrot, Butternut, & Ginger, Bol*	1 Pack/500g	175	8	35	0.5	3.8	1.6	1.4
Carrot, Ginger, & Butternut, Super, Chef Select, Lidl*	½ Pack/300g	111	4.2	37	1	4.4	1.4	1.3
Carrot, Red Lentil & Cumin, Organic, Waitrose*	1 Pack/350g	175	8.8	50	0.2	6.7	2.5	0.5
Carrot, Thai, Skinny, Aldi*	½ Pot/300g	90	4.8	30	0.5	3.3	1.6	0.6
Cauliflower Cheese, Kale, & Cheddar, Yorkshire Provender*	½ Pot/300g	192	12.6	64	2.5	3.4	4.2	0.6
Cauliflower, & Celeriac, Love Life, Waitrose*	1 Pot/350g	79	3.1	23	1.6	1.4	0.9	1.3
Cauliflower, & Wensleydale, Crosse & Blackwell*	1 Can/400g	184	8	46	1.6	5.3	2	0.4
Cauliflower, Chicken, & Turmeric, Waitrose*	1 Pot/400g	221	7.6	55	3	5.8	1.9	1.4
Cauliflower, Chickpea, & Turmeric, Indian, Glorious!*	½ Pot/300g	114	2.4	38	2	4.4	0.8	2.7
Cauliflower, Masala Spiced, Specially Selected, Aldi*	½ Can/200g	106	6.4	53	1.7	4.1	3.2	0.6
Cauliflower, Onion, & Potato, Soup of the Day, Heinz*	½ Carton/200g	76	3.2	38	1.4	4.4	1.6	1
Celeriac, Velvety, Waitrose*	½ Pot/300g	151	11.5	50	0.8	2.8	3.8	0.9
Chicken Arrabbiata, Meal, G&B, Asda*	1 Pot/380g	167	1.9	44	3.6	5.6	0.5	1.8
Chicken Bone, Broth, Borough Broth Co.*	1 Pack/324g	58	1.6	18	2.6	0.6	0.5	0.5
Chicken Jambalaya, Spicy, Waitrose*	½ Pot/300g	156	4.2	52	3.8	5.5	1.4	1
Chicken Noodle, & Vegetable, Waitrose*	1 Can/400g	140	2.4	35	1.6	5.5	0.6	0
Chicken Noodle, Canned, Asda*	1 Can/400g	180	3.2	45	1.5	7.9	0.8	0.3
Chicken Noodle, Canned, Heinz*	1 Can/400g	128	1.2	32	1.3	6.1	0.3	0.2
Chicken Noodle, Canned, Sainsbury's*	½ Can/217g	78	0.7	36	1.7	7.4	0.3	0.7
Chicken Noodle, Chinese, Fresh, Asda*	½ Pot/300g	120	2.1	40	2.3	5.6	0.7	0.8
Chicken Noodle, Clear, Weight Watchers*	1 Can/295g	51	0.6	17	0.8	3.1	0.2	0.2
Chicken Noodle, Dry, Nissin*	1 Pack/85g	364	14.1	428	9.5	62	16.6	3.3
Chicken Noodle, Fresh, Sainsbury's*	½ Pot/300g	132	3.3	44	2.9	5.6	1.1	0.5
Chicken Noodle, In a Cup, BGTY, Sainsbury's*	1 Sachet/219ml	59	1.1	27	1.7	4.9	0.5	0.5
Chicken Noodle, Soup in a Cup, Made Up, Sainsbury's*	1 Serving/200ml	44	0.2	22	0.7	4.7	0.1	0.2
Chicken Noodle, Super Good, Baxters*	1 Can/400g	200	5.2	50	3.1	6.6	1.3	0.5
Chicken Noodle, Super, Dry, Knorr*	1 Pack/56g	182	2.7	325	14.3	56	4.9	1.8
Chicken Noodle, Thai Green, Yorkshire Provender*	½ Pot/300g	159	6	53	2.9	5.6	2	0
Chicken Noodle, with Sweetcorn, Canned, M&S*	1 Can/400g	184	3.2	46	2.8	6.8	0.8	0.4
Chicken, & Bean, Mexican Spiced, Eat Smart, Morrisons*	1 Can/400g	200	2	50	2.9	7.3	0.5	1.9
Chicken, & Leek, Cup a Soup, Made Up, Batchelors*	1 Serving/259g	96	4.7	37	0.5	4.7	1.8	0.7
Chicken, & Lentil, Spinach, & Cumin, Yorkshire Provender*	½ Pot/300g	159	4.8	53	3.9	4.6	1.6	2.1
Chicken, & Multigrain, Finest, Tesco*	½ Pot/298g	125	3.6	42	3.2	3.9	1.2	1.3
Chicken, & Mushroom, Grain Soup , Sainsbury's*	1 Pot/600g	332	14.5	55	3.8	4.4	2.4	0.5
Chicken, & Orzo, Tuscan, Glorious!*	½ Pot/300g	120	1.2	40	2.8	6.2	0.4	0.7
Chicken, & Sweetcorn, Fresh, Average	***1 Serving/300g***	***146***	***3.1***	***48***	***2.4***	***7.3***	***1***	***0.6***
Chicken, & Vegetable, Canned, Average	***1 Can/400g***	***192***	***8.5***	***48***	***2.5***	***4.6***	***2.1***	***0.8***
Chicken, & Vegetable, Chunky, Canned, Soupreme, Aldi*	1 Can/400g	184	2.4	46	3	6.4	0.6	1.3
Chicken, & Vegetable, Chunky, Meal Soup, Tesco*	1 Can/400g	184	7.2	46	2.5	4.6	1.8	1
Chicken, & Vegetable, Fresh, Tesco*	½ Pack/300g	118	3.3	39	3.6	3.2	1.1	1.1
Chicken, & Barley, Broth, Heinz*	½ Can/200g	58	0.4	29	1.4	4.9	0.2	0.9
Chicken, & Bean, Mexican Style, Slimzone, Asda*	½ Can/200g	90	1	45	2.8	6.6	0.5	1.8
Chicken, & Chorizo, Smoky, Waitrose*	½ Pot/300g	123	4.2	41	2.5	3.9	1.4	1.2
Chicken, & Chorizo, Spanish, Extra Special, Asda*	½ Pot/300ml	150	7.5	50	2.5	4.2	2.5	0.5

S

	Measure INFO/WEIGHT	per Measure KCAL	FAT	Nutrition Values per 100g / 100ml KCAL	PROT	CARB	FAT	FIBRE
SOUP								
Chicken, & Grains, Fresh, M&S*	½ Pot/300g	222	7.5	74	3.7	8.1	2.5	2
Chicken, & Leek, Canned, Duncan's, Aldi*	1 Can/400g	108	2.8	27	1.3	3.8	0.7	0.5
Chicken, & Multigrain, Crosse & Blackwell*	1 Can/391g	176	3.1	45	2	4.5	0.8	1.1
Chicken, & Mushroom, Chestnut, Fresh, Finest, Tesco*	1 Pot/600g	282	9.6	47	3	5.1	1.6	0.1
Chicken, & Noodle, Canned, Bramwells, Aldi*	1 Can/400g	148	3	37	1.4	5.5	0.8	1.2
Chicken, & Spelt, Broth, Deluxe, Lidl*	½ Pot/300g	141	3.3	47	3	5.6	1.1	1.5
Chicken, & Sweetcorn, Low Fat, Soupreme*	½ Pot/300g	126	4.5	42	2.3	4.6	1.5	0.9
Chicken, & Vegetable, Broth, Fresh, Sainsbury's*	1 Pot/600ml	216	10.2	36	2.3	2.7	1.7	0.6
Chicken, & Vegetable, Chunky, Canned, Asda*	½ Can/200g	90	2	45	4.3	4.3	1	0.8
Chicken, & Vegetable, Chunky, Fresh, M&S*	½ Pot/300g	165	6.6	55	2.3	6.1	2.2	1
Chicken, & Vegetable, Chunky, Morrisons*	1 Can/400g	184	4.4	46	3.8	4.8	1.1	1
Chicken, & Vegetable, Creamy, Sainsbury's*	1 Pot/400g	220	7.6	55	1.7	6.6	1.9	2.1
Chicken, & Vegetable, Fresh, Morrisons*	1 Pot/600g	318	10.2	53	3.2	5.6	1.7	1.2
Chicken, & Vegetable, Low Fat, Soupreme, Aldi*	½ Pot/303g	100	2.1	33	2	4.5	0.7	0.8
Chicken, & Vegetable, Meal Soup, Sainsbury's*	1 Pot/400g	268	9.6	67	3.8	7	2.4	1.3
Chicken, & Vegetable, Slimming World*	1 Carton/500g	170	2	34	3.7	3.3	0.4	1.1
Chicken, Arrabbiata, Hearty, Bowl, Sainsbury's*	1 Pack/400g	198	4	50	2.5	6.8	1	1.6
Chicken, Balti, Meal, Sainsbury's*	1 Pack/400g	242	7.1	61	3.9	6.3	1.8	1.8
Chicken, Broth, Favourites, Baxters*	1 Can/400g	164	2.8	41	1.6	7.2	0.7	0.7
Chicken, Classic, New Covent Garden*	½ Carton/280g	151	7	54	3.7	4	2.5	0.5
Chicken, Cream Of, Bramwells, Aldi*	1 Can/400g	208	12	52	1.5	4.7	3	0.5
Chicken, Cream of, Canned, Sainsbury's*	1 Can/400g	216	10.8	54	2.1	5	2.7	0.5
Chicken, Cream of, Canned, Tesco*	1 Can/400g	192	12	48	2.5	2.8	3	0.1
Chicken, Cream of, Knorr*	1 Serving/250ml	50	2	20	0.3	2.8	0.8	0
Chicken, Cream Of, No Added Sugar, Heinz*	½ Can/200g	106	6	53	1.6	4.9	3	0.1
Chicken, Cream of, Reduced Salt, Heinz*	1 Can/400g	216	12	54	1.7	4.9	3	0.1
Chicken, Cream of, Soupreme, Aldi*	1 Can/400g	228	15.2	57	1.8	3.8	3.8	0.4
Chicken, Cup A Soup, Knorr*	1 Sachet/170g	139	6.5	82	1.7	10	3.8	0.5
Chicken, Green Thai, Spiced, M&S*	½ Pot/300g	195	11.4	65	2	6.3	3.8	0.6
Chicken, Green Thai, Waitrose*	1 Pot/600g	462	30	77	4.4	3.5	5	1.6
Chicken, Hotpot, Chunky, Big Soup, Heinz*	½ Can/258g	126	3.1	49	2.3	7.4	1.2	0.8
Chicken, Jamaican Jerk, TTD, Sainsbury's*	½ Pot/300g	169	3.6	56	3.5	6.6	1.2	2.5
Chicken, Katsu, Naked, Hearty, Sainsbury's*	1 Pot/397g	258	11.9	65	2.1	6.5	3	1.6
Chicken, Keralan, Sainsburys*	½ Carton/300g	252	15.3	84	3.5	5.5	5.1	1.1
Chicken, Made Up, Cup a Soup, Batchelors*	1 Sachet/253g	91	5.1	36	0.6	4	2	0.5
Chicken, Miso, Noodle, Waitrose*	1 Pot/400g	268	8.8	67	5.9	5.9	2.2	0.9
Chicken, Moroccan Inspired, Finest, Tesco*	½ Pot/300g	156	3.3	52	3.7	4.9	1.1	4
Chicken, Moroccan Inspired, Love Life, Waitrose*	½ Pot/300g	136	2.4	45	2.7	6.1	0.8	1.4
Chicken, Moroccan, Harira, Hearty, Baxters*	1 Can/400g	236	2.8	59	3.2	9.5	0.7	1.9
Chicken, Mulligatawny, Finest, Tesco*	½ Pot/300g	237	9.9	79	5	6.7	3.3	1
Chicken, Multigrain, Hearty, Waitrose*	½ Pot/300g	141	3	47	3.6	4.9	1	2.1
Chicken, Peri Peri, Asda*	½ Can/197g	77	1.8	39	1.8	5.5	0.9	0.6
Chicken, Potato & Bacon, Big Soup, Heinz*	1 Can/515g	294	11.3	57	3	6.1	2.2	0.5
Chicken, Potato & Leek, Weight Watchers*	1 Can/295g	97	2.4	33	1.1	5.1	0.8	0.3
Chicken, Potato, & Bacon, Chunky, Tesco*	½ Can/200g	100	2.6	50	3.6	5.7	1.3	0.7
Chicken, Roast, Cream of, Crosse & Blackwell*	1 Can/400g	214	10.4	54	3.8	3.5	2.6	0.6
Chicken, Thai Style, Canned, Soupreme, Aldi*	1 Can/400g	200	10.8	50	2.5	3.8	2.7	1.1
Chicken, Thai, Deluxe, Lidl*	½ Can/190g	129	6.8	68	1.6	7	3.6	1.5
Chicken, Thai, Fresh, Finest, Tesco*	½ Pot/300g	192	11.7	64	3	3.8	3.9	0.7
Chicken, Tomato, & Grains, Tuscan, Glorious!*	½ Pack/300g	111	2.1	37	2	4.9	0.7	1.5
Chicken, Weight Watchers*	1 Can/295g	97	3	33	1.6	4.4	1	0
Chickpea, & Coconut, Indonesian Style, Lidl*	1 Pot/400g	340	22.8	85	1.4	5.2	5.7	3.3
Chickpea, Albert Heijn*	1 Pack/570ml	450	19.9	79	3	8	3.5	1.5

S

	Measure INFO/WEIGHT	per Measure KCAL	FAT	Nutrition Values per 100g / 100ml KCAL	PROT	CARB	FAT	FIBRE
SOUP								
Chilli, Tomato, & Pasta, COU, M&S*	1 Serving/300g	150	5.7	50	1.3	7.2	1.9	0.9
Chipotle, & Bean, Mexican Inspired, Waitrose*	1 Can/396g	198	5.9	50	1.9	6.3	1.5	1.6
Chorizo, Beans, & Caramelised Onion, TTD, Sainsbury's*	1 Pot/400g	168	5.2	42	2.2	3.9	1.3	3
Chowder, Haddock, Smoked, Scottish, TTD, Sainsbury's*	1 Dish/116g	228	17.2	197	11.8	3.9	14.9	0.5
Chowder, Ham & Sweetcorn, Diet Chef Ltd*	1 Pack/300g	165	3.6	55	1.9	9.2	1.2	0.9
Chowder, Seafood, Waitrose*	1 Can/404g	226	11.3	56	2.2	5.6	2.8	0.6
Chowder, Smoked Haddock & Salmon, Cully & Sully*	1 Pack/400g	232	9.2	58	2.6	6.2	2.3	0.9
Chowder, Sweetcorn, Microwaved, Slimming World*	1 Pot/500g	160	2.5	32	1.1	5.3	0.5	0.7
Cock-A-Leekie, Favourites, Baxters*	1 Can/400g	116	2.4	29	1.1	4.7	0.6	0.3
Coconut, Corn, & Sweet Potato, Creamy, Bol*	1 Pot/500g	280	6	56	1.7	7.8	1.2	3.5
Coconut, Curry, Sri Lankan, Spiced, TTD, Sainsbury's*	½ Pot/300g	195	9.3	65	1.3	7.3	3.1	1.5
Coconut, Lime, & Chilli, Glorious!*	½ Tub/300g	168	2.4	56	3.4	6.7	0.8	4.1
Country Garden, Canned, Vegetarian, Baxters*	1 Can/400g	144	2	36	1	6.2	0.5	1
Country Vegetable, Chunky, Canned, Sainsbury's*	1 Can/400g	152	2.4	38	1	6.5	0.6	1.2
Courgette, & Parmesan, Fresh, Sainsbury's*	1 Pack/300ml	198	16.8	66	1.5	2.5	5.6	0.4
Courgette, & Pea, Creamy, with a Hint of Chilli, BOL*	1 Pot/500g	255	10	51	2.4	4	2	3.7
Crayfish, Deluxe, Lidl*	1 Serving/280g	174	11.8	62	1.3	4.5	4.2	0.5
Daal, Lentil, Bangalore, Glorious!*	1 Pot/600g	294	8.4	49	2	6.1	1.4	2.2
Dahl, Indian Spiced, Asda*	½ Pot/300g	138	3	46	2.2	5.8	1	2.6
Dahl, Lentil, Bangalore, Sainsbury's*	1 Serving/300g	117	2.7	39	1.7	4.7	0.9	2.3
Dhal, Lentil, Co-Op*	1 Pot/600g	324	11.4	54	2.1	6.1	1.9	1.8
Fish, Bouillabaise, Bistro, M&S*	1 Pack/820g	2665	18	325	10	4.3	2.2	1.3
French Onion, & Red Onion, Canned, Waitrose*	1 Can/400g	140	2.4	35	2.2	4.8	0.6	0.6
Game, Royal, Favourites, Baxters*	1 Can/400g	152	0.8	38	1.8	6.9	0.2	0.3
Garden Vegetable, Fresh, Tesco*	½ Pot/300g	117	0.6	39	1.4	7.2	0.2	1.4
Gazpacho, Hacendada*	1 Serving/333ml	250	23.3	75	0.6	2.5	7	0
Golden Vegetable, Cup a Soup, Made Up, Batchelors*	1 Sachet/250ml	80	2.3	32	0.3	5.5	0.9	0.4
Green Veg, Broth, Chinese Style, Veg Pot, Naked Noodle*	1 Pot/300g	216	0.6	72	2.8	13.8	0.2	2
Green Vegetable, & Kale, British, Crosse & Blackwell*	1 Can/394g	130	1.2	33	1.6	5.1	0.3	1.8
Haddock, Smoked, Chowder, M&S*	½ Pot/300g	141	6.6	47	2.1	4.3	2.2	0.6
Ham Hock, & Vegetable, Broth, Crosse & Blackwell*	1 Can/400g	158	2	40	2.7	5.7	0.5	0.8
Ham, Hock, & Sweetcorn, TTD, Sainsbury's*	1 Pack/600g	468	22.8	78	2.6	7.8	3.8	1.1
Highlander's Broth, Favourites, Baxters*	1 Can/400g	192	5.6	48	1.7	6.3	1.4	0.9
Hot & Sour	***1 Serving/233g***	***90***	***2.8***	***39***	***2.6***	***4.3***	***1.2***	***0.5***
Jackfruit, Bean, & Chipotle Chilli, Plant Based, Baxters*	1 Can/380g	201	1.1	53	2.8	8.6	0.3	2.4
Kotosoupa, with Noodles, Greek, Knorr*	½ Pack/505ml	106	2.5	21	0.8	4.2	0.5	0.5
Laksa, Chicken Noodle, Cook*	1 Pack/300g	300	9	100	6.6	12.2	3	0.9
Lamb, & Vegetable, Big Soup, Heinz*	½ Can/200g	120	2.6	60	3	9.1	1.3	1.3
Lamb, Minted, Hot Pot, Big Soup, Heinz*	1 Can/500g	295	6.5	59	2.8	8.5	1.3	1
Leek & Potato, Pot, Chef Select, Lidl*	½ Pot/300g	93	3.6	31	0.6	4	1.2	0.9
Leek & Potato, Canned, Morrisons*	1 Can/400g	156	4	39	0.7	6.5	1	0.6
Leek & Potato, Maris Piper, New Covent Garden Food Co*	½ Carton/280g	162	10.4	58	1.1	5.5	3.7	0.7
Leek, & Chicken, Knorr*	1 Serving/300ml	82	5.2	27	0.6	2.4	1.7	0.1
Leek, & Potato	***1oz/28g***	***15***	***0.7***	***52***	***1.5***	***6.2***	***2.6***	***0.8***
Leek, & Potato, Canned, Asda*	1 Can/400g	160	3.6	40	0.9	6.5	0.9	1
Leek, & Potato, Canned, Sainsbury's*	½ Can/200g	92	3.2	46	1	6.7	1.6	0.3
Leek, & Potato, Classics, Canned, Heinz*	1 Can/400g	196	7.2	49	0.8	7.1	1.8	0.6
Leek, & Potato, Cup a Soup, Batchelors*	1 Sachet/28g	115	4.9	411	7.5	53.9	17.5	3.6
Leek, & Potato, Favourites, Baxters*	1 Can/400g	192	7.2	48	1	6.6	1.8	0.9
Leek, & Potato, Fresh with Cream, Tesco*	½ Tub/300g	146	8.4	49	0.7	4.6	2.8	1.2
Leek, & Potato, Soup in a Mug, HL, Tesco*	1 Serving/16g	54	0.9	336	4.3	67.1	5.6	7.4
Lentil, & Bacon, Canned, Sainsbury's*	½ Can/200g	102	1.4	51	4.1	6.6	0.7	1
Lentil, & Bacon, Canned, Tesco*	1 Serving/200g	96	1.4	48	3.2	7.2	0.7	0.5

S

	Measure INFO/WEIGHT	per Measure KCAL	FAT	Nutrition Values per 100g / 100ml KCAL	PROT	CARB	FAT	FIBRE
SOUP								
Lentil, & Bacon, Chunky, Canned, M&S*	1 Can/400g	204	2.4	51	3.3	7.2	0.6	1.8
Lentil, & Bacon, Classic, Heinz*	1 Can/400g	232	5.6	58	2.7	8.4	1.4	0.7
Lentil, & Bacon, Favourites, Baxters*	1 Can/400g	208	2.8	52	3.4	7.3	0.7	0.8
Lentil, & Barley, Superbean, M&S*	1 Pack /600g	270	9	45	1.8	5.1	1.5	2.1
Lentil, & Chick Pea, Fresh, Organic, Tesco*	1 Serving/300ml	117	2.4	39	1.9	6.1	0.8	0.5
Lentil, & Ham, Red, Waitrose*	½ Pot/300g	147	3.3	49	3.9	5.8	1.1	2
Lentil, & Smoked Bacon, Fresh, Tesco*	1 Pack/600g	420	11.4	70	3.9	8.5	1.9	1.6
Lentil, & Vegetable, LC, Tesco*	1 Can/400g	188	0.8	47	2.5	8.8	0.2	1.1
Lentil, & Vegetable, Spicy, Chilled, M&S*	½ Serving/300g	150	2.4	50	2.7	8	0.8	1.1
Lentil, & Bacon, Smoked, New Covent Garden Soup Co*	½ Pack/280g	182	6.2	65	5.9	4.1	2.2	2.8
Lentil, & Red Pepper, Smoky, Plant Chef, Tesco*	1 Serving/400g	184	2	46	2.8	6.8	0.5	1.2
Lentil, & Spinach, Dahl, Tideford Organics*	½ Pot/300g	117	6.3	39	1.4	3.1	2.1	0.9
Lentil, & Vegetable, Vegetarian, Baxters*	1 Can/400g	160	0.8	40	1.9	7.4	0.2	1.2
Lentil, Asda*	½ Can/202g	89	0.4	44	2.6	8	0.2	0.7
Lentil, Classic, Heinz*	1 Can/400g	180	0.8	45	2.4	8.5	0.2	0.8
Lentil, Maggi*	1 Serving/250ml	68	0.6	27	1.8	4.5	0.2	0.6
Lentil, Red, with Carrots, Potato & Onion, Asda*	1 Can/400g	192	0.8	48	1.4	10.2	0.2	1.2
Lentil, Scotty Brand*	1 Pot/550g	374	1.6	68	3.9	10.4	0.3	3.8
Lentil, Spicy, M&S*	1 Serving/100g	50	1.1	50	2.6	6.3	1.1	2.1
Lobster, Bisque, Waitrose*	½ Carton/300g	201	13.8	67	0.9	5.5	4.6	0.6
Minestrone, & Smoked Bacon, Baxters*	1 Pot/350g	172	6	49	2.2	5.8	1.7	0.7
Minestrone, Canned, Average	***1 Can/400g***	***252***	***12***	***63***	***1.8***	***7.6***	***3***	***0.9***
Minestrone, Chunky, Fresh, Sainsbury's*	½ Pot/300g	93	0.6	31	1.4	6.1	0.2	2.3
Minestrone, Chunky, Love Life, Waitrose*	1 Can/400g	166	0.4	42	1.3	8.7	0.1	1.9
Minestrone, Classic, Heinz*	1 Can/400g	128	0.8	32	1	6.2	0.2	0.8
Minestrone, Favourites, Baxters*	1 Can/400g	168	2.4	42	1.6	7	0.6	1.2
Minestrone, Fresh, Average	***1 Carton/600g***	***244***	***4.9***	***41***	***1.7***	***6.8***	***0.8***	***1.2***
Minestrone, Pack, Dry, Knorr*	1 Pack/61g	204	2.4	335	12	58.8	4	6.9
Minestrone, Pot, Chef Select, Lidl*	½ Pot/300g	138	1.5	46	2.2	7.3	0.5	1.9
Minestrone, Warming, Canned, Asda*	1 Can/400g	148	2	37	1.4	6.3	0.5	1.2
Minestrone, with Croutons in a Mug, Tesco*	1 Sachet/23g	83	1.9	360	9	62.6	8.1	2.7
Minestrone, with Croutons, Cup a Soup, Batchelors*	1 Serving/254g	89	1.8	35	0.6	6.5	0.7	0.5
Minestrone, with Croutons, Dry, Soupreme, Aldi*	1 Serving/27g	94	1.7	349	7.6	65.3	6.4	4.4
Minestrone, with GF Pasta, Tideford*	1 Pot/600g	180	4.8	30	1.3	3.9	0.8	1.4
Miso, Paste, Wakame, Sachets, Yutaka*	1 Sachet/18g	18	0.6	100	7.1	16	3.6	0
Miso, Rainbow, Japanese, Skinny Soup, Glorious!*	½ Pot/300g	81	0.9	27	1.4	4.1	0.3	0.9
Miso, Wakama*	1 Sachet/8g	27	0.6	336	18.7	48.6	7.6	0
Miso, with Tofu, Instant, Kikkoman*	1 Sachet/10g	35	1	350	30	30	10	0
Moroccan Bean, Very Special, Wattie's*	1 Serving/265g	176	0.8	66	3.2	11.4	0.3	2
Moroccan, with Vegan Pieces, Quorn*	½ Pot/283g	136	1.7	48	4.2	4.4	0.6	3.7
Mulligatawny	***1 Serving/220g***	***213***	***15***	***97***	***1.4***	***8.2***	***6.8***	***0.9***
Mulligatawny, Canned, Morrisons*	1 Can/400g	196	6.4	49	1.8	6.5	1.6	0.8
Mulligatawny, Canned, Tesco*	1 Can/400g	188	4	47	1.3	8.1	1	0.3
Mulligatawny, Classic, Heinz*	1 Can/400g	232	7.6	58	1.9	8	1.9	0.5
Multigrain, High Fibre, Waitrose*	1 Pot/400g	232	6	58	2.6	6.8	1.5	3.5
Mushroom, & Chestnut, Fresh, Finest, Tesco*	1 Serving/250g	130	8.2	52	1.1	4.7	3.3	0.7
Mushroom, Canned, HL, Tesco*	1 Can/400g	132	5.6	33	0.5	4.4	1.4	0.2
Mushroom, Cream of, Bramwells, Aldi*	½ Can/200g	106	5.8	53	1.3	5.4	2.9	0.5
Mushroom, Cream of, Canned, Tesco*	½ Can/200g	94	5.8	47	0.7	4.8	2.9	0.2
Mushroom, Cream of, Classics, Heinz*	1 Can/400g	208	11.2	52	1.5	5.2	2.8	0.1
Mushroom, Cream of, Condensed, Batchelors*	1 Can/295g	330	25.1	112	1.3	7.5	8.5	0.2
Mushroom, Cream Of, Tesco*	½ Can/200g	116	7.2	58	1.3	5	3.6	0.4
Mushroom, for One, Heinz*	1 Can/290g	148	7.8	51	1.4	5.1	2.7	0.1

S

	Measure INFO/WEIGHT	per Measure KCAL	FAT	Nutrition Values per 100g / 100ml KCAL	PROT	CARB	FAT	FIBRE
SOUP								
Mushroom, Fresh, Average	***1 Serving/300g***	***146***	***9.3***	***49***	***1.3***	***4***	***3.1***	***0.8***
Mushroom, Risotto, Grain, Meal Soup, Sainsbury's*	1 Pack/400g	257	11.2	64	2	7	2.8	1.5
Mushroom, Wild, Cup, As Prepared, Waitrose*	1 Serving/213g	98	3	46	0.6	7.5	1.4	0.5
Mushroom, with Croutons in a Cup, Waitrose*	1 Sachet/212g	102	4.2	48	0.6	6.8	2	0.5
Mushroom, with Croutons, Soup in a Mug, Tesco*	1 Serving/226ml	115	4.7	51	1	6.8	2.1	0.4
Noodle, Cantonese Hot & Sour, Baxters*	1 Serving/215g	133	2.8	62	1.4	11.1	1.3	0.5
Noodle, Chicken, Chilli, Ramen, Waitrose*	1 Pack/401g	325	8.8	81	7.7	7.1	2.2	1.3
Noodle, Cup, Shin, Nongshim*	1 Cup/75g	326	11.2	435	7	68	15	0
Noodle, Seafood, Ramyun, Nongshim*	1 Pack/125g	522	16.2	418	8.3	67	13	0
Noodle, Sweet & Spicy, Cup Soup, Made Up, Tesco*	1 Sachet/220g	77	0.2	35	0.7	7.5	0.1	0.6
Onion, French	***1oz/28g***	***11***	***0.6***	***40***	***0.2***	***5.7***	***2.1***	***1***
Onion, French, & Cider, Waitrose*	1 Can/425g	94	0.4	22	0.5	4.8	0.1	0.4
Onion, French, Favourites, Baxters*	½ Can/200g	46	1	23	0.7	3.8	0.5	0.3
Oxtail, Average	***1 Can/400g***	***163***	***4.5***	***41***	***2***	***5.8***	***1.1***	***0.4***
Oxtail, Canned	***1 Serving/220g***	***97***	***3.7***	***44***	***2.4***	***5.1***	***1.7***	***0.1***
Oxtail, Classic, Heinz*	1 Can/400g	168	2	42	1.9	7.3	0.5	0.3
Pancetta, & Lentil, Tuscan Style, Aldi*	1 Serving/200g	170	3.6	85	10	6.7	1.8	0
Pancetta, Barley, & Kale, Finest, Tesco*	½ Pot/302g	148	5.4	49	2.6	4.4	1.8	2.6
Parsnip, & Honey, Fresh, Sainsbury's*	½ Carton/300g	192	12.6	64	1.1	5.4	4.2	1.5
Parsnip, Creamy, Waitrose*	1 Can/400g	168	8.4	42	1.2	4	2.1	1
Parsnip, Spicy, Average	***1 Serving/400g***	***212***	***11.2***	***53***	***0.9***	***6***	***2.8***	***1.6***
Parsnip, Spicy, Vegetarian, Baxters*	1 Can/400g	212	9.6	53	1.2	5.9	2.4	1.7
Parsnip, Winter Spiced, Tideford Organics*	1 Pot/600g	216	8.4	36	0.9	4.5	1.4	1.1
Pea, & Ham	***1 Serving/220g***	***154***	***4.6***	***70***	***4***	***9.2***	***2.1***	***1.4***
Pea, & Ham Hock, Cherrywood, Specially Selected, Aldi*	½ Pack/300g	144	4.8	48	3.3	4.1	1.6	1.7
Pea, & Ham, Canned, Favourites, Baxters*	1 Can/400g	218	4	55	3.3	7.1	1	2
Pea, & Ham, Canned, Tesco*	1 Can/400g	184	2	46	3.1	6.1	0.5	2.1
Pea, & Ham, Classic, Heinz*	1 Can/400g	252	3.2	63	2.8	10.1	0.8	1.1
Pea, & Ham, Petit Pois, Fresh, TTD, Sainsbury's*	½ Pot/300g	201	7.8	67	3.8	6.1	2.6	2.2
Pea, & Ham, Split, Asda*	1 Serving/300g	129	0.6	43	3.5	6.9	0.2	0.7
Pea, & Mint, Best of British, Crosse & Blackwell*	1 Can/400g	192	8.4	48	1.7	4.6	2.1	1.9
Pea, & Mint, Fresh, Co-Op*	½ Tub/300g	105	1.7	35	1.7	4.8	0.6	1.8
Pea, & Mint, Fresh, Finest, Tesco*	1 Serving/300g	165	7.2	55	1.3	6	2.4	1.5
Pea, & Mint, Fresh, M&S*	1 Serving/164g	49	0.2	30	1.8	6.3	0.1	1.5
Pea, & Mint, Fresh, Sainsbury's*	½ Pot/300g	102	2.7	34	1.4	5	0.9	1.9
Pea, & Mint, Fresh, Tesco*	½ Pot/300g	145	3.3	48	2.4	6	1.1	2.4
Pea, & Mint, Garden, Vegetarian, Baxters*	½ Can/200g	100	1.6	50	2.5	7.3	0.8	1.9
Pea, & Mint, Slimming World, Iceland*	1 Tub/500g	205	2	41	2.5	5.6	0.4	2.7
Pea, & Mint, with Leek, Fresh, Waitrose*	1 Serving/300g	123	4.5	41	1.7	4.4	1.5	1.5
Pea, & Ham Hock, Fresh, The Best, Morrisons*	½ Pot/300g	180	7.5	60	3	5.5	2.5	1.9
Pea, & Ham, Asda*	½ Can/198g	81	1.4	41	2.4	5.1	0.7	2.1
Pea, & Ham, Rustic, Newgate, Lidl*	1 Can/400g	204	2.8	51	3	6.8	0.7	2.6
Pea, & Ham, Vegan, Suma*	1 Can/400g	196	2.4	49	2.7	7.1	0.6	1.8
Pea, & Mint, Cup, Waitrose*	1 Cup/215ml	103	2.2	48	1.1	8.3	1	0.5
Pea, & Watercress, Daylesford*	½ Pack/250g	125	6.2	50	1.9	5	2.5	1
Pea, Basil, & Lemon, Re:nourish*	1 Serving/500g	205	4	41	2.1	5.3	0.8	3.4
Pea, Coconut, & Tumeric, Tideford Organics*	½ Pot/300g	99	3	33	1.6	3.5	1	1.6
Pea, Edamame, & Spinach, Canned, Waitrose*	1 Can/400g	172	3.6	43	2.4	5.5	0.9	1.4
Pea, Garden, & Ham, Bramwells, Aldi*	1 Can/400g	208	4	52	3.5	6.2	1	2.1
Pea, Hearty, & Wiltshire Cured Ham Hock, Waitrose*	½ Carton/300g	165	4.2	55	3.1	6.6	1.4	1.8
Pea, Split, Yellow, Simply Organic*	1 Pot/600g	354	3	59	4.3	10.4	0.5	2.6
Peas, & Greens, Soupreme, Aldi*	1 Pot/600g	306	7.2	51	1.7	7.5	1.2	1.8
Pepper, & Chorizo, Canned, Sainsbury's*	1 Can/400ml	172	4	43	7	2	1	0

S

	Measure INFO/WEIGHT	per Measure KCAL	FAT	Nutrition Values per 100g / 100ml KCAL	PROT	CARB	FAT	FIBRE
SOUP								
Pepper, with Chilli, Italiamo, Lidl*	1 Can/390ml	222	9.4	57	0.6	7.6	2.4	1.3
Potato, & Leek, Optifast, Nestle*	1 Pack/44g	172	4.8	392	36	34	11	6.5
Prawn, King, & Glass Noodles, Pho, pot	***1 Pot/642g***	***212***	***2.6***	***33***	***1.8***	***5.4***	***0.4***	***0.5***
Prawn, Tom Yum, Cook*	1 Portion/335g	231	3	69	3.5	10.8	0.9	0
Pumpkin, & Sweet Potato, Super-Licious, Baxters*	1 Pot/350g	168	7.4	48	0.9	5.9	2.1	0.8
Pumpkin, Creamy, Very Special, Heinz*	1 Sm Can/290g	188	5.5	65	1.3	9.9	1.9	1.1
Pumpkin, Spicy, Fresh, Sainsbury's*	½ Pot/300g	87	3	29	0.9	4.2	1	1.3
Ramen, Classic, Broth, Brilliant, Itsu*	1 Serving/250ml	138	1.2	55	0.5	12	0.5	0.5
Red Lentil, Apricot, & Chilli, Tideford Organics*	1 Pot/600g	228	8.4	38	1.3	4.6	1.4	1
Red Lentil, Spicy, Waitrose*	1 Pot/600g	270	3.6	45	1.6	8	0.6	0.6
Red Pepper, & Wensleydale, Asda*	1 Carton /600g	306	12.6	51	2.5	5	2.1	0.8
Red Pepper, Canned, Morrisons*	½ Can/198g	117	5.7	59	1	6.7	2.9	1
Red Pepper, Roasted, & Tomato, Canned, Sainsbury's*	1 Can/400g	196	6	49	1	7.5	1.5	0.9
Red Pepper, Roasted, & Tomato, M&S*	1 Serving/150g	105	7.4	70	1.4	5	4.9	0.6
Red Pepper, Roasted, Fresh, Waitrose*	1 Pack/600g	172	9	29	0.8	3	1.5	1
Roasted Tomatoes, & Basil, Love Yourself Diet*	1 Pack/255g	139	9	55	1.6	4.3	3.5	0
Root Vegetable, Roasted, Waitrose*	1 Pot/350g	102	3.2	29	0.6	3.7	0.9	1.7
Scotch Broth, Canned, Tesco*	½ Can/200g	85	2.6	42	1.3	5.9	1.3	0.8
Scotch Broth, Classic, Heinz*	1 Can/400g	156	2.4	39	1.4	6.7	0.6	0.6
Scotch Broth, Favourites, Baxters*	1 Can/400g	168	4	42	1.8	6.8	1	1.4
Scotch Broth, Scotty Brand*	½ Pot/275g	72	0.8	26	1.1	5.8	0.3	2.2
Seafood Chowder, Canned, TTD, Sainsbury's*	½ Can/200g	114	5.6	57	1.9	5.9	2.8	0.5
Spinach, & Green Lentil, Spiced, Asda*	½ Pot/250g	122	5	49	2.7	5	2	0
Spinach, & Olive, Italiamo, Lidl*	1 Can/400g	252	15.2	63	1.2	5.4	3.8	1.1
Spinach, Creme Fraiche, & Nutmeg, Organic, Waitrose*	½ Pot/300g	243	22.8	81	0.9	2.3	7.6	1.1
Split Pea, Organic, Amy's Kitchen*	1 Can/400g	172	1.6	43	2	7.8	0.4	2.4
Spring Veg, Pinch Of Nom*	1 Bowl/300ml	134	2.7	45	1.5	7	0.9	1.4
Squash, & Red Pepper, Spiced, Sainsbury's*	½ Can/200g	78	2.6	39	0.6	5.7	1.3	1.1
Steak, & Potato, Angus, Big Soup, Heinz*	½ Can/250g	120	2	48	3.1	6.8	0.8	0.6
Steak, & Ale, Chunky, Asda*	1 Can/400g	188	4.4	47	3	5.9	1.1	0.6
Steak, & Vegetables, Big Soup, Heinz*	1 Can/498g	294	5	59	3.7	8.3	1	1
Sweet Potato, & Cauliflower, Super Soup, Bol*	½ Pot/250g	142	3.2	57	3.4	10	1.3	3.9
Sweet Potato, & Lentil, Dahl, Yorkshire Provender*	1 Pot/600g	330	16.2	55	2.6	6.9	2.7	0
Sweet Potato, & Red Chilli, Asda*	½ Pot/300g	144	5.4	48	0.5	7.1	1.8	0.8
Sweet Potato, Coconut & Chilli, TTD, Sainsbury's*	½ Pot/300g	176	5.7	59	0.9	8.5	1.9	1.8
Sweet Potato, Coconut, & Chilli, Finest, Tesco*	½ Pot/300g	192	11.7	64	1.1	5.8	3.9	0.6
Sweet Potato, Coconut, & Chilli, The Best, Morrisons*	½ Pot/300g	222	11.7	74	1	8	3.9	1.2
Sweet Potato, Sri Lankan, Plant Based, Baxters*	1 Can/380g	205	6.8	54	0.8	7.9	1.8	1.4
Sweetcorn, & Yellow Pepper, Blended, Heinz*	½ Can/200g	98	4.2	49	0.9	6.6	2.1	0.6
Tarka Dahl, Canned, M&S*	1 Can/400g	260	4.4	65	1.9	8.6	1.1	1.8
Thai Chicken, & Lemongrass, Cup Soup, Ainsley Harriott*	1 Sachet/224g	101	3.4	45	0.6	7.3	1.5	0.1
Thai Green Curry, Vegetable, Heart, Bowl, Sainsbury's*	1 Pack/400g	256	10.8	64	0.8	8.3	2.7	1.6
Thai Green, Vegetable, Naked, Hearty, Sainsbury's*	1 Pot/400g	256	10.8	64	0.8	8.3	2.7	1.6
Thai, Dry Weight, Sachet, Knorr*	1 Sachet/35g	133	4.2	379	10	57	12	3.5
Three Bean, Chilli, Fresh, Tesco*	½ Pot/300g	126	0.3	42	3.3	6	0.1	2.2
Tom Yum, Chicken, Cook*	1 Pack/280g	126	3.1	45	3.8	5.4	1.1	0.7
Tomato, & Basil, CBY, Asda*	½ Pot/297g	89	2.4	30	1	4.3	0.8	0.7
Tomato, & Basil, Creamy, Cully & Sully*	1 Pack/400g	216	18.5	54	0.8	2.5	4.6	0.5
Tomato, & Basil, Cup, Co-Op*	1 Sachet/45g	158	1.8	350	2	76	4	4
Tomato, & Basil, Fresh, Finest, Tesco*	½ Pot/300g	219	14.7	73	1	6.3	4.9	0.6
Tomato, & Basil, Fresh, Low Fat, Sainsbury's*	½ Carton/300ml	75	1.8	25	1.1	4.1	0.6	0.7
Tomato, & Basil, Fresh, M Kitchen, Morrisons*	½ Pot/300g	115	3.6	38	1	5.5	1.2	0.7
Tomato, & Basil, Fresh, M&S*	½ Pot/300g	120	5.1	40	1	5	1.7	1.3

S

	Measure INFO/WEIGHT	per Measure KCAL	FAT	Nutrition Values per 100g / 100ml KCAL	PROT	CARB	FAT	FIBRE
SOUP								
Tomato, & Basil, Italian Plum, Finest, Tesco*	1 Pot/600g	360	13.8	60	1.3	7.2	2.3	0.6
Tomato, & Basil, Italian Style, Co-Op*	1 Pack/500g	200	10	40	1	4	2	0.6
Tomato, & Basil, Italian, Vegetarian, Baxters*	1 Can/415g	170	3.7	41	1.4	5.7	0.9	0.6
Tomato, & Basil, M&S*	½ Pot/300g	105	4.2	35	0.7	4.5	1.4	1
Tomato, & Basil, Rich, Waitrose*	1 Serving/130g	53	1.3	41	1.3	6.3	1	0.7
Tomato, & Basil, Sun Dried, Heinz*	1 Serving/275ml	124	5.2	45	0.6	6.5	1.9	0.1
Tomato, & Brown Lentil, Healthy, Baxters*	1 Can/415g	199	0.8	48	2.6	9	0.2	2.7
Tomato, & Butter Bean, Classic, Heinz*	½ Can/200g	92	1.4	46	1.3	8.1	0.7	0.8
Tomato, & Lentil, Truly Irresistible, Co-Op*	½ Pot/300g	165	2.1	55	3.1	8	0.7	1.2
Tomato, & Red Pepper, Fire Roasted, Asda*	½ Tub/265g	114	6.9	43	0.7	4.1	2.6	1
Tomato, & Three Bean, Canned, BGTY, Sainsbury's*	½ Can/198g	113	1	57	3.4	8.7	0.5	2.2
Tomato, & Three Bean, Eat Smart, Morrisons*	1 Can/400g	228	4	57	2.8	8.2	1	2.2
Tomato, & Thyme, Organic, Duchy, Waitrose*	½ Pot/300g	140	8.9	47	1.2	3.3	3	1
Tomato, & Vegetable, Cup a Soup, Batchelors*	1 Serving/218g	107	2.6	49	1.1	8.5	1.2	0.6
Tomato, & Balsamic, Finest, Tesco*	½ Pot/300g	116	4.2	38	1.2	4.9	1.4	0.7
Tomato, & Basil, Bramwells, Aldi*	1 Can/400g	188	8.8	47	0.8	4.9	2.2	2.1
Tomato, & Basil, Canned, Sainsbury's*	1 Can/400g	228	11.2	57	1	6.5	2.8	0.8
Tomato, & Basil, Jane Plan*	1 Pack/300g	159	8.4	53	0.9	5.6	2.8	1
Tomato, & Basil, New Covent Garden Food Co*	½ Carton/280g	112	4.5	40	1.2	5.4	1.6	0.9
Tomato, & Chorizo, Deluxe, Lidl*	½ Can/200g	168	8.8	84	2.7	8.2	4.4	0.5
Tomato, & Chorizo, Specially Selected, Aldi*	½ Can/200g	168	8.8	84	2.7	8.2	4.4	0.5
Tomato, & Lentil, Super Spicy, M&S*	1 Pot/300g	150	3.3	50	2.6	6.3	1.1	2.1
Tomato, Borlotti Bean & Kale, Fresh, M&S*	1 Pot/600g	318	10.2	53	2	6.3	1.7	2.1
Tomato, Cannellini Beans, & Garlic, Heinz*	½ Can/200g	110	2.2	55	2.4	9.1	1.1	2.4
Tomato, Cream of, & Basil, Canned, Heinz*	1 Can/400g	232	12	58	0.9	6.6	3	0.4
Tomato, Cream of, Canned, Average	***1 Can/400g***	***208***	***12***	***52***	***0.8***	***5.9***	***3***	***0.7***
Tomato, Cream of, Condensed, Batchelors*	1 Can/295g	378	18.3	128	1.4	16.5	6.2	0.4
Tomato, Cream of, Fresh, Sainsbury's*	1 Pot/600g	318	19.2	53	0.8	5.2	3.2	1.3
Tomato, Cream of, Fresh, Waitrose*	½ Pot/300g	167	8.1	56	0.9	6.6	2.7	0.6
Tomato, Cream Of, Pot, Heinz*	1 Pot/280g	135	3.1	48	1.2	8	1.1	0.8
Tomato, Cup, Made Up, Bramwells, Aldi*	1 Sachet/252g	83	1.8	33	0.5	5.8	0.7	0.5
Tomato, Gazpacho, Innocent*	1 Bowl/200g	80	4.6	40	0.6	2.8	2.3	2.4
Tomato, Knorr*	1 Serving/170ml	85	2.3	50	1.1	8.1	1.4	0.5
Tomato, Mediterranean, Vegetarian, Baxters*	1 Can/400g	126	0.4	32	0.9	5.6	0.1	0.8
Tomato, Optifast, Nestle*	1 Pack/44g	172	4.8	392	36	34	11	6.5
Tomato, Organic, Auga*	1 Pack/400g	252	16	63	0.8	5.9	4	1.4
Tomato, Original, Cup a Soup, Batchelors*	1 Sachet/254g	104	2.3	41	0.6	7.3	0.9	0.5
Tomato, Plum, & Basil, Newgate, Lidl*	1 Can/400g	160	6.4	40	0.7	5.4	1.6	0.7
Tomato, Red Lentil & Pepper, CBY, Asda*	½ Pot/300g	177	3.3	59	3	8.8	1.1	0.9
Tomato, Red Pepper, & Lentil, Morrisons*	1 Pot/600g	372	12.6	62	2.2	7.4	2.1	2.3
Tomato, Smart Price, Asda*	1 Can/400g	184	7.6	46	0.6	6.5	1.9	0.9
Tomato, Spicy, Lentil, & Red Pepper, Fresh, Sainsbury's*	1 Pot/600g	390	7.8	65	3.7	8.8	1.3	1.8
Tomato, Spinach, & Lentil, Heinz*	½ Can/200g	85	1.4	43	1.7	7.7	0.7	1.1
Tomato, Stockwell & Co., Tesco*	1 Can/400g	192	6.4	48	0.5	7.5	1.6	0.5
Tomato, Weight Watchers*	1 Can/295g	76	1.5	26	0.7	4.6	0.5	0.3
Turkey, Broth, Canned, Baxters*	½ Can/208g	79	1.5	38	1.3	6.5	0.7	0.7
Vegetable Tagine, Slimming World*	1 Tub/500g	215	2	43	2.6	5.6	0.4	3.1
Vegetable, & Three Bean, Chunky, M&S*	1 Can/400g	228	3.6	57	3	7.7	0.9	3.1
Vegetable, Barley, Amy's Kitchen*	1 Can/400g	152	4.8	38	0.8	5.3	1.2	1.2
Vegetable, Broth, Hearty, Weight Watchers*	1 Can/295g	135	0.6	46	2	8.2	0.2	1.4
Vegetable, Canned	***1oz/28g***	***13***	***0.2***	***48***	***1.4***	***9.9***	***0.6***	***1.5***
Vegetable, Chunky, Canned, Asda*	½ Can/200g	98	1	49	2.1	7.9	0.5	2.4

S

	Measure INFO/WEIGHT	per Measure KCAL	FAT	KCAL	PROT	CARB	FAT	FIBRE
				Nutrition Values per 100g / 100ml				
SOUP								
Vegetable, Chunky, Canned, Sainsbury's*	1 Can/400g	184	2.8	46	1.5	8.3	0.7	1.2
Vegetable, Chunky, Canned, Soupreme, Aldi*	1 Can/400g	172	4	43	1.1	6.4	1	2.3
Vegetable, Chunky, Canned, Tesco*	½ Can/200g	80	1.2	40	1.1	7	0.6	1.3
Vegetable, Chunky, Diet Chef Ltd*	1 Pack/300g	114	0.9	38	1.4	7.4	0.3	1.3
Vegetable, Chunky, Fresh, CBY, Asda*	½ Pot/300g	117	2.1	39	1.6	5.9	0.7	1.1
Vegetable, Chunky, Fresh, Tesco*	½ Pot/300g	138	4.8	46	1.4	5.7	1.6	1.6
Vegetable, Chunky, Fresh, Waitrose*	½ Pot/300g	132	5.4	44	1.3	4.5	1.8	2.1
Vegetable, Chunky, Parsley Box*	1 Pack/300g	108	0.6	36	1.5	7.4	0.2	0.6
Vegetable, Country, Chunky, Baxters*	1 Can/400g	188	2.4	47	1.6	7.2	0.6	2
Vegetable, Country, Chunky, Fresh, M&S*	½ Pot/300g	123	4.8	41	0.8	5.3	1.6	1.2
Vegetable, Country, Fresh, Soupreme, Aldi*	1 Tub/600g	204	3.6	34	1.1	5.1	0.6	1.7
Vegetable, Country, Hearty, Canned, Baxters*	1 Can/400g	192	2.4	48	1.9	7.5	0.6	1.9
Vegetable, Country, Knorr*	1 Pack/500ml	160	3.5	32	0.9	5.5	0.7	1.2
Vegetable, Country, Weight Watchers*	1 Can/295g	97	0.3	33	1.2	6.3	0.1	1
Vegetable, Cully & Sully*	1 Pack/400g	204	14.4	51	0.6	4.2	3.6	0.9
Vegetable, Cup Soup, Dry, Heinz*	1 Sachet/16g	54	1.1	348	5.8	64.5	7.1	3.2
Vegetable, Cup Soup, Made Up, Heinz*	1 Cup/200g	62	0.6	31	0.5	6.3	0.3	0.3
Vegetable, Dry Mix, The Kee Diet*	1 Sachet/40g	138	3.3	344	40.2	27.5	8.3	5.2
Vegetable, Farmhouse, Thick, Co-Op*	1 Can/400g	140	1.6	35	1	7	0.4	0.3
Vegetable, Fresh, Average	***1 Serving/300g***	***118***	***4.1***	***40***	***1.4***	***5.4***	***1.4***	***1.3***
Vegetable, Golden, Cup, GFY, Asda*	1 Sachet/217ml	52	1.1	24	0.5	4.4	0.5	0.2
Vegetable, Golden, Slim a Soup, Batchelors*	1 Sachet/207g	58	1.7	28	0.5	4.7	0.8	0.7
Vegetable, Green, & Grains, Vegan, Waitrose*	1 Pot/400g	248	12	62	3.1	3.8	3	3.6
Vegetable, Hearty, Asda*	½ Can/200g	88	1.2	44	1.1	7.9	0.6	1.3
Vegetable, Instant, Cup, Average	***1 Pack/19g***	***69***	***2***	***362***	***8.7***	***57.1***	***10.5***	***5.5***
Vegetable, No Added Sugar, Canned, Heinz*	½ Can/200g	84	1.4	42	1.2	7.2	0.7	1.2
Vegetable, Pot, Classic, Heinz*	1 Pot/355g	142	3.2	40	1	7.8	0.9	1
Vegetable, Root, & Turmeric, Baxters*	1 Can/400g	164	5.6	41	0.8	6.3	1.4	0.5
Vegetable, Scotty Brand*	½ Pot/275g	118	1	43	2.3	9.2	0.4	3.3
Vegetable, Spring, Classic, Heinz*	1 Can/400g	148	1.6	37	0.8	7	0.4	0.8
Vegetable, Spring, Florida, Dry, Knorr*	1 Pack/36g	104	2	290	7.8	52.2	5.6	5.2
Vegetable, Spring, Sainsbury's*	½ Can/200g	72	0.8	36	0.8	7.4	0.4	0.6
Vegetable, Ten, Broth, Morrisons*	1 Pot/600g	240	7.8	40	1.7	5.8	1.3	1.1
Watercress, M&S*	½ Pot/300g	75	5.1	25	1.3	1.5	1.7	0.6
SOUP MIX								
Broccoli, & Stilton, Knorr*	1 Portion/225ml	101	7.2	45	0.8	3.1	3.2	0.5
Butternut Squash, & Red Pepper, Asda*	½ Pack/178g	57	0.9	32	1	6.1	0.5	1.4
Butternut Squash, & Sweet Potato, COOK!, M&S*	1 Pack/600g	360	1.2	60	1.1	12.3	0.2	2.3
Butternut Squash, Sainsbury's*	¼ Pack/150g	63	2.1	42	0.8	6.3	1.4	0.9
Country, Morrisons*	1 Serving/80g	82	0.6	102	6	13.7	0.8	7.8
Leek & Potato, As Sold, G&B, Asda*	¼ Pack/125g	69	0.4	55	1.7	10.5	0.3	1.7
Potato, & Leek, Sainsbury's*	1 Serving/100g	31	0.5	31	1.4	5.5	0.5	1
Red Pepper, & Carrot, Nature's Pick, Aldi*	1 Serving/100g	16	0.5	16	1.4	1.8	0.5	0.8
Sweet Potato, Nature's Pick, Aldi*	1 Serving/100g	24	0.5	24	0.8	4.1	0.5	1.2
Vegetable, & Lentil, Boiled, Sainsbury's*	¼ Pack/150g	57	0.8	38	1.8	6.2	0.5	2.1
Vegetable, & Lentil, Cook with, M&S*	¼ Pack/150g	75	0.6	50	1.9	8.2	0.4	2.9
Vegetable, Asda*	½ Pack/250g	95	1.2	38	0.9	7.5	0.5	0.7
Vegetable, Kit, Morrisons*	1 Pack/500g	220	3.5	44	1.2	6.6	0.7	3
Winter, Broth, Morrisons*	1 Pack/600g	294	3.6	49	1.5	7.9	0.6	3.1
SOUTHERN COMFORT								
37.5% Volume	***1 Pub Shot/35ml***	***72***	***0***	***207***	***0***	***0***	***0***	***0***
SOYA								
Chunks, Protein, Natural, Nature's Harvest*	1 Serving/50g	172	0.5	345	50	35	1	4

S

	Measure INFO/WEIGHT	per Measure KCAL	FAT	Nutrition Values per 100g / 100ml KCAL	PROT	CARB	FAT	FIBRE
SOYA								
Chunks, Tree Of Life*	1 Serving/34g	123	0.3	361	52	36	1	0
Mince, Dry Weight, Sainsbury's*	1 Serving/50g	164	0.4	328	47.2	33.2	0.8	3.6
Schnitzel, Golden Crumbed, Fry's*	1 Schnitzels/80g	186	12	232	10.3	16	15	6.1
Schnitzel, Like Meat*	1 Pack/180g	436	21.6	242	11	19	12	6.5
Tenderstrips, Roast, Naked Glory*	½ Pack/120g	172	5.5	143	20	4.3	4.6	5.8
Tenderstrips, Smoky BBQ , Naked Glory*	1 Serving/70g	80	0.3	115	18	8	0.4	5.1
Tenderstrips, Tikka, Vegetarian, Naked Glory*	1 Serving/70g	91	1.9	130	20	3.4	2.7	5
SPAGHETTI								
Alphabet, Morrisons*	1 Can/200g	118	0.8	59	1.5	11.9	0.4	0.8
Bare Naked, Barenaked*	1 Serving/100g	17	0.1	17	0.3	0.9	0.1	3.4
Black Bean, Cooked, The Foodie Market, Aldi*	1 Serving/125g	125	2.9	100	15	1.6	2.3	7.9
Black Bean, Organic, Dry, Aldi*	1 Serving/50g	162	2.6	325	46	13	5.3	21
Black Bean, Organic, Dry, Explore Asian*	1 Serving/56g	198	2	353	44	15	3.6	21
Cooked, Average	***1oz/28g***	***33***	***0.2***	***119***	***4.1***	***24.8***	***0.6***	***1.1***
Courgetti, with Chargrilled Chicken, BFY, M&S*	1 Pack/370g	211	7	57	7	2.5	1.9	1
Dry, Average	***1oz/28g***	***98***	***0.4***	***350***	***12.1***	***72.1***	***1.5***	***2.4***
Durum Wheat, Dry, Average	***1oz/28g***	***97***	***0.1***	***348***	***12.4***	***71.8***	***0.4***	***1.4***
Edamame, Organic, Dry, Explore Asian*	1 Serving/56g	204	2	365	45	18	3.6	20
Fresh, Cooked, Average	***1 Serving/125g***	***182***	***2.2***	***146***	***6.1***	***26.9***	***1.7***	***1.8***
Fresh, Dry, Average	***1 Serving/100g***	***278***	***3***	***278***	***10.8***	***53***	***3***	***2.2***
GF, Cooked, Free From, Morrisons*	1 Portion/75g	129	0.4	172	2.8	38.6	0.6	0.9
GF, Free From, Tesco*	1 Serving/75g	266	0.8	355	7	78.4	1	2
Hoops, Canned, Simply, Lidl*	1 Can/410g	234	1.2	57	1.5	11.2	0.3	1.5
Hoops, Canned, Smart Price, Asda*	½ Can/205g	127	0.6	62	1.7	13	0.3	0.4
Hoops, in Tomato Sauce, Heinz*	½ Can/200g	106	0.4	53	1.7	11.1	0.2	0.5
Hoops, in Tomato Sauce, Snap Pot, Heinz*	1 Pot/190g	115	0.4	61	1.7	12.6	0.2	0.6
in Rich Tomato Sauce, Canned, Corale, Aldi*	½ Can/200g	114	1	57	2.1	10	0.5	2.6
in Tomato Sauce with Parsley, Weight Watchers*	1 Sm Can/200g	100	0.4	50	1.8	9.9	0.2	0.6
in Tomato Sauce, Canned	***1oz/28g***	***18***	***0.1***	***64***	***1.9***	***14.1***	***0.4***	***0.7***
Loops, Canned, Simply, Lidl*	½ Can/205g	117	0.6	57	1.5	11.2	0.3	1.5
Marinara	***1 Serving/450g***	***675***	***18.9***	***150***	***8***	***19***	***4.2***	***0.9***
Organic, Cooked, So Organic, Sainsbury's*	1 Serving/200g	318	1.4	159	5.2	32.3	0.7	1.4
Organic, Cooked, Tesco*	1 Serving/150g	190	0.6	127	3.7	25.4	0.4	1.6
Prawn, Chilli, Waitrose*	1 Pack/360g	382	11.5	106	4.4	13.9	3.2	2
Tomato, & Basil, Sainsbury's*	1 Pack/395g	367	7.9	93	3.1	14.6	2	2
Tricolore, Dry, Italiamo, Lidl*	1 Serving/60g	210	0.7	350	12.5	70.5	1.2	0
Whole Wheat, Cooked, Average	***1oz/28g***	***32***	***0.3***	***113***	***4.7***	***23.2***	***0.9***	***3.5***
Whole Wheat, Dry, Average	***1 Serving/100g***	***324***	***2.6***	***324***	***13.5***	***62.2***	***2.6***	***8***
with Sausages, in Tomato Sauce, Heinz*	1 Can/400g	352	14	88	3.4	10.8	3.5	0.5
SPAGHETTI & MEATBALLS								
Beef, with Spiced Tomato & Pepper Sauce, BFY, M&S*	1 Pack/380g	361	9.9	95	7.3	10	2.6	1.2
Discover The Choice*	1 Pack/450g	486	26.6	108	7.7	5.5	5.9	0.8
Shroomballs, Plant Pioneers, Sainsbury's*	1 Pack/387g	375	8.9	97	3.4	14.5	2.3	2.5
Taste of Italy, Tesco*	1 Pack/420g	479	15.1	114	7.2	12.4	3.6	1.7
Veggie, Plant Based, Asda*	1 Pack/378g	473	18.9	125	6.3	12	5	3
SPAGHETTI BOLOGNAISE								
Beef, & Pancetta, Microwaved, Luxury, Iceland*	1 Meal/445g	663	30.7	149	9.1	12	6.9	1.3
Chef Select, Lidl*	1 Serving/450g	477	12.2	106	7	12.7	2.7	1.2
Classic, Bisto*	1 Pack/375g	338	8.6	90	4.4	12.2	2.3	1.2
Meat Free, Plant Based, Asda*	1 Pack/400g	456	13.2	114	5	15	3.3	1.4
Nutriquick*	1 Portion/370g	377	7	102	10	11	1.9	0
SPAGHETTI WITH								
King Prawn, Italian, Cooked, Finest, Tesco*	1 Pack/390g	485	22.9	125	5	12.2	5.9	1.3

	Measure INFO/WEIGHT	per Measure KCAL	FAT	Nutrition Values per 100g / 100ml KCAL	PROT	CARB	FAT	FIBRE
SPAGHETTI WITH								
Tomato, & Basil, Parsley & Parmesan Cheese, M&S*	1 Pack/400g	584	29.2	146	3.8	15.1	7.3	2.2
SPAM*								
Pork & Ham, Chopped, Spam*	1 Serving/100g	289	24.3	289	15	3.2	24.3	0
SPICE MIX								
Baharat, Blends, Bart*	1 Pinch/1g	3	0.1	333	13.7	18.5	13.7	0
Chilli Con Carne, Bramwells, Aldi*	¼ Sachet/13g	41	0.5	318	9.7	55	3.7	13
Creole, Seasoned Pioneers*	1 Tbsp/15g	47	0.8	313	8.3	43.2	5.2	15.1
Dukkha, Cooks' Ingredients, Waitrose*	1 Tsp/5g	17	0.8	349	18.3	30.7	17	19.6
for Fajitas, Old El Paso*	1 Pack/35g	107	2.1	306	9	54	6	0
for Mexican Fajitas, Discovery*	½ Pack/15g	34	1	230	8	35	6.5	17.5
Moroccan, Rub, Schwartz*	1 Serving/3g	9	0.3	309	15	36.4	11.4	19.5
Napoli, Spaghetti, Kania*	1 Serving/22g	68	0.3	311	7.1	63.5	1.4	0
Peri Peri, Medium, Bag & Bake, Nando's*	1 Bag/20g	57	0.2	286	4.6	60	1.2	0
Peri Peri, Pan Fry, Nando's*	1 Sachet/20g	21	1.3	105	3	7	6.5	5.5
Ras El Hanout, Al'fez*	1 Tsp/2g	4	0.2	217	9.8	25.7	8.3	17.5
Ras El Hanout, Blend, Finest, Tesco*	1 Tsp/5g	16	0.5	320	9.4	37.1	9.2	23.6
Rogan Josh, Authentic, Schwartz*	1 Pack/35g	108	3.5	309	11.1	30.3	10	26.7
Smokehouse BBQ, Wrap It, Schwartz*	¼ Pack/8g	24	0.2	317	8.1	59.2	3.2	9.5
Sriracha Seasoning, Schwartz*	1 Tsp/2g	5	0.1	261	6.5	44.6	4.3	0
Zaatar, Waitrose*	1 Serving/10g	42	3	416	14.7	8.2	30.2	26.1
SPINACH								
Baby Leaf, Sainsbury's*	1 Serving/80g	14	0.4	18	2.5	0.6	0.5	1.3
Baby Leaf, Whole, Frozen, Sainsbury's*	1 Serving/80g	18	0.6	22	3.2	0.5	0.7	1.2
Baby, Average	***1 Serving/90g***	***22***	***0.7***	***25***	***2.8***	***1.6***	***0.8***	***2.1***
Boiled or Steamed, Average	***1 Serving/80g***	***17***	***0.6***	***21***	***2.6***	***0.9***	***0.8***	***2.1***
Canned, Average	***1 Serving/80g***	***16***	***0.4***	***20***	***2.8***	***1.3***	***0.5***	***2.7***
Chopped, Heritage*	1 Serving/80g	21	0.6	26	3.1	0.5	0.8	2.1
Creamed, Hacendado*	1 Pack/450g	288	15.8	64	2.8	4.4	3.5	1.9
Creamed, with Macarpone, Finest, Tesco*	½ Pack/121g	94	6	78	4.1	2.8	5	2.7
Leaf, Frozen, Lidl*	1 Serving/80g	37	0.6	46	3.9	4.3	0.8	0
Mornay, Waitrose*	½ Pack/125g	112	8.6	90	3.3	3.6	6.9	1.6
Raw, Average	***1 Serving/80g***	***19***	***0.6***	***24***	***2.9***	***1.4***	***0.7***	***2.2***
SPIRALI								
Dry, Average	***1 Serving/50g***	***176***	***0.8***	***352***	***12.2***	***72.6***	***1.6***	***2.8***
SPIRITS								
40% Volume	***1 Shot/35ml***	***78***	***0***	***222***	***0***	***0***	***0***	***0***
Amaretti, Non Alcoholic, Lyre's*	1 Single/25ml	18	0	70	0	17	0	0
American Malt, Non Alcoholic, Lyre's*	1 Single/25ml	4	0	17	0	3.7	0	0
Aperitif, Dry, Non Alcoholic, Lyre's*	1 Single/25ml	4	0	15	0	2.9	0	0
Aperitif, Rosso, Non Alcoholic, Lyre's*	1 Single/25ml	15	0	59	0	14	0	0
Coffee Originale, Non Alcoholic, Lyre's*	1 Single/25ml	16	0	64	0	15	0	0
Dark Cane, Non Alcoholic, Lyre's*	1 Single/25ml	5	0	20	0	4.5	0	0
Dry London, Non Alcoholic, Lyre's*	1 Single/25ml	2	0	10	0	1.9	0	0
Italian Orange, Non Alcoholic, Lyre's*	1 Single/25ml	19	0	76	0	18	0	0
Italian Spritz, Non Alcoholic, Lyre's*	1 Single/25ml	20	0	80	0	20	0	0
Juniper, & Inca Berry, Non Alcoholic, Caleno*	1 Serve/50ml	20	0	39	0	9	0	0
Licor 43, Diego Zamora*	1 Single/25ml	76	0	304	0.2	36.6	0.1	0
Livener, Alcohol Free, Three Spirit*	1 Serve/50ml	21	0	42	0	10	0	0
Nightcap, Alcohol Free, Three Spirit*	1 Serve/50ml	30	0	60	0	12.8	0	0
Non Alcoholic, Garden, Seedlip Ltd*	1 Serve/50ml	0	0	0	0	0	0	0
Non Alcoholic, Spice 94, Botanical, Seedlip Ltd*	1 Serve/50ml	0	0	0	0	0	0	0
Orange Sec, Non Alcoholic, Lyre's*	1 Single/25ml	15	0	61	0	15	0	0
Social Elixir, Alcohol Free, Three Spirit*	1 Serve/50ml	26	0	52	0	11.2	0	0

S

	Measure INFO/WEIGHT	per Measure KCAL	FAT	Nutrition Values per 100g / 100ml KCAL	PROT	CARB	FAT	FIBRE
SPIRITS								
Spiced Cane, Non Alcoholic, Lyre's*	1 Single/25ml	4	0	18	0	3.9	0	0
Spiced Citrus, Ultra Low Alcohol, Atopia*	1 Single/25ml	6	0	23	0	5	0	0
White Cane, Non Alcoholic, Lyre's*	1 Single/25ml	4	0	15	0	3.4	0	0
SPLIT PEAS								
Dried, Average	***1oz/28g***	***89***	***0.5***	***319***	***22.1***	***57.4***	***1.7***	***3.2***
Green, Dried, Average	***1 Serving/80g***	***261***	***1.3***	***326***	***22.5***	***45***	***1.6***	***20***
Yellow, Cooked, Average	***1 Serving/80g***	***101***	***0.7***	***126***	***9.3***	***15.4***	***0.9***	***9.8***
Yellow, Dry, Average	***1 Serving/40g***	***105***	***0.7***	***263***	***20.1***	***29.3***	***1.8***	***24.6***
SPONGE FINGERS								
Almond Fingers, Tesco*	1 Finger/46g	174	6.1	379	5.3	58.8	13.2	1.7
Boudoir, Sainsbury's*	1 Finger/5g	20	0.2	396	8.1	82.8	3.6	0.4
Tesco*	1 Finger/5g	19	0.2	386	7.6	80.6	3.7	1
Trifle, Average	***1 Sponge/24g***	***77***	***0.5***	***319***	***5.2***	***69.9***	***2.2***	***0.8***
SPONGE PUDDING								
Average	***1 Portion/170g***	***578***	***27.7***	***340***	***5.8***	***45.3***	***16.3***	***1.1***
Blackberry & Apple, HE, Tesco*	1 Pot/103g	159	1.4	155	3.1	32.6	1.4	0.7
Blueberry, & Lemon, Waitrose*	1 Pudding/105g	288	13.6	274	4.4	33.8	13	2.3
Cherry & Almond Flavour, Sainsbury's*	¼ Pudding/110g	334	15.7	304	3.5	40.3	14.3	0.7
Chocolate & Sauce, Co-Op*	1 Pack/225g	608	29.2	270	5	34	13	0.6
Chocolate, M&S*	1 Pudding/105g	401	24.3	382	5.7	36	23.1	3.5
Chocolate, Sainsbury's*	¼ Pudding/110g	464	28.3	422	5.4	42.3	25.7	0.8
Chocolate, Tesco*	1 Serving/115g	430	19.2	374	3.7	50.8	16.7	2.7
Chocolate, Trufree*	1 Serving/115g	374	17.2	325	2.5	44	15	2
Chocolate, Waitrose*	1 Pudding/110g	400	22.5	363	3.6	41.4	20.4	1.7
Golden Syrup, Co-Op*	1 Can/300g	945	39	315	2	47	13	0.6
Golden Syrup, Lyons*	1 Sponge/95g	351	14.2	369	3.2	55.3	14.9	0.6
Honey& Fig, M&S*	¼ Pudding/73g	225	12	310	3.6	34.8	16.6	3.4
Lemon Curd, Heinz*	¼ Can/78g	236	9.1	302	2.6	46.7	11.7	0.6
Lemon, M&S*	1 Pudding/105g	326	16	310	4.3	39.4	15.2	2.3
Lemon, Waitrose*	1 Serving/105g	212	2.5	202	3.4	41.7	2.4	1.4
Milk Chocolate, Sticky Puds, Cadbury*	1 Pudding/95g	390	17.3	360	4.2	48.9	16	0.8
Mixed Berry, BGTY, Sainsbury's*	1 Pudding/110g	189	2.6	172	2.4	33.3	2.4	3.8
Pear & Ginger, COU, M&S*	1 Pudding/100g	175	0.7	175	1.9	39.8	0.7	1.1
Raspberry, Tesco*	1 Serving/100g	377	14.5	377	3.2	58.2	14.5	0.7
Salted Caramel, Specially Selected, Aldi*	1 Pudding/115g	459	20.7	399	3.6	54	18	1
Salted Caramel, Tesco*	1 Pudding/115g	464	21.6	404	3.2	55.2	18.8	0.6
Syrup, BGTY, Sainsbury's*	1 Pudding/110g	338	4.5	307	2.8	64.6	4.1	0.4
Syrup, Finest, Tesco*	1 Pudding/115g	330	9	287	3.1	51.2	7.8	0.6
Syrup, GFY, Asda*	1 Sponge/105g	207	4.3	197	2	38	4.1	2.6
Syrup, Iceland*	1 Pudding/115g	462	18.6	402	3.9	59.3	16.2	1.7
Syrup, Individual, Tesco*	1 Pudding/110g	390	14.5	355	3.1	55.6	13.2	0.5
Syrup, Sainsbury's*	¼ Pudding/110g	408	13	371	2.7	63.5	11.8	0.4
Syrup, Value, Tesco*	1 Serving/100g	307	10.2	307	2.1	51.7	10.2	0.6
Toffee & Pecan	***½ Pudding/100g***	***395***	***18.4***	***395***	***4.3***	***52.3***	***18.4***	***1.4***
Treacle, Heinz*	1 Serving/160g	445	13	278	2.5	48.9	8.1	0.6
Treacle, Waitrose*	1 Pudding/105g	385	13.8	367	2.8	59.5	13.1	0.5
with Custard	***1 Serving/200g***	***521***	***24.9***	***261***	***4.8***	***34.1***	***12.4***	***0.9***
with Jam or Treacle	***1oz/28g***	***93***	***4***	***333***	***5.1***	***48.7***	***14.4***	***1***
SPOTTED DICK								
Average	***1 Serving/105g***	***343***	***17.5***	***327***	***4.2***	***42.7***	***16.7***	***1***
Individual, Tesco*	1 Pudding/121g	417	14.5	345	3.2	55.2	12	1.2
with Custard	***1 Serving/210g***	***438***	***15.6***	***209***	***3.4***	***31.5***	***7.4***	***1.3***

	Measure INFO/WEIGHT	per Measure KCAL	FAT	Nutrition Values per 100g / 100ml KCAL	PROT	CARB	FAT	FIBRE
SPRATS								
Fried	***1oz/28g***	***116***	***9.8***	***415***	***24.9***	***0***	***35***	***0***
Raw	***1oz/28g***	***33***	***2.1***	***117***	***12.4***	***0***	***7.5***	***0***
SPREAD								
Aivar, Pelagonia *	1 Tbsp/20g	32	1.4	161	3.7	20	7	0
Almond, 100%, Sainsbury's*	1 Tbsp/20g	128	10.9	639	29.3	4.3	54.4	7.6
Average	***1 Thin Spread/7g***	***51***	***5.7***	***726***	***0.1***	***0.5***	***81***	***0***
Biscoff, Smooth, Lotus*	1 Tbsp/15g	88	5.7	584	2.9	57	38.1	0.8
Butter Me Up, Light, Tesco*	1 Thin Spread/7g	24	2.7	350	0.3	0.5	38	0
Butter Me Up, Tesco*	1 Thin Spread/7g	35	3.8	503	0.7	1	55	0.5
Butter Style, Average	***1 Thin Spread/7g***	***44***	***4.8***	***627***	***0.7***	***1.1***	***68.9***	***0***
Butterlicious, Vegetable, Sainsbury's*	1 Thin Spread/7g	44	4.8	628	0.6	1.1	69	0
Cashew, Pip & Nut*	1 Serving/15g	87	6.6	580	18	27	44	0
Clover, Light, Dairy Crest Ltd*	1 Thin Spread/7g	32	3.4	455	0.7	2.9	49	0
Enriched Olive, Tesco*	1 Thin Spread/7g	38	4.1	540	0.2	1.2	59	0
Fruit, Apricot, Organic, Meridian Foods*	1 Tsp/5g	6	0	121	0.6	27.1	0.3	2.4
Heart, Cholesterol Reducing, Dairygold	***1 Thin Spread/7g***	***24***	***2.5***	***338***	***0.7***	***2.8***	***36***	***0***
Lactofree Spreadable, Lactofree, Arla*	1 Serving/10g	68	7.5	679	0.5	0.5	75	0
Light, Benecol*	1 Thin Spread/7g	23	2.4	333	2.5	0	35	0
Light, Flora*	1 Thin Spread/7g	28	3.2	398	0.5	0.5	45	0
Low Fat, Average	***1 Thin Spread/7g***	***27***	***2.8***	***390***	***5.8***	***0.5***	***40.5***	***0***
Margerine, Extra Fit, Latta*	1 Thin Spread/7g	19	0.4	265	0.6	3.3	5.5	0
Margerine, Soft, for Cooking, Planta Fin*	1 Serving/10g	54	6	540	0.5	0.5	60	0
Nut Butter, Almond, Pumpkin Spice, Pip & Nut*	1 Tbsp/15g	90	7.4	599	21.7	12.6	49.5	8.2
Nut Butter, Almond, Smooth, Pip & Nut*	1 Tbsp/15g	96	8.2	640	26.7	6	54.7	8
Nut Butter, Almond, Smooth, Whole Earth*	1 Tbsp/15g	94	8	628	30.6	26	53	9.1
Nut Butter, Hazelnut, Bulk Powders*	1 Tbsp/30g	195	19	650	14.1	6	63.5	6.5
Nut Butter, Hazelnut, Dark Chocolate, Active Foods*	1 Serving/10g	60	5.5	602	12	18	55	4.5
Olive Oil, Bertolli*	1 Serving/10g	53	5.9	532	0.5	0.5	59	0
Olive, Light, Tesco*	1 Spread/10g	28	3	278	0.1	0.6	30.5	0.5
Olive, Low Fat, Morrisons*	1 Thin Spread/7g	24	2.7	346	0.9	0	38	0
Olive, Reduced Fat, Asda*	1 Thin Spread/7g	38	4.1	536	0.2	1.1	59	0
Olive, Sainsbury's*	1 Thin Spread/7g	29	3.2	410	0.5	1	45	0.5
Olive, Tesco*	1 Thin Spread/7g	29	3.2	415	0.2	2	45	0.7
Olive, Waitrose*	1 Thin Spread/7g	29	3.2	409	0.5	0.6	45	0.5
Orange, Thick Cut, St Dalfour*	1 Spread/11g	23	0	211	0.6	52	0.1	1.6
Plant Butter, Salted, Flora*	1 Thin Spread/7g	49	5.5	701	0	0.5	79	0
Pro Activ with Olive Oil, Flora*	1 Thin Spread/7g	22	2.4	320	0.5	0.5	35	0
Pro Activ, Light, Flora*	1 Thin Spread/7g	22	2.4	320	0.5	0.5	35	0
Pro Active, Becel*	1 Thin Spread/7g	22	1.8	320	0	0	25	0
Reduced Fat, Average	***1 Thin Spread/7g***	***25***	***2.7***	***356***	***0.6***	***3***	***38***	***0***
Salted Caramel, Tiptree, Wilkin & Sons*	1 Tsp/5g	21	1.2	425	4	50	23	0
Seed Butter, 3, Daylesford*	1 Thick Spread/12g	73	5.8	609	34.7	5.8	48.1	7
Shortening, Vegetable, Kremelta*	1 Tsp/5g	45	5	900	0	0	100	0
Slightly Salted, M&S*	1 Thick Spread/12g	87	9.6	725	0.6	0.6	80	0.3
Soft, Reduced Fat, Smart Price, Asda*	1 Thin Spread/7g	32	3.5	455	0.2	1	50	0
Sunflower, Average	***1 Thin Spread/7g***	***42***	***4.6***	***595***	***0.1***	***0.4***	***65.9***	***0.4***
Sunflower, Dairy Free, Free From, Asda*	1 Thin Spread/7g	36	3.9	510	0.5	0.5	56	0.5
Sunflower, Light, BFY, Morrisons*	1 Thin Spread/7g	24	2.7	342	0	0	38	0
Sunflower, Light, Greenvale, Aldi*	1 Thin Spread/7g	20	2.1	290	5	5	30	5
Sunflower, Light, Reduced Fat, Asda*	1 Thin Spread/7g	24	2.7	347	0.3	1	38	0.1
Sunflower, Low Fat, Aldi*	1 Thin Spread/7g	26	2.7	366	0.2	5.7	38	0
Vegan Block, Organic, Naturli*	1 Thin Spread/7g	47	5.2	670	0.5	0.5	75	0
Vegan, Spreadable, Organic, Naturli*	1 Thin Spread /7g	48	5.2	681	0.5	0.5	75	0

S

	Measure INFO/WEIGHT	per Measure KCAL	FAT	Nutrition Values per 100g / 100ml KCAL	PROT	CARB	FAT	FIBRE
SPREAD								
Vegetable, Soft, Tesco*	1 Thin Spread/7g	46	5.1	661	0.1	1	73	0
Vitalite, Dairy Free, Dairy Crest Ltd*	1 Thin Spread/7g	35	3.9	503	0	0	56	0
with Soya, Dairy Free, Pure Spreads*	1 Thin Spread/7g	34	3.8	490	0.5	1	54	0
with Sunflower, Dairy Free, Organic, Pure Spreads*	1 Thin Spread/7g	38	4.1	537	0.5	1	59	0
SPRING ROLLS								
Chicken, Katsu, Curry, Finest, Tesco*	1 Roll/28g	74	3.7	266	8.8	27.2	13.1	1.9
Chicken, Starter, Asda*	1 Roll/47g	119	6.1	253	11	21	13	2.7
Duck, Asda*	1 Roll/17g	46	2.1	267	7.1	30	12	3.4
Duck, Chinese Takeaway, Morrisons*	1 Roll/40g	97	4.4	243	7	27.8	11.1	2
Duck, Hoisin , Sainsbury's*	1 Roll/20g	57	3	287	5.9	30.6	15.3	1.8
Duck, Mini, Asda*	1 Roll/18g	47	1.9	259	8.7	32.8	10.3	1.9
Duck, Mini, Chef Select, Lidl*	1 Roll/20g	66	3.9	328	6.3	31.1	19.3	2.1
Duck, Party Bites, Sainsbury's*	1 Roll/20g	49	1.8	245	10.1	31.4	8.8	1
Duck, Party, Asda*	1 Roll/18g	47	2	259	7.1	32	11	3.1
Duck, Sainsbury's*	1 Roll/50g	138	7.4	275	9.8	22.8	14.8	5.9
Duck, Waitrose *	1 Roll/36g	92	4.4	256	8.2	26.8	12.1	3.6
From Restaurant, Average	***1 Roll/140g***	***344***	***14.8***	***246***	***11.1***	***23.2***	***10.6***	***0***
M&S*	1 Roll/36g	66	2.3	183	4.6	25.6	6.4	2.2
Mini Vegetable, Co-Op*	1 Roll/18g	40	1.6	220	4.1	30.9	9.1	2.7
Mini, Asda*	1 Roll/20g	35	0.6	175	3.5	33.6	3	1.9
Mini, Sainsbury's*	1 Roll/12g	27	1.2	221	4.2	28.7	9.9	1.6
No Duck, Hoisin, Vegan, Iceland*	1 Roll/20g	40	1.2	201	3.8	31.4	6.1	3.2
No Duck, Plant Chef, Tesco*	1 Roll/18g	43	1.6	239	4.9	33.3	9	2.8
No Duck, Plant Pioneers, Sainsbury's*	1 Roll/46g	90	3.8	195	2.7	25.6	8.3	3.3
No Duck, with Hoisin Dip, Plant Kitchen, M&S*	1 Roll/21g	45	1.1	211	5.7	34	5.3	2.4
Oriental Vegetable, Tesco*	1 Roll/60g	148	7.4	248	3.6	29.7	12.4	1.4
Prawn, Crispy, M&S*	1 Roll/34g	75	3.4	220	10	22.2	9.9	1.3
Thai, Sainsbury's*	1 Roll/30g	69	3.4	229	2.9	28.8	11.3	3.5
Vegetable, Asda*	1 Roll/62g	126	5.6	203	3.5	27	9	2.7
Vegetable, Asda*	1 Roll/18g	46	2.2	254	5.1	30	12	3.1
Vegetable, Cantonese, Large, Sainsbury's*	1 Roll/63g	130	6.3	205	3.6	25.3	9.9	1.5
Vegetable, Chilled, Tesco*	1 Roll/68g	149	7.6	221	4	25.9	11.3	1.6
Vegetable, Chinese Snack Selection, Waitrose*	1 Roll/18g	51	2.2	282	4.2	36.8	12.1	4.4
Vegetable, Chinese Takeaway, Sainsbury's*	1 Roll/59g	100	3.7	170	4	24.4	6.3	2.8
Vegetable, Co-Op*	1 Roll/50g	116	7	232	3.3	23	14	2.4
Vegetable, Iceland*	1 Roll/19g	35	1.3	183	3.3	26.1	6.6	2.8
Vegetable, M&S*	1 Roll/37g	80	3.6	215	4.3	27.8	9.6	2
Vegetable, Mini, Nirvana*	1 Roll/26g	54	2.7	208	3.5	25.1	10.4	1.7
Vegetable, Mini, Occasions, Sainsbury's*	1 Roll/24g	52	2.3	216	4.1	28.2	9.6	2.9
Vegetable, Mini, Party Food, M&S*	1 Roll/20g	40	1.6	200	3.7	26.2	8.1	2.7
Vegetable, Mini, Tesco*	1 Roll/16g	33	1.3	208	4	28.3	8.1	3
Vegetable, Sainsbury's*	1 Roll/53g	129	7	244	4.3	25.3	13.3	2.9
SPRITE*								
Sprite*	1 Bottle/500ml	70	0	14	0	3.3	0	0
Zero, Lemon & Lime, Sprite*	1 Bottle/500ml	6	0	1	0	0	0	0
Zero, Sprite*	1 Can/330ml	3	0	1	0	0	0	0
SPRITZER								
Red Grape, Non-Alcoholic, Extra Special, Asda*	1 Bottle/750ml	330	0	44	0	11	0	0
Rose & Grape, Non Alcoholic, Extra Special, Asda*	1 Bottle/750ml	90	0	12	0	3	0	0
White Wine, Echo Falls*	1 Serving/125ml	78	0	39	0	0	0	0
with White Zinfadel, Echo Falls*	1 Serving/200ml	216	0	108	0	0	0	0
SQUASH								
Apple & Blackcurrant, No Added Sugar, Tesco*	1 Serving/30ml	4	0	15	0.2	2	0	0

S

	Measure INFO/WEIGHT	per Measure KCAL	FAT	Nutrition Values per 100g / 100ml KCAL	PROT	CARB	FAT	FIBRE
SQUASH								
Apple & Mango, High Juice, Diluted , Tesco *	1 Glass/250ml	50	0	20	0	4.8	0	0.1
Apple & Mango, High Juice, Diluted, Sainsbury's*	1 Serving/250ml	88	0	35	0	8.5	0	0.2
Apple, Cherry & Raspberry, High Juice, Robinson's*	1 Serving/25ml	49	0	196	0.2	47.6	0.1	0
Blackcurrant, High Juice, Diluted, M&S*	1 Serving/250ml	10	0.2	4	0.1	0.7	0.1	0.1
Blackcurrant, High Juice, Diluted, Tesco*	1 Serving/250ml	10	0.2	4	0.1	0.7	0.1	0.1
Blackcurrant, No Added Sugar, Tesco*	1 Serving/25ml	4	0	14	0.4	1.7	0	0
Cherries & Berries, Tesco*	1 Serving/25ml	5	0	21	0.2	3.2	0	0
Cherries & Berries, Sugar Free, Diluted, Tesco*	1 Glass/250ml	5	0	2	0	0.3	0	0
Cranberry, & Raspberry, Ocean Spray*	1 Glass/200ml	200	0	100	0	25	0	0
Cranberry, Light, Classic, Undiluted, Ocean Spray*	1 Serving/50ml	32	0	63	0.2	14.1	0	0
Feta Stuffed, with Herby Mixed Grain, Gousto*	1 Serving/583g	560	18.7	96	3.3	11.7	3.2	2
Fruit & Barley Orange, Diluted, Robinson's*	1 Serving/50ml	6	0	12	0.2	1.7	0	0.1
Fruit & Barley, Tropical, No Added Sugar, Robinson's*	1 Serving/60ml	7	0	12	0.2	1.6	0	0
Lemon Barley Water, Made Up, Robinson's*	1 Serving/250ml	48	0	19	0.1	4.4	0	0
Lemon, Double Concentrate, Value, Tesco*	1 Serving/25ml	3	0	11	0.2	0.3	0	0
Lemon, High Juice, Diluted, Sainsbury's*	1 Glass /250ml	98	0.2	39	0.1	9.1	0.1	0.1
Lemon, Real Fruit, Diluted, Robinson's*	1 Serving/250ml	12	0	5	0	0	0	0
Orange & Mango, Low Sugar, Sainsbury's*	1 Serving/250ml	5	0.2	2	0.1	0.2	0.1	0.1
Orange & Mango, Special R, Diluted, Robinson's*	1 Serving/250ml	20	0	8	0.2	0.9	0	0
Orange, & Mango, No Added Sugar, Diluted, Robinson's*	1 Serving/200ml	4	0	2	0	0	0	0
Orange, Fruit & Barley, Undiluted, Sainsbury's*	1 Serving/20ml	4	0	20	2.5	3.5	0	0
Orange, Light, Harboe*	1 Serving/200ml	6	0	3	0	0	0	0
Orange, No Added Sugar, Diluted, Lindhouse, Lidl*	1 Serving/200ml	6	0.2	3	0.1	0.3	0.1	0
Orange, No Added Sugar, High Juice, Sainsbury's*	1 Serving/100ml	6	0.1	6	0.1	1.1	0.1	0.1
Orange, No Added Sugar, Undiluted, Tree Top*	1 Serving/50ml	6	0.2	11	0.5	1.8	0.5	0.5
Pear Drop Flavour, Diluted, Tesco*	1 Serving/50ml	3	0	6	0.1	0.5	0	0
Pink Grapefruit, High Juice, Low Sugar, Tesco*	1 Serving/75ml	12	0.1	16	0.2	3.7	0.1	0
Spaghetti, Baked	***1oz/28g***	***6***	***0.1***	***23***	***0.7***	***4.3***	***0.3***	***2.1***
Spaghetti, Including Pips & Rind, Raw	***1oz/28g***	***5***	***0.1***	***20***	***0.4***	***3.4***	***0.4***	***1.7***
Strawberry, & Kiwi, Creations, Diluted, Robinson's*	1 Serving/200ml	6	0	3	0	0.6	0	0
Summer Fruit, No Added Sugar, Sainsbury's*	1 Serving/250ml	5	0.2	2	0.1	0.2	0.1	0.1
Summer Fruits & Barley, no Added Sugar, Tesco*	1 Serving/50ml	6	0	11	0.2	1.7	0	0
Summer Fruits, No Added Sugar, Sun Quench, Aldi*	1 Serving/25ml	5	0.1	21	0.5	2.9	0.5	0.5
Summer Fruits, Robinson's*	1 Measure/25ml	14	0	56	0.1	13	0	0
Summer, All Varieties	***1 Sm/118g***	***21***	***0.2***	***18***	***1.2***	***3.8***	***0.2***	***1.2***
Winter, Acorn, Baked, Average	***1oz/28g***	***16***	***0***	***56***	***1.1***	***12.6***	***0.1***	***3.2***
Winter, Acorn, Raw, Average	***1oz/28g***	***9***	***0***	***30***	***0.6***	***6.8***	***0.1***	***1.7***
Winter, All Varieties, Flesh Only, Raw, Average	***1oz/28g***	***10***	***0***	***34***	***1***	***8.6***	***0.1***	***1.5***
SQUID								
in Batter, Fried in Blended Oil, Average	***1oz/28g***	***55***	***2.8***	***195***	***11.5***	***15.7***	***10***	***0.5***
Raw, Average	***1oz/28g***	***23***	***0.5***	***81***	***15.4***	***1.2***	***1.7***	***0***
Rings, Salt & Pepper, Smokey, Sainsbury's*	1 Pack/100g	109	3.4	109	18.2	1.5	3.4	0.5
Salt & Pepper Chargrilled, Cooked, Tesco*	1 Pack/80g	78	2.3	98	17.9	0	2.9	0.1
STAR FRUIT								
Average, Tesco*	1oz/28g	9	0.1	31	0.5	7.1	0.3	1.3
STARBURST								
Fruit Chews, Tropical, Mars*	1 Tube/45g	168	3.3	373	0	76.9	7.3	0
Mars*	1 Pack/45g	182	3.3	405	0	83.9	7.3	0
STEAK & KIDNEY PUDDING								
M&S*	1 Pudding/121g	260	13.4	215	9.2	19.4	11.1	3.2
Tesco*	1 Serving/190g	437	22.6	230	10	20.7	11.9	1.2
Waitrose*	1 Pudding/223g	497	26.1	223	8.9	20.4	11.7	1.2

S

	Measure INFO/WEIGHT	per Measure KCAL	FAT	Nutrition Values per 100g / 100ml KCAL	PROT	CARB	FAT	FIBRE
STEW								
Aubergine, & Split Pea, Allplants*	1 Serving/380g	429	17.9	113	4.5	12	4.7	2.7
Bean, Moroccan, V Taste, Morrisons*	1 Pack/301g	256	5.1	85	4	11.6	1.7	3.8
Beef & Dumplings	***1 Serving/652g***	***766***	***32.7***	***117***	***7.4***	***10.7***	***5***	***0.8***
Beef, & Dumplings, Frozen, Tesco*	1 Serving/400g	380	12.8	95	5.7	10.5	3.2	1.5
Beef, Asda*	½ Can/196g	178	4.9	91	10	7	2.5	1.5
Beef, Canned, Asda*	1 Can/392g	353	13.7	90	8.9	5.3	3.5	0.9
Beef, Canned, Princes*	1 Serving/196g	145	5.1	74	8	4	2.6	1.5
Beef, Diet Chef Ltd*	1 Pack/270g	200	3.5	74	7.3	7.8	1.3	1.1
Beef, Meal for One, M&S*	1 Pack/440g	350	8.4	80	7	8.7	1.9	2
Beef, Minced, & Onion, Tesco*	1 Pack/300g	219	7.2	73	3.6	8.8	2.4	0.9
Beef, Value, Tesco*	1 Serving/200g	170	9.8	85	4	6.2	4.9	1
Brazilian, One Pot, Aldi*	1 Pot/381g	373	14.8	98	3.2	11	3.9	3.2
Chicken & Dumplings, Birds Eye*	1 Pack/320g	282	8.6	88	7	8.9	2.7	0.5
Chicken & Dumplings, Tesco*	1 Serving/450g	567	29.7	126	7.6	9.1	6.6	0.7
Chicken, & Dumplings, Oven Baked, Iceland*	1 Serving/467g	500	20.1	107	4.5	11.9	4.3	1.1
Chicken, Catalan, Ready Set Cook!, Aldi*	½ Pack/200g	214	2.2	107	15	7.4	1.1	3.7
Chicken, Morrisons*	1 Pack/400g	492	7.6	123	17.6	8.9	1.9	0.5
Chickpea, Moroccan, Allplants*	½ Pack/380g	551	20.1	145	4.8	17	5.3	3.9
Lamb, with Basmati Rice, Hello Fresh*	1 Serving/369g	336	1	91	3	19	0.3	0
Lentil & Vegetable, Organic, Simply Organic*	1 Pack/400g	284	6	71	3.5	11	1.5	1.3
Lentil, Moroccan, Plant Kitchen, M&S*	1 Pack/300g	282	6	94	3.5	14.2	2	2.5
Moroccan, Vegetable, Slimfree, Aldi*	1 Pack/500g	155	2.5	31	1.2	4.7	0.5	1.9
Peri Peri, & Black Bean, Hello Fresh*	1 Serving/588g	759	29.4	129	7	13	5	0
Rainbow, Roots, & Vegetables, Gro, Co-Op*	1 Pack/400g	232	6.4	58	2.6	8.3	1.6	2.8
Roots, Hearty, Allplants*	½ Pack/380g	433	19.8	114	4.2	11	5.2	3
Sweet Potato, & Bean, Vegan, Waitrose*	½ Pack/220g	152	2.9	69	2.2	9.3	1.3	5.8
Tuscan Bean, Tasty Veg Pot, Innocent*	1 Pot/400g	320	7.6	80	3.1	12.5	1.9	3.6
Vegetable, Moroccan, Lidl*	1 Pack/500g	145	2	29	1.1	4	0.4	2.4
STIR FRY								
Beef, BGTY, Sainsbury's*	½ Pack/125g	156	5.1	125	22	0.1	4.1	0
Beef, Chilli, Noodles, Musclefood*	1 Pack/235g	226	3.8	96	10	11	1.6	1.8
Beef, Chilli, Spicy, Musclefood*	1 Serving/353g	314	8.8	89	13.4	2.5	2.5	1.6
Beef, Steak, The Juicy Meat Co.*	½ Pack/140g	277	9.9	198	31.6	1.6	7.1	0.5
Beef, Teriyaki, Aldi*	½ Pack/196g	214	5.7	109	13	8.2	2.9	0.5
Beef, Teriyaki, M&Ss*	1 Pack/500g	375	3.5	75	10	7.1	0.7	0.1
Butternut Squash, & Edamame, Waitrose*	½ Pack/151g	74	1.5	49	3.1	6.2	1	1.6
Butternut Squash, Mangetout, & Chilli, Asda*	½ Pack/130g	79	3.5	61	1.6	5.8	2.7	3.5
Chicken Chow Mein, Fresh, HL, Tesco*	1 Pack/400g	312	4.8	78	5.7	11.4	1.2	1.3
Chicken, & Broccoli, Hello Fresh*	1 Serving/446g	651	22.3	146	10	15	5	0
Chicken, 387, Oakhouse Foods Ltd*	1 Pack/430g	404	2.6	94	8.4	12.9	0.6	1.8
Chicken, Chinese Style, Kit, Asda*	½ Pack/190g	160	1.9	84	12	6.6	1	0.5
Chicken, Chinese, Meal Kit, Aldi*	½ Pack/211g	278	8.6	132	16	7.6	4.1	1.2
Chicken, Fajita, Kit, Tesco*	½ Pack/230g	288	10.6	122	14.8	4.4	4.5	2.2
Chicken, Fajita, Musclefood*	1 Serving/358g	301	10.4	84	11.4	2	2.9	2.3
Chicken, Fajita, Ready Set Cook!, Aldi*	1 Pack/535g	749	30	140	18	3.6	5.6	0.8
Chicken, Naked, Musclefood*	1 Serving/350g	217	4.2	62	9.9	2.5	1.2	1
Chicken, Teriyaki, Tesco*	½ Pack/250g	315	13.5	126	13.5	5.7	5.4	0.5
Chicken, Thai, Musclefood*	1 Serving/336g	279	8.7	83	11.8	1.9	2.6	2.4
Chicken, Tikka, Biryani, Iceland*	½ Pack/351g	432	17.9	123	5.6	13.4	5.1	0.7
Chinese Chicken, As Consumed, Iceland*	½ Pack/371g	353	2.6	95	6.5	15.2	0.7	1
Chinese Prawn, Iceland*	1 Pack/340g	235	4.4	69	3.1	11.1	1.3	2.1
Chinese Style Rice with Vegetables, Tesco*	1 Serving/550g	495	13.8	90	2.2	14.8	2.5	0.3
Edamame Bean, & Broccoli, Asda*	1 Pack/320g	227	10.2	71	3.9	5.5	3.2	2.3

	Measure INFO/WEIGHT	per Measure KCAL	FAT	Nutrition Values per 100g / 100ml KCAL	PROT	CARB	FAT	FIBRE
STIR FRY								
Edamame Bean, Oaklands, Lidl*	½ Pack/150g	70	2.4	47	3.5	3	1.6	3.3
Green Vegetable, M&S*	1 Pack/220g	165	13	75	3.1	2.5	5.9	2.2
Malaysian Peanut Satay, Kit, Street Kitchen*	1 Pack/255g	477	19.9	187	4.7	25	7.8	0
Meal Kit, Teriyaki Chicken, Go Cook, Asda*	½ Pack/267g	318	6.7	119	13	11	2.5	0.6
Mixed Pepper, Sainsbury's*	1 Pack/300g	188	12.9	70	1.5	4.6	4.8	1.2
Mushroom, Asda*	1 Pack/320g	144	4.2	45	2.5	4.4	1.3	2.5
Mushroom, Morrisons*	¼ Pack/80g	25	0.4	31	2.1	3.5	0.5	2.1
Mushroom, Sweet & Crunchy, Stir Fried, Oaklands, Lidl*	1/3 Pack/86g	25	0.2	29	1.7	3.5	0.2	3.2
Mushroom, Tender, Waitrose*	1 Pack/400g	180	8	45	2.1	2.3	2	4.7
Noodles & Bean Sprouts, Tesco*	½ Pack/125g	131	2.6	105	4.2	16.1	2.1	0.7
Oriental Style Pak Choi, M&S*	1 Pack/220g	165	12.5	75	2.2	3.5	5.7	2.4
Oriental Style, Vegetables, Sainsbury's*	1 Pack/300g	195	14.4	65	1.5	4.1	4.8	2.1
Pork, Super Quick, Hello Fresh*	1 Serving/338g	531	13	157	9.4	20.9	3.8	0
Protein, Green Isle*	1 Serving/100g	185	11	185	7	12	11	6.2
Rice, Quinoa & Vegetable, Waitrose*	½ Pack/134g	199	7.8	148	5.4	15.6	5.8	6
Salmon, Teriyaki, Musclefood *	1 Serving/275g	475	15.4	173	12	17	5.6	2.2
Singapore, Noodle, Iceland*	½ Pack/346g	294	10.7	85	5.4	8.2	3.1	1.5
Sticky Veg Satay, Cook*	1 Pack/289g	335	9	116	3.5	18.9	3.1	1.2
Sweet Mixed Pepper, Waitrose*	½ Pack/150g	111	6.1	74	2.1	4.2	4.1	5.8
Teriyaki, Kit, Co-Op*	½ Pack/170g	104	0.8	61	1.6	12	0.5	1.6
Vegetable & Mushroom, Asda*	½ Pack/160g	59	2.4	37	2.4	3.4	1.5	3.4
Vegetable Mix, As Consumed, Tesco*	½ Pack/128g	72	3	56	1.9	5.5	2.3	3
Vegetable Mix, Chinese Inspired, Tesco*	1 Pack/320g	166	9.3	52	1.5	3.8	2.9	2.3
Vegetable, & Beansprout, Tesco*	½ Pack/160g	95	5	59	2	4.5	3.1	2.7
Vegetable, Chop Suey, Chinese, Sharwood's*	1 Pack/310g	223	3.4	72	1.5	13.9	1.1	0.6
Vegetable, Oriental Mix, Tesco*	½ Pack/126g	88	4.4	70	2.6	5.7	3.5	2.7
Vegetable, Rainbow, Fresh Tastes, Asda*	½ Pack/225g	119	5	53	1.8	4.6	2.2	3.8
Vegetable, Ready Prepared, M&S*	½ Pack/150g	38	0.4	25	2.2	3.5	0.3	2.2
Vegetable, Thai Style, Tesco*	½ Pack/135g	42	0.7	31	2.3	4.2	0.5	2.1
Vegetables, Chinese, Ready to Cook, Morrisons*	¼ Pack/81g	25	0.3	31	1.7	4.2	0.4	2.1
Vegetables, Co-Op*	1 Serving/80g	29	0.4	36	1.8	5	0.5	2.7
Vegetables, Mixed, Frozen, Tesco*	¼ Pack/150g	81	3.8	54	1.5	4.4	2.5	4
Vegetables, Superbright, Waitrose*	½ Pack/150g	129	7.2	86	3.5	4.3	4.8	5.6
Vegetables, Sweet & Crunchy, Stir Fried, Oaklands, Lidl*	1 Serving/87g	33	0.2	38	1.6	5.2	0.2	4.4
STOCK								
Beef Bone, Broth, Ossa*	1 Cup/250ml	45	1.2	18	3.6	0.8	0.5	0.5
Beef, Cooks' Ingredients, Waitrose*	1 Jar/500g	110	2.5	22	3.2	0.9	0.5	0.5
Beef, Fresh, Sainsbury's*	¼ Pot/113g	27	0.6	24	5.1	0.5	0.5	0.5
Beef, Heston from Waitrose, Waitrose*	¼ Pack/125g	34	0.6	27	4.9	0.8	0.5	0.9
Beef, Made Up, Stock Pot, Knorr*	1 Serving/100ml	10	0.4	10	0.2	1	0.4	0
Beef, Pot, Made Up, Tesco*	¼ Pot/125ml	12	0.4	10	0.4	1.3	0.3	0.1
Beef, Rich, Stock Pot, Knorr*	1 Pot/28g	42	1.1	150	3	27	4	0.8
Beef, Slow Cooked, Finest, Tesco*	¼ Pouch/113ml	18	0.2	16	2	1.6	0.2	0
Broth, Beef Bone, 10hr, Daylesford*	1 Serving/250ml	125	2.5	50	5.7	3.7	1	1.7
Chicken, Atkins & Potts*	1 Pack/350g	56	2.1	16	1.3	1.1	0.6	0.1
Chicken, Bone, Broth, Ossa*	1 Cup/250ml	28	1.2	11	2.6	0.2	0.5	0.5
Chicken, Concentrated, M&S*	1 Tsp/5g	16	0.9	315	25.6	12.2	18.1	0.8
Chicken, Cooks' Ingredients, Waitrose*	1 Pack/500ml	75	0.5	15	3.2	0.3	0.1	0.2
Chicken, Fresh, Pot, Tesco*	1/3 Pot/100ml	19	1.2	19	1	1.1	1.2	0.1
Chicken, Fresh, Sainsbury's*	½ Pot/142ml	23	0.1	16	3.7	0.1	0.1	0.3
Chicken, GF, Stock Pot, As Sold, Knorr*	1 Stock Pot/28g	26	1.1	92	4.1	9.1	4	1
Chicken, Granules, Knorr*	1 Tsp/4.5g	10	0.2	232	13.1	36.5	3.7	0.4
Chicken, Home Prepared, Average	***1fl oz/30ml***	***7***	***0.3***	***24***	***3.8***	***0.7***	***0.9***	***0.3***

S

	Measure INFO/WEIGHT	per Measure KCAL	FAT	Nutrition Values per 100g / 100ml KCAL	PROT	CARB	FAT	FIBRE
STOCK								
Chicken, Made Up, Stock Pot, Knorr*	1 Serving/125ml	15	0.3	12	0.2	1.6	0.2	0
Chicken, Rich & Savoury, Pot, As Sold, Tesco*	1 Pot/28g	48	1.6	171	7.1	22.8	5.7	1.4
Fish, Home Prepared, Average	***1 Serving/250ml***	***42***	***2***	***17***	***2.3***	***0***	***0.8***	***0***
Mushroom, Pot, As Sold, Knorr*	1 Pot/28g	41	0.8	148	2.8	28	2.7	1.6
Red Wine, Pot, As Sold, Oxo*	1 Pot/20g	22	0.1	111	0.8	25.6	0.5	2.8
Vegetable, As Sold, Stock Pot, Knorr*	1 Serving/5g	5	0.3	100	6.2	6.4	5.3	1.3
Vegetable, Cooks Ingredients, Waitrose*	1 Pouch/500ml	15	0.5	3	0.2	0.4	0.1	0.5
Vegetable, Fresh, COOK!, M&S*	¼ Pouch/125ml	15	0.1	12	0.3	2.5	0.1	0.1
Vegetable, Made Up, Stock Pot, Knorr*	1 Serving/125ml	8	0.6	6	0.5	0.5	0.5	0.5
Vegetable, Organic, Knorr*	1 Pot/26g	32	2.2	122	5.2	5.2	8.6	1.2
Vegetable, Organic, Pot, Kallo*	1 Pot/24g	23	1.5	96	1.5	7.5	6.1	0
STOCK CUBES								
Beef, Dry Weight, Bovril*	1 Cube/6g	12	0.2	197	10.8	29.3	4.1	0
Beef, Dry Weight, Oxo*	1 Cube/6g	15	0.3	265	17.4	38.4	4.9	4.2
Beef, Knorr*	1 Cube/10g	31	2.3	310	5	19	23	0
Beef, Knorr*	1 Cube/11ml	1	0.1	7	0.5	0.5	0.5	0.5
Beef, Made Up, Oxo*	1 Cube/189ml	17	0.4	9	0.6	1.3	0.2	0.1
Beef, Organic, Kallo*	1 Cube/12g	25	1	208	16.7	16.7	8.3	0
Beef, Reduced Salt, Made Up, Oxo*	1 Cube/500ml	45	2.5	9	0.6	1.3	0.5	0.5
Beef, Tesco*	1 Cube/7g	17	0.2	260	9.7	48.9	2.8	1.3
Chicken	***1 Cube/6g***	***14***	***0.9***	***237***	***15.4***	***9.9***	***15.4***	***0***
Chicken, Dry, Average	***1 Cube/10g***	***29***	***1.8***	***293***	***7.3***	***25.5***	***18***	***0.4***
Chicken, Made Up, Average	***1 Pint/568ml***	***43***	***1***	***8***	***0.4***	***1.1***	***0.2***	***0.1***
Chicken, Reduced Salt, Dry, Oxo*	1 Cube/7g	22	0.3	321	14.6	54.9	3.9	2.8
Chicken, Reduced Salt, Prepared, Oxo*	1 Cube/500ml	50	2.5	10	0.5	1.7	0.5	0.5
Fish, Knorr*	1 Cube/10g	32	2.4	321	8	18	24	1
Fish, Sainsbury's*	1 Cube/11g	31	2.2	282	19.1	7.3	20	0.9
Ham, Knorr*	1 Cube/10g	31	1.9	313	11.8	24.4	18.7	0
Lamb, Made Up, Knorr*	1 Serving/100ml	5	0.6	5	0.3	0.3	0.6	0.1
Vegetable, Average	***1 Cube/7g***	***18***	***1.2***	***253***	***13.5***	***11.6***	***17.3***	***0***
Vegetable, Bouillon, Vegetarian, Amoy*	1 Cube/10g	30	2	300	0	20	20	0
Vegetable, Low Salt, Organic, Made Up, Kallo*	1 Serving/500ml	50	3.5	10	0.3	0.7	0.7	0.2
Vegetable, Organic, Yeast Free, Dry, Kallo*	1 Cube/11g	37	3.1	334	11.4	8.2	27.8	2.3
STOLLEN								
Bites, Marzipan, Holly Lane, Aldi*	1 Bite/27g	111	4.8	412	5.9	55	18	1.9
Bites, with Jamaican Rum, Aldi*	1 Bite/23g	88	3.9	382	6.5	50	17	1.7
Cherry, & Almond, Finest, Tesco*	1 Slice/50g	195	7.8	390	5.9	55.2	15.6	2.6
STOVIES								
Chef Select, Lidl*	1 Pack/412g	346	3.7	84	4.6	13	0.9	2.9
Mckinley's *	1 Serving/390g	351	7.8	90	4.3	13.4	2	0.8
Scottish, Mcintosh Of Strathmore*	1 Pack/300g	231	6.3	77	4	10.8	2.1	2.4
STRAWBERRIES								
Dried, Urban Fresh Fruit*	1 Pack/35g	111	0.1	318	1.6	77	0.4	5.9
Fresh, Raw, Average	***1 Berry/12g***	***3***	***0***	***28***	***0.8***	***6***	***0.1***	***1.4***
Frozen, Average	***1 Serving/100g***	***30***	***0.2***	***30***	***0.8***	***6.3***	***0.2***	***1***
in Fruit Juice, Canned, Average	***1/3 Can/127g***	***58***	***0***	***46***	***0.4***	***11***	***0***	***1***
in Syrup, Canned, Average	***1 Serving/100g***	***63***	***0***	***63***	***0.4***	***15.2***	***0***	***0.6***
STROGANOFF								
Beef, & Rice, Charlie Bigham's*	1 Serving/395 g	675	34.8	171	8.5	13.1	8.8	0
Beef, & Rice, TTD, Sainsbury's*	1 Pack/410g	595	20.9	145	9.6	15.2	5.1	1.7
Beef, & Mushroom, Jane Plan*	1 Pack/300g	339	15.3	113	5.3	10.7	5.1	1.2
Beef, Asda*	1 Serving/120g	276	20.4	230	16	3.3	17	0.6
Beef, Creamy, COOK!, M&S*	½ Pack/250g	292	17	117	10.3	3.5	6.8	0

S

	Measure INFO/WEIGHT	per Measure KCAL	FAT	Nutrition Values per 100g / 100ml KCAL	PROT	CARB	FAT	FIBRE
STROGANOFF								
Beef, Luxury, Iceland*	1 Pack/388g	528	13.6	136	8.2	17.5	3.5	0.9
Beef, Oven Baked, Slimming World*	1 Pack/500g	275	2.5	55	8.6	3.3	0.5	1.5
Beef, with Long Grain Rice, Broccoli, & Peas, BFY, M&S*	1 Pack/361g	361	7.2	100	8.5	10.6	2	2.7
Beef, with Wild Rice, Extra Special, Asda*	1 Pack/389g	451	9.3	116	6	17	2.4	0.9
Chicken, with Rice, BGTY, Sainsbury's*	1 Pack/415g	448	5.4	108	7	17.1	1.3	1.1
Mushroom, Eat Smart, Morrisons*	1 Pack/400g	312	4.4	78	2.6	14.3	1.1	1
Mushroom, Portobello, Charred, Finest, Tesco*	½ Pack/164g	207	14.9	126	3.9	6.1	9.1	2.2
Mushroom, with Rice, BGTY, Sainsbury's*	1 Serving/450g	418	6.8	93	3.3	16.6	1.5	1
Pork, Classic Kitchen, Tesco*	½ Pack/222g	284	13.5	128	12.9	4.6	6.1	1.2
STRUDEL								
Apple with Sultanas, Tesco*	1/6 Strudel/100g	245	12	245	2.9	30.9	12	0.7
Apple, Co-Op*	1 Slice/100g	225	12	225	3	28	12	3
Apple, Dessert Menu, Aldi*	½ Strudel/94g	248	12.2	264	2.9	33	13	2.2
Apple, Ovenbaked, CBY, Asda*	1 Slice/100g	249	12	249	2.7	31.6	12	1.7
Apple, Sainsbury's*	1 Serving/90g	233	11.7	259	2.8	31.6	13	1.9
Apple, Tesco*	1 Serving/94g	226	11.6	241	2.6	28.9	12.4	1.7
Berry, Frozen, Tesco*	1 Serving/94g	220	9.9	234	2.7	31.2	10.5	1.9
STUFFING								
Cranberry, & Orange, Plant Kitchen, M&S*	1 Serving/50g	81	3.4	162	5.7	15.9	6.8	7.1
Oatmeal, & Onion, Speyside Specialities*	1 Pack/440g	1518	74.5	345	8.2	40.8	16.9	0
Olde English Chestnut, Sainsbury's*	1 Serving/110g	216	12.8	196	9.4	13.5	11.6	2.1
Pork, Chestnut & Onion, Cooked, Finest, Tesco*	1/8 Pack/41g	108	6.9	263	12.9	13.6	16.8	2.4
Pork, Sage, & Onion, M&S*	¼ Pack/85g	186	12.7	219	11.7	8.5	14.9	2
Pork, Sausagemeat, Gourmet, Waitrose *	1 Serving/56g	137	10	245	15.9	4.8	17.8	0.8
Sage & Onion, for Chicken, Paxo*	1 Serving/50g	60	0.6	120	3.4	22.8	1.3	1.7
Sage & Onion, Quixo, Aldi*	1 Serving/45g	53	0.5	117	3.3	22	1.2	2
Sausagemeat, Sainsbury's*	1 Serving/100g	175	4.2	175	7	27	4.2	2.3
STUFFING BALLS								
British Pork, Sage & Onion, Cooked, Finest, Tesco*	1 Ball/25g	55	2.5	224	13.9	17.4	10.2	2.2
Pork, Sage, & Onion, Sainsbury's*	1 Ball/24g	63	4.4	258	12	11	18	2.2
Pork, Sausagemeat, Aunt Bessie's*	1 Ball/26g	55	2.1	212	7.2	27.3	8.2	3
Sage & Onion, Aunt Bessie's*	1 Ball/26g	60	1.6	229	5.5	39	6.3	3.1
STUFFING MIX								
Apple & Herb, Special Recipe, Sainsbury's*	1 Serving/41g	68	0.9	165	3.8	32.4	2.2	2.2
Dry, Average	***1 Serving/25g***	***84***	***1***	***338***	***9.6***	***70.1***	***3.8***	***5.3***
Garlic, & Herb, Tesco*	1 Serving/50g	90	1.3	179	4.7	32.8	2.6	2.8
Sage & Onion, Asda*	1 Ball/30g	56	0.7	187	5.3	35	2.2	3.4
Sage & Onion, Co-Op*	1 Serving/28g	94	0.6	335	10	68	2	6
Sage & Onion, Prepared, Tesco*	1 Serving/100g	50	0.4	50	1.5	10.1	0.4	0.9
Sage & Onion, As Prepared, Newgate, Lidl*	1 Serving/45g	52	0.5	116	3.3	22.1	1.2	2
Sage & Onion, Dry Weight, Tesco*	1 Pack/170g	578	4.1	340	10.3	69.3	2.4	6.3
Sage & Onion, Dry, Asda*	1 Serving/11g	56	0.7	527	15.1	94.1	6.6	9.4
Sage & Onion, M&S*	1 Serving/30g	108	1	359	11.4	67.8	3.4	6
Sage & Onion, with Apple, Made Up, Paxo*	1 Serving/50g	69	0.8	138	3.8	26	1.6	2.2
Sage, & Onion, Kania, Lidl*	1 Serving/50g	56	0.8	113	3	21	1.5	1.8
SUET								
Beef, Tesco*	1 Serving/100g	854	91.9	854	0.6	6.2	91.9	0.1
Vegetable, Average	***1oz/28g***	***234***	***24.6***	***836***	***1.2***	***10.1***	***87.9***	***0***
Vegetable, Light, Shredded, As Sold, Atora*	¼ Pack/50g	314	26.4	627	9.9	23.7	52.7	8.9
SUGAR								
Brown, Soft, Average	***1 Tsp/4g***	***15***	***0***	***382***	***0***	***96.5***	***0***	***0***
Brown, Soft, Light, Average	***1 Tsp/5g***	***20***	***0***	***393***	***0.2***	***97.8***	***0.1***	***0***
Caster, Average	***1 Tsp/5g***	***20***	***0***	***399***	***0***	***99.8***	***0***	***0***

S

	Measure INFO/WEIGHT	per Measure KCAL	FAT	Nutrition Values per 100g / 100ml KCAL	PROT	CARB	FAT	FIBRE
SUGAR								
Cubes, Silver Spoon*	1 Cube/4g	16	0	400	0	100	0	0
Dark Brown, Muscovado, Average	***1 Tsp/7g***	***27***	***0***	***380***	***0.2***	***94.8***	***0***	***0***
Dark Brown, Soft, Average	***1 Tsp/5g***	***18***	***0***	***369***	***0.1***	***92***	***0***	***0***
Demerara, Average	***1 Tsp/5g***	***18***	***0***	***368***	***0.2***	***99.2***	***0***	***0***
Golden, Unrefined, Average	***1 Tsp/4g***	***16***	***0***	***399***	***0***	***99.8***	***0***	***0***
Granulated, Organic, Average	***1 Tsp/4g***	***16***	***0***	***398***	***0.2***	***99.7***	***0***	***0***
Icing, Average	***1 Tsp/4g***	***16***	***0***	***394***	***0***	***102.2***	***0***	***0***
Light Or Diet, Average	***1 Tsp/4g***	***16***	***0***	***394***	***0***	***98.5***	***0***	***0***
Muscovado, Light, Average	***1 Tsp/5g***	***19***	***0***	***384***	***0***	***96***	***0***	***0***
White, Granulated, Average	***1 Tsp/5g***	***20***	***0***	***398***	***0***	***100***	***0***	***0***
SULTANAS								
Average	***1oz/28g***	***82***	***0.1***	***291***	***2.8***	***69.2***	***0.4***	***2***
SUNDAE								
Blackcurrant, Holly Lane, Aldi*	1 Sundae/47g	201	8.5	427	3.2	61	18	3.2
Blackcurrant, M&S*	1 Sundae/53g	212	10.2	400	3	54.2	19.2	1.9
Caramel, From Restaurant, Average	***1 Sundae/155g***	***304***	***9.3***	***196***	***4.7***	***31.8***	***6***	***0***
Chocolate & Vanilla, HL, Tesco*	1 Sundae/120g	193	3.1	161	2.8	31.5	2.6	0.6
Chocolate & Vanilla, Tesco*	1 Sundae/70g	140	6	199	2.8	27.5	8.6	0.5
Chocolate Brownie, Tesco*	1 Pot/136g	271	15	199	5.2	18.8	11	1.9
Chocolate Mint, COU, M&S*	1 Pot/90g	108	2.3	120	5.4	17.8	2.6	0.5
Chocolate Nut	***1 Serving/70g***	***195***	***10.7***	***278***	***3***	***34.2***	***15.3***	***0.1***
Chocolate, Sainsbury's*	1 Pot/140g	393	29.8	281	2.5	19.3	21.3	0.6
Chocolate, Triple, Sainsbury's*	1 Pot/125g	253	14.1	203	5.2	18.9	11.3	2.3
Ice Cream	***1 Serving/170g***	***482***	***15.4***	***284***	***5.9***	***45.3***	***9.1***	***0.3***
Strawberry & Vanilla, Tesco*	1 Serving/68g	120	3.9	177	2	29.5	5.7	0.1
Strawberry, & Raspberry, COU, M&S*	1 Pot/110g	154	4.1	140	3.1	23.3	3.7	0.4
Strawberry, M&S*	1 Sundae/45g	173	8	385	3.4	53.3	17.8	1
Toffee & Vanilla, Tesco*	1 Serving/70g	133	4.5	189	2.1	30.7	6.4	0.1
Toffee, Asda*	1 Serving/120g	322	19.2	268	2.1	29	16	0
Toffee, Sainsbury's*	1 Sundae/140g	378	27.2	270	3.1	20.2	19.4	0.9
Vanilla Caramel, Aldi*	1 Sundae/72g	159	7.4	221	2.6	29.2	10.3	0.7
SUPPLEMENT								
Black Edition, Huel*	2 Scoops/90g	390	17.1	433	43	18	19	8.3
Black Edition, Vanilla, Huel black edition *	1 Scoop/45g	199	9	442	44	29	20	7.3
Green Apple, Vitamin Drink, Low Calorie, Vit Hit*	1 Serving/100ml	8	0.1	8	0.1	1.4	0.1	0.1
Impact Whey Isolate, Unflavoured, Myprotein*	1 Scoop/25g	103	1.9	412	82	4	7.5	0
Inulin, Powder, Organic, Real Food Source*	1 Spoon/10g	20	0	204	0	6	0	90
Inulin, Powder, Pure, SimplyGo*	1 Scoop/5g	10	0	210	0	8	0	89
Just Protein, Team Rh*	1 Serving/20g	84	1.1	422	80	13	5.7	0
Milkshake, Sachet, Nualtra Foodlink Complete*	1 Sachet/57g	383	16	672	33.3	71.9	28.1	0
Protein Shake, Coconut, Purition*	1 Serving/40g	192	12.8	480	41	7.8	32	17.2
Protein Shake, Macadamia & Vanilla, Purition*	1 Serving/40g	198	14	495	39.1	8.6	35	15.6
Protein Shake, Vegan Hemp, Chocolate, Purition*	1 Serving/40g	194	12.1	484	35.4	11.3	30.3	27.3
Protein, Hemp, Powder, Funktional Foods*	1 Tbsp/15g	54	1.6	362	49	10	11	13
Protein, Powder, Collagen, Chocolate, Myprotein*	1 Scoop/30g	106	0.2	352	81	47	0.6	1.8
Protein, Pro V-Gain, Vegan, Chocolate, Sci MX*	1 Scoop/15g	53	0.3	353	73	7.4	2.3	5.9
Protein, Pure Whey Isolate, Vanilla, Bulk Powders*	1 Scoop/30g	115	0.6	382	87	4	2	0
Protein, Smart, Peanut Butter Cup, PhD Nutrition*	1 Scoop/30g	116	3	388	62	12	10	1
Protein, Super Shake Powder, Pulsin*	1 Serving/30g	114	2.8	380	65.7	6	9.3	4.7
Protein, Superfood, Amazing Grass*	1 Scoop/29g	113	2.6	390	69	5.2	9	9
Protein, Whey Isolate, R1 Protein*	1 Scoop/29g	109	0	377	85.6	3.4	0	0
Shake, Pea, & Wholegrain Rice, Chocolate, V-protein *	1 Serving/24g	91	0.4	380	80	9.7	1.6	2.7
Shake, Protein, Diet, Slimzest*	1 Scoop/30g	114	1.2	380	80	6	4	0

	Measure INFO/WEIGHT	per Measure KCAL	FAT	Nutrition Values per 100g / 100ml KCAL	PROT	CARB	FAT	FIBRE
SUPPLEMENT								
Smoothie, Golden Milk, Purition*	1 Scoop/10g	48	3.2	480	39	9	32.5	18
Tablet, Berocca*	1 Tablet/4.5g	5	0	109	0	5.7	0.1	0
Vanilla Shake, Michael Mosley*	1 Serving/50g	198	8	396	42.4	12.4	16	14
Whey Protein, Holland & Barrett*	1 Serving/24g	94	1.9	392	73.3	7.1	7.9	0
Whey Protein, Iso:Pro, Myprotein*	1 Scoop/25g	100	0.2	399	97	0	1	0.8
Whey Protein, Pure, Strawberry, Bulk Powders*	1 Scoop/30g	125	2.2	417	76.3	8.7	7.5	0.4
Whey Protein, Salted Caramel, Impact, Myprotein*	1 Serving/50g	205	3.6	410	79	7.1	7.2	0.2
Whey Protein, Strawberry, Natural, Impact, Myprotein*	1 Scoop/25g	98	1.8	391	73	7.3	7.1	0.8
Whey, Protein, Banana, PBN*	1 Scoop/30g	119	1.7	397	78.6	7.1	5.8	0.7
SUSHI								
Big Boy Box, Tanpopo*	1 Pack/506g	906	16.7	179	6	31.6	3.3	0
California Rolls 8 Pack	***1 Pack/206g***	***354***	***9.3***	***172***	***5.1***	***27.5***	***4.5***	***1.4***
Californian Roll & Nigiri, Selection, M&S*	1 Pack/215g	355	5.8	165	7.1	28	2.7	1.1
Chicken, & Duck, Hoisin, Selection, Asda*	1 Pack/167g	278	4.5	166	5	30	2.7	1.3
Chicken, Katsu, & Tempura Rice, Tanpopo*	1 Pack/290g	803	53.9	277	7.6	21	18.6	0.6
Chicken, Katsu, Bento, Taiko Foods*	1 Pack/235g	526	26.1	224	6.2	25.1	11.1	0
Chicken, Katsu, Tesco*	1 Pack/76g	122	2.6	161	4.4	27.4	3.4	1.5
Classic, My Sushi, Lidl*	1 Pack/200g	328	42	164	4.7	31.5	21	0
Dragon Roll, Firecracker Prawn, M&S*	1 Pack/166g	224	4.5	135	4.2	22.9	2.7	0.9
Dragon Roll, Katsu Chicken, M&S*	1 Pack/167g	241	3.3	144	5.1	25.8	2	1.2
Duck, & Chicken, Eat & Go, Aldi*	1 Pack/130g	206	2.6	158	4.7	30	2	1
Fish & Vegetable, Co-Op*	1 Pack/143g	238	3.7	166	4.6	31	2.6	0.7
Fish Roll, Nigiri & Maki Selection, M&S*	1 Pack/210g	315	4.8	150	6.5	25.8	2.3	1
Fish Selection, Large, Tesco*	1 Pack/218g	365	6.8	167	5.3	29	3.1	0.9
Fish Selection, Morrisons*	1 Pack/152g	236	1.5	155	4	32	1	0.9
Fish, Selection, Asda*	1 Pack/153g	242	2.6	158	5.3	30	1.7	0.6
Fish, Snack Pack, On the Go, Sainsbury's*	1 Pack/96g	150	2.4	156	5.5	27.3	2.5	1.2
Fish, Snack, Tesco*	1 Pack/104g	159	2.6	153	4.5	28	2.5	1.5
Futomaki, Veg & Chive, Waitrose*	1 Pack/146g	169	4.5	116	2.6	19	3.1	1.6
Hosomaki, Vegan, Morrisons*	1 Pack/140g	220	1.7	158	3	33	1.2	1.5
Katsu Chicken, Snack, M&S*	1 Pack/63g	96	0.8	153	3.8	31	1.3	1.1
Naniwa, Box, Lidl*	1 Pack/190g	262	3.8	138	4.6	25	2	0.6
Rolls, California, MSC, Taiko Foods*	1 Pack/135g	252	9.7	187	4.4	24	7.2	0
Rolls, Duck, Teriyaki, Taiko Foods*	1 Pack/131g	224	7.5	171	6	20.8	5.7	0
Rolls, Tuna, Crispy, Taiko Foods*	1 Roll/29g	47	1.1	163	5.9	25.8	3.8	0
Rolls, Veggie, Snack, Shapers, Boots*	1 Pack/66g	93	0.6	141	3.5	28.8	0.9	1.4
Salmon & Roll Set, Sainsbury's*	1 Serving/101g	167	2.6	165	4.9	30.4	2.6	0.8
Salmon & Prawn, Nigiri, M&S*	1 Pack/125g	186	1.4	149	7	27.2	1.1	1
Salmon Wrap, Taiko Foods*	1 Pack/200g	284	4.6	142	5.1	24.8	2.3	0
Salmon, & Prawn, Selection, Co-Op*	1 Pack/148g	241	3.8	163	5.2	29	2.6	0.7
Salmon, Smoked, & Tuna, Tesco*	1 Pack/136g	227	3.9	167	4.9	29.8	2.9	0.7
Salmon, Smoked, & Tuna, Tesco*	1 Pack/136g	218	4.4	160	5.9	26.6	3.2	0.7
Salmon, Smoked, Snack Pack, Tesco*	1 Pack/69g	114	1.9	165	5	29.1	2.7	0.9
Salmon, Smoked, Snack, Eat & Go, Aldi*	1 Pack/69g	106	1.4	153	5.8	26	2	0.7
Snack Box, with Soy Sauce, Eat Well, M&S*	1 Box/78g	115	1.1	147	4.5	28.8	1.4	0.6
Taiko, California, Waitrose*	1 Pack/140g	246	10.1	176	4.1	22	7.2	4.1
Taiko, Fuji Set, Waitrose*	1 Pack /332g	515	10	155	5	28	3	1
Tokujo Maki, Taiko*	1 Box/226g	355	9.7	157	4.1	24.5	4.3	0
Tuna, to Snack Selection, Food to Go, M&S*	1 Serving/150g	225	3.9	150	5.2	26.4	2.6	2.3
Vegetable Selection Pack, M&S*	1 Pack/154g	215	2.8	140	2.8	28.1	1.8	1.3
Vegetable, Box, Lidl*	1 Box/210g	353	10.8	168	4.7	24.6	5.1	2
Vegetable, Box, Select & Go*	1 Serving/210g	212	9.4	101	3.8	25.4	4.5	1.6
Vegetable, Morrisons*	1 Pack/75g	126	2.9	168	3.4	29.2	3.9	1.4

	Measure INFO/WEIGHT	per Measure KCAL	FAT	Nutrition Values per 100g / 100ml KCAL	PROT	CARB	FAT	FIBRE
SUSHI								
Vegetable, Selection, Aldi*	1 Pack/149g	238	5.1	160	3.1	29	3.4	1.1
Vegetable, Selection, M&S*	1 Pack/132g	197	1.5	149	4	30.1	1.1	1.1
Vegetable, Taster, Co-Op*	1 Pack/68g	118	3.5	174	3.8	27.9	5.2	1
Vegetarian, Snack Selection, Tesco*	1 Pack/85g	106	2.8	125	3.7	20.1	3.3	0.6
Wrap, Tuna, MSC, Taiko Foods*	1 Wrap/100g	159	3.2	159	4.6	27.6	3.2	0
Yo!, Bento Box, Sainsbury's*	1 Pack/208g	530	6.2	255	8.4	48.7	3	0.9
SWEDE								
Boiled, Average	***1oz/28g***	***3***	***0***	***11***	***0.3***	***2.3***	***0.1***	***0.7***
Raw, Flesh Only, Peeled	***1 Serving/100g***	***24***	***0.3***	***24***	***0.7***	***5***	***0.3***	***1.6***
Raw, Unprepared, Average	***1oz/28g***	***5***	***0.1***	***18***	***0.7***	***3.8***	***0.3***	***1.6***
SWEET & SOUR								
Chicken, & Noodles, Chinese Takeaway, Tesco*	1 Pack/350g	350	0.7	100	5.7	18.8	0.2	0.2
Chicken, Balls, Chinese Takeaway, Iceland*	1 Pack/255g	311	3.3	122	9.9	17.5	1.3	6
Chicken, Breaded, Fried, From Restaurant, Average	***6 Pieces/130g***	***346***	***18***	***266***	***13***	***22.3***	***13.8***	***0***
Chicken, Chinese Favourites Box, M&S*	½ Pack/125g	146	0.8	117	8.1	19.3	0.6	1.1
Chicken, Chinese Takeaway, Sainsbury's*	1 Pack/264g	515	16.9	195	13.1	21.3	6.4	1
Chicken, Crispy, with Sweet & Sour Sauce, Tesco*	½ Pack/165g	354	16.7	214	11.1	19.3	10.1	1
Chicken, in Batter, Cantonese, Chilled, Sainsbury's*	1 Pack/350g	560	21	160	8.9	22.4	6	0.9
Chicken, with Egg Fried Rice, Calorie Controlled, Tesco*	1 Pack/380g	380	3	100	6.9	15.5	0.8	1.6
Chicken, with Noodles, Steamed, HE, Tesco*	1 Pack/370g	289	0.7	78	8.3	10.8	0.2	0.6
Chicken, with Rice, 233, Oakhouse Foods Ltd*	1 Meal/400g	544	12	136	6.3	20.7	3	0.6
Chicken, with Rice, Chilled, BGTY, Sainsbury's*	1 Pack/400g	344	3.6	86	6	13.5	0.9	1
Chicken, with Rice, Weight Watchers, Heinz*	1 Pack/310g	360	3.1	116	5.2	21.2	1	0.4
Pork	***1oz/28g***	***48***	***2.5***	***172***	***12.7***	***11.3***	***8.8***	***0.6***
Pork, Battered, Sainsbury's*	½ Pack/175g	306	8.8	175	7.3	25.1	5	0.6
Sweet & Sour, Stir Fry, Aldi*	½ Pack/199g	310	10.5	156	13	13	5.3	1.2
Sweet & Sour, with Rice, Counted, Morrisons*	1 Pack/303g	358	2.1	118	6.7	20.4	0.7	1.4
Sweet & Sour, with Rice, Oh So Lean*	1 Pack/400g	106	0.8	27	0.8	5.8	0.2	0.5
with Long Grain Rice, Rice Time, Uncle Ben's*	1 Pot/300g	393	2.4	131	1.9	28.4	0.8	0.7
SWEET POTATO								
Baked, Flesh Only, Average	***1 Med/130g***	***150***	***0.5***	***115***	***1.6***	***27.9***	***0.4***	***2.8***
Boiled in Salted Water, Average	***1 Med/200g***	***168***	***0.6***	***84***	***1.1***	***20.5***	***0.3***	***2.3***
Chunks, Ready Prepared, Morrisons*	1 Serving/80g	56	0.2	70	1.3	14.3	0.2	2.7
Mash, Tesco*	½ Pack/200g	181	3.6	90	1.4	16	1.8	2.2
Mashed, Microwaved, Sainsbury's*	½ Pack/200g	144	3.2	72	1.2	12.3	1.6	1.6
Puffs, Frozen, Alexia*	1 Serving/84g	140	4.5	167	1.2	27.4	5.4	3.5
Raw, Peeled, Average	***1 Sm/130g***	***112***	***0.1***	***86***	***1.6***	***20.1***	***0***	***2.1***
Raw, Unprepared, Average	***1 Potato/200g***	***174***	***0.6***	***87***	***1.2***	***21.3***	***0.3***	***3***
Roasted, & Spiced Carrot, M&S*	1 Pack/130g	183	10.3	141	4.1	11.8	7.9	3.3
Steamed, Average	***1 Med/200g***	***168***	***0.6***	***84***	***1.1***	***20.4***	***0.3***	***2.3***
Wedges, BBQ, Oven Baked, Tesco*	¼ Pack/135g	144	0.3	107	1.8	22.9	0.2	3.4
Wedges, Chilled, Cooked, Sainsbury's*	½ Pack/150g	150	3	100	1.7	17.1	2	3.4
Wedges, Eat Well, M&S*	½ Pack/150g	123	2.2	82	1.4	14.5	1.5	2.6
Wedges, Morrisons*	1 Serving/125g	190	6.5	152	1.5	23.4	5.2	2.9
Wedges, Sainsbury's*	1 Serving/125g	186	6.2	149	2.2	21.8	5	3.9
SWEETBREAD								
Lamb, Fried	***1oz/28g***	***61***	***3.2***	***217***	***28.7***	***0***	***11.4***	***0***
SWEETCORN								
Baby, Frozen, Average	***1oz/28g***	***7***	***0.1***	***24***	***2.5***	***2.7***	***0.4***	***1.7***
Boiled, Average	***1oz/28g***	***31***	***0.6***	***111***	***4.2***	***19.6***	***2.3***	***2.2***
Canned with Sugar & Salt, Average	***1 Lge Can/340g***	***369***	***4***	***108***	***3.2***	***21.5***	***1.2***	***1.9***
Cobs, Mini, Iceland*	1 Cob/100g	80	1.9	80	3.6	9.5	1.9	5.1
Frozen, Average	***1 Serving/80g***	***84***	***1.7***	***105***	***3.8***	***17.9***	***2.1***	***1.8***

	Measure INFO/WEIGHT	per Measure KCAL	FAT	Nutrition Values per 100g / 100ml KCAL	PROT	CARB	FAT	FIBRE
SWEETCORN								
No Sugar & Salt, Canned, Average	***½ Can/125g***	***99***	***1.3***	***79***	***2.7***	***15***	***1.1***	***1.6***
with Peppers, Canned, Average	***1 Serving/50g***	***40***	***0.2***	***79***	***2.6***	***16.4***	***0.3***	***0.6***
SWEETENER								
Calorie Free, Truvia*	1 Sachet/1.5g	0	0	0	0	99	0	0
Canderel*	1 Tbsp/2g	8	0	379	24.7	7	0	5.3
Canderel, Spoonful, Canderel*	1 Tsp/0.5g	2	0	384	2.9	93	0	0
Erythritol, 100%, Pure Via*	1 Tsp/5g	0	0	0	0	100	0	0
Granulated, Low Calorie, Splenda*	1 Tsp/0.5g	2	0	391	0	97.7	0	0
Granulated, Silver Spoon*	1 Tsp/0.5g	2	0	387	1	96.8	0	0
Granulated, Tesco*	1 Tsp/1g	4	0	383	1.8	94	0	0
Natural Syrup, Fruit, Dark, Sweet Freedom*	1 Tsp/5g	13	0	292	0	79	0	0
Silver Spoon*	1 Tablet/0.1g	0	0	325	10	71	0	0
Stevia Leaf, Granules, Pure Via*	1 Tsp/5g	0	0	2	0	99	0.5	0
Stevia, & Erythritol, Nkd Living*	1 Tsp/5g	0	0	0	0	99.5	0	0
Tablet, Average	***1 Tablet/0.1g***	***0***	***0***	***355***	***8.7***	***73***	***0***	***0.8***
Tablets, Low Calorie, Canderel*	1 Tablet/0.1g	0	0	342	13	72.4	0	0
Tablets, Splenda*	1 Tablet/0.1g	0	0	345	10	76.2	0	1.6
Tablets, Tesco*	1 Tablet/1g	0	0	20	2	2	0.5	0
The Pantry, Aldi*	1 Tsp1g	4	0	376	0.5	94	0.5	0.5
Xylosweet, Xylitol*	1 Serving/4g	10	0	240	0	100	0	0
SWEETS								
Almonds, Sugared, Dragee*	1 Sweet/4g	17	0.6	472	10	68.3	17.9	2.5
Balla Stixx, Strawberry, Haribo*	1 Stick/25g	93	0.9	373	2.7	82	3.6	0
Big Purple One, Quality Street, Nestle*	1 Sweet/39g	191	9.9	490	4.7	60.5	25.5	0.7
Blackcurrant & Liquorice, M&S*	1 Sweet/8g	32	0.3	400	0.6	89	4.3	0
Blackcurrant Liquorice, Dark, Glacier, Fox's*	1 Sweet/5g	18	0	360	0	90.1	0	0
Blueberry, Bliss, Candy Kittens*	1 Sweet/6g	20	0	335	0.8	81	0.1	0
Boiled, Spiced Pumpkin, Uncle Joe's*	1 Sweet/6g	23	0	387	0	96.4	0.2	0.1
Bon Bons, Raspberry, Tesco*	1 Serving/25g	103	1.5	411	0.1	89.3	5.9	0.5
Butter Candies, Original, Werther's*	1 Sweet/5g	21	0.4	424	0.1	85.7	8.9	0.1
Butter Mintoes, Dominion, Aldi*	3 Sweets/22g	93	1.7	418	0.5	87	7.8	0.5
Candy Cane, Average	***1 Cane/13g***	***50***	***0***	***386***	***0***	***96***	***0***	***0.2***
Candy Cane, Peppermint, Sainsbury's*	1 Cane/12g	48	0	386	0	96.5	0	0
Candy Corn, Brachs*	19 Pieces/39g	140	0	359	0	92.3	0	0
Candy Floss, Asda*	1 Tub/75g	292	0	390	0	100	0	0
Chew	***1oz/28g***	***107***	***1.6***	***381***	***1***	***87***	***5.6***	***1***
Chew Bars, Great British Puds, Swizzles*	1 Sweet/18g	64	1.1	355	0.1	74	6.1	0
Chewits, Blackcurrant, Leaf*	1 Chew/3g	12	0.1	385	0.2	87.5	3	0
Chewits, Cola, Leaf*	1 Chew/3g	12	0.1	385	0.2	87.5	3	0
Chewits, Fruit Salad, Leaf*	1 Chew/3g	12	0.1	385	0.2	87.5	3	0
Chewits, Sour Apple, Xtreme, Chewits*	1 Pack/34g	133	1	391	0	86	3	0
Chewits, Strawberry, Leaf*	1 Chew/3g	12	0.1	385	0.2	87.5	3	0
Chewitts, Blackcurrant	***1 Pack/33g***	***125***	***0.9***	***378***	***0.3***	***86.9***	***2.7***	***0***
Chews, Just Fruit, Fruit-tella*	1 Serving/43g	170	2.8	400	0.9	79.5	6.5	0
Chews, Sour, Infernal, Chupa Chups*	1 Sweet/8g	32	0.5	397	0.9	82	5.9	0
Chews, Spearmint, Victoria, Aldi*	1 Sweet/10g	40	0.8	405	0.3	83.8	7.6	0
Chews, Strawberry Mix, Starburst*	1 Sweet/4g	15	0.3	401	0	83.9	7.3	0
Chewy, Vimto*	1 Pack/30g	115	0.9	384	0	88	3	0
Choco & Mint, Mentos*	1 Pack/38g	156	3.2	410	2.8	79	8.5	0
Chocolate Caramels, Milk, Tesco*	1 Sweet/3g	15	0.5	444	2.7	72.1	16.1	0.1
Chocolate Eclairs, Cadbury*	1 Sweet/8g	36	1.4	455	4.5	68.9	17.9	0
Chocolate Eclairs, Co-Op*	1 Sweet/8g	38	1.6	480	3	71	20	0.6
Chocolate Eclairs, Holland & Barrett*	1 Sweet/6g	18	0.7	306	1.8	81.9	11.3	1.4

S

	Measure INFO/WEIGHT	per Measure KCAL	FAT	Nutrition Values per 100g / 100ml KCAL	PROT	CARB	FAT	FIBRE
SWEETS								
Chocolate Limes, Pascall*	1 Sweet/8g	27	0.2	333	0.3	77.2	2.5	0
Chocolate Limes, Poundland*	1 Sweet/5g	21	0.2	414	0.5	95.5	3.3	0
Cola Bottles, Barratt*	1 Sweet/10g	34	0	337	1.3	82	0.4	0.1
Cola Bottles, Fizzy, M&S*	1 Pack/200g	650	0	325	6.4	75	0	0
Cola Bottles, Giant, Morrisons*	1 Pack/140g	469	0.1	335	8.9	74.3	0.1	0.6
Cola Sherbets, Sugar Free, Dominion, Aldi*	2 Sweets/10g	23	0	238	0.5	96	0.5	0.5
Creamy Strawberry, Sugar Free, Dominion, Aldi*	1 Sweet/4g	11	0.2	266	0.5	87	6.2	0
DipDab, Softies, Barratt*	1 Bag/160g	557	0.3	348	0.4	86.2	0.2	0
Dolly Mix, Bassett's*	1 Bag/45g	171	1.4	380	3	85.1	3.1	0.4
Dolly Mixtures, M&S*	1 Pack/115g	431	1.6	375	1.8	89.2	1.4	0
Dolly Mixtures, Sainsbury's*	1 Serving/10g	40	0.2	401	1.4	94.4	1.9	0.1
Dolly Mixtures, Smart Price, Asda*	1 Sweet/3g	11	0	380	0.5	91	1.6	0
Dolly Mixtures, Tesco*	1 Pack/100g	376	1.5	376	1.6	88.9	1.5	0
Double Lolly, Swizzels Matlow*	1 Lolly/10g	41	0.3	407	0	92.4	3.4	0
Double Lolly, Swizzle*	1 Lolly/10g	41	0.3	411	0	93.7	3.4	0
Dragibus, Haribo*	1 Serving/25g	94	0.1	375	0	93	0.5	0
Drops, Lemon & Orange, M&S*	1 Pack42g	97	0	230	0	61	0	0
Drumstick, Matlow's*	1 Pack/40g	164	2.2	409	0.4	88.3	5.5	0
Drumstick, Squashies, Sour Cherry & Apple, Swizzels*	1 Serving/30g	105	0.1	349	3.4	82	0.2	0
Edinburgh Rock, Gardiners of Scotland*	1 Piece/2g	8	0	380	0.1	94.4	0.3	0.8
Eton Mess, Candy Kittens*	1 Sweet/6g	20	0	340	1.4	82	0.2	0
Fizzy Belts, Multi Coloured, Dominion, Aldi*	1/3 Pack/25g	24	0.1	94	0.9	28.7	0.5	0.5
Fizzy Dummies, Barratt*	1 Pack/200g	688	0	344	0	84.4	0	0
Fizzy Fish, Maynards*	4 Sweets/26g	92	0	352	0.1	87	0.1	0
Fizzy Fruits, Lidl*	5 Sweets/19g	63	0	330	3.9	78.4	0.1	0.5
Fizzy Mix, Tesco*	½ Bag/50g	166	0	332	5.2	75.2	0	0
Fizzy Multicolour Belts, Tesco*	5 Belts/25g	92	0.5	370	2.5	85	1.9	1.4
Fizzy Pop, M&S*	1 Sweet/4g	14	0	352	0.1	88.7	0.5	0.5
Flumps, Bassett's*	1 Serving/5g	16	0	325	4	77	0	0
Foamy Mushrooms, Chewy, Asda*	1 Sweet/2.6g	9	0	347	4.2	82	0.2	0
Fruit Gums & Jellies	***1 Tube/33g***	***107***	***0***	***324***	***6.5***	***79.5***	***0***	***0***
Fruit Pastilles, Sweet Corner, Lidl*	11 Sweets/40g	133	0	333	4	77.6	0.1	3.4
Fruity Chews, Percy Pig, M&S*	¼ Bag/38g	129	0.1	344	0.5	84.4	0.2	1.1
Fruity Chews, Starburst*	1 Sweet/8g	34	0.6	404	0	83.4	7.4	0
Fruity Frogs, Rowntree's*	1 Serving/40g	128	0.1	321	4.7	74.5	0.2	0
Go Bananas, & Monkeys, M&S*	1 Bag/70g	264	0.1	377	2.9	91.3	0.1	0.5
Gummy Bears	***10 Bears/25g***	***80***	***0***	***320***	***8***	***76***	***0***	***0***
Gummy Mix, Tesco*	1 Pack/100g	327	0.1	327	5.9	75.7	0.1	0
Gummy Worms	***10 Worms/74g***	***286***	***0***	***386***	***0***	***98.9***	***0***	***98.9***
Happy Cola Zing, Haribo*	1 Pack/25g	96	1	384	1.8	85	4.2	0
Henry Hippo, Sweet Corner, Lidl*	1 Serving/25g	88	0.1	350	0.8	86.1	0.2	0.5
Ice Cream Sundae, Asda*	1 Sweet/2g	9	0	387	4.9	70	0.5	0.5
Jellies, Fruit, Ringtons*	4 Jellies/44g	150	0.2	341	0.1	84	0.4	0.7
Jellies, Very Berry, Rowntrees*	1 Sweet/4g	12	0	326	5	74.8	0.2	0.1
Jelly Beans, Lucozade*	1 Pack/30g	111	0	370	0	92	0	0
Jelly Beans, Tesco*	¼ Bag/63g	243	0.2	385	0.1	94.5	0.3	0.3
Jelly Bunnies, Bassetts, Maynards*	4 Sweets/26g	87	0	330	3.5	78	0.1	0
Jelly Tots, Rowntree's*	1 Pack/42g	145	0	346	0.1	86.5	0	0
Kisses, Hershey*	1 Sweet/5g	28	1.6	561	7	59	32	0
Laces, Apple Flavour, Tesco*	5 Laces/15g	52	0.5	347	3.6	74.8	3.2	2.1
Laces, Strawberry, Sainsbury's*	1 Serving/25g	94	1.2	377	3.3	76.3	4.6	0.1
Laces, Strawberry, Tesco*	1 Serving/75g	260	2.4	347	3.6	74.8	3.2	2.1
Lances, Strawberry Flavour, Fizzy, Tesco*	½ Pack/50g	177	1.3	354	2.8	79.8	2.6	1.8

	Measure INFO/WEIGHT	per Measure KCAL	FAT	Nutrition Values per 100g / 100ml KCAL	PROT	CARB	FAT	FIBRE
SWEETS								
Lemon, Drops, Cool, Trebor*	1 Sweet/2g	5	0	237	0.1	96	0.1	0
Licorice, Sugar Free, Dominion, Aldi*	1 Serving/25g	56	0.1	224	0.5	77	0.5	1.6
Liquorice, Boiled, Sugar Free, Sula*	1 Sweet/3g	7	0	227	0.2	93	0	0.2
Liquorice, Catherine Wheels, M&S*	1 Wheel/19g	61	0.2	321	4.2	72.2	1.1	2.8
Liquorice, Gums, Lion*	1 Sweet/4g	14	0	351	8.5	77.7	0.6	0.7
Lovehearts, Swizzels*	1 Sweet/2g	7	0	359	0.7	88.2	0	0
Maoam, Maomixx, Haribo*	1 Sweets/25g	98	1.6	394	1	84	6.4	0
Maynards Sours, Bassett's*	1 Pack/52g	169	0	325	6.1	75	0	0
Mentos, Fruit, Mentos*	1 Sweet/3g	12	0.1	388	0	92	1.9	0
Midget Gems, Co-Op*	12 Sweets/28g	100	0.1	356	0.5	89	0.5	0.5
Midget Gems, Maynards*	1 Sweet/1g	3	0	340	8.7	76.2	0	0
Midget Gems, Value, Tesco*	1 Serving/40g	130	0.1	324	4.5	76.1	0.2	0
Milk Chocolate Eclairs, Sainsbury's*	1 Sweet/8g	33	1.1	442	2.1	75.7	14.5	0.5
Milk Chocolate Eclairs, Value, Tesco*	1 Bag/200g	918	32.6	459	2.6	75.2	16.3	1
Milk Duds, Hershey*	13 Pieces/33g	170	6	510	3	84	18	0
Milk Teeth, Barratt*	1 Serving/20g	64	0	318	3.9	75.6	0	0
Mini Macs, CBY, Asda*	1 Pack/200g	437	13.1	218	1	38.8	6.6	0
Mini Marti, Mushrooms, Asda*	1 Sweet/3g	10	0	340	3.8	81.1	0.1	0
Minions, Haribo*	½ Pack/35g	120	0.2	342	6.6	77	0.5	0
Minis, Starburst*	1 Serving/49g	198	2.9	404	0	87	5.9	0
Mint Balls, Uncle Joe's*	1 Sweet/6g	24	0	393	0	97	0.5	0
Mint Humbugs, Dominion, Aldi*	1 Sweet/8g	33	0.2	407	0.5	95	2.7	0.5
Mint Humbugs, Sugar Free, Morrisons*	1 Sweet/3g	9	0.2	287	0.3	92.5	7	0
Mint Humbugs, Sugar Free, Sula*	1 Sweet/3g	8	0.2	280	0.2	87.1	7.7	0
Mint imperial , Dominion, Aldi*	1 Serving/20g	78	0.1	389	0.5	96	0.5	0.5
Mystery Swirl, Laffy Taffy*	1 Rope/23g	80	1.5	349	0	78.6	6.6	0
Nerds, Grape & Strawberry, Wonka*	1 Serving/30g	120	0	400	0	93.3	0	0
Nougat, Caramel, Soft, Lonka*	1 Cube/11g	45	1.1	409	2.3	78	9.6	0
Original, Chocolate Soft Caramel, Speciality, Werther's*	1 Piece/6g	30	1.5	480	5.1	61.5	23.5	1
Paradise Fruits, Dominion, Aldi*	1 Sweet/6g	23	0	382	0	95.5	0	0
Parma Violets, Swizzlers*	1 Sm Tube/10g	41	0.3	414	0	94.9	3.3	0
Party Size, Haribo*	1 Pack/25g	86	0.1	343	6.7	78	0.5	0
Pear Drops, Free From Fellows*	1 Sweet/4g	11	0	273	0	97	0	0
Pencils, Strawberry, Co-Op*	2 Pencils/16g	59	0.5	369	3.1	87.5	3.1	3.1
Percy Pig & Pals, Soft, M&S*	1 Sweet/8g	30	0	344	5.8	80	0.1	0
Percy Pig, 1/3 Less Sugar, M&S*	1 Percy/9g	29	0	320	1	72.5	0.4	11
Pic 'n' Mix, Woolworths*	1 Serving/180g	750	6	417	0	96.7	3.3	0
Pick & Mix, Cup, Asda*	1 Cup/160g	554	1.1	346	3.2	82	0.7	0.6
Pizza, Gummi, Gummy zone*	1 Pack/23g	80	0.1	347	5.8	81	0.5	0.5
Pomegranate Hearts, Biona Organic*	1 Pack/75g	238	0.2	317	0.1	78	0.2	2.3
Rainbow Twists, Haribo*	1 Pack/70g	234	1.8	334	0.5	80	2.5	0
Randoms, 30% Less Sugar, Rowntree's*	9 Sweets/35g	106	0	299	5	63	0.1	13
Randoms, Rowntree's*	1 Pack/50g	164	0.2	328	4.9	75.7	0.3	0.6
Randoms, Sours, Rowntree's*	1 Serving/20g	67	0	334	4	77.3	0	0
Raspberry Flavour Mushrooms, Tesco*	1 Serving/25g	90	0.3	359	3.8	83	1.2	0.6
Refreshers, Candyland, Barratt*	1 Tube/34g	129	0.5	380	0	89.1	1.4	0
Refreshers, Softies, Mini, Barratt*	1 Bag/30g	107	0.2	358	3.2	85	0.6	0.5
Refreshers, Strawberry, Soft Chew, Swizzels*	1 Sweet/5g	44	0.7	873	0.2	185.1	13.3	0
Rhubarb & Custard, Sainsbury's*	1 Sweet/8g	28	0	351	0.1	87.7	0	0
Rhubarb & Custards, Tesco*	1 Sweet/8g	32	0	395	0.1	98.2	0.1	0.5
Rotella, Haribo*	1 Sweet/8g	26	0.1	325	0.5	78	1.6	0
Rowntree's*	1 Tube/49g	170	0.1	344	4.8	81.3	0.2	0
Sherbert Lemons, M&S*	1 Serving/20g	76	0	380	0	93.9	0	0

S

	Measure INFO/WEIGHT	per Measure KCAL	FAT	Nutrition Values per 100g / 100ml KCAL	PROT	CARB	FAT	FIBRE
SWEETS								
Sherbet Lemons, Bassett's*	1 Sweet/7g	25	0	375	0	93.9	0	0
Sherbet Pip, Old Sam's Sweet Shoppe*	12 Pips/9g	35	0.1	394	0.5	95	1.6	0.5
Shockers, Orange Sherbet, Tango*	1 Bar/11g	41	0.4	371	0	79	3.9	0
Shrimps & Bananas, Sainsbury's*	½ Pack/50g	188	0	376	2.5	91.3	0.1	0.5
Shrimps, & Bananas, Barratt*	1 Serving/25g	94	0.1	376	2.9	90.5	0.3	0.5
Shrimps, & Bananas, Tesco*	1 Pack/80g	299	0.2	374	2.8	90.1	0.2	0.6
Snakes, Super Sour, Fizzy, Asda*	½ Pack/20g	70	0.1	350	5.4	82	0.5	0.5
Soft Fruits, Trebor*	1 Roll/45g	165	0	367	0	90.9	0	0
Soft Gums, Sugar Free, Morrisons*	1 Serving/25g	55	0.1	219	0.5	81.8	0.4	0
Soft Jellies, Scary Jellies, Maynards*	1 Pack/17g	54	0	321	3.1	76	0.2	0
Sour Snakes, Gelatine Free, Fruitella*	1 Bag/120g	409	0	341	0	84	0	0
Sour Watermelon, Candy Kittens*	1 Serving/25g	85	0	341	0.8	83	0.1	0
Spogs, Average	***1 Sweet/4g***	***13***	***0***	***332***	***3.9***	***79***	***0.1***	***0***
Squashies, Drumsticks, Raspberry & Milk, Swizzels*	¼ Pack/40g	142	0.1	355	3.4	83.9	0.2	0
Squidglets, Haribo*	1 Sweet/3g	11	0	339	4.5	79	0.5	0
Squidgy Babies, Haribo*	1 Serving/25g	86	0.1	346	5.7	80	0.5	0
Squish'ems, Randoms, Rowntrees*	5 Sweets/20g	68	0	334	4.8	77	0.1	0
Strawberry & Cream, Sugar Free, Sula*	1 Sweet/3g	9	0.2	267	0.2	90.5	5.4	0
Strawberry Straws, Fizzy, Sainsburys*	1 Straw/8g	30	0.2	373	2.8	85	2.2	1.2
Strawberry Trunks, Bebito*	1 Stick/15g	57	0.2	381	2.1	90	1.4	0
Strawberry, Wild, Candy Kittens*	1 Sweet/6g	20	0	334	0.8	81	0.1	0
Sugar Free, Sula*	1 Sweet/3g	7	0	231	0	96.1	0	0
Summer Fruits, 30% Less Sugar, Fruit-tella*	1 Sweet/4g	14	0.2	350	1.6	69	5.6	0
Tangfastics, Mini, Haribo*	1 Pack/16g	55	0.1	346	6.6	80	0.5	0
Tangfastics, Stixx, Haribo*	1 Stick/25g	95	0.8	381	1.3	87	3.3	0
Terrific Turtles, Haribo*	1 Serving/30g	104	0.2	345	5.8	79	0.5	0
Tic Tac, Cool Cherry, Ferrero*	1 Pack/18g	69	0.1	382	0.2	92.2	0.7	0
Tooty Frooties, Rowntree's*	1 Bag/28g	111	1	397	0.1	91.5	3.5	0
Twists, Hawaiian Punch, Kenny's*	4 Twists/27g	80	0	296	3.7	77.8	0	0
Wendy the Worm, Veggie, Dominion, Aldi*	1 Sweet/13g	44	0.1	339	0.5	85	0.5	0.7
Wine Gummies, Matlow, Swizzels*	1 Pack/16g	52	0	324	0	58.7	0	0
Wine Gums, Free From Fellows*	1 Sweet/6g	12	0	217	0	81	0.3	0
Yo Yo's, All Flavours, 100% Fruit, We Are Bear*	1 Roll/10g	28	0	275	1.9	63.4	0.2	12
SWORDFISH								
Grilled, Average	***1oz/28g***	***39***	***1.5***	***139***	***22.9***	***0***	***5.2***	***0***
Raw, Average	***1oz/28g***	***42***	***2***	***149***	***21.1***	***0***	***7.2***	***0***
SYRUP								
Black Forest, Premium, Monin*	1 Serving/30ml	100	0	334	0	82	0	0
Butterscotch, Monin*	1 Serving/30ml	100	0	333	0	80	0	0
Caramel, for Coffee, Lyle's*	2 Tsps/10ml	33	0	329	0	83	0	0
Caramel, Sugar Free, Monin*	1 Serving/30ml	0	0	0	0	13.3	0	0
Chocolate Mint, Monin*	1 Serving/30ml	100	0	333	0	80	0	0
Cinnamon, Monin*	1 Serving/30ml	100	0	333	0	80	0	0
Cinnamon, Sweet Freedom*	1 Tsp/5g	14	0	283	0	71	0	5
Fire, Gold, Sukrin*	1 Serving	600	0	2000	0	8	0	69
Gingerbread, Monin*	1 Serving/30ml	90	0	300	0	76.7	0	0
Gingerbread, Sugar Free, Monin*	1 Serving/20g	3	0	14	0	0.6	0	0
Golden, Average	***1 Tbsp/20g***	***61***	***0***	***304***	***0.4***	***78.2***	***0***	***0***
Golden, Zero Calorie, The Skinny Food Co.*	1 Tbsp/15ml	1	0	4	0	0.2	0	1.1
Hazelnut, Monin*	1 Serving/30ml	90	0	300	0	73.3	0	0
Maple, Average	***1 Tbsp/20g***	***52***	***0***	***262***	***0***	***67.2***	***0.2***	***0***
Maple, Skinny Syrup, Zero Calorie, The Skinny Food Co.*	1 Tbsp/15ml	1	0	4	0	0.2	0	1.1
Organic Rice Malt, Clearspring*	2 Tbsp/42g	133	0.2	316	1.5	76.8	0.4	0

	Measure INFO/WEIGHT	per Measure KCAL	FAT	Nutrition Values per 100g / 100ml KCAL	PROT	CARB	FAT	FIBRE
SYRUP								
Passion Fruit, Premium, Monin*	1 Serving/30ml	103	0	343	0	84.9	0	0
Passionfruit, Tasti*	1 Tbsp/15ml	28	0.2	188	1	46.1	1	0
Stem Ginger, Average	***1 Tbsp/15ml***	***45***	***0***	***300***	***0***	***76.7***	***0***	***0***
Sugar	***1 Tbsp/20g***	***64***	***0***	***319***	***0***	***83.9***	***0***	***0***
Vanilla, Monin*	1 Shot/35ml	119	0	340	0	84.4	0	0

S

	Measure INFO/WEIGHT	per Measure KCAL	FAT	Nutrition Values per 100g / 100ml KCAL	PROT	CARB	FAT	FIBRE
TABOULEH								
Average	***1oz/28g***	***33***	***1.3***	***119***	***2.6***	***17.2***	***4.6***	***0***
TACO								
10 Min Beany Avo, Gousto*	1 Serving	688	27	688	21	81	27	12
Halloumi, Ten Min, Gousto*	1 Serving/454g	676	32.7	149	7.8	14.6	7.2	1.7
Prawn, & Chorizo, Hello Fresh*	1 Serving/506g	875	40.5	173	8	14	8	0
TACO KIT								
Crispy Chicken, Soft, Stand 'N' Stuff, Old El Paso*	1 Taco/44g	100	1.5	227	7	41.1	3.4	2.5
Enchilada, Open, Stand 'N' Stuff, Old El Paso *	1 Enchilada/50g	102	2	204	5.5	34.7	4	3.4
Garlic & Paprika, Crunchy, As Sold, Old El Paso *	1 Taco/26g	77	3.6	296	3.8	37.3	13.8	2.7
Mexican, Street Food, Wahaca*	½ Pack/205g	441	7.2	215	5.8	40.9	3.5	3.2
TACO SHELLS								
Corn, Crunchy, Old El Paso*	1 Taco/13g	66	3.5	509	5.4	59.2	27	3.6
Old El Paso*	1 Taco/12g	57	2.7	478	7.4	60.8	22.8	0
TAGINE								
Aubergine, Spiced, Allplants*	1 Pack/380g	429	9.5	113	3.8	17	2.5	3.1
Beef, Slow Cooked, Cook*	1 Serving/325g	462	15.6	142	13.5	11.2	4.8	1.3
Chickpea, Jane Plan*	1 Pack/300g	135	4.2	45	1.5	6.7	1.4	1.6
Lamb, & Couscous, Finest, Tesco*	1 Pack/422g	570	16	135	7.2	17.1	3.8	1.8
Lamb, Moroccan Style with Couscous, M&S*	1 Pack/400g	340	5.6	85	8.9	8.3	1.4	1.6
Lamb, Slow Cooked, M&S*	½ Pack/234g	290	9.1	124	15.6	5.8	3.9	1.6
Moroccan, Quorn*	1 Pack/376g	361	4.1	96	4.7	15.2	1.1	3.3
Moroccan, Veggie Bowl, Birds Eye*	1 Serving/380g	433	11.4	114	4.9	15	3	3.3
TAGLIATELLE								
Chicken, & Mushroom, BFY, M&S*	1 Pack/370g	407	8.9	110	8.1	13	2.4	1.8
Dry, Average	***1 Serving/100g***	***356***	***1.8***	***356***	***12.6***	***72.4***	***1.8***	***1***
Egg, Dry, Average	***1 Serving/75g***	***272***	***2.5***	***362***	***14.2***	***68.8***	***3.3***	***2.3***
Egg, Fresh, Dry, Average	***1 Serving/125g***	***345***	***3.5***	***276***	***10.6***	***53***	***2.8***	***2.1***
Fresh, Dry, Average	***1 Serving/75g***	***211***	***2***	***281***	***11.4***	***53.3***	***2.6***	***2.6***
Ham & Mushroom, BGTY, Sainsbury's*	1 Pack/400g	371	7.4	95	5.1	13.8	1.9	1.2
Ham & Mushroom, Italian, Waitrose*	1 Pack/400g	585	24	151	7.1	16.3	6.2	1
Ham, & Mushroom, Counted, Morrisons*	1 Pack/323g	284	7.1	88	4.1	12.5	2.2	1
Ham, & Mushroom, Creamy, Meal for One, M&S*	1 Pack/400g	564	20.4	141	7.4	15.8	5.1	1.1
Ham, & Mushroom, Sainsbury's*	1 Pack/396g	570	20.2	144	6.6	17.4	5.1	1.1
Lamb Ragu, Slow Cooked, Finest, Tesco*	1 Pack/400g	560	19.2	140	8.5	14.9	4.8	1.1
Prawn, King, Mussels, & Clams, Waitrose*	1 Pack/255g	395	12.7	155	8.1	18.4	5	2
Salmon, & Broccoli, Calorie Counted, Asda*	1 Pack/331g	278	6.6	84	4.9	11	2	1.3
Verdi, Fresh, Average	***1 Serving/125g***	***171***	***1.8***	***137***	***5.5***	***25.5***	***1.5***	***1.8***
Wholewheat, Cooked, Co-Op*	1 Serving/100g	138	1.1	138	5.1	24	1.1	5.9
TAHINI PASTE								
Average	***1 Tbsp/15g***	***97***	***8.9***	***649***	***23***	***8.1***	***59.3***	***8.1***
Dark, Meridian Foods*	1 Serving/10g	61	6	608	18.2	0.9	60	7.9
TANGERINES								
Fresh, Raw	***1 Sm/50g***	***18***	***0***	***35***	***0.9***	***8***	***0.1***	***1.3***
Fresh, Raw, Weighed with Peel, Average	***1 Med/70g***	***13***	***0.1***	***18***	***0.5***	***4.2***	***0.1***	***0.7***
TANGO*								
Cherry, Britvic*	1 Bottle/500ml	55	0	11	0	2.4	0	0
Orange, Britvic*	1 Can/330ml	63	0	19	0.1	4.4	0	0
Orange, Sugar Free, Britvic*	1 Can/330ml	13	0	4	0	0	0	0
Strawberry & Watermelon, Sugar Free, Britvic*	1 Can/330ml	10	0	3	0	0	0	0
Tropical, Sugar Free, Britvic*	1 Can/330ml	13	0	4	0	0.5	0	0
TAPENADE								
Olive, Black, Antipasti, Belazu*	1 Serving/25g	105	10.8	420	1.9	3.6	43	4.9
Olive, Black, M&S*	¼ Jar/33g	122	12.8	374	1.2	0.1	39.5	6.8

T

	Measure INFO/WEIGHT	per Measure KCAL	FAT	Nutrition Values per 100g / 100ml KCAL	PROT	CARB	FAT	FIBRE
TAPENADE								
Olive, Black, Specially Selected, Aldi*	1 Tbsp/20g	46	4.6	231	1.4	2.7	23	4.4
Olive, Green, Belazu*	1 Serving/25g	66	6.8	265	0.9	2.7	27.2	2.2
Olive, Kalamata, Sainsbury's*	1 Serving/25g	63	6.6	253	1.6	1.4	26.2	2.8
TAPIOCA								
Creamed, Ambrosia*	½ Can/213g	159	3.4	75	2.6	12.6	1.6	0.2
Raw	***1oz/28g***	***101***	***0***	***359***	***0.4***	***95***	***0.1***	***0.4***
TARAMASALATA								
Average	***1 Tbsp/30g***	***143***	***14.4***	***478***	***4.2***	***7.9***	***47.9***	***1.1***
Smoked, Co-Op*	¼ Pack/42g	199	20.2	474	3.1	7.6	48	0.6
TARRAGON								
Dried, Ground	***1 Tsp/2g***	***5***	***0.1***	***295***	***22.8***	***42.8***	***7.2***	***0***
Fresh, Average	***1 Tbsp/3.8g***	***2***	***0***	***49***	***3.4***	***6.3***	***1.1***	***0***
TART								
Almond, & Blueberry, Bakery in Store, M&S*	1 Tart/90g	335	17	372	5.6	43.3	18.9	1.1
Apple & Custard, Asda*	1 Tart/84g	227	11	270	3.1	35	13.1	0.1
Apple, & Salted Caramel, Tesco*	1 Slice/83g	222	7.9	267	3.1	41.5	9.5	1.9
Bacon, Maple, & Extra Mature Cheddar, Finest, Tesco*	½ Pack/200g	642	42.8	321	10.5	21	21.4	1.4
Bakewell, Average	***1 Tart/50g***	***228***	***14.8***	***456***	***6.3***	***43.5***	***29.7***	***1.9***
Bakewell, Lemon, Average	***1 Tart/46g***	***206***	***9.7***	***447***	***3.7***	***60.9***	***21.1***	***0.9***
Blackcurrant, Sundae, Tesco*	1 Tart/55g	240	11	436	3	60	19.9	2.2
Butternut Squash, Mascarpone, & Sage, Finest, Tesco*	¼ Tart/100g	281	17.5	281	6.7	23.3	17.5	1.6
Caramel, Salted, & Chocolate, Waitrose*	1/12 Tart/79g	349	18.5	443	5.1	52.2	23.5	1.2
Caramelised Onion, & Goats Cheese, M&S*	1 Tart/600g	405	27	68	1.3	4.7	4.5	0
Cheese, & Asparagus, Oven Baked, Asda*	1 Tart/100g	271	17	271	7.9	20	17	1.8
Chocolate, Co-Op*	1 Tart/22g	102	6.8	465	4	42	31	0.7
Chorizo, Cheddar, & Mixed Pepper, Sainsbury's*	1 Tart/150g	384	27.4	256	7.2	15.2	18.3	1.2
Coconut, & Raspberry, Holly Lane, Aldi*	1 Tart/48g	191	8.2	397	4.4	56	17	3.3
Courgette, & Pecorino, Finest, Tesco*	¼ Tart/100g	302	21.6	302	5.8	20.5	21.6	1.3
Custard, Egg, Classic, Co-Op*	1 Tart/87g	246	10.4	283	6.5	36	12	0.6
Custard, Individual, Average	***1 Tart/94g***	***260***	***13.6***	***277***	***6.3***	***32.4***	***14.5***	***1.2***
Custard, Portuguese, Tesco*	1 Tart/55g	160	7.2	290	4.4	38.4	13	1
Date, Pecan & Almond, Sticky, Sainsbury's*	1/8 Tart/75g	298	10.3	397	5	63.5	13.7	1.7
Egg Custard, Asda*	1 Tart/80g	215	10.4	269	9	29	13	1.2
Egg Custard, Free Range, Sainsbury's*	1 Tart/85g	232	10	273	6.3	35	11.8	0.9
Egg Custard, Twin Pack, Tesco*	1 Tart/86g	244	10.6	284	6.8	35.9	12.3	1.3
Feta Cheese & Spinach, Puff Pastry, Tesco*	1 Tart/108g	306	19.2	283	7.1	23.5	17.8	0.9
Jam, Average	***1 Slice/90g***	***342***	***13.4***	***380***	***3.3***	***62***	***14.9***	***1.6***
Jam, Real Fruit, Mr Kipling*	1 Tart/35g	139	4.7	396	3.5	64.5	13.4	1.5
Jam, Real Fruit, Sainsbury's*	1 Tart/37g	142	5.2	383	3.4	60.9	14	1.4
Lemon Curd, Asda*	1 Tart/30g	121	4.5	402	2.8	64	15	2.2
Lemon Curd, Tesco*	1 Tart/30g	128	4.7	428	3.4	67	15.8	2
Lemon, & Raspberry, Finest, Tesco*	1 Tart/120g	360	16.8	300	5.2	38.4	14	2.9
Lemon, M&S*	1/6 Tart/50g	208	14.6	415	5	32.7	29.3	0.9
Lemon, Sicilian, All Butter, The Best, Morrisons*	1/6 Tart/72g	222	9	308	5.7	42.6	12.5	1.1
Lemon, Zesty, Tesco*	1/6 Tart/64g	260	15.5	405	5.3	41	24.2	0.7
Mixed Fruit, Fresh, Waitrose*	1 Tart/129g	351	17.4	272	4.2	32.8	13.5	1.5
Passion Fruit, & Raspberry, Finest, Tesco*	1 Slice/75g	286	14.6	382	4.3	47.1	19.5	0.7
Pecan, Free From, Sainsbury's*	1 Tart/50g	239	13.2	477	4.7	54.4	26.4	1.7
Pineapple, Individual, Waitrose*	1 Tart/54g	216	6.1	400	2.2	77.2	11.3	0.5
Plum, Continental, Specially Selected, Aldi*	1 Slice/75g	196	6.7	262	3.6	40	9	3.1
Plum, Seriously Fruity, Waitrose*	1/6 Tart/95g	183	5.9	192	2.9	30.2	6.2	1.9
Rhubarb, & Custard, Crumble, Deluxe, Lidl*	1 Slice/90g	297	14	330	4.3	42.2	15.6	2
Spinach, & Ricotta, Individual, TTD, Sainsbury's*	1 Tart/170g	466	33.7	274	7.5	16.5	19.8	1.4

T

	Measure INFO/WEIGHT	per Measure KCAL	per Measure FAT	Nutrition Values per 100g / 100ml KCAL	PROT	CARB	FAT	FIBRE
TART								
Strawberry, & Fresh Cream, Finest, Tesco*	1 Tart/129g	350	19.1	271	3.3	31.1	14.8	1.2
Strawberry, British Cream, Asda*	1 Tart/127g	348	17.8	274	3.6	33	14	0.6
Strawberry, Custard, Asda*	1 Tart/100g	335	15	335	3.1	47	15	0
Strawberry, Fresh, M&S*	1 Tart/120g	305	18.4	255	3.1	26.4	15.4	2.4
Tomato, & Mascarpone, Cherry, Asda*	1 Tart/160g	290	18	181	4.4	15.6	11.2	1.1
Treacle, Average	***1 Serving/125g***	***460***	***17.6***	***368***	***3.7***	***60.4***	***14.1***	***1.1***
Treacle, with Custard	***1 Serving/251g***	***586***	***23.5***	***233***	***3.1***	***36.1***	***9.4***	***0.8***
Vegetable & Feta, Deli, M&S*	½ Tart/115g	315	18.4	274	5	20	16	6
Vegetable, Roasted, Finest, Tesco*	¼ Tart/113g	213	10.4	188	2.9	22.5	9.2	2.1
TARTE								
Au Chocolat, Seriously Chocolatey, Waitrose*	1/6 Tarte/70g	348	22.8	497	6	43.8	32.6	2.6
Au Citron, Frozen, TTD, Sainsbury's*	1/6 Tarte/80g	232	13.4	290	4.7	40.7	16.8	7.7
Au Citron, Waitrose*	1 Tarte/100g	325	18.1	325	4.9	35.7	18.1	1
Bacon, Leek & Roquefort, Bistro, Waitrose*	¼ Tarte/100g	277	18.2	277	8.4	19.8	18.2	0.6
Mixed Berry, Crumble, Frozen, Waitrose*	1/6 Tarte/76g	224	8.3	296	3.3	44.8	11	2.2
Tatin, 1, Waitrose*	1 Tarte/50g	106	4.6	212	1.9	29.9	9.1	1.6
TARTLETS								
All Butter, Sweet, TTD, Sainsbury's*	1 Tartlet/23g	116	5.5	504	6.3	64.8	24.1	1.7
Brie & Cranberry, Filo, Waitrose*	1 Tartlet/16g	44	2.2	275	8.9	26.9	13.9	3.5
Brie, & Cranberry, Party Food, M&S*	1 Tartlet/19g	56	3.2	295	7.8	26.9	17.1	1.3
Cauliflower, & Kale, Curried, Lidl*	1 Tartlet/110g	330	19.8	300	5.4	27.9	18	2.4
Cheese, Goats, & Caramelised Onion, Aldi*	1 Tartlet/150g	402	26	268	7.3	20.7	17.3	1.2
Raspberry, Mini, M&S*	1 Tartlet/27g	90	5.4	330	4.3	34.4	19.6	0.5
Tomato, & Goats Cheese, Waitrose*	1 Tartlet/130g	295	19	227	6.6	17.4	14.6	2
TEA								
Assam, Blended, TTD, Sainsbury's*	1 Serving/2g	0	0	0	0	0	0	0
Blackberry & Nettle, Twinings*	1 Mug/250ml	5	0	2	0	0.3	0	0
Camomile, Pure, Classic Herbal, Twinings*	1 Serving/200ml	4	0	2	0	0.3	0	0
Chai, Latte, Spiced, Drink Me*	1 Sachet/15g	68	2.3	452	7.6	70.5	15.3	1.2
Chai, Twinings*	1 Mug/200ml	2	0	1	0.1	0	0	0
Choco, Yogi Tea*	1 Mug/200ml	8	0	4	0	1	0	0
Cranberry & Elderflower, Boost, Tetley*	1 Mug/225ml	5	0	2	0.1	0.6	0	0
Cranberry, & Blood Orange, Twinings*	1 Cup/250ml	5	0	2	0	0	0	0
Damask, Rose, Chinese, Choi Time*	1 Mug/500ml	0	0.3	0	0	0	0.1	0
Decaf, Tetley*	1 Mug/100ml	1	0	1	0	0.3	0	0
Earl Grey, Infusion with Water, Average	***1 Mug/250ml***	***2***	***0***	***1***	***0***	***0.2***	***0***	***0***
Fennel, Three, Pukka Herbs*	1 Serving/200ml	8	0	4	0	0	0	0
Fruit Or Herbal, Made with Water, Twinings*	1 Mug/200ml	8	0	4	0	1	0	0
Fruit, Twinings*	1 Mug/227ml	4	0	2	0	0.4	0	0
Ginger, Herbal, Brit & Tang*	1 Tea Bag/2g	5	0	278	0	55.6	0	0
Green, Matcha, Twinings*	1 Mug/250ml	2	0	1	0	0	0	0
Green, Pure, Tetley*	1 Mug/250ml	2	0	1	0	0.3	0	0
Green, Rooibos, Naturally Caffeine Free, Tick Tock*	1 Mug/250ml	0	0	0	0	0	0	0
Green, with Jasmine, Twinings*	1 Mug/100ml	1	0	1	0	0.2	0	0
Green, with Lemon, Knightsbridge, Lidl*	1 Mug/200ml	1	0	0	0	0	0	0
Green, with Mint, Whittards of Chelsea*	1 Mug/100ml	1	0	1	0.2	0.1	0	0
Green, with Pomegranate, Twinings*	1 Mug/200ml	2	0	1	0	0.2	0	0
Ice, with Lemon, Lipton*	1 Bottle/325ml	91	0	28	0	6.9	0	0
Ice, with Mango, Lipton*	1 Bottle/500ml	165	0	33	0	8.1	0	0
Ice, with Peach, Lipton*	1 Bottle/500ml	140	0	28	0	6.8	0	0
Iced, Green, Lipton*	1 Can/253ml	38	1.3	15	0.5	3.6	0.5	0
Iced, Peach, Low Calories, Lipton*	1 Bottle/505ml	96	2.5	19	0.5	4.7	0.5	0
Iced, Peach, Twinings*	1 Mug/200ml	60	0.2	30	0.1	7.3	0.1	0

	Measure INFO/WEIGHT	per Measure KCAL	FAT	Nutrition Values per 100g / 100ml KCAL	PROT	CARB	FAT	FIBRE
TEA								
Iced, Peach, Zero, Freeway*	1 Serving/300ml	6	0	2	0.1	0.4	0	0
Iced, Raspberry, Bottle, Lipton*	1 Mug/250ml	48	1.3	19	0.5	4.6	0.5	0
Instant, Typhoo*	1 Tsp/3g	14	0.8	457	5.6	51.4	25.4	0
Lemon, & Ginger, Lipton*	1 Cup/200ml	8	0	4	0.5	0.5	0	0
Lemon, & Ginger, Lazy Days, Tea Pigs*	1 Mug/200ml	2	0	1	0	0	0	0
Lemon, Ginger, & Manuka Honey, Pukka Herbs*	1 Mug/200ml	6	0	3	0	0	0	0
Lemon, Iced, Diet, Nestea*	1 Glass/250ml	3	0	1	0	0	0	0
Lemon, Instant, Original, Lift*	2 Tsp/7g	23	0	324	1.4	79.6	0	0
Lemon, Instant, Tesco*	1 Serving/7g	23	0	326	1	80.5	0	0
Made with 1% Milk, Average	***1 Mug/250ml***	***12***	***0.2***	***5***	***0.4***	***0.8***	***0.1***	***0***
Made with Water	***1 Mug/227ml***	***0***	***0***	***0***	***0.1***	***0***	***0***	***0***
Made with Water with Semi-Skimmed Milk, Average	***1 Mug/200ml***	***14***	***0.4***	***7***	***0.5***	***0.7***	***0.2***	***0***
Made with Water with Skimmed Milk, Average	***1 Mug/270ml***	***16***	***0.5***	***6***	***0.5***	***0.7***	***0.2***	***0***
Made with Water with Whole Milk, Average	***1 Mug/200ml***	***16***	***0.8***	***8***	***0.4***	***0.5***	***0.4***	***0***
Morning Detox, Twinings*	1 Mug/200ml	5	0	2	0	0.3	0	0
Nettle & Peppermint, Twinings*	1 Mug/200ml	2	0	1	0	0.2	0	0
Nettle & Sweet Fennel, Twinings*	1 Mug/200ml	4	0	2	0	0.3	0	0
Oolong, Average	***1 Mug/200ml***	***5***	***0.2***	***2***	***0.1***	***0.2***	***0.1***	***0.2***
Peppermint, Made with Water, Average	***1 Mug/200ml***	***3***	***0***	***2***	***0***	***0.2***	***0***	***0***
Raspberry & Cranberry, T of Life, Tetley*	1 Mug/100ml	36	0	36	0	9	0	0
Red Berries, Brewed, PG Tips*	1 Mug/200ml	5	0	2	0	0.6	0	0
Red Bush, Made with Water, Tetley*	1 Mug/250ml	2	0	1	0	0.1	0	0
Red, ChariTea*	1 Bottle/330ml	53	0	16	0	3.4	0	0
Sleep, Herbal Infusion, Brewed, Twinings*	1 Mug/200ml	4	0	2	0	0.3	0	0
Strawberry Lemonade, Cold Infuse, Twinings*	1 Mug/200ml	4	0	2	0	0	0	0
Super Fruits, Blueberry, & Rasberry, Boost, Tetley*	1 Mug/250ml	5	0	2	0.1	0.6	0	0
Turmeric, Orange, & Star Anise, Superblends, Twinings*	1 Mug/200ml	2	0	1	0	0.5	0	0
Wild Berry, Made Up, Asda*	1 Mug/250ml	2	0	1	0	0	0	0
TEACAKES								
Average	***1 Teacake/60g***	***178***	***4.5***	***296***	***8***	***52.5***	***7.5***	***0***
Black Forest, Co-Op*	1 Teacake/22g	94	3.6	427	4.6	63.6	16.4	2.3
Chocolate, & Orange, M&S*	1 Teacake/18g	80	3.1	445	5.4	66.4	17.1	2.1
Fruited, Free From, Waitrose*	1 Teacake/67g	176	2.4	263	3	50.9	3.6	7.5
Fruited, Iceland*	1 Teacake/60g	171	2.4	285	8.8	51.6	4	3.5
Fruity, Warburton's*	1 Teacake/63g	164	1.9	262	8.7	48	3	3.2
Jam, Lees*	1 Teacake/19g	82	2.9	443	4.2	69.8	15.8	2.5
Large, Sainsbury's*	1 Teacake/73g	212	3.6	291	7.6	52.4	4.9	3.4
Marshmallow, Milk Chocolate, Tunnock's*	1 Teacake/24g	106	4.6	440	4.9	61.9	19.2	2.4
Mini Bites, M&S*	1 Bite/6g	29	1.2	484	3.2	72.6	20.3	2.1
Richly Fruited, Waitrose*	1 Teacake/72g	205	2.7	285	7.8	55	3.7	2.2
Salted Caramel, M&S*	1 Teacake/18g	80	3.2	448	5.3	65.3	17.9	1.4
Toasted, Average	***1 Teacake/60g***	***197***	***5***	***329***	***8.9***	***58.3***	***8.3***	***0***
Toasted, Henllan Bakery*	1 Teacake/60g	144	1.7	240	7.1	46.7	2.8	0
Wagon Wheel, Burton's*	1 Teacake/15g	66	2.6	440	3.3	66	17.3	2
Wholemeal, Potts Bakers *	1 Teacake/100g	215	2.2	215	9.6	36.3	2.2	5.9
with Orange Filling, M&S*	1 Teacake/20g	80	2.8	410	4.5	66.6	14.2	0.9
TEMPEH								
Average	***1oz/28g***	***46***	***1.8***	***166***	***20.7***	***6.4***	***6.4***	***4.3***
Barbecue, Slices, Oasis*	1 Serving/30g	58	4.2	193	12.4	2.9	14	0
Curry Flavoured, Pieces, Plant Power*	½ Pack/90g	331	27	368	21	3.5	30	7.7
Lupin, Organic, Better Nature*	1 Pack/170g	245	8.2	144	17	3.5	4.8	10
Original, Organic, Plant Power*	1 Pack/198g	364	19.2	184	19	2	9.7	6.5
The Tofoo Co.*	1 Serving/67g	139	7.3	208	21.3	1.8	10.9	6.1

T

	Measure INFO/WEIGHT	per Measure KCAL	FAT	Nutrition Values per 100g / 100ml KCAL	PROT	CARB	FAT	FIBRE
TEQUILA								
Average	***1 Pub Shot/35ml***	***78***	***0***	***224***	***0***	***0***	***0***	***0***
TERRINE								
Crab, & King Prawn, M&S*	1 Pack/120g	244	17.6	203	8.9	8.6	14.7	0.1
Ham Hock, M&S*	1 Slice/70g	98	4.1	140	22.5	0.1	5.8	0.5
Raspberry Jelly, Plant Kitchen, M&S*	¼ Pack/137g	81	0.3	59	0.5	13.5	0.2	0.7
Salmon & King Prawn, Waitrose*	1 Serving/75g	98	4	130	19.3	1.3	5.3	0
Salmon, Pate, Sainsbury's*	1 Terrine/50g	116	9.7	233	11.8	2.5	19.4	0.5
Salmon, Scottish, M&S*	1 Terrine/58g	116	8.3	200	14	3.7	14.3	0.5
Vegetable, Waitrose *	1 Serving/60g	86	5.1	143	3.5	11.7	8.4	3.7
THYME								
Dried, Average	***1 Tsp/1g***	***3***	***0.1***	***276***	***9.1***	***45.3***	***7.4***	***0***
Fresh, Average	***1 Tsp/1g***	***1***	***0***	***95***	***3***	***15.1***	***2.5***	***0***
TIA MARIA								
Original	***1 Pub Shot/35ml***	***105***	***0***	***300***	***0***	***0***	***0***	***0***
TIC TAC								
Extra Strong Mint, Ferrero*	2 Tic Tacs/1g	4	0	381	0	95.2	0	0
Fresh Mint, Ferrero*	2 Tic Tacs/1g	4	0	390	0	97.5	0	0
Lime & Orange, Ferrero*	2 Tic Tacs/1g	4	0	386	0	95.5	0	0
TIKKA MASALA								
Cauliflower, Fire Roasted, Bol*	1 Serving/405g	413	15	102	3.5	12.3	3.7	2.5
Cheeky, Wicked Kitchen, Tesco*	1 Pack/353g	487	15.2	138	5.9	17.6	4.3	3
Chicken, & Rice, Ready Meal, Healthy Range, Average	***1 Serving/400g***	***390***	***6.4***	***98***	***6.6***	***14.3***	***1.6***	***1.1***
Chicken, & Pilau Rice, BGTY, Sainsbury's*	1 Pack/364g	400	6.5	110	6.8	15.2	1.8	2.5
Chicken, & Pilau Rice, Meal for One, M&S*	1 Pack/400g	592	20.4	148	8.9	15.3	5.1	2.7
Chicken, A Taste of India, Tesco*	½ Pack/218g	318	19.2	146	11.1	4.6	8.8	2
Chicken, Calorie Counted, Asda*	1 Pack/399g	395	6	99	6.7	15	1.5	0.5
Chicken, Frozen, Asda*	1 Pack/390g	581	13.3	149	6.7	22	3.4	1.1
Chicken, Hot, Sainsbury's*	1 Pack/400g	604	37.2	151	13.2	3.6	9.3	1.5
Chicken, Hot, Takeaway, Tesco*	½ Pack/194g	244	13.9	126	9	5.3	7.2	2
Chicken, Slim Choice, Sainsbury's*	1 Pack/346g	246	5.9	71	11.1	3.7	1.7	0.8
Chicken, Slim Cook, Tesco*	1 Pack/477g	367	4.8	77	11.8	4.5	1	1.3
Chicken, Slow Cooked, British, Sainsburys*	½ Pack/225g	367	20	163	17.6	3	8.9	0.6
Chicken, with Pilau Rice, Serves 1, Sainsbury's*	1 Pack/450g	724	24.8	161	7.5	18.7	5.5	3.3
Chicken, with Rice, Free From, Sainsbury's*	1 Pack/375g	435	12.8	116	7.2	12.5	3.4	3.1
Meal Kit, Pataks*	½ Pack/157g	221	15.7	141	2.4	7.8	10	0
Paneer, Co-Op*	1 Pack/400g	320	12.4	80	4.5	7.5	3.1	2.1
Prawn, with Fragrant Pilau Rice, Finest, Tesco*	1 Pack/398g	474	15.5	119	4.4	16.2	3.9	0.8
Tasty Bite*	1 Serving/142g	126	6	89	2.7	7.8	4.2	4.4
Vegetarian, Chef's Selection, Quorn*	½ Pack/170g	274	17	161	6	10	10	3.5
TILAPIA								
Raw, Average	***100g***	***95***	***1***	***95***	***20***	***0***	***1***	***0***
Roasted, Spiced, with Tomatoes, & Lentils, Hello Fresh*	1 Serving/483g	261	3	54	7	4.3	0.6	0
TIME OUT								
Break Pack, Cadbury*	1 Serving/20g	108	6.3	530	6.2	58.3	30.7	0
Chocolate Fingers, Cadbury*	2 Fingers/35g	186	10.6	530	7.1	57.3	30.3	1.1
TIRAMISU								
Asda*	1 Pot/100g	252	11	252	4.3	34	11	0.5
Classic, Individual, Sainsbury's*	1 Pot/100g	242	9.9	242	3.8	30.6	9.9	1.2
Classic, Sainsbury's*	1 Serving/84g	209	8.5	250	4.2	31.7	10.2	1.1
Dessert Menu, Aldi*	¼ Pack/125g	340	15	272	4.3	32	12	1.4
Dine in Dessert, M&S*	½ Dessert/145g	515	36.7	355	2.6	28.8	25.3	0.7
Envia*	1 Pot/80g	243	12.9	304	3.2	33	16.1	0
Family Size, Tesco*	1 Serving/125g	356	18.1	285	4.3	34.5	14.5	4.3

T

	Measure INFO/WEIGHT	per Measure KCAL	per Measure FAT	KCAL	PROT	CARB	FAT	FIBRE
				Nutrition Values per 100g / 100ml				
TIRAMISU								
Morrisons*	1 Pot/90g	248	9.9	276	4	38	11	0
Single Size, Tesco*	1 Pot/100g	290	12.9	290	3.8	35.1	12.9	4.5
Waitrose*	1 Pot/90g	221	11.2	246	6.4	27.2	12.4	0
TOAD IN THE HOLE								
Aunt Bessie's*	1 Serving/158g	419	23	265	11.4	22.2	14.6	0.9
Average	***1 Serving/231g***	***640***	***40.2***	***277***	***11.9***	***19.5***	***17.4***	***1.1***
Frozen, Cooked, CBY, Asda*	1 Slice/72g	168	7.5	232	9.2	24.2	10.4	2.6
Mini, Aunt Bessie's*	1 Serving/62g	118	6.8	191	11	12	11	3.6
with Three Sausages, Asda*	1 Pack/150g	435	27	290	10	22	18	1
TOASTIE								
All Day Breakfast, M&S*	1 Toastie/174g	375	13.8	215	11.2	25	7.9	1.7
Cheese & Pickle, M&S*	1 Toastie/136g	320	9.1	235	10.4	33.5	6.7	2.6
Cheese & Onion, Ginsters*	1 Toastie/122g	330	12.3	269	10.9	33.1	10	1.5
Cheese, & Tomato , Real Wrap Co.*	1 Toastie/164g	364	11.8	222	10.2	28.4	7.2	0
Ham & Cheese, White Bread	***1 Toastie/150g***	***409***	***14.9***	***273***	***14.5***	***31.3***	***9.9***	***0.9***
TOFFEE APPLE								
Average	***1 Apple/141g***	***188***	***3***	***133***	***1.2***	***29.2***	***2.1***	***2.3***
TOFFEE CRISP								
Biscuit, Nestle*	1 Biscuit/19g	99	5.3	519	3.9	62.3	27.8	1.4
Bitesize, Nestle*	1 Serving/20g	101	5.4	518	3.8	63	27.6	1.3
TOFFEES								
Assorted, Bassett's*	1 Toffee/8g	35	1.1	434	3.8	73.1	14	0
Assorted, Sainsbury's*	1 Toffee/8g	37	1.3	457	2.2	76.5	15.8	0.2
Butter, Smart Price, Asda*	1 Toffee/8g	37	1.3	440	1.3	75	15	0
Chewy, Werther's*	1 Toffee/5g	22	0.8	436	3.5	71.3	15.2	0.1
Dairy, Waitrose*	1 Toffee/8g	37	1.1	458	2	80.2	14.3	0.5
Dark Chocolate, Riesen*	1 Toffee/30g	135	5.5	449	4.1	66.3	18.3	0
Devon Butter, Thorntons*	1 Toffee/9g	40	1.5	444	1.7	72.2	16.7	0
English Butter, Co-Op*	1 Toffee/8g	38	1.6	470	2	71	20	0
Everyday Value, Tesco*	1 Toffee/8g	34	1.1	450	2.1	77.3	14.8	0.3
Liquorice, Thorntons*	1 Bag/100g	506	29.4	506	1.9	58.8	29.4	0
Mixed, Average	***1oz/28g***	***119***	***5.2***	***426***	***2.2***	***66.7***	***18.6***	***0***
Original, Cartwright & Butler*	1 Toffee/8g	36	1	445	1.5	80	13	0.5
Original, Thorntons*	1 Bag/100g	514	30.1	514	1.8	59.3	30.1	0
TOFU								
Average	***1 Pack/250g***	***297***	***16.5***	***119***	***13.4***	***1.4***	***6.6***	***0.1***
Deep Fried, Tofu King*	½ Pack/115g	384	31.3	334	21.2	0.7	27.2	0
Fried, Average	***1oz/28g***	***75***	***4***	***268***	***28.6***	***9.3***	***14.1***	***0***
J-basket*	1 Serving/100g	69	3.9	69	5.7	2.6	3.9	0
Nature, Bjorg*	1 Pack/200g	330	19.8	165	17	1.1	9.9	1.5
Organic, Block, Cauldron Foods*	½ Pack/198g	234	14.1	118	12.6	1	7.1	1.9
Pieces, Marinated, Organic, Cauldron Foods*	1 Pack/160g	363	27.2	227	17.5	1	17	2.7
Smoked, Edeka*	1 Serving/100g	164	9.5	164	18.2	0.7	9.5	0
Smoked, Organic, Clearspot*	1/3 Pack/75g	103	5.7	137	15.2	2	7.6	0.6
Super Firm, Organic, Plant Kitchen, M&S*	1 Pack/300g	369	19.8	123	15	0.3	6.6	1.1
Sweet Chilli, Spicy, Bites, Cooked, The Tofoo Co.*	½ Pack/113g	356	16.6	316	12.9	31.8	14.7	2.3
Teriyaki, Organic, Cauldron Foods*	½ Pack/80g	168	12	210	16	2.8	15	2.1
Teriyaki, Organic, The Tofoo Co.*	1/3 Pack/70g	109	5.5	156	15.6	5.9	7.8	0.5
TOMATILLOS								
Raw	***1 Med/34g***	***11***	***0.3***	***32***	***1***	***5.8***	***1***	***1.9***
TOMATO PASTE								
Average	***1 Tbsp/20g***	***19***	***0***	***96***	***5***	***19.2***	***0.2***	***1.5***
Sun Dried, Average	***1 Hpd Tsp/10g***	***38***	***3.5***	***385***	***3.2***	***13.8***	***35.2***	***0***

T

	Measure INFO/WEIGHT	per Measure KCAL	FAT	Nutrition Values per 100g / 100ml KCAL	PROT	CARB	FAT	FIBRE
TOMATO PUREE								
Average	***1 Tbsp/15g***	***11***	***0***	***76***	***4.5***	***14.1***	***0.2***	***2.3***
Double Concentrate, Average	***1 Tbsp/15g***	***13***	***0***	***85***	***4.9***	***14.9***	***0.2***	***3.6***
Garlic, Double Concentrate, Morrisons*	1 Tbsp/15g	13	0	86	3.9	14.9	0.3	3.8
Tomato & Garlic, GIA*	1 Tbsp/15g	14	0.1	91	3.3	17.6	0.4	0
TOMATOES								
Cherry, Average	***1 Tomato/15g***	***3***	***0***	***18***	***0.7***	***3***	***0.3***	***0.5***
Cherry, on the Vine, Average	***1 Serving/80g***	***15***	***0.3***	***18***	***0.7***	***3.1***	***0.3***	***1.2***
Chopped, Canned, Branded Average	***1 Serving/130g***	***27***	***0.2***	***21***	***1.1***	***3.8***	***0.1***	***0.8***
Chopped, Italian, Average	***½ Can/200g***	***47***	***0.2***	***23***	***1.3***	***4.4***	***0.1***	***0.9***
Chopped, with Chilli, & Peppers, Asda*	1 Can/400g	96	2	24	1.3	4.2	0.5	0.6
Chopped, with Garlic, Average	***½ Can/200g***	***43***	***0.3***	***21***	***1.2***	***3.8***	***0.1***	***0.8***
Chopped, with Herbs, Average	***½ Can/200g***	***42***	***0.3***	***21***	***1.1***	***3.8***	***0.1***	***0.8***
Diced, Fire Roasted, Hunt's*	½ Can/123g	30	0	24	0.8	4.9	0	1.6
Fresh, Raw, Average	***1 Med/123g***	***22***	***0.2***	***18***	***0.9***	***3.9***	***0.2***	***1.2***
Fried in Blended Oil	***1 Med/85g***	***77***	***6.5***	***91***	***0.7***	***5***	***7.7***	***1.3***
Grilled, Average	***1 Med/85g***	***17***	***0.3***	***20***	***0.8***	***3.5***	***0.3***	***1.5***
Heritage, Jewel, TTD, Sainsbury's*	1 Pack/250g	62	1.2	25	1.1	3.4	0.5	1.2
Marinated, with Garlic & Oregano, The Deli, Aldi*	½ Pack/75g	68	3.5	90	2.8	7.8	4.7	2.7
Marmonde, Raw, Waitrose*	1 Tomato/120g	24	0.4	20	0.7	3.1	0.3	1
Mix, Summer Selection, Eat Well, M&S*	¼ Pack/70g	15	0.4	22	1.1	3.6	0.5	1.3
Plum, Baby, Average	***1 Serving/50g***	***9***	***0.2***	***18***	***1.5***	***2.3***	***0.3***	***1***
Plum, in Tomato Juice, Average	***1 Can/400g***	***71***	***0.4***	***18***	***1***	***3.3***	***0.1***	***0.7***
Plum, in Tomato Juice, Premium, Average	***1 Can/400g***	***93***	***1.2***	***23***	***1.3***	***3.8***	***0.3***	***0.7***
Pome Dei Moro, Waitrose*	1 Serving/80g	16	0.2	20	0.7	3.1	0.3	1.2
Pomodorino, TTD, Sainsbury's*	1 Tomato/8g	2	0	25	1.1	3.4	0.5	1.2
Ripened on the Vine, Average	***1 Med/123g***	***22***	***0.4***	***18***	***0.7***	***3.1***	***0.3***	***0.7***
Ruby Jewel, Raw, Sainsbury's*	1 Tomato/45g	9	0.2	20	0.7	3.1	0.5	1
Salad, Raw, Tesco*	1 Tomato/80g	14	0.1	17	0.5	3	0.1	1
Santini, M&S*	1 Serving/80g	16	0.2	20	0.7	3.1	0.3	1
Semi-Dried, Cooks' Ingredients, Waitrose*	1 Serving/50g	58	0.4	115	4.5	19.5	0.8	6.1
Stuffed with Rice Based Filling, Average	***1oz/28g***	***59***	***3.8***	***212***	***2.1***	***22.2***	***13.4***	***1.1***
Sugardrop, Finest, Tesco*	1 Tomato/14g	3	0	20	0.7	3.1	0.3	1
Sun Dried in Oil	***100g***	***301***	***24.8***	***301***	***5.8***	***13.5***	***24.8***	***7***
Sun Dried, Average	***3 Pieces/20g***	***43***	***3.2***	***214***	***4.7***	***13***	***15.9***	***3.3***
Sun Dried, Marinated, Antipasti, Cypressa*	1 Serving/30g	45	1.8	150	5.8	15.9	6	5.6
Sunsoaked, in Oil, Drained, TTD, Sainsbury's*	¼ Pot/33g	48	2.8	146	3.9	11.2	8.4	5.1
Sweet, Baby, Mixed, Finest, Tesco*	½ Pack/125g	25	0.4	20	0.7	3.1	0.3	1
Tri-Colour, On the Vine, Finest, Tesco*	8 Tomatoes/80g	21	0.4	26	1.1	3.6	0.5	1.2
TONGUE								
Lunch, Average	***1oz/28g***	***51***	***3***	***181***	***20.1***	***1.8***	***10.6***	***0***
Ox, British, Waitrose*	1 Slice/32g	68	4.9	213	17	1.7	15.4	0
Ox, Deli Counter, Sainsbury's*	1 Serving/100g	195	13.3	195	18.3	0.5	13.3	0.1
Pork, Lunch, Slices, Iceland*	1 Pack/80g	184	12	230	22.4	0.9	15	1
Slices, Average	***1oz/28g***	***56***	***3.9***	***201***	***18.7***	***0***	***14***	***0***
TONIC WATER								
Average	***1 Glass/250ml***	***82***	***0***	***33***	***0***	***8.8***	***0***	***0***
Clementine, Refreshingly Light, Fever-Tree*	1 Serving/250ml	48	0	19	0	4.7	0	0
Cucumber, Light, Fever-Tree*	1 Serving/250ml	48	0	19	0	4.8	0	0
Diet, Asda*	1 Glass/200ml	2	0	1	0	0	0	0
Indian, Diet, Schweppes*	1 Glass/100ml	1	0	1	0	0	0	0
Indian, Low Calorie, Vive, Aldi*	1 Glass/250ml	3	0	1	0	0	0	0
Indian, Premium, Fever-Tree*	1 Can/150ml	42	0	28	0	7.1	0	0
Indian, Schweppes*	1 Glass/250ml	55	0	22	0	5.1	0	0

	Measure INFO/WEIGHT	per Measure KCAL	FAT	Nutrition Values per 100g / 100ml KCAL	PROT	CARB	FAT	FIBRE
TONIC WATER								
Indian, Slimline, Schweppes*	1 Serving/188ml	3	0	2	0.4	0	0	0
Lemon, Refreshingly Light, Fever Tree*	½ Bottle/250ml	42	0	17	0	4.2	0	0.5
Lemon, Sicilian, Fever-Tree*	1 Bottle/200ml	70	0	35	0	8.7	0	0
Light, Refreshingly, Fever-Tree*	1 Can/150ml	22	0	15	0	3.8	0	0
Low Calorie, Tesco*	1 Glass/200ml	4	0	2	0	0.5	0	0
Mediterranean, Refreshingly Light, Fever-Tree*	1 Serving/250ml	48	0	19	0	4.8	0	0
TOPIC								
Mars*	1 Bar/47g	234	12.3	498	6.2	59.6	26.2	1.7
TORTE								
Cherry Bakewell, No.1, Waitrose*	1 Slice/85g	252	12.6	297	4.5	36.2	14.8	0.5
Chocolate Fondant, Gu*	1 Slice/62g	264	18.9	423	5.7	32	30.2	1.8
Chocolate, Luxury, Kirstys*	1 Slice/83g	301	18.3	363	3	36.4	22.1	3.4
Chocolate, Plant Kitchen, M&S*	1 Torte/70g	312	21.1	445	4.5	37.4	30.1	3.3
Chocolate, Tesco*	1 Slice/50g	126	6	251	3.6	32.3	11.9	1
Lemon & Mango, Waitrose*	1 Slice/80g	142	2.4	177	3.9	33.6	3	0.6
TORTELLINI								
Arrabbiata, Spicy, Morrisons*	½ Pack/210g	489	13.6	233	7.3	35.4	6.5	2.1
Beef, & Red Wine, Italian, Asda*	½ Pack/150g	242	4.2	161	9	25	2.8	0
Cheese, & Ham, Italiano, Tesco*	½ Pack/150g	396	12.3	264	12.8	34.8	8.2	3
Chicken, & Pancetta, Smoked, Rana La Famiglia*	1 Serving/125g	354	13.8	283	16	29	11	0
Ham, & Cheese, Fresh, Asda*	½ Pack/150g	255	9	170	6	23	6	1.7
Meat, Italian, Tesco*	1 Serving/125g	332	9.5	266	10.6	38.9	7.6	2.3
Mushroom, Asda*	1 Serving/125g	218	5.2	174	6	28	4.2	2.3
Pepperoni, Spicy, Asda*	½ Pack/150g	252	6	168	7	26	4	0
Sausage, & Ham, Italiano, Tesco*	1 Pack/300g	816	27.9	272	13.1	34	9.3	3.7
Spinach, & Ricotta, Italian, Asda*	½ Pack/150g	189	3.6	126	5	21	2.4	0.6
Spinach, & Ricotta, Filled, Aldi*	½ Pack/150g	252	3	168	7.5	29	2	2.3
Spinach, & Ricotta, Italian, Morrisons*	½ Pack/210g	286	5.9	136	4.9	22.1	2.8	1.5
Tomato, & Mozzarella, Fresh, Sainsbury's*	½ Pack/150g	291	12	194	7.5	23	8	3.4
TORTELLONI								
Arrabiata, Sainsbury's*	½ Pack/210g	407	11.8	194	7.1	28.8	5.6	2.6
Beef, & Red Wine, Sainsbury's*	½ Pack/150g	256	5.8	171	7.4	25.9	3.9	1.7
Cheese, & Smoked Ham, As Consumed, Tesco*	½ Pack/270g	535	17.3	198	8.4	25.8	6.4	1.8
Cheese, & Tomato, Cucina, Aldi*	1 Pack/250g	555	12	222	8.1	36	4.8	2
Cheese, & Tomato, Italian, Cooked, Asda*	½ Pack/209g	454	13.4	217	7.9	31	6.4	2.1
Cheese, & Tomato, Tesco*	½ Pack/195g	404	10.3	207	8.2	30	5.3	3
Chicken & Bacon, As Consumed, Italiano, Tesco*	½ Pack/280g	567	14	202	6.8	30.7	5	3.7
Chicken, & Bacon, Italian, Cooked, Morrisons*	½ Pack/210g	399	8.2	190	6.8	31	3.9	2.1
Chicken, & Mushroom, Italian, Cooked, Asda*	½ Pack/209g	427	8.6	204	7.5	33	4.1	2.3
Chicken, & Prosciutto, Buitoni*	1 Serving/109g	330	9	302	14.7	42.2	8.2	1.8
Chorizo, Smoky, Fresh, Sainsbury's*	½ Pack/203g	398	12.8	196	8.5	25.6	6.3	1.5
Ham & Cheese, Italian Cuisine, Aldi*	½ Pack/150g	340	10.2	227	9.3	31	6.8	1.6
Ham, & Cheese, Chef Select, Lidl*	1 Pack/250g	545	14.8	218	7.3	33.1	5.9	1.6
Ham, & Cheese, Cooked, Morrisons*	½ Pack/210g	389	9.5	185	7.5	27.9	4.5	1.6
Mushroom, Fresh, Sainsbury's*	1 Pack/400g	656	10.8	164	5.9	27.9	2.7	2.3
Mushroom, Porcini, & Ricotta, Chef Select, Lidl*	½ Pack/125g	278	6.8	222	11.2	31.3	5.4	1.5
Spinach, & Ricotta Cheese, Co-Op*	½ Pack/126g	315	6.3	250	10	41	5	4
Spinach, & Ricotta, Fresh, Waitrose*	½ Pack/150g	239	5.3	159	6.3	24.4	3.5	2.5
Spinach, & Ricotta, Sainsbury's*	½ Pack/150g	326	10.8	217	7.8	30.2	7.2	2.4
Spinach, & Ricotta, Chef Select, Lidl*	1 Serving/125g	288	11.9	230	9.5	24.4	9.5	4.6
Spinach, & Ricotta, Cooked, HFC, Tesco*	½ Pack/175g	326	5.8	186	6.1	31.5	3.3	3.2
Wild Mushroom, Italian, Sainsbury's*	½ Pack/150g	309	12.3	206	7.7	25.4	8.2	2.3

T

	Measure INFO/WEIGHT	per Measure KCAL	FAT	Nutrition Values per 100g / 100ml KCAL	PROT	CARB	FAT	FIBRE
TORTIGLIONI								
Beef Ragu, No.1, Waitrose*	1 Pack/373g	656	17.9	176	11.4	20.8	4.8	1.8
Dry, Average	***1 Serving/75g***	***266***	***1.4***	***355***	***12.5***	***72.2***	***1.9***	***2.1***
TORTILLA								
Chorizo, & Roasted Vegetables, Morrisons*	1 Tortilla/130g	238	15.2	183	9.1	10	11.7	1
Mozzarella, & Cherry Tomato, M&S*	¼ Serving/90g	151	9.8	168	6.6	9.7	10.9	2.5
Pockets, Old El Paso*	1 Tortilla/28g	94	3	339	9.3	50.6	10.7	1.4
Potato, & Onion, Vegan, Ready to Eat, Squeaky Bean*	½ Pack/125g	170	5.9	136	3.9	18	4.7	3.4
Red Pepper & Chorizo, Slices, Waitrose*	1 Slice/113g	180	10.3	160	10	8.6	9.2	1.6
Vegetable, Roasted, Mediterranean, M&S*	½ Pack/110g	138	5.9	125	6.9	11.1	5.4	2.3
TORTILLA CHIPS								
Chorizo & Red Pepper, M&S*	1 Serving/25g	122	5	487	5.9	68.2	20.2	4.3
Cool Flavour, BGTY, Sainsbury's*	1 Pack/22g	94	2.7	425	7.1	71.4	12.3	4.5
Cool Flavour, Sainsbury's*	1 Serving/50g	232	9.4	463	5.7	68.1	18.7	3.7
Cool Original, Snaktastic, Lidl*	1 Serving/25g	116	5.3	466	5.9	60.6	21.2	4.5
Cool, Tesco*	1 Serving/40g	202	10	505	6.1	62.6	25	2.7
Lightly Salted, M&S*	1 Serving/20g	98	4.8	490	7.2	61.5	24.1	4.5
Lightly Salted, Tesco*	1 Serving/50g	248	13.8	495	4.8	56.8	27.6	7.5
Lightly Salted, Waitrose*	1 Serving/40g	187	8.6	468	7.1	61.2	21.6	6.5
Lighty Salted, Basics, Sainsbury's*	½ Pack/50g	242	11.9	483	6.5	60.7	23.8	5.3
Lime Salsa, Tortilla Scoops, M&S*	1 Serving/30g	147	6.9	491	5.7	61.9	23.1	6.1
Nachips, Original, Old El Paso*	1 Serving/50g	250	13.4	500	6.2	56.4	26.7	4.7
Plain	***1 Serving/100g***	***486***	***21.1***	***486***	***6.8***	***62***	***21.1***	***4.2***
Rainbow, Sainsbury's*	1 Pack/20g	96	4.3	479	5.5	62.1	21.5	7.6
Turkey, & Stuffing, Free From, Tesco*	½ Pack/75g	370	16.9	494	6.2	65.2	22.5	2.9
Veggie, Lightly Salted, Co-Op*	1 Serving/33g	165	8.3	499	5.9	60	25	4.8
with Guacamole	***1 Serving/100g***	***515***	***30.8***	***515***	***6***	***53***	***30.8***	***6.3***
TREACLE								
Black, Average	***1 Tbsp/20g***	***51***	***0***	***257***	***1.2***	***67.2***	***0***	***0***
TRIFLE								
Average	***1 Serving/170g***	***272***	***10.7***	***160***	***3.6***	***22.3***	***6.3***	***0.5***
Berry, Mixed, Waitrose*	1 Pot/120g	200	13	167	2.2	15	10.8	0.7
Chocolate, Milbona, Lidl*	1 Pot/90g	202	12.8	224	4.4	19	14.2	1.1
Fruit Cocktail, Individual, M&S*	1 Pot/135g	205	9.2	150	2.7	19.3	6.7	0.7
Fruit Cocktail, Individual, Tesco*	1 Pot/113g	175	8.8	155	1.7	19.6	7.8	0.6
Fruit, Cocktail, Morrisons*	1 Pot/135g	167	7.2	124	1.7	17	5.3	0.8
Peach & Zabaglione, COU, M&S*	1 Glass/130g	150	3	115	2.8	20.6	2.3	0.8
Raspberry & Sherry, Waitrose*	1 Pot/120g	223	14.3	186	2.5	16.9	11.9	0.7
Raspberry, Large, Tesco*	¼ Pack/150g	207	10.2	138	1.8	17.1	6.8	0.6
Raspberry, Pot, Sainsbury's*	1 Pot/125g	181	7.6	145	2.1	19.9	6.1	1.3
Raspberry, Tesco*	1 Pot/145g	188	8.8	130	1.7	16.8	6.1	0.6
Strawberry Jelly, M&S*	1 Pot/135g	167	6.5	124	2.6	17.2	4.8	0.6
Strawberry, Aldi*	1/3 Trifle/153g	193	8	126	1.9	18	5.2	0.7
Strawberry, Co-Op*	1 Pot/125g	146	5.5	117	1.7	17	4.4	0.7
Strawberry, Everyday Value, Tesco*	¼ Trifle/118g	157	6.4	133	1.4	18.5	5.4	2.4
Strawberry, Individual, Morrisons*	1 Pot/135g	173	7.3	128	1.7	17.7	5.4	0.9
Strawberry, Individual, Pots, Tesco*	1 Pot/135g	174	6.1	129	1.8	20	4.5	0.6
Strawberry, Individual, Sainsbury's*	1 Pot/125g	168	8.2	134	2.1	16.2	6.6	0.6
Strawberry, Individual, Waitrose*	1 Pot/150g	206	8.6	137	1.8	19.7	5.7	1
Strawberry, Low Fat, COU, M&S*	1 Pot/140g	148	3.5	106	2.9	17.6	2.5	0.8
Strawberry, Milbona, Lidl*	1 Trifle/125g	196	11.2	157	1.9	16.8	9	0
Strawberry, Tesco*	¼ Pack/150g	213	10.8	142	1.7	17.2	7.2	0.6
TRIPE								
& Onions, Stewed	***1oz/28g***	***26***	***0.8***	***93***	***8.3***	***9.5***	***2.7***	***0.7***

T

	Measure INFO/WEIGHT	per Measure KCAL	FAT	Nutrition Values per 100g / 100ml KCAL	PROT	CARB	FAT	FIBRE
TRIPE								
Ox, Real Lancashire*	1 Serving/100g	36	0.7	36	7.2	0.1	0.7	0
TROUT								
Brown, Steamed, Average	***1 Serving/120g***	***162***	***5.4***	***135***	***23.5***	***0***	***4.5***	***0***
Fillet, Loch, Scottish, Roasted, M&S*	1 Fillet/90g	176	10.4	196	22.5	0.4	11.6	0.6
Fillets, Loch, Scottish, M&S*	1 Fillet/110g	226	13.2	205	24.2	0	12	0
Fillets, Loch, Scottish, Skin On, Aldi*	1 Fillet/95g	192	10.5	202	26	0.5	11	0.5
Fillets, with Juniper Berries, Ocean Sea, Lidl*	1 Serving/63g	87	3.5	138	22	0	5.5	0
Grilled, Weighed with Bones & Skin	***1 Serving/100g***	***98***	***3.9***	***98***	***15.7***	***0***	***3.9***	***0***
Rainbow, Grilled, Average	***1 Serving/120g***	***162***	***6.5***	***135***	***21.5***	***0***	***5.4***	***0***
Rainbow, Raw, Average	***1oz/28g***	***33***	***1.3***	***118***	***19.1***	***0***	***4.7***	***0***
Rainbow, Smoked, Average	***1 Pack/135g***	***190***	***7.6***	***140***	***21.7***	***0.8***	***5.6***	***0***
Raw, Average	***1 Serving/120g***	***159***	***6.5***	***132***	***20.6***	***0***	***5.4***	***0***
Smoked, Average	***2 Fillets/135g***	***187***	***7.1***	***138***	***22.7***	***0.3***	***5.2***	***0.1***
TUMS								
Reg, Tums*	1 Tablet/2g	2	0	125	0	25	0	0
TUNA								
Albacore, in Extra Virgin Olive Oil, Drained, Waitrose*	½ Jar/75g	194	13.1	258	25.2	0	17.5	0
Bluefin, Cooked, Dry Heat, Average	***1 Serving/100g***	***184***	***6.3***	***184***	***29.9***	***0***	***6.3***	***0***
Chilli, & Garlic, Fusions, Fishmonger, Aldi*	1 Can/80g	142	7.4	177	21	2.5	9.2	0.5
Chipotle, No Drain, Infusions, John West*	1 Pot/80g	165	8.4	206	24.4	3.3	10.5	0
Chunks, in Brine, Average, Drained	***1 Can/130g***	***141***	***0.7***	***108***	***25.9***	***0***	***0.5***	***0***
Chunks, in Brine, Drained, Average	***1 Can/130g***	***141***	***0.7***	***108***	***25.9***	***0***	***0.5***	***0***
Chunks, in Spring Water, Average, Drained	***1 Sm Can/56g***	***60***	***0.4***	***108***	***25.4***	***0***	***0.6***	***0.1***
Chunks, in Sunflower Oil, Average, Drained	***1 Can/138g***	***260***	***12.6***	***188***	***26.5***	***0***	***9.2***	***0***
Chunks, Skipjack, in Brine, Average	***1 Can/138g***	***141***	***0.8***	***102***	***24.3***	***0***	***0.6***	***0***
Flakes, in Brine, Average	***1oz/28g***	***29***	***0.2***	***104***	***24.8***	***0***	***0.6***	***0***
Flakes, in Coronation Dressing, Sainsbury's*	1 Can/80g	72	0.4	90	15	5.7	0.5	1.2
in Water, Average	***1 Serving/120g***	***126***	***1***	***105***	***24***	***0.1***	***0.8***	***0***
Jalapeno, Infusions, John West*	1 Can/80g	142	6.1	177	24.1	3	7.6	0
Lemon, & Thyme, Fusions, Drained, Fishmonger, Aldi*	1 Tin/80g	170	11.2	212	20	1.9	14	0.5
Lime & Black Pepper, John West*	1 Serving/85g	134	7	158	18	2	8.2	2.1
Soy, & Ginger, Fusions, Fishmonger, Aldi*	1 Can/80g	152	8	190	21	3.2	10	0.5
Steak, Albacore, Pan Fried, Waitrose*	1 Steak/92g	128	1.5	139	30.8	0.5	1.6	0.5
Steaks, in Brine, Average	***1 Sm Can/99g***	***106***	***0.5***	***107***	***25.6***	***0***	***0.6***	***0***
Steaks, in Olive Oil, Average	***1 Serving/111g***	***211***	***10.7***	***190***	***25.8***	***0***	***9.6***	***0***
Steaks, in Sunflower Oil, Average	***1 Can/150g***	***269***	***12.6***	***179***	***26***	***0***	***8.4***	***0***
Steaks, Raw, Average	***1 Serving/140g***	***179***	***2.7***	***128***	***27.6***	***0.1***	***1.9***	***0.2***
Steaks, Skipjack, in Brine, Average	***½ Can/75g***	***73***	***0.4***	***98***	***23.2***	***0***	***0.6***	***0***
Yellowfin, Cooked, Dry Heat, Average	***1 Serving/100g***	***139***	***1.2***	***139***	***30***	***0***	***1.2***	***0***
TURBOT								
Grilled	***1oz/28g***	***34***	***1***	***122***	***22.7***	***0***	***3.5***	***0***
Raw	***1oz/28g***	***27***	***0.8***	***95***	***17.7***	***0***	***2.7***	***0***
TURKEY								
Breast, Butter Basted, Average	***1 Serving/75g***	***110***	***3.6***	***146***	***23.7***	***1.9***	***4.9***	***0.4***
Breast, Diced, Healthy Range, Average	***1oz/28g***	***30***	***0.4***	***108***	***23.8***	***0***	***1.3***	***0***
Breast, Diced, Tikka, Tesco*	1 Serving/125g	186	4.1	149	28.8	0.6	3.3	0.7
Breast, Honey Roast, Sliced, Average	***1 Serving/50g***	***57***	***0.7***	***114***	***24***	***1.6***	***1.4***	***0.2***
Breast, Joint, Raw, Average	***1 Serving/125g***	***134***	***2.6***	***108***	***21.3***	***0.7***	***2.1***	***0.6***
Breast, Joint, Wrapped in Bacon, Iceland*	1 Serving/100g	182	8.5	182	27.9	0.3	8.5	0
Breast, Pieces, Tikka, Bernard Matthews*	1 Pack/90g	97	1.5	108	20.2	2.4	1.7	0.1
Breast, Raw, Average	***1oz/28g***	***33***	***0.6***	***117***	***24.1***	***0.5***	***2***	***0.1***
Breast, Roasted, Average	***1oz/28g***	***37***	***0.9***	***131***	***24.6***	***0.7***	***3.3***	***0.1***
Breast, Roll, Cooked, Average	***1 Slice/10g***	***9***	***0.1***	***92***	***17.6***	***3.5***	***0.8***	***0***

T

	Measure INFO/WEIGHT	per Measure KCAL	FAT	Nutrition Values per 100g / 100ml KCAL	PROT	CARB	FAT	FIBRE
TURKEY								
Breast, Slices, Cooked, Average	***1 Slice/20g***	***23***	***0.3***	***114***	***24***	***1.2***	***1.4***	***0.3***
Breast, Smoked, Sliced, Average	***1 Slice/20g***	***23***	***0.4***	***113***	***23.4***	***0.7***	***2***	***0***
Breast, Steaks, in Crumbs, Average	***1 Steak/76g***	***217***	***14.1***	***286***	***13.7***	***16.4***	***18.5***	***0.2***
Breast, Steaks, Raw, Average	***1oz/28g***	***30***	***0.3***	***107***	***24.3***	***0***	***1.1***	***0***
Breast, Strips, for Stir Fry, Average	***1 Serving/175g***	***205***	***2.7***	***117***	***25.6***	***0.1***	***1.6***	***0***
Dark Meat, Raw, Average	***1oz/28g***	***29***	***0.7***	***104***	***20.4***	***0***	***2.5***	***0***
Leg, Dark Meat, Raw , Average, Weighed with Bone	***1 Serving/100g***	***73***	***1.8***	***73***	***14.3***	***0***	***1.8***	***0***
Light Meat, Raw, Average	***1oz/28g***	***29***	***0.2***	***105***	***24.4***	***0***	***0.8***	***0***
Light Meat, Roasted	***1 Cup/140g***	***163***	***3.3***	***116***	***22.1***	***0***	***2.4***	***0***
Mince, Average	***1oz/28g***	***45***	***2***	***161***	***23.9***	***0***	***7.2***	***0***
Mince, Lean, Healthy Range, Average	***1oz/28g***	***33***	***1.1***	***118***	***20.3***	***0***	***4.1***	***0***
Rashers, Average	***1 Rasher/26g***	***26***	***0.4***	***101***	***19.1***	***2.3***	***1.6***	***0***
Rashers, Smoked, Average	***1 Serving/75g***	***76***	***1.4***	***101***	***19.8***	***1.5***	***1.8***	***0***
Roast, Meat & Skin, Average	***1oz/28g***	***48***	***1.8***	***171***	***28***	***0***	***6.5***	***0***
Roast, Meat Only, Average	***1 Serving/100g***	***157***	***3.2***	***157***	***29.9***	***0***	***3.2***	***0***
Schnitzel, Garlic & Herb, Bernard Matthews*	1 Serving/130g	354	15.7	272	17.5	22.6	12.1	1.3
Smoked, Applewood, 1, Waitrose*	½ Pack/40g	48	0.4	121	27.3	0.5	1.1	0.1
Strips, Stir-Fried, Average	***1oz/28g***	***46***	***1.3***	***164***	***31***	***0***	***4.5***	***0***
Thigh, Diced, Average	***1oz/28g***	***33***	***1.2***	***117***	***19.6***	***0***	***4.3***	***0***
Wafer Thin, Honey Roast, Average	***1 Slice/10g***	***11***	***0.2***	***109***	***19.2***	***4.2***	***1.7***	***0.2***
TURKEY DINNER								
& Ham, Irish Classics, Tesco*	1 Pack/500g	481	12.5	96	7.3	10.4	2.5	1.6
Roast, Asda*	1 Pack/400g	344	6.4	86	7	11	1.6	2
Roast, Meal for One, M&S*	1 Pack/435g	492	17.8	113	8.1	9.6	4.1	2.4
Roast, Sainsbury's*	1 Pack/450g	354	9	79	6.8	8.4	2	1.9
TURKEY HAM								
Average	***1 Serving/75g***	***81***	***2.9***	***108***	***15.6***	***2.8***	***3.9***	***0***
TURKISH DELIGHT								
Fry's*	1 Bar/51g	185	3.4	363	1.2	74	6.7	1.2
Milk Chocolate, M&S*	1 Pack/55g	220	4.7	400	1.6	79	8.5	0
Rose, & Lemon, Sainsbury's*	2 Pieces/34g	117	0.2	343	0.5	85.5	0.5	0.5
TURMERIC								
Powder	***1 Tsp/3g***	***11***	***0.3***	***354***	***7.8***	***58.2***	***9.9***	***0***
TURNIP								
Boiled, Average	***1oz/28g***	***3***	***0.1***	***12***	***0.6***	***2***	***0.2***	***1.9***
Raw, Unprepared, Average	***1oz/28g***	***5***	***0.1***	***17***	***0.7***	***3.5***	***0.2***	***1.8***
TURNOVER								
Apple, Bramley & Cream, Sainsbury's*	1 Turnover/78g	243	13.6	312	3.9	34.3	17.4	1.3
Apple, Bramley, & Cream, Waitrose*	1 Turnover/82g	254	15	309	4.1	31	18.3	2.3
Apple, Co-Op*	1 Turnover/77g	308	20.8	400	4	35	27	1
Apple, Puff Pastry, Bakery, Tesco*	1 Turnover/83g	263	13	317	4.3	38.6	15.7	1.8
Raspberry, Fresh Cream, Asda*	1 Turnover/100g	411	23	411	6	45	23	2.1
Raspberry, Fresh Cream, Tesco*	1 Turnover/74g	244	15.6	330	4.4	29.9	21.1	1.6
Raspberry, with Cream, Sainsbury's*	1 Turnover/65g	222	13.1	342	4.5	34.7	20.2	1.7
TWIGLETS								
Original, Jacob's*	1 Sm Bag/25g	104	3	414	13.3	57.3	12	11.5
TWIRL								
Cadbury*	1 Finger/22g	118	6.8	535	7.6	56	30.9	0.8
Treat Size, Cadbury*	1 Bar/21g	115	6.6	535	7.6	56	30.9	0.8
TWIX								
'Xtra, Mars*	1 Pack/85g	416	20.1	490	4.7	65.5	23.7	1.5
Fun Size, Mars*	1 Bar/20g	99	4.8	495	4.5	64.6	24	1.5
Salted Caramel, Mars*	1 Bar/23g	113	5.5	491	4.3	65	24	0

	Measure INFO/WEIGHT	per Measure KCAL	FAT	Nutrition Values per 100g / 100ml KCAL	PROT	CARB	FAT	FIBRE
TWIX								
Standard, Mars*	1 Pack/58g	284	13.7	490	4.7	65.5	23.7	1.5
Top, Mars*	1 Bar/28g	143	7.8	511	5.2	60.2	27.7	0
White, Fingers, Mars*	1 Bar/23g	115	5.8	502	4.8	64	25	0
White, Mars*	1 Pack/46g	231	11.5	502	4.8	64	25	0
TZATZIKI								
Average	***1 Tbsp/15g***	***11***	***0.8***	***76***	***3.4***	***3.4***	***5.5***	***0.2***

T

	Measure INFO/WEIGHT	per Measure KCAL	FAT	Nutrition Values per 100g / 100ml KCAL	PROT	CARB	FAT	FIBRE
VANILLA EXTRACT								
Average	***1 Tbsp/13g***	***37***	***0***	***288***	***0.1***	***12.6***	***0.1***	***0***
VEAL								
Chop, Loin, Raw, Weighed with Bone, Average	***1 Chop/195g***	***317***	***17.8***	***163***	***18.9***	***0***	***9.1***	***0***
Escalope, Fried, Average	***1oz/28g***	***55***	***1.9***	***196***	***33.7***	***0***	***6.8***	***0***
Mince, Raw, Average	***1oz/28g***	***40***	***2***	***144***	***20.3***	***0***	***7***	***0***
Shoulder, Lean Only, Roasted, Average	***1oz/28g***	***35***	***1.3***	***125***	***19.9***	***0***	***4.4***	***0***
Sirloin, Lean & Fat, Roasted, Average	***1oz/28g***	***43***	***2.2***	***152***	***18.9***	***0***	***7.8***	***0***
Sirloin, Lean Only, Roasted, Average	***1oz/28g***	***33***	***1.2***	***118***	***18.4***	***0***	***4.4***	***0***
Steak, Osso Bucco, Rose, M&S*	1 Steak/250g	262	5.7	105	21	0.1	2.3	0
VEGAN								
Festive Wreath, Plant Kitchen, M&S*	¼ Pack/180g	432	29.9	240	7.1	10.9	16.6	9.1
Fillets, Quorn*	1 Fillet/63g	58	0.4	92	14.2	3.5	0.6	7.8
Mexican, Ready Meal, Lazy Vegan*	1 Pack/350g	434	15	124	7.7	12	4.3	3.3
Pieces, Vegan, Quorn*	¼ Pack/70g	79	2	113	15.3	3.9	2.8	5.3
Seitan Pieces, Ginger & Soy Marinated, Biona Organic*	1 Serving/100g	92	0.4	92	18.3	3.9	0.4	0.3
Seitan, Original, Alberts*	1 Slice/66g	92	0.5	139	26.6	6	0.7	0
Steak, Plant Pioneers, Sainsbury's*	1 Steak/101g	171	5.8	170	13.8	13.1	5.8	4.9
Veggie, Balls, Waitrose*	4 Balls/80g	118	3.9	148	8.5	15.1	4.9	5.3
VEGEMITE								
Australian, Kraft*	1 Tsp/5g	9	0	173	23.5	19.7	0	0
VEGETABLE CHIPS								
Cassava, Average	***1oz/28g***	***99***	***0.1***	***353***	***1.8***	***91.4***	***0.4***	***4***
Oven Cooked, Aunt Bessie's*	1 Serving/125g	205	11.9	164	2.2	14	9.5	5.8
VEGETABLE FINGERS								
Crispy, Birds Eye*	2 Fingers/60g	107	4.8	179	3.2	23.5	8	2.3
Crispy, Gro, Co-Op*	1 Finger/28g	57	2.3	202	3.9	26	8.3	3.2
Sainsbury's*	3 Fingers/79g	191	8.4	243	4.6	30	10.7	4.1
Tesco*	1 Finger/25g	52	2.2	206	4.1	26.4	8.6	3.3
VEGETABLE MEDLEY								
Broccoli, Carrot, & Brussel Sprout, Nature's Pick, Aldi*	1 Serving/80g	27	0.8	34	2.3	4	1	2.5
Broccoli, Carrot, Babycorn, & Sugar Snap, Aldi*	1 Serving/100g	31	0.5	31	2.1	3.6	0.5	2.2
Broccoli, Cauliflower, & Carrot, Chef's Larder*	1 Serving/80g	22	0	28	1.8	3.5	0	1.8
Broccoli, Romanesco, Peas, & Spinach, Birds Eye*	1 Bag/150g	76	0.8	51	4	5.4	0.5	4.3
Buttery, Asda*	½ Pack/143g	86	4.1	60	2.3	4.5	2.9	3.2
Chargrilled, Waitrose*	1 Serving/100g	77	3	77	2.5	8.3	3	3.3
Colourful, Waitrose*	½ Pack/171g	60	0.9	35	1.9	5.1	0.5	1.6
Country Mix, As Sold, Morrisons*	1 Serving/80g	30	0.1	37	2.5	4.7	0.1	3.5
Five, Tesco*	¼ Pack/115g	45	0.6	39	1.9	5.1	0.5	3.4
Floret, & Carrot, Mix, Boiled, Iceland*	1 Serving/80g	9	0.2	11	0.7	1.4	0.2	0.8
Four Seasons, Aldi*	1 Serving/80g	38	0.7	48	3.1	5.6	0.9	2.6
Frozen, M&S*	1 Pack/500g	175	4	35	3.4	3.9	0.8	3.1
Green Grocers, Lidl*	1 Serving/80g	22	0.4	28	1.6	2.8	0.5	2.7
Green, Frozen, Morrisons*	1 Serving/80g	45	1	56	4.6	4.9	1.2	3.5
Green, Microwaved, Extra Special, Asda*	½ Pack/74g	53	3.1	72	3.1	2.8	4.2	5.1
Green, with Bouillon Butter, Co-Op*	1 Serving/80g	54	2.4	67	3.5	4.8	3	3.2
Grilled, Essential, Waitrose*	1 Serving/81g	38	0.2	47	1.8	8.1	0.3	2.4
Hearty Farmhouse Mix, SteamFresh, Birds Eye*	1 Bag/135g	46	0.8	34	1.8	4.2	0.6	2.5
Mange Tout, Corn, Broccoli, Spring Onion, Chilli, Tesco*	½ Pack/110g	38	0.3	35	2.7	4.4	0.3	2.1
Medley, Tender, Green, Sainsbury's*	1 Pack/160g	62	0.8	39	2.9	4.3	0.5	3.6
Mixed, Tesco*	½ Pack/112g	46	0.6	41	2.3	4.9	0.5	3.8
Potatoes, Green Beans, & Peas, with Dressing, Tesco*	½ Pack/175g	156	2.8	89	2.7	14.9	1.6	2.4
Roasted, Waitrose*	½ Pack/200g	282	15.6	141	1.2	16.4	7.8	3.7
Runner Bean, & Mixed Veg Selection, M&S*	½ Pouch/100g	36	0.5	36	2.9	3.1	0.5	3.6

V

	Measure INFO/WEIGHT	per Measure KCAL	FAT	Nutrition Values per 100g / 100ml KCAL	PROT	CARB	FAT	FIBRE
VEGETABLES								
& Bean, Stew Mix, Cooks' Ingredients, Waitrose*	½ Pack/200g	166	3.8	83	4.2	10.2	1.9	4.3
Balls, Mushroom, & Lentil, Vegetarian, Tesco*	½ Pack/131g	173	4.5	132	7.2	15	3.4	6.4
Carrots, & Peas, Chilled, Fresh Tastes, Asda*	1 Serving/200g	76	0.8	38	2.4	4.8	0.4	2.9
Casserole, Cooks' Ingredients, Waitrose*	¼ Pack/138g	48	0.4	35	0.9	6	0.3	2.5
Collard Greens, Raw, Average*	1 Serving/80g	26	0.5	32	3	5	0.6	4
Crudites, & Beetroot Dip, Aldi*	1 Pack/110g	59	2.8	54	1.3	6	2.5	1.3
Green, Petit Pois & Beans, Parsley, Mint & Butter, Tesco*	½ Pack/129g	106	6.6	82	3.4	2.6	5.1	6.1
Grilled, Frozen, Sainsbury's*	1 Serving/80g	42	2.9	52	1.2	3.8	3.6	1.5
Indian Spiced, HL, Tesco*	1 Pack/347g	267	5.5	77	3	11.5	1.6	2.7
Layered, Super Green, with Minted Butter, M&S*	1 Serving/80g	51	2.2	64	3.6	4.4	2.7	3.6
Layered, with Butter, Waitrose*	1 Pack/280g	207	16.2	74	1.7	3.6	5.8	2.4
Mashed Carrot & Swede, Frozen, As Sold, Aunt Bessie's*	1 Serving/125g	61	2.5	49	0.5	5.7	2	2.9
Mediterranean Style, Roast, Nature's Pick, Aldi*	½ Pack/200g	114	6.4	57	1.2	5.2	3.2	1.5
Mediterranean, Chunky, Cooked, Sainsbury's*	¼ Pack/119g	56	2	47	1.1	5.9	1.7	2
Mediterranean, Frozen, Netto*	1 Serving/80g	90	3.8	113	3.2	10.4	4.7	8.3
Mediterranean, Roasting, Waitrose*	½ Pack/200g	96	4.6	48	1.4	4.9	2.3	1.4
Mediterranean, Roasting, with Dressing, M&S*	¼ Pack/165g	58	1.5	35	1	4.7	0.9	2.1
Pea, & Leeks, Cook*	1 Serving/145g	149	9.9	103	3.5	9.7	6.8	0
Peas, Spinach, Spring Greens, & Samphire, M&S*	½ Pack/105g	85	4.4	81	3.8	4.7	4.2	4.6
Pepper, Red, & Carrot, Mash, Smoky, M&S*	1 Pack/300g	162	9.3	54	0.5	4.4	3.1	3.2
Peppers, Mixed, Stir Fry, Tesco*	1 Pack/320g	173	9	54	1.6	4.4	2.8	2.4
Rice, Cauliflower, Broccoli, Squash, & Carrot, Asda *	½ Pack/150g	45	0.8	30	1.6	4.6	0.5	1.5
Roasted, in Herb, & Honey Glaze, Farmfoods*	1 Serving/100g	65	1.9	65	1.2	9.3	1.9	0
Roasted, Italian, M&S*	1 Serving/95g	218	20	230	1.8	7.1	21	1.7
Roasted, Summer, Tesco*	1 Serving/80g	46	1.7	58	1.5	7.5	2.1	1.6
Roasting, Rustic, Chunky, Oven Baked, Iceland*	1/16 Pack/68g	77	3.2	113	1.5	13.4	4.7	5.5
Roasting, with Rosemary, & Thyme, Tesco*	1 Serving/100g	119	3.1	119	1.3	18	3.1	7
Root, for Mashing, Eat Fresh, Tesco*	1 Pack/720g	238	2.9	33	0.7	5.4	0.4	2.7
Root, for Roasting, Frozen, M&S*	1 Serving/150g	135	8.8	90	1	6.7	5.9	3.1
Root, Mashed, Microwaved, Growers Selection, Asda*	½ Pack/200g	116	4.4	58	0.7	7.2	2.2	2.7
Root, Parmentier, Cooked, Sainsbury's*	½ Pack/117g	122	3.7	104	1.6	15.5	3.2	3.4
Root, Rainbow, Collection, M&S*	½ Pack/176g	67	2.5	38	0.7	3.9	1.4	3.6
Root, Roasted, Extra Special, Asda*	½ Pack/205g	160	3.1	78	1.1	15	1.5	6
Root, Roasted, Ready to Roast, Mash Direct*	1 Pack/350g	200	7.4	57	0.8	5.8	2.1	5.9
Salsifis, Canned, Notre Jardin*	1 Can/400g	124	0.8	31	1.3	4.7	0.2	2.7
Selection, Lightly Buttered & Seasoned, M&S*	½ Pack/150g	122	7.5	81	1.5	6.2	5	2.6
Selection, Roasted, COU, M&S*	1 Pack/250g	88	2	35	1.2	6.1	0.8	0.6
Shredded Leaf, Steamers, Waitrose*	1 Bag/160g	43	0.8	27	2.3	2.5	0.5	2.8
Soup Mix, Winter, Sainsbury's*	1 Serving/149g	61	0.3	41	1.1	7.9	0.2	1.7
Spicy, & Rice, Plant Chef, Tesco*	1 Pack/344g	365	10.3	106	2.3	16.1	3	2.8
Stir Fry, Frozen, Sainsbury's*	1 Serving/80g	19	0.2	24	1.3	3.9	0.3	2
Stir Fry, Hot, & Spicy, Natures Pick, Aldi*	1 Serving/100g	37	0.5	37	1.6	5.3	0.5	2.3
Stir Fry, Oriental, Nature's Pick, Aldi*	1 Pack/300g	123	1.5	41	1.8	6.8	0.5	2
Stir Fry, Oriental, Oaklands*	1 Pack/300g	60	1.5	20	1.1	3	0.5	1.8
Stir Fry, Tesco*	1 Serving/150g	38	0.2	25	0.9	5	0.1	1.4
Swede, & Carrot, Cubed, Ready to Cook, M&S*	¼ Pack/120g	40	0.5	33	0.7	5.4	0.4	2.7
Tempura, Nests, Specially Selected, Aldi*	2 Nests/62g	153	6.2	246	3.4	33	10	3.4
Thai Style, Frozen, Four Seasons, Aldi*	1 Serving/100g	57	2.2	57	1.9	6.1	2.2	2.4
VEGETABLES MIXED								
Asian, Cooks' Ingredients, Waitrose*	¼ Pack/100g	42	0.5	42	1.8	7.2	0.5	2
Asian, Wok, Frozen, Iglo Foods Group*	1 Serving/150g	45	0.8	30	1.4	4.1	0.5	1.9
Baby Corn, & Vegetable Selection, Eat Well, M&S*	½ Pack/100g	38	0.5	38	2.3	4.5	0.5	3.3
Broccoli, Peas & Green Beans, Mixed, Co-Op*	1 Serving/80g	36	0.3	45	4.8	3.8	0.4	3.6

	Measure INFO/WEIGHT	per Measure KCAL	FAT	Nutrition Values per 100g / 100ml KCAL	PROT	CARB	FAT	FIBRE
VEGETABLES MIXED								
Bruschetta Topping, Tesco*	¼ Jar/48g	97	8.5	201	2	7.2	17.6	3
Buttergemuse, Freshona, Lidl*	1 Serving/152g	147	8	97	2.7	7.8	5.3	0
Carrot, Broccoli & Sweetcorn, Steam Bags, Sainsbury's*	1 Bag/131g	68	1.6	52	2.1	7.5	1.2	1.8
Carrot, Broccoli, & Sweetcorn, Iceland*	1 Pack/300g	150	3	50	2.5	6.1	1	3.6
Carrot, Cauliflower & Broccoli, Mixed, Waitrose*	1 Serving/80g	32	0.5	40	2.4	4.9	0.6	2.9
Carrot, Cauliflower & Broccoli, Prepared, Mixed, Co-Op*	1 Pack/250g	100	1.5	40	2.4	5	0.6	2.7
Carrot, Cauliflower, & Broccoli, Fresh, Mixed, Tesco*	1 Serving/80g	26	0.2	32	2.6	3.9	0.2	2.8
Carrot, Cauliflower, & Broccoli, Meadow Fresh, Lidl*	1 Serving/80g	213	2.7	266	13.3	38	3.3	14
Carrots, Peas, Cauliflower, & Broccoli, Frozen, Tesco*	1 Serving/80g	36	0.6	45	2.4	5.4	0.8	3.1
Carrots, Peas, Green Beans & Sweetcorn, Mixed, Tesco*	1 Serving/80g	47	0.8	58	3.3	6.9	1	4.3
Casserole with Baby Potatoes, Fresh, Mixed, M&S*	½ Pack/350g	140	1	40	1.2	7.8	0.3	2.1
Casserole, Mixed, Tesco*	1 Serving/80g	35	0.2	44	1	7.9	0.3	2.6
Casserole, Nature's Pick, Aldi*	¼ Pack/150g	62	0.8	41	1.1	7.8	0.5	2
Chargrilled, Frozen, as Consumed, Morrisons*	1 Serving/80g	34	0.9	42	1.2	5.5	1.1	2.6
Chinese, Wok, with Edamame, Jumbo*	¼ Pack/100g	37	0.7	37	2.5	4.1	0.7	2.1
Coleslaw, Crunchy, Kit, Morrisons*	½ Pack/150g	217	2.1	145	0.7	2	1.4	3.6
Fajita, Ready to Cook, Tesco*	½ Pack/139g	82	2.4	59	1.1	8.5	1.7	2.4
Farmhouse, Mixed, Frozen, Boiled in Salted Water, Tesco*	1 Serving/80g	41	0.7	51	3.2	5.7	0.9	3.5
Fine Cut, Steamers, Waitrose*	1 Pouch/160g	77	1	48	3.2	5.5	0.6	4.1
Frozen, Organic, Duchy, Waitrose*	1 Serving/80g	41	0.7	51	3	6	0.9	3.6
Greens, & Corn, Mixed, Steam Bags, Tesco*	1 Bag/160g	90	1.9	56	3.9	5.4	1.2	4
Italian Style, Seasoned, Frozen, Freshona, Lidl*	¼ Pack/188g	90	5.6	48	1.6	2.8	3	1.9
Mediterranean, & Potatoes, Morrisons*	1 Serving/125g	176	7.1	141	2.3	18.1	5.7	4
Mediterranean, Chargrilled, Frozen, Sainsbury's*	1 Serving/80g	73	4.3	91	1.5	8	5.3	2.7
Mediterranean, Oven Baked, Asda*	½ Pack/200g	126	7	63	0.7	6.2	3.5	1.7
Mediterranean, Roasting, Cooked, Tesco*	½ Pack/200g	56	0.4	28	1	5.2	0.2	0.9
Mediterranean, Slimming World*	1 Pack/320g	106	0.3	33	1.9	5.2	0.1	1.5
Mediterranean, Tray, Oven Baked, Asda*	½ Pack/133g	57	1.5	43	1.4	6	1.1	1.4
Microwave Bags, Co-Op*	1 Bag/160g	87	1.6	54	2.7	7.5	1	2.2
Mix, Steamer, Love Life, Waitrose*	1 Bag/160g	83	1.8	52	2.8	7.7	1.1	2.8
Mixed, Baby, Steam, Fresh, Tesco*	1 Pack/160g	72	1.3	45	2.7	6.7	0.8	3.8
Mixed, Bag, M&S*	1 Serving/200g	70	0.4	35	2.9	5.6	0.2	0
Mixed, Freshly Frozen, Asda*	1 Serving/80g	42	0.6	52	3.2	8	0.8	3
Mixed, Freshly Frozen, Iceland*	1 Serving/100g	54	0.8	54	3.3	8.3	0.8	3.7
Mixed, Frozen, Cooked, Sainsbury's*	1 Serving/80g	45	0.6	56	2.9	7.5	0.7	4
Mixed, Layered, Classics, M&S*	½ Pack/160g	112	6.2	70	1.2	7.3	3.9	1.2
Mixed, Roast, Four Seasons*	1 Serving/187g	79	0.4	42	1.2	8.8	0.2	0
Mixed, Special, Sainsbury's*	1 Serving/120g	68	1.2	57	3.2	8.9	1	2.9
Peas & Carrots, Buttery & Tender, Mixed, Tesco*	½ Pack/150g	138	6.1	92	3.7	7.9	4.1	4.5
Peas, Cabbage, & Tenderstem, Layers, Waitrose*	1/3 Pack/83g	85	4.2	103	6.2	6.2	5	4
Peas, Carrots, & Sweetcorn, Pepper & Butter, Tesco*	½ Pack/178g	128	4.4	72	2.8	7.6	2.5	3.9
Peas, Courgette, & Spring Greens Selection, Tesco*	½ Pack/122g	78	3.7	64	3.4	3.3	3	5.1
Pickled, Drained, Cypressa*	1 Serving/100g	13	0.6	13	0.5	0	0.6	2
Roasting Tray, Quick Cook, Tesco*	½ Pack/200g	144	5	72	2.5	8.6	2.5	2.5
Roasting, in Herb, & Honey Glaze, Farmfoods*	1 Serving/80g	52	1.5	65	1.2	9.3	1.9	0
Roasting, Selection, Sweet & Colourful, Waitrose*	½ Pack/300g	147	3	49	1	7.5	1	2.8
Root, Diced, Tesco*	1/3 Pack/240g	120	0.7	50	0.6	9.3	0.3	3.6
Soup, Chopped, The Greengrocers*	1 Bag/350g	98	1.8	28	1.4	3.3	0.5	2.4
Stew Pack, Slow cooker, Raw, Market St, Morrisons*	1/6 Pack/167g	90	0.5	54	1.3	10.4	0.3	2.3
Stir Fry, Peppers, Mixed, Nature's Pick, Aldi*	1 Serving/80g	27	0.4	34	1.7	5	0.5	1.8
Tenderstem, & Mixed Vegetables, Tesco*	½ Pack/80g	54	0.6	34	2.1	4.2	0.4	2.6
Winter Greens, Raw, Morrisons*	1/3 Pack/100g	22	0.4	22	1.5	2.1	0.4	2.1
Winter, Maple Roasted, Waitrose*	½ Pack/168g	294	11.3	175	2.1	24.1	6.7	5.1

V

	Measure INFO/WEIGHT	per Measure KCAL	FAT	Nutrition Values per 100g / 100ml KCAL	PROT	CARB	FAT	FIBRE
VEGETARIAN								
Chunks, Pulled, Pea Protein, Vegini*	1 Pack/140g	308	14	220	26	4.2	10	4.5
Galette, Vegetale, le Bistrot, Sojasun*	1 Galette/90g	189	8	210	17	13	8.9	5
Roast, Nut & Date, with Gravy, Asda*	1 Serving/196g	300	12.7	153	4.7	16.1	6.5	5.5
Schnitzel, Breaded, Tivall*	1 Schnitzel/100g	202	9.5	202	16	11	9.5	4
Schnitzel, Cheese, Jumbo Lekker Veggie*	1 Schnitzel/100g	229	10.2	229	10.1	23.9	10.2	0.7
Slices, Sage & Onion, VBites Foods Ltd*	1 Slice/10g	23	1.4	234	21.3	5.2	14.1	0.6
Slices, Sage & Onion, Vegi Deli, The Redwood Co*	1 Slice/10g	23	1.4	233	21.4	5	14.1	0.5
Steak, Beef Style, Quorn*	1 Steak/86g	126	4.5	146	16	5.3	5.2	6.9
Steak, Soya, & Wheat, Barbecue, Cereal*	1 Veg Steak/80g	160	7.7	200	19	6.3	9.6	6.2
Steak, Vivera*	1 Steak/100g	195	10	195	18	6.3	10	4.6
Strips, BBQ, Quorn*	½ Pack/140g	183	4.1	131	14.3	8.4	2.9	6.8
Strips, Sweet, & Smoky, Quorn*	3 Strips/92g	171	3.3	186	10.6	25.1	3.6	5.5
VEGETARIAN MINCE								
Beefless, Alt*	¼ Pack/90g	140	3.9	156	24	2.1	4.4	5.6
Cooked, Meat Free, Tesco*	¼ Pack/113g	112	0.9	99	15.1	5.8	0.8	4
Hack, Incredible, Garden Gourmet*	½ Pack/100g	165	7.9	165	17.2	3.6	7.9	5
Meat Free, As Sold, The Meatless Farm Co*	1 Pack/400g	796	40.8	199	19.3	7.8	10.2	4.9
Meat Free, Improved Recipe, Frozen Sainsbury's*	1 Serving/77g	131	3.9	170	18.6	11.7	5	2
Meat Free, Plant Chef, Tesco*	¼ Pack/91g	236	12.4	259	20.7	10.7	13.6	5.7
Mushroom, Meat Free, Bolognese, Aldi*	½ Pack/85g	56	3.7	66	2.5	3.3	4.4	1.6
No Meat, Plant Kitchen, M&S*	½ Pack/90g	110	2.9	122	16.1	4.3	3.2	5.7
Plant Based, 100%, Naturli*	¼ Pack/100g	210	11	210	18	9.6	11	3.2
Plant Based, Without Meat, Lidl*	½ Pack/138g	308	19.9	224	17.9	4.8	14.5	3.7
Savoury, Soya Protein, Neal's Yard*	1 Serving/100g	342	1	342	50	39	1	5
Simply, Garden Gourmet*	1 Serving/80g	119	2.4	149	19.3	6.9	3	8.8
Sunflower, Organic, Dry, Just Wholefoods*	1 Serving/18g	55	0.4	305	51	9	2	20
Vegan, Meat Free, Ocado*	¼ Pack/128g	115	0.6	90	15	3.7	0.5	5.8
Vegan, Plant, Vivera*	1 Pack/220g	277	1.3	126	20	7.2	0.6	5.8
Vegemince, Realeat*	1 Serving/125g	218	12.5	174	18	3	10	3
Vegetarian, Mince, Frozen & Chilled, Quorn*	1 Serving/87g	91	1.7	105	14.5	4.5	2	5.5
VENISON								
Grill Steak, Average	***1 Steak/150g***	***178***	***3.8***	***119***	***19***	***5***	***2.5***	***1***
in Red Wine & Port, Average	***1oz/28g***	***21***	***0.7***	***76***	***9.8***	***3.5***	***2.6***	***0.4***
Minced, Cooked, Average	***1 Serving/100g***	***187***	***8.2***	***187***	***26.4***	***0***	***8.2***	***0***
Minced, Raw, Average	***1 Serving/100g***	***157***	***7.1***	***157***	***21.8***	***0***	***7.1***	***0***
Raw, Haunch, Meat Only, Average	***1 Serving/100g***	***103***	***1.6***	***103***	***22.2***	***0***	***1.6***	***0***
Roasted, Average	***1oz/28g***	***46***	***0.7***	***165***	***35.6***	***0***	***2.5***	***0***
Steak, Raw, Average	***1oz/28g***	***30***	***0.5***	***108***	***22.8***	***0***	***1.9***	***0***
VERMICELLI								
Dry	***1oz/28g***	***99***	***0.1***	***355***	***8.7***	***78.3***	***0.4***	***0***
Egg, Cooked, Average	***1 Serving/185g***	***239***	***2.6***	***129***	***5***	***24***	***1.4***	***1***
VERMOUTH								
Alcohol Free, Versin*	1 Serve/50ml	32	0	64	0	16	0	0
Dry	***1 Shot/50ml***	***54***	***0***	***109***	***0.1***	***3***	***0***	***0***
Sweet	***1 Shot/50ml***	***76***	***0***	***151***	***0***	***15.9***	***0***	***0***
VIMTO*								
Cordial, No Added Sugar, Undiluted, Vimto*	1 Serving/50ml	2	0	4	0	0.7	0	0
Grape, Blackcurrant & Raspberry Drink, Fizzy, Vimto*	1 Can/330ml	147	0	44	0	11	0	0
Mango, Strawberry & Pineapple, Remix, Diluted, Vimto*	1 Serving/200ml	4	0	2	0	0.2	0	0
Raspberry, Orange & Passionfruit, Remix, Diluted, Vimto*	1 Serving/200ml	4	0	2	0	0.2	0	0
VINAIGRETTE								
Balsamic Vinegar & Pistachio, Finest, Tesco*	1 Tbsp/15ml	56	5.9	370	0.2	2.8	39.2	0
Balsamic, Hellmann's*	1 Tbsp/15ml	12	0.4	82	0.1	9.6	2.7	0.6

	Measure INFO/WEIGHT	per Measure KCAL	FAT	Nutrition Values per 100g / 100ml KCAL	PROT	CARB	FAT	FIBRE
VINAIGRETTE								
Balsamic, Specially Selected, Aldi*	1 Tbsp/15ml	44	3.9	293	0.5	15	26	0.5
Classic, Mellow Yellow, Farrington's*	1 Tbsp/15ml	92	9.9	614	1.1	3.9	66.1	0
Fat Free, Hellmann's*	1 Tbsp/15ml	8	0.1	48	0.5	11	0.5	0
French Style, Finest, Tesco*	1 Tbsp/15ml	93	9.8	620	0.6	6.3	65.3	0.2
Garlic, & Chives, Fat Free, Hellmann's*	1 Tbsp/15ml	5	0.1	36	0.5	7.7	0.5	0
Light, Dressing, Asda*	1 Tbsp/15ml	6	0.1	38	0.5	7.2	0.6	1.7
Olive Oil & Lemon, Amoy*	1 Tbsp/15ml	38	3.6	250	0.3	3	24	0
PB, Waitrose*	1 Tbsp/15ml	13	0.1	89	0.4	20.9	0.4	0.5
Rhubarb, & Vinegar, The Little Herb Farm*	1 Tbsp/15ml	21	0	139	0.3	33.9	0	0.5
VINDALOO								
Chicken, Average	***1 Serving/410g***	***787***	***51.2***	***192***	***18.5***	***2.6***	***12.5***	***0.3***
Volcanic, Takeaway, Morrisons*	½ Pack/175g	205	9.8	117	10.7	5.1	5.6	2
VINE LEAVES								
Stuffed with Rice	***1oz/28g***	***73***	***5***	***262***	***2.8***	***23.8***	***18***	***0***
VINEGAR								
Apple Cider, Garden Of England*	1 Tbsp/15ml	1	0	8	0.1	1.8	0.1	0.1
Apple Cider, Raw & Unpasteurised, Willy's*	1 Serving/25ml	7	0	29	0	3.2	0	0
Apple Cyder, with Honey, Aspall*	1 Servingl/30ml	46	0.1	154	0.2	35	0.3	0
Balsamic, Average	***1 Tsp/5ml***	***6***	***0***	***115***	***0.9***	***26***	***0***	***0***
Balsamic, with Garilc, Heinz*	1 Serving/15ml	12	0.6	82	0.4	10.3	4.3	0
Cider	***1 Tbsp/15ml***	***2***	***0***	***14***	***0***	***5.9***	***0***	***0***
Cider, Apple, Organic, with Mother, Natural Umber*	1 Serving/15ml	20	0	133	0.7	31.9	0	0.5
Malt, Average	***1 Tbsp/15g***	***1***	***0***	***4***	***0.4***	***0.6***	***0***	***0***
Red Wine, Average	***1 Tbsp/15ml***	***3***	***0***	***19***	***0***	***0.3***	***0***	***0***
VODKA								
& Diet Coke, Average	***1 Serving/150ml***	***68***	***0***	***45***	***0***	***0***	***0***	***0***
& Tonic, Ready Mixed, M&S*	1 Can/250ml	202	0	81	0	6.3	0	0
37.5% Volume	***1 Pub Shot/35ml***	***72***	***0***	***207***	***0***	***0***	***0***	***0***
40% Volume	***1 Pub Shot/35ml***	***78***	***0***	***222***	***0***	***0***	***0***	***0***
Cookies & Cream, Sidekick, Halewood International Ltd*	1 Serving/30ml	48	0.5	160	0.3	7.7	1.6	0
Rhubarb, Average	***1 Single/25ml***	***57***	***0***	***229***	***0***	***0***	***0***	***0***
Smirnoff & Cranberry, Premixed, Canned, Diageo*	1 Can/250ml	175	0	70	0	8.5	0	0
Smirnoff & Diet Cola, Premixed, Canned, Diageo*	1 Can/250ml	100	0	40	0	0	0	0
Smirnoff & Schweppes Tonic, Premixed, Canned, Diageo*	1 Can/250ml	158	0	63	0	6.4	0	0
VOL AU VENTS								
Deluxe, Lidl*	1 Pastry/7g	40	2.8	567	7.8	41.5	40.7	1.5
Mushroom, Sainsbury's*	1 Serving/14g	49	3.1	350	6.9	30.8	22.1	1.4
Seafood, Party, Youngs*	1 Serving/17g	60	4.2	354	8.3	26	24.8	1

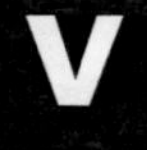

	Measure INFO/WEIGHT	per Measure KCAL	FAT	Nutrition Values per 100g / 100ml KCAL	PROT	CARB	FAT	FIBRE
WAFERS								
Banana, Kiddylicious*	1 Pack/4g	16	0	397	5.3	91.5	0.8	1.1
Caramel, Dark Chocolate, Tunnock's*	1 Wafer/30g	148	7.6	492	5.2	60.7	25.4	0
Caramel, Log, Tunnock's*	1 Wafer/32g	150	6.7	468	4.2	65.7	21	3.4
Caramel, Tunnock's*	1 Wafer/30g	134	5.2	448	3.6	69.2	17.4	2.5
Chocolate, Sugar Free, Gullon*	1 Wafer/9g	39	2	434	4.4	68	22	3.4
for Ice Cream, Askeys*	1 Wafer/2g	6	0	388	11.4	79	2.9	0
Hazelnut, Milky, Slices, Sondey, Lidl*	1 Slice/25g	135	8.3	539	6.3	52	33	3.7
Ice Cream, Jacob's*	1 Pack/15g	60	0.5	402	10.7	80.1	3.5	3.4
Rolls, Double Chocolate, Thorntons*	3 Rolls/18g	92	4.6	511	6.3	62.3	25.8	2.5
Timeout, Cadbury*	1 Bar/21g	111	6	524	6.7	60	28.3	2.1
WAFFLES								
Belgian, Sugar, Aldi*	1 Waffle/55g	249	12.6	452	5.7	54	23	2
Belgian, TTD, Sainsbury's*	1 Waffle/25g	122	7.3	490	6	50.6	29.3	1.2
Caramel, Asda*	1 Waffle/8g	37	1.8	459	3.3	62	22	1.1
Caramel, M&S*	1 Waffle/33g	154	6.2	473	3.3	71.7	18.9	1.2
Classic, Frozen, Hello Morning, Birds Eye*	1 Waffle/30g	97	4.3	319	7	40	14	2.6
Filled, Chocolate & Hazelnut, Village Bakery, Aldi*	1 Waffle/34g	169	9.9	497	6.2	52.9	29.1	1.5
GF, Schar*	1 Waffle/25g	120	7	478	4.8	52	28	1.1
Stroop, Caramel, Mini, Daelmans*	1 Waffle/7g	29	1.1	421	3.5	65	16	1.5
Stroopwafel, Caramel, Daelmans*	1 Wafel/29g	131	6.1	452	3	62	21	1.5
Sugar, Rowan Hill Bakery, Lidl*	1 Waffle/55g	246	12.7	447	6.2	53	23	1.7
Sweet, American Style, Sainsbury's*	1 Waffle/35g	160	8.9	457	7.2	50.6	25.3	1.1
Toasting, McVitie's*	1 Waffle/25g	115	6.3	461	5.7	52.6	25.5	0.8
WAGON WHEEL								
Jammie, Burton's*	1 Biscuit/40g	168	5.6	420	5.1	67.7	14.1	1.9
WALNUT WHIP								
Classic, M&S*	1 Whip/28g	144	8.1	515	6.8	55.8	28.9	2
Nestle*	1 Whip/35g	173	8.8	494	5.3	61.3	25.2	0.7
WALNUTS								
Average	**_1 Nut/7g_**	**_48_**	**_4.8_**	**_688_**	**_14.7_**	**_3.3_**	**_68.5_**	**_3.5_**
Halves, Average	**_1 Half/3g_**	**_23_**	**_2.3_**	**_669_**	**_17.4_**	**_6.3_**	**_65_**	**_4.7_**
Pickled, in Malt Vinegar, Drained, Opies*	1 Walnut/25g	23	0	92	0.8	23	0	3.4
WASABI								
Paste, Ready Mixed, Japanese, Yutaka*	1 Tsp/5g	14	0.4	286	2.7	53	7	0
WATER								
Apple, & Raspberry, Sparkling, Spring, Tesco*	1 Glass/330ml	7	0	2	0	0.5	0	0
Apple, & Strawberry, Flavoured, Morrisons*	1 Serving/200ml	3	0	2	0.2	0.1	0	0
Cherry, & Plum, Flavoured, Asda*	1 Serving/250ml	2	0	1	0	0.5	0	0
Cranberry, & Raspberry, Flavoured, Morrisons*	1 Serving/200ml	3	0	2	0.2	0.1	0	0
Elderflower, Presse, Sparkling, M&S*	1 Bottle/330ml	99	0.3	30	0.1	7.4	0.1	0.5
Fruity, Lemon & Lime, Just Bee*	1 Serving/200ml	40	0	20	0	4.6	0	0
Lemon & Lime, Flavoured, Sparkling, Spring, Sainsbury's*	1 Glass/250ml	4	0.2	2	0.1	0.1	0.1	0.1
Lemon & Lime, Sugar Free, Touch of Fruit, Volvic*	1 Bottle/150ml	2	0	1	0	0	0	0
Lemon & Lime, Sparkling, M&S*	1 Bottle/500ml	15	0	3	0	0.4	0	0
Lemon & Lime, Still, M&S*	1 Bottle/500ml	5	0	1	0	0.2	0	0
Lemon, & Lime, Still, Tesco*	1 Bottle/500ml	4	0	1	0	0	0	0
Lemon, Lively, Sparkling, Pure Life, Nestle*	1 Bottle/1L	10	0	1	0	0	0	0
Mineral Or Tap	**_1 Glass/200ml_**	**_0_**	**_0_**	**_0_**	**_0_**	**_0_**	**_0_**	**_0_**
Peach, & Raspberry, Still, M&S*	1 Bottle/500ml	10	0	2	0	0	0	0
Peach, & Passion Fruit, Sparkling, Tesco*	1 Glass/250ml	5	0	2	0	0.3	0	0
Sparkling, Lemon & Lime, Aquaroma*	1 Glass/250ml	2	0	1	0	0	0	0
Sparkling, San Pellegrino*	1 Glass/200ml	0	0	0	0	0	0	0
Sparkling, Smart Price, Asda*	1 Glass/300ml	0	0	0	0	0	0	0

W

	Measure INFO/WEIGHT	per Measure KCAL	FAT	Nutrition Values per 100g / 100ml KCAL	PROT	CARB	FAT	FIBRE
WATER								
Sparkling, Triple Berry, Ugly Brands Inc*	1 Can/330ml	3	0	1	0	0	0	0
Spring, Strawberry & Kiwi, Rubicon*	1 Bottle/500ml	12	0	2	0	0.1	0	0
Still, Highland Spring*	1 Bottle/750ml	0	0	0	0	0	0	0
Strawberry, & Guava, Still, M&S*	1 Glass/250ml	5	0	2	0	0.1	0	0
Strawberry, & Kiwi, Still, Shapers, Boots*	1 Glass/250ml	2	0	1	0	0.1	0	0.9
Strawberry, & Kiwi, Still, Sainsbury's*	1 Serving/200ml	8	0	4	1	0	0	0
Strawberry, Original, Touch of Fruit, Volvic*	1 Bottle/500ml	99	0	20	0	4.8	0	0
Strawberry, Sparkling, Spring, Tesco*	1 Bottle/1000g	20	0	2	0	0.2	0	0
Strawberry, Sugar Free, Touch of Fruit, Volvic*	1 Bottle/500ml	7	0	1	0	0.1	0	0
Vitamineral, Power, Ale Coq*	1 Bottle/750ml	150	0	20	0	4.8	0	0
Watermelon Flavour, Protein, Vieve*	1 Bottle/500ml	80	0	16	4	0	0	0
Watermelon, What A Melon*	1 Pack/330ml	79	0	24	0.6	5.4	0	0
WATER CHESTNUTS								
Raw, Average	***1oz/28g***	***8***	***0***	***29***	***0.8***	***6.6***	***0***	***0.1***
with Bamboo Shoots, Sainsbury's*	1 Serving/50g	29	0.1	58	2	12	0.2	1.1
WATERCRESS								
Raw, Trimmed, Average	***1 Sprig/2.5g***	***1***	***0***	***22***	***3***	***0.4***	***1***	***1.5***
WATERMELON								
Flesh Only, Average	***1 Serving/250g***	***75***	***0.8***	***30***	***0.4***	***7***	***0.3***	***0.4***
Raw	***1 Wedge/286g***	***48***	***0.6***	***17***	***0.3***	***3.7***	***0.2***	***0.3***
Raw, Weighed with Skin, Average	***1 Wedge/286g***	***49***	***0.5***	***17***	***0.2***	***4***	***0.2***	***0.2***
WELLINGTON								
Beef, Christmas, M&S*	1 Serving/150g	315	13.4	210	13.6	18	8.9	1.5
Beetroot, Vegan, Waitrose*	1 Wellington/187g	411	23.2	220	4.2	21.5	12.4	2.6
Mushroom, Creamy, The Best, Morrisons*	1 Wellington/169g	439	27.9	260	5.8	20.8	16.5	2.6
Mushroom, M&S*	½ Pack/305g	805	52.8	264	4.8	21	17.3	2.3
Portabello Mushroom, Vegetarian, Tesco*	¼ Pack/117g	268	12.2	229	5.1	27.6	10.4	2
WHEAT BRAN								
Average	***1 Tbsp/7g***	***14***	***0.4***	***206***	***14.1***	***26.8***	***5.5***	***36.4***
WHISKY								
& Cola, Premixed, White Label, 500ml, Jim Beam*	1 Bottle /500ml	254	0	51	0	4.5	0	0
37.5% Volume	***1 Pub Shot/35ml***	***72***	***0***	***207***	***0***	***0***	***0***	***0***
40% Volume	***1 Pub Shot/35ml***	***78***	***0***	***222***	***0***	***0***	***0***	***0***
Scots, 37.5% Volume	***1 Pub Shot/35ml***	***72***	***0***	***207***	***0***	***0***	***0***	***0***
Scots, 40% Volume	***1 Pub Shot/35ml***	***78***	***0***	***224***	***0***	***0***	***0***	***0***
Tennessee Apple, 35%, Jack Daniel's*	1 Pub Shot/35ml	86	0	245	0	0	0	0
Tennessee Fire, 35%, Jack Daniel's*	1 Pub Shot/35ml	86	0	245	0	0	0	0
Tennessee Honey, 35%, Jack Daniel's*	1 Pub Shot/35ml	86	0	245	0	13.3	0	0
WHITE PUDDING								
Average	***1oz/28g***	***126***	***8.9***	***450***	***7***	***36.3***	***31.8***	***0***
WHITEBAIT								
in Flour, Fried	***1oz/28g***	***147***	***13.3***	***525***	***19.5***	***5.3***	***47.5***	***0.2***
Raw, Average	***1 Serving/100g***	***172***	***11***	***172***	***18.3***	***0***	***11***	***0***
WHITING								
in Crumbs, Fried in Blended Oil	***1 Serving/180g***	***344***	***18.5***	***191***	***18.1***	***7***	***10.3***	***0.2***
Raw	***1oz/28g***	***23***	***0.2***	***81***	***18.7***	***0***	***0.7***	***0***
Steamed	***1 Serving/85g***	***78***	***0.8***	***92***	***20.9***	***0***	***0.9***	***0***
WIENER SCHNITZEL								
Average	***1oz/28g***	***62***	***2.8***	***223***	***20.9***	***13.1***	***10***	***0.4***
WINE								
0% Alcohol, Freixenet*	1 Glass/125ml	31	0	25	0	6	0	0
Cava Rosado, Tesco*	1 Glass/125ml	139	0	111	0	0	0	0
Fruit, Average	***1 Glass/125ml***	***115***	***0***	***92***	***0***	***5.5***	***0***	***0***

	Measure INFO/WEIGHT	per Measure KCAL	FAT	Nutrition Values per 100g / 100ml KCAL	PROT	CARB	FAT	FIBRE
WINE								
Madeira, Henriques & Henriques*	1 Glass/125ml	162	0	130	0	0	0	0
Mead, Average	***1 Glass/125ml***	***193***	***0***	***155***	***0***	***17.4***	***0***	***0***
Mulled, Homemade, Average	***1 Glass/125ml***	***245***	***0***	***196***	***0.1***	***25.2***	***0***	***0***
Mulled, Sainsbury's*	1 Glass/125ml	112	0	90	0	8.6	0	0
Mulled, Tesco*	1 Glass/125ml	120	0	96	0	0	0	0
Nosecco , Alcohol Free, Asda*	1 Glass/125ml	35	0.6	28	0.5	7	0.5	0
Original, Lambrini*	1 Glass/125ml	88	0	70	0	0	0	0
Red, Amarone, Average*	***1 Glass/125ml***	***120***	***0***	***96***	***0.1***	***3***	***0***	***0***
Red, Australian, 13.5%, 19 Crimes*	1 Glass/125ml	110	0	88	0	0	0	0
Red, Average	***1 Glass/125ml***	***104***	***0***	***83***	***0***	***2***	***0***	***0***
Red, Beaujolais Villages, Louis Jadot*	1 Glass/125ml	156	0	125	0	4	0	0
Red, Burgundy, 12.9% Abv, Average	***1 Glass/125ml***	***110***	***0***	***88***	***0.1***	***3.7***	***0***	***0***
Red, Cabernet Sauvignon, 13.1% Abv, Average	***1 Glass/125ml***	***105***	***0***	***84***	***0.1***	***2.6***	***0***	***0***
Red, Cabernet Sauvignon, Alcohol Free, Lindemans*	1 Glass/125ml	21	0	17	0	3.5	0	0
Red, Cabernet Tempranillo, Low Alcohol, Tesco*	1 Glass/125ml	78	0	62	0	14.7	0	0
Red, Claret, 12.8% Abv, Average	***1 Glass/125ml***	***105***	***0***	***84***	***0.1***	***3***	***0***	***0***
Red, De-Alcoholised, 0.0%, Sangre De Toro*	1 Glass/125ml	29	0	23	0	3.5	0	0
Red, Gamay, 12.3% Abv, Average	***1 Glass/125ml***	***99***	***0***	***79***	***0.1***	***2.4***	***0***	***0***
Red, Garnacha Syrah, De-Alcoholised, Natureo, Torres*	1 Glass/125ml	29	0	23	0	3.5	0	0
Red, Merlot, 13.3% Abv, Average	***1 Glass/125ml***	***105***	***0***	***84***	***0.1***	***2.5***	***0***	***0***
Red, Merlot, Alcohol Free, Vintense*	1 Glass/125ml	21	0	17	0	3.9	0	0
Red, Merlot, Red Grape, Alcohol Free, M&S*	1 Glass/125ml	55	0.1	44	0.2	10.7	0.1	0.1
Red, Non Alcoholic, Ame*	1 Glass/125ml	42	0	34	0	5.7	0	0
Red, Petit Sirah, 13.5% Abv, Average	***1 Glass/125ml***	***108***	***0***	***86***	***0.1***	***2.7***	***0***	***0***
Red, Pinot Noir, 13% Abv, Average	***1 Glass/125ml***	***104***	***0***	***83***	***0.1***	***2.3***	***0***	***0***
Red, Sangiovese, 13.6% Abv, Average	***1 Glass/125ml***	***109***	***0***	***87***	***0.1***	***2.6***	***0***	***0***
Red, Shiraz, 10.8%, Fair Trade, Co-Op*	1 Glass/125ml	96	0	77	0	0	0	0
Red, Shiraz, Alcohol Free, Zero, McGuigan*	1 Glass/125ml	36	0.2	29	0.3	7	0.2	0
Red, Shiraz, Sumika, M&S*	1 Glass/125ml	65	0	52	0	0	0	0
Red, Shiraz, Unvined, Alcohol Removed, Jacob's Creek*	1 Glass/150ml	25	0	17	0	3.7	0	0
Red, Syrah, 13.1% Abv, Average	***1 Glass/125ml***	***105***	***0***	***84***	***0.1***	***2.6***	***0***	***0***
Red, Zinfandel, 13.9% Abv, Average	***1 Glass/125ml***	***111***	***0***	***89***	***0.1***	***2.9***	***0***	***0***
Rose, Alcohol Free, Eisberg*	1 Glass/125ml	32	0	26	0	5.9	0	0
Rose, Dealcoholised, Delight, McGuigan*	1 Glass/125ml	34	0.1	27	0.2	6	0.1	0
Rose, Fizzero, Sparkling, Zero Alcohol, M&S*	1 Glass/125ml	28	0	22	0	5.2	0	0
Rose, Garnacha, Low Alcohol, Tesco*	1 Glass/125ml	78	0	62	0	14.7	0	0
Rose, Medium, Average	***1 Glass/125ml***	***98***	***0***	***79***	***0***	***2.1***	***0***	***0***
Rose, Muscat, Non Alcoholic, Co-Op*	1 Glass/125ml	55	0	44	0	11	0	0
Rose, Sparkling, Average	***1 Glass/125ml***	***102***	***0***	***82***	***0***	***2.5***	***0***	***0***
Rose, The Pink Chill, Co-Op*	1 Glass/125ml	85	0	68	0	0	0	0
Rose, White Grenache, Blossom Hill*	1 Glass/125ml	105	0	84	0	3.2	0	0
Rose, White Zinfandel, Barefoot*	1 Glass/125ml	74	0	60	0	0	0	0
Rose, White Zinfandel, Ernest & Julio Gallo*	1 Glass/125ml	101	0	81	0.2	2.7	0	0
Sangria, Average	***1 Glass/125ml***	***95***	***0***	***76***	***0.1***	***9.9***	***0***	***0.1***
Vie, Rose, Low Alcohol, Blossom Hill*	1 Glass/125ml	66	0	53	0	3.9	0	0
White, Average	***1 Glass/125ml***	***95***	***0***	***76***	***0***	***2.4***	***0***	***0***
White, Chardonnay, Alcohol Free, Vintense*	1 Glass/125ml	22	0	18	0	4.1	0	0
White, Chardonnay, Alcohol Removed, Fre*	1 Glass/125ml	33	0	26	0	7.5	0	0
White, Chenin Blanc, 12% Abv, Average	***1 Glass/125ml***	***101***	***0***	***81***	***0.1***	***3.3***	***0***	***0***
White, Cotes De Gascogne Blanc, Tesco*	1 Glass/125ml	80	0	64	0	0.3	0	0
White, De-Alcoholised, 0.0%, Sangre De Toro*	1 Glass/125ml	25	0	20	0	3.6	0	0
White, Dry, Average	***1 Glass/125ml***	***88***	***0***	***70***	***0.1***	***0.6***	***0***	***0***
White, Fume Blanc, 13.1% Abv, Average	***1 Glass/125ml***	***104***	***0***	***83***	***0.1***	***2.3***	***0***	***0***

W

	Measure INFO/WEIGHT	per Measure KCAL	FAT	Nutrition Values per 100g / 100ml KCAL	PROT	CARB	FAT	FIBRE
WINE								
White, Gewurztraminer, 12.6% Abv, Average	***1 Glass/125ml***	***102***	***0***	***82***	***0.1***	***2.6***	***0***	***0***
White, Late Harvest, 10.6% Abv, Average	***1 Glass/125ml***	***141***	***0***	***113***	***0.1***	***13.4***	***0***	***0***
White, Medium, Average	***1 Glass/125ml***	***92***	***0***	***74***	***0.1***	***3***	***0***	***0***
White, Moscato, Blanco, Low Alcohol, 5.5%, Lidl*	1 Glass/125ml	62	0	50	0	0	0	0
White, Muller-Thurgau, 11.3% Abv, Average	***1 Glass/125ml***	***96***	***0***	***77***	***0.1***	***3.5***	***0***	***0***
White, Muscat, 11% Abv, Average	***1 Glass/125ml***	***104***	***0***	***83***	***0.1***	***5.2***	***0***	***0***
White, Pinot Blanc, 13.3% Abv, Average	***1 Glass/125ml***	***102***	***0***	***82***	***0.1***	***0***	***0***	***0***
White, Pinot Grigio, 13.4% Abv, Average	***1 Glass/125ml***	***105***	***0***	***84***	***0.1***	***2.1***	***0***	***0***
White, Riesling, 11.9% Abv, Average	***1 Glass/125ml***	***101***	***0***	***81***	***0.1***	***3.7***	***0***	***0***
White, Sauvignon Blanc, 13.1% Abv, Average	***1 Glass/125ml***	***102***	***0***	***82***	***0.1***	***2***	***0***	***0***
White, Sauvignon Blanc, Alcohol Free, Vintense*	1 Glass/125ml	20	0	16	0	4.5	0	0
White, Sauvignon Blanc, Dealcoholised, Tesco*	1 Glass/125ml	41	0	33	0.7	9.9	0	0
White, Sauvignon Blanc, Low Alcohol, Tesco*	1 Glass/125ml	66	0	53	0	12.6	0	0
White, Sauvignon, Alcohol Free, Eisberg*	1 Glass/125ml	28	0	22	0	4.9	0	0
White, Semillon, 12.5% Abv, Average	***1 Glass/125ml***	***104***	***0***	***83***	***0.1***	***3.1***	***0***	***0***
White, Sparkling, Alcohol Free, Zero, McGuigan*	1 Glass/125ml	41	0.2	33	0.1	8	0.2	0
White, Sparkling, Average	***1 Glass/125ml***	***92***	***0***	***74***	***0.3***	***5.1***	***0***	***0***
White, Sparkling, ICE Edition, J.P.Chenet*	1 Glass/125ml	92	0	74	0	0	0	0
White, Sparkling, Low Alcohol, Tesco*	1 Glass/125ml	39	0	31	0	10.2	0	0
White, Sweet, Average	***1 Glass/125ml***	***118***	***0***	***94***	***0.2***	***5.9***	***0***	***0***
WINE GUMS								
Average	***1 Sweet/6g***	***19***	***0***	***315***	***5***	***73.4***	***0.2***	***0.1***
Haribo*	1 Pack/175g	609	0.4	348	0.1	86.4	0.2	0.4
Maynards*	4 Sweets/24g	79	0	329	4.8	76	0.2	0
Tangy, Maynards*	1 Serving/30g	100	0.1	334	4.3	78	0.2	0
WISPA								
Cadbury*	1 Bar/40g	220	13.6	550	7.3	52.5	34	1
Gold, Cadbury*	1 Bar/52g	265	15.1	510	5.3	56	29	0.7
WONTON								
Chicken, Massaman, Cups, Finest, Tesco*	1 Wonton/19g	52	3.1	274	8.7	22	16.5	1.3
Prawn, Oriental Selection, Waitrose*	1 Wonton/18g	45	2	252	9.1	29.2	11	1.1
Prawn, Oriental Snack Selection, Sainsbury's*	1 Wonton/20g	77	5.1	384	9.6	26.8	25.6	4.3
Vegetable, Sweet & Sour, Tesco*	1 Wonton/14g	39	1.9	281	4.5	33.6	13.5	3.6
WOTSITS								
Baked, Really Cheesy, Walkers*	1 Bag/23g	123	7.4	546	5.5	56	33	1.1
Flamin Hot, Giants, Walkers*	1 Serving/30g	160	9.3	533	5.7	57.4	31	1.7
Flaming Hot, Wotsits*	1 Bag/16g	85	4.8	534	5.5	60	30	1.1
Really Cheesy, Big Eat, Walkers*	1 Bag/36g	197	11.9	547	5.5	56	33	1.1
Sizzling Steak, Wotsits*	1 Bag/14g	69	3.3	511	6.7	65.6	24.3	1.7
WRAP								
BBQ Chicken, One Stop*	1 Pack/154g	339	7.2	220	12	31.6	4.7	1.7
Bean, Spicy, with Cheese, Tesco*	1 Pack/198g	423	15.8	213	7.6	25.8	8	3.9
Bean, Three, Mexican Style, Sainsbury's*	1 Pack/190g	435	12.2	229	5.8	35.5	6.4	3.3
Breakfast Scramble, Amy's kitchen *	1 Pack/100g	287	13	287	10	31	13	3
Buffalo Chicken, Tesco*	1 Pack/181g	370	10.2	204	11.8	26	5.6	1
Caesar, Wicked Kitchen, Tesco*	1 Pack/240g	602	28.5	251	7.2	27.5	11.9	2.5
Cauliflower, Coronation, Plant Chef, Tesco*	1 Pack/220g	426	20.5	194	4	22	9.3	3
Chicken, & Bacon, Caesar, COU, M&S*	1 Pack/205g	607	31	296	13.3	26	15.1	1.3
Chicken, BBQ, & Coleslaw, Tesco*	1 Pack/221g	417	12.6	189	9.2	24.4	5.7	1.5
Chicken, BBQ, No Mayo, Tesco*	1 Pack/154g	353	8.6	229	12.2	31.7	5.6	1.7
Chicken, BBQ, On the Go, Sainsbury's*	1 Pack/199g	418	8.6	210	11.5	30.7	4.3	1.2
Chicken, BBQ, Shapers, Boots*	1 Pack/156g	278	4.5	178	11	26	2.9	1.8
Chicken, Cajun, Tesco*	1 Pack/175g	310	10	177	6.3	24.6	5.7	1.1

W

	Measure INFO/WEIGHT	per Measure KCAL	FAT	Nutrition Values per 100g / 100ml KCAL	PROT	CARB	FAT	FIBRE
WRAP								
Chicken, Coronation , Waitrose*	1 Pack/164g	283	8.3	173	10.1	21.3	5.1	2.2
Chicken, Fajita, M&S*	1 Pack/213g	394	15.1	185	8.8	20.1	7.1	2.5
Chicken, Fajita, Morrisons*	1 Pack/214g	430	16.5	201	9.5	22.5	7.7	1.9
Chicken, Fajita, PB, Waitrose*	1 Pack/218g	368	5.7	169	10.5	26	2.6	1.9
Chicken, Fillets, with Cheese, & Bacon, Asda*	1 Pack/164g	366	21.3	223	25	1.4	13	0
Chicken, Jerk, Tesco*	1 Pack/218g	473	16.1	217	9.4	26.2	7.4	4
Chicken, Korma, Rainbow, Co-Op*	1 Pack/198g	348	8.5	176	8.6	24	4.3	2.4
Chicken, Lemon, & Garlic, Tesco*	1 Pack/185g	411	14.6	222	10.1	27.2	7.9	1.1
Chicken, M&S*	1 Pack/247g	530	24.9	215	8.2	23.4	10.1	1.6
Chicken, Mexican Style, Co-Op*	1 Pack/163g	367	14.7	225	11	26	9	3
Chicken, Piri Piri, Aldi*	1 Pack/168g	324	10.6	193	9.3	24	6.3	1.6
Chicken, Salad, Roast, Sainsbury's*	1 Pack/214g	443	19.9	207	10	20.9	9.3	2.5
Chicken, Southern Fried, CBY, Asda*	1 Pack/210g	452	17	215	7.1	27	8.1	2.7
Chicken, Sweet Chilli , Sainsbury's*	1 Pack/209g	434	11.5	208	8.5	30.1	5.5	1.8
Chicken, Tikka, Average	***1 Wrap/200g***	***403***	***15.1***	***202***	***9.5***	***23.6***	***7.6***	***4.4***
Chicken, Tikka, with Onion Bhaji, Tesco*	1 Pack/192g	435	15.9	227	10.3	26.6	8.3	2.2
Duck, Hoisin, GF, M&S*	1 Pack/183g	285	6	156	10.2	17.5	3.3	7.6
Duck, Hoisin, M&S*	1 Pack/225g	405	8.3	180	8.4	27.7	3.7	1.5
Duck, Hoisin, No Mayo, Tesco*	1 Pack/178g	361	10	203	9.8	27.7	5.6	1.2
Falafel, & Spinach, Aldi*	1 Pack/207g	486	24.8	235	6.7	25	12	2.9
Falafel, Spiced, & Feta, with Mint, & Coriander, Waitrose*	1 Pack/223g	484	22.7	217	6	24	10.2	2.6
Hoisin, Plant Chef, Tesco*	1 Pack/175g	387	6.8	221	11	34.8	3.9	1.4
Mozzarella, & Pesto, M&S*	1 Pack/243g	559	27.9	230	7.8	23	11.5	1.7
Mozzarella, & Tomato, Asda*	1 Pack/198g	457	21.8	231	8.4	23	11	2.2
Pork, Mexican, Tesco*	1 Pack/237g	448	17.3	189	7.9	22	7.3	1.6
Prawn, Sweet Chilli, King, M&S*	1 Pack/155g	225	3.1	145	8	24.2	2	2.1
Salmon, & Cream Cheese, Akis at AB*	1 Pack/185g	381	14.2	206	10.1	23.4	7.7	1
Smokehouse No Chicken, Plant Kitchen, M&S*	1 Pack/248g	498	15.6	201	7	29.7	6.3	3
Soft Cheese, & Spinach, to Go*	1 Pack/250g	278	6.7	111	4.5	17.4	2.7	0
Tuna, Sweetcorn, & Red Pepper, BGTY, Sainsbury's*	1 Pack/178g	306	8.2	172	11.5	21.2	4.6	2.1
Turkey, Bacon, & Cranberry, COU, M&S*	1 Pack/144g	230	2.2	160	9.6	27.1	1.5	2.3
Turkey, Feast, Sainsbury's*	1 Pack/212g	502	18.2	237	11.3	27.6	8.6	1.8
Vegetable, Roasted, & Pesto, Plant Chef, Tesco*	1 Pack/168g	351	15.1	209	3.8	26.5	9	3.5

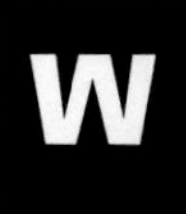

	Measure INFO/WEIGHT	per Measure KCAL	FAT	Nutrition Values per 100g / 100ml KCAL	PROT	CARB	FAT	FIBRE
YAM								
Baked	***1oz/28g***	***43***	***0.1***	***153***	***2.1***	***37.5***	***0.4***	***1.7***
Boiled, Average	***1oz/28g***	***37***	***0.1***	***133***	***1.7***	***33***	***0.3***	***1.4***
YEAST								
Extract	***1 Tsp/9g***	***16***	***0***	***180***	***40.7***	***3.5***	***0.4***	***0***
Extract, Reduced Salt, Sainsbury's*	1 Tsp/4g	10	0	246	41.2	17.6	0.5	4.3
Flakes, Nutritional, Whole Food Earth*	1 Tbsp/5g	17	0.2	341	53	34.8	5	21
Fresh, Average	***1 Serving/30g***	***32***	***0.6***	***105***	***8.4***	***18***	***1.9***	***0***
Quick, Doves Farm*	1 Serving/8g	28	0.5	355	43.5	19	5.7	27
YOGHURT								
0% Fat, Active, Brooklea, Aldi*	1 Pot/125g	59	0.6	47	4.2	7.3	0.5	0.5
0% Fat, Envia*	1 Pot/125g	45	0.1	36	4.3	4.5	0.1	0
3.8% Fat, Alnatura Bioland*	1 Pot/150g	111	5.7	74	4.2	5	3.8	0.1
Activia, Danone*	1 Pot/132g	125	4.2	94	3.5	12.8	3.2	2
All Flavours, Smooth, Ski, Nestle*	1 Pot/120g	100	3.1	83	3.3	11.6	2.6	0
Apple Crumble, West Country, Luxury , M&S*	1 Pot/150g	201	9.9	134	2.7	16	6.6	0.5
Apple, & Pear, Low Fat, Sainsbury's*	1 Pot/125g	115	1.9	92	4.3	15.2	1.5	0.2
Apricot, Bio Activia, Danone*	1 Pot/125g	121	4	97	3.7	13.3	3.2	1.7
Apricot, Fat Free, Weight Watchers*	1 Pot/110g	45	0.1	41	4	5	0.1	0.2
Apricot, Low Fat, Brooklea, Aldi*	1 Pot/125g	99	1	79	2.8	15.1	0.8	0
Apricot, Low Fat, Sainsbury's*	1 Pot/124g	108	1.6	87	4.2	14.3	1.3	0.5
Apricot, Low Fat, Tesco*	1 Pot/125g	112	2.2	90	4.3	14.1	1.8	0
Banana, & Custard, Smooth, Mullerlight, Muller*	1 Pot/175g	94	0.2	54	4.1	8.6	0.1	0.6
Banana, & Custard, Milbona, Lidl*	1 Pot/165g	99	0.2	60	4.4	10	0.1	0.5
Banana, Choco Flakes, Crunch Corner, Muller*	1 Pot/130g	177	6.2	136	4.5	18	4.8	0
Banana, Fat Free, Light, Sainsbury's*	1 Pot/100g	54	0.5	54	5.2	7.5	0.5	0.5
Banana, Low Fat, Average	***1 Serving/100g***	***98***	***1.4***	***98***	***4.6***	***16.7***	***1.4***	***0.1***
Banoffee, Snackpot, Activia, Danone*	1 Pot/155g	116	0.2	75	5	13.3	0.1	0.3
Banoffee, Thick & Creamy, Specially Selected, Aldi*	1 Pot/150g	191	10	127	2.8	14	6.7	0
Berry, Five, Greek Style, Reduced Fat, M&S*	1 Pot/205g	322	17	157	6.7	12.6	8.3	2.5
Berry, Lite, Hansells Foods*	1 Serving/222g	151	0.2	68	5.1	11.8	0.1	0
Black Cherry, Low Fat, Live, M&S*	1 Serving/100g	81	1	81	3.8	14.1	1	0
Black Cherry, West Country, Extra Special, Asda*	1 Pot/150g	200	10.2	133	2.8	15	6.8	0.5
Black Cherry, West Country, TTD, Sainsbury's*	1 Pot/150g	186	9.3	124	3	13.7	6.2	0.5
Black Country, West Country, Sainsbury's*	1 Pot/150g	186	9.3	124	3	13.7	6.2	0.5
Blackberry, Soya, Alpro*	1 Pot/125g	94	2.4	75	3.6	9.7	1.9	1.1
Blackcurrant, & Elderflower, Soya, Alpro*	1 Pot/125g	92	2.4	74	3.6	9.5	1.9	1.1
Blackcurrant, Garden Fruits, Low Fat, Tesco*	1 Pot/125g	120	2.4	95	3.8	15.1	1.9	0.3
Blackcurrant, Soya, Go On, Alpro*	1 Pot/150g	122	4.2	81	5.1	7.5	2.8	2
Blueberry, Fruit Corner, Muller*	1 Pot/150g	156	5.7	104	3.8	12.9	3.8	0.4
Blueberry, Greek Style, Alpro*	1 Pot/150g	123	4	82	4.7	8.6	2.7	1.7
Blueberry, Icelandic Style, Isey Skyr*	1 Pot/180g	157	0.4	87	9.7	12	0.2	0
Blueberry, Icelandic Style, Skyr, Brooklea, Aldi*	1 Pot/150g	122	0.8	81	7.7	12	0.5	0.5
Blueberry, Protein, Arla*	1 Pot/200g	140	0.4	70	10	6.5	0.2	0
Blueberry, Soya, Alpro*	1 Pot/125g	91	2.5	73	3.6	9.4	2	1.2
Blueberry, SoYummy, Aldi*	1 Serving/150g	111	2	74	3.5	11.5	1.3	0
Cafe Vanille, Isey Skyr*	1 Serving/170g	126	3.6	74	9.6	4.2	2.1	0
Caramel, Indulgent Layered, Specially Selected, Aldi*	1 Pot/150g	276	16.5	184	2.3	19	11	1.4
Caramel, Salted, Cheesecake, Greek, Whipped, Muller*	1 Pot/100g	180	7.9	180	4.2	21.8	7.9	0
Caramel, Salted, Greek Style, Luxury, Oykos, Danone*	1 Pot/110g	172	9.2	157	2.7	17.6	8.4	0
Cereals, Fibre, Bio Activia, Danone*	1 Pot/120g	119	4.1	99	3.7	13.5	3.4	3
Cherry, Biopot, Onken*	1 Serving/150g	153	4	102	3.8	14	2.7	0
Cherry, Black, & Cream, The Best, Morrisons*	1 Pot/150g	218	9.4	146	3.2	19	6.3	0
Cherry, Black, Average	***1 Serving/100g***	***96***	***2.2***	***96***	***3.4***	***16.5***	***2.2***	***0.1***

YOGHURT	Measure INFO/WEIGHT	per Measure KCAL	FAT	Nutrition Values per 100g / 100ml KCAL	PROT	CARB	FAT	FIBRE
Cherry, Black, Greek Style, Corner, Muller*	1 Pot/150g	172	4.5	115	5	16.2	3	0.1
Cherry, Black, Low Fat, Average	***1 Serving/100g***	***69***	***0.6***	***69***	***3.8***	***12.2***	***0.6***	***0.3***
Cherry, Greek Style, Layered, Brooklea, Aldi*	1 Pot/125g	89	0.6	71	5.7	11	0.5	0.5
Cherry, Greek Style, Light & Free, Danone*	1 Pot/115g	55	0.1	48	4.3	7.4	0.1	0.1
Cherry, Light, Fat Free, Muller*	1 Pot/175g	88	0.2	50	3.9	7.9	0.1	0.2
Cherry, Luscious, Intensely Creamy, Activia, Danone*	1 Pot/110g	109	3.3	99	5	12.8	3	0.2
Cherry, Mascarpone Style, Bliss, Muller*	1 Pack/110g	131	5.3	119	3.1	15	4.8	0
Cherry, Red, Fruit Corner, Muller*	1 Pot/150g	158	5.8	105	3.8	13	3.9	0.5
Cherry, Soya, Alpro*	1 Pot/125g	91	2.5	73	3.6	9.4	2	1.2
Chocolate Orange, Protein, Arla*	1 Pot/200g	150	1.4	75	10	7.6	0.7	0
Coconut, & Vanilla, Greek Style, Fat Free, Brooklea, Aldi*	1 Pot/125g	74	0.6	59	5.9	7.6	0.5	0.5
Coconut, Greek Style, Brooklea, Aldi*	1 Serving/150g	212	12.9	141	3.7	12	8.6	0.5
Coconut, Greek Style, Milbona, Lidl*	1 Pot/150g	236	14.7	157	3.9	13	9.8	0.5
Coconut, Low Fat, Tesco*	1 Serving/150g	150	4	100	5	13.8	2.7	0.1
Coconut, Protein, Arla*	1 Pot/200g	144	1	72	10	6.2	0.5	0
Fat Free, Activia, Danone*	1 Pot/120g	107	3.4	89	3.9	11.8	2.8	0
Fat Free, Smooth, Milbona, Lidl*	1 Pot/175g	88	0.2	50	4.4	7.3	0.1	0.1
Fig, Bio, Activia, Danone*	1 Pot/125g	124	4.2	99	3.6	13.4	3.4	0.2
Framboise, Siggi's, Skyr*	1 Pot/140g	123	2.7	88	8.9	8.9	1.9	0
French, Set, Low Fat, Iceland*	1 Pot/125g	100	1.5	80	3.6	13.6	1.2	0
Fruit, Low Fat, Average	***1 Pot/125g***	***112***	***0.9***	***90***	***4.1***	***17.9***	***0.7***	***0***
Fudge, Deluxe, Lidl*	1 Pot/150g	226	11	151	3.1	17.9	7.3	0.5
Fudge, Devonshire Style, Finest, Tesco*	1 Pot/150g	206	9.2	137	4	16.4	6.1	0.4
Gin & Tonic, Inspired, Mullerlight, Muller*	1 Pot/160g	72	0.7	45	4.4	6	0.5	0
Ginger, Greek Style, Bio, Live, Rachel's Organic*	1 Serving/100g	137	7.4	137	3.2	14.4	7.4	0
Gingerbread, Mullerlight, Muller*	1 Pot/160g	80	0.8	50	4.8	6.7	0.5	0
Goat's Milk, Natural, St Helen's Farm*	1 Serving/150g	158	11	105	5.5	4.3	7.3	0
Goats Whole Milk	***1 Carton/150g***	***94***	***5.7***	***63***	***3.5***	***3.9***	***3.8***	***0***
Gooseberry, & Elderflower, Fragrant, Creamy, Waitrose*	1 Pot/150g	188	9.9	125	2.6	13.8	6.6	0.5
Gooseberry, & Elderflower, West Country, M&S*	1 Pot/150g	190	10.2	127	3	13.5	6.8	0
Gooseberry, Low Fat, Average	***1 Serving/100g***	***90***	***1.4***	***90***	***4.5***	***14.5***	***1.4***	***0.2***
Gourmet, Live, Deluxe, Lidl*	1 Serving/150g	206	8.4	137	5	16.4	5.6	0.5
Greek Style, 0% Fat, Eat Well, M&S*	1 Pot/200g	116	0.4	58	10.1	3.4	0.2	1.1
Greek Style, Fat Free, Brooklea, Aldi*	1 Serving/150g	100	0.8	67	7	9.2	0.5	0.5
Greek Style, Fat Free, Country Farm*	1 Serving/125g	76	0.5	61	6.1	8.4	0.4	0.5
Greek Style, Fat Free, County Farms*	1 Serving/150g	92	0.6	61	6.1	8.4	0.4	0.5
Greek Style, Fat Free, Morrisons*	¼ Pot/125g	68	0.2	54	6.7	6.3	0.2	0
Greek Style, Free From, Tesco*	¼ Pot/100g	54	3.3	54	5.8	0	3.3	0.7
Greek Style, Honey, Easiyo*	1 Serving/250g	250	9.8	100	3.6	12.5	3.9	0
Greek Style, Layered, Light, Brooklea, Aldi*	1 Pot/125g	69	0.6	55	5.7	7.5	0.5	0.5
Greek Style, Low Fat, M&S*	1 Serving/100g	71	2.6	71	5.2	6.6	2.6	0.5
Greek Style, Low Fat, Milbona, Lidl*	1 Serving/150g	88	3	59	6	4	2	0
Greek Style, Morrisons*	1 Serving/125g	158	12.4	126	5.2	4	9.9	0
Greek Style, Strained, 0%, Glenisk Organic Dairy Co*	1 Pot/150g	84	0	56	10	4	0	0
Greek Style, with Banana, M&S *	1 Pack/171g	220	7.2	129	5.5	16.8	4.2	1.2
Greek Style, with Coconut, Tesco*	1 Serving/150g	184	11.4	123	3.3	10.1	7.6	0.7
Greek Style, with Honey, Brooklea, Aldi*	1/3 Pot/150g	206	11	137	3.3	15	7.3	0.5
Greek Style, with Honey, Tesco*	1 Pot/100g	144	8	144	4.2	13.7	8	0
Greek, 0% Fat, Strained, Authentic, Total, Fage*	1 Pot/170g	92	0	54	10.3	3	0	0
Greek, 0% Fat, with Honey, Total, Fage*	1 Pot/170g	180	0	106	8.3	18	0	0
Greek, 2% Fat, Strained, Authentic, Total, Fage*	1 Pot/170g	119	3.4	70	9.9	3	2	0
Greek, 5% Fat, Brooklea, Aldi*	1 Serving/200g	208	11.2	104	8.7	4.8	5.6	0.5
Greek, Authentic, 0% Fat, Milbona, Lidl*	1 Serving/150g	84	0	56	9	4.8	0	0

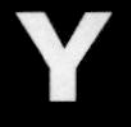

	Measure INFO/WEIGHT	per Measure KCAL	FAT	Nutrition Values per 100g / 100ml KCAL	PROT	CARB	FAT	FIBRE
YOGHURT								
Greek, Authentic, 10% Fat, The Best, Morrisons*	¼ Pot/125g	164	12.5	131	6	4.3	10	0
Greek, Authentic, Delta*	1 Serving/125g	168	12.5	134	6.5	3.8	10	0
Greek, Authentic, Fat Free, TTD, Sainsbury's*	¼ Pot/125g	81	0.6	65	9.9	6	0.5	0.5
Greek, Authentic, Natural, Strained, Waitrose*	1 Serving/125g	164	12.8	131	5.9	3.7	10.2	0.3
Greek, Authentic, TTD, Sainsbury's*	1 Serving/100g	137	10.7	137	6	4.1	10.7	0
Greek, Creamy, Authentic, Milbona, Lidl*	1 Serving/100g	132	10	132	6	4.5	10	0
Greek, Natural, Strained, Fat Free, No.1, Waitrose*	1 Serving/125g	81	0.6	65	9.6	5.5	0.5	0.5
Greek, with Blueberries, Total 0%, Total, Fage*	1 Serving/150g	123	0	82	8.3	12.3	0	0
Greek, with Espresso, Finest, Tesco*	1 Pot/150g	133	0.2	88	8.6	13.1	0.2	0
Hazelnut, Greek, Brooklea, Aldi*	1 Pot/150g	144	0.8	96	8.2	14	0.5	0.5
Hazelnut, Light, Amore, Muller*	1 Pot/130g	82	0.6	63	8	6.7	0.5	0
Hazelnut, Longley Farm*	1 Pot/150g	201	8.5	134	5.5	16	5.7	0
Hazelnut, Low Fat, Deliciously Nutty, Waitrose*	1 Pot/150g	153	4.2	102	6.1	12.9	2.8	0.5
Hazelnut, Sainsbury's*	1 Serving/150g	183	3.4	122	5	20.3	2.3	0.2
Honey, Breakfast Pot, Activia, Danone*	1 Pot/160g	192	4.2	120	4.9	18.8	2.6	0.7
Honey, Greek Style, 0% Fat, Tesco*	1/3 Pot/150g	122	0.3	81	6.8	13.1	0.2	0
Honey, Greek Style, Hansell*	1 Serving/222g	233	9.5	105	4.1	12.3	4.3	0
Honey, Greek Style, Milbona, Lidl*	1 Pot/100g	145	8.3	145	3.8	13.5	8.3	0.5
Honey, Greek Style, Morrisons*	1/3 Pot/150g	236	14.3	157	4.1	13.5	9.5	0.7
Honey, Greek Style, Strained, 0% Fat, Liberte, Yoplait*	1 Pot/100g	92	0.1	92	7.7	14.1	0.1	0.1
Irish, Indulgent, Deluxe, Lidl*	1 Serving/150g	246	11.6	164	3.5	19.5	7.7	1.3
Kefir, Coconut, & Honey, The Great Dairy Collective*	1 Serving/250g	143	6.5	57	3	8.2	2.6	0
Kefir, Mixed Berry, Morrisons*	1 Pot/149g	130	2.8	87	4.3	13.1	1.9	0
Kefir, Natural, Organic, Yeo Valley*	1 Pot/350g	224	7.4	64	4.7	6.4	2.1	0
Kefir, Natural, The Great Dairy Collective*	1 Serving/150g	155	8.3	103	5	8.7	5.5	0
Kefir, Nature, Coop Naturaplan*	1 Pot/150g	117	5.2	79	4.5	6	3.5	0
Kefir, Strawberry, Organic, Yeo Valley*	½ Pot/175g	138	3.3	79	4.2	11.1	1.9	0
Kefir, Vanilla, Morrisons*	1 Pot/151g	122	3	81	3.8	11.7	2	0.5
Kiwi, Bio, Activia, Danone*	1 Pot/125g	122	4.2	98	3.6	12.9	3.4	0.3
Kiwi, Mixed Fruit, Activia, Danone*	1 Pot/120g	109	3.5	91	3.9	12.2	2.9	0
Lactose Free, Sainsbury's*	1 Serving/100g	108	7.2	108	5.3	5.6	7.2	0.5
Layered, Brooklea, Aldi*	1 Pot/125g	69	0.6	55	5.5	7.7	0.5	0.5
Lemon Curd, Luxury, Extra Special, Asda*	1 Pot/150g	242	13.2	161	3.2	17	8.8	0.5
Lemon Curd, Whole Milk, Yeo Valley*	1 Pot/120g	149	5.3	124	4.7	16.3	4.4	0
Lemon, Greek Style, Fat Free, Brooklea, Aldi*	1 Pot/125g	71	0.6	57	5.8	8	0.5	0.5
Lemon, Greek Style, Fat Free, Country Farm, Lidl*	¼ Pot/250g	152	1	61	6.1	8.4	0.4	0.5
Lemon, Greek Style, Fat Free, Muller*	1 Pot/120g	72	0.2	60	6.3	7.5	0.2	0
Lemon, Greek Style, Light & Free, Danone*	1 Pot/115g	53	0.1	46	4.5	6.8	0.1	0
Lemon, Greek Style, Whipped, Bliss Corner, Muller*	1 Pot/110g	177	6.5	161	4	22.2	5.9	0
Lemon, Italian Inspired, Light, Amore, Muller*	1 Pot/130g	78	0.6	60	8.5	6.4	0.5	0
Lemon, Lavish, Greek Style, Light & Free, Danone*	1 Pot/115g	56	0.1	49	4.9	7.1	0.1	0.1
Lemon, Luscious, Greek Style, Mullerlight, Muller*	1 Serving/150g	82	0.8	55	5.8	6.9	0.5	0
Lemon, Sicilain, The Best, Morrisons*	1 Pot/150g	235	12.1	157	3.4	17.5	8.1	0
Lemon, Soya, Free From, Asda*	1 Pot/100g	77	2	77	3.7	11	2	0.5
Mandarin, Fat Free, Mullerlight, Muller*	1 Pot/175g	95	0.2	54	4.2	8.5	0.1	0
Mandarin, Llaeth Y Llan, Village Dairy*	1 Pot/125g	130	3.5	104	5.6	14.3	2.8	0.1
Mango, & Honey, Kefir, M&S*	1 Pack/140g	98	2.4	70	3.8	9.9	1.7	0.5
Mango, & Passion Fruit, Finest, Tesco*	1 Pot/150g	166	7.6	111	3.8	12.3	5.1	0.2
Mango, & Passion Fruit, Low Fat, Morrisons *	1 Pot/125g	96	1.4	77	4.5	12.2	1.1	0.4
Mango, & Passion Fruit, Skyr, M&S*	1 Serving/75g	62	0.3	83	10.3	9.3	0.4	0.5
Mango, Bio, Activia, Danone*	1 Pot/125g	124	4.2	99	3.5	13.5	3.4	0.2
Mango, Carrot, Banana, Simply Fruit & Veg, Danone*	1 Pot/110g	78	2.8	71	4.3	7.6	2.5	0
Mango, Papaya, & Passion Fruit, Bio, Morrisons*	1 Serving/150g	156	5.1	104	3.1	14.9	3.4	0.5

Y

	Measure INFO/WEIGHT	per Measure KCAL	per Measure FAT	KCAL	PROT	CARB	FAT	FIBRE
				Nutrition Values per 100g / 100ml				
YOGHURT								
Mango, Papaya, & Passion Fruit, Onken*	1 Serving/150g	144	4	96	3.8	13	2.7	0.2
Mango, Soya, Go On, Alpro*	1 Pot/150g	129	4.2	86	5	9.1	2.8	1.3
Milky Bar, Mixup, Nestle*	1 Pot/65g	98	3.8	150	4.5	18.5	5.9	0
Muesli, Bircher Style, M&S*	1 Pot/190g	230	5.9	121	5.4	17	3.1	1.6
Muesli, Bircher, Summer Berry, M&S*	1 Pot/195g	277	13.1	142	3.7	15	6.7	3.4
Myrtille, Siggi's, Skyr*	1 Pot/140g	126	2.8	90	9	9	2	0
Natural, Bio Activia, Individual Pots, Danone*	1 Pot/125g	86	4.2	69	4.2	5.5	3.4	0
Natural, Bio Live, Low Fat, Organic, Waitrose*	¼ Pot/125g	81	1.2	65	5.8	8.3	1	0
Natural, Bio Set, Low Fat, Sainsbury's*	1 Pot/150g	78	2.2	52	3.9	5.7	1.5	0
Natural, Bio, Lancashire Farm*	3 Dstsps/40g	32	1.4	80	5.2	7	3.5	0.5
Natural, Biopot, Onken*	1 Serving/125g	82	4.4	66	4.5	4.1	3.5	0
Natural, Fat Free, Lancashire Farm Dairies*	1 Serving/100g	48	0.1	48	5	7.3	0.1	0.9
Natural, Fat Free, Llaeth Y Llan, Village Dairy*	1 Serving/100g	57	0.2	57	5.7	7.9	0.2	0.1
Natural, Fat Free, Morrisons*	1 Serving/100g	47	0.2	47	5	6.4	0.2	0
Natural, Fat Free, Onken*	1 Serving/150g	63	0	42	5.6	3.1	0	0
Natural, Fat Free, Riverford Organic Farmers Ltd*	1 Serving/75ml	40	0.2	54	5.4	8.2	0.2	0
Natural, Greek Style, Average	***1 Serving/100g***	***138***	***10.6***	***138***	***4.7***	***6.1***	***10.6***	***0***
Natural, Greek Style, Low Fat, Average	***1 Serving/100g***	***77***	***2.7***	***77***	***6.1***	***7.3***	***2.7***	***0.2***
Natural, Icelandic Style, Strained, Fat Free, Skyr, Arla*	1 Serving/150g	98	0.3	65	11	4	0.2	0
Natural, Isey Skyr*	1 Serving/170g	104	0.3	61	11	3.7	0.2	0
Natural, Kerned, Super Thick, 0% Fat, Yeo Valley*	1 Serving/113g	64	0.6	57	10	3.5	0.5	0
Natural, Kerned, Super Thick, 5% Fat, Yeo Valley*	1 Serving/150g	142	7.5	95	9	3.5	5	0
Natural, Live, 0% Fat, Eat Well, M&S*	1 Serving/125g	68	0.2	54	5.6	7.5	0.2	0.5
Natural, Low Fat, Average	***1 Med Pot/125g***	***75***	***1.6***	***60***	***5.4***	***7***	***1.3***	***0***
Natural, Low Fat, Live, Waitrose*	1 Pot/175g	114	1.8	65	5.8	8.2	1	0
Natural, Organic, Daylesford*	1 Serving/150g	118	4.5	79	5.7	7.8	3	0
Natural, Probiotic, Organic, Yeo Valley*	1 Pot/120g	98	5.4	82	5.1	5.6	4.5	0
Natural, Scottish, Mccallums*	1 Serving/150g	116	4.8	78	4.9	7.2	3.2	0
Natural, Simplesmente, Pingo Doce*	1 Pot/125g	62	1.9	50	3.9	5.2	1.5	0
Natural, Whole Milk, Set, Biopot, Onken*	1 Serving/125g	85	4.4	68	4.5	4.1	3.5	0
Natural, with Honey, Greek Style, Sainsbury's*	1 Sm Pot/125g	174	9.8	139	3.7	13.4	7.8	0.5
Oat Based, Light & Free, Danone*	1 Serving/150g	69	0.6	46	0.6	9.6	0.4	0
Oat-Gurt, Plain, Oatly*	¼ Pot/100g	84	3.5	84	1.5	11	3.5	1
Orange, & Pink Grapefruit, Finest, Tesco*	1 Pot/150g	162	7.8	108	4	11.2	5.2	0.4
Orange, Sprinkled with Dark Chocolate, Light, Muller*	1 Pot/165g	91	0.8	55	4.3	7.4	0.5	0.1
Passion Fruit, Gourmet, Live, The Great Dairy Collective*	1 Pot/150g	190	8.2	127	5.1	14.2	5.5	0
Passion Fruit, Greek Style, Luxury, Oykos, Danone*	1 Pot/110g	163	9.1	148	2.9	15.4	8.3	0.1
Passion Fruit, Soya, Go On, Alpro*	1 Pot/150g	126	4.4	84	5.2	8.5	2.9	1.4
Paturages*	1 Pot/125g	42	0.6	34	4.4	4.2	0.5	0.5
Peach, & Apricot, Fruit Corner, Muller*	1 Pot/150g	160	5.7	107	3.9	13.5	3.8	0.5
Peach, & Apricot, HL, Tesco*	1 Bottle/100g	70	1.2	70	2.3	12.4	1.2	0.2
Peach, & Cream, Intensely Creamy, Activia, Danone*	1 Pot/120g	118	3.6	98	4.8	13	3	0.3
Peach, & Mango, Thick & Creamy, Waitrose*	1 Pot/125g	136	3.1	109	3.7	17.8	2.5	0.3
Peach, & Passion Fruit, Fat Free, Milbona, Lidl*	1 Pot/180g	122	0.7	68	12.4	3.5	0.4	0.5
Peach, & Pineapple, Fat Free, Mullerlight, Muller*	1 Pot/175g	89	0.2	51	4.3	7.7	0.1	0.2
Peach, & Mango, Ann Forshaw's*	1 Pot/150g	196	8.8	131	4.1	15.4	5.9	0
Peach, & Pear, Soya, No Bits, Alpro*	1 Pot/125g	99	2.5	79	3.7	10.7	2	1
Peach, Bio, Activia, Fat Free, Danone*	1 Pot/125g	71	0.1	57	4.7	9.3	0.1	1
Peach, Greek Style, Luxury, Oykos, Danone*	1 Pot/110g	154	8.9	140	3.1	13.4	8.1	0.3
Peach, Low Fat, Average	***1 Serving/100g***	***86***	***1.1***	***86***	***4.5***	***14.6***	***1.1***	***0.2***
Peach, Melba, Low Fat, Average	***1 Serving/100g***	***75***	***0.7***	***75***	***2.6***	***14.5***	***0.7***	***0***
Peach, No Added Sugar, Zero, Yoplait*	1 Pot/125g	58	0.1	46	4.5	5.8	0.1	0.2
Peach, Proviact, Lidl*	1 Pot/66g	35	0.1	53	3.4	9.4	0.1	0.4

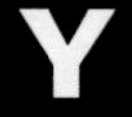

	Measure INFO/WEIGHT	per Measure KCAL	per Measure FAT	KCAL	PROT	CARB	FAT	FIBRE
				Nutrition Values per 100g / 100ml				
YOGHURT								
Peach, Simply Fruit, Danone*	1 Pot/110g	78	2.8	71	4.3	7.4	2.5	0
Pear, & Blackcurrant, M&S*	1 Pot/150g	183	9.6	122	2.8	12.9	6.4	0.8
Pear, Irish, 0% Fat, Duneen, Aldi*	1 Carton/125g	66	0.6	53	4.7	7.5	0.5	0.5
Pineapple, & Peach, Fruity, Mullerlight, Muller*	1 Pot/175g	89	0.2	51	4.2	7.7	0.1	0.2
Plain, Coconut, Dairy Free, Just Free, Lidl*	1 Pot/125g	85	4.4	68	0.5	8.4	3.5	0.2
Plain, Greek Style, Alpro*	1 Serving/50g	34	1.6	68	5.8	2.6	3.3	1.5
Plain, Half Fat, Bio, Jumbo*	1 Serving/150ml	75	2.2	50	4.2	4.3	1.5	0
Plain, Low Fat, Average	***1 Serving/100g***	***63***	***1.6***	***63***	***5.2***	***7***	***1.6***	***0***
Plain, Skyr, Lidl*	1 Pack/150g	93	0.3	62	11	4	0.2	0
Plain, Soya, Average	***1oz/28g***	***20***	***1.2***	***72***	***5***	***3.9***	***4.2***	***0***
Plain, Soya, Simply, Alpro*	1 Tbsp/20g	10	0.5	50	4	2.1	2.3	1
Plain, Whole Milk, Average	***1oz/28g***	***22***	***0.8***	***79***	***5.7***	***7.8***	***3***	***0***
Plain, with Almond, Soya, Alpro*	1 Tbsp/20g	11	0.6	54	3.9	2.3	2.8	1.1
Plain, with Coconut, Soya, Alpro*	1 Tbsp/20g	11	0.6	55	3.9	2.3	3	0.8
Pomegranate, Soya, Alpro*	1 Pot/125g	92	2.4	74	3.6	9.5	1.9	1.1
Pouring, Court Lodge Organic*	1 Serving/125g	91	5.9	73	3	4.7	4.7	0
Proviact, Milbona, Lidl*	1 Pot/125g	59	0.1	47	3.1	8.2	0.1	0.5
Prune, Bio, Activia, Danone*	1 Pot/125g	122	4.1	98	3.6	13.1	3.3	0.8
Prune, Live, M&S*	1 Pack/159g	254	6.5	160	5.4	24.4	4.1	1.7
Quark, Plain, Muller*	1 Pot/150g	176	9.2	117	7.1	8.3	6.1	0
Quark, Strawberry, Muller*	1 Pot/150g	186	7.2	124	5.5	13.7	4.8	0
Quark, Vanilla, Muller*	1 Pot/150g	186	7.4	124	6.4	13.4	4.9	0
Raspberry, & Cranberry, Fat Free, Milbona, Lidl*	1 Pot/174g	87	0.2	50	4.2	7.8	0.1	0.5
Raspberry, & Cranberry, Fat Free, Mullerlight, Muller*	1 Pot/175g	91	0.2	52	4.3	7.8	0.1	0.5
Raspberry, & Cream, The Best, Morrisons*	1 Pot/150g	205	9.7	137	3.2	16.2	6.5	0.3
Raspberry, & Apple, No Added Sugar, Alpro*	½ Pot/200g	116	3.8	58	3.6	4.8	1.9	1.3
Raspberry, & Cranberry, Soya, Alpro*	1 Pot/125g	94	2.4	75	3.6	9.7	1.9	1.1
Raspberry, Fat Free, Average	***1 Serving/100g***	***64***	***0.1***	***64***	***4.9***	***11***	***0.1***	***1.7***
Raspberry, Greek Style, Bio-Live, Rachel's Organic*	1 Serving/150g	194	10.6	129	3.1	13.1	7.1	0
Raspberry, Greek Style, Brooklea, Aldi*	1 Pot/150g	124	0.8	83	8.3	12	0.5	0.5
Raspberry, Greek Style, Easiyo*	1 Serving/180g	198	6.7	110	3.9	15.3	3.7	0
Raspberry, Greek Style, Light, Fat Free, Brooklea, Aldi*	1 Pot/125g	72	0.6	58	5.8	8.2	0.5	0.5
Raspberry, Greek Style, Oykos, Danone*	1 Serving/110g	156	9	142	2.7	13.9	8.2	0.5
Raspberry, Greek Style, Tim's Dairy*	1 Pot/125g	179	10.5	143	4.6	12.4	8.4	0.4
Raspberry, High Protein, Fat Free, Milbona, Lidl*	1 Pot/180g	223	0.7	124	12.6	3.4	0.4	0.5
Raspberry, Intensely Creamy, Juicy, Activia, Danone*	1 Pot/110g	109	3.3	99	4.8	12.7	3	0.6
Raspberry, Low Fat, Average	***1 Serving/100g***	***83***	***1.1***	***83***	***4.1***	***14.1***	***1.1***	***0.8***
Raspberry, Onken*	1 Serving/150g	142	4	95	3.8	13	2.7	0.5
Raspberry, Organic, Yeo Valley*	1 Pot/150g	152	5.8	101	4.2	12.3	3.9	0.4
Raspberry, Pouring, Icelandic Style, Skyr, Arla*	1 Serving/150g	96	0.8	64	6	9.1	0.5	0.1
Raspberry, Protein, Arla*	1 Pot/200g	126	0.4	63	10	5.6	0.2	0
Raspberry, Protein, Milbona, Lidl*	1 Pot/180g	124	0.7	69	12.6	3.4	0.4	0.5
Raspberry, Protein, Thick, Eat Well, M&S*	1 Pot/200g	154	0.4	77	11.7	6.9	0.2	0.5
Raspberry, Razzle, Greek Style, Light & Free, Danone*	1 Pot/115g	61	0.1	53	4.7	7.8	0.1	1.1
Raspberry, River Cottage*	1 Jar/160g	85	3.1	53	2.6	7.6	1.9	0.1
Raspberry, Skyr, Icelandic, Siggi's*	1 Pot/150g	108	0	72	10	7.7	0	0
Raspberry, Skyr, Milbona, Lidl*	½ Pot/175g	100	0.4	57	8.9	4.6	0.2	0.5
Raspberry, Squidgy Pouches, Brooklea, Aldi*	1 Pouch/80g	67	2.3	84	3.4	11	2.9	0.5
Raspberry, Summer Fruits, Benecol*	1 Pot/120g	90	2	75	0.2	9.7	1.7	3.7
Raspberry, Summer, Biopot, Onken*	1/5 Pot/90g	91	2.4	101	3.8	15	2.7	0.6
Rhubarb, & Vanilla, Greek Style, Fat Free, Asda*	1 Pot/125g	60	0.6	48	5.8	5.3	0.5	0.6
Rhubarb, Champagne, Scottish, Deluxe, Lidl*	1 Pot/150g	198	9.3	132	4	14.7	6.2	0.5
Rhubarb, Crumble, Inspired, Mullerlight, Muller*	1 Pot/172g	86	0.2	50	4.1	7.5	0.1	0

	Measure	per Measure		Nutrition Values per 100g / 100ml				
	INFO/WEIGHT	KCAL	FAT	KCAL	PROT	CARB	FAT	FIBRE
YOGHURT								
Rhubarb, Fruity, Mullerlight, Muller*	1 Pot/175g	91	0.2	52	4.2	7.9	0.1	0
Rhubarb, Layer, Bonne Maman*	1 Pot/125g	134	5.1	107	2.3	15	4.1	0.6
Rhubarb, Live, Thick & Creamy, Manor Farm*	1 Pot/128g	166	9.3	130	5	13.4	7.3	0
Rhubarb, Longley Farm*	1 Pot/150g	165	5.6	110	4.9	14.3	3.7	0
Rhubarb, Low Fat, Average	***1 Serving/100g***	***83***	***1.2***	***83***	***4.6***	***13.3***	***1.2***	***0.2***
Rhubarb, Spiced, Thick & Creamy, COU, M&S*	1 Pot/170g	68	0.2	40	4.3	5.8	0.1	0.5
Rhubarb, SuperValu*	1 Jar/140g	161	8.1	115	3.4	12	5.8	0
Rhubarb, Timperley, TTD, Sainsbury's*	1 Pot/150g	170	9.9	113	3.2	10.1	6.6	0.5
Rhubarb, West Country, Finest, Tesco*	1 Pot/150g	147	6.8	98	3.5	10.9	4.5	0
Roasted Hazelnut, Low Fat, Super Nutty, M&S*	1 Pot/150g	153	4.2	102	6.1	12.9	2.8	0.4
Salted Caramel, Protein, Arla*	1 Pot/200g	146	1.2	73	10	7.5	0.6	0
Salted Caramel, Thick & Creamy, Live, Nomadic*	1 Pot/160g	181	6.7	113	5.4	13.4	4.2	0.5
Skyr, Apple, Baked, Isey Skyr*	1 Serving/75g	40	0.2	54	9	4.1	0.2	0
Skyr, Icelandic, Raspberry Granola, Corner, Muller*	1 Pot/180g	256	11.9	142	7.4	12.2	6.6	0
Skyr, Mango & Passion Fruit, Fat Free, Tesco*	1 Pot/150g	114	0	76	8.5	10.2	0	0.4
Skyr, Natural, Icelandic Style, M&S*	1/3 Pot/150g	99	0.2	66	12.2	3.7	0.1	0.5
Skyr, Natural, Migros*	1 Pot/170g	104	0.2	61	11	4	0.1	0
Skyr, Raspberry, Fat Free, Tesco*	1 Pot/150g	110	0	73	8.3	9.7	0	0.4
Smooth Toffee, Fat Free, Mullerlight, Muller*	1 Pot/160g	78	0.8	49	4.8	6.6	0.5	0
Soya, Mercadona*	1 Pot/125g	54	3.4	43	4.6	0	2.7	0
Soya, Natural, SoYummy, Aldi*	1 Serving/100g	48	1.5	48	4.2	4.2	1.5	0
Soya, Plain, Just Free, Lidl*	1 Serving/100g	51	1.5	51	4.2	5	1.5	0.5
Soya, Plain, No Sugars, Alpro*	1 Tbsp/30g	13	0.7	42	4	0	2.3	0.9
Stracciatella, Kvarg, Lindahls, Nestle*	1 Pot/151g	95	0.9	63	11	3.4	0.6	0
Strained, 2% Fat, Olympos*	1 Serving/200g	140	4	70	9	4	2	0
Strawberry, & Acai, Skyr, Light, Muller*	1 Pot/150g	90	0.8	60	9.5	4.3	0.5	0
Strawberry, & Cream, Finest, Tesco*	1 Pot/150g	206	10.4	137	3.4	15.4	6.9	0.5
Strawberry, & Cream, Scottish, Deluxe, Lidl*	1 Pot/150g	198	9	132	4.1	15.1	6	0.5
Strawberry, & Vanilla, Double Up, Munch Bunch, Nestle*	1 Pot/86g	85	2.3	99	6.1	12.6	2.7	0
Strawberry, & Banana, Soya, No Bits, Alpro*	1 Pot/125g	99	2.5	79	3.7	10.7	2	1
Strawberry, & Raspberry, Greek Style, High Protein, Alpro*	1 Pot/150g	123	4	82	4.7	8.8	2.7	1.5
Strawberry, Active, Brooklea, Aldi*	1 Pot/125g	118	3.9	94	3	13	3.1	0.5
Strawberry, Active, Fat Free, Optifit, Aldi*	1 Pot/125g	54	0.5	43	3	7.1	0.4	0.4
Strawberry, Activia, Danone*	1 Pot/120g	107	3.4	89	3.9	11.8	2.8	0
Strawberry, Benecol*	1 Pot/120g	85	2.3	71	3.8	9.6	1.9	0
Strawberry, Bio, Activia, Danone*	1 Pot/125g	124	4.1	99	3.6	13.6	3.3	0.2
Strawberry, Breakfast Crunch, Corner, Muller*	1 Pot/135g	163	3.5	121	5.5	0	2.6	0
Strawberry, Creamy, Milbona, Lidl*	1 Pot/150g	204	11.1	136	3.1	14	7.4	0.5
Strawberry, Fat Free, Average	***1 Serving/100g***	***66***	***0.1***	***66***	***4.9***	***11.1***	***0.1***	***0.6***
Strawberry, Finest, Tesco*	1 Pot/150g	155	7.5	103	3.5	10.7	5	0
Strawberry, Fruit Corner, Corner, Muller*	1 Pot/128g	134	5	105	5.7	10.3	3.9	0.1
Strawberry, Greek Style, 0% Fat, Liberte, Yoplait*	1 Pot/100g	79	0.2	79	8	11	0.2	0.4
Strawberry, Greek Style, Almarai*	1 Pot/150g	220	10.6	147	5.7	15.2	7.1	0
Strawberry, Greek Style, Bio Live, Activia, Danone*	1 Pot/110g	109	3.3	99	5	12.9	3	0.2
Strawberry, Greek Style, Fat Free, Brooklea, Aldi*	1 Pot/125g	72	0.3	57	4.9	8.8	0.2	0.2
Strawberry, Greek Style, Fat Free, Milbona, Lidl*	1 Pot/125g	78	0.6	62	5.9	8.4	0.5	0.5
Strawberry, Greek Style, Fat Free, Morrisons*	1 Pot/125g	64	0.2	51	4.8	7.5	0.2	0.1
Strawberry, Greek Style, Fruitopolis, Mullerlight, Muller*	1 Pot/130g	84	0.1	65	4.8	10.8	0.1	0
Strawberry, Greek Style, Luxury, Oykos, Danone*	1 Pot/110g	159	8.9	145	3.2	14.6	8.1	0.3
Strawberry, Greek Style, Milbona, Lidl*	1 Pot/125g	160	7.8	128	2.4	15.5	6.2	0.5
Strawberry, Greek Style, Whipped, Bliss, Corner, Muller*	1 Pot/110g	142	6.5	129	4.1	14.3	5.9	0
Strawberry, Greek, Brooklea, Aldi*	1 Pot/150g	118	0.8	79	8.3	11	0.5	0.5
Strawberry, Greek, Lactose Free, Morrisons *	1 Pot/150g	100	1.8	67	6.1	7.7	1.2	0.7

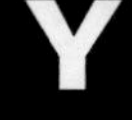

	Measure INFO/WEIGHT	per Measure KCAL	FAT	Nutrition Values per 100g / 100ml KCAL	PROT	CARB	FAT	FIBRE
YOGHURT								
Strawberry, Icelandic Style, Strained, Fat Free, Skyr, Arla*	1 Pot/150g	109	0.7	73	9.6	7.4	0.5	0.1
Strawberry, Icelands*	1 Serving/125g	96	0.2	77	4.3	14.2	0.2	0.5
Strawberry, Irish, Coolree Creamery*	1 Pot/125g	121	4.2	97	5.3	11	3.4	0.5
Strawberry, Jogobella, Zott*	1 Serving/125g	112	3.4	90	3.5	12	2.7	0
Strawberry, Jogurtpur Erdbeer, Emmi*	1 Becher/150g	147	4.2	98	4.5	13	2.8	0
Strawberry, Lactose Free, Lactofree, Arla*	1 Pot/125g	126	3.2	101	3.5	15.9	2.6	0.4
Strawberry, Layer, Bonne Maman*	1 Pot/125g	139	5.1	111	2.3	16	4.1	0.4
Strawberry, Low Fat, Average	***1 Serving/100g***	***81***	***1***	***81***	***4.5***	***13.6***	***1***	***0.2***
Strawberry, Milbona, Lidl*	1 Pot/175g	175	5.2	100	3	15	3	0
Strawberry, Mullerlight, Muller*	1 Pot/160g	83	0.8	52	4.9	7	0.5	0
Strawberry, Naked, Good to Go, Onken*	1 Pack/100g	88	2.8	88	4	11	2.8	0
Strawberry, Organic, Bio Live, Yeo Valley*	1 Serving/150g	147	6	98	4.5	10.9	4	0
Strawberry, Probiotic, Organic, Yeo Valley*	1 Pot/125g	125	5	100	4.4	11.7	4	0.1
Strawberry, Protein 20g, Arla*	1 Pot/200g	140	0.4	70	10	6.5	0.2	0
Strawberry, Protein, Grahams*	1 Pot/190g	148	0.8	78	11.4	7.2	0.4	0
Strawberry, Protein, Thick, M&S*	1 Pot/200g	154	0.4	77	11.7	6.9	0.2	0.5
Strawberry, Rice, Low Fat, Muller*	1 Pot/180g	193	4.1	107	3.2	18.4	2.3	0.4
Strawberry, Shortcake, Crunch Corner, Muller*	1 Pot/130g	192	7.3	148	4.5	19.3	5.6	0.1
Strawberry, Simply Fruit, Danone*	1 Serving/150g	106	3.8	71	4.6	7.1	2.5	0
Strawberry, Skyr, High Protein, Isey Skyr*	1 Pot/170g	143	0.3	84	9.2	11	0.2	0
Strawberry, Soya, Alpro*	¼ Pot/125g	92	2.4	74	3.6	9.4	1.9	1
Strawberry, Split Pot, Asda*	1 Pot/151g	134	3.6	89	3	14	2.4	0.5
Strawberry, Summer Fruits, Benecol*	1 Pot/120g	90	2	75	0.2	9.7	1.7	3.7
Strawberry, Thick & Creamy, Brooklea, Aldi*	1 Pot/150g	206	11.1	137	3.1	14	7.4	0.5
Strawberry, Thick & Creamy, Golden Acre*	1 Pot/150g	219	11.7	146	2.3	16.5	7.8	0.5
Strawberry, Thick & Creamy, Lichfields*	1 Pot/125g	174	9.2	139	2.7	15	7.4	0.7
Strawberry, TruBlend, Fage*	1 Cup/150g	114	2.4	76	8	4.8	1.6	0
Strawberry, Yoplait*	1 Pack/125g	112	2.9	90	3.3	13	2.3	0.2
Strawberry, Zero Fat, Yoplait*	1 Pot/125g	56	0.1	45	4.5	5.6	0.1	0.2
Taillefine aux Fruits, Danone*	1 Pot/125g	58	0.1	46	4.5	6.7	0.1	0
Toffee, Cheesecake, Inspired, Goodies, Mullerlight, Muller*	1 Pot/107g	97	2	91	4.5	13.4	1.9	0
Toffee, Creamfields*	1 Pot/125g	86	1.2	69	2	13	1	0
Toffee, Greek Style, Fat Free, Light, Asda*	1 Pot/125g	68	0.6	54	5.7	7	0.5	0.5
Toffee, Low Fat, Deliciously Silky, Waitrose*	1 Pot/151g	143	3	95	4.6	14.5	2	0.5
Toffee, Smooth, Milbona, Lidl*	1 Pot/175g	105	0.4	60	4.5	9.7	0.2	0.5
Toffee, Smooth, Mullerlight, Muller*	1 Pot/120g	73	1.3	61	6.3	8.5	1.1	0
Toffee, Tempting, Greek Style, Muller Light *	1 Pot/120g	84	0.1	70	6.3	10.1	0.1	0
Tropical, Granola, Duo, Brooklea, Aldi*	1 Pot/135g	177	6.2	131	3.6	18.5	4.6	0.8
Unsweetened, Easiyo*	1 Serving/200g	101	0.3	50	5.1	7	0.2	0
Unsweetened, Greek Style, Hansells Foods*	1 Serving/200g	214	13.2	107	6.6	6.9	6.6	0
Vanilla, & Chocolate Sprinkles, Fat Free, Milbona, Lidl*	1 Pot/175g	93	0.9	53	3.9	7.6	0.5	0.1
Vanilla, & Granola, Low Fat, Activia, Danone*	1 Pot/165g	185	3.3	112	5.3	18.2	2	1.8
Vanilla, 0% Fat, Yeo Valley*	1 Serving/150g	122	0	81	5.8	14.1	0	0
Vanilla, Average	***1 Serving/120g***	***100***	***5.4***	***83***	***4.5***	***12.4***	***4.5***	***0.8***
Vanilla, Bio Live, Luscious, Organic, Rachel's Organic*	1 Serving/150g	164	8.1	109	3.3	11.8	5.4	0
Vanilla, Choco Balls, Crunch Corner, Snack Size, Muller*	1 Pot/85g	118	4.1	139	3.8	20.2	4.8	0
Vanilla, Creamy, with Mini Smarties, Nestle*	1 Pot/120g	182	6.5	152	3.6	21.5	5.4	0
Vanilla, Fat Free, Light, Sainsbury's*	1 Pot/100g	52	0.5	52	5.1	7.2	0.5	0.5
Vanilla, Fat Free, Onken*	½ Pot/225g	166	0.2	74	4.4	12.6	0.1	0.3
Vanilla, Greek Style, 0% Fat, COU, M&S*	1 Pot/140g	81	0.3	58	6.8	7.2	0.2	0.5
Vanilla, Greek Style, Light & Free, Danone*	1 Pot/115g	58	0.1	50	4.5	6.8	0.1	2
Vanilla, Greek Style, Tesco*	¼ Pot/112g	140	9	125	2.6	12.7	8	0

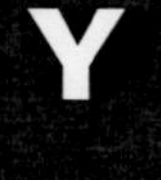

	Measure INFO/WEIGHT	per Measure KCAL	per Measure FAT	Nutrition Values per 100g / 100ml KCAL	PROT	CARB	FAT	FIBRE
YOGHURT								
Vanilla, Greek, 0% Fat, Brooklea, Aldi*	1 Pot/150g	122	0.8	81	8.3	11	0.5	0.5
Vanilla, Greek, Lactose Free, Morrisons*	1 Pot/150g	105	0.9	70	5.6	10.5	0.6	0
Vanilla, Isey Skyr*	1 Pot/170g	94	0.3	55	9.7	3.5	0.2	0
Vanilla, Light, Fat Free, Milbona, Lidl*	1 Serving/165g	92	0	56	4.7	8.9	0	0
Vanilla, Low Fat, Probiotic, Organic, M&S*	1 Serving/100g	85	1.8	85	6.2	10.9	1.8	0
Vanilla, Madagascan, West Country, TTD, Sainsbury's*	1 Pot/150g	197	11.8	132	3.1	11.9	7.9	0.5
Vanilla, Pouring, Icelandic Style, Skyr, Arla*	1 Serving/150g	92	0.8	61	6.3	8.1	0.5	0
Vanilla, Protein, Milbona, Lidl*	1 Pot/180g	121	0.7	67	12.5	3	0.4	0.5
Vanilla, Smooth, Light, Fat Free, Mullerlight, Muller*	1 Pot/175g	88	0.2	50	4.3	7.2	0.1	0
Vanilla, Soya, Alpro*	1 Sm Pot/125g	82	2.8	66	3.7	7.5	2.2	0.9
Vanilla, SoYummy, Aldi*	1 Serving/150g	106	2	71	3.5	10.9	1.3	0
Vanilla, TruBlend, Fage*	1 Pot/150g	111	2.4	74	8	4.1	1.6	0
Vanilla, Vibe, Light & Free, Danone*	1 Pot/115g	61	0.1	53	4.9	7.1	0.1	0
Vanilla, with Oreo Pieces, Muller*	1 Pot/120g	186	7.1	155	3.5	21.3	5.9	0
with Apricot Layer, Bonne Maman*	1 Pot/125g	140	5.1	112	2.4	16	4.1	0.5
with Raspberry Layer, Bonne Maman*	1 Pot/125g	136	5.1	109	2.4	15	4.1	1
YOGHURT DRINK								
Actimel, Blueberry, Danone*	1 Bottle/100g	74	1.5	74	2.6	11.8	1.5	0.5
Average	***1fl oz/30ml***	***19***	***0***	***62***	***3.1***	***13.1***	***0***	***0***
Blueberry, & Blackcurrant, Skyr, Arla*	1 Bottle/350ml	214	0.7	61	5.8	8.1	0.2	0
Blueberry, Cholesterol Lowering, Tesco*	1 Bottle/100g	49	1.5	49	2.5	6.2	1.5	0.1
Blueberry, Cholesterol Reducing, Morrisons*	1 Bottle/100g	36	1.1	36	2.7	3.9	1.1	0.1
Cholesterol Lowering, Asda*	1 Bottle/100g	76	1.4	76	2.9	13	1.4	1
Fruit, Mixed, Actimel, Danone*	1 Bottle/100ml	88	1.5	88	2.7	16	1.5	0
Lemon, 0% Fat, No Added Sugar, Actimel, Danone*	1 Bottle/100g	27	0.1	27	2.6	3.2	0.1	0.2
Light, Benecol*	1 Bottle/68g	40	1.4	60	2.8	7.3	2.1	0.1
Light, Yakult*	1 Bottle/65ml	27	0	42	1.4	10.2	0	1.8
Multi Fruit, Actimel, Danone*	1 Bottle/100g	85	1.5	85	2.7	14.4	1.5	0.1
Multifruit, Brooklea, Aldi*	1 Bottle/100g	71	1.3	71	2.5	12	1.3	0.5
Original, 0.1% Fat, Actimel, Danone*	1 Bottle/100g	27	0.1	27	2.7	3	0.1	0.2
Original, Cholesterol Lowering, Sainsbury's*	1 Bottle/100g	36	1.1	36	2.7	3.4	1.1	0.5
Original, Cholesterol Reducing, Tesco*	1 Bottle/100ml	51	1.6	51	2.7	6.1	1.6	0.8
Original, No Added Sugar, Benecol*	1 Bottle/68g	32	1.4	47	2.8	4.3	2	0
Peach, & Apricot, Benecol*	1 Bottle/68g	33	1.4	49	2.9	4.8	2	0
Strawberry, Actimel, Danone*	1 Bottle/100g	74	1.5	74	2.9	11.5	1.5	0
Strawberry, Benecol*	1 Bottle/68g	38	1.4	56	3.2	6.2	2	0
Strawberry, Cholesterol Lowering, Brooklea, Aldi*	1 Bottle/100g	37	1.2	37	2.4	3.9	1.2	0.6
Strawberry, Cholesterol Lowering, Milbona, Lidl*	1 Bottle/100g	53	1.4	53	3.3	6.6	1.4	0
Strawberry, Cholesterol Lowering, Sainsbury's*	1 Bottle/100g	37	1.2	37	2.4	3.9	1.2	0.6
Strawberry, Cholesterol Reducing, Morrisons*	1 Bottle/100ml	36	1.2	36	2.4	3.9	1.2	0.1
Strawberry, Cholesterol Reducing, Tesco*	1 Bottle/100g	46	1.7	46	2.7	4.7	1.7	0.8
Strawberry, Fat Free, Actimel, Danone*	1 Bottle/100ml	27	0.1	27	2.6	3.2	0.1	0.2
Yakult*	1 Bottle/65ml	43	0.1	66	1.3	14.7	0.1	0
YORKIE								
Original, Nestle*	1 Bar/55g	302	17.4	546	6.2	57.9	31.5	1.9
Raisin & Biscuit, Duo, Nestle*	1 Bar/33g	165	8.3	505	6.2	60.2	25.4	2
Raisin & Biscuit, Nestle*	1 Bar/67g	338	16.9	508	5.3	61.9	25.4	1.7
YORKSHIRE PUDDING								
12, Frozen, Asda*	1 Pudding/18g	45	1.4	246	9	35	7.4	2.2
Average	***1 Pudding/30g***	***62***	***3***	***208***	***6.6***	***24.7***	***9.9***	***0.9***
Batters, in Foils, Ready to Bake, Frozen, Aunt Bessie's*	1 Pudding/17g	47	1.8	276	9.1	32.6	10.8	1.4
Beef Dripping, Cooked, Specially Selected, Aldi*	1 Pudding/44g	129	5.7	293	9.4	32	13	3
Beef Dripping, Oven Baked, Extra Special, Asda*	1 Pudding/46g	132	5.1	287	9.2	3.6	11	3

Y

	Measure INFO/WEIGHT	per Measure KCAL	per Measure FAT	Nutrition Values per 100g / 100ml KCAL	PROT	CARB	FAT	FIBRE
YORKSHIRE PUDDING								
Beef Dripping, Oven Baked, Luxury, Iceland*	1 Yorkshire/44g	122	5.3	276	10.1	30.8	12	2.4
Beef, Mini, Waitrose*	1 Pudding/14g	33	1.3	234	13.5	23.2	9.4	1.3
Carvery, Aunt Bessie's*	1 Pudding/57g	140	4.2	244	9.1	34	7.3	3.3
Chicken, with Potatoes, Stuffing, & Chipolatas, M&S*	1 Serving/365g	646	31.4	177	9.5	14.7	8.6	1.2
Extra Large, Aunt Bessie's*	1 Yorkshire/42g	113	3.6	266	8.2	39	8.4	1.5
Frozen, Oven Baked, Tesco*	1 Pudding/27g	79	2.8	294	11.9	36.2	10.4	4.2
Frozen, Ovenbaked, Iceland*	1 Pudding/20g	53	1.8	262	7.4	36.8	8.8	3.1
Giant, Aunt Bessie's*	1 Pudding/97g	260	7.5	269	8.6	42	7.8	2.6
Mini, Co-Op*	1 Pudding/16g	50	2	312	6.2	43.8	12.5	2.5
Mini, Farmfoods*	1 Pudding/3g	8	0.2	281	9.6	43.2	7.7	1.9
Original, Golden, As Consumed, Aunt Bessie's*	1 Pudding/19g	53	1.6	279	8.4	41.6	8.4	2.6
with Chicken, & Pigs in Blankets, Filled, Morrisons*	1 Pack/375g	578	21	154	8.1	16.8	5.6	1.7
YULE LOG								
Chocolate, Belgian, Finest, Tesco*	1 Slice/93g	294	14.6	316	4.7	38.2	15.7	1.8
Chocolate, Festive Food To Order, Tesco *	1 Serving/76g	261	11.1	343	5.7	46.4	14.6	1.8
Chocolate, Frozen, Tesco*	1 Slice/80g	251	14.6	315	7.5	28.8	18.3	2.3
Chocolate, Sainsbury's*	1 Slice/35g	153	7.7	432	5	51.6	21.8	4.6
Chocolate, Tesco*	1 Slice/30g	133	6.7	439	5.3	52.6	22.2	3.6
Mini, M&S*	1 Cake/36g	165	8.4	460	5.7	56.9	23.3	1.1

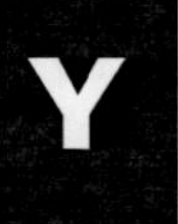

	KCAL
ALL BAR ONE	
BEEF	
Steak, & Frites	1089
Steak, Ribeye, 8oz, with Peppercorn Sauce, & Fries	1069
BEETROOT	
Carpaccio	313
BREAD	
Rustic, with Olive Oil	711
BREAKFAST	
Vegan	745
Vegetarian	801
Vegetarian, Sm Appetites	499
BREAKFAST - FULL ENGLISH	
& Toasted Sourdough	1098
with Spinach & Potato Hash, & Toasted Sourdough	1419
Sausage, Egg, Beans, & Toast, Sm Appetites	629
BREAKFAST - POT	
Chorizo, Egg	610
Egg, Protein	725
BREAKFAST - PROTEIN POWER UP	
Salmon, Egg, Avocado, & Grapefruit, with Salad	372
BREAKFAST - SHAKSHUKA	
Standard	589
with Avocado	1017
with Halloumi	1017
with Sourdough	748
with Streaky Bacon	702
BREAKFAST CEREAL	
Bircher, Blueberry	528
BROWNIES	
Chocolate, with Bourbon Vanilla Ice Cream	582
Chocolate, with Vanilla Ice Cream, Sm Appetites	389
BRUSCHETTA	
Avocado, & Tomato, Crushed	545
BURGERS	
Beef, Bacon & Cheese	921
Beef, Classic	543
Beef, Dirty	914
Beef, Sliders, Sm Appetites	445
Beef, The Californian	1267
Beef, The French	1166
Beef, The Hipster	1243
Beef, The Skinny	549
Beef, The Smoky	1399
Beef, The Spanish	1205
Beef, The Wagyu	1403
Chicken, Grilled, Classic	496
BURGERS VEGAN	
Plant Based	755
BURGERS VEGETARIAN	
Tomato, Beetroot, & Mozzarella	905
Tomato, Beetroot, & Mozzarella, The Californian	1205
Tomato, Beetroot, & Mozzarella, The French	1104
Tomato, Beetroot, & Mozzarella, The Hipster	1181

	KCAL
ALL BAR ONE	
BURGERS VEGETARIAN	
Tomato, Beetroot, & Mozzarella, The Skinny	487
Tomato, Beetroot, & Mozzarella, The Smoky	1337
Tomato, Beetroot, & Mozzarella, The Spanish	1144
BURRITO	
Chicken	776
Chicken, with Fries	1179
Chicken, with House Salad	967
CAKE	
Chocolate, Mascarpone, & Orange, Mousse	250
Raspberry, & Pistachio, Traybake	150
CHEESECAKE	
Biscoff, with Banana, & Caramel	849
Lemon, Sicilian, with Blueberry Compote, Baked	558
CHICKEN	
Katsu, Main	702
Piri Piri, Half	450
Piri Piri, Half, with Fries	853
Piri Piri, Half, with House Salad	641
Karaage, Sticky, Bites	477
Schnitzel, with Fries, & Garlic Cream	694
Skewers, Teriyaki, Ginger	335
Wings, BBQ	586
Wings, Buttermilk	657
CROISSANT	
with Butter, & Jam	661
DOUGHNUTS	
Churros	582
DUMPLINGS	
Duck, Crispy	400
EGGS	
Benedict, Standard	750
Benedict, with Avocado	1178
Florentine, Standard	748
Florentine, with Avocado	1176
Poached, with Mushrooms, on Toasted Sourdough	461
Royale, Standard	824
Royale, with Avocado	1252
Scrambled, & Salmon, on Toasted Sourdough	722
FISH	
Cod, & Mushy Peas, & Tartare Sauce, Sm Appetites	301
Goujons, with Aioli	349
Goujons, with Tartare Sauce, Sm Appetites	278
FISH & CHIPS	
Main	758
FISH CAKES	
Haddock, Smoked, & Mustard	291
Haddock, Smoked, & Mustard, with Fries	694
Haddock, Smoked, & Mustard, with House Salad	482
FLATBREAD	
Garlic, Stonebaked	1054
Houmous, & Kale	615

ALL BAR ONE	KCAL
FRIES	
Halloumi, Standard	460
Potato, Standard	399
Potato, Sm Appetites	177
Potato, with Parmesan, Truffle Oil, & Rosemary	482
Potato, with Smoked Paprika & Saffron Aioli	482
Trio, Standard	1125
FRUIT	
Strawberries, & Bananas, Fresh, Sm Appetites	253
HASH	
Potato, Spinach, & Onion, Pan Fried	582
HOUMOUS	
Duo	715
ICE CREAM	
Trio	318
Vanilla, 2 Scoops, Sm Appetites	244
KEBAB	
Chorizo, & Halloumi, Skewers	601
LAMB	
Kibbeh	553
LASAGNE	
Plant Based	747
MACARONI CHEESE	
Main	430
MEATBALLS	
Lamb, Spiced	499
MELT	
Chicken, BBQ, Bacon, & Cheese	774
MEZZE	
Little, Sm Appetites	738
MUFFIN	
Blueberry	547
Blueberry Cheesecake	463
Carrot Cake	459
Chocolate, Triple	505
Lemon, & White Chocolate	462
NACHOS	
Original	997
Vegan	831
with BBQ Pulled Pork	1425
NOODLES	
Pad Thai	606
Pad Thai, Little, Sm Appetites	313
Pad Thai, with Chicken Breast	808
Pad Thai, with Pan Fried King Prawns	703
Pad Thai, with Sliced Beef Fillet	775
PAIN AU CHOCOLAT	
Pastry	425
PANCAKES - BUTTERMILK	
with Maple Syrup, Banana, & Berries	491
with Maple Syrup, & Smoked Bacon	568
PASTRY	
Spinach & Feta, Bourek	303

ALL BAR ONE	KCAL
PIE	
Pecan, Bourbon, with Cinnamon Ice Cream	540
PLATTER	
Brunch Board, for Two, Breakfast, Ã,½ Board	1137
Deli Board, Sharing, Whole Board	1826
Grazing Board, Sharing, Whole Board	2170
Mezze Board, Sharing, Whole Board	2016
POTATOES	
Patatas Bravas	283
PRAWN CRACKERS	
Portion	58
PRAWNS	
King, Pan Fried, Add On	104
King, Pan Fried	292
QUESADILLA	
Chicken	514
Lentil, & Chickpea	460
RIBS	
BBQ, Smoked	1494
RICE	
Miso, Bowl	474
Miso, Bowl, with Chicken Breast	670
Miso, Bowl, with Pan Fried King Prawns	585
Miso, Bowl, with Sliced Beef Fillet	726
Steamed, Sm Appetites	179
ROLL	
Bacon, Sour Cream, Chilli Tomato Jam, & Coriander	716
SALAD	
Chicken, & Avocado, Chargrilled	905
Chicken, & Avocado, Chargrilled, Sm Appetites	427
Duck, Crispy	568
Feta, Beetroot, & Walnut	509
Feta, Carrot, & Quinoa	626
House	202
Rocket, & Parmesan	234
Side	202
Small Appetites	96
Superfood	440
Superfood, with Chicken Breast	634
Superfood, with Garlic & Lemon Marinated Halloumi	634
Superfood, with Pan Fried King Prawns	654
SANDWICH	
Bacon, with Sliced Tomatoes, & Tomato Sauce	670
Chicken, Grilled, Focaccia	610
Club	1454
Sausage	939
Sausage, Veggie	685
Steak, Fillet	606
SAUCE	
Katsu Curry	156
SAUSAGE	
Cocktail, Maple Glazed	572

	KCAL
ALL BAR ONE	
SORBET	
Raspberry, 2 Scoops, Sm Appetites	255
Raspberry	546
SOUP	
Tomato, Vegetable, & Quinoa	122
SQUID	
Calamari, Salt & Pepper	404
TACO	
Chilli Non Carne	503
TOAST	
Sourdough, with Avocado, & Feta	732
TORTE	
Chocolate, Salted Caramel, with Hazelnut Ice Cream	535
TORTILLA	
Huevos Rancheros	585
VEGETABLES	
Tempura	351
WAFFLES	
Belgian, with Maple Syrup, Fruit, & Yoghurt	1028
WRAP	
Fish Finger	534

	KCAL
ASK ITALIAN	
ANTIPASTO	
The Mixed One, Classico	6479
ARANCINI	
Spinach & Ricotta, with Tomato Dip	387
BEEF	
in Chianti Sauce, Slow Cooked	876
BREAD	
Garlic	588
Garlic, with Mozzarella	784
Rosemary, & Olive Oil	499
BREADSTICKS	
& Tomato, Dip, Little Tums, Kids Menu	159
BROCCOLI	
Side, Kids Menu	13
BRUSCHETTA	
BLANK	365
CALZONE	
Con Carne Piccante	970
Goats Cheese, & Spinach	991
Pollo	899
CANNELLONI	
Sausage, Ragu, Baked, with Creme Fraiche	658
CARBONARA	
Asparagus & Pancetta, Fresca	882
Asparagus & Pancetta, Light, with Salad	541
Linguine	814
CHEESE	
Fonduta, with Dough Sticks	864
CHEESECAKE	
Honeycomb. with Vanilla Gelato	719
Passion Fruit, & Raspberry	481
CHICKEN	
with Tomato Dip, & Garlic Mayo, Lecca-Lecca	675
Pollo, Milanese	753
Pollo, Milanese, with Chips	1009
CHIPS	
Garlic, & Cheese, Side	892
with Mayo, Side	863
COURGETTE	
Zucchine Fritti	328
DESSERT	
Chocolate Etna	851
Gelato, Warm Cookie, & Salted Caramel	968
Gelato Gondola, Salted Caramel	516
DESSERT PIZZA	
Chocolate, Kids Menu	160
DESSERT RAVIOLI	
Rhubarb & Custard	445
DOUGH BALLS	
Cheese, Fontal, & Chilli	711
Plain	550
FETTUCCINE	
Bolognese	692

	KCAL
ASK ITALIAN	
FETTUCCINE	
Con Melanzane, Vegan	843
Con Verdure, Vegan	1042
FRIES	
Sweet Potato, Rosemary	300
FRUIT MIX	
Kids Menu	14
GIRASOLE	
Spinach, & Ricotta	743
GNOCCHI	
Chocolate, Baked	473
ICE CREAM	
Gelato, Chocolate, 3 Scoops	268
Gelato, Hazelnut, 3 Scoops	332
Gelato, Salted Caramel, 3 Scoops	308
Gelato, Vanilla, 3 Scoops	283
ICE LOLLY	
Apple, & Raspberry, Kids Menu	43
Orange, & Apple, Kids Menu	45
LASAGNE	
Beef, & Pork, Ragu	717
Grande	1021
LINGUINE	
Seafood, Con Frutti Di Mare	828
MEATBALLS	
Pork, & Beef, Picante, in Spicy, Tomato Sauce	718
MUSHROOMS	
Al Forno	540
OLIVES	
Italian	204
PANNA COTTA	
Portion	191
PASTA	
Crab & Ricotta, Half Moon	692
in Tomato Sauce, Little Tums, Kids Menu	201
King Prawn, & Crayfish, Fresca	708
Sausage, & Truffle Infused Olive Oil, Fresca	940
with Butter, Little Tums, Kids Menu	245
PASTA SAUCE	
Bolognese, Choose Your Favourite, Kids Menu	137
Cheese, Choose Your Favourite, Kids Menu	217
Tomato, Choose Your Favourite, Kids Menu	109
PENNE	
Arrabiata	759
Arrabiata, with Chicken	869
Beef, Meatballs, Ragu, Mozzarella, Manzo Piccante	718
Chicken, Al Pollo Della Casa	842
Plain, Choose Your Favourite, Kids Menu	346
PIZZA	
Caprina, Light, Prima (Pizza Only)	382
Caprina, Prima	863
Fiorentina, Two Egg, Prima	903
Margherita, Classic	733

	KCAL
ASK ITALIAN	
PIZZA	
Margherita, Four Cheese	738
Margherita, No Topping, Kids Menu	423
Margherita, Vegan, Prima	535
Pollo E Funghi, Classic	764
Pollo Picante Con Pancetta, Light, Prima (Pizza Only)	435
Pollo Picante Con Pancetta, Prima	914
Salami, Misti, Prima	1011
Salsiccia, Sausage, Spicy, Prima	1116
Stromboli, Classic	881
Super Green, Prima	691
Verdure, Classic	793
PIZZA TOPPING	
Cheese, Extra, Top Your Own, Kids Menu	158
Chicken, Top Your Own, Kids Menu	44
Ham, Top Your Own, Kids Menu	34
Mushrooms, Top Your Own, Kids Menu	14
Olives, Black, Top Your Own, Kids Menu	13
Pepperoni, Top Your Own, Kids Menu	93
Red Peppers, Roasted, Top Your Own, Kids Menu	8
PORK	
Belly, Porchetta	1143
PRAWNS	
King, Butterfly, Light	114
King, Butterfly, on Italian Bread	416
PROFITEROLES	
Ice Cream, Chocolate Sauce	325
RAVIOLI	
Beef, & Chianti	728
Ravioli, Four Cheese, & Beef Ragu	571
RISOTTO	
Con Pollo E Funghi	818
SALAD	
Caesar, Chicken, Kale	571
Cheese, Burrata, Tomatoes, Rocket, Caprese	303
Insalata Di Pollo E Pancetta	743
Mixed, Side	18
Rainbow, Side	66
Rainbow, Vegan	243
Side, Kids Menu	44
SEA BASS	
Al Forno	465
SNACKS	
Nibbles, Spicy	167
SORBET	
Sorbetti, Mango, 3 Scoops	154
Sorbetti, Raspberry, 3 Scoops	196
SOUFFLE	
Cheese, Twice Baked	376
SPAGHETTI	
Al Pomodoro	672
Lentil, Ragu, Vegan	849
Plain, Choose Your Favourite, Kids Menu	346

	KCAL
ASK ITALIAN	
SPAGHETTI	
Pomodoro, Vegan	765
SQUID	
Calamari, Breaded	476
SUNDAE	
Ice Cream, Chocolate, Make Your Own, Kids Menu	89
Ice Cream, Vanilla, Make Your Own, Kids Menu	94
TAGLIATELLE	
Pesto, Genovese, Purple	926
Pesto, Genovese, Purple, Light, with Salad	486
TART	
Chocolate, & Blood Orange	310
Pear	333
TIRAMISU	
Portion	419
TOMATOES	
Plum, Side, Kids Menu	4
TOPPING	
Grapes, Make Your Own Sundae	8
Marshmallow & Sprinkles, Make your Own Sundae	25
Meringue, Plain, Make Your Own Sundae,	40
Strawberries, Make Your Own Sundae	8
White Chocolate Swirl, Make Your Own Sundae	55
TORTELLINI	
Cheese, & Vegetable, Dip & Tip	281
VEGETABLES	
Sticks, with Bread, & Dip, Kids Menu	175
WHITEBAIT	
Breaded	683

	KCAL
BEEFEATER RESTAURANT	
BEANS	
Baked, in Tomato Sauce, Side, Kids Menu	51
BBQ, Spiced, Side	157
BEEF	
Duo	1437
Slow Cooked, Kids, Sunday Lunch Menu	697
Slow Cooked, Sunday Lunch Menu	1351
Steak, & Frites	686
Steak, & Frites, Daytime Saver	629
Steak, Fillet, 8oz, & Chips	813
Steak, Fillet, 8oz, & Chips, & Salad	831
Steak, Fillet, 8oz, & Side Salad	461
Steak, Fillet, 8oz, with Veg Medley	505
Steak, Flat Iron, 6oz, & Chips	747
Steak, Flat Iron, 6oz, & Chips, & Salad	765
Steak, Flat Iron, 6oz, & Side Salad	395
Steak, Flat Iron, 6oz, with Veg Medley	439
Steak, Porterhouse, 18oz, & Chips	1503
Steak, Porterhouse, 18oz, & Chips, & Salad	1521
Steak, Porterhouse, 18oz, & Side Salad	1151
Steak, Porterhouse, 18oz, with Veg Medley	1197
Steak, Rib-eye, 10oz, & Chips	988
Steak, Rib-eye, 10oz, & Chips, & Salad	993
Steak, Rib-eye, 10oz, & Side Salad	624
Steak, Rib-eye, 10oz, with Veg Medley	668
Steak, Ribs, & Prawn, Combo	1720
Steak, Rump, 10oz, & Chips	941
Steak, Rump, 10oz, & Chips, & Peas, Daytime Saver	844
Steak, Rump, 10oz, & Chips, & Salad	966
Steak, Rump, 10oz, & Chips, & Salad, Daytime Saver	832
Steak, Rump, 10oz, with Veg Medley	651
Steak, Rump. 10oz, & Side Salad	595
Steak, Sirloin, 8oz, & Chips	802
Steak, Sirloin, 8oz, & Chips, & Peas, Daytime Saver	705
Steak, Sirloin, 8oz, & Chips, & Salad	808
Steak, Sirloin, 8oz, & Chips, & Salad, Daytime Saver	693
Steak, Sirloin, 8oz, & Salad	437
Steak, Sirloin, 8oz, with Veg Medley	482
Steak, with Chips, Kids Menu	461
BREAD	
Brown, Buttered, Extra	257
Flatbread, Garlic, & Dips	912
Flatbread, Garlic, Strips	1013
Garlic	218
Garlic, Kids Menu	112
White, Buttered, Extra	254
BROWNIES	
Chocolate	555
Chocolate, Daytime Saver Menu	555
BURGERS	
Beef, Bacon & Cheese, Triple	1697
Beef, Kids Menu	587
Steak, Daytime Saver Menu	863

BEEFEATER RESTAURANT	KCAL
BURGERS	
Steak, Double, Daytime Saver Menu	1152
Steak, with Cheese & Bacon, Daytime Saver Menu	1080
Beef, Bacon & Cheese, Double	1530
Steak, with Cheese & Bacon	1187
Chicken, Tabasco, Crispy	1059
Steak, Smoky BBQ, Summer BBQ Specials	1463
BURGERS VEGAN	
with BBQ Pulled Soya	938
BURGERS VEGETARIAN	
Main	910
CAKE	
Trio of Sponges, with Custard	695
CAULIFLOWER CHEESE	
Sunday Lunch Menu	283
CHEESE	
Halloumi, Battered, & Chips, Daytime Saver Menu	983
CHEESECAKE	
Vanilla, Baked	675
CHICKEN	
BBQ, with Half Rack Of Ribs	1025
BBQ, with Whole Rack Of Ribs	1432
Breast, Kids, Sunday Lunch Menu	453
Breast, Plain	693
Breast, Smoky Paprika, Grilled	729
Breast, Smoky Paprika, Grilled, Daytime Saver Menu	578
Escalope, Breast, Breaded	1309
Goujons, Buttermilk, Summer BBQ Specials	742
Half, Roasted, Sunday Lunch Menu	1486
Melt, BBQ Sauce, Grilled	858
Poppin, with Chips, & Beans, Kids Menu	400
Wings, with BBQ, Spicy, 3, Side	160
Wings, with BBQ, Crispy, 5	260
Wings, with BBQ, Crispy, 8	401
Wings, with Piri Piri, Crispy, 5	252
Wings, with Piri Piri, Crispy, 8	394
Wings, with Piri Piri, Spicy, 3, Side	153
CHIPS	
Cheesy, & Gravy	726
Side, Kids Menu	187
Triple Cooked, Side	418
Triple Cooked, Spicy, Side	420
COD	
Bites, Breaded, Kids Menu	517
CORN	
Cob, Mini, Side	61
Cob, Mini, Side, Kids Menu	29
CRUMBLE	
Apple, Toffee, Salted	596
DESSERT	
Caramel Apple Betty, with Custard	496
Caramel Apple Betty, with Ice Cream	462

BEEFEATER RESTAURANT	KCAL
DESSERT	
Caramel Apple Betty, with Pouring Cream	531
Caramel Apple Betty, with Whipped Cream	455
Chocolate Challenge, Mini, Kids Menu	342
Mississippi Mud Pie	991
DOUGHNUTS	
Mini, Kids Menu	249
FISH & CHIPS	
Beer Battered, Daytime Saver Menu	886
FRIES	
Potato, Skinny, Side	328
Potato, Skinny, Spicy, Side	329
FROZEN YOGHURT	
Strawberry	235
Strawberry, Kids Menu	197
FRUIT SALAD	
Mixed, Kids Menu	49
GAMMON	
Blackened, with Egg, Daytime Saver Menu	751
Blackened, with Pineapple, Daytime Saver Menu	729
Steak, Blackened, in Spicy Rub	1034
Steak, Chargrilled, with Egg & Pineapple	1026
Steak, with Egg, Daytime Saver Menu	746
Steak, with Pineapple, Daytime Saver Menu	723
HADDOCK - BEER BATTERED	
with Chips, Ultimate, Daytime Saver Menu	920
with Chips & Mushy Peas	958
with Chips & Peas	920
ICE CREAM	
Vanilla, with Caramel Sauce, Kids Menu	254
Vanilla, with Chocolate Sauce, Kids Menu	253
Vanilla, with Raspberry Sauce, Kids Menu	253
with Chocolate Sauce	279
with Chocolate Sauce, Sunday Lunch Menu	275
KEBAB	
Pork & Beef, Kofta, Grilled	444
LAMB	
Rump, Minted, Grilled	720
Rump, Sunday Lunch Menu	1270
LASAGNE	
Beef & Pork, with Chips, Daytime Saver	872
Beef & Pork, with Salad, Daytime Saver	595
Sweet Potato & Feta, with Chips	975
Sweet Potato & Feta, with Chips, Daytime Saver	937
Sweet Potato & Feta, with Salad	697
Sweet Potato & Feta, with Salad, Daytime Saver	659
LINGUINE	
Roast Vegetable, in Tomato Sauce	563
Roast Vegetable, In Tomato Sauce, with Chicken	718
Roast Vegetable, in Tomato Sauce, with Salmon	1010
MACARONI CHEESE	
Daytime Saver Menu	888

	KCAL
BEEFEATER RESTAURANT	
MAKHANI	
Chicken, Daytime Saver Menu	998
MEATBALLS	
Arrabiata, Linguine	821
MIXED GRILL	
Rump Steak, Chicken Breast, Gammon, Sausage	1741
Flat Iron Steak, Chicken Breast, Gammon, Sausage	1498
Sirloin Steak, Chicken Breast, Gammon, Sausage	1583
MUSHROOMS	
Crispy, Flat Cap, in Breadcrumbs	489
NACHOS	
with Cheesy Yoghurt Dip, Kids Menu	235
ONION RINGS	
Beer Battered, Crispy, Side	221
PASTA	
Penne, in Tomato Sauce, Kids Menu	347
PATE	
Duck, with Ciabatta	430
PEAS	
Side, Kids Menu	47
PIE	
Banoffee	701
Beef, & Cheddar, with Mash & Gravy	1397
Chicken & Ham, Daytime Saver Menu	1114
PLATTER	
The Beefeater, Sharing	700
The Beefeater, with Ribs, Sharing	904
POTATO MASH	
Side, Kids Menu	131
POTATOES	
Crushed, Garlic, Side	344
Dauphinoise, Sunday Lunch Menu	320
Dippers, With Cheese, & Bacon, Loaded	587
Dippers, with Cheese, Loaded	492
Dippers, with Cheese, Sharing	1262
Dippers, with Cheese & Spring Onion, Loaded	517
Jacket, Side	438
PRAWN COCKTAIL	
Classic, with Ciabatta	340
PRAWNS	
Garlic, with Ciabatta	371
King, Garlic, 3, Side	151
PROFITEROLES	
Main Menu	465
Daytime Saver Menu	465
PUDDING	
Apple Crisp	299
RIBS - BBQ	
Sticky, Summer BBQ Specials	451
Half Rack, & Chips, Daytime Saver Menu	946
Sticky Bourbon, Grill	1320
RISOTTO	
Chicken, & Mushroom, Creamy	833

	KCAL
BEEFEATER RESTAURANT	
RISOTTO	
Chicken, & Mushroom, Daytime Saver Menu	831
Mushroom, Creamy	678
Mushroom, Daytime Saver Menu	676
BLT, with Egg, Daytime Saver Menu	328
SALAD	
Caesar, Chicken, Goujons, Summer BBQ Specials	986
Caesar, Chicken, Grilled, Daytime Saver Menu	463
Caesar, Salmon, Blackened, Summer BBQ Specials	1076
Caesar, Summer BBQ Specials	421
Chicken, Jerk, Mango, Summer BBQ Specials	323
Chunky Slaw, Side	149
Greek, Crunchy, Side	173
Halloumi, Jerk, Mango, Summer BBQ Specials	421
Mixed, Large, Side	68
Mixed Bean	604
Salmon, Jerk, Mango, Summer BBQ Specials	621
Side, Kids Menu	6
Steak, with Pear	778
SALMON	
Grilled	1014
SANDWICH	
Chicken Goujons, Buttermilk, Daytime Saver Menu	1054
Steak, Open, with Fries, Daytime Saver Menu	986
SAUCE	
Bearnaise, Steak Sauces	135
Beef, Rich, Steak Sauces	42
Cheddar, Pulled Ham, & Mushroom, Steak Sauces	98
Peppercorn, Triple, Steak Sauces	41
Prawn & Lobster, Steak Sauces	67
SAUSAGE & MASH	
Bangers, Kids Menu	391
Main	902
Quorn	729
Vegetarian, Bangers, Kids Menu	361
SEA BASS	
Oven Baked, with Crunchy Greek Salad	451
SORBET	
Lemon Curd	242
SOUP	
Tomato	351
SPAGHETTI BOLOGNESE	
Kids Menu	345
SPINACH	
Creamy, Side	123
SUNDAE	
Cookie Dough	694
Funny Face, Kids Menu	265
Rocky Road	688
TRIFLE	
Strawberry, Pimms, Summer BBQ Specials	699
VEGETABLES	
Medley, Side	112

	KCAL
BEEFEATER RESTAURANT	
VEGETABLES	
Sticks, Side, Kids Menu	28
Sticks, with Yoghurt Dip	51
WAFFLES	
Apple, Salted, Toffee, Summer BBQ Specials	881
WELLINGTON	
Vegetable, Sunday Lunch Menu	1646
WRAP	
Chicken Breast, Cheese, Vegetables, Kids Menu	540
Quorn Sausage, Cheese, Vegetables, Kids Menu	540
Salmon, Cheese, Vegetables, Kids Menu	605
YOGHURT	
Strawberry, Kids Menu	127

	KCAL
BELLA ITALIA	
ANTIPASTI	
Board, Starter	806
ARANCINI	
Starter	477
BEANS	
Green, Side	42
BEEF - STEAK	
Sirloin, with Chips	1453
Sirloin, with Salad	525
BOLOGNESE	
Penne, GF	756
Penne, GF, Vegan	944
Spaghetti	688
Spaghetti, Vegan	668
BREAD	
Pane Bella	801
BROWNIES	
Chocolate	396
BRUSCHETTA	
GF, with Tomatoes, & Red Onion, Starter	343
with Tomatoes, & Red Onion, Starter	674
BURGERS	
Americano, GF	664
Bean, Cannellini, No Sides	593
Beef, Black Angus, No Sides	664
Chicken, Pollo, No Sides	659
Vegan, No Sides	472
CALZONE	
Carne	1102
Diavola	1162
Verdure, Pesto	1312
CARBONARA	
Main	792
GF	1035
CHEESE	
Goats, Extra	120
Mozzarella, Carrozza, Starter	849
CHEESECAKE	
Strawberry	675
CHICKEN	
Breast, Grilled, with Fries	1284
Breast, Grilled, with Salad	356
Breast, Grilled, with Salad, GF	737
Extra	168
Half, Barbecue, Fries, Onion Rings, & Coleslaw	1579
Half, Piri Piri, Fries, Onion Rings, & Coleslaw	1634
Half, Sweet & Sour, Fries, Onion Rings, & Coleslaw	3019
Pollo, Lenticchie, Lighter	335
Pollo Funghi	681
Pollo Milanese	848
Wings, Barbecue	372
Wings, Piri Piri	434
Wings, Sweet & Sour	469

BELLA ITALIA	KCAL
COLESLAW	
Side	109
DESSERT	
Cookie Dough, Al Forno	867
Cookie Dough, Vegan, Al Forno	864
Dolcetti, Sharing	956
DOUGH BALLS	
Bites, with Basil Pesto	520
Bites, with Garlic & Rosemary Dip	473
DOUGHNUTS	
with Chocolate Sauce, Mini	516
FLATBREAD	
GF, with Caramelised Onion, Vegan	915
GF, with Garlic Butter	677
GF, with Mozzarella, & Garlic Butter	867
GF, with Pomodoro, & Pesto	611
GF, with Sausage, 'Nduja, & Mozzarella	657
with Garlic Butter	723
with Mozzarella, & Garlic Butter	907
with Onion, Caramelised, & Mozzarella	976
with Pomodoro, & Pesto	732
with Sausage, 'Nduja, & Mozzarella	808
FRIES	
Potato, Side	1116
Potato, Side	458
Sweet Potato, Side	335
ICE CREAM	
Bubblegum	292
Cherry, Amarena	347
Chocolate Chip	305
Hazelnut	291
Honeycomb	335
Limoncello	209
Mint Chocolate Chip	332
Raspberry	118
Strawberry	205
Vanilla	258
LASAGNE	
Traditional, Al Forno	836
MEATBALLS	
Pork, & Beef, Polpette, Starter	511
Vegan, GF, Polpette, Starter	316
Vegan, Polpette, Starter	454
MUSHROOMS	
Funghi, Arrosto, GF, Starter	332
Funghi, Arrosto, Starter	440
OLIVES	
Sicilain	196
ONION RINGS	
Side	667
PANNA COTTA	
Coconut	378

BELLA ITALIA	KCAL
PASTA	
Bolognese Spirali, Lighter	283
Cacio E Pepe	1193
Cacio E Pepe, GF	1476
Calabrese	774
Calabrese, GF	1388
Carne Festa, Al Forno	1029
Gamberoni Spirali, Lighter	259
Lenticchie Spirali, Lighter	299
Marco Polo	1006
Marco Polo, GF	1070
Marco Polo, Vegan, & GF	1093
Marco Polo, Vegan	1002
Penne, Pomodoro, GF	423
Pollo Alla Crema, Al Forno	1043
Pollo Pesto	1037
Pollo Pesto, GF	1205
Pollo Pesto, Vegan, & GF	1089
Pollo Pesto, Vegan	1318
Pomodoro Rustica	574
PIZZA	
Campagna, Standard	869
Campagna, GF	1029
Campagna, Ripiena Crust	1461
Campagna, Roma	869
Carne Mista, Standard	1006
Carne Mista, GF	1171
Carne Mista, Ripiena Crust	1541
Carne Mista, Roma	1006
Cotto, Standard	801
Cotto, GF	873
Cotto, Ripiena Crust	1233
Cotto, Roma	801
Diavola Forte, Standard	1255
Diavola Forte, GF	1523
Diavola Forte, Ripiena Crust	1871
Diavola Forte, Roma	1255
Funghi Luganica, Standard	1404
Funghi Luganica, GF	1454
Funghi Luganica, Ripiena Crust	1788
Funghi Luganica, Roma	1435
Gamberoni, Standard	895
Gamberoni, GF	1065
Gamberoni, Ripiena Crust	1289
Gamberoni, Roma	910
Margherita, Standard	764
Margherita, GF	911
Margherita, Ripiena Crust	1187
Margherita, Roma	764
Vegan Cheese, Standard	931
Milli Colori, Lighter	525
Parma Bufala, Standard	1039
Parma Bufala, GF	1334

BELLA ITALIA	KCAL
PIZZA	
Parma Bufala, Ripiena Crust	1388
Parma Bufala, Roma	1110
Pepperoni Piccante, Standard	963
Pepperoni Piccante, Roma	963
Pepperoni Piccante, GF	1065
Pepperoni Piccante, Ripiena Crust	1408
Pollo, Barbecue, Standard	979
Pollo, Barbecue, GF	1167
Pollo, Barbecue, Ripiena Crust	1596
Pollo, Barbecue, Roma	979
Pollo, Sapori, Lighter	533
Pollo, Vesuvio, Standard	924
Pollo, Vesuvio, GF	1144
Pollo, Vesuvio, Ripiena Crust	1311
Pollo, Vesuvio, Roma	924
Margherita, Queen, Standard	1085
Margherita, Queen, GF	989
Margherita, Queen, Ripiena Crust	1514
Margherita, Queen, Roma	1085
Barbecue, Vegan, Standard	930
Barbecue, Vegan, GF	987
Barbecue, Vegan, Roma	930
PIZZA BASE	
Create Your Own	832
GF, Create Your Own	726
Ripiena, Create Your Own	1328
Roma, Create Your Own	844
Vegan, GF, Create Your Own	935
PIZZA TOPPING	
Black Olives	30
Chicken	358
Cotto Ham	112
Goats Cheese	155
Green Chilli	4
Mozzarella, Buffalo	106
Mushrooms, Garlic	48
Pancetta	68
Pepperoni	127
Red Onion	42
Roast Peppers	55
Rocket	1
Salami	64
Sausage, 'Nduja	146
Sausage, Luganica	101
Spinach	6
Spring Onion	12
Tuna	66
POTATOES	
New, Crushed, with Spring Onions, Side	249
PRAWNS	
King, Gamberi, GF, Starter	332
King, Gamberi, Starter	303

BELLA ITALIA	KCAL
RIBS - RACK, BARBECUE	
& Chicken, Half, with Coleslaw, Onion Rings, & Fries	1391
Slow Roasted, with Coleslaw, Onion Rings, & Fries	1609
RIBS - RACK, PIRI PIRI	
& Chicken, Half, with Coleslaw, Onion Rings, & Fries	1352
Slow Roasted, with Coleslaw, Onion Rings, & Fries	1532
RIBS - RACK, SWEET & SOUR	
& Chicken, Half, with Coleslaw, Onion Rings, & Fries	2932
Slow Roasted, with Coleslaw, Onion Rings, & Fries	3028
RIGATONI	
Funghi Crema	654
Funghi Crema, GF	896
RISOTTO	
Pescatore	570
Pollo Funghi	620
Verdura	560
SALAD	
Insalata Caesar	432
Insalata Caesar, with Pollo, & Pancetta	561
Insalata Caprese, Starter	339
Insalata di Verona	875
Insalata Giardiniera	265
Insalata Parma Bufala	655
Mixed, Side	98
Side	188
SALMON	
Extra	342
Salmone Al Forno	906
Salmone Al Forno, GF	946
SAUCE	
Garlic Butter, Steak Sauce	65
Mushroom, Creamy, Steak Sauce	226
Peppercorn, Steak Sauce	83
SOUP	
Seasonal, GF, Starter	294
Seasonal, Starter	410
SPAGHETTI	
Gamberoni, Arrabiata	692
Gamberoni, Arrabiata, GF	526
Marinara	653
Marinara, GF	965
SPAGHETTI & MEATBALLS	
Polpette American, Vegan	797
Polpette Americano	760
SQUID	
Calamari, Starter	282
SUNDAE	
Banoffee	1192
Eton Mess	499
Rocky Road	1023
TAGLIATELLE	
Capra	906
Capra, GF	908

	KCAL
BELLA ITALIA	
TIRAMISU	
Portion	463
TOPPING	
Banana	79
Biscuits, Amaretti	45
Chocolate Tagliatelle	40
Ice Cream Cone, Crushed	39
Marshmallows	33
Popping Candy	59
Sprinkles	41
Whipped Cream	92
VEGETABLES	
Mediterranean, Roasted, Side	65

	KCAL
BILL'S	
ASPARAGUS	
& Baby Spinach, Side	154
BEEF - STEAK	
Flat Iron	694
Minute, with Chips, & Egg, & Garlic Butter	968
no Chips, Kids	359
Ribeye, 14oz	650
Sirloin, 10oz	617
with Chips, Kids	534
BREAD	
& Houmous, For 2	392
Basket, with Butters, Ã,½ Basket	730
Basket, without Butters, Whole Basket	956
Flatbread, Smoky, Italian, Ã,½ Bread	333
Focaccia, for Soup	130
Focaccia, with Houmous, & Olives	392
Garlic, & Herb, Flatbread, Ã,½ Bread	290
Sourdough, Rosemary, Pea Houmous, & Garlic	632
Sourdough, Rosemary & Garlic, Grilled, & Eggs	960
Stone Baked, with Balsamic, & Olive Oil, For 2	264
Tortilla, Corn, Spiced, with Guacamole	516
Tortilla, Corn, Spiced, without Guacamole	441
BREAKFAST	
Eggs, Baked, with Spicy Beans, & Chorizo	444
Eggs, Baked, Spicy Beans, & Chorizo, & Flatbread	564
Full English, Brunch, with Toast	1317
Full English, with Toast	887
Full English, Veggie, with Toast	807
Garden, No Hollandaise	707
Garden, Plate, No Hollandaise	951
Kids	558
Vegan, Full	626
BREAKFAST CEREAL	
Porridge, Oat	600
BROCCOLI	
Long Stem, Side	179
BROWNIES	
Chocolate, Warm, no Ice Cream	569
Chocolate, Warm, no Ice Cream, Kids	218
Chocolate, Warm, with Ice Cream	676
Chocolate, Warm, with Ice Cream, Kids	325
BUNS	
Bacon, Breakfast	667
Sausage, Cumberland, Breakfast	563
BURGERS	
Chicken, Buttermilk, no Chipotle Mayo	592
Chicken, Buttermilk, with Chipotle Mayo	822
Chicken, Fillet, Kids	365
Halloumi, with Lime Mayo	939
Halloumi	684
Hamburger	696
Hamburger, with Mayo, Kids	372
Lamb, no Tzatziki	804

	KCAL
BILL'S	
BURGERS	
Lamb, with Tzatziki	833
Naked, with Salad, & Tzatziki, no Bun	525
CAKE	
Carrot, no Whipped Cream	198
Carrot, with Whipped Cream	312
Victoria Sponge	598
CAULIFLOWER CHEESE	
for Two, Ã,½ Portion	119
CHEESE	
Halloumi, Sticks, Crispy, no Lemon Garlic Mayo	578
CHEESECAKE	
Banana, & Honeycomb	827
CHICKEN	
Half, Paprika, Garlic, & Chilli, with Fries	1302
Milanese, with Salad	738
Paillard	596
Pan Fried, with Wild Mushrooms	705
Skewers, Devilled	452
Skewers, Mojo Marinated, no Dressing	1057
Skewers, Mojo Marinated, with Dressing	1154
CHOCOLATES	
Truffles, Salted Caramel, 3 Truffles	168
COD - BEER BATTERED	
with Pea Puree, Tartare Sauce, & Fries	1123
CRAB CAKES	
Baked, with Tartare Sauce	567
Baked, without Tartare Sauce	417
with Egg, & Asparagus	655
CREME BRULEE	
Coconut, & Orange Rice	344
CRUMBLE	
Apple, & Salted Caramel	613
CURRY	
Chicken, Thai Green, with Rice	734
Chicken, Thai Green, without Rice	507
DESSERT	
Chocolate Bombe, Meltin	937
Eton Mess, Mango, & Passion Fruit	477
DHAL - AUBERGINE	
Lentil, & Chickpea, Roasted	543
Lentil, & Chickpea, Roasted, with Flatbread	695
DOUGHNUTS	
Cinnamon, Mini, no Sauce	483
Cinnamon, Mini, Salted Caramel & Chocolate Sauce	649
Strawberry Dusted, Warm	711
DUMPLINGS	
Chicken, Sesame, with Chutney	336
Pork, Sesame, Golden Fried, with Dipping Sauce	451
EGGS	
Benedict, with Hollandaise	468
Benedict, without Hollandaise	244
Florentine, with Hollandaise	680

	KCAL
BILL'S	
EGGS	
Florentine, without Hollandaise	456
on Toast, Kids	337
Royale, with Hollandaise	534
Royale, without Hollandaise	310
Scrambled, on Toast	731
Scrambled, on Toast, with Bacon	745
Scrambled, on Toast, with Salmon	698
FISH FINGERS	
Cod, Kids	271
FRIES	
Potato, Kids, Side	175
Potato, Side	349
Sweet Potato, Side	510
FRUIT	
Strawberries, & Banana, no Sauce, Kids	93
Strawberries, & Banana, Chocolate Sauce, Kids	198
GNOCCHI	
Diablo	928
ICE CREAM	
Vanilla, Kids	107
KALE	
Sauteed	104
MACARONI CHEESE	
Kids	429
with Focaccia	1290
with Mushroom, & Leek	1167
MACARONI CHEESE	
with Side Salad, & Dressing	1269
with Side Salad, No Dressing	1172
without Sides	1160
MASH	
Potato, Side	194
MAYONNAISE	
Chipotle	216
Truffle, Side	347
MERINGUE	
Eton Mess, Lemon	847
MEZZE	
Halloumi, & Houmous, for 4	377
Sharing, for 4, Ã,¼ Mezze	429
Veggie, Sharing, for 4, Ã,¼ Mezze	343
MOUSSE	
Chocolate, & Hazelnut, Kids	202
MUSHROOMS	
Garlic, Sauteed, Chestnut	180
NUTS	
Spiced, & Roasted Corn, For 2	303
OLIVES	
Green, Giant, Gordal	161
OMELETTE	
Summer	488

BILL'S	KCAL
PANCAKES - BUTTERMILK	
Kids	375
with Bacon, & Syrup, 3 Stack	803
with Bacon, & Syrup, 5 Stack	1271
with Banana, Berries, with Syrup, 3 Stack	542
with Banana, Berries, with Syrup, 5 Stack	845
PATE	
Chicken Liver, Oak Smoked, Parfait, with Toast	809
Chicken Liver, Oak Smoked, Parfait, without Toast	528
PIE	
Fish	794
PRAWN COCKTAIL	
BLANK	356
RIBS	
BBQ, Kids	305
Main	791
RISOTTO	
Crab, & Courgette	620
SALAD	
Caesar, Chicken, without Dressing	627
Chicken, with Turmeric, & Freekeh	1292
Feta, Crispy, & Watermelon	425
Glow Bowl	1133
Halloumi, Grilled, & Pesto Toast, with Dressing	706
Halloumi, Grilled, with Dressing	548
Halloumi, Grilled, no Dressing	356
Halloumi, Grilled, & Pesto Toast, no Dressing	514
Kale, Chickpea, & Miso, Houmous	755
Mixed, no Dressing	24
Mixed, with Dressing	121
Rainbow, Side	137
Salmon, Seared	728
Summer	695
Summer, with Flatbread	815
SANDWICH	
Bacon, Kids	512
Fish Finger	884
Sausage, Kids	482
SAUCE	
Bearnaise, for Steak	158
Garlic Butter, for Steak	193
Hollandaise	224
Mushroom, for Steak	69
Peppercorn, for Steak	46
SAUSAGE	
Cumberland, Kids	427
Cumberland, Mini, Glazed	294
SCONE	
Cream Tea, No Clotted Cream	552
Cream Tea, with Clotted Cream	728
with Jam, & Clotted Cream, Warm	709
with Jam, Warm	562

BILL'S	KCAL
SEA BASS	
Pan Fried, with Rosti	523
SOUP	
Pea, & Watercress, without Focaccia	161
Salad, & Half Sandwich	676
Tomato, Roasted, with Cream	209
Tomato, Roasted, with Cream & Pesto Toast	367
Tomato, Roasted, with Pesto Toast	250
Tomato, Roasted, without Cream & Pesto Toast	92
SQUID	
Calamari, Crispy, with lemon Garlic Mayonnaise	624
Calamari, Crispy, without lemon Garlic Mayonnaise	369
SUNDAE	
Granola, Breakfast	467
Banoffee, Melting	658
Ice Cream, Vanilla, Kids	292
TART	
Ricotta, Red Pepper, & Cheddar, no Dressing	664
Ricotta, Red Pepper, & Cheddar, with Dressing	761
TEACAKES	
Toasted, no Butter	267
Toasted, with Butter	527
TOAST	
& Butter, Bloomer	356
with Avocado, & Bacon	687
with Avocado, & Poached Eggs	426
with Avocado, & Salmon	640
with Avocado	497
with Beans, Kids	219
with Butter, Kids	180
TOASTIE	
Ham, & Cheese, Kids	478
TORTILLA CHIPS	
Corn, Crispy, Kids	247
Spiced, For 2	258
WELLINGTON	
Carrot, & Cashew Nut	715
YOGHURT	
Strawberries, Banana, & Honey, Kids	108

	KCAL
BREWERS FAYRE	
BACON	
Back, Rasher, Breakfast	165
BEANS	
Baked, Breakfast	91
Baked, in Tomato Sauce, Side, Kids Menu	51
BEEF	
Steak, Rib-eye, with Hollandaise Sauce	1250
Steak, Rib-eye, with Peppercorn Sauce	1199
Steak, Rump, Grilled	874
Steak, Sirloin, Grilled	886
Steak, & Eggs	1041
Yorkshire, Wrap, with Chips, & Gravy	1129
BHAJI	
Sweet Potato	58
BITES	
Hog Roast, with Apple Sauce	263
Mac 'N' Cheese	442
BREAD	
Flatbread, Garlic	312
Flatbread, Garlic, with Cheese	379
Garlic, Kids Menu	110
Garlic, Side, Kids Menu	106
Garlic, with Cheese, Side	318
BROWNIES	
Chocolate, with Ice Cream	755
BUBBLE & SQUEAK	
Side	348
BURGERS	
Chicken, Breaded, The South Western	925
Beef, Bash Street, Kids Menu	697
Beef, Black & Blue, with Chips	1328
Beef, Cheese, & Mushroom	988
Beef, Cheese, & Mushroom, Double	1308
Beef, Extra	327
Beef, Ultimate, with Chips	1741
Chicken, Extra	211
Cluck 'N' Ale, with Chips	1517
Cluck 'N' Ale, with Sweet Potato Fries	1564
Halloumi, Heaven, with Chips	1136
Halloumi Heaven, with Sweet Potato Fries	1069
The New Yorker	1139
Vegan, with Chips	899
BURRITO	
Bowl, with Salad	555
Chicken, Bowl	710
CAKE	
Chocolate, & Orange, Mousse, Mini	220
Chocolate, Fudge, Luxury	810
CAULIFLOWER CHEESE	
Side	281
CHEESE	
& Bacon, Extra	115
Brie, Breaded, Bites	326

	KCAL
BREWERS FAYRE	
CHEESE	
Halloumi, & Chips, with Mushy Peas	1035
Halloumi, & Chips, with Peas	997
Mozzarella, Sticks, Side	330
CHEESECAKE	
Raspberry, & Prosecco	502
Vanilla, with Blackcurrant & Prosecco Compote	375
CHICKEN	
& Ribs, Combo, Full Rack, Chips, Coleslaw, Salad	1628
& Ribs, Combo, Half Rack, Chips, Coleslaw, & Salad	1248
Bites, Breaded, Kids Menu	525
Bites, Buffalo, Poppin	246
Breast, Garlic, Breaded	1326
Breast, Smoky Paprika, Grilled	430
Smothered, BBQ Sauce,	914
Smothered, BBQ Sauce, Double Up	1271
Smothered, BBQ Sauce, with Mac 'N' Cheese	1213
Buttermilk, & Cheesy Nachos	750
Katsu Curry	1037
Combo	1344
Forestiere, with Crushed Potatoes, & Green Beans	441
Goujons, Combo Feast	1849
Goujons, with Chicken Wings, Combo Feast	2269
Goujons, Southern Fried	406
Half, Roasted, Lemon & Thyme, with Chips	1600
Half, Roasted, with Chips	799
Half, Roasted, BBQ, with Chips	436
Stuffed, Mozzarella, with Bacon, & Chips	886
Stuffed, Mozzarella, with Bacon, & Roast Potatoes	746
Skewers, Honey & Mustard	212
Skewers, Jerk	292
Wings, Buffalo	463
Tikka, with Rice	851
CHILLI	
Bean, Three, with Rice, & Tortilla Chips	537
Beef, Mexican, with Rice	716
CHIPS	
Side	363
Smothered, Creamy Cheese Sauce, Side	551
Smothered, Curry Sauce, Side	467
Smothered, Gravy, Side	436
COD	
Bites, Breaded, Kids Menu	642
Loin, Baked, with Ratatouille, & Roast Potatoes	447
COLESLAW	
Side	138
Side, Kids Menu	40
CORN	
Cob, Mini, Side, Kids Menu	29
CRUMBLE	
Apple, Toffee, Salted	670
DESSERT	
Caramel Apple Betty	496

BREWERS FAYRE	KCAL
DESSERT	
Chocolate, Mini, Mash Up, Kids Menu	344
Dirty Mud Pie	995
Fondue, Chocolate Fudge, Sharing	854
DIP	
Dessicated Coconut	158
DOUGHNUTS	
Cinnamon	547
EGGS	
Breakfast	311
EMPANADAS	
Cheese	401
FISH & CHIPS	
with Mushy Peas	939
with Peas	901
FISH CAKES	
Single	126
FRIES	
Furious, Side	409
Tiger, Side	381
FROZEN YOGHURT	
Strawberry	274
FRUIT SALAD	
Kids Menu	49
GAMMON - STEAK	
With Egg, Grilled	903
with Egg & Pineapple, Grilled	833
with Pineapple, Grilled	764
HADDOCK - BATTERED	
with Chips & Mushy Peas, Atlantic, Giant	1093
with Chips & Peas, Atlantic, Giant	1055
HOT DOG	
The Big Bad Dog, Kids Menu	612
ICE CREAM	
Vanilla, with Caramel Sauce, Kids Menu	259
Vanilla, with Chocolate Sauce, Kids Menu	256
Vanilla, with Raspberry Sauce, Kids Menu	256
LAMB	
Shank, Slow Cooked, in Gravy	760
LASAGNE	
Beef & Pork, Main	580
Beef & Pork, with Side Salad	713
Sweet Potato & Feta, with Side Salad	744
MEATBALLS	
Chicken, Tikka	261
MIXED GRILL	
Flat Iron Steak, Gammon, Chicken, & Sausage	1412
Mediterranean	1355
Mediterranean, with Rice	1199
Rump Steak, Gammon, Chicken, & Sausage	1485
Ultimate, Summer	1781
Ultimate, Summer, with Prawns	1983

BREWERS FAYRE	KCAL
MOUSSE	
Lemon	730
Lemon, Mini	151
MUSHROOMS	
Closed Cup, Breakfast, Brewers Fayre*	169
Garlic, & Herb, Breaded	303
NACHOS	
with Cheesy Yoghurt Dip, Kids Menu	230
ONION RINGS	
Battered, Side	467
PASTA	
in Tomato Sauce, Kids Menu	344
Mac 'N' Cheese, Side	301
Mac 'N' Cheese, with Garlic Bread, & Salad	896
Penne, Tomato, & Roasted Vegetable, with Chicken	731
PATE	
Chicken Liver, with Toast	388
PEAS	
Side, Kids Menu	47
PEPPERS	
Jalapeno, Cheesy, Poppers, Side	378
PIE	
Apple, with Custard	316
Beef, & Stout, with Mash, Beans, & Gravy	1171
Chicken, & Chorizo, Creamy Sauce	516
Fish	747
Lemon Meringue, with Cream	606
PIZZA	
Chocolate, Kids Menu	375
PLATTER	
Chip Shop	1327
POPPADOMS	
Single	32
POTATO DIPPERS	
Crispy	483
Loaded, Sharing	526
Spicy Cheese Sauce, Loaded, Sharing	494
PRAWN COCKTAIL	
Starter	369
PRAWNS	
Crispy, with Garlic Mayo	488
King, Tempura, with Sweet Chilli	475
PROFITEROLES	
with Salted Caramel Sauce	422
PUDDING	
Beef, & Doom Bar Ale	1300
Bread & Butter, Summer Berry	587
Jaffa, Sharing	1034
Sticky Toffee, with Custard	753
Sticky Toffee	719
QUICHE	
Cheese, Three, Crustless	572

	KCAL
BREWERS FAYRE	
RIBS - RACK	
Full, BBQ	1297
Full, in Whisky Glaze	1160
SALAD	
Caesar, Chicken & Bacon	536
Chicken, & Bacon, Grilled	434
Chicken, Coronation	549
Cobb, Brewers	567
Mixed, Side	51
Ploughmans	480
Prawn, Sweet Chilli, Battered	718
Salmon	384
SALMON	
Baked, with Hollandaise Sauce	727
SAMOSAS	
Vegetable	191
SANDWICH	
Chicken, Strips, Spicy, Brown Bread	688
Chicken, Strips, Spicy, White Bread	682
Fish, Goujons, Brown Bread	682
Fish, Goujons, White Bread	676
Ham & Cheese, Brown Bread	630
Ham & Cheese, White Bread	624
Prawn, Brown Bread	589
Prawn, White Bread	583
SAUCE	
Blue Cheese	39
Hollandaise	81
Peppercorn	29
Tennessee Whisky Glaze, Jack Daniels	89
SAUSAGE	
Egg, & Chips	1012
Pork, Battered	159
Premium, Breakfast	137
Vegetarian, Egg, & Chips	858
SAUSAGES & MASH	
Bangers, Kids Menu	391
Vegetarian, Bangers, Kids Menu	364
SCAMPI	
Wholetail, Breaded, with Mushy Peas	868
Wholetail, Breaded, with Peas	830
SOUP	
Tomato	251
SPAGHETTI BOLOGNESE	
Beano-ese, Kids Menu	320
SUNDAE	
Choc-A-Block, Caramel, Cadbury	583
Choc-a-block, Cadbury	639
Funny Face, Kids Menu	268
Oreo	919
Salted Caramel, Brownie, & Popcorn	714
TOAST	
with Creamy Mushrooms	210

	KCAL
BREWERS FAYRE	
TOMATOES	
Grilled, Halved, Breakfast	28
TRIFLE	
Strawberry Pimms	634
VEGETABLES	
Green, Medley, Side	112
Sticks, & Cucumber Yoghurt Dip, Kids Menu	49
Sticks, Side, Kids Menu	28
WAFFLES - BELGIAN	
with Chocolate Honeycomb Ice Cream	497
with Salted Caramel Ice Cream	468
WRAP	
Chicken, Build Your Own, Kids Menu	491
Salmon, Build Your Own, Kids Menu	495
Sausage, Quorn, Build Your Own, Kids Menu	491
YORKSHIRE PUDDING	
with Sausage & Mash, Giant	1329
with Sausage & Mash, Vegetarian, Ultimate	1093

BURGER KING	KCAL
BITES	
Cheese, Chilli, 6	302
BURGERS	
Bacon, Double Cheese, XL	905
Bacon King	1064
Veggie Bean	668
Cheeseburger. Bacon, Double	431
Cheeseburger, Kids	282
Chicken, Royale, Bacon, & Cheese	703
Chicken, Royale, with Cheese	671
Chicken Royale	596
Crispy Chicken	605
Halloumi Bacon King	704
Halloumi King	616
Hamburger, Kids	244
Steakhouse	748
Veggie, Kids	289
Whopper	635
Whopper, Double	881
CHICKEN	
Fries	212
Fries, Jalapeno	218
Nuggets, 6	249
Nuggets, Kids	166
FRIES	
Reg	282
ONION RINGS	
Reg, 5	300

CAFFE NERO	KCAL
BARS	
Chocolate, Dark, & Hazelnut	196
BEANS	
Protein Mix, Savoury	121
BISCUITS	
Biscotti, Almond	147
Stem Ginger	133
BREAKFAST CEREAL	
Porridge, with Semi Skimmed Milk, no Topping	234
Porridge, with Skimmed Milk, no Topping	210
Porridge, with Soya Milk, no Topping	232
BROWNIES	
Chocolate, Belgian	241
Chocolate, Caramel & Sea Salt	257
Chocolate, GF	252
CAKE	
Banana & Walnut Loaf	345
Billionaires	514
Cappuccino, Coffee, & Caramel	444
Cappuccino, Individual	553
Carrot	541
Chocolate Fudge	420
Ginger Spiced, Vegan, Loaf	321
Lemon Drizzle, Loaf	372
Raspberry, & Coconut, Slice	248
Raspberry & Amaretti, Crumble	338
CHEESECAKE	
Lemon, Sicilian	343
Salted Caramel, & Chocolate, Vegan	350
CHOCOLATE	
Coins	109
Milk, Stracciatella	200
COFFEE	
Americano, Grande	23
Americano, Iced	15
Americano, Reg	15
Cappuccino, Coconut Milk, Grande	88
Cappuccino, Coconut Milk, Reg	50
Cappuccino, Iced	24
Cappuccino, Oat Milk, Grande	106
Cappuccino, Oat Milk, Reg	64
Cappuccino, Semi Skimmed, Grande	107
Cappuccino, Semi Skimmed, Reg	65
Cappuccino, Skimmed Milk, Grande	83
Cappuccino, Skimmed Milk, Reg	52
Cappuccino, Soya Milk, Grande	97
Cappuccino, Soya Milk, Reg	59
Latte, Caramel, Coconut Milk	380
Latte, Caramel, Oat Milk	417
Latte, Caramel, Semi Skimmed Milk	420
Latte, Caramel, Skimmed Milk	388
Latte, Caramel, Soya Milk	406
Cortado, Standard	49

	KCAL
CAFFE NERO	
COFFEE	
Espresso, Single	7
Espresso, Con Panna	56
Espresso, Tonic, Original	52
Espresso, Tonic, Ultimate	95
Flat White, Whole Milk	95
Latte, Coconut Milk, Grande	86
Latte, Coconut Milk, Reg	49
Latte, Gingerbread, Coconut Milk, Grande	148
Latte, Gingerbread, Coconut Milk, Reg	90
Latte, Gingerbread, Oat Milk, Grande	110
Latte, Gingerbread, Oat Milk, Reg	110
Latte, Gingerbread, Semi Skimmed, Grande	352
Latte, Gingerbread, Semi Skimmed, Reg	280
Latte, Gingerbread, Skimmed Milk, Grande	323
Latte, Gingerbread, Skimmed Milk, Reg	263
Latte, Gingerbread, Soya Milk, Grande	175
Latte, Gingerbread, Soya Milk, Reg	105
Latte Gingerbread, Whole Milk, Grande	391
Latte, Gingerbread, Whole Milk, Reg	301
Latte, Iced, Coconut	142
Latte, Iced, Semi Skimmed	155
Latte, Oat Milk, Grande	123
Latte, Oat Milk, Reg	70
Latte, Caramel, Salted, Coconut Milk, Grande	155
Latte, Caramel, Salted, Coconut Milk, Reg	95
Latte, Caramel, Salted, Oat Milk, Grande	191
Latte, Caramel, Salted, Oat Milk, Reg	116
Latte, Caramel, Salted, Semi Skimmed, Grande	191
Latte, Caramel, Salted, Semi Skimmed, Reg	116
Latte, Caramel, Salted, Skimmed Milk, Grande	160
Latte, Caramel, Salted, Soya Milk, Grande	183
Latte, Caramel, Salted, Soya Milk, Reg	111
Latte, Caramel, Salted, Whole Milk, Grande	233
Latte, Caramel, Salted, Whole Milk, Reg	140
Latte, Semi Skimmed, Grande	131
Latte, Semi Skimmed, Reg	72
Latte, Skimmed Milk, Grande	97
Latte, Skimmed Milk, Reg	55
Latte, Soya Milk, Grande	115
Latte, Soya Milk, Reg	66
Macchiato, Standard	9
Mocha, Coconut Milk, Grande	171
Mocha, Coconut Milk, Reg	117
Mocha, Oat Milk, Grande	188
Mocha, Oat Milk, Reg	131
Mocha, Semi Skimmed, Grande Milk	363
Mocha, Semi Skimmed, Reg	305
Mocha, Skimmed Milk, Grande	339
Mocha, Skimmed Milk, Reg	292
Mocha, Soya Milk, Grande	179
Mocha, Soya Milk, Reg	126
Mocha, White Chocolate, Coconut Milk	368

	KCAL
CAFFE NERO	
COFFEE	
Mocha, White Chocolate, Oat Milk	405
Mocha, White Chocolate, Semi Skimmed milk	397
Mocha, White Chocolate, Skimmed milk	365
Mocha, White Chocolate, Soya Milk	384
COFFEE BEANS	
Chocolate Coated	133
CONSERVE	
Raspberry	72
Strawberry	72
COOKIES	
Caramel, Chocolate	330
Chocolate, Belgian	314
Oat & Raisin	301
CREAM	
Clotted	234
Whipped, for Coffee	171
CRISPS	
Mature Cheddar, & Red Onion, Kettle	202
Sea Salt, Kettle	205
Sea Salt & Balsamic Vinegar, Kettle	201
CROISSANT	
Almond	343
Apricot	251
Butter	219
Ham, & Mature Cheddar	325
Raspberry, Vegan	296
DRIED FRUIT & NUTS	
Mix	192
FLAPJACK	
Fruit, Vegan	315
FRUIT	
Rolls, Bear Yo Yo's	54
FRUIT SALAD	
Seasonal	106
GINGERBREAD	
Man, Ginnie	289
Man, Gino	289
HONEY	
Topping, for Porridge	97
HOT CHOCOLATE	
Coconut Milk, Grande	260
Coconut Milk, Reg	164
Milano, Standard	458
Mint, Coconut Milk, Grande	327
Mint, Coconut Milk, Reg	214
Mint, Oat Milk, Grande	362
Mint, Oat Milk, Reg	236
Mint, Semi Skimmed, Grande	532
Mint, Semi Skimmed, Reg	406
Mint, Skimmed Milk, Grande	502
Mint, Skimmed Milk, Reg	387
Mint, Soya Milk, Grande	355

	KCAL
CAFFE NERO	
HOT CHOCOLATE	
Mint, Soya Milk, Reg	231
Mint, Whole Milk, Grande	573
Mint, Whole Milk, Reg	431
Oat Milk, Grande	298
Oat Milk, Reg	186
Roasted Hazelnut, Coconut Milk, Grande	323
Roasted Hazelnut, Coconut Milk, Reg	207
Roasted Hazelnut, Oat Milk, Grande	362
Roasted Hazelnut, Oat Milk, Reg	229
Roasted Hazelnut, Semi Skimmed, Grande	532
Roasted Hazelnut, Semi Skimmed, Reg	399
Roasted Hazelnut, Skimmed Milk, Grande	499
Roasted Hazelnut, Skimmed Milk, Reg	380
Roasted Hazelnut, Soya Milk, Grande	354
Roasted Hazelnut, Soya Milk, Reg	224
Roasted Hazelnut, Whole Milk, Grande	575
Roasted Hazelnut, Whole Milk, Reg	424
Semi Skimmed Milk, Grande	524
Semi Skimmed Milk, Reg	398
Skimmed Milk, Grande	484
Skimmed Milk, Reg	374
Soya Milk, Grande	290
Soya Milk, Reg	182
JUICE	
Mango & Passionfruit, Booster	196
Raspberry & Peach, Booster	220
LEMONADE	
Garden Mint	96
MARSHMALLOWS	
for Hot Chocolate	20
MILK SHAKE	
Frappe, Belgian Chocolate	215
Frappe Creme, Espresso & Caramel	503
Frappe, Latte, Semi Skimmed Milk	229
Frappe Creme, Salted Caramel & Pistachio	480
Frappe, Strawberry, Semi Skimmed	245
Frappe, Strawberry, Soya Milk	234
Frappe Creme, Triple Belgian Chocolate	435
Frappe, Vanilla, Semi Skimmed	240
Frappe, Vanilla, Soya Milk	230
MUFFIN	
Blueberry	376
Chocolate Filled	448
Cranberry, Seeds, & Oat	387
Lemon, with Lemon Curd Filling	398
PAIN AU CHOCOLAT	
Single	268
PAIN AU RAISIN	
Single	296
PANINI	
Brie, Bacon, & Cranberry	536
Festive Feast, Vegan	436

	KCAL
CAFFE NERO	
PANINI	
Ham, & Mozzarella	414
Mozzarella, & Tomato	480
Tuna Melt	513
Turkey Feast	490
PARCELS	
Tomato, & Caramelised Onion, with Mozzarella	374
Vegetables, Roasted, & Spanish Chorizo	390
PASTRY	
Chocolate Twist	280
Cinnamon Swirl	350
PIE	
Mince, Star Topped	354
POPCORN	
Sea Salt	87
Sweet & Salty	114
RICE CAKES	
Chocolate	81
ROULADE	
Black Forest, Luxury	414
SALAD	
Chicken, & Mozzarella, Italian Style	246
Falafel, & Houmous	305
SANDWICH	
Bacon, Coffee Cured, Ciabatta, Roll	348
BLT, Classic	496
Chicken Salad, Chargrilled	441
Egg Mayonnaise, Free Range	449
Sausage, Ciabatta Roll	413
Tuna, Red Pepper, & Rocket	333
SAUSAGE ROLL	
Pork, & Pancetta	467
Vegetable, Vegan	354
SCONE	
Fruit, Sultana	287
SHORTBREAD	
Caramel, with Belgian Chocolate	377
Crunchy, All Butter	264
SYRUP	
Vanilla	97
TEA	
Black, & Peach	84
Chai Latte, Coconut Milk	188
Chai Latte, Oat Milk	230
Chai Latte, Semi Skimmed Milk	232
Chai Latte, Skimmed Milk	195
Chai Latte, Soya Milk	216
Green, & Mango	76
TEACAKES	
Rich Fruit, Toasted, with Butter	272
TOASTIE	
Mozzarella, & Roasted Tomato, Melt, Tostati	406
Mushroom, & Mascarpone, Melt, Tostati	388

CAFFE NERO

	KCAL
TOASTIE	
Pigs in Blankets, Melt, Tostati	588
Tomato, Roasted, & Pesto, Tostati	362
WAFFLES	
Caramel	332
YOGHURT	
Raspberry	249

COSTA

	KCAL
BARS	
Granola, Square, Traybake	329
Raspberry, & Coconut, GF	287
BISCUITS	
Biscotti, Almond	155
Fruit, & Oat	228
Ginger, Stem	234
Gingerbread	176
BITES	
Mallow, Millionaire	84
BREAD	
Baguette, Half, SOTF	188
BREAKFAST	
All Day, Protein, Meal Pot	198
Bacon, Smoked, Sourdough, Roll	389
Bircher, Berry	259
Croissant, Ham, & Emmenthal	358
Granola, & Coconut, Sprinkle	85
Muffin, Scrambled Egg, & Mushroom	298
Oats, Instant, Porridge Pot	294
Porridge, Wholegrain, GF	231
Sausage, Pork, Sourdough, Roll	488
Veggie, Egg, Pot	198
BROWNIES	
Chocolate, GF	309
BUNS	
Brioche, Cinnamon	332
Chocolate, & Caramel, Sticky	396
CAKE	
Banana, & Pecan, Loaf	325
Caramel, Crisp, Traybake	410
Carrot, Layered	576
Chocolate, Seriously	572
Chocolate, Tiffin	402
Coffee, Walnut, & Pecan	591
Iced Slice, Vegan, GF	320
Lemon, Drizzle, Loaf	365
Lemon, Drizzle, Slices, Wrapped	350
Raspberry, & Almond, Traybake	465
Raspberry & Blackcurrant Ripple	512
CHEESECAKE	
New York, SOTF	564
Vanilla, Baked, Individual	384
CHILLI	
Bean, Smoky, & Rice, Pot	291
CHOCOLATE	
Coins	380
Dark, Bar	178
Flake	44
Milk, Bar	176
Truffle, Lindt	85

COSTA	KCAL
COFFEE - AMERICANO	
No Milk, Massimo	10
No Milk, Medio	8
No Milk, Primo	6
White, 12oz, Express	60
White, 16oz, Express	55
White, 8oz, Express	49
COFFEE - BABYCHINO	
Almond Milk	22
Coconut Milk	30
Semi Skimmed Milk	41
Semi Skimmed Milk, Lactofree	35
Skimmed Milk	29
Soya Milk	38
Whole Milk	59
COFFEE - BLACK	
Cold Brew	1
Flat	4
COFFEE - CAPPUCCINO	
Almond Milk, Massimo	90
Almond Milk, Massimo, Takeaway	94
Almond Milk, Medio	72
Almond Milk, Medio, Takeaway	72
Almond Milk, Primo	49
Almond Milk, Primo, Takeaway	56
Coconut Milk, Massimo	115
Coconut Milk, Massimo, Takeaway	122
Coconut Milk, Medio	92
Coconut Milk, Medio, Takeaway	92
Coconut Milk, Primo	62
Coconut Milk, Primo, Takeaway	71
Semi Skimmed Milk, Lactofree, Massimo	133
Semi Skimmed Milk, Lactofree, Massimo, Takeaway	140
Semi Skimmed Milk, Lactofree, Medio	106
Semi Skimmed Milk, Lactofree, Medio, Takeaway	106
Semi Skimmed Milk, Lactofree, Primo	71
Semi Skimmed Milk, Lactofree, Primo, Takeaway	82
Semi Skimmed Milk, Massimo	153
Semi Skimmed Milk, Massimo, Takeaway	162
Semi Skimmed Milk, Medio	122
Semi Skimmed Milk, Medio, Takeaway	122
Semi Skimmed Milk, Primo	81
Semi Skimmed Milk, Primo, Takeaway	94
Shaken, Almond Milk, Iced, Medio	65
Shaken, Almond Milk, Iced, Primo	48
Shaken, Coconut Milk, Iced, Medio	73
Shaken, Coconut Milk, Iced, Primo	56
Shaken, Semi Skimmed Milk, Iced, Medio	85
Shaken, Semi Skimmed Milk, Iced, Primo	69
Shaken, Skimmed Milk, Iced, Medio	72
Shaken, Skimmed Milk, Iced, Primo	55
Shaken, Soya Milk, Iced, Medio	82
Shaken, Soya Milk, Iced, Primo	65

COSTA	KCAL
COFFEE - CAPPUCCINO	
Shaken, Whole Milk, Iced, Medio	104
Shaken, Whole Milk, Iced, Primo	88
Skimmed Milk, Massimo	111
Skimmed Milk, Massimo, Takeaway	120
Skimmed Milk, Medio	90
Skimmed Milk, Medio, Takeaway	90
Skimmed Milk, Primo	60
Skimmed Milk, Primo, Takeaway	70
Soya Milk, Massimo	139
Soya Milk, Massimo, Takeaway	150
Soya Milk, Medio	112
Soya Milk, Medio, Takeaway	112
Soya Milk, Primo	74
Soya Milk, Primo, Takeaway	87
Whipped Milk, Almond Milk, Iced, Medio	98
Whipped Milk, Almond Milk, Iced, Primo	62
Whipped Milk, Coconut Milk, Iced, Medio	104
Whipped Milk, Coconut Milk, Iced, Primo	66
Whipped Milk, Semi Skimmed Milk, Iced, Medio	113
Whipped Milk, Semi Skimmed Milk, Iced, Primo	73
Whipped Milk, Skimmed Milk, Iced, Medio	103
Whipped Milk, Skimmed Milk, Iced, Primo	66
Whipped Milk, Soya Milk, Iced, Medio	110
Whipped Milk, Soya Milk, Iced, Primo	71
Whipped Milk, Whole Milk, Iced, Medio	127
Whipped Milk, Whole Milk, Iced, Primo	83
Whole Milk, Massimo	209
Whole Milk, Massimo, Takeaway	223
Whole Milk, Medio	168
Whole Milk, Medio, Takeaway	168
Whole Milk, Primo	109
Whole Milk, Primo, Takeaway	129
COFFEE - COLD BREW	
Bonfire Spiced, Medio	88
Bonfire Spiced, Medio, Takeaway	88
Bonfire Spiced, Primo	63
Bonfire Spiced, Primo, Takeaway	63
with Whipped Milk, Semi Skimmed Milk, Medio	19
with Whipped Milk, Semi Skimmed Milk, Primo	16
COFFEE - CORTADO	
Caramel, Almond Milk	64
Caramel, Almond Milk, Takeaway	72
Caramel, Coconut Milk, Takeaway	85
Caramel, Semi Skimmed Milk	89
Caramel, Semi Skimmed Milk, Lactofree	81
Caramel, Semi Skimmed Milk, Lactofree, Takeaway	94
Caramel, Semi Skimmed Milk, Takeaway	104
Caramel, Skimmed Milk	73
Caramel, Skimmed Milk, Takeaway	84
Caramel, Soya Milk	84
Caramel, Soya Milk, Takeaway	98
Caramel, Whole Milk	111

COSTA

COFFEE - CORTADO	KCAL
Caramel, Whole Milk, Takeaway	132
Almond Milk, Solo	32
Almond Milk, Solo, Iced	39
Almond Milk, Solo, Takeaway	40
Coconut Milk, Solo, Iced	47
Semi Skimmed Milk, Lactofree, Solo	51
Semi Skimmed Milk, Lactofree, Solo, Takeaway	64
Semi Skimmed Milk, Solo	60
Semi Skimmed Milk, Solo, Iced	58
Semi Skimmed Milk, Solo, Takeaway	76
Skimmed Milk, Solo	42
Skimmed Milk, Solo, Iced	46
Skimmed Milk, Solo, Takeaway	53
Soya Milk, Solo	55
Soya Milk, Solo, Iced	56
Soya Milk, Solo, Takeaway	69
Whole Milk, Solo	85
Whole Milk, Solo, Iced	75
Whole Milk, Solo, Takeaway	108
COFFEE - ESPRESSO	
Character Roast, Colombian	3
con Pana, Doppio	139
con Pana, Solo	136
Decaff, Solo	3
Ristretto, Doppio	8
Ristretto, Solo	2
Shot	3
COFFEE - FILTER	
Massimo	6
Medio	4
Primo	3
COFFEE - FLAT WHITE	
Almond Milk, Primo	57
Almond Milk, Primo, Takeaway	67
Coconut Milk, Primo	78
Coconut Milk, Primo, Takeaway	91
Semi Skimmed Milk, Primo	107
Semi Skimmed Milk, Lactofree, Primo	92
Semi Skimmed Milk, Lactofree, Primo, Takeaway	107
Semi Skimmed Milk, Primo, Takeaway	126
Skimmed Milk, Primo	75
Skimmed Milk, Primo, Takeaway	89
Soya Milk, Primo	98
Soya Milk, Primo, Takeaway	116
Whole Milk, Primo	152
Whole Milk, Primo, Takeaway	178
COFFEE - ICED	
Americano, Medio	57
Americano, Primo	40
Cortado, Semi Skimmed Milk, Lactofree, Solo	52
Espresso, Doppio	39
Espresso, Ristretto, Doppio	38

COSTA

COFFEE - ICED	KCAL
Espresso, Ristretto, Solo	19
Espresso, Solo	20
Espresso Macchiato, Almond Milk, Doppio	40
Espresso Macchiato, Almond Milk, Solo	20
Espresso Macchiato, Coconut Milk, Doppio	40
Espresso Macchiato, Coconut Milk, Solo	20
Espresso Macchiato, Semi Skimmed Milk, Doppio	41
Espresso Macchiato, Semi Skimmed Milk, Solo	21
Espresso Macchiato, Skimmed Milk, Doppio	40
Espresso Macchiato, Skimmed Milk, Solo	20
Espresso Macchiato, Soya Milk, Doppio	40
Espresso Macchiato, Soya Milk, Solo	20
Espresso Macchiato, Whole Milk, Doppio	41
Espresso Macchiato, Whole Milk, Solo	21
Flat White, Almond Milk	57
Flat White, Coconut Milk	68
Flat White, Semi Skimmed Milk	81
Flat White, Semi Skimmed Milk, Lactofree	75
Flat White, Skimmed Milk	67
Flat White, Soya Milk	79
Flat White, Whole Milk	107
Latte, Almond Milk, Medio	95
Latte, Almond Milk, Primo	65
Latte, Coconut Milk, Medio	116
Latte, Coconut Milk, Primo	81
Latte, Semi Skimmed Milk, Medio	146
Latte, Semi Skimmed Milk, Primo	103
Latte, Semi Skimmed Milk, Lactofree, Medio	129
Latte, Semi Skimmed Milk, Lactofree, Primo	91
Latte, Skimmed Milk, Massimo	179
Latte, Skimmed Milk, Medio	113
Latte, Skimmed Milk, Primo	79
Latte, Soya Milk, Massimo	200
Latte, Soya Milk, Medio	136
Latte, Soya Milk, Primo	96
Latte, Whole Milk, Medio	192
Latte, Whole Milk, Primo	138
Mocha, Almond Milk, Medio	134
Mocha, Almond Milk, Primo	94
Mocha, Coconut Milk, Medio	149
Mocha, Coconut Milk, Primo	105
Mocha, Cortado, Semi Skimmed, Lactofree, Medio	159
Mocha, Cortado, Semi Skimmed, Lactofree, Primo	113
Mocha, Semi Skimmed Milk, Medio	171
Mocha, Semi Skimmed Milk, Primo	121
Mocha, Skimmed Milk, Medio	148
Mocha, Skimmed Milk, Primo	104
Mocha, Soya Milk, Medio	164
Mocha, Soya Milk, Primo	116
Mocha, Whole Milk, Primo	204
Mocha, Whole Milk, Primo	146
Mocha, Cortado, Almond Milk, Solo	73

	KCAL
COSTA	
COFFEE - ICED	
Mocha, Cortado, Coconut Milk, Solo	79
Mocha, Cortado, Semi Skimmed Milk, Solo	83
Mocha, Cortado, Semi Skimmed Milk, Solo	65
Mocha, Cortado, Skimmed Milk, Solo	55
Mocha Cortado, Soya Milk, Solo	85
Mocha, Cortado, Whole Milk, Solo	80
COFFEE - LATTE	
Almond Milk, Massimo	102
Almond Milk, Massimo, Takeaway	108
Almond Milk, Medio	79
Almond Milk, Medio, Takeaway	79
Almond Milk, Primo	50
Almond Milk, Primo, Takeaway	58
Coconut Milk, Massimo	137
Coconut Milk, Massimo, Takeaway	145
Coconut Milk, Medio	106
Coconut Milk, Medio, Takeaway	106
Coconut Milk, Primo	68
Coconut Milk, Primo, Takeaway	77
Semi Skimmed Milk, Lactofree, Massimo	161
Semi Skimmed Milk, Lactofree, Massimo, Takeaway	170
Semi Skimmed Milk, Lactofree, Medio	125
Semi Skimmed Milk, Lactofree, Medio, Takeaway	125
Semi Skimmed Milk, Lactofree, Primo	79
Semi Skimmed Milk, Lactofree, Primo, Takeaway	90
Semi Skimmed Milk, Massimo	188
Semi Skimmed Milk, Massimo, Takeaway	199
Semi Skimmed Milk, Medio	146
Semi Skimmed Milk, Medio, Takeaway	146
Semi Skimmed Milk, Primo	93
Semi Skimmed Milk, Primo, Takeaway	105
Skimmed Milk, Massimo	132
Skimmed Milk, Massimo, Takeaway	139
Skimmed Milk, Medio	102
Skimmed Milk, Medio, Takeaway	102
Skimmed Milk, Primo	66
Skimmed Milk, Primo, Takeaway	75
Soya Milk, Massimo	175
Soya Milk, Massimo, Takeaway	184
Soya Milk, Medio	135
Soya Milk, Medio, Takeaway	135
Soya Milk, Primo	86
Soya Milk, Primo, Takeaway	97
Whole Milk, Massimo	269
Whole Milk, Massimo, Takeaway	283
Whole Milk, Medio	207
Whole Milk, Medio, Takeaway	207
Whole Milk, Primo	133
Whole Milk, Primo, Takeaway	149
COFFEE - LATTE, BONFIRE SPICED	
Almond Milk, Medio	160
Almond Milk, Primo	110

	KCAL
COSTA	
COFFEE - LATTE, BONFIRE SPICED	
Coconut Milk, Medio	186
Coconut Milk, Primo	127
Semi Skimmed Milk, Lactofree, Medio	198
Semi Skimmed Milk, Lactofree, Primo	137
Semi Skimmed Milk, Medio	221
Semi Skimmed Milk, Primo	152
Skimmed Milk, Medio	182
Skimmed Milk, Primo	126
Soya Milk, Medio	210
Soya Milk, Primo	144
Whole Milk, Medio	277
Whole Milk, Primo	190
COFFEE - LATTE, GINGERBREAD	
Almond Milk, Medio	207
Almond Milk, Medio, Takeaway	235
Almond Milk, Primo	187
Almond Milk, Primo, Takeaway	213
Coconut Milk, Medio	230
Coconut Milk, Medio, Takeaway	267
Coconut Milk, Primo	203
Coconut Milk, Primo, Takeaway	238
Semi Skimmed Milk, Lactofree, Medio	242
Semi Skimmed Milk, Lactofree, Medio, Takeaway	285
Semi Skimmed Milk, Lactofree, Primo	212
Semi Skimmed Milk, Lactofree, Primo, Takeaway	251
Semi Skimmed Milk, Medio	262
Semi Skimmed Milk, Medio, Takeaway	315
Semi Skimmed Milk, Primo	226
Semi Skimmed Milk, Primo, Takeaway	273
Skimmed Milk, Medio	227
Skimmed Milk, Medio, Takeaway	264
Skimmed Milk, Primo	201
Skimmed Milk, Primo, Takeaway	235
Soya Milk, Medio	252
Soya Milk, Medio, Takeaway	300
Soya Milk, Primo	219
Soya Milk, Primo, Takeaway	262
Whole Milk, Medio	312
Whole Milk, Medio, Takeaway	387
Whole Milk, Primo	262
Whole Milk, Primo, Takeaway	329
COFFEE - LATTE, HAZELNUT PRALINE	
Almond Milk, Massimo	315
Almond Milk, Massimo, Takeaway	359
Almond Milk, Medio	284
Almond Milk, Medio, Takeaway	311
Almond Milk, Primo	250
Almond Milk, Primo, Takeaway	276
Coconut Milk, Medio	306
Coconut Milk, Medio, Takeaway	344
Coconut Milk, Primo	266
Coconut Milk, Primo, Takeaway	301

	KCAL
COSTA	
COFFEE - LATTE, HAZELNUT PRALINE	
Semi Skimmed Milk, Lactofree, Medio	319
Semi Skimmed Milk, Lactofree, Medio, Takeaway	362
Semi Skimmed Milk, Lactofree, Primo	275
Semi Skimmed Milk, Lactofree, Primo, Takeaway	314
Semi Skimmed Milk, Medio	339
Semi Skimmed Milk, Medio, Takeaway	391
Semi Skimmed Milk, Primo	289
Semi Skimmed Milk, Primo, Takeaway	337
Skimmed Milk, Medio	304
Skimmed Milk, Medio, Takeaway	340
Skimmed Milk, Primo	264
Skimmed Milk, Primo, Takeaway	298
Soya Milk, Medio	329
Soya Milk, Medio, Takeaway	377
Soya Milk, Primo	282
Soya Milk, Primo, Takeaway	326
Whole Milk, Medio	389
Whole Milk, Medio, Takeaway	464
Whole Milk, Primo	325
Whole Milk, Primo, Takeaway	392
COFFEE - MACCHIATTO	
Almond Milk, Solo	8
Coconut Milk, Solo	9
Semi Skimmed Milk, Lactofree, Solo	10
Semi Skimmed Milk, Solo	11
Skimmed Milk, Solo	9
Soya Milk, Solo	10
Whole Milk, Solo	13
COFFEE - MOCHA	
Almond Milk, Massimo	194
Almond Milk, Massimo, Takeaway	208
Almond Milk, Medio	155
Almond Milk, Medio, Takeaway	160
Almond Milk, Primo	87
Almond Milk, Primo, Takeaway	102
Coconut Milk, Massimo	219
Coconut Milk, Massimo, Takeaway	234
Coconut Milk, Medio	174
Coconut Milk, Medio, Takeaway	180
Coconut Milk, Primo	99
Mocha, Coconut Milk, Primo, Takeaway	116
Semi Skimmed Milk, Lactofree, Massimo	236
Semi Skimmed Milk, Massimo, Lactofree, Takeaway	248
Semi Skimmed Milk, Lactofree, Medio	184
Semi Skimmed Milk, Medio, Lactofree, Takeaway	190
Semi Skimmed Milk, Lactofree, Primo	105
Semi Skimmed Milk, Lactofree, Primo, Takeaway	123
Semi Skimmed Milk, Massimo	257
Semi Skimmed Milk, Massimo, Takeaway	270
Semi Skimmed Milk, Medio	200
Semi Skimmed Milk, Medio, Takeaway	209
Semi Skimmed Milk, Primo	115

	KCAL
COSTA	
COFFEE - MOCHA	
Semi Skimmed Milk, Primo, Takeaway	137
Skimmed Milk, Massimo	219
Skimmed Milk, Massimo, Takeaway	230
Skimmed Milk, Medio	171
Skimmed Milk, Medio, Takeaway	177
Skimmed Milk, Primo	97
Skimmed Milk, Primo, Takeaway	114
Soya Milk, Massimo	245
Soya Milk, Massimo, Takeaway	261
Soya Milk, Medio	193
Soya Milk, Medio, Takeaway	199
Soya Milk, Primo	109
Soya Milk, Primo, Takeaway	130
Whole Milk, Massimo	312
Whole Milk, Massimo, Takeaway	332
Whole Milk, Medio	244
Whole Milk, Medio, Takeaway	252
Whole Milk, Primo	141
Whole Milk, Primo, Takeaway	167
Cortado, Almond Milk	50
Cortado, Almond Milk, Takeaway	81
Cortado, Coconut Milk	57
Cortado, Coconut Milk, Takeaway	93
Cortado, Skimmed Milk	56
Cortado, Semi Skimmed Milk	61
Cortado, Semi Skimmed Milk, Takeaway	99
Cortado, Skimmed Milk, Takeaway	91
Cortado, Skimmed Milk	67
Cortado, Skimmed Milk, Takeaway	109
Cortado, Soya Milk, New Recipe	64
Cortado, Soya Milk, Takeaway	104
Cortado, Whole Milk	83
Cortado, Whole Milk, Takeaway	135
COOKIES	
Chocolate, Caramel, & Hazelnut	333
Chocolate Chunk, Bake Off, SOTF	306
Chocolate Chunk	306
Toffee, & Pecan, Vegan	334
CREAM	
Whipping, Extras	133
CROISSANT	
Almond	321
Almond, SOTF	374
Butter	213
Butter, SOTF	267
Chocolate, & Hazelnut, SOTF	372
Cup, with Nutella	305
CUPCAKES	
Banoffee	431
CURRY	
Thai, Red, Pot	275

COSTA	KCAL
DOUGHNUTS	
Chocolatey, SOTF	309
Pineapple, & Coconut, SOTF	359
DRIED FRUIT	
Mango	96
FLAPJACK	
Fruity, Vegan, GF	251
FROSTINO - BELGIAN CHOCOLATE	
Almond Milk, Medio	348
Almond Milk, Medio, Takeaway	348
Almond Milk, Primo	292
Almond Milk, Primo, Takeaway	292
Coconut Milk, Medio	363
Coconut Milk, Medio, Takeaway	363
Coconut Milk, Primo	303
Coconut Milk, Primo, Takeaway	303
Semi Skimmed Milk, Lactofree, Medio	374
Semi Skimmed Milk, Lactofree, Medio, Takeaway	374
Semi Skimmed Milk, Lactofree, Primo	311
Semi Skimmed Milk, Lactofree, Primo, Takeaway	311
Semi Skimmed Milk, Medio	386
Semi Skimmed Milk, Medio, Takeaway	386
Semi Skimmed Milk, Primo	320
Semi Skimmed Milk, Primo, Takeaway	320
Skimmed Milk, Medio	362
Skimmed Milk, Medio, Takeaway	362
Skimmed Milk, Primo	302
Skimmed Milk, Primo, Takeaway	302
Soya Milk, Medio	379
Soya Milk, Medio, Takeaway	379
Soya Milk, Primo	315
Soya Milk, Primo, Takeaway	315
Whole Milk, Medio	420
Whole Milk, Medio, Takeaway	420
Whole Milk, Primo	346
Whole Milk, Primo, Takeaway	346
Coffee, Almond Milk, Medio	354
Coffee, Almond Milk, Medio, Takeaway	354
Coffee, Almond Milk, Primo	295
Coffee, Almond Milk, Primo, Takeaway	295
Coffee, Coconut Milk, Medio	369
Coffee, Coconut Milk, Medio, Takeaway	369
Coffee, Coconut Milk, Primo	306
Coffee, Coconut Milk, Primo, Takeaway	306
Coffee, Semi Skimmed, Lactofree, Medio	380
Coffee, Semi Skimmed, Lactofree, Medio, Takeaway	380
Coffee, Semi Skimmed, Lactofree, Primo	314
Coffee, Semi Skimmed, Lactofree, Primo, Takeaway	314
Coffee, Semi Skimmed Milk, Medio	392
Coffee, Semi Skimmed Milk, Medio, Takeaway	392
Coffee, Semi Skimmed Milk, Primo	323
Coffee, Semi Skimmed Milk, Primo, Takeaway	323
Coffee, Skimmed Milk, Medio	368

COSTA	KCAL
FROSTINO - BELGIAN CHOCOLATE	
Coffee, Skimmed Milk, Medio, Takeaway	368
Coffee, Skimmed Milk, Primo	305
Coffee, Skimmed Milk, Primo, Takeaway	305
Coffee, Soya Milk, Medio	385
Coffee, Soya Milk, Medio, Takeaway	385
Coffee, Soya Milk, Primo	318
Coffee, Soya Milk, Primo, Takeaway	318
Coffee, Whole Milk, Medio	426
Coffee, Whole Milk, Medio, Takeaway	426
Coffee, Whole Milk, Primo	349
Coffee, Whole Milk, Primo, Takeaway	349
FROSTINO - COFFEE	
Almond Milk, Medio	101
Almond Milk, Medio, Takeaway	101
Almond Milk, Primo	70
Almond Milk, Primo, Takeaway	70
Coconut Milk, Medio	116
Coconut Milk, Medio, Takeaway	116
Coconut Milk, Primo	82
Coconut Milk, Primo, Takeaway	82
Semi Skimmed Milk, Lactofree, Medio	126
Semi Skimmed Milk, Lactofree, Medio, Takeaway	126
Semi Skimmed Milk, Lactofree, Primo	90
Semi Skimmed Milk, Lactofree, Primo, Takeaway	90
Semi Skimmed Milk, Medio	138
Semi Skimmed Milk, Medio, Takeaway	138
Semi Skimmed Milk, Primo	99
Semi Skimmed Milk, Primo, Takeaway	99
Skimmed Milk, Medio	114
Skimmed Milk, Medio, Takeaway	114
Skimmed Milk, Primo	81
Skimmed Milk, Primo, Takeaway	81
Soya Milk, Medio	131
Soya Milk, Medio, Takeaway	131
Soya Milk, Primo	94
Soya Milk, Primo, Takeaway	94
Whole Milk, Medio	172
Whole Milk, Medio, Takeaway	172
Whole Milk, Primo	125
Whole Milk, Primo, Takeaway	125
FROSTINO - MINT CHOC CHIP	
Almond Milk, Medio	406
Almond Milk, Medio, Takeaway	407
Almond Milk, Primo	329
Almond Milk, Primo, Takeaway	329
Coconut Milk, Medio	421
Coconut Milk, Medio, Takeaway	422
Coconut Milk, Primo	341
Coconut Milk, Primo, Takeaway	341
Semi Skimmed Milk, Lactofree, Medio	431
Semi Skimmed Milk, Lactofree, Medio, Takeaway	432
Semi Skimmed Milk, Lactofree, Primo	349

	KCAL
COSTA	
FROSTINO - MINT CHOC CHIP	
Semi Skimmed Milk, Lactofree, Primo, Takeaway	349
Semi Skimmed Milk, Medio	442
Semi Skimmed Milk, Medio, Takeaway	444
Semi Skimmed Milk, Primo	358
Semi Skimmed Milk, Primo, Takeaway	358
Skimmed Milk, Medio	419
Skimmed Milk, Medio, Takeaway	421
Skimmed Milk, Primo	340
Skimmed Milk, Primo, Takeaway	340
Soya Milk, Medio	435
Soya Milk, Medio, Takeaway	438
Soya Milk, Primo	353
Soya Milk, Primo, Takeaway	353
Whole Milk, Medio	475
Whole Milk, Medio, Takeaway	478
Whole Milk, Primo	384
Whole Milk, Primo, Takeaway	384
FROSTINO - SALTED CARAMEL CRUNCH	
Almond Milk, Medio	322
Almond Milk, Medio, Takeaway	322
Almond Milk, Primo	274
Almond Milk, Primo, Takeaway	274
Coconut Milk, Medio	337
Coconut Milk, Medio, Takeaway	337
Coconut Milk, Primo	285
Coconut Milk, Primo, Takeaway	285
Semi Skimmed Milk, Lactofree, Medio	347
Semi Skimmed Milk, Lactofree, Medio, Takeaway	347
Semi Skimmed Milk, Lactofree, Primo	293
Semi Skimmed Milk, Lactofree, Primo, Takeaway	293
Semi Skimmed Milk, Medio	359
Semi Skimmed Milk, Medio, Takeaway	359
Semi Skimmed Milk, Primo	302
Semi Skimmed Milk, Primo, Takeaway	302
Skimmed Milk, Medio	335
Skimmed Milk, Medio, Takeaway	335
Skimmed Milk, Primo	284
Skimmed Milk, Primo, Takeaway	284
Soya Milk, Medio	352
Soya Milk, Medio, Takeaway	352
Soya Milk, Primo	297
Soya Milk, Primo, Takeaway	297
Whole Milk, Medio	393
Whole Milk, Medio, Takeaway	393
Whole Milk, Primo	328
Whole Milk, Primo, Takeaway	328
Coffee, Almond Milk, Medio	328
Coffee, Almond Milk, Medio, Takeaway	328
Coffee, Almond Milk, Primo	277
Coffee, Almond Milk, Primo, Takeaway	277
Coffee, Coconut Milk, Medio	343
Coffee, Coconut Milk, Medio, Takeaway	343

	KCAL
COSTA	
FROSTINO - SALTED CARAMEL CRUNCH	
Coffee, Coconut Milk, Primo	288
Coffee, Coconut Milk, Primo, Takeaway	288
Coffee, Semi Skimmed, Lactofree, Medio	353
Coffee, Semi Skimmed, Lactofree, Medio, Takeaway	353
Coffee, Semi Skimmed, Lactofree, Primo	296
Coffee, Semi Skimmed, Lactofree, Primo, Takeaway	296
Coffee, Semi Skimmed Milk, Medio	365
Coffee, Semi Skimmed Milk, Medio, Takeaway	365
Coffee, Semi Skimmed Milk, Primo	305
Coffee, Semi Skimmed Milk, Primo, Takeaway	305
Coffee, Skimmed Milk, Medio	341
Coffee, Skimmed Milk, Medio, Takeaway	341
Coffee, Skimmed Milk, Primo	287
Coffee, Skimmed Milk, Primo, Takeaway	287
Coffee, Soya Milk, Medio	358
Coffee, Soya Milk, Medio, Takeaway	358
Coffee, Soya Milk, Primo	300
Coffee, Soya Milk, Primo, Takeaway	300
Coffee, Whole Milk, Medio	399
Coffee, Whole Milk, Medio, Takeaway	399
Coffee, Whole Milk, Primo	331
Coffee, Whole Milk, Primo, Takeaway	331
FROSTINO - STRAWBERRY	
Almond Milk, Medio	384
Almond Milk, Primo	318
Coconut Milk, Medio	400
Coconut Milk, Primo	330
Semi Skimmed Milk, Lactofree, Medio	410
Semi Skimmed Milk, Lactofree, Primo	338
Semi Skimmed Milk, Medio	422
Semi Skimmed Milk, Primo	347
Skimmed Milk, Medio	398
Skimmed Milk, Primo	329
Soya Milk, Medio	415
Soya Milk, Primo	342
Whole Milk, Medio	456
Whole Milk, Primo	373
FRUIT COMPOTE	
Berry, Hedgerow, SOTF	76
Mixed Berry, Topping	38
FRUIT SALAD	
Breakfast	67
Snack Box, Kids	258
HOT CHOCOLATE	
Almond Milk, Massimo	294
Almond Milk, Massimo, Takeaway	316
Almond Milk, Medio	207
Almond Milk, Medio, Takeaway	226
Almond Milk, Primo	118
Almond Milk, Primo, Takeaway	152
Coconut Milk, Massimo	331
Coconut Milk, Massimo, Takeaway	355

COSTA	KCAL
HOT CHOCOLATE	
Coconut Milk, Medio	236
Coconut Milk, Medio, Takeaway	257
Coconut Milk, Primo	138
Coconut Milk, Primo, Takeaway	176
Luxury, Eat In	113
Luxury, Takeaway	150
Almond Milk, Mini, with Flake	83
Almond Milk, Mini, with Marshmallow	69
Coconut Milk, Mini, with Flake	97
Coconut Milk, Mini, with Marshmallow	81
Semi Skimmed, Mini, Lactofree, with Flake	101
Semi Skimmed, Mini, Lactofree, with Marshmallow	85
Semi Skimmed Milk, Mini, with Flake	124
Semi Skimmed Milk, Mini, with Marshmallow	108
Skimmed Milk, Mini, with Flake	108
Skimmed Milk, Mini, with Marshmallow	92
Soya Milk, Mini, with Flake	104
Soya Milk, Mini, with Marshmallow	88
Whole Milk, Mini, with Flake	96
Whole Milk, Mini, with Marshmallow	80
Semi Skimmed Milk, Lactofree, Massimo	352
Semi Skimmed Milk, Lactofree, Massimo, Takeaway	377
Semi Skimmed Milk, Lactofree, Medio	252
Semi Skimmed Milk, Lactofree, Medio, Takeaway	274
Semi Skimmed Milk, Lactofree, Primo	148
Semi Skimmed Milk, Lactofree, Primo, Takeaway	190
Semi Skimmed Milk, Massimo	384
Semi Skimmed Milk, Massimo, Takeaway	413
Semi Skimmed Milk, Medio	277
Semi Skimmed Milk, Medio, Takeaway	302
Semi Skimmed Milk, Primo	165
Semi Skimmed Milk, Primo, Takeaway	212
Skimmed Milk, Massimo	327
Skimmed Milk, Massimo, Takeaway	351
Skimmed Milk, Medio	232
Skimmed Milk, Medio, Takeaway	254
Skimmed Milk, Primo	135
Skimmed Milk, Primo, Takeaway	174
Soya Milk, Massimo	368
Soya Milk, Massimo, Takeaway	395
Soya Milk, Medio	264
Soya Milk, Medio, Takeaway	288
Soya Milk, Primo	157
Soya Milk, Primo, Takeaway	201
Whole Milk, Massimo	467
Whole Milk, Massimo, Takeaway	501
Whole Milk, Medio	341
Whole Milk, Medio, Takeaway	372
Whole Milk, Primo	208
Whole Milk, Primo, Takeaway	267
HOT CHOCOLATE - BLACK FOREST	
Almond Milk, Medio	314

COSTA	KCAL
HOT CHOCOLATE - BLACK FOREST	
Almond Milk, Medio, Takeaway	333
Almond Milk, Primo	249
Almond Milk, Primo, Takeaway	272
Coconut Milk, Medio	333
Coconut Milk, Medio, Takeaway	355
Coconut Milk, Primo	262
Coconut Milk, Primo, Takeaway	289
Semi Skimmed Milk, Lactofree, Medio	344
Semi Skimmed Milk, Lactofree, Medio, Takeaway	367
Semi Skimmed Milk, Lactofree, Primo	269
Semi Skimmed Milk, Lactofree, Primo, Takeaway	298
Semi Skimmed Milk, Medio	361
Semi Skimmed Milk, Medio, Takeaway	387
Semi Skimmed Milk, Primo	281
Semi Skimmed Milk, Primo, Takeaway	313
Skimmed Milk, Medio	331
Skimmed Milk, Medio, Takeaway	353
Skimmed Milk, Primo	261
Skimmed Milk, Primo, Takeaway	287
Soya Milk, Medio	352
Soya Milk, Medio, Takeaway	377
Soya Milk, Primo	275
Soya Milk, Primo, Takeaway	306
Whole Milk, Medio	403
Whole Milk, Medio, Takeaway	435
Whole Milk, Primo	310
Whole Milk, Primo, Takeaway	351
HOT CHOCOLATE - BONFIRE SPICED	
Almond Milk, Medio	267
Almond Milk, Medio, Takeaway	286
Almond Milk, Primo	165
Almond Milk, Primo, Takeaway	198
Coconut Milk, Medio	292
Coconut Milk, Medio, Takeaway	314
Coconut Milk, Primo	181
Coconut Milk, Primo, Takeaway	220
Semi Skimmed Milk, Lactofree, Medio	306
Semi Skimmed Milk, Lactofree, Medio, Takeaway	329
Semi Skimmed Milk, Lactofree, Primo	191
Semi Skimmed Milk, Lactofree, Primo, Takeaway	233
Semi Skimmed Milk, Medio	329
Semi Skimmed Milk, Medio, Takeaway	354
Semi Skimmed Milk, Primo	205
Semi Skimmed Milk, Primo, Takeaway	252
Skimmed Milk, Medio	289
Skimmed Milk, Medio, Takeaway	311
Skimmed Milk, Primo	180
Skimmed Milk, Primo, Takeaway	218
Soya Milk, Medio	317
Soya Milk, Medio, Takeaway	341
Soya Milk, Primo	198
Soya Milk, Primo, Takeaway	242

COSTA	KCAL
HOT CHOCOLATE - BONFIRE SPICED	
Whole Milk, Medio	384
Whole Milk, Medio, Takeaway	415
Whole Milk, Primo	242
Whole Milk, Primo, Takeaway	301
HOT CHOCOLATE - CARAMEL	
Luxury	121
Luxury, Takeaway	159
HOT CHOCOLATE - GINGERBREAD & CREAM	
Almond Milk, Medio	290
Almond Milk, Medio, Takeaway	309
Almond Milk, Primo	233
Coconut Milk, Medio	309
Coconut Milk, Medio, Takeaway	331
Coconut Milk, Primo	246
Coconut Milk, Primo, Takeaway	273
Semi Skimmed Milk, Lactofree, Medio	320
Semi Skimmed Milk, Lactofree, Medio, Takeaway	343
Semi Skimmed Milk, Lactofree, Primo	253
Semi Skimmed Milk, Lactofree, Primo, Takeaway	282
Semi Skimmed Milk, Medio	337
Semi Skimmed Milk, Medio, Takeaway	363
Semi Skimmed Milk, Primo	264
Semi Skimmed Milk, Primo, Takeaway	297
Skimmed Milk, Medio	307
Skimmed Milk, Medio, Takeaway	329
Skimmed Milk, Primo	244
Skimmed Milk, Primo, Takeaway	271
Soya Milk, Medio	328
Soya Milk, Medio, Takeaway	353
Soya Milk, Primo	259
Soya Milk, Primo, Takeaway	289
Whole Milk, Medio	379
Whole Milk, Medio, Takeaway	411
Whole Milk, Primo	293
Whole Milk, Primo, Takeaway	334
Almond Milk, Primo, Takeaway	256
HOT CHOCOLATE - HAZELNUT PRALINE	
Almond Milk, Medio	355
Almond Milk, Medio, Takeaway	374
Almond Milk, Primo	284
Almond Milk, Primo, Takeaway	307
Coconut Milk, Medio	374
Coconut Milk, Medio, Takeaway	396
Coconut Milk, Primo	297
Coconut Milk, Primo, Takeaway	324
Semi Skimmed Milk, Lactofree, Medio	385
Semi Skimmed Milk, Lactofree, Medio, Takeaway	408
Semi Skimmed Milk, Lactofree, Primo	304
Semi Skimmed Milk, Lactofree, Primo, Takeaway	333
Semi Skimmed Milk, Medio	402
Semi Skimmed Milk, Medio, Takeaway	428
Semi Skimmed Milk, Primo	316

COSTA	KCAL
HOT CHOCOLATE - HAZELNUT PRALINE	
Semi Skimmed Milk, Primo, Takeaway	348
Skimmed Milk, Medio	372
Skimmed Milk, Medio, Takeaway	484
Skimmed Milk, Primo	295
Skimmed Milk, Primo, Takeaway	322
Soya Milk, Medio	393
Soya Milk, Medio, Takeaway	418
Soya Milk, Primo	310
Soya Milk, Primo, Takeaway	341
Whole Milk, Medio	430
Whole Milk, Medio, Takeaway	476
Whole Milk, Primo	345
Whole Milk, Primo, Takeaway	385
HOT CHOCOLATE - WHITE	
Almond Milk, Massimo	276
Almond Milk, Massimo, Takeaway	300
Almond Milk, Medio	208
Almond Milk, Medio, Takeaway	234
Almond Milk, Primo	137
Almond Milk, Primo, Takeaway	164
Coconut Milk, Massimo	315
Coconut Milk, Massimo, Takeaway	348
Coconut Milk, Medio	237
Coconut Milk, Medio, Takeaway	274
Coconut Milk, Primo	156
Coconut Milk, Primo, Takeaway	194
Semi Skimmed Milk, Lactofree, Massimo	341
Semi Skimmed Milk, Lactofree, Massimo, Takeaway	380
Semi Skimmed Milk, Lactofree, Medio	256
Semi Skimmed Milk, Lactofree, Medio, Takeaway	300
Semi Skimmed Milk, Lactofree, Primo	168
Semi Skimmed Milk, Lactofree, Primo, Takeaway	213
Semi Skimmed Milk, Massimo	371
Semi Skimmed Milk, Massimo, Takeaway	417
Semi Skimmed Milk, Medio	279
Semi Skimmed Milk, Medio, Takeaway	331
Semi Skimmed Milk, Primo	183
Semi Skimmed Milk, Primo, Takeaway	236
Skimmed Milk, Massimo	310
Skimmed Milk, Massimo, Takeaway	342
Skimmed Milk, Medio	234
Skimmed Milk, Medio, Takeaway	269
Skimmed Milk, Primo	154
Skimmed Milk, Primo, Takeaway	190
Soya Milk, Massimo	353
Soya Milk, Massimo, Takeaway	395
Soya Milk, Medio	266
Soya Milk, Medio, Takeaway	313
Soya Milk, Primo	175
Soya Milk, Primo, Takeaway	223
White, Whole Milk, Massimo	457
Whole Milk, Massimo, Takeaway	523

COSTA	KCAL
HOT CHOCOLATE - WHITE	
Whole Milk, Medio	344
Whole Milk, Medio, Takeaway	418
Whole Milk, Primo	225
Whole Milk, Primo, Takeaway	301
ICE CREAM	
Vanilla, Individual Tubs, SOTF	159
ICE CREAM CONE	
Gingerbread	224
JUICE DRINK	
Coconut, & Watermelon, Fruit Cooler, Medio	117
Coconut, & Watermelon, Fruit Cooler, Primo	88
Mango & Passionfruit, Fruit Cooler, Medio	149
Mango & Passionfruit, Fruit Cooler, Primo	112
Red Summer Berries, Fruit Cooler, Medio	198
Red Summer Berries, Fruit Cooler, Primo	150
LEMONADE	
Peach	87
MACARONI CHEESE	
Bolognese	481
Box	597
MARSHMALLOWS	
Portion	20
MERINGUE	
Pink Swirl	183
Pink Swirl, SOTF	183
MILK DRINK - CHOCOLATE	
Almond Milk, Medio, Iced	200
Almond Milk, Medio, Iced, Takeaway	208
Almond Milk, Primo, Iced	143
Almond Milk, Primo, Iced, Takeaway	146
Coconut Milk, Medio, Iced	221
Coconut Milk, Medio, Iced, Takeaway	232
Coconut Milk, Primo, Iced	161
Coconut Milk, Primo, Iced, Takeaway	165
Semi Skimmed, Lactofree, Medio, Iced	235
Semi Skimmed, Lactofree, Medio, Iced, Takeaway	249
Semi Skimmed, Lactofree, Primo, Iced	172
Semi Skimmed, Lactofree, Primo, Iced, Takeaway	177
Semi Skimmed Milk, Medio, Iced	252
Semi Skimmed Milk, Medio, Iced, Takeaway	267
Semi Skimmed Milk, Primo, Iced	186
Semi Skimmed Milk, Primo, Iced, Takeaway	192
Skimmed Milk, Medio, Iced	219
Skimmed Milk, Medio, Iced, Takeaway	230
Skimmed Milk, Primo, Iced	159
Skimmed Milk, Primo, Iced, Takeaway	163
Soya Milk, Medio, Iced	242
Soya Milk, Medio, Iced, Takeaway	257
Soya Milk, Primo, Iced	178
Soya Milk, Primo, Iced, Takeaway	184
Whole Milk, Medio, Iced	299
Whole Milk, Medio, Iced, Takeaway	321

COSTA	KCAL
MILK DRINK - CHOCOLATE	
Whole Milk, Primo, Iced	226
Whole Milk, Primo, Iced, Takeaway	234
MILK WHIP	
Strawberry, Medio	168
Strawberry, Primo	117
Vanilla, Medio	104
Vanilla, Primo	74
MUFFIN	
Banana & Pecan Breakfast Loaf	442
Blueberry	389
Caramel, Salted	391
Chocolate	485
Chocolate, with Flake	405
Lemon	399
Lotus Biscoff	467
Mini	76
Raspberry, & White Chocolate	364
Raspberry Rainbow	425
NUTS	
Natural, Mixed	187
ORANGES	
Easy Peeler	59
PANETTONE	
Classic	377
PANINI	
Brie, & Bacon	530
Goats Cheese, & Grilled Pepper, Focaccia	491
Ham, British, & Cheddar	438
Mozzarella, Tomato, & Basil	508
Tuna, Melt	471
PASTRY	
Cheese, Twist	327
Chocolate, Twist	305
Pain Aux Raisins	274
POPCORN	
Sweet & Salty	137
PRETZELS	
Salted, Bites, Baked	97
RAISINS	
Chocolate, Milk	161
RISOTTO	
Butternut Squash	301
SALAD	
Chicken, Roast	196
Cous Cous, Moroccan Styles	392
Pasta, Mozzarella, & Sun-Dried Tomato	529
SANDWICH	
Chicken, Roast, & Bacon	454
Chicken, Salad, Roast	427
Egg, Free Range	342
Ham, & Cheddar Cheese, Baguette, SOTF	716
Mozzarella, & Tomato, Baguette, SOTF	670

	KCAL
COSTA	
SANDWICH	
Tuna, & Sweetcorn	395
Tuna & Cucumber, SOTF	566
SAUSAGE ROLL	
Single	400
SCONE	
Cheese	391
SHORTBREAD	
Bites, Mini	47
Chocolate Chunk, Milk	344
Jammy	238
Millionaire	396
SOUP	
Carrot & Coriander	167
SWEETS	
Cola Bottles, Sugar Free, Vegan	87
Gummy Bears, Sugar Free, Vegan	87
SYRUP	
Caramel	14
Caramel, Sugar Free	1
Cinnamon	16
Gingerbread, Sugar Free	1
Roasted Hazelnut	15
Vanilla	17
TART	
Apple, Glazed, SOTF	193
Bakewell, Cherry	389
Bakewell, Mini	273
Custard, Portugese	169
Lemon	347
Mince, Vegan, GF	322
TEA	
English, Breakfast	1
English, Breakfast, Decaff	3
Green, Jasmine	1
Green, Simply Sencha	3
Fruit, Superfruity	2
Earl Grey, The Earl	3
Mint, Thoroughly Minted	3
TEA - CHAI LATTE	
Almond Milk, Massimo	192
Almond Milk, Massimo, Takeaway	192
Almond Milk, Medio	160
Almond Milk, Medio, Takeaway	160
Almond Milk, Primo	105
Almond Milk, Primo, Takeaway	123
Coconut Milk, Massimo	225
Coconut Milk, Massimo, Takeaway	225
Coconut Milk, Medio	190
Coconut Milk, Medio, Takeaway	190
Coconut Milk, Primo	125
Coconut Milk, Primo, Takeaway	149
Semi Skimmed Milk, Lactofree, Massimo	244

	KCAL
COSTA	
TEA - CHAI LATTE	
Semi Skimmed Milk, Lactofree, Massimo, Takeaway	244
Semi Skimmed Milk, Lactofree, Medio	207
Semi Skimmed Milk, Lactofree, Medio, Takeaway	207
Semi Skimmed Milk, Lactofree, Primo	135
Semi Skimmed Milk, Lactofree, Primo, Takeaway	164
Semi Skimmed Milk, Massimo	273
Semi Skimmed Milk, Massimo, Takeaway	273
Semi Skimmed Milk, Medio	234
Semi Skimmed Milk, Medio, Takeaway	234
Semi Skimmed Milk, Primo	153
Semi Skimmed Milk, Primo, Takeaway	187
Skimmed Milk, Massimo	221
Skimmed Milk, Massimo, Takeaway	221
Skimmed Milk, Medio	187
Skimmed Milk, Medio, Takeaway	187
Skimmed Milk, Primo	123
Skimmed Milk, Primo, Takeaway	147
Soya Milk, Massimo	259
Soya Milk, Massimo, Takeaway	259
Soya Milk, Medio	221
Soya Milk, Medio, Takeaway	221
Soya Milk, Primo	144
Soya Milk, Primo, Takeaway	176
Whole Milk, Massimo	348
Whole Milk, Massimo, Takeaway	348
Whole Milk, Medio	302
Whole Milk, Medio, Takeaway	302
Whole Milk, Primo	196
Whole Milk, Primo, Takeaway	245
TEA - ICED	
Peach, Medio	95
Peach, Medio, Takeaway	97
Peach, Primo	67
Peach, Primo, Takeaway	67
Strawberry, Infusion, Medio	123
Strawberry, Infusion, Medio, Takeaway	123
Strawberry, Infusion, Primo	83
Strawberry, Infusion, Primo, Takeaway	83
Chai Latte, Almond Milk, Medio	116
Chai Latte, Almond Milk, Primo	82
Chai Latte, Coconut Milk, Medio	132
Chai Latte, Coconut Milk, Primo	95
Chai Latte, Semi Skimmed Milk, Lactofree, Medio	143
Chai Latte, Semi Skimmed Milk, Lactofree, Primo	103
Chai Latte, Semi Skimmed Milk, Medio	156
Chai Latte, Semi Skimmed Milk, Primo	113
Chai Latte, Skimmed Milk, Medio	131
Chai Latte, Skimmed Milk, Primo	93
Chai Latte, Soya Milk, Medio	149
Chai Latte, Soya Milk, Primo	107
Chai Latte, Whole Milk, Medio	192
Chai Latte, Whole Milk, Primo	141

COSTA

	KCAL
TEACAKES	
Fruit, No Butter, Breakfast	312
Fruit, Vegan, No Butter, Breakfast	295
TOAST	
Brown, Seeded	382
Fruit	298
White, No Butter	275
TOASTIE	
Cheddar, & Tomato, Slow Roasted	446
Chicken, & Bacon	418
Emmenthal, & Mushroom	436
Ham, & Cheese	307
Ham, Wiltshire, & Mature Cheddar	409
Turkey, & Trimmings	474
WAFERS	
Cocoa, Snack	223
Vanilla, Snack	230
WAFFLES	
Belgian, SOTF	462
WRAP	
Chicken, & Bacon, Caesar	532
Chicken, Fajita, Roast	439
Chickpea & Mango, Spiced, Vegan, SOTF	412
Tomato, & Mozzarella	400
YOGHURT	
Granola, Berry, Hedgerow, SOTF	299
Greek Style, 0% Fat, Organic	68

DOMINO'S PIZZA

	KCAL
BREAD	
Garlic, Dippers	243
Garlic, Pizza	311
CHICKEN	
Chick 'n' Mix	386
Kickers, Combo Box	178
Kickers	186
Strippers, Combo Box	218
Strippers	268
Wings, Combo Box	195
Wings	222
Wings, Red Hot, Franks	224
Wings, Spicy BBQ	250
COLESLAW	
Side	146
COOKIES	
Serving	183
DESSERT	
Cinni Dippers	200
DIP	
BBQ, Big	188
BBQ	47
Garlic & Herb, Big	676
Garlic & Herb	169
Honey & Mystard	109
Red Hot, Franks, Big	23
Red Hot, Franks	6
Salsa, Tangy	43
Sweet Chilli	54
DOUGH BALLS	
Twisted, with Cheese	339
Twisted, with Ham	341
Twisted, with Pepperoni	373
NACHOS	
no Jalapenos	263
with Jalapenos	264
PIZZA - AMERICAN HOT	
Classic Crust, Delight Mozzarella, Large	195
Classic Crust, Delight Mozzarella, Medium	174
Classic Crust, Delight Mozzarella, Personal	136
Classic Crust, Delight Mozzarella, Small	254
Classic Crust, Large	208
Classic Crust, Medium	189
Classic Crust, Personal	147
Classic Crust, Small	261
Italian Style Crust, Delight Mozzarella, Large	159
Italian Style Crust, Delight Mozzarella, Medium	140
Italian Style Crust, Delight Mozzarella, Small	209
Italian Style Crust, Large	172
Italian Style Crust, Medium	152
Italian Style Crust, Small	228
Stuffed Crust, Delight Mozzarella, Large	229
Stuffed Crust, Delight Mozzarella, Medium	207

	KCAL
DOMINO'S PIZZA	
PIZZA - AMERICAN HOT	
Stuffed Crust, Large	224
Stuffed Crust, Medium	218
Stuffed Crust, Tabasco, Delight Mozzarella, Large	229
Stuffed Crust, Tabasco, Delight Mozzarella, Medium	212
Stuffed Crust, Tabasco, Large	238
Stuffed Crust, Tabasco, Medium	221
Thin & Crispy, Delight Mozzarella, Large	143
Thin & Crispy, Delight Mozzarella, Medium	136
Thin & Crispy, Large	160
Thin & Crispy, Medium	150
PIZZA - AMERICANO	
Classic Crust, Delight Mozzarella, Large	232
Classic Crust, Delight Mozzarella, Medium	206
Classic Crust, Delight Mozzarella, Personal	155
Classic Crust, Delight Mozzarella, Small	272
Classic Crust, Large	234
Classic Crust, Medium	214
Classic Crust, Small	274
Italian Style Crust, Delight Mozzarella, Large	189
Italian Style Crust, Delight Mozzarella, Medium	199
Italian Style Crust, Delight Mozzarella, Small	226
Italian Style Crust, Large	202
Italian Style Crust, Medium	219
Italian Style Crust, Small	238
Stuffed Crust, Delight Mozzarella, Large	261
Stuffed Crust, Delight Mozzarella, Medium	237
Stuffed Crust, Large	273
Stuffed Crust, Medium	251
Stuffed Crust, Tabasco, Delight Mozzarella, Large	266
Stuffed Crust, Tabasco, Delight Mozzarella, Medium	238
Stuffed Crust, Tabasco, Large	276
Stuffed Crust, Tabasco, Medium	247
Thin & Crispy, Delight Mozzarella, Large	167
Thin & Crispy, Delight Mozzarella, Medium	158
Thin & Crispy, Large	179
Thin & Crispy, Medium	247
Classic Crust, Personal	332
PIZZA - BACON DOUBLE CHEESE	
Classic Crust, Delight Mozzarella, Large	201
Classic Crust, Delight Mozzarella, Medium	177
Classic Crust, Delight Mozzarella, Personal	145
Classic Crust, Delight Mozzarella, Small	254
Classic Crust, Large	219
Classic Crust, Medium	195
Classic Crust, Personal	104
Classic Crust, Small	266
Italian Style Crust, Delight Mozzarella, Large	165
Italian Style Crust, Delight Mozzarella, Medium	143
Italian Style Crust, Delight Mozzarella, Small	210
Italian Style Crust, Large	182
Ã‚Â Italian Style Crust, Medium	159
Italian Style Crust, Small	233

	KCAL
DOMINO'S PIZZA	
PIZZA - BACON DOUBLE CHEESE	
Stuffed Crust, Delight Mozzarella, Large	236
Stuffed Crust, Delight Mozzarella, Medium	210
Stuffed Crust, Large	234
Stuffed Crust, Medium	224
Stuffed Crust, Tabasco, Delight Mozzarella, Large	236
Stuffed Crust, Tabasco, Delight Mozzarella, Medium	215
Stuffed Crust, Tabasco, Large	248
Stuffed Crust, Tabasco, Medium	227
Thin & Crispy, Delight Mozzarella, Large	149
Thin & Crispy, Delight Mozzarella, Medium	139
Thin & Crispy, Large	170
Thin & Crispy, Medium	157
PIZZA - BUFFALO CHICKEN	
Classic Crust, Delight Mozzarella, Large	178
Classic Crust, Delight Mozzarella, Medium	155
Classic Crust, Delight Mozzarella, Personal	124
Classic Crust, Delight Mozzarella. Small	223
Classic Crust, Large	192
Classic Crust, Medium	169
Classic Crust, Personal	135
Classic Crust, Small	231
Italian Style Crust, Delight Mozzarella, Large	142
Italian Style Crust, Delight Mozzarella, Medium	121
Italian Style Crust, Delight Mozzarella, Small	179
Italian Style Crust, Large	155
Italian Style Crust, Medium	133
Italian Style Crust, Small	198
Stuffed Crust, Delight Mozzarella, Large	223
Stuffed Crust, Delight Mozzarella, Medium	188
Stuffed Crust, Large	229
Stuffed Crust, Medium	199
Stuffed Crust, Tabasco, Delight Mozzarella, Large	212
Stuffed Crust, Tabasco, Delight Mozzarella, Medium	200
Stuffed Crust, Tabasco, Large	221
Stuffed Crust, Tabasco, Medium	209
Thin & Crispy, Delight Mozzarella, Large	126
Thin & Crispy, Delight Mozzarella, Medium	200
Thin & Crispy, Large	143
Thin & Crispy, Medium	131
PIZZA - CHEESE & TOMATO	
Classic Crust, Delight Mozzarella, Large	176
Classic Crust, Delight Mozzarella, Medium	153
Classic Crust, Delight Mozzarella, Personal	119
Classic Crust, Delight Mozzarella, Small	219
Classic Crust, Large	193
Classic Crust, Medium	171
Classic Crust, Personal	131
Classic Crust, Small	230
GF Crust, Delight Mozzarella, Small	188
GF Crust, Small	201
Italian Style Crust, Delight Mozzarella, Large	140
Italian Style Crust, Delight Mozzarella, Medium	120

DOMINO'S PIZZA

	KCAL
PIZZA - CHEESE & TOMATO	
Italian Style Crust, Delight Mozzarella, Small	174
Ã‚Â Italian Style Crust, Large	157
Italian Style Crust, Medium	135
Ã‚Â Italian Style Crust, Small	194
Stuffed Crust, Delight Mozzarella, Large	211
Stuffed Crust, Delight Mozzarella, Medium	186
Stuffed Crust, Large	209
Stuffed Crust, Medium	201
Stuffed Crust, Tabasco, Delight Mozzarella, Large	211
Stuffed Crust, Tabasco, Delight Mozzarella, Medium	192
Stuffed Crust, Tabasco, Large	223
Stuffed Crust, Tabsaco, Medium	204
Thin & Crispy, Delight Mozzarella, Large	124
Thin & Crispy, Delight Mozzarella, Medium	115
Thin & Crispy, Large	145
Thin & Crispy, Medium	133
PIZZA - CHICKEN FEAST	
Classic Crust, Delight Mozzarella, Large	184
Classic Crust, Delight Mozzarella, Medium	162
Classic Crust, Delight Mozzarella, Personal	128
Classic Crust, Delight Mozzarella, Small	231
Classic Crust, Large	198
Classic Crust, Medium	177
Classic Crust, Personal	139
Classic Crust, Small	238
Italian Style Crust, Delight Mozzarella, Lge	148
Italian Style Crust, Delight Mozzarella, Medium	128
Italian Style Crust, Delight Mozzarella, Small	186
Italian Style Crust, Lge	161
Italian Style Crust, Medium	140
Italian Style Crust, Small	206
Stuffed Crust, Delight Mozzarella, Large	219
Stuffed Crust, Delight Mozzarella, Medium	195
Stuffed Crust, Large	214
Stuffed Crust, Medium	206
Stuffed Crust, Tabasco, Delight Mozzarella, Large	219
Stuffed Crust, Tabasco, Delight Mozzarella, Medium	200
Stuffed Crust, Tabasco, Large	228
Stuffed Crust, Tabasco, Medium	209
Thin & Crispy, Delight Mozzarella, Large	132
Thin & Crispy, Delight Mozzarella, Medium	124
Thin & Crispy, Large	149
Thin & Crispy, Medium	138
PIZZA - CHOCOLATE	
Lotta	211
PIZZA - DELIGHT CHICKEN	
Delight Mozzarella, Large	148
Delight Mozzarella, Medium	122
Delight Mozzarella, Small	151
PIZZA - DELIGHT VEGI	
Delight Mozzarella, Large	146
Delight Mozzarella, Medium	120

DOMINO'S PIZZA

	KCAL
PIZZA - DELIGHT VEGI	
Delight Mozzarella, Small	149
PIZZA - DELUXE	
Classic Crust, Delight Mozzarella, Large	193
Classic Crust, Delight Mozzarella, Medium	173
Classic Crust, Delight Mozzarella, Personal	135
Classic Crust, Delight Mozzarella, Small	251
Classic Crust, Large	207
Classic Crust, Medium	187
Classic Crust, Personal	145
Classic Crust, Small	258
Italian Style Crust, Delight Mozzarella, Large	158
Italian Style Crust, Delight Mozzarella, Medium	139
Italian Style Crust, Delight Mozzarella, Small	206
Italian Style Crust, Large	171
Italian Style Crust, Medium	151
Italian Style Crust, Small	226
Stuffed Crust, Delight Mozzarella, Large	228
Stuffed Crust, Delight Mozzarella, Medium	206
Stuffed Crust, Large	223
Stuffed Crust, Medium	217
Stuffed Crust, Tabasco, Delight Mozzarella, Large	228
Stuffed Crust, Tabasco, Delight Mozzarella, Medium	211
Stuffed Crust, Tabasco, Large	237
Stuffed Crust, Tabasco, Medium	220
Thin & Crispy, Delight Mozzarella, Large	142
Thin & Crispy, Delight Mozzarella, Medium	138
Thin & Crispy, Large	159
Thin & Crispy, Medium	153
PIZZA - FARMHOUSE	
Classic Crust, Delight Mozzarella, Large	170
Classic Crust, Delight Mozzarella, Medium	149
Classic Crust, Delight Mozzarella, Personal	120
Classic Crust, Delight Mozzarella, Small	216
Classic Crust, Large	184
Classic Crust, Medium	164
Classic Crust, Personal	130
Classic Crust, Small	223
Italian Style Crust, Delight Mozzarella, Large	134
Italian Style Crust, Delight Mozzarella, Medium	115
Italian Style Crust, Delight Mozzarella, Small	171
Italian Style Crust, Large	147
Italian Style Crust, Medium	128
Italian Style Crust, Small	190
Stuffed Crust, Delight Mozzarella, Large	205
Stuffed Crust, Delight Mozzarella, Medium	182
Stuffed Crust, Large	199
Stuffed Crust, Medium	193
Stuffed Crust, Tabasco, Delight Mozzarella, Large	205
Stuffed Crust, Tabasco, Delight Mozzarella, Medium	187
Stuffed Crust, Tabasco, Large	214
Stuffed Crust, Tabasco, Medium	196
Thin & Crispy, Delight Mozzarella, Large	118

DOMINO'S PIZZA

PIZZA - FARMHOUSE

	KCAL
Thin & Crispy, Delight Mozzarella, Medium	111
Thin & Crispy, Large	136
Thin & Crispy, Medium	126

PIZZA - FIERY VEGI SIZZLER

	KCAL
Classic Crust, Delight Mozzarella, Large	160
Classic Crust, Delight Mozzarella, Medium	139
Classic Crust, Delight Mozzarella, Personal	113
Classic Crust, Delight Mozzarella, Small	202
Classic Crust, Large	174
Classic Crust, Medium	154
Classic Crust, Personal	124
Classic Crust, Small	209
Italian Style Crust, Delight Mozzarella, Large	124
Italian Style Crust, Delight Mozzarella, Medium	106
Italian Style Crust, Delight Mozzarella, Small	157
Italian Style Crust, Large	138
Italian Style Crust, Medium	118
Italian Style Crust, Small	177
Stuffed Crust, Delight Mozzarella, Large	195
Stuffed Crust, Delight Mozzarella, Medium	172
Stuffed Crust, Large	190
Stuffed Crust, Medium	184
Stuffed Crust, Tabasco, Delight Mozzarella, Large	195
Stuffed Crust, Tabasco, Delight Mozzarella, Medium	178
Stuffed Crust, Tabasco, Large	204
Stuffed Crust, Tabasco, Medium	187
Thin & Crispy, Delight Mozzarella, Large	108
Thin & Crispy, Delight Mozzarella, Medium	101
Thin & Crispy, Large	126
Thin & Crispy, Medium	116

PIZZA - FOUR VEGI

	KCAL
Classic Crust, Delight Mozzarella, Large	165
Classic Crust, Delight Mozzarella, Medium	145
Classic Crust, Delight Mozzarella, Personal	118
Classic Crust, Delight Mozzarella, Small	209
Classic Crust, Large	179
Classic Crust, Medium	159
Classic Crust, Personal	128
Classic Crust, Small	216
Italian Style Crust, Delight Mozzarella, Large	129
Italian Style Crust, Delight Mozzarella, Medium	111
Italian Style Crust, Delight Mozzarella, Small	164
Italian Style Crust, Large	143
Italian Style Crust, Medium	123
Italian Style Crust, Small	737
Stuffed Crust, Delight Mozzarella, Large	200
Stuffed Crust, Delight Mozzarella, Medium	178
Stuffed Crust, Large	195
Stuffed Crust, Medium	189
Stuffed Crust, Tabasco, Delight Mozzarella, Large	200
Stuffed Crust, Tabasco, Delight Mozzarella, Medium	183
Stuffed Crust, Tabasco, Large	209

DOMINO'S PIZZA

PIZZA - FOUR VEGI

	KCAL
Stuffed Crust, Tabasco, Medium	192
Thin & Crispy, Delight Mozzarella, Large	114
Thin & Crispy, Delight Mozzarella, Medium	107
Thin & Crispy, Large	131
Thin & Crispy, Medium	121

PIZZA - FULL HOUSE

	KCAL
Classic Crust, Delight Mozzarella, Large	197
Classic Crust, Delight Mozzarella, Medium	174
Classic Crust, Delight Mozzarella, Personal	145
Classic Crust, Delight Mozzarella, Small	253
Classic Crust, Large	211
Classic Crust, Medium	189
Classic Crust, Personal	155
Classic Crust, Small	260
Italian Style Crust, Delight Mozzarella, Large	161
Italian Style Crust, Delight Mozzarella, Medium	141
Italian Style Crust, Delight Mozzarella, Small	208
Italian Style Crust, Large	174
Italian Style Crust, Medium	153
Italian Style Crust, Small	228
Stuffed Crust, Delight Mozzarella, Large	228
Stuffed Crust, Delight Mozzarella, Medium	207
Stuffed Crust, Large	226
Stuffed Crust, Medium	219
Stuffed Crust, Tabasco, Delight Mozzarella, Large	231
Stuffed Crust, Tabasco, Delight Mozzarella, Medium	213
Stuffed Crust, Tabasco, Large	240
Stuffed Crust,Tabasco,Ã,Â Medium	221
Thin & Crispy, Delight Mozzarella, Large	145
Thin & Crispy, Delight Mozzarella, Medium	136
Thin & Crispy, Large	162
Thin & Crispy, Medium	151

PIZZA - HAM & PINEAPPLE

	KCAL
Classic Crust, Delight Mozzarella, Large	170
Classic Crust, Delight Mozzarella, Medium	149
Classic Crust, Delight Mozzarella, Personal	120
Classic Crust, Delight Mozzarella, Small	216
Classic Crust, Large	183
Classic Crust, Medium	164
Classic Crust, Personal	130
Classic Crust, Small	223
Italian Style Crust, Delight Mozzarella, Large	201
Italian Style Crust, Delight Mozzarella, Medium	115
Italian Style Crust, Delight Mozzarella, Small	171
Italian Style Crust, Large	147
Italian Style Crust, Medium	127
Italian Style Crust, Small	190
Stuffed Crust, Delight Mozzarella, Large	204
Stuffed Crust, Delight Mozzarella, Medium	182
Stuffed Crust, Large	199
Stuffed Crust, Medium	193
Stuffed Crust, Tabasco, Delight Mozzarella, Large	204

	KCAL
DOMINO'S PIZZA	
PIZZA - HAM & PINEAPPLE	
Stuffed Crust, Tabasco, Delight Mozzarella, Medium	187
Stuffed Crust, Tabasco, Large	213
Stuffed Crust, Tabasco, Medium	196
Thin & Crispy, Delight Mozzarella, Large	118
Thin & Crispy, Delight Mozzarella, Medium	111
Thin & Crispy, Large	135
Thin & Crispy, Medium	125
PIZZA - HOT & SPICY	
Classic Crust, Delight Mozzarella, Large	171
Classic Crust, Delight Mozzarella, Medium	149
Classic Crust, Delight Mozzarella, Personal	120
Classic Crust, Delight Mozzarella, Small	215
Classic Crust, Large	185
Classic Crust, Medium	164
Classic Crust, Personal	131
Classic Crust, Small	193
Italian Style Crust, Delight Mozzarella, Large	135
Italian Style Crust, Delight Mozzarella, Medium	115
Italian Style Crust, Delight Mozzarella, Small	171
Italian Style Crust, Large	149
Italian Style Crust, Medium	128
Italian Style Crust, Small	190
Stuffed Crust, Delight Mozzarella, Large	206
Stuffed Crust, Delight Mozzarella, Medium	182
Stuffed Crust, Large	201
Stuffed Crust, Medium	193
Stuffed Crust, Tabasco, Delight Mozzarella, Large	206
Stuffed Crust, Tabasco, Delight Mozzarella, Medium	187
Stuffed Crust, Tabasco, Large	215
Stuffed Crust, Tabasco, Medium	196
Thin & Crispy, Delight Mozzarella, Large	119
Thin & Crispy, Delight Mozzarella, Medium	111
Thin & Crispy, Large	137
Thin & Crispy, Medium	126
PIZZA - HOUSE SPECIAL TANDOORI	
Classic Crust, Delight Mozzarella, Large	224
Classic Crust, Delight Mozzarella, Medium	200
Classic Crust, Delight Mozzarella, Personal	167
Classic Crust, Delight Mozzarella, Small	288
Classic Crust, Large	241
Classic Crust, Medium	218
Classic Crust, Personal	180
Classic Crust, Small	300
Italian Style Crust, Delight Mozzarella, Large	188
Italian Style Crust, Delight Mozzarella, Medium	167
Italian Style Crust, Delight Mozzarella, Small	244
Italian Style Crust, Large	205
Italian Style Crust, Medium	182
Italian Style Crust, Small	267
Stuffed Crust, Delight Mozzarella, Large	259
Stuffed Crust, Delight Mozzarella, Medium	233
Stuffed Crust, Large	257

	KCAL
DOMINO'S PIZZA	
PIZZA - HOUSE SPECIAL TANDOORI	
Stuffed Crust, Medium	248
Stuffed Crust, Tabasco, Delight Mozzarella, Large	259
Stuffed Crust, Tabasco, Delight Mozzarella, Medium	239
Stuffed Crust, Tabasco, Large	271
Stuffed Crust, Tabasco, Medium	250
Thin & Crispy, Delight Mozzarella, Large	172
Thin & Crispy, Delight Mozzarella, Medium	162
Thin & Crispy, Large	257
Thin & Crispy, Medium	180
PIZZA - MEAT LOVERS	
Classic Crust, Delight Mozzarella, Large	211
Classic Crust, Delight Mozzarella, Medium	189
Classic Crust, Delight Mozzarella, Personal	148
Classic Crust, Delight Mozzarella, Small	276
Classic Crust, Large	225
Classic Crust, Medium	204
Classic Crust, Personal	159
Classic Crust, Small	283
Italian Style Crust, Delight Mozzarella, Large	263
Italian Style Crust, Delight Mozzarella, Medium	155
Italian Style Crust, Delight Mozzarella, Small	231
Italian Style Crust, Large	225
Italian Style Crust, Medium	167
Italian Style Crust, Small	251
Stuffed Crust, Delight Mozzarella, Large	246
Stuffed Crust, Delight Mozzarella, Medium	222
Stuffed Crust, Large	241
Stuffed Crust, Medium	233
Stuffed Crust, Tabasco, Delight Mozzarella, Large	246
Stuffed Crust, Tabasco, Delight Mozzarella, Medium	227
Stuffed Crust, Tabasco, Large	255
Stuffed Crust, Tabasco, Medium	236
Thin & Crispy, Delight Mozzarella, Large	159
Thin & Crispy, Delight Mozzarella, Medium	151
Thin & Crispy, Large	176
Thin & Crispy, Medium	165
PIZZA - MEATEOR	
Classic Crust, Delight Mozzarella, Large	246
Classic Crust, Delight Mozzarella, Medium	220
Classic Crust, Delight Mozzarella, Personal	184
Classic Crust, Delight Mozzarella, Small	294
Classic Crust, Large	249
Classic Crust, Medium	228
Classic Crust, Personal	194
Classic Crust, Small	296
Italian Style Crust, Delight Mozzarella, Large	204
Italian Style Crust, Delight Mozzarella, Medium	213
Italian Style Crust, Delight Mozzarella, Small	248
Italian Style Crust, Large	216
Italian Style Crust, Medium	233
Italian Style Crust, Small	260
Stuffed Crust, Delight Mozzarella, Large	276

DOMINO'S PIZZA	KCAL
PIZZA - MEATEOR	
Stuffed Crust, Delight Mozzarella, Medium	251
Stuffed Crust, Large	288
Stuffed Crust, Medium	266
Stuffed Crust, Tabasco, Delight Mozzarella, Large	280
Stuffed Crust, Tabasco, Delight Mozzarella, Medium	252
Stuffed Crust, Tabasco, Large	291
Stuffed Crust, Tabasco, Medium	261
Thin & Crispy, Delight Mozzarella, Large	182
Thin & Crispy, Delight Mozzarella, Medium	172
Thin & Crispy, Large	193
Thin & Crispy, Medium	179
PIZZA - MEATILICIOUS	
Classic Crust, Delight Mozzarella, Large	202
Classic Crust, Delight Mozzarella, Medium	180
Classic Crust, Delight Mozzarella, Personal	155
Classic Crust, Delight Mozzarella, Small	263
Classic Crust, Large	216
Classic Crust, Medium	195
Classic Crust, Personal	166
Classic Crust, Small	271
Italian Style Crust, Delight Mozzarella, Large	166
Italian Style Crust, Delight Mozzarella, Medium	146
Italian Style Crust, Delight Mozzarella, Small	219
Italian Style Crust, Large	179
Italian Style Crust, Medium	158
Italian Style Crust, Small	238
Stuffed Crust, Delight Mozzarella, Large	237
Stuffed Crust, Delight Mozzarella, Medium	213
Stuffed Crust, Large	232
Stuffed Crust, Medium	224
Stuffed Crust, Delight Mozzarella, Large	237
Stuffed Crust, Tabasco, Delight Mozzarella, Medium	218
Stuffed Crust, Tabasco, Large	245
Stuffed Crust, Tabasco, Medium	227
Thin & Crispy, Delight Mozzarella, Large	150
Thin & Crispy, Delight Mozzarella, Medium	142
Thin & Crispy, Large	165
Thin & Crispy, Medium	156
PIZZA - MEATZZA	
Classic Crust, Delight Mozzarella, Large	207
Classic Crust, Delight Mozzarella, Medium	185
Classic Crust, Delight Mozzarella, Personal	142
Classic Crust, Delight Mozzarella, Small	270
Classic Crust, Large	221
Classic Crust, Medium	200
Classic Crust, Personal	153
Classic Crust, Small	277
Italian Style Crust, Delight Mozzarella, Large	171
Italian Style Crust, Delight Mozzarella, Medium	151
Italian Style Crust, Delight Mozzarella, Small	225
Italian Style Crust, Large	184
Italian Style Crust, Medium	164

DOMINO'S PIZZA	KCAL
PIZZA - MEATZZA	
Italian Style Crust, Small	244
Stuffed Crust, Delight Mozzarella, Large	241
Stuffed Crust, Delight Mozzarella, Medium	218
Stuffed Crust, Large	236
Stuffed Crust, Medium	230
Stuffed Crust, Tabasco, Large	251
Stuffed Crust, Tabasco, Medium	232
Thin & Crispy, Delight Mozzarella, Large	169
Thin & Crispy, Delight Mozzarella, Medium	158
Thin & Crispy, Large	172
Thin & Crispy, Medium	162
PIZZA - MEXICAN HOT	
Classic Crust, Delight Mozzarella, Large	202
Classic Crust, Delight Mozzarella, Medium	179
Classic Crust, Delight Mozzarella, Personal	135
Classic Crust, Delight Mozzarella, Small	257
Classic Crust, Large	219
Classic Crust, Medium	197
Classic Crust, Personal	147
Classic Crust, Small	268
Italian Style Crust, Delight Mozzarella, Large	166
Italian Style Crust, Delight Mozzarella, Medium	145
Italian Style Crust, Delight Mozzarella, Small	212
Ã‚Â Italian Style Crust, Large	182
Italian Style Crust, Medium	160
Italian Style Crust, Small	236
Stuffed Crust, Delight Mozzarella, Large	236
Stuffed Crust, Delight Mozzarella, Medium	212
Stuffed Crust, Large	235
Stuffed Crust, Medium	226
Stuffed Crust, Tabasco, Delight Mozzarella, Large	236
Stuffed Crust, Tabasco, Delight Mozzarella, Medium	217
Stuffed Crust, Tabasco, Large	249
Stuffed Crust, Tabasco, Medium	229
Thin & Crispy, Delight Mozzarella, Large	150
Thin & Crispy, Delight Mozzarella, Medium	141
Thin & Crispy, Large	170
Thin & Crispy, Medium	159
PIZZA - MIGHTY MEATY	
Classic Crust, Delight Mozzarella, Large	211
Classic Crust, Delight Mozzarella, Medium	188
Classic Crust, Delight Mozzarella, Personal	144
Classic Crust, Delight Mozzarella, Small	273
Classic Crust, Large	224
Classic Crust, Medium	203
Classic Crust, Personal	155
Classic Crust, Small	281
Italian Style Crust, Delight Mozzarella, Large	175
Italian Style Crust, Delight Mozzarella, Medium	154
Italian Style Crust, Delight Mozzarella, Small	228
Italian Style Crust, Large	188
Italian Style Crust, Medium	167

	KCAL
DOMINO'S PIZZA	
PIZZA - MIGHTY MEATY	
Italian Style Crust, Small	248
Stuffed Crust, Delight Mozzarella, Large	245
Stuffed Crust, Delight Mozzarella, Medium	221
Stuffed Crust, Large	240
Stuffed Crust, Medium	232
Stuffed Crust, Tabasco, Delight Mozzarella, Large	245
Stuffed Crust, Tabasco, Delight Mozzarella, Medium	226
Stuffed Crust, Tabasco, Large	254
Stuffed Crust, Tabasco, Medium	235
Thin & Crispy, Delight Mozzarella, Large	159
Thin & Crispy, Delight Mozzarella, Medium	150
Thin & Crispy, Large	176
Thin & Crispy, Medium	165
PIZZA - MIXED GRILL	
Classic Crust, Delight Mozzarella, Large	199
Classic Crust, Delight Mozzarella, Medium	177
Classic Crust, Delight Mozzarella, Personal	145
Classic Crust, Delight Mozzarella, Small	260
Classic Crust, Large	212
Classic Crust, Medium	192
Classic Crust, Personal	156
Classic Crust, Small	267
Italian Style Crust, Delight Mozzarella, Large	163
Italian Style Crust, Delight Mozzarella, Medium	143
Italian Style Crust, Delight Mozzarella, Small	215
Italian Style Crust, Large	176
Italian Style Crust, Medium	156
Italian Style Crust, Small	235
Stuffed Crust, Delight Mozzarella, Large	233
Stuffed Crust, Delight Mozzarella, Medium	210
Stuffed Crust, Large	228
Stuffed Crust, Medium	221
Stuffed Crust, Tabasco, Delight Mozzarella, Large	234
Stuffed Crust, Tabasco, Delight Mozzarella, Medium	215
Stuffed Crust, Tabasco, Large	243
Stuffed Crust, Tabasco, Medium	224
Thin & Crispy, Delight Mozzarella, Large	147
Thin & Crispy, Delight Mozzarella, Medium	139
Thin & Crispy, Large	164
Thin & Crispy, Medium	154
PIZZA - NEW YORKER	
Classic Crust, Delight Mozzarella, Large	200
Classic Crust, Delight Mozzarella, Medium	179
Classic Crust, Delight Mozzarella, Personal	142
Classic Crust, Delight Mozzarella, Small	263
Classic Crust, Large	214
Classic Crust, Medium	194
Classic Crust, Personal	152
Classic Crust, Small	270
GF Crust, Delight Mozzarella, Small	232
GF Crust, Small	241
Italian Style Crust, Delight Mozzarella, Large	164

	KCAL
DOMINO'S PIZZA	
PIZZA - NEW YORKER	
Italian Style Crust, Delight Mozzarella, Medium	145
Italian Style Crust, Delight Mozzarella, Small	218
Italian Style Crust, Large	178
Italian Style Crust, Medium	158
Italian Style Crust, Small	237
Stuffed Crust, Delight Mozzarella, Large	235
Stuffed Crust, Delight Mozzarella, Medium	212
Stuffed Crust, Large	230
Stuffed Crust, Medium	223
Stuffed Crust, Tabasco, Delight Mozzarella, Large	235
Stuffed Crust, Tabasco, Delight Mozzarella, Medium	217
Stuffed Crust, Tabasco, Large	244
Stuffed Crust, Tabasco, Medium	226
Thin & Crispy, Delight Mozzarella, Large	149
Thin & Crispy, Delight Mozzarella, Medium	141
Thin & Crispy, Large	166
Thin & Crispy, Medium	156
PIZZA - PEPPERONI PASSION	
Classic Crust, Delight Mozzarella, Large	223
Classic Crust, Delight Mozzarella, Medium	200
Classic Crust, Delight Mozzarella, Personal	157
Classic Crust, Delight Mozzarella, Small	292
Classic Crust, Large	240
Classic Crust, Medium	218
Classic Crust, Personal	169
Classic Crust, Small	303
GF Crust, Delight Mozzarella, Small	261
Italian Style Crust, Delight Mozzarella, Large	187
Italian Style Crust, Delight Mozzarella, Medium	166
Italian Style Crust, Delight Mozzarella, Small	247
Italian Style Crust, Large	203
Italian Style Crust, Medium	182
Italian Style Crust, Small	271
Stuffed Crust, Delight Mozzarella, Large	257
Stuffed Crust, Delight Mozzarella, Medium	233
Stuffed Crust, Large	256
Stuffed Crust, Medium	247
Stuffed Crust, Tabasco, Delight Mozzarella, Large	257
Stuffed Crust, Tabasco, Delight Mozzarella, Medium	238
Stuffed Crust, Tabasco, Large	270
Stuffed Crust, Tabasco, Medium	250
Thin & Crispy, Delight Mozzarella, Large	171
Thin & Crispy, Delight Mozzarella, Medium	162
Thin & Crispy, Large	191
Thin & Crispy, Medium	180
PIZZA - RANCH BBQ	
Classic Crust, Delight Mozzarella, Large	241
Classic Crust, Delight Mozzarella, Medium	212
Classic Crust, Delight Mozzarella, Personal	159
Classic Crust, Delight Mozzarella, Small	279
Classic Crust, Large	243
Classic Crust, Medium	220

DOMINO'S PIZZA

	KCAL
PIZZA - RANCH BBQ	
Classic Crust, Personal	170
Classic Crust, Small	282
Italian Style Crust, Delight Mozzarella, Large	198
Italian Style Crust, Delight Mozzarella, Medium	205
Italian Style Crust, Delight Mozzarella, Small	233
Italian Style Crust, Large	211
Italian Style Crust, Medium	225
Italian Style Crust, Small	245
Stuffed Crust, Delight Mozzarella, Large	270
Stuffed Crust, Delight Mozzarella, Medium	243
Stuffed Crust, Large	282
Stuffed Crust, Medium	257
Stuffed Crust, Tabasco, Delight Mozzarella, Large	274
Stuffed Crust, Tabasco, Delight Mozzarella, Medium	244
Stuffed Crust, Tabasco, Large	285
Stuffed Crust, Tabasco, Medium	253
Thin & Crispy, Delight Mozzarella, Large	176
Thin & Crispy, Delight Mozzarella, Medium	164
Thin & Crispy, Large	188
Thin & Crispy, Medium	171
PIZZA - SCRUMMY	
Classic Crust, Delight Mozzarella, Large	229
Classic Crust, Delight Mozzarella, Medium	205
Classic Crust, Delight Mozzarella, Personal	173
Classic Crust, Delight Mozzarella, Small	299
Classic Crust, Large	242
Classic Crust, Medium	220
Classic Crust, Personal	184
Classic Crust, Small	306
Italian Style Crust, Delight Mozzarella, Large	193
Italian Style Crust, Delight Mozzarella, Medium	172
Italian Style Crust, Delight Mozzarella, Small	254
Italian Style Crust, Large	206
Italian Style Crust, Medium	184
Italian Style Crust, Small	273
Stuffed Crust, Delight Mozzarella, Large	263
Stuffed Crust, Delight Mozzarella, Medium	238
Stuffed Crust, Large	258
Stuffed Crust, Medium	250
Stuffed Crust, Tabasco, Delight Mozzarella, Large	263
Stuffed Crust, Tabasco, Delight Mozzarella, Medium	244
Stuffed Crust, Tabasco, Large	272
Stuffed Crust, Tabasco, Medium	252
Thin & Crispy, Delight Mozzarella, Large	177
Thin & Crispy, Delight Mozzarella, Medium	167
Thin & Crispy, Large	194
Thin & Crispy, Medium	182
PIZZA - SIZZLER	
Classic Crust, Delight Mozzarella, Large	205
Classic Crust, Delight Mozzarella, Medium	183
Classic Crust, Delight Mozzarella, Personal	140
Classic Crust, Delight Mozzarella, Small	309

DOMINO'S PIZZA

	KCAL
PIZZA - SIZZLER	
Classic Crust, Large	220
Classic Crust, Medium	194
Classic Crust, Personal	151
Classic Crust, Small	333
Italian Style Crust, Delight Mozzarella, Large	171
Italian Style Crust, Delight Mozzarella, Medium	153
Italian Style Crust, Delight Mozzarella, Small	211
Italian Style Crust, Large	184
Italian Style Crust, Medium	159
Italian Style Crust, Small	230
Stuffed Crust, Delight Mozzarella, Large	232
Stuffed Crust, Delight Mozzarella, Medium	224
Stuffed Crust, Large	242
Stuffed Crust, Medium	232
Stuffed Crust, Tabasco, Delight Mozzarella, Large	244
Stuffed Crust, Tabasco, Delight Mozzarella, Medium	215
Stuffed Crust, Tabasco, Large	251
Stuffed Crust, Tabasco, Medium	234
Thin & Crispy, Delight Mozzarella, Large	148
Thin & Crispy, Delight Mozzarella, Medium	146
Thin & Crispy, Large	163
Thin & Crispy, Medium	153
PIZZA - TANDOORI HOT	
Classic Crust, Delight Mozzarella, Large	171
Classic Crust, Delight Mozzarella, Medium	149
Classic Crust, Delight Mozzarella, Personal	120
Classic Crust, Delight Mozzarella, Small	215
Classic Crust, Large	185
Classic Crust, Medium	164
Classic Crust, Personal	130
Classic Crust, Small	222
Italian Style Crust, Delight Mozzarella, Large	135
Italian Style Crust, Delight Mozzarella, Medium	115
Italian Style Crust, Delight Mozzarella, Small	170
Italian Style Crust, Large	148
Italian Style Crust, Medium	127
Italian Style Crust, Small	189
Stuffed Crust, Delight Mozzarella, Large	205
Stuffed Crust, Delight Mozzarella, Medium	182
Stuffed Crust, Large	200
Stuffed Crust, Medium	193
Stuffed Crust, Tabasco, Delight Mozzarella, Large	205
Stuffed Crust, Tabasco, Delight Mozzarella, Medium	188
Stuffed Crust, Tabasco, Large	214
Stuffed Crust, Tabasco, Medium	204
Thin & Crispy, Delight Mozzarella, Large	119
Thin & Crispy, Delight Mozzarella, Medium	111
Thin & Crispy, Large	136
Thin & Crispy, Medium	126
PIZZA - TANDOORI SIZZLER	
Classic Crust, Delight Mozzarella, Large	170
Classic Crust, Delight Mozzarella, Medium	147

	KCAL
DOMINO'S PIZZA	
PIZZA - TANDOORI SIZZLER	
Classic Crust, Delight Mozzarella, Personal	119
Classic Crust, Delight Mozzarella, Small	213
Classic Crust, Large	183
Classic Crust, Medium	162
Classic Crust, Personal	129
Classic Crust, Small	220
Italian Style Crust, Delight Mozzarella, Large	134
Italian Style Crust, Delight Mozzarella, Medium	114
Italian Style Crust, Delight Mozzarella, Small	168
Italian Style Crust, Large	147
Italian Style Crust, Medium	126
Italian Style Crust, Small	188
Stuffed Crust, Delight Mozzarella, Large	204
Stuffed Crust, Delight Mozzarella, Medium	180
Stuffed Crust, Large	199
Stuffed Crust, Medium	192
Stuffed Crust, Tabasco, Delight Mozzarella, Large	204
Stuffed Crust, Tabasco, Delight Mozzarella, Medium	186
Stuffed Crust, Tabasco, Large	194
Stuffed Crust, Tabasco, Medium	213
Thin & Crispy, Delight Mozzarella, Large	118
Thin & Crispy, Delight Mozzarella, Medium	109
Thin & Crispy, Large	135
Thin & Crispy, Medium	124
PIZZA - TEXAS BBQ	
Classic Crust, Delight Mozzarella, Large	208
Texas BBQ, Classic Crust, Delight Medium	182
Texas BBQ, Classic Crust, Delight Personal	144
Classic Crust, Delight Mozzarella, Small	236
Classic Crust, Large	211
Classic Crust, Medium	190
Classic Crust, Personal	155
Classic Crust, Small	239
GF Crust, Delight Mozzarella, Small	197
GF Crust, Small	206
Italian Style Crust, Delight Mozzarella, Large	166
Italian Style Crust, Delight Mozzarella, Medium	176
Italian Style Crust, Delight Mozzarella, Small	191
Italian Style Crust, Large	178
Italian Style Crust, Medium	195
Italian Style Crust, Small	202
Stuffed Crust, Delight Mozzarella, Large	238
Stuffed Crust, Delight Mozzarella, Medium	214
Stuffed Crust, Large	250
Stuffed Crust, Medium	228
Stuffed Crust, Tabasco, Delight Mozzarella, Large	242
Stuffed Crust, Tabasco, Delight Mozzarella, Medium	214
Stuffed Crust, Tabasco, Large	253
Stuffed Crust, Tabasco, Medium	223
Thin & Crispy, Delight Mozzarella, Large	144
Thin & Crispy, Delight Mozzarella, Medium	134
Thin & Crispy, Large	156

	KCAL
DOMINO'S PIZZA	
PIZZA - TEXAS BBQ	
Thin & Crispy, Medium	142
PIZZA - THE CHEESEBURGER	
Classic Crust, Delight Mozzarella, Large	197
Classic Crust, Delight Mozzarella, Medium	173
Classic Crust, Delight Mozzarella, Personal	137
Classic Crust, Delight Mozzarella, Small	248
Classic Crust, Large	211
Classic Crust, Medium	188
Classic Crust, Personal	146
Classic Crust, Small	255
Italian Style Crust, Delight Mozzarella, Large	161
Italian Style Crust, Delight Mozzarella, Medium	139
Italian Style Crust, Delight Mozzarella, Small	203
Italian Style Crust, Large	175
Italian Style Crust, Medium	151
Italian Style Crust, Small	223
Stuffed Crust, Delight Mozzarella, Large	232
Stuffed Crust, Delight Mozzarella, Medium	206
Stuffed Crust, Large	227
Stuffed Crust, Medium	217
Stuffed Crust, Tabasco, Delight Mozzarella, Large	232
Stuffed Crust, Tabasco, Delight Mozzarella, Medium	211
Stuffed Crust,Tabasco, Large	241
Stuffed Crust, Tabasco, Medium	220
Thin & Crispy, Delight, Medium	134
Thin & Crispy, Delight Mozzarella, Large	146
Thin & Crispy, Large	163
Thin & Crispy, Medium	149
PIZZA - TUNA SUPREME	
Classic Crust, Delight Mozzarella, Large	177
Classic Crust, Delight Mozzarella, Medium	152
Classic Crust, Delight Mozzarella, Personal	123
Classic Crust, Delight Mozzarella, Small	221
Classic Crust, Large	191
Classic Crust, Medium	167
Classic Crust, Personal	134
Classic Crust, Small	228
Italian Style Crust, Delight Mozzarella, Large	141
Italian Style Crust, Delight Mozzarella, Medium	119
Italian Style Crust, Delight Mozzarella, Small	176
Italian Style Crust, Large	154
Italian Style Crust, Medium	131
Italian Style Crust, Small	196
Stuffed Crust, Delight Mozzarella, Large	212
Stuffed Crust, Delight Mozzarella, Medium	185
Stuffed Crust, Large	206
Stuffed Crust, Medium	197
Stuffed Crust, Tabasco, Delight Mozzarella, Large	212
Stuffed Crust, Tabasco, Delight Mozzarella, Medium	191
Stuffed Crust, Tabasco, Large	220
Stuffed Crust, Tabasco, Medium	199
Thin & Crispy, Delight Mozzarella, Large	125

	KCAL
DOMINO'S PIZZA	
PIZZA - TUNA SUPREME	
Thin & Crispy, Delight Mozzarella, Medium	114
Thin & Crispy, Large	142
Thin & Crispy, Medium	129
PIZZA - ULTIMATE BACON CHEESEBURGER	
Classic Crust, Delight Mozzarella, Large	217
Classic Crust, Delight Mozzarella, Medium	193
Classic Crust, Delight Mozzarella, Personal	156
Classic Crust, Delight Mozzarella, Small	278
Classic Crust, Large	231
Classic Crust, Medium	207
Classic Crust, Personal	167
Classic Crust, Small	285
Italian Style Crust, Delight Mozzarella, Large	181
Italian Style Crust, Delight Mozzarella, Medium	159
Italian Style Crust, Delight Mozzarella, Small	233
Italian Style Crust, Large	195
Italian Style Crust, Medium	171
Italian Style Crust, Small	253
Stuffed Crust, Delight Mozzarella, Large	262
Stuffed Crust, Delight Mozzarella, Medium	226
Stuffed Crust, Large	269
Stuffed Crust, Medium	237
Stuffed Crust, Tabasco, Delight Mozzarella, Large	252
Stuffed Crust, Tabasco, Delight Mozzarella, Medium	231
Stuffed Crust, Tabasco, Large	264
Stuffed Crust, Tabasco, Medium	240
Thin & Crispy, Delight Mozzarella, Large	165
Thin & Crispy, Delight Mozzarella, Medium	155
Thin & Crispy, Large	193
Thin & Crispy, Medium	169
PIZZA - VEG-A-ROMA	
Classic Crust, Delight Mozzarella, Large	174
Classic Crust, Delight Mozzarella, Medium	153
Classic Crust, Delight Mozzarella, Personal	124
Classic Crust, Delight Mozzarella, Small	265
Classic Crust, Large	190
Classic Crust, Medium	164
Classic Crust, Personal	135
Classic Crust, Small	289
Italian Style Crust, Delight Mozzarella, Large	140
Italian Style Crust, Delight Mozzarella, Medium	123
Italian Style Crust, Delight Mozzarella, Small	166
Italian Style Crust, Large	153
Italian Style Crust, Medium	129
Italian Style Crust, Small	186
Stuffed Crust, Delight Mozzarella, Large	201
Stuffed Crust, Delight Mozzarella, Medium	194
Stuffed Crust, Large	211
Stuffed Crust, Medium	201
Stuffed Crust, Tabasco, Delight Mozzarella, Large	213
Stuffed Crust, Tabasco, Delight Mozzarella, Medium	185
Stuffed Crust, Tabasco, Large	220

	KCAL
DOMINO'S PIZZA	
PIZZA - VEG-A-ROMA	
Stuffed Crust, Tabasco, Medium	203
Thin & Crispy, Delight Mozzarella, Large	118
Thin & Crispy, Large	132
Thin & Crispy, Medium	123
PIZZA - VEGI CLASSIC	
Classic Crust, Delight Mozzarella, Large	162
Classic Crust, Delight Mozzarella, Medium	140
Classic Crust, Delight Mozzarella, Personal	114
Classic Crust, Delight Mozzarella, Small	203
Classic Crust, Large	176
Classic Crust, Medium	155
Classic Crust, Personal	124
Classic Crust, Small	210
Italian Style Crust, Delight Mozzarella, Large	126
Italian Style Crust, Delight Mozzarella, Medium	107
Italian Style Crust, Delight Mozzarella, Small	158
Italian Style Crust, Large	139
Italian Style Crust, Medium	119
Italian Style Crust, Small	178
Stuffed Crust, Delight Mozzarella, Large	196
Stuffed Crust, Delight Mozzarella, Medium	173
Stuffed Crust, Large	191
Stuffed Crust, Medium	185
Stuffed Crust, Tabasco, Delight Mozzarella, Large	205
Stuffed Crust, Tabasco, Delight Mozzarella, Medium	179
Stuffed Crust, Tabasco, Large	205
Stuffed Crust, Tabasco, Medium	187
Thin & Crispy, Delight Mozzarella, Large	110
Thin & Crispy, Delight Mozzarella, Medium	102
Thin & Crispy, Large	127
Thin & Crispy, Medium	117
PIZZA - VEGI SIZZLER	
Classic Crust, Delight Mozzarella, Large	161
Classic Crust, Delight Mozzarella, Medium	140
Classic Crust, Delight Mozzarella, Personal	114
Classic Crust, Delight Mozzarella, Small	202
Classic Crust, Large	175
Classic Crust, Medium	154
Classic Crust, Personal	124
Classic Crust, Small	210
Italian Style Crust, Delight Mozzarella, Large	125
Italian Style Crust, Delight Mozzarella, Medium	106
Italian Style Crust, Delight Mozzarella, Small	158
Italian Style Crust, Large	138
Italian Style Crust, Medium	118
Italian Style Crust, Small	177
Stuffed Crust, Delight Mozzarella, Large	173
Stuffed Crust, Delight Mozzarella, Medium	173
Stuffed Crust, Large	190
Stuffed Crust, Medium	184
Stuffed Crust, Tabasco, Delight Mozzarella, Large	195
Stuffed Crust, Tabasco, Delight Mozzarella, Medium	178

	KCAL
DOMINO'S PIZZA	
PIZZA - VEGI SIZZLER	
Stuffed Crust, Tabasco, Large	204
Stuffed Crust, Tabasco, Medium	187
Thin & Crispy, Delight Mozzarella, Large	109
Thin & Crispy, Delight Mozzarella, Medium	102
Thin & Crispy, Large	126
Thin & Crispy, Medium	116
PIZZA - VEGI SUPREME	
Classic Crust, Delight Mozzarella, Large	165
Classic Crust, Delight Mozzarella, Medium	144
Classic Crust, Delight Mozzarella, Personal	116
Classic Crust, Delight Mozzarella, Small	208
Classic Crust, Large	179
Classic Crust, Medium	159
Classic Crust, Personal	127
Classic Crust, Small	215
GF Crust, Delight Mozzarella, Small	177
GF Crust, Small	186
Italian Style Crust, Delight Mozzarella, Large	129
Italian Style Crust, Delight Mozzarella, Medium	110
Italian Style Crust, Delight Mozzarella, Small	163
Italian Style Crust, Large	143
Italian Style Crust, Medium	122
Italian Style Crust, Small	183
Stuffed Crust, Delight Mozzarella, Large	200
Stuffed Crust, Delight Mozzarella, Medium	177
Stuffed Crust, Large	195
Stuffed Crust, Medium	188
Stuffed Crust, Tabasco, Delight Mozzarella, Large	200
Stuffed Crust, Tabasco, Delight Mozzarella, Medium	182
Stuffed Crust, Tabasco, Large	209
Stuffed Crust, Tabasco, Medium	191
Thin & Crispy, Delight Mozzarella, Large	114
Thin & Crispy, Delight Mozzarella, Medium	106
Thin & Crispy, Large	131
Thin & Crispy, Medium	122
PIZZA - VEGI VOCLANO	
Classic Crust, Delight Mozzarella, Medium	165
Stuffed Crust, Delight Mozzarella, Large	215
Classic Crust, Delight Mozzarella, Large	188
Classic Crust, Delight Mozzarella, Personal	130
Classic Crust, Delight Mozzarella, Small	247
Classic Crust, Large	207
Classic Crust, Medium	179
Classic Crust, Personal	143
Classic Crust, Small	307
Italian Style Crust, Delight Mozzarella, Large	154
Italian Style Crust, Delight Mozzarella, Medium	135
Italian Style Crust, Delight Mozzarella, Small	180
Italian Style Crust, Large	170
Italian Style Crust, Medium	144
Italian Style Crust, Small	203
Stuffed Crust, Delight Mozzarella, Medium	206

	KCAL
DOMINO'S PIZZA	
PIZZA - VEGI VOLCANO	
Stuffed Crust, Large	228
Stuffed Crust, Medium	216
Stuffed Crust, Tabasco, Delight Mozzarella, Large	214
Stuffed Crust, Tabasco, Delight Mozzarella, Medium	197
Stuffed Crust, Tabasco, Large	248
Stuffed Crust, Tabasco, Medium	218
Thin & Crispy, Delight Mozzarella, Large	131
Thin & Crispy, Delight Mozzarella, Medium	128
Thin & Crispy, Large	149
Thin & Crispy, Medium	138
POTATO WEDGES	
Portion	169
WRAP	
Chicken, & Bacon, Wrapzz	403
Meatball Feast, Wrapzz	526
Pepperoni Passion, Wrapzz	453
Tandoori Hot, Wrapzz	332
Texas BBQ, Wrapzz	417
Vegi Supreme, Wrapzz	301

FARMHOUSE INNS	KCAL
BACON	
Cheese, & BBQ Sauce, Hunters, Steak Topper	440
Extra	106
BEANS	
BBQ, Combo Feast	127
Extra	129
BEEF	
Steak, Rib-eye, 9oz, Naked	771
Steak, Rib-eye, 9oz, with Sides	1597
Steak, Rump, 4oz, Extra	144
Steak, Rump, 8oz, Naked	415
Steak, Rump, 8oz, with Sides	1241
Steak, Sirloin, 8oz, Naked	474
Steak, Sirloin, 8oz, with Sides	1300
BHAJI	
Onion, Extra	361
BREAD	
Ciabatta, Garlic, Cheesy	655
Ciabatta, Garlic, Sides	450
Garlic, Combo Feast	225
Malted, & Butter, Sides	337
White, & Butter, Sides	374
BREAKFAST	
All Day, with Malted Bread	1696
All Day, with White Bread	1733
BURGERS - BEEF	
Patty Only, Extra	357
BURGERS - BEEF - SIGNATURE CARVERY	
Double Up, with Chips, & Coleslaw	2118
with Chips, & Coleslaw	1761
BURGERS - BEEF, FARMHOUSE BBQ	
Mac Stack, Double Up, with Chips, & Coleslaw	2307
Mac Stack, with Chips, & Coleslaw	1950
BURGERS - BEEF, GIANT	
The Farm, with Chips, & Coleslaw	2252
BURGERS - CHEESEBURGER	
Double Up, with Chips, & Coleslaw	1751
Smoked Bacon, Double Up, with Chips, & Coleslaw	1816
Smoked Bacon, with Chips, & Coleslaw	1459
with Chips, & Coleslaw	1394
BURGERS - CHICKEN	
Bombay Bird, Double Up, with Chips, & Coleslaw	2481
Bombay Bird, with Chips, & Coleslaw	2121
Dirty Hunters, Double Up, with Chips, & Coleslaw	2071
Dirty Hunters, with Chips, & Coleslaw	1749
Tex Mex, Double Up, with Chips, & Coleslaw	2192
Tex Mex, with Chips, & Coleslaw	1870
BURGERS - CHICKPEA & RED PEPPER	
Double Up, with Chips, & Coleslaw	1550
with Chips, & Coleslaw	1366
CHEESE	
Extra	165
Parmigiana, Topper	151

FARMHOUSE INNS	KCAL
CHICKEN	
Breast, Curried, Skewer	1092
Breast, Extra	89
Breast, Kebab, Skewer, Combo Feast	189
Breast, Kebab, Skewer, Extra	189
Fillets, Roast, Combo Feast	179
Goujons, Southern Fried, with BBQ Dip	596
Hunters	1401
Medley, Crispy, no Sauce	1739
Smothered	1850
Southern Fried, Curried, Skewer	1325
Southern Fried, Extra	322
Southern Fried, Skewer, Combo Feast	422
Southern Fried, Skewer, Extra	422
Strips, Fully Loaded	1601
Strips, Louisiana, Combo Feast	280
Wings, Combo Feast	538
Wings, no Sauce	1015
CHIPS	
Combo Feast	655
Curry Sauce, Topped, Side	796
Hunters, Topped, Side	1023
Side	655
COD	
Battered, with Chips, & Garden Peas, Large	1685
Battered, with Chips, & Mushy Peas, Large	1736
COLESLAW	
Combo Feast	306
Sides	205
CORN	
Cob, Combo Feast	161
Cob, Side	161
EGGS	
Fried, 2, Steak Topper	240
Fried, Extra	120
FISH	
Battered, Atlantic, with Chips, & Mushy Peas	1817
Battered, Atlantic, with Chips, & Peas	1766
FISH & CHIPS	
Chip Shop Supper	2330
GAMMON - STEAK	
4oz, Extra	198
Naked	486
Naked, with Egg, & Pineapple	672
Naked, with Fried Egg	726
Naked, with Pineapple	618
with Chips, & Peas	1302
GRAVY	
Chip Shop Supper	42
Extra	42
GRILLS	
Mixed, Farmhouse	2202

FARMHOUSE INNS	KCAL
GUACAMOLE	
Portion	93
HAM	
Hand Carved, & Eggs, with Chips, & Peas	1126
HASH BROWNS	
Extra	78
JACKET POTATO	
with Baked Beans	431
with Cheese, & Baked Beans	510
with Mozzarella, & Cheddar Cheese	424
with Tuna Mayonnaise	483
LAMB	
Shank, Minted, with Mash, & Veg	1213
LASAGNE	
Beef, Naked	584
Beef, with Chips, & Garlic Bread	1381
MACARONI CHEESE	
Combo Feast	232
Luxury	778
MAYONNAISE	
Garlic	190
MUSHROOMS	
Button, Breaded, Garlic, with Garlic Mayonnaise	655
Button, Sides	283
NACHOS	
Cheesy, Big	888
ONION RINGS	
Combo Feast	327
Sides	654
PATE	
Chicken, Liver, with Bread, Onion Chutney, & Salad	474
PEAS	
Garden, Chip Shop Supper	56
Mushy, Chip Shop Supper	107
PIE	
Beef & Ale, Slow Cooked, No Sides	1184
Beef & Ale, Slow Cooked, with Chips	1839
Beef & Ale, Slow Cooked, with Mashed Potato	1436
Chicken & Mushroom, No Sides	1215
Chicken & Mushroom, with Chips	1870
Chicken & Mushroom, with Mashed Potato	1467
PLATTER	
Chicken, Sharer	2459
RIBS	
Rack, Mini, Extra	204
SALAD	
Chicken, & Bacon, Hot	884
Chicken, Skewer	467
Side, Combo Feast	45
Side	45
SALMON	
Fillet, Scottish, Grilled	431
Fillet, Scottish, Grilled, with Hollandaise Sauce	538

FARMHOUSE INNS	KCAL
SALSA	
Portion	56
SANDWICH	
Carvery, Bap	1149
Cheese & Chutney, Ciabatta Roll	1042
Cheese & Chutney, Floured Bap	1027
Chicken, Bacon, Tomato, Melt, Ciabatta Roll	1180
Chicken, Bacon Tomato, Melt, Floured Bap	1165
Chicken Goujons, & Mayo, Ciabatta Roll	1318
Chicken Goujons, & Mayo, Floured Bap	1303
Hunters Chicken, Melt, Ciabatta Roll	1170
Hunters Chicken, Melt, Floured Bap	1155
Fish Fingers, & Tartare Sauce, Ciabatta Roll	1148
Fish Fingers, & Tartare Sauce, Floured Bap	1133
Tuna, Melt, Ciabatta Roll	989
Tuna, Melt, Floured Bap	974
SAUCE	
BBQ, Texan	144
BBQ, Texan, for Chicken Wings	72
Char Sui, Combo Feast	195
Char Sui, for Chicken Wings	130
Curry, Chip Shop Supper	141
Diane	425
Peppercorn	101
Piri Piri, Combo Feast	30
Piri Piri	40
Piri Piri, for Chicken Wings	20
Sour Cream	165
Sweet Chilli, Combo Feast	98
Sweet Chilli	131
Texan BBQ, Combo Feast	108
SAUSAGE	
Extra	181
Pigs in Blanket, Extra	209
SAUSAGE & MASH	
Main	1447
SCAMPI	
Wholetail, Breaded	1251
Wholetail, Breaded, Naked	550
TART	
Vegetable, no Sides	483
Vegetable, with Chips	1138
Vegetable, with Mashed Potato	735
TIKKA MASALA - CHICKEN	
no Sides	1100
with Chips	1755
with Pilau Rice, & Chips	1699
with Pilau Rice	1534
YORKSHIRE PUDDING	
& Pigs in Blanket, Extra	309
Extra	100
Giant, Extra	490
Wrap, All The Meats, Giant	1604

	KCAL
FARMHOUSE INNS	
Wrap, Beef, & Horseradish, Giant	1684
Wrap, Turkey, & Cranberry, Giant	1611

	KCAL
FIVE GUYS	
BACON	
Rashers, 2	78
BANANA	
Milkshake Mix-in	148
BISCUITS	
Oreo, Pieces, Milkshake Mix-in	62
BUNS	
Burger	238
Hot Dog	215
BURGERS	
Beef, Patty Only	195
CHOCOLATE	
Milkshake Mix-in	201
COFFEE	
Milkshake Mix-in	5
CREAM	
Whipped, Milkshake Mix-in	88
EGGS	
Extra	119
FRIES	
Large	1491
Little	694
Reg	1019
HOT DOG	
Sausage Only	192
MILK	
Malted, Mlkshake Mix-in	59
MILK SHAKE	
Base, No Mix-in	714
PEANUT BUTTER	
Milkshake Mix-in	348
SEASONING MIX	
Cajun, for Fries	20
SPREAD	
Lotus Biscoff, Milkshake Mix-in	145
STRAWBERRIES	
Milkshake Mix-in	94
SUGAR	
Caramel, Salted, Milkshake Mix-in	113
TOPPING	
BBQ Sauce	20
Brown Sauce, HP	10
Cheese, Slice	64
Hot Sauce	2
Jalapeno Peppers	1
Lettuce	3
Mayonnaise	113
Mushrooms, Grilled	12
Mustard	4
Onions	9
Onions, Grilled	11
Peppers, Green	2
Pickles	2

FIVE GUYS

	KCAL
TOPPING	
Relish	15
Tomato Ketchup	14
Tomatoes	6

GOURMET BURGER KITCHEN

	KCAL
BITES	
Falafel	343
BURGERS	
Beef, Avocado, & Bacon	875
Beef, Cheese, & Bacon, with American Cheese	942
Beef, Classic	692
Beef, Classic, Small	533
Beef, Major Tom	922
Beef, Taxidriver	875
Californian, Vegan	503
Chicken, Chick Chick Boom, Panko	638
Chicken, Classic	445
Chicken, Classic, Panko	627
Chicken, Classic, Small	360
Chicken, Hey Pesto, Panko	1076
Chicken, Satay	552
Chicken, Satay, Panko	795
Falafel, Vegetarian	508
Lamb, Classic	578
Lamb, Lamburghini	644
Special, Jumpin Jack	642
Veggie, Classic	513
Veggie, Classic, Small	406
Veggie, Classic, with American Cheese	635
Veggie, Classic, with American Cheese, Small	468
Veggie, Classic, with Cheddar	676
Veggie, Classic, with Cheddar, Small	488
Veggie, Classic, with Smoked Applewood	676
Veggie, Classic, with Smoked Applewood, Small	489
Veggie, Jack-in-a-Bun	465
CHEESE ALTERNATIVE	
Vegan, Extra	95
CHICKEN	
Wings, Spicy	696
COFFEE	
Americano	56
Cappuccino	122
Flat White	118
Latte	118
DRINK	
Elderflower, Fizz	81
Ginger & Lemongrass, Fizz	82
Rhubarb & Vanilla, Fizz	83
Strawberry & Elderflower, Fizz	82
FRIES	
Chunky, Small, Junior	429
Skinny, Small, Junior	454
LEMONADE	
Cloudy	84
MILK SHAKE	
Banana	627
Cheesecake, Strawberry & Oreo	815

GOURMET BURGER KITCHEN	KCAL
PEPPERS	
Jalapeno, Extras	22
SALAD	
Caesar	267
Simple	83
SAUCE	
Mayo, Beetroot, Vegan	146
Mayo, Harissa, Vegan	236

GREGGS	KCAL
BAGUETTE	
Bacon, & Egg, Omelette, Free Range, Hot	555
Bacon, & Sausage, Hot	598
Sausage, Lorne, & Bacon	644
Bacon, Hot	509
Cheese, Cheddar, Mature, & Salad	482
Chicken, Mexican	526
Chicken, Roast, & Bacon, Club	500
Chicken, Southern Fried, Hot	602
Chicken, Tandoori	505
Chicken Mayonnaise, Roast	499
Ham, & Cheese	528
Ham, Honey Roast, & Chicken Melt, Hot	539
Ham, & Salad	438
Omelette, Hot	515
Sausage, & Egg, Omelette, Free Range, Hot	625
Sausage, Hot	600
Sausage, Lorne, & Omelette	695
Sausage, Lorne	691
Tuna, Crunch	459
BAKE	
Beef, Corned	409
Cheese, & Onion	437
Chicken	422
Nacho Chilli Cheese	434
Steak	408
Steak, Vegan	380
Vegetable	424
Cake, Chocolate	359
BISCUITS	
Empire	280
Gingerbread, Man	173
Jammy Heart	273
Shortbread, Chocolate, Chunks	161
Shortbread, Caramel	293
BREAD	
Baguette	318
Brown, Half Malted, Bloomer	134
Rolls, Corn Topped	201
Rolls, Whtite, Floured	197
Stottie, Cheese, & Onion	507
Stottie, Tuna Mayonnaise	462
BREAKFAST	
Beans, Omelette, & Hash Browns, Veggie Box	327
Beans, Omelette, Sausages, & Hash Browns, Box	357
BREAKFAST CEREAL	
Porridge, Apple, & Cinnamon, GF	232
Porridge, Creamy Oats, Simply, GF	210
Porridge, Golden Syrup, GF	244
BROWNIES	
Chocolate, Triple, GF	97
BUNS	
Belgian	390

GREGGS	KCAL
BUNS	
Iced, Finger, Cream	407
Iced, Finger	244
Iced, Split	392
CAKE	
Fondant Fancy	278
Pineapple	273
Tottenham	389
CHEESECAKE	
London	447
CHERRYADE	
Sparkling, No Added Sugar	20
CHICKEN	
Bites, Spicy BBQ	290
Goujons, Southern Fried	394
COFFEE	
Americano, Large	11
Americano, Reg	9
Americano, Soya Milk, Large	20
Americano, Soya Milk, Reg	19
Decaf, Large	11
Decaf, Reg	9
Decaf, Soya Milk, Large	16
Decaf, Soya Milk, Reg	16
Cappuccino, Large	114
Cappuccino, Reg	94
Cappuccino, Soya Milk, Large	106
Cappuccino, Soya Milk, Reg	83
Espresso, Shot	11
Flat White, Reg	71
Flat White, Soya Milk	59
Latte, Caramel, Iced, Reg	170
Latte, Caramel, Large	248
Latte, Caramel, Reg	223
Latte, Iced, Reg	111
Latte, Large	133
Latte, Pumpkin Spice, Large	253
Latte, Pumpkin Spice, Reg	228
Latte, Reg	111
Latte, Soya Milk, Large	106
Latte, Soya Milk, Reg	83
Latte, Vanilla, Iced, Reg	170
Latte, Vanilla, Large	248
Latte, Vanilla, Reg	223
Mocha, Large	296
Mocha, Mint, Reg	343
Mocha, Reg	233
White, Large	45
White, Reg	34
White, Soya Milk, Large	25
White, Soya Milk, Reg	19
COOKIES	
Chocolate, Chunk, Triple	346

GREGGS	KCAL
COOKIES	
Chocolate, Milk	358
Chocolate, White	359
CRISPS	
Cheese Puffs	201
Mature Cheddar & Onion	198
Salt & Vinegar, Crunchy Sticks	175
Sea Salt, & Cider Vinegar	194
Thai Sweet Chilli	203
Tortilla, Chilli	193
CROISSANT	
All Butter	306
DOUGHNUTS	
Caramel Custard	303
Chocolate, Milk, Filled	295
Chocolate, Milk, Ring	234
Chocolate, Triple	343
Coconut, Cream, Finger	393
Cream, Finger	369743
Cream	363
Devon	239156
Glazed, Ring	195
Iced, Ring	231
Jam	237
Pink, Jammie	317
Vanilla	300
Yum Yum	300
Yum Yum, Mini	131
DRIED FRUIT	
Tropical Mix	108
DRINK	
Mango, & Pineapple, Sparkling, No Added Sugar	15
ECLAIR	
with Cream Filling	344
FRUIT	
Medley	82
Tropical, Pot	72
GRAPES	
Mixed	99
HOT CHOCOLATE	
Large	281
Mint, Reg	334
Reg	219
JUICE	
Apple, Fairtrade	70
Orange, Fairtrade	69
LEMONADE	
Cloudy, Sparkling	15
Raspberry, Sparkling	10
MELT	
Sausage, Bean, & Cheese	453
MUFFIN	
Chocolate, Triple	462

	KCAL
GREGGS	
NUTS	
Naked, Mixed	157
PAIN AU CHOCOLAT	
Single	312
PASTA SALAD	
Chicken, & Bacon	450
Feta, & Slow Roasted Tomato	380
Tuna, Crunch	378
PASTRY	
Chocolate Twist	306
PASTY	
Beef, & Vegetable	459
PIE	
Haggis	352
Mince, Savoury	417
Scotch	367
PIZZA	
Cheese, Three	552
Pepperoni, Three Cheese	617
POTATO WEDGES	
Southern Fried	278
RAISINS	
Chocolate, & Yoghurt, Mix	128
ROLL	
Bacon, & Egg, Omelette, Free Range, Hot	395
Bacon, & Sausage, Hot	438
Bacon, & Sausage, Lorne	483
Bacon, Hot	348
Chicken, Chargrill	351
Chicken, Roast, & Salad, Sub	350
Ham, Honey Roast, & Egg Salad, Sub	337
Omelette, Hot	398
Sausage, & Egg, Omelette, Free Range	441
Sausage, Hot	416
Omelette, & Sausage, Lorne	487
Sausage, Lorne	395
Tuna Mayonnaise, Sub	343
SALAD	
Ham, & Egg, Honey Roast	332
SANDWICH	
BLT	387
Cheese, & Onion	356
Cheese, & Pickle	396
Cheese, & Tomato	396
Chicken, & Bacon	473
Chicken, Chargrill, Oval Bite	444
Chicken, Mexican	347
Chicken, Mexican, Oval Bite	492
Chicken, Roast, & Salad	348
Chicken, Tandoori	348
Egg Mayonnaise, & Tomato	373
Egg Mayonnaise, Free Range, Malted Brown Bread	356
Egg Salad, Free Range	316

	KCAL
GREGGS	
SANDWICH	
Ham, & Egg, with Salad, Honey Roast	335
Ham, Honey Roast	316
Ploughmans, Cheddar Cheese, Mature, Oval Bite	504
Tuna, Crunch, Bloomer	329
Tuna Mayonnaise, & Cucumber, Malted Brown Bread	340
SAUSAGE ROLL	
Freshly Baked	329
Vegan	311
SCONE	
Cheese	343
Fruit	298
SLICES	
Bavarian	389
Custard, Vanilla	332
SNACKS	
BBQ, Smoky, Crunch	104
SOUP	
Chicken, Spicy, & Red Pepper	120
Tomato, Cream of	216
TEA	
Green, Reg	0
Peppermint, Reg	0
Soya Milk, Reg	9
White, Large	12
White, Reg	9
TOASTIE	
Cheese, Cheddar, & Chutney, Greggs*	455
Chicken, BBQ, & Bacon	510
Ham, & Cheddar Cheese	464
TURNOVER	
Apple, Fresh Cream	461
Apple, Iced, Danish	339
WATER	
Lemon, & Lime	5
WRAP	
Bacon, & Cheese	385
Chicken, Chargrilled	446
Chicken, Chipotle Chilli, Mexican	469

HARVESTER RESTAURANT	KCAL
AVOCADO	
Smashed, Build Your Own Breakfast	349
BACON	
Back, Build Your Own Breakfast	83
Extra	94
BEANS	
Baked, Extra	63
Baked, Heinz, Build Your Own Breakfast	63
Baked, Side, Kids Menu	51
BEEF - BRISKET	
Hickory Smoked, with Mash, & Veg	1001
BEEF - STEAK, FILLET	
8oz, for Mixed Grill	287
8oz, with Fries, Mushroom, Tomato, & Onion Rings	432
BEEF - STEAK, RUMP	
4oz, Build Your Own Breakfast	224
4oz, Extra, Breakfast	224
4oz, for Mixed Grill	164
4oz, Kids Menu	164
8oz, & Fries, Mushroom, Tomato, & Onion Rings	475
8oz, for Mixed Grill	329
BEEF - STEAK, SIRLOIN	
10oz, Ancho Chilli	970
10oz, for Mixed Grill	521
10oz, with Fries, Mushroom, Tomato, & Onion Rings	666
BISCUITS	
Oreo, Crumb, Extra	145
Oreo, Extra	93
BITES	
Quorn, Southern Fried, Kids Menu	199
Quorn, Southern Fried, Starter	327
BLACK PUDDING	
Build Your Own Breakfast	81
Extra	81
BREAD	
Garlic, Cheesy, Side	354
Garlic, Cheesy, Tapas	633
Garlic, Side	165
Garlic, Tapas	331
BREAKFAST	
Signature, Kids, No Egg	300
The Classic, No Egg	838
The Vegan	1002
The Vegan, Kids	310
The Veggie, No Egg	572
The Veggies, Kids, No Egg	378
BROCCOLI	
Tenderstem, Chargrilled, Side	37
Tenderstem, Chargrilled, Side, Kids Menu	28
BROWNIES - CHOCOLATE	
Belgian, with Chocolate Sauce, & Ice Cream	673
with Chocolate Sauce, Belgian, Mini	287

HARVESTER RESTAURANT	KCAL
BURGERS	
Bean, Beyond, Vegan	666
Bean, Patty, Extra	241
Beef, Mini, Kids Menu	330
Beef, Patty, Extra	391
Beef, The Classic	971
Chicken, Mini, Kids Menu	213
Chicken, Southern Fried, Extra	438
Chicken, The Classic	731
Vegan, Plant Based, Moving Mountains, Extra	302
The Big One	1808
The Cowboy	993
Vegan, The Purist	1432
The True Blue	1099
CAKE	
Chocolate, Fudge, Chocolate Sauce, & Ice Cream	922
CAULIFLOWER	
Buffalo, with Garlic Mayo, Starter	470
CHEESE	
Halloumi, Battered, & Chips, No Peas	877
Halloumi, Extra	179
Monterey Jack, Extra	65
Stilton, Long Clawson, Extra	164
CHEESE ALTERNATIVE	
Mature, Slice, Violife, Extra	57
CHEESECAKE	
Vanilla, Baked	622
Vanilla, Baked, Mini	260
CHICKEN - BBQ	
Breast, Grilled, Kids Menu	298
BBQ	833
CHICKEN - BURGER	
Breast, Extra	176
CHICKEN - BUTTERMILK	
Fried, Kids Menu	253
Tenders, Fried, Starter	395
CHICKEN - CAJUN	
Breast, Extra	176
CHICKEN - CAJUN, SURF & TURF	
Rump Steak, Prawns, Corn, Apple & Fennel Slaw	723
CHICKEN - CARIBBEAN	
with Golden Rice & Beans, Grilled Pineapple	469
CHICKEN - GRILLED	
Breast, Kids Menu	176
Breast, with Jacket Potato, Simply	282
CHICKEN - ROTISSERIE	
Half	510
Half, Jerk, Grilled, with Coconut Rice, & Beans	1065
Half, with Half Rack Ribs, Combo	931
Quarter, Extra	200
Quarter, Kids Menu	359
Quarter, Triple, Combo	715
Quarter, with Ribs, Original Combo	732

HARVESTER RESTAURANT	KCAL
CHICKEN - SKEWERS	
with Chorizo, Churrasco	964
CHICKEN - STRIPS	
Kids Menu, Sm Bites	88
CHICKEN - VEGETARIAN	
Quorn, Stack, BBQ	697
CHICKEN - WINGS	
Sticky, Tapas	296
with BBQ, Sticky	530
CHILLI	
Beef, Chipotle, Pulled	328
Non Carne, Kids Menu	545
Non Carne, Vegan, for Nachos	136
Non Carne, with Rice	542
CHIPS - TRIPLE COOKED	
Chunky, Build Your Own Breakfast	484
Chunky, Nashville Hot, Side	484
Chunky, Sage & Onion, Side	500
Chunky, Side	484
Chunky, Side, Kids Menu	218
COD	
Fillet, Battered, Kids Menu	308
& Chips, with Mushy Peas	688
& Chips, with Peas	675
CORN	
Buttered, Side	207
Cobette, Side, Kids Menu	58
CREAM	
Fluffy, Extra	103
CURRY	
Vegetable, Thai Green	628
CUSTARD	
Extra	90
DESSERT	
Cherry Blizzard	534
Chocolate Orange, Slice	329
Mini Combo, Brownie, Blackcurrant, & Cheesecake	751
EGGS	
Benedict, Portion	668
Fried, Free Range, Build Your Own Breakfast	130
Fried, Free Range, Extra	85
Mediterranean, Portion	599
Poached, Free Range, Build Your Own Breakfast	86
Scrambled, Free Range, Build Your Own Breakfast	108
Scrambled, on Toast, Kids Menu, Sm Bites	265
FISH CAKES	
Salmon, with Watercress, Melting Middle	638
FISH FINGERS	
Kids Menu	220
Kids Menu, Sm Bites	166
FRIES	
Halloumi, with Green Devil Sauce	427
Sweet Potato, Side	503

HARVESTER RESTAURANT	KCAL
FRIES	
Sweet Potato, Side, Kids Menu	201
FRITTERS - SWEETCORN	
Smoked Cheddar, & Chilli, Build Your Own Breakfast	135
Spicy, with Avocado, & Eggs	614
FRUIT SALAD	
Tutti Frutti, with Strawberry Yoghurt, Kids Menu	107
GAMMON - STEAK	
7oz, No Topping	611
7oz, Double Up	1076
7oz, Double Up, with Egg, & Pineapple	1189
7oz, Double Up, with Egg	1161
7oz, Double Up, with Pineapple	1103
7oz, Egg, & Pineapple	724
7oz, for Mixed Grill	273
7oz, with Egg	696
7oz, with Pineapple	638
GRAVY	
Chicken, Specialty, Extra	29
HASH	
Potato, & Spinach	334
HASH BROWNS	
Build Your Own Breakfast	91
HOUMOUS	
Build Your Own Breakfast	844
ICE CREAM	
Extra	101
Non Dairy, Extra	223
JELLY	
Peach, Fruitypot, Kids Menu	72
LAMB	
Shank, Moroccan Style	1197
MACARONI CHEESE	
Bites, with Smokey Ketchup	428
Cauliflower, Kids Menu	313
Extra	279
Side	279
MIXED GRILL	
Excludes Steak	961
Ultimate, Excludes Steak	1999
The Pitmaster	3389
MOUSSAKA	
Feta, & Butternut Squash	654
MOUSSE	
Blackcurrant	295
Blackcurrant, Kids Menu	164
Blackcurrant, Mini	164
MUSHROOMS	
Breaded, with Garlic Mayo Dip, Starter	501
Flat, Build Your Own Breakfast	12
Garlic, Oven Baked, with Garlic Bread, Starter	272
NACHOS	
Starter	529

HARVESTER RESTAURANT	KCAL
NACHOS	
Vegan, Starter	523
ONION RINGS	
Side	487
PANCAKES	
Buttermilk, & Bacon, with Syrup	752
Buttermilk, with Fruit, & Syrup, Kids	192
Buttermilk, with Fruit, & Syrup	623
Butttermilk, Side	106
PASTA	
In Tomato Sauce, Kids Menu, Sm Bites	237
Spinach, & Ricotto, in Tomato & Basil Sauce	831
PEAS	
Chilli & Garlic, Kickin', Side	124
Garden, Side	60
Mushy, Side	73
Side, Kids Menu	60
PIE	
Cherry, Sugar Dusted	563
Cookies, & Cream	315
Fish, Cheddar Mash Topped	440
PORK	
Bell, Glazed, with Hash Potatoes, Mac & Cheese	1646
Pulled, BBQ, Extra	239
Pulled, BBQ, for Nachos	239
POTATOES	
Skins, Cheese, & Bacon, Tapas	407
Skins, Cheese, Tapas	313
Jacket, Side	273
Jacket, Side, Kids Menu	273
Jacket, with Sour Cream, Side	348
Mashed, Side	212
Mash, Side, Kids Menu	94
PRAWNS	
Crackerjack, with Green Devil Sauce, Starter	293
Garlic, King, & Chilli, Extra	172
Garlic, King, & Chilli Butter, with Garlic Bread, Starter	358
RIBS - FULL RACK	
Jerk BBQ, with Chicken Wings, Corn, Slaw, & Chips	1828
Jerk BBQ, with Chips, Slaw, & Corn	1516
Slow Cooked, BBQ Sauce, with Chips, Slaw, & Corn	1000
RIBS - HALF RACK	
BBQ, Extra	403
Kids Menu	348
RIBS - KILO	
Kiln Smoked, Bourbon Sauce	509
RICE	
Chicken, Katsu, Bowl	505
Golden, & Beans, Side	229
Vegetable, Sunshine, Kids Menu	190
SALAD	
Feel Good	307
Feel Good, with Cajun Chicken	503

HARVESTER RESTAURANT	KCAL
SALAD	
Feel Good, with Chicken Breast	483
Feel Good, with Quorn Fillets, Cajun	850
Feel Good, with Salmon	699
Feel Good, with Steak, Rump, 8oz	644
Feel Good, with Tofu Skewers, Peri Peri	544
SALMON	
Grilled, Spiked Sticky, with Golden Rice, & Beans	674
Grilled, Kids Menu	218
SANDWICH	
Steak	591
SAUCE	
Caribbean Curry, Steak Sauce	250
Chasseur, Steak Sauce	30
Chocolate, Belgian, Dessert	58
Chocolate, Belgian, Dessert, Kids Menu	29
Craft Ale, Bacon, & Mushroom, Steak Sauce	67
Katsu, Steak Sauce	92
Peppercorn, Steak Sauce	46
Raspberry, Dessert	57
Salted Caramel, Dessert	51
Strawberry, Dessert	57
Toffee, Fudge, Dessert	64
Toffee, Fudge, Dessert, Kids Menu	32
SAUSAGE	
& Yorkie, Kids Menu	275
& Yorkie, Kids Menu, Sm Bites	192
Pork, Build Your Own Breakfast	217
Pork, Extra	217
Pork, Cheddar, Jalapeno, with BBQ Sauce	452
Vegan	80
Vegetarian, & Yorkie, Kids Menu	265
Vegetarian, & Yorkie, Kids Menu, Sm Bites	185
SCAMPI	
Extra	139
Wholetail, Whitby, Excluding Peas	425
SEA BASS	
Grilled, Meal, Simply	518
SOUP	
Tomato, & Basil	193
SPINACH	
Build Your Own Breakfast	12
SPONGE PUDDING	
Lemon	493
Treacle	941
SQUID	
Calamari, Strips, with Garlic Mayo, Starter	278
SUNDAE	
Best	255
Best, Kids Menu	239
Best, Vegan	673
Best, Vegan, Kids Menu	448
Blueberry, Eton Mess	530

HARVESTER RESTAURANT	KCAL
SUNDAE	
Build Your Own, Kids Menu	453
Caramel, Salted, Rocky Road	618
Chocolate, Brownie, Rocky Horror	683
Chocolate, Brownie, Rocky Horror, Kids Menu	446
Passion Fruit, & White Chocolate	678
Strawberry Cheesecake	619
TAGINE	
Aubergine, & Red Lentil	1077
TART	
Camembert, & Cherry Tomato, Puff Pastry	635
TOFU	
Skewers, Peri Peri	641
TOMATOES	
Build Your Own Breakfast	6
TOPPING	
Cheese, Stilton, & Bacon	352
VEGETABLES	
Steamed, Side	77
Steamed, Side, Kids Menu	46
Sticks, Side, Kids Menu	44
WAFFLES	
Belgian, Extra	390
Chicken, Buttermilk Fried, & Bacon, with Syrup	1323
WRAP	
Chicken, Breast, Cajun, Grilled	467
Chicken, Breast, Grilled	448
Chicken, Build Your Own, Kids Menu	415
Chicken, Buttermilk Fried	525
Halloumi	629
Quorn, Fillet, Cajun	390
Quorn, Southern Fried	475

HUNGRY HORSE	KCAL
BACON	
Streaky, Side, Extra	66
BAGUETTE	
Cheesy Melt	755
Chicken, Club	889
Chicken, Mayo, Southern Fried	663
Fish Fingers, & Mayo	661
BEANS	
Baked, Jacket Potato Topping	73
Baked, Side, Extra	73
BEEF	
Dinner, Roast, Sunday	967
Rump Steak, 12oz, Big Plate Specials	1344
Rump Steak, 12oz, Naked, Big Plate Specials	520
Rump Steak, 12oz, Side, Extra	435
Rump Steak, 4oz	821
Rump Steak, 4oz, Naked	230
Rump Steak, 8oz	966
Rump Steak, 8oz, Mix it Up, Big Plate Specials	289
Rump Steak, 8oz, Naked	375
Sirloin Steak, 9oz, Big Plate Specials	1304
Sirloin Steak, 9oz, Naked, Big Plate Specials	480
Steak, Smothered, 8oz, Sizzler, Big Plate Specials	1364
Dinner, Sunday Roast, Big Plate Specials	1597
Dinner, Sunday Roasts, Kids	523
BHAJI	
Onion, Extra Portion	541
BREAD	
Baguette, Ã,½, & Butter, Extra	197
Brown, & Butter, Side	337
Garlic, Ciabatta, Cheesy	522
Garlic, Ciabatta	358
Naan, Extra	345
White, & Butter, Side	374
Wrap, Tortilla, Soft, Mix it Up, Big Plate Specials	329
BREAKFAST	
All Day, Big Plate Specials	1561
Full English, Classics	845
BURGERS	
Beef, & Chicken, Quadzilla	2768
Beef, Bacon, & Egg, Sunny Stacker	1308
Beef, Bacon, Chicken, & Pulled Pork, Carni-Four	2368
Beef, Classic, Double	1527
Beef, Classic	1170
Beef, Double Daddy	2219
Beef, Extra Patty	357
Beef, Sizzler, Combo, Big Plate Specials	2412
Beef, Smokin' Jack	1539
Beef, with Cheese, & Bacon, Double	1619
Beef, with Cheese, & Bacon	1262
Beef, with Cheese, Double	1553
Beef, with Cheese	1196
Chicken, Bombay Bird	1828

	KCAL
HUNGRY HORSE	
BURGERS	
Chicken, Extra Fillet	290
Chicken, Southern Fried, Double	1534
Chicken, Southern Fried, Extra Patty	360
Chicken, Southern Fried	1174
Veggie, Chinese, Double	1251
Veggie, Chinese	1021
Veggie, Hoisin, Extra Patty	185
BUTTER	
Portion	29
CAKE	
Chocolate, Fudge, Warm	905
CHEESE	
Grated, Side, Extra	165
Halloumi, Battered, & Chips	1183
Halloumi, Battered, & Chips, with Baked Beans	1256
Halloumi, Battered, & Chips, with Garden Peas	1263
Halloumi, Battered, & Chips, with Mushy Peas	1303
Halloumi, Battered, & Chips, with Salad	1195
Halloumi, Battered, Mix It Up, Big Plate Specials	764
Halloumi, Extra	800
Halloumi, Fingers	886
Mozzarella, Mature Cheddar, Jacket Potato Topping	165
CHEESECAKE	
Millionaires	593
CHICKEN	
Breast, Extra Portion	179
Skewers, Breast, Kebab, Mix It Up, Big Plate Special	378
Roast, Breast, Sunday, Kids Menu	508
Skewers, Breast, Extra	189
Crispy, Jumbo, with Curry Sauce, Big Plate Specials	1709
Roast, Fillet, Sunday	864
Roast, Fillet, Sunday, Big Plate Special	1436
Fingers, Battered, Mix it Up, Big Plate Specials	660
Fingers, Battered, Plain, Starter	607
New Yorker, & Salad, Live Well	449
New Yorker, Big Plate Specials	1721
New Yorker, Classics	1168
Parmigiana, Big Plate Specials	1179
Roast, Half, Flattened, Mix it Up, Big Plate Special	304
Skewers, Southern Fried, Mix It Up, Big Plate Special	844
Skewers, Southern Fried, Extra	422
Wings, Plain, Starter	766
Wings, with Caribbean Dressing, Starter	916
Wings, with Caribbean Dressing, Starter	757
Wings, with Char Sui Sauce, Starter	929
Wings, with Char Sui Sauce, Starter	770
Wings, with Fajita Seasoning, Starter	801
Wings, with Fajita Seasoning, Starter	642
Wings, with Garlic & Parmesan Sauce, Starter	965
Wings, with Garlic & Parmesan Sauce, Starter	806
Wings, with Hot Sauce, Starter	834
Wings, with Hot Sauce, Starter	675

	KCAL
HUNGRY HORSE	
CHICKEN	
Wings, with Lemon & Pepper Sauce, Starter	959
Wings, with Lemon & Pepper Sauce, Starter	800
Wings, with Piri Piri Hot Sauce, Starter	791
Wings, with Piri Piri Hot Sauce, Starter	632
Wings, with Texan BBQ Sauce, Starter	856
Wings, with Texan BBQ Sauce, Starter	697
CHILLI	
Con Carne, Jacket Potato Topping	162
CHIPS	
Cheesy, Side	583
Mix it Up, Big Plate Specials	574
Side	418
COD & CHIPS	
Jumbo, No Sides Big Plate Specials	1605
Jumbo, with Baked Beans, Big Plate Specials	1678
Jumbo, with Garden Peas, Big Plate Specials	1665
Jumbo, with Mushy Peas, Big Plate Specials	1725
Jumbo, with Salad, Big Plate Specials	1617
COLESLAW	
Jacket Potato Topping	75
Mix it Up, Big Plate Specials	100
Side	75
CORN	
Cobs, Mini, Mix it Up, Big Plate Specials	39
on the Cob, Side	72
CRUMBLE	
Apple	515
CURRY	
Chickpea, & Sweet Potato, Big Plate Specials	2247
Chickpea, & Sweet Potato, Classics	691
CUSTARD	
Extra	89
DESSERT	
Piecaken, Black Forest	967
Piecaken, Black Forest, Vegan	1024
DRESSING	
Caribbean, Mix It Up, Big Plate Specials	300
EGGS	
Fried, Side, Extra	118
FISH & CHIPS	
Vegan, Fillets, No Sides, Classics	696
Vegan, Fillets, with Baked Beans, Classics	769
Vegan, Fillets, with Garden Peas, Classics	756
Vegan, Fillets, with Mushy Peas, Classics	816
Vegan, Fillets, with Salad, Classics	708
No Sides, Classics	1337
Battered, with Baked Beans, Classics	1410
Battered, with Garden Peas, Classics	1397
Battered, with Mushy Peas, Classics	1457
Battered, with Salad, Classics	1349
FRIES	
Dirty, Mac & Bacon, Side	910

	KCAL
HUNGRY HORSE	
FRIES	
Dirty, Mac & Cheese, Side	778
Dirty, Nacho Cheese, & Bacon, Side	760
Dirty, Pizza Topper, Side	691
Dirty, Tikka, Side	1034
Mix it Up, Big Plate Specials	546
Side	546
Sweet Potato, Mix it Up, Big Plate Specials	410
Sweet Potato, Side	410
GAMMON	
Grilled, 15oz, Big Plate Specials	1503
Grilled, 5oz, Classics	782
Grilled, 5oz, Mix It Up, Big Plate Specials	498
ICE CREAM	
Bubblegum, Extra	120
Chocolate, Extra	99
Vanilla, Extra	97
LASAGNE	
& Salad, Live Well	543
Beef, Classics	687
MACARONI CHEESE	
Classics	756
Side	281
MAYONNAISE	
Muddy, Extra	286
MIXED GRILL	
Full Monty, Big Plate Special	1878
Mini	1308
MUSHROOMS	
Breaded, Garlic	686
Side, Extra	57
NACHOS	
Muchos Nachos Grande	1101
ONION RINGS	
5, Side	389
Horseshoe Stacker, 20, Ã,½	892
Mix it Up, Big Plate Specials	311
PASTA	
Deli, Live Well	401
Deli, with Halloumi, Live Well	600
Deli, with Roast Chicken, Live Well	580
Deli, with Rump Steak, Live Well	545
Deli, with Salmon Fillet, Live Well	771
PEAS	
Mushy, Side, Extra	120
Side, Extra	60
PIE	
Steak & Ale, No Sides	1111
Steak & Ale, with Chips	1529
Steak & Ale, with Mash	1360
Chicken & Mushroom, Woodland, No Sides	1142
Chicken & Mushroom, Woodland, with Chips	1560
Chicken & Mushroom, Woodland, with Mash	1391

	KCAL
HUNGRY HORSE	
PINEAPPLE	
Slice, Side, Extra	14
PIZZA	
Margherita, Classics	903
Meat Feast, Classics	1229
Pepperoni, Classics	1067
PLATTER	
Ultimate, Big Combo, Starter	2568
POPPADOMS	
& Chutney, Extra Portion	190
POTATOES	
Jacket, Mix it Up, Big Plate Specials	194
Jacket, Plain, Add Toppings Seperately	259
Jacket, Plain, Side	194
Mashed, Side, Extra	249
Roast, Extra	335
RICE	
Dirty, Mix it Up, Big Plate Specials	191
ROULADE - RED CABBAGE & APPLE	
Sunday Roast, Vegetarian, Big Plate Specials	1750
Sunday Roast, Vegetarian	950
Sunday Roast, Vegetarian, Kids	687
SALAD	
Classic, Live Well	58
Classic, with Halloumi, Live Well	254
Classic, with Roast Chicken, Live Well	233
Classic, with Rump Steak, Live Well	198
Classic, with Salmon Fillet, Live Well	424
Dressed, Side	33
Side, Mix It Up, Big Plate Specials	49
SALMON	
Fillet, Mix It Up, Big Plate Specials	370
SANDWICH	
Chicken, Crispy, Big Plate Specials	2531
Chicken, Southern Fried, Steak, Big Plate Specials	2472
Halloumi, Big Plate Specials	3060
SAUCE	
BBQ, Texan, Extra	90
BBQ, Texan, Mix it Up, Big Plate Specials	180
BBQ, with Jack Daniels, Steak Sauce	146
Char Sui, Mix It Up, Big Plate Specials	325
Curry	141
Garlic, & Parmesan, Mix it Up, Big Plate Specials	199
Hot, Mix it Up, Big Plate Specials	68
Lemon, & Pepper, Mix It Up, Big Plate Specials	386
Lemon, & Garlic, Steak Sauce	160
Parmigiana, Extra	35
Peppercorn, Steak Sauce	52
Piri Piri, Extra	25
Piri Piri, Hot, Mix it Up, Big Plate Specials	50
Sour Cream	103
Sweet Chilli	82

HUNGRY HORSE	KCAL
SAUSAGE	
Side, Extra	348
SAUSAGE & MASH	
Vegetarian, Quorn*, Classics	541
SCAMPI	
Breaded, Wholetail, & Salad, Live Well	481
Breaded, Wholetail, No Sides, Classics	939
Breaded, Wholetail, with Baked Beans, Classics	1012
Breaded, Wholetail, with Garden Peas, Classics	999
Breaded, Wholetail, with Mushy Peas, Classics	1059
Breaded, Wholetail, with Salad, Classics	951
Jumbo, No Sides, Big Plate Specials	1310
Jumbo, with Baked Beans, Big Plate Specials	1383
Jumbo, with Garden Peas, Big Plate Specials	1370
Jumbo, with Mushy Peas, Big Plate Specials	1430
Jumbo, with Salad, Big Plate Specials	1322
SOUP	
Tomato, Roasted	283
Tomato, Roasted, Vegan	171
SPICES	
Fajita Seasoning, Mix It Up, Big Plate Specials	52
SPONGE PUDDING	
Syrup	665
SUNDAE	
Candymania, Big, The Ultimate	1853
Candymania	841
Trifle-tastic	412
TIKKA MASALA	
Chicken, Big Plate Specials	2366
Chicken, Classics	810
TOMATOES	
Side, Extra	8
TOPPING	
Hot, Steak Topper	71
New Yorker, Steak Topper	177
Sunny, Steak Topper	235
Surf, Steak Topper	172
WRAP	
Cheesy Melt	646
Chicken, Club	780
Chicken, Mayo, Southern Fried	554
Fish Fingers, & Mayo	552
YORKSHIRE PUDDING	
Extra	100

ITSU	KCAL
BARS	
Brownie, Cocoa Butter	185
Chocolate, Pie, Raw	167
Coconut, Crushed, & Chocolate	293
Pecan, Cashew, & Date, Glazed	184
BEANS	
Edamame, Chocolate Coated	152
Edamame	192
BROWNIES	
Cocoa Butter, with Caramelised Miso	185
BUNS	
Bao, Duck, Hoisin	294
Bao, Spicy Veg	262
CHICKEN	
Katsu, Klean, Rice Bowl	574
Korean, Rice Bowl, Spicy	556
Teriyaki, Rice Bowl	596
Thai, Rice Bowl	765
CHOCOLATE	
Bar, Crushed Coconut, & Matcha	293
Pie, with Pink Himalayan Salt, Raw	167
DESSERT	
Mochi, Chocolate Ganache	230
Mochi, Mango Cheesecake	208
Salted Caramel, Pot, The Coconut Collaborative	127
DUMPLINGS - GYOZA	
Beef, Korean BBQ	352
Chicken, & Spring Onion	251
Chicken, Frozen	157
King Prawn	216
Vegetable, Fusion	240
Veggie, Steamed	192
JERKY	
Beef Twerky	97
JUICE	
Orange, Press	118
Veg Press	113
JUICE DRINK	
Ginger, Detox, Zinger, Super Tonic	56
Goji, Mandarin, & Lime, Super Tonic	33
KOMBUCHA	
Ginger, & Lemon	27
Original	26
Passionfruit	28
MOUSSE	
Chocolate	248
NOODLES	
Udon, Chicken, Chargrilled	507
Udon, Chicken, Chilli	559
Udon, I'thai, Stir Fry Style	669
Udon, with Gyoza, Veggie	496
PEAS	
Dried, Wasabi	111

ITSU	KCAL
PRAWN CRACKERS	
Peking Duck	96
Salt, & Vinegar	98
Wasabi, Mild	95
PUDDING	
Lemon Zinger	234
White Chocolate Dream	293
RICE CAKES	
Chocolate, Dark	85
Chocolate, Milk	83
Yoghurt	80
SALAD	
Chicken, Sesame, No Dressing	369
Chicken, Teriyaki, On a Bed, No Dressing	471
Salmon, Poke, On a Bed, No Dressing	541
Salmon, Teriyaki, On a Bed, No Dressing	501
Sushi, Japanese	203
Tofu, No Meat Mondays, No Dressing	406
SEAWEED	
Crispy Thins, Sea Salt Flavour	24
Crispy Thins, Sweet Soy & Sea Salt Flavour	22
Crispy Thins, Wasabi Flavour	22
SMOOTHIE	
Raw Fruitifix, Beauty	258
Raw Veg, Beauty	232
SOUP	
Chicken Noodle	293
Coconut, with Veggie Meatballs	506
Miso	36
Miso, Noodle, Detox	177
Paste, Miso, Chilli, Easy	31
SUSHI	
Avocado, Baby, Rolls	259
California Rolls	292
Festival	517
Health & Happiness, Box	575
Itsu Classics	616
Salmon, & Avo, Dragon Roll	422
Salmon, Avocado, Rolls	287
Salmon, Full House	636
Salmon	299
Salmon, Sashimi	240
Salmon, Super, Light	402
Tuna, Line Caught, Bento	333
Tuna, Spicy, Dragon Roll	373
Veggie, Collection	476
Veggie, Dragon Roll	358
WATER	
Ginger, Low	65
Lemon, Low	66
Zen, Cucumber, & Mint	3
Zen, Peach, & Lychee	4

J D WETHERSPOON	KCAL
APPLES	
Slices, Kids Menu	43
AVOCADO	
Side or Add On	84
BACON	
Maple Cured, & American Style Cheese, Extra	168
Maple Cured, & Cheddar Cheese, Extra	170
Maple Cured, Extra	86
Rashers, Extra or Add On	103
BANANA	
Extra or Add On	105
BEANS	
Baked, Extra or Add On	126
Baked, No Added Sugar, Kids Menu	63
Baked, on Toast, White	543
Baked, on Toast, White, Small	240
Baked, on Toast, Wholewheat	546
Baked, on Toast, Wholewheat Small	242
BEEF - STEAK, RUMP	
10oz, Eggs, & Chips, Sunday Brunch	1225
10oz, with Chips, & Cheese & Leek Sauce	1426
10oz, with Chips, & Peppercorn Sauce	1413
10oz, with Chips, & Jack Daniels Honey Glaze	1413
10oz, with Chips, & Whisky Sauce	1406
10oz, with Chips	1086
10oz, with Jacket Potato, & Cheese & Leek Sauce	1129
10oz, with Jacket Potato, & Peppercorn Sauce	1116
10oz, with Jacket Potato, & Jack Daniels Glaze	1115
10oz, with Jacket Potato, & Whisky Sauce	1108
10oz, with Jacket Potato	789
10oz, with Rainbow Quinoa Salad	668
10oz, with Side Salad	558
BEEF - STEAK, SIRLOIN	
8oz, Eggs, & Chips, Sunday Brunch	1199
8oz, with Chips, & Cheese & Leek Sauce	1395
8oz, with Chips, & Peppercorn Sauce	1382
8oz, with Chips, & Jack Daniels Honey Glaze	1382
8oz, with Chips, & Whisky Sauce	1375
8oz, with Chips	1055
8oz, with Jacket Potato, & Cheese & Leek Sauce	1120
8oz, with Jacket Potato, & Peppercorn Sauce	1085
8oz, with Jacket Potato, & Jack Daniels Honey Glaze	1085
8oz, with Jacket Potato, & Whisky Sauce	1100
8oz, with Jacket Potato	758
8oz, with Rainbow Quinoa Salad	638
8oz, with Side Salad	527
BHAJI	
Onion, 2, Curry Club	330
BITES	
Macaroni Cheese, with Salsa, Side or Add On	276
BLACK PUDDING	
Extra or Add On	352

J D WETHERSPOON	KCAL
BLUEBERRIES	
Extra or Add On	17
BOLOGNESE	
Spaghetti, Kids Menu	285
BREAD	
Naan, Garlic	281
Naan, Plain	224
Two Slices, & Butter, Extra or Add On	191
Two Slices, & Lurpak Spreadable	442
BREAKFAST	
All Day, Brunch, Pub Classics	1238
All Day, Brunch, Small, Pub Classics	678
All Day, Brunch, Vegetarian, Pub Classics	1175
All Day, Brunch, Vegetarian, Small, Pub Classics	709
American	1368
American, Small	684
Freedom	447
Large	1420
Small	460
Traditional	819
Vegan	879
Vegetarian	932
Vegetarian, Large	1357
Vegetarian, Small	374
BREAKFAST CEREAL	
Porridge, Moma	250
BROWNIES	
Chocolate, with Ice Cream, Warm	797
Chocolate, with Ice Cream, Warm, Mini	424
BURGERS - BEEF	
6oz, Extra	346
6oz Classic	1171
BBQ, with Chips, & Onion Rings	1679
Caledonian, with Chips, & Onion Rings	1758
Empire State, with Chips, & Onion Rings	1949
Tennessee, with Chips, & Onion Rings	1585
Ultimate, with Chips, & Onion Rings	1703
BURGERS - CHICKEN, BUTTERMILK	
BBQ, with Chips, & Onion Rings	1683
Breaded, Fried	1175
Tennessee, with Chips, & Onion Rings	1590
with Brie, & Chilli Jam, with Chips, & Onion Rings	1616
BURGERS - CHICKEN, GRILLED	
Breast, BBQ, with Chips, & Onion Rings	1539
Breast	1031
Breast, Skinny	453
Breast, Tennessee, with Chips, & Onion Rings	1446
with Brie, & Chilli Jam, with Chips, & Onion Rings	1472
BURGERS - VEGAN	
Beyond, Meat Free	1112
Beyond, Meat Free, Patty, Extra or Add On	287
Gourmet, with Chips, & Onion Rings	1464

J D WETHERSPOON	KCAL
BURGERS - VEGETABLE	
Breaded	1082
Breaded, Patty, Extra or Add On	257
with Brie, & Chilli Jam, with Chips, & Onion Rings	1523
CARROTS	
Bag, Kids Menu	30
CHEESE	
American, Burger Topping	82
Brie, Extra or Add On	150
Cheddar, Burger Topping	83
Halloumi, Grilled, Extra or Add On	477
CHICKEN - BREAST	
Bites, 5, with Sticky Soy Sauce, Extra or Add On	251
Buttermilk Fried, Extra or Add On	350
Grilled, Extra or Add On	206
Grilled, Kids Menu	206
CHICKEN - GRILLED, & RIBS	
Half Rack, BBQ, with Onion Rings, & Chips	1721
Half Rack, BBQ, with Onion Rings, & Jacket Potato	1446
CHICKEN - MELT, BBQ	
with Peas, Tomato, & Mushrooms, Chips	1146
with Peas, Tomato, & Mushrooms, Jacket Potato	871
CHICKEN - NUGGETS	
Breast, Kids Menu	155
Quorn*, Kids Menu	238
CHICKEN - STRIPS, SOUTHERN FRIED	
with Smoky Chipotle Mayo, Sm Plates	653
& Chips, Small	625
with Jack Daniels Honey Glaze, Extra or Add On	406
with Jack Daniels Honey Glaze, & Chips	1225
CHICKEN - WINGS	
5, with Sriracha Hot Sauce, Extra or Add On	588
Sriracha Hot Sauce, & Blue Cheese Dip, Sm Plates	1289
CHICKEN - WINGS, & RIBS	
Half Rack, BBQ, with Onion Rings, & Chips	2020
Half Rack, BBQ, with Onion Rings, & Jacket Potato	1745
CHILLI	
Beef, Burger Topping	178
Beef, Rice, Tortilla Chips, & Sour Cream	780
Five Bean, Burger Topping	119
Five Bean, with Rice, & Tortilla Chips, Pub Classics	587
Five Bean, with Rice, Kids Menu	322
Vegan, Smoky, with Rice, Kids Menu	342
CHIPS	
Bowl, Side	955
Bowl, with Curry Sauce, Side	1073
Kids Menu	326
Side	597
CHIPS - TOPPED	
Curry Sauce, Chip Shop Style, Sm Plates	1073
Loaded, Cheese, Bacon, & Sour Cream, Sm Plates	1281
COD	
Battered, Kids Menu	376

	KCAL
J D WETHERSPOON	
CORN	
Cob, Mini, Kids Menu	55
Cobs, Mini, Two, Extra or Add on	101
CRUMBLE	
Apple, Bramley, with Ice Cream	633
CUCUMBER	
Sticks, & Tomato Wedges, Kids Menu	12
CURRY - CAULIFLOWER & SPINACH MANGALOREAN	
with Chips, Simple	1069
with Pilau Rice, Naan Bread, & Poppadoms	944
with Pilau Rice, Simple	672
CURRY - FLAMING DRAGON	
Chicken, Curry Club	918
CURRY - PRAWN & FISH SRI LANKAN	
with Rice, Naan Bread, & Poppadoms	1233
CURRY - SWEET POTATO, CHICKPEA & SPINACH	
Curry Club	878
DESSERT	
Cookie Dough Sandwich, & Ice Cream, Warm	705
DIP	
Garlic & Herb, Extra	177
EGGS - BENEDICT	
Standard	519
Miners	760
with Mushroom	484
EGGS - FRIED	
Extra	72
EGGS - POACHED	
Extra or Add On	63
EGGS - SCRAMBLED	
Extra or Add On	167
on Toast	533
on Toast, Wholemeal	536
FISH & CHIPS	
Cod, Fillet, Battered, & Mushy Peas	1384
Cod, Fillet, Battered, & Peas	1312
Cod, Fillet, Battered, & Mushy Peas, Small	827
Cod, Fillet, Battered, & Peas, Small	758
Haddock, Fillet, Battered, & Mushy Peas	1357
Haddock, Fillet, Battered, & Mushy Peas, Small	815
Haddock, Fillet, Battered, & Peas	1288
Haddock, Fillet, Battered, & Peas, Small	746
FRIES	
Halloumi, Side or Add On	475
Halloumi, with Sweet Chilli Sauce, Sm Plates	475
FRUIT	
Fresh, & Ice Cream	304
Fresh, Breakfast	178
GAMMON	
10oz, with Egg, & Chips	1310
10oz, with Egg, & Jacket Potato	1035
5oz, with Egg, & Chips	1048
5oz, with Egg, & Jacket Potato	773

	KCAL
J D WETHERSPOON	
GARLIC BREAD	
Pizza, 11"	707
Pizza, 11", Sm Plates	707
Pizza, 8", Side	354
Pizza, with Cheese, 11"	853
Pizza, with Cheese, 8", Side	427
HADDOCK	
Battered, Kids Menu	364
HAGGIS	
Scottish, Neeps, & Tatties, Pub Classics	923
HAM	
& Egg, Wiltshire Cured, Kids Menu	125
Egg, & Chips, Wiltshire Cured, Pub Classics	847
Egg, & Chips, Wiltshire Cured, Small, Pub Classics	453
HASH BROWNS	
Two, Extra or Add On	216
HONEY	
Extra or Add On	92
ICE CREAM	
Vanilla, Extra or Add On	125
Vanilla, with Raspberry Sauce, Pot, Childrens	119
Vegan, Extra or Add On	162
JACKET POTATO	
Plain, Kids Menu	225
with Beans, & Salad, Deli Deals	483
with Beans, Kids Menu	288
with Cheese, & Salad	531
with Five Bean Chilli, & Salad	413
with Five Bean Chilli, Kids Menu	344
with Roasted Vegetables, & Salad	374
with Roasted Vegetables, Kids Menu	305
with Smoky Vegan Chilli, Kids Menu	364
with Tuna Mayo, & Salad, Deli Deals	532
JALFREZI	
Chicken, Curry Club	908
JAM	
Smoky Chilli, Burger Topping	41
Strawberry, Extra or Add On	76
KORMA	
Chicken, Curry Club	1066
LASAGNE	
Beef, British, with Dressed Side Salad	756
Vegetable, Mediterranean, with Dressed Side Salad	603
MADRAS	
Beef, Curry Club	1077
MARMALADE	
Extra or Add On	75
MIXED GRILL	
with Chips	1454
with Chips, Large	1949
with Jacket Potato	1179
with Jacket Potato, Large	1674

J D WETHERSPOON	KCAL
MUFFIN	
Breakfast	499
Egg, & Bacon, Breakfast	331
Egg, & Cheese, Breakfast	279
Egg, & Sausage, Breakfast	448
MUSHROOMS	
Extra or Add On	126
NACHOS	
Sm Plates	627
ONION RINGS	
Six, Extra or Add On	255
Twelve, Side	510
PANCAKES - AMERICAN	
Small, with Maple Flavour Syrup	295
Small, with Maple Flavour Syrup, & Bacon	338
with Ice Cream, Mini	420
with Bacon, & Maple Flavour Syrup, Breakfast	676
Maple Flavour Syrup, & Ice Cream	715
Maple Flavour Syrup, Breakfast	590
PANINI	
Chicken, Bacon, & Cheese, BBQ, Deli Deals	637
Brie, Bacon, & Smoky Chilli Jam, Deli Deals	624
Cheese, & Tomato, Deli Deals	587
Ham, & Cheese, Wiltshire Cured, Deli Deals	552
Tuna, Cheese, & Mayo, Melt, Deli Deals	731
PASTA	
Alfredo	645
Tomato, & Mascarpone, Kids Menu	243
PEAS	
Extra or Add On	110
Kids Menu	55
Mushy, Side	248
PIZZA	
Chicken, BBQ, 11"	1103
Chicken, BBQ, 8"	559
Ham & Mushroom, 11"	1002
Ham & Cheese, Kids Menu	420
Ham & Mushroom, 8"	501
Hawaiian, 11"	1033
Hawaiian, 8"	516
Hawaiian, Kids Menu	443
Margherita, 11"	931
Margherita, 8"	466
Margherita, Kids Menu	392
Meat Feast, Spicy, 11"	1227
Meat Feast, Spicy, 8", Sm Plates	622
Pepperoni, 11"	1186
Pepperoni, 8"	593
Vegetable, Roasted, 11"	1024
Vegetable, Roasted, 8"	512
Vegetable, Roasted, Kids Menu	432
Vegetable, Roasted, Vegan, 11"	710
Vegetable, Roasted, Vegan, 8", Sm Plates	355

J D WETHERSPOON	KCAL
PIZZA	
Vegetable, Roasted, Vegan, Kids Menu	348
PIZZA TOPPING	
Avocado, Half	84
Bacon, Maple Cured	86
BBQ Sauce	69
Chicken, Breast	103
Chillies, Sliced	7
Ham	56
Mozzarella	169
Mushrooms	8
Onion, Red	10
Pepperoni	128
Pineapple	24
Tomato, Slices	13
Vegetables, Roasted	80
POPPADOMS	
Side	95
POTATO	
Rosti, Two, Extra or Add On	165
POTATOES	
Mashed, Kids Menu	134
PRAWNS	
King, Spicy Coated, with Sweet Chilli Sauce	474
PUDDING - STEAK & KIDNEY	
with Chips, Peas, & Gravy, Pub Classics	1261
RIBS - PORK, BBQ	
Half Rack, Extra or Add on	581
Half Rack, with Onion Rings, Sm Plates	836
with Coleslaw, Onions Rings, & Chips	2013
with Coleslaw, Onions Rings, & Jacket Potato	1738
RICE	
Mexican, Side	203
Pilau, Side	225
RISOTTO	
Mushroom, Creamy, Pub Classics	470
ROGAN JOSH	
Lamb, Curry Club	980
SALAD	
Chicken, Pulled, Avocado, & Bacon	444
Quinoa, Rainbow	407
Quinoa, Side or Add on	179
Quinoa, with Grilled Halloumi, & Kale Dressing	823
Side	72
SAMOSAS	
Vegetable, 2, Curry Club	209
SANDWICH	
Bacon, Butty, White	509
Bacon Butty, Wholewheat	512
Sausage, Butty, Quorn* White	605
Sausage, Butty, White	691
Sausage, Butty, Wholewheat	694
Sausage, Quorn*, Butty, Wholewheat	608

J D WETHERSPOON	KCAL
SAUCE	
BBQ, Burger Topping	83
Bearnaise, Beef Dripping	123
Chocolate, Belgian, Extra or Add On	58
Curry, Chip Shop Style	118
Honey Glaze, Jack Daniels	73
Peppercorn, Creamy	74
Toffee, Extra or Add On	72
SAUSAGE	
Extra or Add On	168
Pork, Kids Menu	336
Quorn, Vegan, Extra or Add On	125
Quorn, Vegan, Kids Menu	251
SCAMPI - BREADED	
Extra or Add On	222
Kids Menu	205
Whitby, with Chips, & Mushy Peas	1037
Whitby, with Chips, & Mushy Peas, Small	655
Whitby, with Chips, & Peas	971
Whitby, with Chips, & Peas, Small	588
SCONE	
Potato, Extra or Add On	80
STRAWBERRIES	
Extra or Add On	14
SYRUP	
Maple Flavoured, Extra or Add On	97
TART	
Chocolate, & Salted Caramel	855
TIKKA MASALA - CHICKEN	
with Chips, Simple	1291
with Pilau Rice, Naan Bread, Poppadoms	1166
with Pilau Rice, Simple	895
TOAST	
& Preserves, Marmalade, White	458
& Preserves, Marmalade, Wholewheat	461
& Preserves	459
& Preserves, Strawberry Jam, Wholewheat	461
TOMATOES	
Halves, Grilled, Extra or Add On	16
VEGETABLES	
Roasted, Extra	80
Roasted, Kids Menu	80
Roasted, Side	120
Tomatoes, Mushrooms, & Peas, Extra or Add On	126
VINDALOO	
Chicken, Curry Club	920
WRAP	
Breakfast	721
Breakfast, Vegetarian	861
Chicken, & Avocado, with Mayonnaise	688
Chicken, Breast, Pulled, & Sweet Chilli Sauce	478
Chicken, Southern Fried, Smokey Chipotle May	637
Halloumi, Grilled, with Sweet Chilli Sauce	698

KFC	KCAL
BEANS	
Baked, BBQ, Large	250
Baked, BBQ, Reg	105
BITES	
Sweet Chilli	355
BURGERS	
BBQ Bacon, Tower, 1 PC, Box Meal	1245
BBQ Bacon, Tower, 2 Hot Wings, Box Meal	1170
BBQ Bacon, Tower	690
BBQ Bacon, Tower, Meal	925
Chicken, Big Daddy, Box Meal	1260
Chicken, Big Daddy, Burger Only	685
Double Down, Box Meal	1145
Double Down, Burger Only	575
Double Down, Meal	825
Chicken Fillet, Bacon & Cheese	585
Chicken Fillet, Box Meal	1045
Chicken Fillet, Burger Only	475
Chicken Fillet, Meal	720
Chicken Fillet, Mini	290
Chicken Fillet, Tower	620
Chicken Fillet, Tower, Meal	870
Chicken, Kids	265
Chicken, Meal, Kids	455
Chicken Zinger, Box Meal	945
Chicken Zinger, Burger Only	450
Chicken Zinger, Meal	700
Chicken Zinger, Stacker, Box Meal	1280
Chicken Zinger, Stacker	780
Chicken Zinger, Stacker, Meal	1030
Chicken Zinger, Tower	595
Chicken Zinger, Tower, Meal	845
Trilogy, Box Meal, with Lipton	1200
Trilogy, Box Meal, with Pepsi Max	1145
Vegan, Burger Only	450
CHICKEN	
Allstars, BBQ, Meal	685
Allstars, Flamin', Meal	720
Boneless, 3 Piece, Dips Meal	705
Boneless, 4 Piece, Dips Meal	835
Boneless, Banquet, Box Meal	920
Boneless, Feast, Dipping, 12 Piece	910
Boneless, Feast, Dipping, 8 Piece	780
Bucket, Bargain, 10 Piece	850
Bucket, Bargain, 14 Piece	1090
Bucket, Bargain, 6 Piece	610
Bucket, Mighty, For One	1155
Bucket, Party, 14 Piece	1225
Colonel, 2 Piece, Meal	730
Colonel, 3 Piece, Meal	970
Colonel, 4 Piece, Meal	1210
Drumstick, Original Recipe	170
Family Feast, 10 Piece	930

	KCAL
KFC	
CHICKEN	
Family Feast, 6 Piece	690
Fillet, Mini	130
Fillet, Mini, Snackbox	475
Fillet, Original Redcipe	220
Fillet, Zinger	200
Fillets, Mini, 10	655
Keel, Original recipe	265
Megabox, with Gravy	930
Original Recipe, Mini Fillet, Meal, Kids	345
Original Recipe, Snackbox	585
Popcorn, Large	465
Popcorn, Meal	535
Popcorn, Meal, Kids	330
Popcorn, Meal, Large	710
Popcorn, Reg	285
Popcorn, Small	135
Popcorn, Snackbox	480
Rib, Original Recipe	325
Thigh, Original Recipe	285
Variety, 2 Piece, Meal	1025
Variety, 3 Piece, Meal	1265
Wicked Variety, 10 Piece	1145
Wicked Variety, 6 Piece	905
Wing, Original Recipe	175
Wings, Hot, 6, Meal	740
Wings, Hot	85
Wings, Hot, Snackbox	510
COFFEE	
Americano, Black, Reg	15
Americano, White, Reg	80
Cafe Mocha, Reg	180
Cappuccino, Reg	125
Espresso, Double	12
Espresso, Single	10
Latte, Caramel, Reg	195
Latte, Reg	140
Latte, Vanilla, Reg	195
COLA	
Pepsi*, Diet or Max, Kids	5
Pepsi*, Diet or Max, Large	15
Pepsi*, Diet or Max, Reg	10
Pepsi*, Kids	100
Pepsi*, Large	180
Pepsi*, Max Cherry, Kids	5
Pepsi*, Max Cherry, Large	10
Pepsi*, Max Cherry, Reg	5
Pepsi*, Reg	130
COLESLAW	
Large	320
Reg	160
COOKIES	
Chocolate, Milk	325

	KCAL
KFC	
COOKIES	
Chocolate, White	335
CORN	
Cobette	85
Cobette, Lge Portion	165
DESSERT	
Krushems, Malteser	225
Krushems, Milky Bar	325
Krushems, Oreo	280
Krushems, Salted Caramel, Soft Serve	375
FRIES	
Large	345
Reg	250
GRAVY	
Large	110
Reg	45
HOT CHOCOLATE	
Reg	180
JUICE	
Orange, Tropicana*	120
JUICE DRINK	
Apple, & Blackcurrant, Robinsons*, Kids	5
Apple, & Blackcurrant, Robinsons*, Reg	5
Blackcurrant, & Apple, Fruit Shoot	10
Club Orange*, Kids	125
Club Orange*, Large	230
Club Orange*, Reg	160
Club Orange*, Zero, Kids	10
Club Orange*, Zero, Large	15
Club Orange*, Zero, Reg	10
Orange, Fruit Shoot	10
LEMONADE	
7up*, Free, Kids	5
7up*, Free, Large	10
7up*, Free, Reg	5
MUFFIN	
Chocolate	555
Lemon	470
ONION RINGS	
BLANK	400
PINEAPPLE	
Sticks	30
POTATOES	
Mashed	110
RICE	
Chicken, Fillet, Ricebox	490
Chicken, Fillet, Ricebox, Meal	740
Chicken, Fillet, Ricebox, with Sugar Free Drink	500
Chicken, Zinger, Ricebox	480
Chicken, Zinger, Ricebox, Meal	725
Chicken, Zinger, Ricebox, with Sugar Free Drink	480
Southern	210
Veggie, Ricebox	365

KFC	KCAL
RICE	
Veggie, Ricebox, Meal	615
Veggie, Ricebox, with Sugar Free Drink	365
SALAD	
Chicken, Fillet	370
Chicken, Fillet, Meal	620
Chicken, Fillet, with Sugar Free Drink	375
Chicken, Zinger	350
Chicken, Zinger, Meal	600
Chicken, Zinger, with Sugar Free Drink	350
Garden, Side	75
Veggie	235
Veggie, Meal	485
Veggie, with Sugar Free Drink	235
SAUCE	
BBQ, Kentucky Smoky, Dip Pot	50
Curry, Large	175
Curry, Reg	75
Hot, Original, Dip Pot	40
HP, BBQ, Heinz, Sachet	15
HP, Brown, Heinz, Sachet	15
Ketchup, Heinz, Sachet	10
Mayo, Garlic Buttermilk, Dip Pot	110
Mayonnaise, Light, Heinz, Sachet	30
Supercharger, Spicy, Dip Pot	150
Sweet Chilli, Sticky, Dip Pot	75
Tomato Sauce, Real, Dip Pot	40
SUNDAE	
Cherry	220
Cherry, Mini	145
Chocolate	230
Chocolate, Mini	150
TANGO*	
Orange, Kids	45
Orange, Large	80
Orange, Reg	60
TEA	
Black, Reg	0
Iced, Lipton*, Kids	20
Iced, Lipton*, Large	60
Iced, Lipton*, Reg	45
WRAP	
Chicken, BBQ	300
Chicken, Flamin'	335
Chicken, Twister, Kentucky Mayo, Box Meal	965
Chicken, Twister, Kentucky Mayo	500
Chicken, Twister, Kentucky Mayo, Meal	750
Chicken, Twister, Nashville Hot, Box Meal	950
Chicken, Twister, Nashville Hot	490
Chicken, Twister, Nashville Hot, Meal	735
Chicken, Twister, Smoky BBQ, Box Meal	935
Chicken, Twister, Smoky BBQ	475
Chicken, Twister, Smoky BBQ, Meal	725

KFC	KCAL
WRAP	
Chicken, Twister, Sweet Chilli, Box Meal	945
Chicken, Twister, Sweet Chilli	485
Chicken, Twister, Sweet Chilli, Meal	735
YOGHURT	
Much Bunch	100

KRISPY KREME	KCAL
COFFEE	
Americano, Black, 12oz	34
Americano, Black, 16oz	46
Cappuccino, 12oz	111
Cappuccino, 16oz	133
Flat White, 8oz	88
Latte, 12oz	132
Latte, 16oz	169
Mocha, 12oz	192
Mocha, 16oz	247
DOUGHNUTS	
Apple Pie	296
Bites	138
Caramel, Iced, Ring	257
Chocolate, Double, Duoghnut	485
Chocolate, White, Dreamcake	405
Chocolate Dreamcake	351
Chocolate Iced, Custard Filled	289
Chocolate Iced, Ring	237
Chocolate Iced, with Sprinkles	262
Chocolate Praline, Cheesecake, Duoghnut	384
Glazed, Original	200
Glazed, with a Creme Filling	371
Lemon Meringue	346
Lotus Biscoff	396
Nutty Chocolatta	379
Raspberry, Glazed	324
Reese's Peanut Butter	395
Salted Caramel, Cheesecake	367
Strawberries & Kreme	326
Strawberry Gloss	244
Vimto, Shimmer	389
HOT CHOCOLATE	
12oz	234
16oz	359
ICE CREAM	
Solo	240
with Caramel Sauce, & Shortbread	319
with Caramel Sauce, Shortbread, & Bites	453
with Caramel Sauce, Shortbread, & Doughnut	369
with Chocolate Sauce, & Shortbread	313
with Chocolate Sauce, Shortbread, & Bites	448
ICE CREAM	
with Chocolate Sauce, Shortbread, & Doughnut	363
MILK SHAKE	
Chocolate Kreme	515
Lotus Biscoff	521
Strawberries, & Kreme	515

LOCH FYNE	KCAL
BEANS	
Edamame, with Ginger, & Chilli	189
BEEF	
Steak, Ribeye, with Chimichurri Sauce	1703
BREAD	
Basket, with Balsamic Oil	797
Garlic, Starter, Kids	349
BURGERS - BEEF	
Chargrilled, Pancetta, Cheese, & Burger Sauce	1669
Gruyere Cheese, No Sides, Kids	459
BUTTER	
Garlic, Fish Bar	188
Garlic	188
Harissa, Fish Bar	207
Harissa	208
Lobster, Fish Bar	131
Lobster	132
Paprika, Smoked, & Sunblush Tomato, Fish Bar	192
Paprika, Smoked, & Sunblush Tomato	192
Salted	221
CABBAGE	
Savoy, Shallot, & Chestnuts, Fish Bar	257
Savoy, Shallot, & Chestnuts	257
Savoy, Shallot, & Chestnuts, Side, Kids	128
CARROTS	
Rainbow, with Harissa Butter, Fish Bar	109
Rainbow, with Harissa Butter	126
CHEESE	
Plate, Scottish	595
CHIPS	
Twice Cooked, Fish Bar	526
Twice Cooked	526
COD	
Fillet, Panko Crusted, No Sides, Kids	380
Fillet, Roasted, Pancetta, & Red Wine Lentils	883
Grilled, Line Caught, Fish Bar	325
Pan Fried, Line Caught, Fish Bar	399
Steamed, Line Caught, Fish Bar	319
CREME BRULEE	
Dessert	621
CRUDITES	
Starter, Kids	166
CRUMBLE	
Plum, Granola, Baked	691
CURRY	
Cauliflower, & Squash, Goan, Spiced	460
Malabar, King Prawn, Kids	303
Seafood, Goan	565
DESSERT	
Chocolate, Fondant	568
DUCK	
Smoked, Gressingham, Fig, & Goats Cheese	241

LOCH FYNE	KCAL
FISH	
Megrim, Whole, Grilled, Fish Bar	415
Megrim, Whole, Pan Fried, Fish Bar	490
Megrim, Whole, Steamed, Fish Bar	415
FISH & CHIPS	
Cod, Battered	1620
Haddock, Battered	1373
Haddock, Takeaway	1437
Portion	1624
FISH CAKES	
Haddock, No Sides, Kids	407
Haddock, Smoked, with Mustard Leeks	733
FRIES	
French, Fish Bar	616
French	560
French, Side, Kids	420
Halloumi, with Chimichurri	743
FRUIT	
Plate, Kids	34
GNOCCHI	
Spinach, Mushroom, Cheese, Leek, & Artichoke	1114
HADDOCK	
Smoked, Poached	643
ICE CREAM	
Amaretti Amaretto, Luxury	136
Chocolate Split, Luxury	129
Mint Chocolate, Luxury	122
Strawberry, Luxury	82
Vanilla, 3 Scoops, Luxury	305
Vanilla, Luxury	110
Vanilla, Vegan, Luxury	102
Walnut, Luxury	130
ICE LOLLY	
Apple, Organic, Kids	17
Rainbow, Organic, Kids	18
Tropical, Organic, Kids	20
KETCHUP	
Portion	20
LANGOUSTINE	
Grilled, with Romesco Sauce, Premium	823
LINGUINE	
Pomodoro, Kids	234
Prawn, & Chilli	729
LOBSTER	
Thermidor, Whole, with Basmiti Rice	688
Thermidor, Whole, with French Fries	1211
MACKEREL - FILLET, CURED	
Red Cabbage, & Apple, with Honey Mustard, Main	474
Red Cabbage, & Apple, with Honey Mustard, Starter	346
MACKEREL - WHOLE	
Grilled, Fish Bar	849
Pan Fried, Fish Bar	923
Steamed, Fish Bar	849

LOCH FYNE	KCAL
MAYONNAISE	
Portion	113
MONKFISH	
Roast, Smoked Pancetta, & Red Wine Lentils	1033
MUSSELS	
Scottish, Rope Grown, Main	1186
Scottish, Rope Grown, Starter	375
OIL	
& Balsamic Vinegar	323
Chilli, Roasted, Fish Bar	114
Chilli, Roasted	152
OLIVES	
Nocellara	186
OYSTERS	
Fyne Vinegar, 1	62
Fyne Vinegar, 12	674
Fyne Vinegar, 3	173
Fyne Vinegar, 6	339
My First Oyster	61
Soy & Ginger, 1	68
Soy & Ginger, 12	680
Soy & Ginger, 3	179
Soy & Ginger, 6	345
Wasabi & Cucumber, 1	71
Wasabi & Cucumber, 12	683
Wasabi & Cucumber, 3	182
Wasabi & Cucumber, 6	348
PAKORA	
Samphire, & Sweet Potato, with Date Chutney	404
PEAS	
Mushy	68
PEPPERS	
Padron, with Smoked Sea Salt	199
PETIT POIS	
Side, Kids	29
PIE	
Apple, No Ice Cream	314
PLATTER	
Shellfish, with Lobster, & Crab	1420
PORK	
Belly, Black Pudding Mash, Spinach, & Apple Puree	748
POTATOES	
Dauphinoise, Fish Bar	615
Dauphinoise	615
Mashed, Creamed, with Chives, Fish Bar	248
Mashed, Creamed, with Chives	248
Mashed, Side, Kids	74
New, Sauteed, Fish Bar	191
New, Sauteed	191
New, with Butter, Fish Bar	238
New, with Butter	239
New, with Butter, Side, Kids	119

LOCH FYNE	KCAL
PRAWNS	
Karagee, with Soy & Ginger Sauce	325
King, Chilli & Garlic, Pan Fried	857
PUDDING	
Sticky Toffee, with Tablet Ice Cream	1194
SALAD - GREEN	
Fish Bar	126
Side	126
SALAD - WARM WINTER	
Puy Lentil & Red Pepper Dressing, Main	603
Puy Lentil & Red Pepper Dressing, Starter	311
SALMON	
Fillet, No Sides, Kids	199
Grilled, Scottish, Fish Bar	536
Pan Fried, Scottish, Fish Bar	611
Smoked, Plate, Classic	337
Steamed, Scottish, Fish Bar	536
SALSA	
Verde	176
SAMPHIRE	
with Lemon, Fish Bar	11
with Lemon	11
SAUCE	
Chimichurri, Fish Bar	114
Chimichurri	114
Cream Anglaise	62
Pesto, Wild Garlic	54
Pesto, Wild Garlic	54
Soy, & Ginger, Fish Bar	23
Soy, & Ginger	23
SAUSAGE	
Chorizo, in Parsley & White Wine	393
SAUSAGE ROLL	
Mini	244
SCALLOPS	
with Chickpea, & Nduja Stew	311
SCOTCH EGG	
Haggis, Curried Potato Cream, & Turnip	773
SEA BASS	
Fillet, No Sides, Kids	250
Whole, Grilled, Fish Bar	596
Whole, Pan Fried, Fish Bar	670
Whole, Steamed, Fish Bar	593
SEA BREAM	
Gilt Head, Grilled, Fish Bar	274
Gilt Head, Pan Fried, Fish Bar	311
Gilt Head, Steamed, Fish Bar	274
SEAFOOD	
Clams, Cockles, & Chorizo, on Sourdough	353
Grill	1003
SORBET	
Lemon, Luxury	62
Pear, Luxury	63

LOCH FYNE	KCAL
SORBET	
Raspberry, Luxury	65
SOUP	
Fish	468
SPINACH	
Buttered, Fish Bar	50
Buttered	50
SQUID	
Salt & Pepper	490
SUNDAE	
Popcorn	564
SWEET POTATO	
Wedges, Side, Kids	283
TART	
Squash. & Ricotta, with Beetroot	140
TORTELLONI	
Beetroot, & Ricotta, Goats Cheese Cream, Main	566
Beetroot, & Ricotta, Goats Cheese Cream, Starter	321
Crab, Devonshire, with Lemon Oil	731
Crab, Devonshire, with Lemon Oil, Premium	712
TRIFLE	
Black Forest	788
TUNA	
Chargrilled, Fish Bar	396
Grilled, Fish Bar	392
Pan Fried, Fish Bar	433
TURBOT	
Whole, Grilled, Fish Bar	604
Whole, Pan Fried, Fish Bar	589
Whole, Steamed, Fish Bar	604
VEGETABLES	
Sticks, Side, Kids	166

	KCAL
MCDONALD'S	
BITES	
Wedges, Nacho Cheese, 5 Pieces	233
Wedges, Nacho Cheese, Sharebox, 15 Pieces	699
BREAKFAST	
Muffin, with Jam	211
BREAKFAST CEREAL	
Porridge, Oat So Simple, Plain	194
BROWNIES	
Chocolate	273
BURGERS	
Big Mac	508
Cheeseburger, Bacon, Double	495
Cheeseburger, Double	445
Cheeseburger	301
Cheeseburger, Triple	588
Chicken, Bacon, Mayo	370
Chicken Legend, with BBQ Sauce	484
Chicken Legend, with Cool Mayo	529
Chicken Legend, with Hot & Spicy Mayo	519
Filet-O-Fish	329
Hamburger	250
Mayo Chicken, Bacon	370
Mayo Chicken	319
McChicken, BLT	489
McChicken Sandwich	388
Quarter Pounder, Deluxe	553
Quarter Pounder, Double, with Cheese	750
Quarter Pounder, Spicy, with Cheese	518
Quarter Pounder, with Cheese	518
Vegetable, Deluxe	380
CARROTS	
Sticks	34
CHEESE	
Melt, Dippers, 12 Pieces	765
Melt, Dippers, 4 Pieces	255
CHICKEN	
McNuggets, 4 Pieces	173
McNuggets, 6 Pieces	259
McNuggets, 9 Pieces	388
Nuggets, Sharebox, 20	863
Selects, 3 Pieces	359
Selects, 5 Pieces	599
COFFEE	
Black, Large	8
Black, Medium	6
Cappuccino, Large	128
Cappuccino, Medium	97
Flat White, Semi Skimmed Milk	86
Latte, Iced	94
Latte, Large	197
Latte, Medium	145
Latte, Salted Caramel, Large	206
Latte, Salted Caramel, Medium	164

	KCAL
MCDONALD'S	
COFFEE	
Latte, Toffee, Large	232
Latte, Toffee, Medium	187
White, Large	74
White, Medium	54
COLA	
Coca-Cola, Diet	1
Coca-Cola	170
Coke, Zero	1
COOKIES	
Triple Chocolate	320
DOUGHNUTS	
Millionaires	250
Sugar	195
FANTA	
Orange	76
FLATBREAD	
Cheesy, Bacon	298
FRIES	
French, Large	444
French, Medium	337
French, Small	237
FRUIT	
Bag, Apple & Grape	46
FRUIT SHOOT	
Apple & Blackcurrant, Robinsons	10
HAPPY MEAL	
Carrot Sticks	34
Cheeseburger, No Sides	301
Chicken Nuggets, 4, No Sides	173
Fish Fingers, No Sides	194
Fries, Small	237
Hamburger, No Sides	250
Veggie Dippers, 2 Pieces	160
Wrap, Chicken, Crispy, No Sides	248
Wrap, Chicken, Grilled, No Sides	181
HASH BROWNS	
Single	136
HOT CHOCOLATE	
Large	231
Medium	173
ICE CREAM CONE	
Single	142
with Flake	185
IRN BRU	
Medium	80
JUICE	
Orange, Tropicana	108
JUICE DRINK	
Oasis	67
LEMONADE	
Sprite, Zero	4

MCDONALD'S	KCAL
MCFLURRY	
Celebrations	343
Celebrations, Mini	171
Dairy Milk, Caramel	346
Dairy Milk, Caramel, Mini	173
Dairy Milk	342
Dairy Milk, Mini	171
Maltesers	266
Maltesers, Mini	133
Oreo	258
Oreo, Mini	129
Smarties	273
Smarties, Mini	137
MCMUFFIN	
Bacon, & Egg, Double	401
Bacon, & Egg	348
Egg, & Cheese	295
Sausage, & Egg, Double	565
Sausage, & Egg	430
MILK	
Organic	125
MILK SHAKE	
Banana, Large	459
Banana, Medium	357
Banana, Small	188
Chocolate, Large	468
Chocolate, Medium	364
Chocolate, Small	192
Strawberry, Large	458
Strawberry, Medium	356
Strawberry, Small	188
Vanilla, Large	469
Vanilla, Medium	366
Vanilla, Small	192
MUFFIN	
Mixed Berry	298
PANCAKE	
& Syrup	477
& Sausage, with Syrup	612
PIE	
Apple, Hot	250
ROLL	
Bacon, with Brown Sauce	356
Bacon, with Tomato Ketchup	351
Breakfast, with Brown Sauce	517
Breakfast, with Ketchup	513
SALAD	
Chicken, Crispy, & Bacon	311
Chicken, Crispy	261
Chicken, No Bacon, Grilled	133
Chicken, with Bacon, Grilled	183
Side	15

MCDONALD'S	KCAL
SMOOTHIE	
Mango & Pineapple, Iced, Large	241
Mango & Pineapple, Iced, Medium	187
TEA	
with Milk	6
VEGETARIAN	
Dippers, 4 Pieces	321
WRAP	
Chicken, Spicy, Snack	322
The BBQ & Bacon Chicken One, Crispy	500
The BBQ & Bacon Chicken One, Grilled	366
The Fajita Chicken One, Crispy	479
The Fajita Chicken One, Grilled	345
The Garlic Mayo Chicken One, Crispy	479
The Garlic Mayo Chicken One, Grilled	345
The Sweet Chilli Chicken One, Crispy	474
The Sweet Chilli Chicken One, Grilled	340
The Veggie One, Spicy	364

NANDO'S	KCAL
AVOCADO	
Ã,¼, Extra	85
Ã,½, Salad Extra	170
BREAD	
Garlic, Kids Menu	218
Garlic, Large, Side	698
Garlic, Reg, Side	349
Pitta, Toasted, with Butter, Extra	246
BROCCOLI	
Long Stem, Large, Side	48
Long Stem, Reg, Side	24
Long Stem, Side, Kids Menu	12
BROWNIES	
Salted Caramel	389
BURGERS	
Beanie, Peri Peri, Extra Hot	593
Beanie, Peri Peri, Hot	552
Beanie, Peri Peri, Lemon & Herb	521
Beanie, Peri Peri, Mango & Lime	534
Beanie, Peri Peri, Medium	531
Beanie, Plain	511
Chicken, Breast, Peri-Peri, Extra Hot	469
Chicken, Breast, Peri-Peri, Hot	428
Chicken, Breast, Peri-Peri, Lemon & Herb	397
Chicken, Breast, Peri-Peri, Mango & Lime	410
Chicken, Breast, Peri-Peri, Medium	407
Chicken, Breast, Plain, Kids Menu	296
Chicken, Breast, Plain	387
Chicken, Butterfly, Peri Peri, Extra Hot	663
Chicken, Butterfly, Peri Peri, Hot	622
Chicken, Butterfly, Peri Peri, Lemon & Herb	591
Chicken, Butterfly, Peri Peri, Mango & Lime	604
Chicken, Butterfly, Peri Peri, Medium	601
Chicken, Butterfly, Plain	581
Chicken, Double, Peri Peri, Extra Hot	607
Chicken, Double, Peri Peri, Hot	566
Chicken, Double, Peri Peri, Lemon & Herb	535
Chicken, Double, Peri Peri, Mango & Lime	548
Chicken, Double, Peri Peri, Medium	545
Chicken, Double, Plain	525
Chicken, Sunset, Peri Peri, Extra Hot	680
Chicken, Sunset, Peri Peri, Hot	639
Chicken, Sunset, Peri Peri, Lemon & Herb	608
Chicken, Sunset, Peri Peri, Mango & Lime	621
Chicken, Sunset, Peri Peri, Medium	618
Chicken, Sunset, Plain	598
Mushroom & Halloumi, Peri Peri, Extra Hot	743
Mushroom & Halloumi, Peri Peri, Hot	702
Mushroom & Halloumi, Peri Peri, Lemon & Herb	671
Mushroom & Halloumi, Peri Peri, Mango & Lime	684
Mushroom & Halloumi, Peri Peri, Medium	681
Mushroom & Halloumi, Plain	661
Supergreen, Peri Peri, Extra Hot	487

NANDO'S	KCAL
BURGERS	
Supergreen, Peri Peri, Hot	446
Supergreen, Peri Peri, Lemon & Herb	415
Supergreen, Peri Peri, Mango & Lime	428
Supergreen, Peri Peri, Medium	425
Supergreen, Plain	405
Sweet Potato & Butternut, Kids Menu	333
Sweet Potato & Butternut, Pattie Only, Kids Menu	219
Sweet Potato & Butternut, Peri Peri, Extra Hot	511
Sweet Potato & Butternut, Peri Peri, Hot	470
Sweet Potato & Butternut, Peri Peri, Lemon & Herb	439
Sweet Potato & Butternut, Peri Peri, Mango & Lime	452
Sweet Potato & Butternut, Peri Peri, Medium	449
Sweet Potato & Butternut, Plain	429
CAKE	
Carrot	737
Choc-A-Lot	582
CHEESE	
Feta, Extra	138
Halloumi, Grilled, Extra	177
Halloumi, Sticks, & Dip	441
CHEESECAKE	
Caramel, Gooey	415
White Chocolate, & Raspberrry	446
CHICKEN	
Breast, Fillet, Peri-Peri, Extra Hot	220
Breast, Fillet, Peri-Peri, Hot	179
Breast, Fillet, Peri-Peri, Lemon & Herb	148
Breast, Fillet, Peri-Peri, Mango & Lime	161
Breast, Fillet, Peri-Peri, Med	158
Breast, Fillet, Plain, Salad Extra	138
Breast, Fillet, Plain, Kids Menu	138
Butterfly, Crispy, Peri Peri, Extra Hot	414
Butterfly, Crispy, Peri Peri, Hot	373
Butterfly, Crispy, Peri Peri, Lemon & Herb	342
Butterfly, Crispy, Peri Peri, Mango & Lime	355
Butterfly, Cripsy, Peri Peri, Medium	352
Butterfly, Crispy, Plain	332
Half, Peri-Peri, Extra Hot	650
Half, Peri-Peri, Hot	609
Half, Peri-Peri, Lemon & Herb	578
Half, Peri-Peri, Mango & Lime	591
Half, Peri-Peri, Medium	588
Half, Plain	568
Breast, Quarter, Peri-Peri, Extra Hot	405
Breast, Quarter, Peri-Peri, Hot	364
Breast, Quarter, Peri-Peri, Lemon & Herb	333
Breast, Quarter, Peri-Peri, Mango & Lime	346
Breast, Quarter, Peri-Peri, Medium	343
Breast, Quarter, Plain	323
Leg, Quarter, Peri-Peri, Extra Hot	327
Leg, Quarter, Peri-Peri, Hot	286
Leg, Quarter, Peri-Peri, Lemon & Herb	255

	KCAL
NANDO'S	
CHICKEN	
Leg, Quarter, Peri-Peri, Mango & Lime	268
Leg, Quarter, Peri-Peri, Medium	265
Leg, Quarter, Plain	245
Thighs, Deboned, Peri-Peri, Extra Hot	637
Thighs, Deboned, Peri-Peri, Hot	596
Thighs, Deboned, Peri-Peri, Lemon & Herb	565
Thighs, Deboned, Peri-Peri, Mango & Lime	578
Thighs, Deboned, Peri-Peri, Medium	575
Thighs, Deboned, Plain	555
Thighs, 2, Salad Extra, Peri Peri, Extra Hot	359
Thighs, 2, Salad Extra, Peri Peri, Hot	318
Thighs, 2, Salad Extra, Peri Peri, Lemon & Herb	287
Thighs, 2, Salad Extra, Peri Peri, Mango & Lime	300
Thighs, 2, Salad Extra, Peri Peri, Medium	297
Thighs, 2, Salad Extra, Plain	277
Whole, Peri-Peri, Extra Hot	1218
Whole, Peri-Peri, Hot	1177
Whole, Peri-Peri, Lemon & Herb	1146
Whole, Peri-Peri, Mango & Lime	1159
Whole, Peri-Peri, Medium	1156
Whole, Plain	1136
Wings, Peri-Peri, Extra Hot, 10	868
Wings, Peri-Peri, Extra Hot, 3	318
Wings, Peri-Peri, Extra Hot, 5	475
Wings, Peri-Peri, Hot, 10	827
Wings, Peri-Peri, Hot, 3	277
Wings, Peri-Peri, Hot, 5	434
Wings, Peri-Peri, Lemon & Herb, 10	796
Wings, Peri-Peri, Lemon & Herb, 3	246
Wings, Peri-Peri, Lemon & Herb, 5	403
Wings, Peri-Peri, Mango & Lime, 10	809
Wings, Peri-Peri, Mango & Lime, 3	259
Wings, Peri-Peri, Mango & Lime, 5	416
Wings, Peri-Peri, Medium, 10	806
Wings, Peri-Peri, Medium, 3	256
Wings, Peri-Peri, Medium, 5	413
Wings, Plain, 10	786
Wings, Plain, Kids Menu, 3	236
Wings, Plain, 3	236
Wings, Plain, 5	393
CHIPS	
Kids Menu	336
Large, Side	1256
Peri Salted, Large, Side	1260
Peri Salted, Reg, Side	467
Reg, Side	465
COFFEE	
Americano	0
Cappuccino	73
Espresso	0
Latte	63

	KCAL
NANDO'S	
COLESLAW	
Large, Side	526
Reg, Side	263
CORDIAL	
Green, Kids Menu	26
CORN	
Cob, Kids Menu	72
Cob, Large, Side	288
Cob, Reg, Side	144
DIP	
Red Pepper, & Chilli, with Pitta	464
FROZEN YOGHURT	
Chocolate	79
Mango	71
Strawberry	70
HOT CHOCOLATE	
BLANK	291
HOUMOUS	
Peri Drizzle, & Pitta	819
Salad Extra	204
ICE CREAM	
Chocolate	145
Coconut	157
Mango	99
Vanilla, Kids Menu	158
Vanilla	161
ICE LOLLY	
Chilly Billy	30
JUICE	
Apple, Pressed	134
Orange	118
JUICE DRINK	
Mango Quencher	120
LEMONADE	
Cloudy	143
MASH	
Creamy, Large, Side	496
Creamy, Reg, Side	248
MILK	
Organic, Kids Menu	113
MUSHROOMS	
Portabello, Extra	105
NUTS	
Peri-Peri	793
OLIVES	
Mixed, Spicy	138
PEAS	
Macho, Large, Side	283
Macho, Reg, Side	141
PEPPER	
Chargrilled, Extra	39
PINEAPPLE	
Slice, Grilled, Extra	37

NANDO'S	KCAL
RELISH	
Chilli, Jam, Extra	149
RICE	
Spicy, Large, Side	492
Spicy, Reg, Side	246
ROLL - CHICKEN, LIVERS	
Portuguese, Peri Peri, Extra Hot	622
Portuguese, Peri Peri, Hot	581
Portuguese, Peri Peri, Lemon & Herb	550
Portuguese, Peri Peri, Mango & Lime	563
Portuguese, Peri Peri, Medium	560
Portuguese, Plain	540
ROLL - STEAK, FILLET	
Prego, Peri Peri, Extra Hot	487
Prego, Peri Peri, Hot	446
Prego, Peri Peri, Lemon & Herb	415
Prego, Peri Peri, Mango & Lime	428
Prego, Peri Peri, Medium	425
Prego, Plain	405
SALAD - CAESAR	
Side	285
with Chicken Breast, Peri Peri, Extra Hot	504
with Chicken Breast, Peri Peri, Hot	463
with Chicken Breast, Peri Peri, Lemon & Herb	432
with Chicken Breast, Peri Peri, Mango & Lime	445
with Chicken Breast, Peri Peri, Med	442
with Chicken Breast, Plain	422
SALAD - GRAINS N GREENS	
Side, Kids Menu	104
Large, Side	356
Side	189
with Chicken Breast, Peri Peri, Extra Hot	409
with Chicken Breast, Peri Peri, Hot	368
with Chicken Breast, Peri Peri, Lemon & Herb	337
with Chicken Breast, Peri Peri, Mango & Lime	350
with Chicken Breast, Peri Peri, Medium	347
with Chicken Breast, Plain	327
SALAD - HOUSE	
Side	126
with Chicken Breast, Peri Peri, Extra Hot	345
with Chicken Breast, Peri Peri, Hot	304
with Chicken Breast, Peri Peri, Lemon & Herb	273
with Chicken Breast, Peri Peri, Mango & Lime	286
with Chicken Breast, Peri Peri, Medium	283
with Chicken Breast, Plain	263
SALAD - MIXED LEAF	
Large, Side	25
Reg, Side	13
with Chicken Breast, Peri Peri, Extra Hot	244
with Chicken Breast, Peri Peri, Hot	203
with Chicken Breast, Peri Peri, Lemon & Herb	172
with Chicken Breast, Peri Peri, Mango & Lime	185
with Chicken Breast, Peri Peri, Medium	182

NANDO'S	KCAL
SALAD - MIXED LEAF	
with Chicken Breast, Plain	162
SANDWICH - PITTA	
Beanie, Pitta, Peri Peri, Extra Hot	602
Beanie, Pitta, Peri Peri, Hot	561
Beanie, Peri Peri, Lemon & Herb	530
Beanie, Peri Peri, Mango & Lime	543
Beanie, Peri Peri, Medium	540
Beanie, Plain	520
Chicken, Breast, Peri-Peri, Extra Hot	478
Chicken, Breast, Peri-Peri, Hot	437
Chicken, Breast, Peri-Peri, Lemon & Herb	406
Chicken, Breast, Peri-Peri, Mango & Lime	419
Chicken, Breast, Peri-Peri, Medium	416
Chicken, Breast, Plain	396
Chicken, Double, Peri Peri, Extra Hot	616
Chicken, Double, Peri Peri, Hot	575
Chicken, Double, Peri Peri, Lemon & Herb	544
Chicken, Double, Peri Peri, Mango & Lime	557
Chicken, Double, Peri Peri, Medium	554
Chicken, Double, Plain	534
Chicken, Thigh, Fino, Peri Peri, Extra Hot	838
Chicken, Thigh, Fino, Peri Peri, Hot	797
Chicken, Thigh, Fino, Peri Peri, Lemon & Herb	766
Chicken, Thigh, Fino, Peri Peri, Mango & Lime	779
Chicken, Thigh, Fino, Peri Peri, Medium	776
Chicken, Thigh, Fino, Plain	756
Mushroom & Halloumi, Peri Peri, Extra Hot	727
Mushroom & Halloumi, Peri Peri, Hot	686
Mushroom & Halloumi, Peri Peri, Lemon & Herb	655
Mushroom & Halloumi, Peri Peri, Mango & Lime	668
Mushroom & Halloumi, Peri Peri, Medium	665
Mushroom & Halloumi, Plain	645
Steak, Fillet, & Veg, Peri Peri, Extra Hot	531
Steak, Fillet, & Veg, Peri Peri, Hot	490
Steak, Fillet, & Veg, Peri Peri, Lemon & Herb	459
Steak, Fillet, & Veg, Peri Peri, Mango & Lime	472
Steak, Fillet, & Veg, Peri Peri, Medium	469
Steak, Fillet, & Veg, Plain	449
Supergreen, Peri Peri, Extra Hot	536
Supergreen, Peri Peri, Hot	495
Supergreen, Peri Peri, Lemon & Herb	464
Supergreen, Peri Peri, Mango & Lime	477
Supergreen, Peri Peri, Medium	474
Supergreen, Plain	454
Sweet Potato & Butternut, Peri Peri, Extra Hot	560
Sweet Potato & Butternut, Peri Peri, Hot	519
Sweet Potato & Butternut, Peri Peri, Lemon Herb	488
Sweet Potato & Butternut, Peri Peri, Mango Lime	501
Sweet Potato & Butternut, Peri Peri, Medium	498
Sweet Potato & Butternut, Plain	478

NANDO'S	KCAL
SAUCE	
Peri Peri Drizzle, Side	97
Perinaise, Condiments	159
SPINACH	
Saucy, Large, Side	195
Saucy, Reg, Side	98
STEW	
Cataplana, Veggie	515
SWEET POTATO	
& Butternut Squash, Fino Side	174
& Butternut Squash, Side, Kids Menu	71
Mash, Fino Side	97
Mash, Kids Menu	48
TART	
Custard, Naughty Natas	169
TEA	
Infusions, All Flavours	0
Organic, Everyday	23
Rubro, Iced	57
TOMATOES	
Kids Menu	13
VEGETABLES	
Chargrilled, Fino Side	93
WRAP	
Beanie, Peri Peri, Extra Hot	736
Beanie, Peri Peri, Hot	695
Beanie, Peri Peri, Lemon & Herb	664
Beanie, Peri Peri, Mango & Lime	677
Beanie, Peri Peri, Medium	674
Beanie, Plain	654
Chicken, Breast, Peri-Peri, Extra Hot	613
Chicken, Breast, Peri-Peri, Hot	572
Chicken, Breast, Peri-Peri, Lemon & Herb	541
Chicken, Breast, Peri-Peri, Mango & Lime	554
Chicken, Breast, Peri-Peri, Medium	551
Chicken, Breast, Plain	531
Chicken, Double, Peri Peri, Extra Hot	750
Chicken, Double, Peri Peri, Hot	709
Chicken, Double, Peri Peri, Lemon & Herb	678
Chicken, Double, Peri Peri, Mango & Lime	691
Chicken, Double, Peri Peri, Medium	688
Chicken, Double, Plain	668
Chicken, Mozam, Grilled, Peri Peri, Extra Hot	546
Chicken, Mozam, Grilled, Peri Peri, Hot	505
Chicken, Mozam, Grilled, Peri Peri, Lemon & Herb	474
Chicken, Mozam, Grilled, Peri Peri, Mango & Lime	487
Chicken, Mozam, Grilled, Peri Peri, Medium	484
Chicken, Mozam, Grilled, Plain	464
Mushroom & Halloumi, Peri-Peri, Extra Hot	802
Mushroom & Halloumi, Peri-Peri, Hot	761
Mushroom & Halloumi, Peri-Peri, Lemon & Herb	730
Mushroom & Halloumi, Peri-Peri, Mango & Lime	743
Mushroom & Halloumi, Peri-Peri, Medium	740

NANDO'S	KCAL
WRAP	
Mushroom & Halloumi, Plain	720
Steak, Fillet, & Veg, Peri Peri, Extra Hot	623
Steak, Fillet, & Veg, Peri Peri, Hot	582
Steak, Fillet, & Veg, Peri Peri, Lemon & Herb	551
Steak, Fillet, & Veg, Peri Peri, Mango & Lime	564
Steak, Fillet, & Veg, Peri Peri, Medium	561
Steak, Fillet, & Veg, Plain	541
Supergreen, Peri Peri, Extra Hot	670
Supergreen, Peri Peri, Hot	629
Supergreen, Peri Peri, Lemon & Herb	598
Sipergreen, Peri Peri, Mango & Lime	611
Supergreen, Peri Peri, Medium	608
Supergreen, Plain	588
Sweet Potato & Butternut, Peri Peri, Extra Hot	694
Sweet Potato & Butternut, Peri Peri, Hot	653
Sweet Potato & Butternut, Peri Peri, Lemon & Herb	622
Sweet Potato & Butternut, Peri Peri, Mango & Lime	635
Sweet Potato & Butternut, Peri Peri, Medium	632
Sweet Potato & Butternut, Plain	612

	KCAL
PIZZA EXPRESS	
BITES	
Halloumi	351
BOLOGNESE	
Penne, Al Forno	674
Penne, Piccolo	353
BREAD	
Garlic	280
Garlic, Vegan	345
Garlic, with Mozzarella	356
Garlic, with Vegan Mozzarella	330
BROWNIES	
Chocolate, Dolcetti	206
Chocolate, Piccolo	206
Chocolate, with Ice Cream	519
BRUSCHETTA	
Originale	362
CAKE	
Carrot, Vegan, Dolcetti	336
Chocolate, Fudge	312
CALZONE	
'Nduja	1196
Verdure	906
CANNELLONI	
Spinach, & Ricotta, Al Forno	705
CHEESE	
Mascarpone, Side	118
CHEESECAKE	
Raspberry, Honeycomb, Cream, Slice	578
Lotus Biscoff, Dolcetti	319
Vanilla, Reduced Fat & Sugar	384
White Chocolate & Raspberry	440
CHICKEN	
Wings, Lemon & Herb	556
CHIPS	
Polenta	454
COULIS	
Fruit, Side	25
CREAM	
Side	139
DESSERT	
Chocolate Fondant, with Vanilla Ice Cream	657
DIP	
Trio, Vegan	270
DOUGH BALLS	
Doppio	828
GF, with Garlic Butter	370
Piccolo	115
Plain	396
Sticks, Side	263
Vegan	336
with Balsamic Vinegar, & Olive Oil, Piccolo	153
with Garlic Butter, & Salad, Piccolo	233
with Butter, Piccolo	54

	KCAL
PIZZA EXPRESS	
DOUGH BALLS	
with Houmous, & Salad, Piccolo	193
with Houmous, Piccolo	130
without Butter	230
DRESSING	
Caesar	157
Honey & Mustard	196
House, Classic	191
House, Light	135
FIGS	
Caffe Reale, Dolcetti	208
ICE CREAM	
Chocolate, & Chocolate Straw, Coppa Gelato	246
Caramel, Salted, & Chocolate Straw, Coppa Gelato	287
Strawberry, & Chocolate Straw, Coppa Gelato	211
Vanilla, & Chocolate Straw, Coppa Gelato	247
Vanilla, Gelato, Side	114
ICE LOLLY	
Fruit, Organic, Pip	18
Rainbow, Organic, Pip	20
JUICE DRINK	
Apple, & Pear, Cawston	54
Apple, & Summer Berries, Cawston	50
LASAGNE	
Classica, Al Forno	712
OLIVES	
Marinate	137
PENNE	
Bianca, Piccolo	355
Napoletana, Piccolo	284
PESTO	
Pollo, Al Forno, GF	1082
PIZZA	
American, Classic	978
American hot, Romana	1010
American, Piccolo	482
American Hot, Leggera, Wholemeal	548
Barbacoa, Leggera, Wholemeal	547
Barbacoa, Romana	1118
Calbrese, Classic	1275
Diavolo, Leggera, Wholemeal	556
Diavolo, Romana	1167
Fiorentina, Classic	942
Giardiniera, Vegan, Classic	843
Giardiniera, Vegan, Leggera, Wholemeal	556
Giardiniera, Vegan, Romana	970
La Reine, Classic	898
La Reine, Leggera, Wholemeal	498
La Reine, Piccolo	437
Margherita, Bufala, Romana	1152
Margherita, Classic	834
Margherita, Vegan, Classic	711
Margherita, Leggera, Wholemeal	440

PIZZA EXPRESS

	KCAL
PIZZA	
Margherita, Vegan, Leggera, Wholemeal	452
Margherita, Piccolo	435
Mezze, Leggera, Wholemeal	522
Mezze, Vegan, Romana	932
Padana, Leggera, Wholemeal	587
Padana, Vegan, Leggera, Wholemeal	560
Padana, Romana	1108
Padana, Vegan, Romana	911
Pollo, Ad Astra, Leggera, Wholemeal	599
Pollo, Ad Astra, Romana	1145
Pollo, Forza, Leggera, Wholemeal	578
Pollo, Forza, Romana	1253
Pollo, Piccolo, Classic	458
Sloppy Giuseppe, Classic	897
Sloppy Giuseppe, Leggera, Wholemeal	490
Veneziana, Classic	938
Veneziana, Vegan, Classic	815
Veneziana, Leggera, Wholemeal	517
Veneziana, Vegan, Leggera, Wholemeal	544
PRAWNS	
King, Garlic	289
PROFITEROLES	
Salted Caramel, Dolcetti	257
SALAD	
Mixed, Side, no Dressiing	74
Mixed, Side, with House Dressing	202
Mozzarella, & Tomato, Buffalo	336
Nicoise, no Dressing	366
Nicoise, with Dressing, & Dough Sticks	820
Nicoise, with Dressing	558
Pollo, no Dressing	502
Pollo, with Dough Balls, Piccolo	283
Pollo, with Dressing, & Dough Sticks	954
Pollo, with Dressing	693
Pollo, with Polenta Chips, Piccolo	265
Rucola	140
Side, Piccolo	16
Superfood, Leggera	171
Superfood, Leggera, with Dressing	424
SORBET	
Coconut, Coppa Gelato	201
Raspberry, Leggera	122
SQUID	
Calamari	504
SUNDAE	
Ic Cream, with Chocolate Sauce, Piccolo	149
Ice Cream, with Fruit Sauce, Piccolo	131
TIRAMISU	
Classic	412
TOMATOES	
Roasted	67

PIZZA HUT

	KCAL
APPLES	
Salad Station	10
BACON	
Bits, Salad Station	104
BEETROOT	
Diced, Salad Station	10
BITES	
Cheesy	469
Cinnamon, Hot	472
Cinnamon, Kids	248
Hot Dog	404
BOLOGNESE	
Spaghetti, Little Boss	198
BREAD	
Garlic	511
Garlic, with Mozzarella	689
BREADSTICKS	
Salad Station	245
BROWNIES	
Chocolate, Hot	600
Chocolate, Kids	394
CARROTS	
Shredded, Salad Station	10
CHEESE TRIANGLES	
Fried	425
Oven Baked	396
CHEESECAKE	
Chocolate, Honeycomb	639
I Can't Believe It's Not	513
Strawberries, & Cream	537
CHICKEN	
Bites	397
Breaded, & Fries, Fried, Big Boss	619
Breaded, & Fries, Fried, Little Boss	548
Breaded, & Fries, Oven Baked, Big Boss	472
Breaded, & Fries, Oven Baked, Little Boss	400
Breaded, & Seasoned Fries, Fried, Big Boss	704
Breaded, & Seasoned Fries, Fried, Little Boss	563
Breaded, & Seasoned Fries, Oven Baked, Big Boss	533
Breaded, & Seasoned Fries, Oven Baked, Little Boss	421
Melt, BBQ Americano	396
Melt, Garlic Mushroom	447
Melt, Naked	246
Melt, Pepperoni	423
Nuggets, Southern Fried	248
Wings	379
CHOCOLATE	
Beans, Ice Cream Factory	460
Chips, Ice Cream Factory	516
Toffee, Crunch, Ice Cream Factory	465
Tricolor, Pieces, Ice Cream Factory	542
COLESLAW	
Salad Station	38

PIZZA HUT	KCAL
COOKIES	
Dough, Chocolate Chip, Hot	651
Dough, S'mores, Hot	691
Dough, Salted Caramel, Hot	631
CORN	
Cob, 3, Side	203
Cob, 5, Side	328
Cob, Mini, Side	328
CROUTONS	
Salad Station	85
CUCUMBER	
Salad Station	2
DIP	
BBQ	35
Blue Cheese, Salad Station	75
Garlic Sauce	89
Sour Cream, & Chive, Dressing	102
DRESSING	
French, Low Fat, Salad Station	15
Olive Oil, & Balsamic Vinegar, Salad Station	124
Ranch, Salad Station	79
Thousand Island, Salad Station	54
FLATBREAD	
BBQ Steak, & Chicken	535
Chicken Delight	440
Ham, & Garlic Mushroom	459
Tuna, & Sweetcorn	457
Virtuous Veg	375
Virtuous Veg, Vegan	332
FRIES	
Cheesy, Fried, Side	854
Cheesy, Oven Baked, Side	680
Fried, Side	673
Oven Baked, Side	355
Seasoned, Fried, Side	702
Seasoned, Oven Baked, Side	384
Sweet Potato, Side	772
ICE CREAM	
Vanilla, Ice Cream Factory, Kids	192
Vanilla, Ice Cream Factory	329
ICE CREAM FLOAT	
Cream Soda, Black Cherry	300
Cream Soda	300
ICE LOLLY	
Orange	69
KETCHUP	
Portion	99
LASAGNE	
Beef	790
Beef, with Garlic Bread, Big Boss	523
LETTUCE	
Mix, Salad Station	2

PIZZA HUT	KCAL
MACARONI CHEESE	
Big Boss	412
Portion	824
with Chicken, Pulled	867
with Garlic Mushrooms	894
MAYONNAISE	
Garlic, Salad Station	92
Light, Salad Station	77
MILK SHAKE	
Chocoholic, Kids	273
Chocoholic	622
Oreo, Kids	309
Oreo	775
Salted Caramel, Kids	328
Salted Caramel	679
Strawberry, Kids	287
Strawberry	698
Vanilla, Kids	263
Vanilla	581
OIL	
Garlic, & Chilli, Salad Station	180
ONION RINGS	
Fried, Side	236
Oven Baked, Side	154
ONIONS	
Crispy, Salad Station	125
Red, Salad Station	7
PASTA	
Cheesy, Little Boss	385
PASTA BAKE	
Cheese, 4, & Spinach, Buffet	245
Marinara, Buffet	273
PASTA SAUCE	
Cheese, Buffet	128
Marinara, Buffet	87
PENNE	
Buffet	265
PEPPERS	
Jalapeno, Poppers, Fried	438
Jalapeno, Poppers, Oven Baked	354
Jalapeno, Salad Station	2
Mixed, Salad Station	3
PIZZA	
All About Mushrooms, Cheesy Bites Crust	2224
All About Mushrooms, Deep Pan, Large	2072
All About Mushrooms, Deep Pan, Reg	1014
All About Mushrooms, GF	918
All About Mushrooms, Stuffed Crust, Individual	1224
All About Mushrooms, Stuffed Crust, Large	2224
All About Mushrooms, Thin Crust, Individual	894
All About Mushrooms, Thin Crust, Large	1472
All About Mushrooms, Vegan, Deep Pan, Large	1979
All About Mushrooms, Vegan, Deep Pan, Reg	964

PIZZA HUT	KCAL
PIZZA	
All About Mushrooms, Vegan, GF	959
All About Mushrooms, Vegan, Thin Crust, Individual	827
All About Mushrooms, Vegan, Thin Crust, Large	1378
Americano, BBQ, Cheesy Bites Crust	2584
Americano, BBQ, Deep Pan, Large	2432
Americano, BBQ, Deep Pan, Reg	1158
Americano, BBQ, GF	1068
Americano, BBQ, Stuffed Crust, Individual	1374
Americano, BBQ, Stuffed Crust, Large	2584
Americano, BBQ, Thin Crust, Individual	1038
Americano, BBQ, Thin Crust, Large	1840
BBQ Jack N Cheese, Cheesy Bites Crust	2296
BBQ Jack N Cheese, Deep Pan, Large	2144
BBQ Jack N Cheese, Deep Pan, Reg	1038
BBQ Jack N Cheese, GF	942
BBQ Jack N Cheese, Stuffed Crust, Individual	1248
BBQ Jack N Cheese, Stuffed Crust, Large	2296
BBQ Jack N Cheese, Thin Crust, Individual	912
BBQ Jack N Cheese, Thin Crust, Large	1536
Chicken, Supreme, Cheesy Bites Crust	2344
Chicken, Supreme, Deep Pan, Large	2192
Chicken, Supreme, Deep Pan, Reg	1050
Chicken, Supreme, GF	954
Chicken, Supreme, Stuffed Crust, Individual	1260
Chicken, Supreme, Stuffed Crust, Large	2344
Chicken, Supreme, Thin Crust, Individual	930
Chicken, Supreme, Thin Crust, Large	1592
Hawaiian, Cheesy Bites Crust	2216
Hawaiian, Deep Pan, Large	2072
Hawaiian, Deep Pan, Reg	1008
Hawaiian, GF	912
Hawaiian, Stuffed Crust, Individual	1212
Hawaiian, Stuffed Crust, Large	2216
Hawaiian, Thin Crust, Individual	888
Hawaiian, Thin Crust, Large	1472
Hot N Spicy, Vagen, Deep Pan, Large	1976
Hot N Spicy, Vegan, Deep Pan, Reg	966
Hot N Spicy, Vegan, GF	870
Hot N Spicy, Vegan, Thin Crust, Individual	840
Hot N Spicy, Vegan, Thin Crust, Large	1368
Chicken, Hot N Spicy, Cheesy Bites Crust	2408
Chicken, Hot N Spicy, Deep Pan, Large	2256
Chicken, Hot N Spicy, Deep Pan, Reg	1092
Chicken, Hot N Spicy, GF	996
Chicken, Hot N Spicy, Stuffed Crust, Individual	1302
Chicken, Hot N Spicy, Stuffed Crust, Large	2408
Chicken, Hot N Spicy, Thin Crust, Individual	972
Chicken, Hot N Spicy, Thin Crust, Large	1656
Veg, Hot N Spicy, Cheesy Bites Crust	2296
Veg, Hot N Spicy, Deep Pan, Large	2152
Veg, Hot N Spicy, Deep Pan, Reg	1050
Veg, Hot N Spicy, GF	954

PIZZA HUT	KCAL
PIZZA	
Veg, Hot N Spicy, Stuffed Crust, Individual	1260
Veg, Hot N Spicy, Stuffed Crust, Large	2296
Veg, Hot N Spicy, Thin Crust, Individual	924
Veg, Hot N Spicy, Thin Crust, Large	1536
Jack N Ch**se, Vegan, Deep Pan, Large	2058
Jack N Ch**se, Vegan, Deep Pan, Reg	994
Jack N Ch**se, Vegan, GF	984
Jack N Ch**se, Vegan, Thin Crust, Individual	873
Jack N Ch**se, Vegan, Thin Crust, Large	1457
Margherita, Cheesy Bites Crust	2280
Margherita, Deep Pan, Big Boss	453
Margherita, Deep Pan, Large	2128
Margherita, Deep Pan, Little Boss	423
Margherita, Deep Pan, Reg	1038
Margherita, GF, Big Boss	433
Margherita, GF, Little Boss	412
Margherita, GF	942
Margherita, Stuffed Crust, Individual	1248
Margherita, Stuffed Crust, Large	2280
Margherita, Thin Crust, Big Boss	374
Margherita, Thin Crust, Individual	918
Margherita, Thin Crust, Large	1528
Margherita, Thin Crust, Little Boss	327
Margherita, Vegan, Deep Pan, Large	2163
Margherita, Vegan, Deep Pan, Reg	1056
Margherita, Vegan, GF	958
Margherita, Vegan, Thin Crust, Individual	935
Margherita, Vegan, Thin Crust, Large	1563
Meat Feast, Cheesy Bites Crust	2528
Meat Feast, Deep Pan, Large	2376
Meat Feast, Deep Pan, Reg	1140
Meat Feast, Epic, Cheesy Bites Crust	2592
Meat Feast, Epic, Deep Pan, Large	2448
Meat Feast, Epic, Deep Pan, Reg	1188
Meat Feast, Epic, GF	1170
Meat Feast, Epic, Stuffed Crust, Individual	1398
Meat Feast, Epic, Stuffed Crust, Large	2592
Meat Feast, Epic, Thin Crust, Individual	1068
Meat Feast, Epic, Thin Crust, Large	1848
Meat Feast, GF	1044
Meat Feast, Stuffed Crust, Individual	1350
Meat Feast, Stuffed Crust, Large	2528
Meat Feast, Thin Crust, Individual	1020
Meat Feast, Thin Crust, Large	1776
New York Hot Dog, Cheesy Bites Crust	2720
New York Hot Dog, Deep Pan, Large	2568
New York Hot Dog, Deep Pan, Reg	1248
New York Hot Dog, GF	1152
New York Hot Dog, Stuffed Crust, Individual	1458
New York Hot Dog, Stuffed Crust, Large	2720
New York Hot Dog, Thin Crust, Individual	1128
New York Hot Dog, Thin Crust, Large	1968

PIZZA HUT	KCAL
PIZZA	
Pepperoni, Cheesy Bites Crust	2384
Peperoni, Deep Pan, Large	2232
Pepperoni, Deep Pan, Reg	1092
Pepperoni, Epic, Cheesy Bites Crust	2760
Pepperoni, Epic, Deep Pan, Large	2616
Pepperoni, Epic, Deep Pan, Reg	1266
Pepperoni, Epic, GF	1170
Pepperoni, Epic, Stuffed Crust, Individual	1476
Pepperoni, Epic, Stuffed Crust, Large	2760
Pepperoni, Epic, Thin Crust, Individual	1146
Pepperoni, Epic, Thin Crust, Large	2008
Pepperoni, GF	996
Pepperoni, Stuffed Crust, Individual	1296
Pepperoni, Stuffed Crust, Large	2384
Pepperoni, Thin Crust, Individual	972
Pepperoni, Thin Crust, Large	1632
Philly Cheese Steak, Cheesy Bites Crust	3000
Philly Cheese Steak, Deep Pan, Large	2848
Philly Cheese, Steak, Deep Pan, Reg	1392
Philly Cheese Steak, GF	1302
Philly Cheese Steak, Stuffed Crust, Individual	1602
Philly Cheese Steak, Stuffed Crust, Large	3000
Philly Cheese Steak, Thin Crust, Individual	1278
Philly Cheese Steak, Thin Crust, Large	2248
Supreme, Cheesy Bites Crust	2600
Supreme, Deep Pan, Large	2440
Supreme, Deep Pan, Reg	1158
Supreme, GF	1068
Supreme, Stuffed Crust, Individual	1368
Supreme, Stuffed Crust, Large	2600
Supreme, Thin Crust, Individual	1038
Supreme, Thin Crust, Large	1840
Texas Meat Meltdown, Cheesy Bites Crust	2880
Texas Meat Meltdown, Deep Pan, Large	2728
Texas Meat Meltdown, Deep Pan, Reg	1308
Texas Meat Meltdown, GF	1014
Texas Meat Meltdown, Stuffed Crust, Individual	1524
Texas Meat Meltdown, Stuffed Crust, Large	2880
Texas Meat Meltdown, Thin Crust, Individual	1188
Texas Meat Meltdown, Thin Crust, Large	2256
The G.O.A.T, Cheesy Bites Crust	2456
The G.O.A.T, Deep Pan, Large	2312
The G.O.A.T, Deep Pan, Reg	1134
The G.O.A.T, GF	1032
The G.O.A.T, Stuffed Crust, Individual	1338
The G.O.A.T, Stuffed Crust, Large	2456
The G.O.A.T, Thin Crust, Individual	1002
The G.O.A.T, Thin Crust, Large	1696
Veggie, Cheesy Bites Crust	2184
Veggie, Deep Pan, Large	2032
Veggie, Deep Pan, Reg	984
Veggie, Epic, Cheesy Bites Crust	2320

PIZZA HUT	KCAL
PIZZA	
Veggie, Epic, Deep Pan, Large	2176
Veggie, Epic, Deep Pan, Reg	1062
Veggie, Epic, GF	966
Veggie, Epic, Stuffed Crust, Individual	1272
Veggie, Epic, Stuffed Crust, Large	2320
Veggie, Epic, Thin Crust, Individual	942
Veggie, Epic, Thin Crust, Large	1568
Veggie, GF	888
Veggie, Stuffed Crust, Individual	1194
Veggie, Stuffed Crust, Large	2184
Veggie, Thin Crust, Individual	864
Veggie, Thin Crust, Large	1432
Veggie, Vegan, Deep Pan, Large	1932
Veggie, Vegan, Deep Pan, Reg	933
Veggie, Vegan, GF	929
Veggie, Vegan, Thin Crust, Individual	812
Veggie, Vegan, Thin Crust, Large	1332
PIZZA TOPPING	
Chicken	20
Ham	13
Pepperoni	34
Peppers	2
Pineapple	21
Sweetcorn	15
Tuna	14
POTATO SALAD	
Salad Station	27
RIBS	
Pork, BBQ	582
Pork, Rack, All American	787
ROLLS	
Jack 'N' Roll, Vegan	305
SALSA	
Salad Station	12
SAUCE	
BBQ	119
Chocolate, Ice Cream Factory, Kids	32
Chocolate, Ice Cream Factory	59
Hot & Spicy	65
Hut House Seasoning	322
Raspberry, Ice Cream Factory	263
Sweet Chilli	175
SULTANAS	
Salad Station	55
SWEETCORN	
Salad Station	15
TOMATOES	
Cherry, Salad Station	3
TOPPING	
Gold Crunch, Ice Cream Factory	681
Lemon Crunch, Ice Cream Factory	382
Sprinkles, Ice Cream Factory	421

PIZZA HUT

	KCAL
TOPPING	
Strawberry Crunch, Ice Cream Factory	382
TORTILLA CHIPS	
Salad Station	96
VINEGAR	
Sarsons	21
WRAP	
Chicken, & Cheese, Little Boss	535
Chicken, & Sweetcorn, Little Boss	426
Chicken, Big Boss	396
Tuna, & Cheese	350
Tuna, & Sweetcorn	245
Tuna	210

PRET A MANGER

	KCAL
ALMONDS	
Chocolate, Dark	217
APPLES	
Portion	85
BAGUETTE	
Avocado, Olives, & Tomato, with Rocket	511
Brie, Pistachio, & Cranberry	589
Brie, Tomato, & Basil, White	466
Cheddar, & Pickle, Posh	620
Chicken, & Bacon, Caesar	592
Christmas Lunch	707
Christmas Lunch, Vegan	579
Egg Mayonnaise, & Bacon, Breakfast	358
Egg Mayonnaise, & Roasted Tomatoes, Breakfast	333
Egg Mayonnaise, Free Range, & Avocado, Breakfast	395
Ham, & Pickles, Jambon Beurre, White	354
Ham, Wiltshire Cured, & Greve	615
Prosciutto, Italian	536
Salmon, Smoked, Soft Cheese, & Dill	451
Salmon, Smoked, with Egg Mayo, Breakfast	358
Tuna Mayo, & Cucumber, Pole & Line Caught, White	560
BANANA	
Portion	62
BARS	
Choc	348
Chocolate Brownie	291
Love Bar	325
Pret Bar	279
BISCUITS	
Ginger Snap	240
Gingerbread	197
Shortbread	419
BREAD	
Baguette, Losange, for Soup	188
Focaccia, Brie, & Bacon	577
Focaccia, Firecracker Chicken	490
Focaccia, Mozzarella, Pesto & Roasted Tomato	491
Focaccia, Pizza, Mixed	913
Focaccia, Pizza, Prosciutto & Mozzarella	848
Focaccia, Pizza, Tomato, Mozzarella, & Pesto	1086
BREAKFAST	
Fruit, Yoghurt, & Granola, Bowl	250
Mango, & Banana, Sunshine, Bowl	253
Poached Egg, & Beans, Power Pot	224
Roll, Bacon, Breakfast	455
Roll, Bacon & Egg	410
Roll, Ham, & Egg, Breakfast	405
Roll, Sausage, & Egg, Breakfast	408
Roll, Veggie, Breakfast	332
BREAKFAST CEREAL	
Bircher Muesli, Bowl	305
Porridge, No Topping	216

	KCAL
PRET A MANGER	
BROWNIE	
Hazelnut & Carmel, Vegan	452
CAKE	
Tiffin, Christmas	395
CHOCOLATE	
Dark, with Sea Salt	136
Milk	145
COFFEE	
American, Black, Iced	1
Americano, Black	0
Cappuccino	92
Espresso	0
Filter Coffee	3
Flat White	80
Frappe, Chocolate	439
Frappe, Classic	251
Latte, Gingerbread	312
Latte, Iced	120
Latte, Salted Caramel	642
Latte, Skimmed Milk	118
Macchiato	5
Mocha, Semi Skimmed Milk	185
COOKIES	
Chocolate, Chunk	370
Chocolate, Dark, & Almond Butter	377
Chocolate Praline	311
Fruit, Oat & Spelt	347
Pecan, & Caramel	391
CORN CAKES	
Chocolate Covered, Dark	239
CRANBERRIES	
& Seeds, Topping, for Breakfast	122
in Coats, Yoghurt Coating	234
CRISPS	
Mature Cheddar, & Red Onion	200
Sea Salt, & Cider Vinegar	196
Sea Salt	203
Smokey Chipotle	203
Vegetable, Carrot, Beetroot, & Parsnip	202
CROISSANT	
Almond	374
Butter, French	291
Chocolate	350
Ham, Cheese, Tomato & Bacon	338
Jam, Very Berry	299
Mozzarella & Tomato	322
CURRY	
Aubergine, Sticky, Thai Red	829
DANISH PASTRY	
Cinnamon	489
DRESSING	
French, Large	294
French, Small	165

	KCAL
PRET A MANGER	
DRESSING	
Tamari, & Ginger, 2oz	63
DRIED FRUIT	
Mango	119
ENCHILADAS	
Chicken, Spicy	665
FRUIT	
Mango & Lime	92
Melon, & Blueberry	38
FRUIT & NUT MIX	
with Chocolate Covered Raisins	177
FRUIT COMPOTE	
Topping, for Breakfast	24
FRUIT SALAD	
Portion	111
Superfruit Salad, Pot	109
GINGER BEER	
Pure Pret	129
GRATIN	
Butternut Squash, & Cauliflower	514
HOT CHOCOLATE	
S'mores	418
Semi SKimmed	256
JUICE	
Apple	120
Daily Greens	144
Ginger, Shot	55
Hot Shot	47
Orange, Fresh	105
Orange, Large	168
JUICE DRINK	
Apple, Fizz, Sparkling, Pure	112
Cranberry & Raspberry, Still, Pure Pret	175
Grape & Elderflower, Sparkling, Pure Pret	109
Green Tea, & Peach, Pure Pret	88
Green Tea Yoga Bunny, Sparkling, Pure Pret	116
Orange, & Passion Fruit, Still, Pure Pret	135
KOMBUCHA	
Ginger	43
LEMONADE	
Lemon & Ginger, Still, Pure Pret	153
Rhubarb, Pure	118
MACARONI CHEESE	
Fish Pie	754
Kale, & Cauliflower	549
Lasagne	572
Pigs in Blankets	896
Prosciutto	586
MILK	
Babyccino, with Chocolate Sprinkles	14
Cold, for Kids	94
Rice-Coconut	150

	KCAL
PRET A MANGER	
MILK SHAKE	
Choc Chunk Cookie	671
Chocolate	427
Five Berry	415
MUFFIN	
Double Berry	441
OMELETTE	
Squash, Soft Cheese, & Feta	201
PAIN AU RAISIN	
BLANK	394
PIE	
Mince	312
POPCORN	
Sea Salt	143
Sweet, & Salt	163
SALAD	
Aubergine, Sticky, Rice Bowl	441
Chicken, Chipotle, Burrito Bowl	442
Chicken, Chipotle, Hot, Burrito Bowl	581
Chicken, Italian, Chef's, without Dressing	612
Chicken, Tamari & Ginger, Bowl	335
Chicken Curry, Thai Red, Hot, Rice Bowl	763
Crayfish, & Avocado, No Bread	352
Egg, & Spinach, Protein Pot	104
Houmous, & Falafel, Mezze	712
Rocket, & Italian Cheese, Side	316
Salmon, & Pickles, Rice Bowl	419
Salmon, & Egg, Smoked, Protein Pot	134
Salmon, & Mango, Bowl	357
Sweet Potato, Chipotle, Bowl	454
Sweet Potato Chilli, Hot, Rice Bowl	625
Tuna, Nicoise, with Dressing	455
SANDWICH	
Avocado, Smashed, Open	293
Cheddar, Mature, & Pret Pickle, Veggie Pret	515
Cheese, Kids	422
Chicken, Avocado, & Basil	482
Christmas Nut Roast, Vegan	600
Club, Classic Super	526
Egg Mayo, Free-Range	363
Ham, & Cheese	534
Ham, Kids	303
Pret's Christmas Lunch	531
Roll, Christmas Lunch, Vegan, Hot	426
Roll, Pigs in Blankets, Hot	521
Salmon, Scottish, Smoked	421
Salmon, Smoked, & Soft Cheese, Open	303
Tuna, & Cucumber	401
SAUCE	
Ketchup, Chipotle, Dip Pot	50
Mayo, Caesar, Dip Pot	291
Pesto, Basil, Dip Pot	229

	KCAL
PRET A MANGER	
SAUSAGE	
Pigs in Blankets, Pot	251
SAUSAGE ROLL	
Portion	376
SMOOTHIE	
Berry Blast	239
Mango, & Pineapple	209
Mango	143
Strawberry, & Banana	211
Vitamin Volcano	137
SOUP	
Chicken, & Butternut, Risotto, Heat at Home	229
Chicken, Broccoli, & Brown Rice	85
Chicken, Broccoli, & Brown Rice, Side	51
Chicken, Katsu	208
Chicken, Katsu, Side	124
Chicken, Laksa	291
Chicken, Laksa, Side	176
Chicken Pot Pie, EAT	280
Chicken Pot Pie, EAT, Side	169
Miso	38
Mushroom, Risotto, Heat at Home	110
Mushroom, Risotto	116
Mushroom, Risotto, Side	69
Pea, & Mint, Heat at Home	233
Pea, & Mint	183
Pea, & Mint, Side	108
Tomato, Souper	207
Tomato, Souper, Side	123
Vegetable, Red Thai	184
Vegetable, Red Thai, Side	110
SPREAD	
Nut Butter, Almond, Easy Peasy Almond Squeezy	191
TEA	
Ceylon, Breakfast	14
Earl Grey, Semi Skimmed	14
Green, Tropical	0
Latte, Chai, Organic	218
Latte, Matcha	205
Latte, Turmeric	198
Peppermint, Peace	0
TOASTIE	
Cheese, Classic	610
Ham, Cheese, & Mustard	605
Tuna Melt	572
TOPPING	
Soup, Pot Pie	91
WRAP	
Avocado, & Herb Salad	506
Chicken, Spicy, Hot	491
Duck, Hoisin, Salad	449
Falafel, & Halloumi, Hot	624
Houmous, & Chipotle	469

PRET A MANGER	KCAL
WRAP	
Ragu, & Red Pepper, Vegan, Hot	420
Swedish Meatball, Hot	661
YOGHURT	
Five Berry, Pot	347

PREZZO	KCAL
ANTIPASTI	
Meats, Cured, Sharers	979
BITES	
Pizza, Sharers	860
Pizza, Spicy, Sharers	860
Pizza, Spicy, Starter	356
Pizza, Starter	356
BOLOGNESE	
Spaghetti	589
Spaghetti, with King Prawns	564
BREAD	
Garlic, Pizza, Large, Sharers	892
Garlic, Starter	271
Garlic, with Balsamic Onions, & Mozzarella, Starter	520
Garlic, with Mozzarella, Starter	386
BROCCOLI	
Tenderstem, & Cauliflower	88
BROWNIE	
Chocolate, Dome	467
BRUSCHETTA	
Tomato, Starter	415
BURGER	
Calabrese, with Fries	1382
CALZONE	
Spicy Carne	898
Tre Carni	930
CARBONARA	
Spaghetti, Chicken, Al Forno	1033
Spaghetti	662
CHEESE	
Mozzarella, Breaded, Starter	561
CHEESECAKE	
Honeycomb Smash, Mini	219
Honeycomb Smash	500
Vanilla, with Caramel Sauce, Mini	203
Vanilla, with Raspberries, Mini	242
CHICKEN	
Breast, Chargrilled, with Mushrooms	384
DESSERT	
Affogato	320
FLATBREAD	
Sharers	849
FRIES	
House, Side	582
Truffle Oil Infused, Side	671
HOUMOUS	
Italian, Starter	667
ICE CREAM	
Chocolate	194
Strawberry	171
Vanilla	171
LASAGNE	
Traditional, Al Forno	687

	KCAL
PREZZO	
MEATBALLS	
Giant, Starter	453
MUSHROOMS	
Stuffed, Baked, Starter	395
OLIVES	
Marinated	102
PANNA COTTA	
with Fruit Compote, Mini	126
with Fruit Compote	375
PASTA - PENNE	
Alla Rusticana	756
Arrabbiata	501
Aubergine	554
Goats Cheese, Al Forno	1033
Gorgonzola	633
Pancetta, Pea, & Mushroom, Light	492
Pesto & Pea	681
Prawn, Spicy, & Basil Pesto, Light	506
Salmon, Oak Smoked	840
PASTRY	
Cannoli, Mini	282
PIZZA	
Chicken, & Roasted Pepper, Large	1111
Chicken, & Roasted Pepper, Reg	923
Chicken, Primavera, Light	524
Fiorentina, Large	1016
Fiorentina, Reg	699
Goats Cheese, & Aubergine, Light	554
Goats Cheese, & Red Pepper, Large	1053
Goats Cheese, & Red Pepper, Reg	910
Margherita, Large	837
Margherita, Reg	705
Margherita, Royale, Premium	979
Garlic Mushroom, Large	725
Garlic Mushroom, Reg	595
Pepperoni, Posh, Premium	1242
Tre Gusti, Large	1339
Tre Gusti, Reg	929
Tropicana, Large	1018
Tropicana, Reg	783
Vesuvio, Large	1052
Vesuvio, Reg	872
PRAWNS	
King, Starter	406
PUDDING	
Sticky Toffee	631
RAVIOLI	
Lobster, & Crab	510
RISOTTO	
Chicken, & Asparagus	787
Mushroom	725
Prawn, King, & Salmon	471

	KCAL
PREZZO	
SALAD	
Caesar, Chicken, no Garlic Bread	737
Caprese, Starter	241
Chicken, Bacon & Avocado, no Garlic Bread	512
Lentil, Beetroot, & Butternut, no Garlic Bread	321
Mix, Side	103
Rocket, with Italian Cheese, Side	93
SALMON	
Fillet, Roast, with Vegetables	483
SEA BASS	
with Vegetables, & Pesto	506
SORBET	
Raspberry	13
SPAGHETTI & MEATBALLS	
Al Forno	903
SQUID	
Calamari, Starter	702
TART	
Chocolate, Salted Caramel	599
TIRAMISU	
Portion	323

STARBUCKS	KCAL
BANANA	
Fairtrade	108
BARS	
Caramel, Stick, Crispy	185
Granola	326
Pistachio, Vegan	326
Raspberry, Stick, Crispy	181
Rocky Road	333
BREAD	
Banana	381
Ciabatta, Cheese, & Marmite, Mini	355
Focaccia, Brie, & Cran-Merry	384
BREAKFAST	
Eggs, Scrambled, Tomato, & Spinach, Hot Box	262
BREAKFAST CEREAL	
Berry Good Bircher	286
Porridge, 5 Grain	285
Porridge, Oatmeal, Classic	303
BROWNIES	
Chocolate, Christmas Tree	372
BURRITO	
Breakfast, All Day, Vegan	388
CAKE	
Carrot, Loaf	323
Chocolate, Christmas Bauble, Loaf	392
Lemon, Loaf	352
CHILLI	
Beef, Pulled, & Rice	310
COFFEE - AMERICANO	
Grande	16
Short	5
Tall	11
Venti	22
COFFEE - AMERICANO, ICED	
Grande	16
Tall	11
Venti	22
COFFEE - CAPPUCCINO	
Almond Milk, Grande	74
Almond Milk, Short	35
Almond Milk, Tall	67
Almond Milk, Venti	104
Coconut Milk, Grande	120
Coconut Milk, Short	57
Coconut Milk, Tall	108
Coconut Milk, Venti	168
Oat Milk, Grande	213
Oat Milk, Short	100
Oat Milk, Tall	191
Oat Milk, Venti	297
Semi Skimmed Milk, Grande	143
Semi Skimmed Milk, Short	68
Semi Skimmed Milk, Tall	129

STARBUCKS	KCAL
COFFEE - CAPPUCCINO	
Semi Skimmed Milk, Venti	201
Skimmed Milk, Grande	103
Skimmed Milk, Short	49
Skimmed Milk, Tall	93
Skimmed Milk, Venti	144
Soy, Grande	119
Soy, Short	56
Soy, Tall	107
Soy, Venti	167
Whole Milk, Grande	181
Whole Milk, Short	85
Whole Milk, Tall	163
Whole Milk, Venti	253
COFFEE - CAPPUCCINO, ICED	
Almond Milk, Grande	70
Almond Milk, Tall	58
Almond Milk, Venti	83
Coconut Milk, Grande	113
Coconut Milk, Tall	92
Coconut Milk, Venti	131
Oat Milk, Grande	201
Oat Milk, Tall	162
Oat Milk, Venti	230
Semi Skimmed Milk, Grande	136
Semi Skimmed Milk, Tall	110
Semi Skimmed Milk, Venti	156
Skimmed Milk, Grande	97
Skimmed Milk, Tall	80
Skimmed Milk, Venti	113
Soy, Grande	113
Soy, Tall	92
Soy, Venti	131
Whole Milk, Grande	171
Whole Milk, Tall	138
Whole Milk, Venti	196
with Cold Foam, Skimmed Milk, Grande	69
with Cold Foam, Skimmed Milk, Tall	57
with Cold Foam, Skimmed Milk, Venti	93
COFFEE - COLD BREW	
Grande	1
Short	0
Tall	1
Venti	1
COFFEE - COLD BREW, LATTE	
Almond Milk, Grande	53
Almond Milk, Tall	40
Almond Milk, Venti	63
Coconut Milk, Grande	91
Coconut Milk, Tall	69
Coconut Milk, Venti	108
Oat Milk, Grande	169
Oat Milk, Tall	127

	KCAL
STARBUCKS	
COFFEE - COLD BREW, LATTE	
Oat Milk, Venti	199
Semi Skimmed Milk, Grande	110
Semi Skimmed Milk, Tall	83
Semi Skimmed Milk, Venti	130
Skimmed Milk, Grande	77
Skimmed Milk, Tall	58
Skimmed Milk, Venti	91
Soy, Grande	91
Soy, Tall	69
Soy, Venti	107
Whole Milk, Grande	142
Whole Milk, Tall	108
Whole Milk, Venti	168
COFFEE - COLD BREW, NITRO	
10oz	4
Tall	4
with Caramel Cold Foam, Skimmed Milk, 10oz	23
with Caramel Cold Foam, Skimmed Milk, Tall	28
with Cold Foam, Skimmed Milk, 10oz	21
with Cold Foam, Skimmed Milk, Tall	26
COFFEE - CORTADO	
Almond Milk	34
Coconut Milk	50
Oat Milk	84
Semi Skimmed Milk	59
Skimmed Milk	44
Soy	50
Whole Milk	72
COFFEE - ESPRESSO	
Con Panna, Doppio	80
Con Panna, Solo	64
Doppio	11
Solo	6
COFFEE - ESPRESSO MACCHIATO	
Almond Milk, Doppio	15
Almond Milk, Solo	7
Coconut Milk, Doppio	17
Coconut Milk, Solo	8
Oat Milk, Doppio	23
Oat Milk, Solo	9
Semi Skimmed Milk, Doppio	19
Semi Skimmed Milk, Solo	7
Skimmed Milk, Doppio	16
Skimmed Milk, Solo	7
Soy, Doppio	17
Soy, Solo	8
Whole Milk, Doppio	21
Whole Milk, Solo	9
COFFEE - FILTER	
Grande	3
Tall	2
Venti	4

	KCAL
STARBUCKS	
COFFEE - FLAT WHITE	
Almond Milk, Short	47
Coconut Milk, Short	73
Oat Milk, Short	126
Semi Skimmed Milk, Short	87
Ã‚Â Skimmed Milk, Short	63
Soy, Short	73
Whole Milk, Short	108
COFFEE - LATTE	
Almond Milk, Grande	92
Almond Milk, Short	43
Almond Milk, Tall	74
Almond Milk, Venti	121
Coconut Milk, Grande	164
Coconut Milk, Short	77
Coconut Milk, Tall	130
Coconut Milk, Venti	214
Oat Milk, Grande	269
Oat Milk, Short	127
Oat Milk, Tall	212
Oat Milk, Venti	350
Semi Skimmed Milk, Grande	180
Semi Skimmed Milk, Short	85
Semi Skimmed Milk, Tall	143
Semi Skimmed Milk, Venti	235
Skimmed Milk, Grande	128
Skimmed Milk, Short	60
Skimmed Milk, Tall	102
Skimmed Milk, Venti	168
Soy, Grande	149
Soy, Short	70
Soy, Tall	119
Soy, Venti	195
Whole Milk, Grande	228
Whole Milk, Short	108
Whole Milk, Tall	181
Whole Milk, Venti	298
COFFEE - LATTE, CARDAMOM VANILLA	
Coconut Milk, Grande	148
Coconut Milk, Short	77
Coconut Milk, Tall	118
Coconut Milk, Venti	207
Oat Milk, Grande	269
Oat Milk, Short	137
Oat Milk, Tall	213
Oat Milk, Venti	366
Semi Skimmed Milk, Grande	179
Semi Skimmed Milk, Short	93
Semi Skimmed Milk, Tall	143
Semi Skimmed Milk, Venti	248
Skimmed Milk, Grande	127
Skimmed Milk, Short	67
Skimmed Milk, Tall	101

	KCAL
STARBUCKS	
COFFEE - LATTE, CARDAMOM VANILLA	
Skimmed Milk, Venti	180
Soy, Grande	148
Soy, Short	77
Soy, Tall	118
Soy, Venti	207
Whole Milk, Grande	228
Whole Milk, Short	117
Whole Milk, Tall	181
Whole Milk, Venti	312
COFFEE - LATTE, EGGNOG	
Grande	344
Short	170
Tall	272
Venti	366
COFFEE - LATTE, GINGERBREAD	
Almond Milk, Grande	254
Almond Milk, Short	143
Almond Milk, Tall	197
Almond Milk, Venti	300
Coconut Milk, Grande	327
Coconut Milk, Short	177
Coconut Milk, Tall	247
Coconut Milk, Venti	392
Oat Milk, Grande	432
Oat Milk, Short	225
Oat Milk, Tall	318
Oat Milk, Venti	523
Semi Skimmed Milk, Grande	343
Semi Skimmed Milk, Short	184
Semi Skimmed Milk, Tall	258
Semi Skimmed Milk, Venti	412
Skimmed Milk, Grande	290
Skimmed Milk, Short	160
Skimmed Milk, Tall	222
Skimmed Milk, Venti	346
Soy, Grande	312
Soy, Short	170
Soy, Tall	236
Soy, Venti	373
Whole Milk, Grande	391
Whole Milk, Short	207
Whole Milk, Tall	291
Whole Milk, Venti	472
COFFEE - LATTE, GINGERBREAD, ICED	
Almond Milk, Grande	227
Almond Milk, Tall	185
Almond Milk, Venti	261
Coconut Milk, Grande	276
Coconut Milk, Tall	224
Coconut Milk, Venti	316
Oat Milk, Grande	347
Oat Milk, Tall	280

	KCAL
STARBUCKS	
COFFEE - LATTE, GINGERBREAD, ICED	
Oat Milk, Venti	397
Semi Skimmed Milk, Grande	287
Semi Skimmed Milk, Tall	233
Semi Skimmed Milk, Venti	329
Skimmed Milk, Grande	252
Skimmed Milk, Tall	205
Skimmed Milk, Venti	289
Soy, Grande	266
Soy, Tall	216
Soy, Venti	305
Whole Milk, Grande	320
Whole Milk, Tall	259
Whole Milk, Venti	366
COFFEE - LATTE, ICED	
Almond Milk, Grande	65
Almond Milk, Tall	54
Almond Milk, Venti	78
Coconut Milk, Grande	105
Coconut Milk, Tall	85
Coconut Milk, Venti	123
Oat Milk, Grande	185
Oat Milk, Tall	149
Oat Milk, Venti	214
Semi Skimmed Milk, Grande	125
Semi Skimmed Milk, Tall	102
Semi Skimmed Milk, Venti	146
Skimmed Milk, Grande	90
Skimmed Milk, Tall	74
Skimmed Milk, Venti	106
Soy, Grande	104
Soy, Tall	85
Soy, Venti	122
Whole Milk, Grande	158
Whole Milk, Tall	128
Whole Milk, Venti	183
Eggnog, Grande	237
Eggnog, Tall	191
Eggnog, Venti	332
COFFEE - LATTE, MACCHIATO	
Almond Milk, Grande	78
Almond Milk, Short	34
Almond Milk, Tall	78
Almond Milk, Venti	102
Coconut Milk, Grande	119
Coconut Milk, Short	54
Coconut Milk, Tall	89
Coconut Milk, Venti	163
Oat Milk, Grande	195
Oat Milk, Short	97
Oat Milk, Tall	162
Oat Milk, Venti	272
Semi Skimmed Milk, Grande	132

STARBUCKS	KCAL
COFFEE - LATTE, MACCHIATO	
Semi Skimmed Milk, Short	66
Semi Skimmed Milk, Tall	110
Semi Skimmed Milk, Venti	184
Skimmed Milk, Grande	94
Skimmed Milk, Short	47
Skimmed Milk, Tall	79
Skimmed Milk, Venti	133
Soy, Grande	110
Soy, Short	55
Soy, Tall	92
Soy, Venti	154
Whole Milk, Grande	166
Whole Milk, Short	83
Whole Milk, Tall	138
Whole Milk, Venti	232
COFFEE - LATTE, TOFFEE NUT	
Almond Milk, Grande	256
Almond Milk, Short	146
Almond Milk, Tall	200
Almond Milk, Venti	302
Coconut Milk, Grande	314
Coconut Milk, Short	172
Coconut Milk, Tall	239
Coconut Milk, Venti	374
Oat Milk, Grande	434
Oat Milk, Short	228
Oat Milk, Tall	321
Oat Milk, Venti	524
Semi Skimmed Milk, Grande	345
Semi Skimmed Milk, Short	187
Semi Skimmed Milk, Tall	260
Semi Skimmed Milk, Venti	413
Skimmed Milk, Grande	293
Skimmed Milk, Short	163
Skimmed Milk, Tall	224
Skimmed Milk, Venti	347
Soy, Grande	314
Soy, Short	173
Soy, Tall	239
Soy, Venti	374
Whole Milk, Grande	393
Whole Milk, Short	209
Whole Milk, Tall	293
Whole Milk, Venti	473
COFFEE - LATTE, TOFFEE NUT, ICED	
Almond Milk, Grande	230
Almond Milk, Tall	188
Almond Milk, Venti	262
Coconut Milk, Grande	278
Coconut Milk, Tall	227
Coconut Milk, Venti	317
Oat Milk, Grande	349

STARBUCKS	KCAL
COFFEE - LATTE, TOFFEE NUT	
Oat Milk, Tall	283
Oat Milk, Venti	398
Semi Skimmed Milk, Grande	289
Semi Skimmed Milk, Tall	235
Semi Skimmed Milk, Venti	330
Skimmed Milk, Grande	254
Skimmed Milk, Tall	207
Skimmed Milk, Venti	290
Soy, Grande	268
Soy, Tall	219
Soy, Venti	306
Whole Milk, Grande	322
Whole Milk, Tall	261
Whole Milk, Venti	367
COFFEE - LATTE, VANILLA	
Almond Milk, Grande	164
Almond Milk, Short	79
Almond Milk, Tall	127
Almond Milk, Venti	210
Coconut Milk, Grande	222
Coconut Milk, Short	107
Coconut Milk, Tall	172
Coconut Milk, Venti	285
Oat Milk, Grande	342
Oat Milk, Short	162
Oat Milk, Tall	265
Oat Milk, Venti	438
Semi Skimmed Milk, Grande	253
Semi Skimmed Milk, Short	121
Semi Skimmed Milk, Tall	196
Semi Skimmed Milk, Venti	324
Skimmed Milk, Grande	201
Skimmed Milk, Short	96
Skimmed Milk, Tall	155
Skimmed Milk, Venti	257
Soy Milk, Grande	222
Soy Milk, Short	106
Soy Milk, Tall	172
Soy Milk, Venti	284
Whole Milk, Grande	301
Whole Milk, Short	143
Whole Milk, Tall	233
Whole Milk, Venti	386
COFFEE - MACCHIATO, CARAMEL	
Almond Milk, Grande	155
Almond Milk, Short	74
Almond Milk, Tall	122
Almond Milk, Venti	193
Coconut Milk, Grande	205
Coconut Milk, Short	98
Coconut Milk, Tall	161
Coconut Milk, Venti	253

	KCAL
STARBUCKS	
COFFEE - MACCHIATO, CARAMEL	
Oat Milk, Grande	308
Oat Milk, Short	145
Oat Milk, Tall	243
Oat Milk, Venti	377
Semi Skimmed Milk, Grande	229
Semi Skimmed Milk, Short	109
Semi Skimmed Milk, Tall	180
Semi Skimmed Milk, Venti	281
Skimmed Milk, Grande	187
Skimmed Milk, Short	89
Skimmed Milk, Tall	146
Skimmed Milk, Venti	231
Soy, Grande	205
Soy, Short	97
Soy, Tall	161
Soy, Venti	253
Whole Milk, Grande	273
Whole Milk, Short	129
Whole Milk, Tall	215
Whole Milk, Venti	335
COFFEE - MACCHIATO, CARAMEL, ICED	
Almond Milk, Grande	140
Almond Milk, Tall	110
Almond Milk, Venti	171
Coconut Milk, Grande	179
Coconut Milk, Tall	141
Coconut Milk, Venti	216
Oat Milk, Grande	259
Oat Milk, Tall	205
Oat Milk, Venti	307
Semi Skimmed Milk, Grande	199
Semi Skimmed Milk, Tall	157
Semi Skimmed Milk, Venti	239
Skimmed Milk, Grande	164
Skimmed Milk, Tall	129
Skimmed Milk, Venti	199
Soy, Grande	178
Soy, Tall	141
Soy, Venti	215
Whole Milk, Grande	232
Whole Milk, Tall	183
Whole Milk, Venti	276
COFFEE - MISTO	
Almond Milk, Grande	48
Almond Milk, Short	24
Almond Milk, Tall	33
Almond Milk, Venti	64
Coconut Milk, Grande	81
Coconut Milk, Short	41
Coconut Milk, Tall	56
Coconut Milk, Venti	109
Oat Milk, Grande	149

	KCAL
STARBUCKS	
COFFEE - MISTO	
Oat Milk, Short	76
Oat Milk, Tall	102
Oat Milk, Venti	200
Semi Skimmed Milk, Grande	98
Semi Skimmed Milk, Short	50
Semi Skimmed Milk, Tall	67
Semi Skimmed Milk, Venti	132
Skimmed Milk, Grande	69
Skimmed Milk, Short	35
Skimmed Milk, Tall	47
Skimmed Milk, Venti	92
Soy, Grande	81
Soy, Short	41
Soy, Tall	55
Soy, Venti	108
Whole Milk, Grande	126
Whole Milk, Short	64
Whole Milk, Tall	86
Whole Milk, Venti	169
COFFEE - MOCHA	
Almond Milk, Grande	225
Almond Milk, Short	128
Almond Milk, Tall	179
Almond Milk, Venti	256
Coconut Milk, Grande	263
Coconut Milk, Short	143
Coconut Milk, Tall	206
Coconut Milk, Venti	300
Oat Milk, Grande	342
Oat Milk, Short	174
Oat Milk, Tall	261
Oat Milk, Venti	389
Semi Skimmed Milk, Grande	283
Semi Skimmed Milk, Short	151
Semi Skimmed Milk, Tall	220
Semi Skimmed Milk, Venti	322
Skimmed Milk, Grande	249
Skimmed Milk, Short	137
Skimmed Milk, Tall	196
Skimmed Milk, Venti	283
Soy, Grande	263
Soy, Short	143
Soy, Tall	205
Soy, Venti	299
Whole Milk, Grande	315
Whole Milk, Short	163
Whole Milk, Tall	242
Whole Milk, Venti	359
COFFEE - MOCHA, ICED	
with Whipped Cream, Almond Milk, Grande	277
with Whipped Cream, Almond Milk, Tall	210
with Whipped Cream, Almond Milk, Venti	310

	KCAL
STARBUCKS	
COFFEE - MOCHA, ICED	
with Whipped Cream, Coconut Milk, Grande	317
with Whipped Cream, Coconut Milk, Tall	241
with Whipped Cream, Coconut Milk, Venti	354
with Whipped Cream, Oat Milk, Grande	397
with Whipped Cream, Oat Milk, Tall	305
with Whipped Cream, Oat Milk, Venti	446
with Whipped Cream, Semi Skimmed Milk, Grande	337
with Whipped Cream, Semi Skimmed Milk, Tall	257
with Whipped Cream, Semi Skimmed Milk, Venti	378
with Whipped Cream, Skimmed Milk, Grande	302
with Whipped Cream, Skimmed Milk, Tall	229
with Whipped Cream, Skimmed Milk, Venti	338
with Whipped Cream, Soy, Grande	316
with Whipped Cream, Soy, Tall	241
with Whipped Cream, Soy, Venti	354
with Whipped Cream, Whole Milk, Grande	370
with Whipped Cream, Whole Milk, Tall	283
with Whipped Cream, Whole Milk, Venti	415
COFFEE - MOCHA, ICED, WHITE	
with Whipped Cream, Almond Milk, Grande	387
with Whipped Cream, Almond Milk, Tall	290
with Whipped Cream, Almond Milk, Venti	458
with Whipped Cream, Coconut Milk, Grande	415
with Whipped Cream, Coconut Milk, Tall	314
with Whipped Cream, Coconut Milk, Venti	497
with Whipped Cream, Oat Milk, Grande	474
with Whipped Cream, Oat Milk, Tall	361
with Whipped Cream, Oat Milk, Venti	577
with Whipped Cream, Semi Skimmed Milk, Grande	430
with Whipped Cream, Semi Skimmed Milk, Tall	326
with Whipped Cream, Semi Skimmed Milk, Venti	517
with Whipped Cream, Skimmed Milk, Grande	405
with Whipped Cream, Skimmed Milk, Tall	305
with Whipped Cream, Skimmed Milk, Venti	483
with Whipped Cream, Soy, Grande	415
with Whipped Cream, Soy, Tall	313
with Whipped Cream, Soy, Venti	497
with Whipped Cream, Whole Milk, Grande	454
with Whipped Cream, Whole Milk, Tall	345
with Whipped Cream, Whole Milk, Venti	550
COFFEE - MOCHA, WHITE CHOC	
Almond Milk, Grande	350
Almond Milk, Short	188
Almond Milk, Tall	276
Almond Milk, Venti	426
Coconut Milk, Grande	388
Coconut Milk, Short	204
Coconut Milk, Tall	306
Coconut Milk, Venti	479
Oat Milk, Grande	466
Oat Milk, Short	235
Oat Milk, Tall	369

	KCAL
STARBUCKS	
COFFEE - MOCHA, WHITE CHOC	
Oat Milk, Venti	588
Semi Skimmed Milk, Grande	408
Semi Skimmed Milk, Short	212
Semi Skimmed Milk, Tall	322
Semi Skimmed Milk, Venti	507
Skimmed Milk, Grande	374
Skimmed Milk, Short	198
Skimmed Milk, Tall	295
Skimmed Milk, Venti	459
Soy, Grande	387
Soy, Short	203
Soy, Tall	306
Soy, Venti	478
Whole Milk, Grande	440
Whole Milk, Short	225
Whole Milk, Tall	347
Whole Milk, Venti	551
COOKIES	
Chocolate, Milk, Chunk	363
Chocolate, Triple	372
Oat, & Raisin	321
CROISSANT	
Almond	339
Butter	255
CUPCAKES	
Salted Caramel, Twinkle & Sprinkle	437
FRAPPUCCINO - CARAMEL	
with Whipped Cream, Almond Milk, Grande	363
with Whipped Cream, Almond Milk, Mini	191
with Whipped Cream, Almond Milk, Tall	264
with Whipped Cream, Almond Milk, Venti	420
with Whipped Cream, Coconut Milk, Grande	379
with Whipped Cream, Coconut Milk, Mini	200
with Whipped Cream, Coconut Milk, Tall	277
with Whipped Cream, Coconut Milk, Venti	438
with Whipped Cream, Oat Milk, Grande	413
with Whipped Cream, Oat Milk, Mini	218
with Whipped Cream, Oat Milk, Tall	305
with Whipped Cream, Oat Milk, Venti	475
with Whipped Cream, Semi Skimmed Milk, Grande	388
with Whipped Cream, Semi Skimmed Milk, Mini	205
with Whipped Cream, Semi Skimmed Milk, Tall	284
with Whipped Cream, Semi Skimmed Milk, Venti	431
with Whipped Cream, Skimmed Milk, Grande	373
with Whipped Cream, Skimmed Milk, Mini	197
with Whipped Cream, Skimmed Milk, Tall	272
with Whipped Cream, Skimmed Milk, Venti	431
with Whipped Cream, Soy, Grande	379
with Whipped Cream, Soy, Mini	200
with Whipped Cream, Soy, Tall	277
with Whipped Cream, Soy, Venti	438
with Whipped Cream, Whole Milk, Grande	402

STARBUCKS	KCAL
FRAPPUCCINO - CARAMEL	
with Whipped Cream, Whole Milk, Mini	212
with Whipped Cream, Whole Milk, Tall	296
with Whipped Cream, Whole Milk, Venti	463
Light, No Whip, Skimmed Milk, Grande	127
Light, No Whip, Skimmed Milk, Mini	72
Light, No Whip, Skimmed Milk, Tall	93
Light, No Whip, Skimmed Milk, Venti	156
FRAPPUCCINO - CARAMEL CREAM	
with Whipped Cream, Almond Milk, Grande	305
with Whipped Cream, Almond Milk, Mini	167
with Whipped Cream, Almond Milk, Tall	227
with Whipped Cream, Almond Milk, Venti	358
with Whipped Cream, Coconut Milk, Grande	327
with Whipped Cream, Coconut Milk, Mini	178
with Whipped Cream, Coconut Milk, Tall	245
with Whipped Cream, Coconut Milk, Venti	385
with Whipped Cream, Oat Milk, Grande	373
with Whipped Cream, Oat Milk, Mini	202
with Whipped Cream, Oat Milk, Tall	283
with Whipped Cream, Oat Milk, Venti	441
with Whipped Cream, Semi Skimmed Milk, Grande	339
with Whipped Cream, Semi Skimmed Milk, Mini	185
with Whipped Cream, Semi Skimmed Milk, Tall	319
with Whipped Cream, Semi Skimmed Milk, Venti	399
with Whipped Cream, Skimmed Milk, Grande	319
with Whipped Cream, Skimmed Milk, Mini	174
with Whipped Cream, Skimmed Milk, Tall	239
with Whipped Cream, Skimmed Milk, Venti	375
with Whipped Cream, Soy, Grande	327
with Whipped Cream, Soy, Mini	178
with Whipped Cream, Soy, Tall	245
with Whipped Cream, Soy, Venti	385
with Whipped Cream, Whole Milk, Grande	358
with Whipped Cream, Whole Milk, Mini	194
with Whipped Cream, Whole Milk, Tall	270
with Whipped Cream, Whole Milk, Venti	422
FRAPPUCCINO - CHAI TEA	
with Whipped Cream, Almond Milk, Grande	313
with Whipped Cream, Almond Milk, Mini	159
with Whipped Cream, Almond Milk, Tall	215
with Whipped Cream, Almond Milk, Venti	354
with Whipped Cream, Coconut Milk, Grande	334
with Whipped Cream, Coconut Milk, Mini	171
with Whipped Cream, Coconut Milk, Tall	232
with Whipped Cream, Coconut Milk, Venti	380
with Whipped Cream, Oat Milk, Grande	377
with Whipped Cream, Oat Milk, Mini	195
with Whipped Cream, Oat Milk, Tall	267
with Whipped Cream, Oat Milk, Venti	433
with Whipped Cream, Semi Skimmed Milk, Grande	345
with Whipped Cream, Semi Skimmed Milk, Mini	177
with Whipped Cream, Semi Skimmed Milk, Tall	241

STARBUCKS	KCAL
FRAPPUCCINO - CHAI TEA	
with Whipped Cream, Semi Skimmed Milk, Venti	393
with Whipped Cream, Skimmed Milk, Grande	326
with Whipped Cream, Skimmed Milk, Mini	166
with Whipped Cream, Skimmed Milk, Tall	226
with Whipped Cream, Skimmed Milk, Venti	370
with Whipped Cream, Soy, Grande	334
with Whipped Cream, Soy, Mini	170
with Whipped Cream, Soy, Tall	232
with Whipped Cream, Soy, Venti	379
with Whipped Cream, Whole Milk, Grande	363
with Whipped Cream, Whole Milk, Mini	186
with Whipped Cream, Whole Milk, Tall	255
with Whipped Cream, Whole Milk, Venti	415
FRAPPUCCINO - CHOCOLATE CREAM	
with Whipped Cream, Almond Milk, Grande	293
with Whipped Cream, Almond Milk, Mini	154
with Whipped Cream, Almond Milk, Tall	210
with Whipped Cream, Almond Milk, Venti	340
with Whipped Cream, Coconut Milk, Grande	316
with Whipped Cream, Coconut Milk, Mini	166
with Whipped Cream, Coconut Milk, Tall	228
with Whipped Cream, Coconut Milk, Venti	367
with Whipped Cream, Oat Milk, Grande	362
with Whipped Cream, Oat Milk, Mini	190
with Whipped Cream, Oat Milk, Tall	263
with Whipped Cream, Oat Milk, Venti	421
with Whipped Cream, Semi Skimmed Milk, Grande	327
with Whipped Cream, Semi Skimmed Milk, Mini	172
with Whipped Cream, Semi Skimmed Milk, Tall	237
with Whipped Cream, Semi Skimmed Milk, Venti	381
with Whipped Cream, Skimmed Milk, Grande	307
with Whipped Cream, Skimmed Milk, Mini	162
with Whipped Cream, Skimmed Milk, Tall	221
with Whipped Cream, Skimmed Milk, Venti	357
with Whipped Cream, Soy, Grande	315
with Whipped Cream, Soy, Mini	166
with Whipped Cream, Soy, Tall	227
with Whipped Cream, Soy, Venti	366
with Whipped Cream, Whole Milk, Grande	327
with Whipped Cream, Whole Milk, Mini	182
with Whipped Cream, Whole Milk, Tall	251
with Whipped Cream, Whole Milk, Venti	403
FRAPPUCCINO - COFFEE	
No Whip, Almond Milk, Grande	192
No Whip, Almond Milk, Mini	89
No Whip, Almond Milk, Tall	138
No Whip, Almond Milk, Venti	239
No Whip, Coconut Milk, Grande	208
No Whip, Coconut Milk, Mini	98
No Whip, Coconut Milk, Tall	152
No Whip, Coconut Milk, Venti	257
No Whip, Oat Milk, Grande	242

STARBUCKS

FRAPPUCCINO - COFFEE

	KCAL
No Whip, Oat Milk, Mini	116
No Whip, Oat Milk, Tall	180
No Whip, Oat Milk, Venti	294
No Whip, Semi Skimmed Milk, Grande	217
No Whip, Semi Skimmed Milk, Mini	103
No Whip, Semi Skimmed Milk, Tall	159
No Whip, Semi Skimmed Milk, Venti	217
No Whip, Skimmed Milk, Grande	202
No Whip, Skimmed Milk, Mini	95
No Whip, Skimmed Milk, Tall	147
No Whip, Skimmed Milk, Venti	250
No Whip, Soy, Grande	208
No Whip, Soy, Mini	98
No Whip, Soy, Tall	152
No Whip, Soy, Venti	257
No Whip, Whole Milk, Grande	231
No Whip, Whole Milk, Mini	110
No Whip, Whole Milk, Tall	170
No Whip, Whole Milk, Venti	282
Coffee Light, No Whip, Skimmed Milk, Grande	118
Coffee Light, No Whip, Skimmed Milk, Mini	59
Coffee Light, No Whip, Skimmed Milk, Tall	83
Coffee Light, No Whip, Skimmed Milk, Venti	129

FRAPPUCCINO - COOKIE & CREAM

	KCAL
with Whipped Cream, Almond Milk, Grande	368
with Whipped Cream, Almond Milk, Mini	179
with Whipped Cream, Almond Milk, Tall	266
with Whipped Cream, Almond Milk, Venti	429
with Whipped Cream, Coconut Milk, Grande	397
with Whipped Cream, Coconut Milk, Mini	193
with Whipped Cream, Coconut Milk, Tall	288
with Whipped Cream, Coconut Milk, Venti	463
with Whipped Cream, Oat Milk, Grande	439
with Whipped Cream, Oat Milk, Mini	214
with Whipped Cream, Oat Milk, Tall	320
with Whipped Cream, Oat Milk, Venti	512
with Whipped Cream, Semi Skimmed Milk, Grande	404
with Whipped Cream, Semi Skimmed Milk, Mini	196
with Whipped Cream, Semi Skimmed Milk, Tall	293
with Whipped Cream, Semi Skimmed Milk, Venti	470
with Whipped Cream, Skimmed Milk, Grande	383
with Whipped Cream, Skimmed Milk, Mini	186
with Whipped Cream, Skimmed Milk, Tall	277
with Whipped Cream, Skimmed Milk, Venti	446
with Whipped Cream, Soy, Grande	391
with Whipped Cream, Soy, Mini	190
with Whipped Cream, Soy, Tall	284
with Whipped Cream, Soy, Venti	456
with Whipped Cream, Whole Milk, Grande	423
with Whipped Cream, Whole Milk, Mini	206
with Whipped Cream, Whole Milk, Tall	308
with Whipped Cream, Whole Milk, Venti	493

FRAPPUCCINO - DOUBLE CHOC CHIP CREAM

	KCAL
with Whipped Cream, Almond Milk, Grande	365
with Whipped Cream, Almond Milk, Mini	187
with Whipped Cream, Almond Milk, Tall	263
with Whipped Cream, Almond Milk, Venti	444
with Whipped Cream, Coconut Milk, Grande	394
with Whipped Cream, Coconut Milk, Mini	201
with Whipped Cream, Coconut Milk, Tall	286
with Whipped Cream, Coconut Milk, Venti	478
with Whipped Cream, Oat Milk, Grande	435
with Whipped Cream, Oat Milk, Mini	222
with Whipped Cream, Oat Milk, Tall	318
with Whipped Cream, Oat Milk, Venti	528
with Whipped Cream, Semi Skimmed Milk, Grande	400
with Whipped Cream, Semi Skimmed Milk, Mini	204
with Whipped Cream, Semi Skimmed Milk, Tall	291
with Whipped Cream, Semi Skimmed Milk, Venti	486
with Whipped Cream, Skimmed Milk, Grande	379
with Whipped Cream, Skimmed Milk, Mini	194
with Whipped Cream, Skimmed Milk, Tall	275
with Whipped Cream, Skimmed Milk, Venti	461
with Whipped Cream, Soy, Grande	388
with Whipped Cream, Soy, Mini	198
with Whipped Cream, Soy, Tall	281
with Whipped Cream, Soy, Venti	471
with Whipped Cream, Whole Milk, Grande	419
with Whipped Cream, Whole Milk, Mini	214
with Whipped Cream, Whole Milk, Tall	306
with Whipped Cream, Whole Milk, Venti	509

FRAPPUCCINO - ESPRESSO

	KCAL
No Whip, Almond Milk, Grande	185
No Whip, Almond Milk, Mini	93
No Whip, Almond Milk, Tall	128
No Whip, Almond Milk, Venti	230
No Whip, Coconut Milk, Grande	201
No Whip, Coconut Milk, Mini	101
No Whip, Coconut Milk, Tall	140
No Whip, Coconut Milk, Venti	247
No Whip, Oat Milk, Grande	233
No Whip, Oat Milk, Mini	119
No Whip, Oat Milk, Tall	165
No Whip, Oat Milk, Venti	282
No Whip, Semi Skimmed Milk, Grande	209
No Whip, Semi Skimmed Milk, Mini	106
No Whip, Semi Skimmed Milk, Tall	146
No Whip, Semi Skimmed Milk, Venti	256
No Whip, Skimmed Milk, Grande	195
No Whip, Skimmed Milk, Mini	98
No Whip, Skimmed Milk, Tall	135
No Whip, Skimmed Milk, Venti	241
No Whip, Soy, Grande	200
No Whip, Soy, Mini	101
No Whip, Soy, Tall	140

STARBUCKS	KCAL
FRAPPUCCINO - ESPRESSO	
No Whip, Soy, Venti	247
No Whip, Whole Milk, Grande	222
No Whip, Whole Milk, Mini	113
No Whip, Whole Milk, Tall	157
No Whip, Whole Milk, Venti	270
Light, No Whip, Skimmed Milk, Grande	112
Light, No Whip, Skimmed Milk, Mini	63
Light, No Whip, Skimmed Milk, Tall	79
Light, No Whip, Skimmed Milk, Venti	128
FRAPPUCCINO - GINGERBREAD	
with Whipped Cream, Almond Milk, Grande	342
with Whipped Cream, Almond Milk, Mini	175
with Whipped Cream, Almond Milk, Tall	246
with Whipped Cream, Almond Milk, Venti	399
with Whipped Cream, Coconut Milk, Grande	363
with Whipped Cream, Coconut Milk, Mini	186
with Whipped Cream, Coconut Milk, Tall	262
with Whipped Cream, Coconut Milk, Venti	421
with Whipped Cream, Oat Milk, Grande	392
with Whipped Cream, Oat Milk, Mini	201
with Whipped Cream, Oat Milk, Tall	287
with Whipped Cream, Oat Milk, Venti	454
with Whipped Cream, Semi Skimmed Milk, Grande	367
with Whipped Cream, Semi Skimmed Milk, Mini	188
with Whipped Cream, Semi Skimmed Milk, Tall	266
with Whipped Cream, Semi Skimmed Milk, Venti	426
with Whipped Cream, Skimmed Milk, Grande	352
with Whipped Cream, Skimmed Milk, Mini	180
with Whipped Cream, Skimmed Milk, Tall	254
with Whipped Cream, Skimmed Milk, Venti	410
with Whipped Cream, Soy, Grande	358
with Whipped Cream, Soy, Mini	183
with Whipped Cream, Soy, Tall	259
with Whipped Cream, Soy, Venti	417
with Whipped Cream, Whole Milk, Grande	381
with Whipped Cream, Whole Milk, Mini	195
with Whipped Cream, Whole Milk, Tall	277
with Whipped Cream, Whole Milk, Venti	441
Light, No Whip, Skimmed Milk, Grande	155
Light, No Whip, Skimmed Milk, Mini	76
Light, No Whip, Skimmed Milk, Tall	114
Light, No Whip, Skimmed Milk, Venti	191
FRAPPUCCINO - GINGERBREAD CREME	
with Whipped Cream, Almond Milk, Grande	288
with Whipped Cream, Almond Milk, Mini	150
with Whipped Cream, Almond Milk, Tall	208
with Whipped Cream, Almond Milk, Venti	330
with Whipped Cream, Coconut Milk, Grande	317
with Whipped Cream, Coconut Milk, Mini	164
with Whipped Cream, Coconut Milk, Tall	230
with Whipped Cream, Coconut Milk, Venti	363
with Whipped Cream, Oat Milk, Grande	358

STARBUCKS	KCAL
FRAPPUCCINO - GINGERBREAD CREME	
with Whipped Cream, Oat Milk, Mini	186
with Whipped Cream, Oat Milk, Tall	262
with Whipped Cream, Oat Milk, Venti	410
with Whipped Cream, Semi Skimmed Milk, Grande	323
with Whipped Cream, Semi Skimmed Milk, Mini	168
with Whipped Cream, Semi Skimmed Milk, Tall	235
with Whipped Cream, Semi Skimmed Milk, Venti	370
with Whipped Cream, Skimmed Milk, Grande	302
with Whipped Cream, Skimmed Milk, Mini	157
with Whipped Cream, Skimmed Milk, Tall	219
with Whipped Cream, Skimmed Milk, Venti	346
with Whipped Cream, Soy, Grande	311
with Whipped Cream, Soy, Mini	161
with Whipped Cream, Soy, Tall	226
with Whipped Cream, Soy, Venti	356
with Whipped Cream, Whole Milk, Grande	342
with Whipped Cream, Whole Milk, Mini	177
with Whipped Cream, Whole Milk, Tall	250
with Whipped Cream, Whole Milk, Venti	392
FRAPPUCCINO - JAVA CHIP	
with Whipped Cream, Almond Milk, Grande	433
with Whipped Cream, Almond Milk, Mini	222
with Whipped Cream, Almond Milk, Tall	311
with Whipped Cream, Almond Milk, Venti	509
with Whipped Cream, Coconut Milk, Grande	413
with Whipped Cream, Coconut Milk, Mini	211
with Whipped Cream, Coconut Milk, Tall	295
with Whipped Cream, Coconut Milk, Venti	487
with Whipped Cream, Oat Milk, Grande	462
with Whipped Cream, Oat Milk, Mini	238
with Whipped Cream, Oat Milk, Tall	335
with Whipped Cream, Oat Milk, Venti	541
with Whipped Cream, Semi Skimmed Milk, Grande	438
with Whipped Cream, Semi Skimmed Milk, Mini	225
with Whipped Cream, Semi Skimmed Milk, Tall	315
with Whipped Cream, Semi Skimmed Milk, Venti	514
with Whipped Cream, Skimmed Milk, Grande	423
with Whipped Cream, Skimmed Milk, Mini	217
with Whipped Cream, Skimmed Milk, Tall	303
with Whipped Cream, Skimmed Milk, Venti	498
with Whipped Cream, Soy, Grande	429
with Whipped Cream, Soy, Mini	220
with Whipped Cream, Soy, Tall	308
with Whipped Cream, Soy, Venti	504
with Whipped Cream, Whole Milk, Grande	451
with Whipped Cream, Whole Milk, Mini	232
with Whipped Cream, Whole Milk, Tall	326
with Whipped Cream, Whole Milk, Venti	528
Light, No Whip, Skimmed Milk, Grande	192
Light, No Whip, Skimmed Milk, Mini	104
Light, No Whip, Skimmed Milk, Tall	137
Light, No Whip, Skimmed Milk, Venti	228

STARBUCKS	KCAL
FRAPPUCCINO - MARSHMALLOW	
with Whipped Cream, Almond Milk, Grande	307
with Whipped Cream, Almond Milk, Mini	162
with Whipped Cream, Almond Milk, Tall	220
with Whipped Cream, Almond Milk, Venti	357
with Whipped Cream, Coconut Milk, Grande	336
with Whipped Cream, Coconut Milk, Mini	177
with Whipped Cream, Coconut Milk, Tall	242
with Whipped Cream, Coconut Milk, Venti	389
with Whipped Cream, Oat Milk, Grande	377
with Whipped Cream, Oat Milk, Mini	198
with Whipped Cream, Oat Milk, Tall	274
with Whipped Cream, Oat Milk, Venti	437
with Whipped Cream, Semi Skimmed Milk, Grande	342
with Whipped Cream, Semi Skimmed Milk, Mini	180
with Whipped Cream, Semi Skimmed Milk, Tall	247
with Whipped Cream, Semi Skimmed Milk, Venti	397
with Whipped Cream, Skimmed Milk, Grande	321
with Whipped Cream, Skimmed Milk, Mini	169
with Whipped Cream, Skimmed Milk, Tall	231
with Whipped Cream, Skimmed Milk, Venti	373
with Whipped Cream, Soy, Grande	330
with Whipped Cream, Soy, Mini	174
with Whipped Cream, Soy, Tall	237
with Whipped Cream, Soy, Venti	383
with Whipped Cream, Whole Milk, Grande	361
with Whipped Cream, Whole Milk, Mini	190
with Whipped Cream, Whole Milk, Tall	262
with Whipped Cream, Whole Milk, Venti	419
FRAPPUCCINO - MATCHA TEA	
with Whipped Cream, Almond Milk, Grande	323
with Whipped Cream, Almond Milk, Mini	160
with Whipped Cream, Almond Milk, Tall	228
with Whipped Cream, Almond Milk, Venti	365
with Whipped Cream, Coconut Milk, Grande	347
with Whipped Cream, Coconut Milk, Mini	172
with Whipped Cream, Coconut Milk, Tall	247
with Whipped Cream, Coconut Milk, Venti	392
with Whipped Cream, Oat Milk, Grande	396
with Whipped Cream, Oat Milk, Mini	196
with Whipped Cream, Oat Milk, Tall	284
with Whipped Cream, Oat Milk, Venti	447
with Whipped Cream, Semi Skimmed Milk, Grande	359
with Whipped Cream, Semi Skimmed Milk, Mini	178
with Whipped Cream, Semi Skimmed Milk, Tall	256
with Whipped Cream, Semi Skimmed Milk, Venti	406
with Whipped Cream, Skimmed Milk, Grande	338
with Whipped Cream, Skimmed Milk, Mini	167
with Whipped Cream, Skimmed Milk, Tall	240
with Whipped Cream, Skimmed Milk, Venti	382
with Whipped Cream, Soy, Grande	346
with Whipped Cream, Soy, Mini	172
with Whipped Cream, Soy, Tall	246

STARBUCKS	KCAL
FRAPPUCCINO - MATCHA TEA	
with Whipped Cream, Soy, Venti	392
with Whipped Cream, Whole Milk, Grande	379
with Whipped Cream, Whole Milk, Mini	188
with Whipped Cream, Whole Milk, Tall	272
with Whipped Cream, Whole Milk, Venti	428
FRAPPUCCINO - MOCHA	
with Whipped Cream, Almond Milk, Grande	330
with Whipped Cream, Almond Milk, Mini	174
with Whipped Cream, Almond Milk, Tall	240
with Whipped Cream, Almond Milk, Venti	394
with Whipped Cream, Coconut Milk, Grande	345
with Whipped Cream, Coconut Milk, Mini	183
with Whipped Cream, Coconut Milk, Tall	253
with Whipped Cream, Coconut Milk, Venti	412
with Whipped Cream, Oat Milk, Grande	376
with Whipped Cream, Oat Milk, Mini	201
with Whipped Cream, Oat Milk, Tall	280
with Whipped Cream, Oat Milk, Venti	449
with Whipped Cream, Semi Skimmed Milk, Grande	353
with Whipped Cream, Semi Skimmed Milk, Mini	188
with Whipped Cream, Semi Skimmed Milk, Tall	260
with Whipped Cream, Semi Skimmed Milk, Venti	421
with Whipped Cream, Skimmed Milk, Grande	339
with Whipped Cream, Skimmed Milk, Mini	180
with Whipped Cream, Skimmed Milk, Tall	249
with Whipped Cream, Skimmed Milk, Venti	405
with Whipped Cream, Soy, Grande	345
with Whipped Cream, Soy, Mini	183
with Whipped Cream, Soy, Tall	253
with Whipped Cream, Soy, Venti	412
with Whipped Cream, Whole Milk, Grande	366
with Whipped Cream, Whole Milk, Mini	195
with Whipped Cream, Whole Milk, Tall	271
with Whipped Cream, Whole Milk, Venti	436
Light, No Whip, Skimmed Milk, Grande	135
Light, No Whip, Skimmed Milk, Mini	72
Light, No Whip, Skimmed Milk, Tall	91
Light, No Whip, Skimmed Milk, Venti	159
FRAPPUCCINO - MOCHA, WHITE CHOC	
with Whipped Cream, Almond Milk, Grande	358
with Whipped Cream, Almond Milk, Mini	181
with Whipped Cream, Almond Milk, Tall	252
with Whipped Cream, Almond Milk, Venti	424
with Whipped Cream, Coconut Milk, Grande	374
with Whipped Cream, Coconut Milk, Mini	190
with Whipped Cream, Coconut Milk, Tall	265
with Whipped Cream, Coconut Milk, Venti	424
with Whipped Cream, Oat Milk, Grande	406
with Whipped Cream, Oat Milk, Mini	208
with Whipped Cream, Oat Milk, Tall	292
with Whipped Cream, Oat Milk, Venti	460
with Whipped Cream, Semi Skimmed Milk, Grande	382

STARBUCKS	KCAL
FRAPPUCCINO - MOCHA, WHITE CHOC	
with Whipped Cream, Semi Skimmed Milk, Mini	194
with Whipped Cream, Semi Skimmed Milk, Tall	272
with Whipped Cream, Semi Skimmed Milk, Venti	433
with Whipped Cream, Skimmed Milk, Grande	368
with Whipped Cream, Skimmed Milk, Mini	187
with Whipped Cream, Skimmed Milk, Tall	260
with Whipped Cream, Skimmed Milk, Venti	418
with Whipped Cream, Soy, Grande	374
with Whipped Cream, Soy, Mini	190
with Whipped Cream, Soy, Tall	265
with Whipped Cream, Soy, Venti	424
with Whipped Cream, Whole Milk, Grande	395
with Whipped Cream, Whole Milk, Mini	202
with Whipped Cream, Whole Milk, Tall	283
with Whipped Cream, Whole Milk, Venti	448
Light, White Choc, No Whip, Skimmed Milk, Grande	155
Light, White Choc, No Whip, Skimmed Milk, Mini	78
Light, White Choc, No Whip, Skimmed Milk, Tall	99
Light, White Choc, No Whip, Skimmed Milk, Venti	166
FRAPPUCCINO - ROOBIOS TEA	
with Whipped Cream, Almond Milk, Grande	305
with Whipped Cream, Almond Milk, Mini	152
with Whipped Cream, Almond Milk, Tall	216
with Whipped Cream, Almond Milk, Venti	343
with Whipped Cream, Coconut Milk, Grande	329
with Whipped Cream, Coconut Milk, Mini	164
with Whipped Cream, Coconut Milk, Tall	235
with Whipped Cream, Coconut Milk, Venti	370
with Whipped Cream, Oat Milk, Grande	378
with Whipped Cream, Oat Milk, Mini	188
with Whipped Cream, Oat Milk, Tall	272
with Whipped Cream, Oat Milk, Venti	425
with Whipped Cream, Semi Skimmed Milk, Grande	341
with Whipped Cream, Semi Skimmed Milk, Mini	170
with Whipped Cream, Semi Skimmed Milk, Tall	244
with Whipped Cream, Semi Skimmed Milk, Venti	384
with Whipped Cream, Skimmed Milk, Grande	320
with Whipped Cream, Skimmed Milk, Mini	160
with Whipped Cream, Skimmed Milk, Tall	228
with Whipped Cream, Skimmed Milk, Venti	360
with Whipped Cream, Soy, Grande	329
with Whipped Cream, Soy, Mini	164
with Whipped Cream, Soy, Tall	234
with Whipped Cream, Soy, Venti	370
with Whipped Cream, Whole Milk, Grande	361
with Whipped Cream, Whole Milk, Mini	180
with Whipped Cream, Whole Milk, Tall	259
with Whipped Cream, Whole Milk, Venti	406
FRAPPUCCINO - STARWBERRIES & CREAM	
with Whipped Cream, Soy, Venti	402
with Whipped Cream, Almond Milk, Grande	402
with Whipped Cream, Almond Milk, Mini	173

STARBUCKS	KCAL
FRAPPUCCINO - STARWBERRIES & CREAM	
with Whipped Cream, Almond Milk, Tall	235
with Whipped Cream, Almond Milk, Venti	378
with Whipped Cream, Coconut Milk, Grande	344
with Whipped Cream, Coconut Milk, Mini	185
with Whipped Cream, Coconut Milk, Tall	252
with Whipped Cream, Coconut Milk, Venti	402
with Whipped Cream, Oat Milk, Grande	387
with Whipped Cream, Oat Milk, Mini	209
with Whipped Cream, Oat Milk, Tall	287
with Whipped Cream, Oat Milk, Venti	452
with Whipped Cream, Semi Skimmed Milk, Grande	355
with Whipped Cream, Semi Skimmed Milk, Mini	191
with Whipped Cream, Semi Skimmed Milk, Tall	261
with Whipped Cream, Semi Skimmed Milk, Venti	415
with Whipped Cream, Skimmed Milk, Grande	337
with Whipped Cream, Skimmed Milk, Mini	181
with Whipped Cream, Skimmed Milk, Tall	246
with Whipped Cream, Skimmed Milk, Venti	393
with Whipped Cream, Soy, Grande	344
with Whipped Cream, Soy, Mini	185
with Whipped Cream, Soy, Tall	252
with Whipped Cream, Whole Milk, Grande	373
with Whipped Cream, Whole Milk, Mini	201
with Whipped Cream, Whole Milk, Tall	275
with Whipped Cream, Whole Milk, Venti	435
FRAPPUCCINO - TOFFEE NUT	
with Whipped Cream, Almond Milk, Grande	350
with Whipped Cream, Almond Milk, Mini	180
with Whipped Cream, Almond Milk, Tall	252
with Whipped Cream, Almond Milk, Venti	406
with Whipped Cream, Coconut Milk, Grande	371
with Whipped Cream, Coconut Milk, Mini	191
with Whipped Cream, Coconut Milk, Tall	268
with Whipped Cream, Coconut Milk, Venti	429
with Whipped Cream, Oat Milk, Grande	350
with Whipped Cream, Oat Milk, Mini	207
with Whipped Cream, Oat Milk, Tall	293
with Whipped Cream, Oat Milk, Venti	462
with Whipped Cream, Semi Skimmed Milk, Grande	375
with Whipped Cream, Semi Skimmed Milk, Mini	193
with Whipped Cream, Semi Skimmed Milk, Tall	272
with Whipped Cream, Semi Skimmed Milk, Venti	434
with Whipped Cream, Skimmed Milk, Grande	360
with Whipped Cream, Skimmed Milk, Mini	185
with Whipped Cream, Skimmed Milk, Tall	260
with Whipped Cream, Skimmed Milk, Venti	418
with Whipped Cream, Soy, Grande	366
with Whipped Cream, Soy, Mini	188
with Whipped Cream, Soy, Tall	265
with Whipped Cream, Soy, Venti	424
with Whipped Cream, Whole Milk, Grande	389
with Whipped Cream, Whole Milk, Mini	200

STARBUCKS	KCAL
FRAPPUCCINO - TOFFEE NUT	
with Whipped Cream, Whole Milk, Tall	283
No Whip, Skimmed Milk, Grande	155
No Whip, Skimmed Milk, Mini	76
No Whip, Skimmed Milk, Tall	114
No Whip, Skimmed Milk, Venti	191
FRAPPUCCINO - TOFFEE NUT CREME	
with Whipped Cream, Almond Milk, Grande	296
with Whipped Cream, Almond Milk, Mini	155
with Whipped Cream, Almond Milk, Tall	214
with Whipped Cream, Almond Milk, Venti	337
with Whipped Cream, Coconut Milk, Grande	325
with Whipped Cream, Coconut Milk, Mini	170
with Whipped Cream, Coconut Milk, Tall	236
with Whipped Cream, Coconut Milk, Venti	370
with Whipped Cream, Oat Milk, Grande	366
with Whipped Cream, Oat Milk, Mini	191
with Whipped Cream, Oat Milk, Tall	268
with Whipped Cream, Oat Milk, Venti	418
with Whipped Cream, Semi Skimmed Milk, Grande	331
with Whipped Cream, Semi Skimmed Milk, Mini	173
with Whipped Cream, Semi Skimmed Milk, Tall	241
with Whipped Cream, Semi Skimmed Milk, Venti	377
with Whipped Cream, Skimmed Milk, Grande	310
with Whipped Cream, Skimmed Milk, Mini	162
with Whipped Cream, Skimmed Milk, Tall	225
with Whipped Cream, Skimmed Milk, Venti	354
with Whipped Cream, Soy, Grande	319
with Whipped Cream, Soy, Mini	167
with Whipped Cream, Soy, Tall	232
with Whipped Cream, Soy, Venti	363
with Whipped Cream, Whole Milk, Grande	350
with Whipped Cream, Whole Milk, Mini	183
with Whipped Cream, Whole Milk, Tall	256
with Whipped Cream, Whole Milk, Venti	399
FRAPPUCCINO - VANILLA CREAM	
with Whipped Cream, Almond Milk, Grande	291
with Whipped Cream, Almond Milk, Mini	149
with Whipped Cream, Almond Milk, Tall	206
with Whipped Cream, Almond Milk, Venti	336
with Whipped Cream, Coconut Milk, Grande	315
with Whipped Cream, Coconut Milk, Mini	160
with Whipped Cream, Coconut Milk, Tall	224
with Whipped Cream, Coconut Milk, Venti	363
with Whipped Cream, Oat Milk, Grande	362
with Whipped Cream, Oat Milk, Mini	184
with Whipped Cream, Oat Milk, Tall	260
with Whipped Cream, Oat Milk, Venti	419
with Whipped Cream, Semi Skimmed Milk, Grande	327
with Whipped Cream, Semi Skimmed Milk, Mini	166
with Whipped Cream, Semi Skimmed Milk, Tall	233
with Whipped Cream, Semi Skimmed Milk, Venti	377
with Whipped Cream, Skimmed Milk , Tall	217

STARBUCKS	KCAL
FRAPPUCCINO - VANILLA CREAM	
with Whipped Cream, Skimmed Milk, Grande	306
with Whipped Cream, Skimmed Milk, Mini	156
with Whipped Cream, Skimmed Milk, Venti	353
with Whipped Cream, Soy, Grande	314
with Whipped Cream, Soy, Mini	160
with Whipped Cream, Soy, Tall	215
with Whipped Cream, Soy, Tall	223
with Whipped Cream, Soy, Venti	363
with Whipped Cream, Whole Milk, Grande	346
with Whipped Cream, Whole Milk, Mini	176
with Whipped Cream, Whole Milk, Tall	248
with Whipped Cream, Whole Milk, Venti	400
FRAPPUCCINO - WHITE CHOC CREAM	
with Whipped Cream, Almond Milk, Grande	313
with Whipped Cream, Almond Milk, Mini	156
with Whipped Cream, Almond Milk, Tall	218
with Whipped Cream, Almond Milk, Venti	352
with Whipped Cream, Coconut Milk, Grande	335
with Whipped Cream, Coconut Milk, Mini	168
with Whipped Cream, Coconut Milk, Tall	236
with Whipped Cream, Coconut Milk, Venti	378
with Whipped Cream, Oat Milk, Grande	380
with Whipped Cream, Oat Milk, Mini	192
with Whipped Cream, Oat Milk, Tall	273
with Whipped Cream, Oat Milk, Venti	432
with Whipped Cream, Semi Skimmed Milk, Grande	346
with Whipped Cream, Semi Skimmed Milk, Mini	174
with Whipped Cream, Semi Skimmed Milk, Tall	246
with Whipped Cream, Semi Skimmed Milk, Venti	392
with Whipped Cream, Skimmed Milk, Grande	326
with Whipped Cream, Skimmed Milk, Mini	164
with Whipped Cream, Skimmed Milk, Tall	230
with Whipped Cream, Skimmed Milk, Venti	368
with Whipped Cream, Soy, Grande	334
with Whipped Cream, Soy, Mini	168
with Whipped Cream, Soy, Tall	236
with Whipped Cream, Soy, Venti	378
with Whipped Cream, Whole Milk, Grande	365
with Whipped Cream, Whole Milk, Mini	184
with Whipped Cream, Whole Milk, Tall	261
with Whipped Cream, Whole Milk, Venti	414
FRUIT SALAD	
Pot	72
HOT CHOCOLATE - BERRY	
Almond Milk, Grande	341
Almond Milk, Short	200
Almond Milk, Tall	241
Almond Milk, Venti	449
Coconut Milk, Grande	366
Coconut Milk, Short	213
Coconut Milk, Tall	259
Coconut Milk, Venti	485

STARBUCKS	KCAL
HOT CHOCOLATE - BERRY	
Oat Milk, Short	233
Oat Milk, Grande	402
Oat Milk, Tall	283
Oat Milk, Venti	537
Semi Skimmed Milk, Grande	371
Semi Skimmed Milk, Short	216
Semi Skimmed Milk, Tall	262
Semi Skimmed Milk, Venti	493
Skimmed Milk, Grande	353
Skimmed Milk, Short	207
Skimmed Milk, Tall	250
Skimmed Milk, Venti	467
Soya Milk, Grande	360
Soya Milk, Short	210
Soya Milk, Tall	255
Soya Milk, Venti	477
Whole Milk, Grande	388
Whole Milk, Short	225
Whole Milk, Tall	274
Whole Milk, Venti	517
HOT CHOCOLATE - CARAMEL	
with Whipped Cream, Almond Milk, Grande	486
with Whipped Cream, Almond Milk, Short	302
with Whipped Cream, Almond Milk, Tall	361
with Whipped Cream, Almond Milk, Venti	633
with Whipped Cream, Coconut Milk, Grande	517
with Whipped Cream, Coconut Milk, Short	319
with Whipped Cream, Coconut Milk, Tall	381
with Whipped Cream, Coconut Milk, Venti	674
with Whipped Cream, Oat Milk, Grande	582
with Whipped Cream, Oat Milk, Short	355
with Whipped Cream, Oat Milk, Tall	422
with Whipped Cream, Oat Milk, Venti	758
with Whipped Cream, Semi Skimmed Milk, Grande	534
with Whipped Cream, Semi Skimmed Milk, Short	328
with Whipped Cream, Semi Skimmed Milk, Tall	392
with Whipped Cream, Semi Skimmed Milk, Venti	695
with Whipped Cream, Skimmed Milk, Grande	506
with Whipped Cream, Skimmed Milk, Short	313
with Whipped Cream, Skimmed Milk, Tall	374
with Whipped Cream, Skimmed Milk, Venti	659
with Whipped Cream, Soy, Grande	517
with Whipped Cream, Soy, Short	319
with Whipped Cream, Soy, Tall	381
with Whipped Cream, Soy, Venti	674
with Whipped Cream, Whole Milk, Grande	560
with Whipped Cream, Whole Milk, Short	343
with Whipped Cream, Whole Milk, Tall	408
with Whipped Cream, Whole Milk, Venti	729
HOT CHOCOLATE - CLASSIC	
with Whipped Cream, Almond Milk, Grande	221
with Whipped Cream, Almond Milk, Tall	181

STARBUCKS	KCAL
HOT CHOCOLATE - CLASSIC	
with Whipped Cream, Almond Milk, Venti	263
with Whipped Cream, Coconut Milk, Grande	263
with Whipped Cream, Coconut Milk, Short	144
with Whipped Cream, Coconut Milk, Tall	216
with Whipped Cream, Coconut Milk, Venti	320
with Whipped Cream, Oat Milk, Grande	347
with Whipped Cream, Oat Milk, Short	178
with Whipped Cream, Oat Milk, Tall	286
with Whipped Cream, Oat Milk, Venti	436
with Whipped Cream, Semi Skimmed Milk, Grande	284
with Whipped Cream, Semi Skimmed Milk, Short	152
with Whipped Cream, Semi Skimmed Milk, Tall	234
with Whipped Cream, Semi Skimmed Milk, Venti	350
with Whipped Cream, Skimmed Milk, Grande	247
with Whipped Cream, Skimmed Milk, Short	137
with Whipped Cream, Skimmed Milk, Tall	203
with Whipped Cream, Skimmed Milk, Venti	299
with Whipped Cream, Soy, Grande	262
with Whipped Cream, Soy, Short	143
with Whipped Cream, Soy, Tall	215
with Whipped Cream, Soy, Venti	319
with Whipped Cream, Whole Milk, Grande	318
with Whipped Cream, Whole Milk, Short	167
with Whipped Cream, Whole Milk, Tall	262
with Whipped Cream, Whole Milk, Venti	397
with Whipped Cream, Almond Milk, Short	127
HOT CHOCOLATE - HAZELNUT	
with Whipped Cream, Almond Milk, Grande	464
with Whipped Cream, Almond Milk, Short	285
with Whipped Cream, Almond Milk, Tall	341
with Whipped Cream, Almond Milk, Venti	609
with Whipped Cream, Coconut Milk, Grande	495
with Whipped Cream, Coconut Milk, Short	302
with Whipped Cream, Coconut Milk, Tall	362
with Whipped Cream, Coconut Milk, Venti	650
with Whipped Cream, Oat Milk, Grande	560
with Whipped Cream, Oat Milk, Short	337
with Whipped Cream, Oat Milk, Tall	403
with Whipped Cream, Oat Milk, Venti	733
with Whipped Cream, Semi Skimmed Milk, Short	311
with Whipped Cream, Whole Milk, Tall	389
with Whipped Cream, Whole Milk, Venti	705
with Whipped Cream, Semi Skimmed Milk, Grande	512
with Whipped Cream, Semi Skimmed Milk, Tall	372
with Whipped Cream, Semi Skimmed Milk, Venti	671
with Whipped Cream, Skimmed Milk, Grande	484
with Whipped Cream, Skimmed Milk, Short	295
with Whipped Cream, Skimmed Milk, Tall	354
with Whipped Cream, Skimmed Milk, Venti	634
with Whipped Cream, Soy, Grande	495
with Whipped Cream, Soy, Short	302
with Whipped Cream, Soy, Venti	649

STARBUCKS	KCAL
HOT CHOCOLATE - HAZELNUT	
with Whipped Cream, Whole Milk, Grande	538
with Whipped Cream, Whole Milk, Short	325
HOT CHOCOLATE - MARSHMALLOW	
with Whipped Cream, Almond Milk, Grande	302
with Whipped Cream, Almond Milk, Short	168
with Whipped Cream, Almond Milk, Tall	238
with Whipped Cream, Almond Milk, Venti	363
with Whipped Cream, Coconut Milk, Grande	375
with Whipped Cream, Coconut Milk, Short	204
with Whipped Cream, Coconut Milk, Tall	296
with Whipped Cream, Coconut Milk, Venti	459
with Whipped Cream, Oat Milk, Grande	482
with Whipped Cream, Oat Milk, Short	257
with Whipped Cream, Oat Milk, Tall	379
with Whipped Cream, Oat Milk, Venti	597
with Whipped Cream, Semi Skimmed Milk, Grande	392
with Whipped Cream, Semi Skimmed Milk, Short	212
with Whipped Cream, Semi Skimmed Milk, Tall	308
with Whipped Cream, Semi Skimmed Milk, Venti	480
with Whipped Cream, Skimmed Milk, Grande	339
with Whipped Cream, Skimmed Milk, Short	186
with Whipped Cream, Skimmed Milk, Tall	267
with Whipped Cream, Skimmed Milk, Venti	411
with Whipped Cream, Soy, Grande	360
with Whipped Cream, Soy, Short	197
with Whipped Cream, Soy, Tall	284
with Whipped Cream, Soy, Venti	439
with Whipped Cream, Whole Milk, Grande	441
with Whipped Cream, Whole Milk, Short	237
with Whipped Cream, Whole Milk, Tall	347
with Whipped Cream, Whole Milk, Venti	544
HOT CHOCOLATE - SIGNATURE	
with Whipped Cream, Almond Milk, Grande	383
with Whipped Cream, Almond Milk, Short	242
with Whipped Cream, Almond Milk, Tall	280
with Whipped Cream, Almond Milk, Venti	509
with Whipped Cream, Coconut Milk, Grande	415
with Whipped Cream, Coconut Milk, Short	259
with Whipped Cream, Coconut Milk, Tall	300
with Whipped Cream, Coconut Milk, Venti	550
with Whipped Cream, Oat Milk, Grande	479
with Whipped Cream, Oat Milk, Short	294
with Whipped Cream, Oat Milk, Tall	341
with Whipped Cream, Oat Milk, Venti	634
with Whipped Cream, Semi Skimmed Milk, Grande	431
with Whipped Cream, Semi Skimmed Milk, Short	268
with Whipped Cream, Semi Skimmed Milk, Tall	310
with Whipped Cream, Semi Skimmed Milk, Venti	571
with Whipped Cream, Skimmed Milk, Grande	403
with Whipped Cream, Skimmed Milk, Short	253
with Whipped Cream, Skimmed Milk, Tall	292
with Whipped Cream, Skimmed Milk, Venti	535

STARBUCKS	KCAL
HOT CHOCOLATE - SIGNATURE	
with Whipped Cream, Soy, Grande	414
with Whipped Cream, Soy, Short	259
with Whipped Cream, Soy, Tall	299
with Whipped Cream, Soy, Venti	550
with Whipped Cream, Whole Milk, Grande	457
with Whipped Cream, Whole Milk, Short	282
with Whipped Cream, Whole Milk, Tall	327
with Whipped Cream, Whole Milk, Venti	605
HOT CHOCOLATE - WHITE	
with Whipped Cream, Almond Milk, Grande	348
with Whipped Cream, Almond Milk, Short	185
with Whipped Cream, Almond Milk, Tall	273
with Whipped Cream, Almond Milk, Venti	422
with Whipped Cream, Coconut Milk, Grande	391
with Whipped Cream, Coconut Milk, Short	201
with Whipped Cream, Coconut Milk, Tall	307
with Whipped Cream, Coconut Milk, Venti	481
with Whipped Cream, Oat Milk, Grande	480
with Whipped Cream, Oat Milk, Short	235
with Whipped Cream, Oat Milk, Tall	378
with Whipped Cream, Oat Milk, Venti	601
with Whipped Cream, Semi Skimmed Milk, Grande	414
with Whipped Cream, Semi Skimmed Milk, Short	210
with Whipped Cream, Semi Skimmed Milk, Tall	325
with Whipped Cream, Semi Skimmed Milk, Venti	511
with Whipped Cream, Skimmed Milk, Grande	375
with Whipped Cream, Skimmed Milk, Short	195
with Whipped Cream, Skimmed Milk, Tall	295
with Whipped Cream, Skimmed Milk, Venti	459
with Whipped Cream, Soy, Grande	391
with Whipped Cream, Soy, Short	201
with Whipped Cream, Soy, Tall	307
with Whipped Cream, Soy, Venti	480
with Whipped Cream, Whole Milk, Grande	450
with Whipped Cream, Whole Milk, Short	223
with Whipped Cream, Whole Milk, Tall	354
with Whipped Cream, Whole Milk, Venti	560
MACARONI CHEESE	
Vegan, Hot Box	470
MUFFIN	
Bacon, & Egg	394
Blueberry	409
Chocolate, Triple	470
Cran-Merry Cheesecake	438
Halloumi, & Avocado	436
Lemon	424
PAIN AU CHOCOLAT	
BLANK	258
PAIN AU RAISIN	
BLANK	293
PANINI	
Festive Feast	534

STARBUCKS	KCAL
PANINI	
Ham, & Cheese, GF	341
Ham, & Cheese	424
Tomato, & Mozzarella	409
Tuna Melt	414
PASTRY	
Cinnamon Swirl	482
Twist, Chocolate	275
PIE	
Mince	403
ROLL	
Bacon, Smoked	334
Breakfast, All Day	463
SALAD	
Chicken	269
Vegetables, Roasted, Vegan	270
SANDWICH	
Chicken, & Hickory Bacon	380
Chicken, Roast, Salad	493
Egg Mayonnaise, Free Range	492
Sausage	478
Turkey, Tis' the Season	534
SHORTBREAD	
Chocolate Caramel	368
Chocolate Chunk, Fairtrade	493
SLICE	
Caramel, Nut	383
SUB	
Turkey, & Swiss Style Cheese, Pretzel	382
TEA - CHAI	
Grande	0
Short	0
Tall	0
Venti	0
TEA - CHAI LATTE	
Almond Milk, Grande	186
Almond Milk, Short	92
Almond Milk, Tall	143
Almond Milk, Venti	241
Coconut Milk, Grande	221
Coconut Milk, Short	109
Coconut Milk, Tall	170
Coconut Milk, Venti	289
Oat Milk, Grande	292
Oat Milk, Short	143
Oat Milk, Tall	227
Oat Milk, Venti	389
Semi Skimmed Milk, Grande	239
Semi Skimmed Milk, Short	117
Semi Skimmed Milk, Tall	185
Semi Skimmed Milk, Venti	315
Skimmed Milk, Grande	208
Skimmed Milk, Short	103

STARBUCKS	KCAL
TEA - CHAI LATTE	
Skimmed Milk, Tall	160
Skimmed Milk, Venti	271
Soy, Grande	220
Soy, Short	109
Soy, Tall	170
Soy, Venti	289
Whole Milk, Grande	268
Whole Milk, Short	131
Whole Milk, Tall	208
Whole Milk, Venti	355
TEA - CHAMOMILE	
Grande	0
Short	0
Tall	0
Venti	0
TEA - EARL GREY	
Grande	0
Short	0
Tall	0
Venti	0
TEA - EMPEROR'S CLOUD	
Ã‚Â Short	0
Grande	0
Tall	0
Venti	0
TEA - ENGLISH BREAKFAST	
Grande	0
Tall	0
Venti	0
Short	0
TEA - GREEN	
Mint Citrus, Grande	0
Mint Citrus, Short	0
Mint Citrus, Tall	0
Mint Citrus, Venti	0
Pineapple, Grande	64
Pineapple, Tall	48
Pineapple, Unsweetened, Grande	0
Pineapple, Unsweetened, Tall	0
Pineapple, Unsweetened, Venti	0
Pineapple, Venti	80
TEA - HIBISCUS	
Grande	0
Short	0
Tall	0
Venti	0
TEA - ICED	
Hibiscus, , Shaken, Grande	0
Hibiscus, , Shaken, Tall	0
Hibiscus, , Shaken, Venti	0
Lemonade, Black, Shaken, Grande	46
Lemonade, Black, Shaken, Tall	35

	KCAL
STARBUCKS	
TEA - ICED	
Lemonade, Black, Shaken, Venti	56
Lemonade, Blackberry Mojito, Shaken, Grande	89
Lemonade, Blackberry Mojito, Shaken, Tall	67
Lemonade, Blackberry Mojito, Shaken, Venti	110
Lemonade, Green, Shaken, Grande	46
Lemonade, Green, Shaken, Tall	35
Lemonade, Green, Shaken, Venti	56
Lemonade, Hibiscus, Shaken, Grande	46
Lemonade, Hibiscus, Shaken, Tall	35
Lemonade, Hibiscus, Shaken, Venti	56
Lemonade, Mango, Black Tea, Shaken, Grande	110
Lemonade, Mango, Black Tea, Shaken, Tall	83
Lemonade, Mango, Black Tea, Shaken, Venti	137
Mango, Tropical, Grande	135
Mango, Tropical, Tall	104
Mango, Tropical, Venti	170
Matcha, Almond Milk, Grande	68
Matcha, Almond Milk, Tall	53
Matcha, Almond Milk, Venti	80
Matcha, Coconut Milk, Grande	117
Matcha, Coconut Milk, Tall	91
Matcha, Coconut Milk, Venti	136
Matcha, Oat Milk, Tall	148
Matcha, Oat Milk, Venti	216
Matcha, Semi Skimmed Milk, Grande	128
Matcha, Semi Skimmed Milk, Tall	100
Matcha, Semi Skimmed Milk, Venti	148
Matcha, Skimmed Milk, Grande	93
Matcha, Skimmed Milk, Tall	72
Matcha, Skimmed Milk, Venti	108
Matcha, Soy, Grande	107
Matcha, Soy, Tall	83
Matcha, Soy, Venti	124
Matcha, Whole Milk, Grande	161
Matcha, Whole Milk, Tall	126
Matcha, Whole Milk, Venti	185
Peach Citrus, Grande	64
Peach Citrus, Tall	48
Peach Citrus, Unsweetened, Grande	0
Peach Citrus, Unsweetened, Tall	0
Peach Citrus, Unsweetened, Venti	0
Peach Citrus, Venti	80
Rooibos, Latte, Almond Milk, Grande	59
Rooibos, Latte, Almond Milk, Tall	46
Rooibos, Latte, Almond Milk, Venti	67
Rooibos, Latte, Coconut Milk, Grande	108
Rooibos, Latte, Coconut Milk, Tall	85
Rooibos, Latte, Coconut Milk, Venti	123
Rooibos, Latte, Oat Milk, Grande	178
Rooibos, Latte, Oat Milk, Tall	141
Rooibos, Latte, Oat Milk, Venti	203
Rooibos, Latte, Semi Skimmed Milk, Grande	118

	KCAL
STARBUCKS	
TEA - ICED	
Rooibos, Latte, Semi Skimmed Milk, Tall	94
Rooibos, Latte, Semi Skimmed Milk, Venti	135
Rooibos, Latte, Skimmed Milk, Grande	83
Rooibos, Latte, Skimmed Milk, Tall	66
Rooibos, Latte, Skimmed Milk, Venti	95
Rooibos, Latte, Soy, Grande	97
Rooibos, Latte, Soy, Tall	77
Rooibos, Latte, Soy, Venti	111
Rooibos, Latte, Whole Milk, Grande	151
Rooibos, Latte, Whole Milk, Tall	119
Rooibos, Latte, Whole Milk, Venti	172
TEA - JASMINE PEARLS	
Grande	0
Short	0
Tall	0
Venti	0
TEA - MATCHA LATTE	
Almond Milk, Grande	276
Almond Milk, Short	45
Almond Milk, Tall	73
Almond Milk, Venti	125
Coconut Milk, Grande	155
Coconut Milk, Short	74
Coconut Milk, Tall	120
Coconut Milk, Venti	202
Oat Milk, Grande	276
Oat Milk, Short	134
Oat Milk, Tall	214
Oat Milk, Venti	360
Semi Skimmed Milk, Grande	186
Semi Skimmed Milk, Short	89
Semi Skimmed Milk, Tall	144
Semi Skimmed Milk, Venti	242
Skimmed Milk, Grande	133
Skimmed Milk, Short	63
Skimmed Milk, Tall	102
Skimmed Milk, Venti	174
Soy, Grande	154
Soy, Short	74
Soy, Tall	119
Soy, Venti	201
Whole Milk, Grande	235
Whole Milk, Short	113
Whole Milk, Tall	182
Whole Milk, Venti	306
TEA - MINT	
Grande	0
Short	0
Tall	0
Venti	0
TEA - ROOIBOS LATTE	
Almond Milk, Grande	86

STARBUCKS	KCAL
TEA - ROOIBOS LATTE	
Almond Milk, Short	42
Almond Milk, Tall	67
Almond Milk, Venti	112
Coconut Milk, Grande	145
Coconut Milk, Short	71
Coconut Milk, Tall	113
Coconut Milk, Venti	189
Oat Milk, Grande	266
Oat Milk, Short	130
Oat Milk, Tall	208
Oat Milk, Venti	347
Semi Skimmed Milk, Grande	176
Semi Skimmed Milk, Short	86
Semi Skimmed Milk, Tall	137
Semi Skimmed Milk, Venti	229
Skimmed Milk, Grande	123
Skimmed Milk, Short	60
Skimmed Milk, Tall	96
Skimmed Milk, Venti	161
Soy, Grande	144
Soy, Short	71
Soy, Tall	113
Soy, Venti	188
Whole Milk, Grande	225
Whole Milk, Short	110
Whole Milk, Tall	175
Whole Milk, Venti	293
TEA - STRAWBERRY	
Black, Grande	64
Black, Tall	48
Black, Unsweetened, Grande	0
Black, Unsweetened, Tall	0
Black, Unsweetened, Venti	0
Black, Venti	80
TEA - YOUTHBERRY	
Grande	0
Youthberry, Short	0
Youthberry, Tall	0
Youthberry, Venti	0
TOAST	
Fruit, Luxury	455
TOASTIE	
Cheese, Five	482
Chicken, & Bacon, BBQ	480
Ham, Hickory, & Cheese	479
WAFFLES	
Caramel, Mini	40
WRAP	
Chicken, & Avocado	390
Vegan, Very Merry	543
YOGHURT	
Berry Crunch, Pot	250

SUBWAY	KCAL
BACON	
2 Strips, Portion	40
BEEF	
Patty, Big, Portion	142
Steak, Portion	94
BREAD	
Garlic, Cheesy, Savers Menu	275
CHEESE	
Cheddar, Peppered	39
Cheddar, Processed	40
Monterey Cheddar	57
CHICKEN	
Breast, Portion	85
Strips, Teriyaki Glazed, Portion	101
Tikka, Portion	89
COOKIES	
Chocolate Chip Candy	211
Chocolate Chunk	216
Double Choc Chip	215
Oatmeal Raisin	195
Raspberry Cheesecake	207
White Chip Macadamia Nut	213
DANISH PASTRY	
Apricot Crown	419
Cinnamon Swirl	207
Vanilla Crown	329
DOUGHNUTS	
Chocolate	351
Sugared	352
EGGS	
Patty, Portion	55
FLATBREAD	
Bacon, Egg, & Cheese, with Salad, Breakfast	296
Bacon, with Salad, Breakfast	293
Chicken, & Bacon, Ranch Melt, with Salad	515
Chicken, BBQ, Pizza, with Salad	366
Chicken, Breast, with Salad	321
Chicken, Pizziola, with Salad	457
Chicken, Teriyaki, with Salad	321
Chicken, Tikka, with Salad	325
Egg, & Cheese, wiith Salad, Breakfast	260
Ham, with Salad	307
Italian BMT, with Salad	428
Meatball Marinara, with Salad	454
Mega Melt, with Salad, Breakfast	473
Pepperoni, Spicy, Pizza, with Salad	359
Sausage, Egg, & Cheese, with Salad, Breakfast	436
Sausage, with Salad, Breakfast	396
Spicy Italian, with Salad	497
Steak, & Cheese, with Salad	369
Subway Melt, with Cheese, & Salad	386
Tuna, with Salad	371
Turkey, & Ham, with Salad	309

SUBWAY	KCAL
FLATBREAD	
Turkey, Breast, with Salad	292
Vegan, with Salad	236
Veggie Delite, with Salad	236
Veggie Supreme, Pizza Sub, with Salad	253
GARLIC BREAD	
Cheesy, with Steak, Ultimate, 6"	527
HASH BROWNS	
Savers Menu	169
MEATBALLS	
Marinara, Portion	218
MUFFIN	
Blueberry	394
Chocolate Chunk	243
Double Chocolate Chip	351
Raspberry, & White Chocolate	389
NACHOS	
with Salsa, Cheese, & Jalapenos, Savers Menu	347
PEPPERONI	
Salami, & Cheese, Spicy Italian, Portion	262
Salami, & Ham, Italian BMT, Portion	192
SALAD	
Chicken, & Bacon, Ranch Melt, without Dressing	334
Chicken, Breast, without Dressing	138
Chicken, Chipotle Melt, without Dressing	268
Chicken, Pizziola, without Dressing	274
Chicken, Rotisserie-Style, without Dressing	160
Chicken, Teriyaki, without Dressing	153
Chicken, Thai, without Salad	218
Chicken Tikka, without Dressing	142
Ham, without Dressing	124
Italian BMT, without Dressing	246
Meatball, Marinara, without Dressing	270
Spicy Italian, without Dressing	314
Steak, & Cheese, without Dressing	186
Subway Melt, with Cheese, without Dressing	205
Tuna, without Dressing	188
Tuna Nicoise, without Dressing	347
Turkey, & Ham, without Dressing	126
Turkey, Breast, without Dressing	109
Vegan, without Dressing	205
Veggie Delite, without Dressing	52
Veggie Patty, without Dressing	212
SANDWICH	
Cheese, Toasted, Bite, Roll, Standard	169
Ham, & Cheese, Toasted, Bite, Roll, Standard	156
Steak, & Cheese, Toasted, Bite, Roll, Standard	120
Tuna Melt, Toasted, Bite, Roll, Standard	171
SAUCE	
Barbecue	39
Chilli, Hot	48
Chilli, Sweet	46
Chipotle Southwest	90

SUBWAY	KCAL
SAUCE	
Deli Mustard	23
Honey Mustard	32
Ketchup	22
Mayonnaise, Lite	50
Ranch	43
Sriracha	27
Sweet Onion	34
SAUSAGE	
Portion	176
SUBS - B.L.T.	
Standard 6"	283
SUBS - BACON	
9 Grain Honey Oat Bread, Breakfast, 6"	291
9 Grain Wheat Bread, Breakfast, 6"	277
Hearty Italian Bread, Breakfast, 6"	278
Italian Herb & Cheese Bread, Breakfast, 6"	310
Italian White Bread, Breakfast, 6"	265
SUBS - BACON, EGG & CHEESE	
9 Grain Honey Oat Bread, Breakfast, 6"	294
9 Grain Wheat Bread, Breakfast, 6"	336
Hearty Italian Bread, Breakfast, 6"	282
Italian Herb & Cheese Bread, Breakfast, 6"	313
Italian White Bread, Breakfast, 6"	269
SUBS - CHICKEN & BACON, RANCH MELT	
with Salad, 9 Grain Honey Oat Bread, 6"	513
with Salad, 9 Grain Wheat Bread, 6"	499
with Salad, Hearty Italian Bread, 6"	500
with Salad, Italian Herb & Cheese Bread, 6"	532
with Salad, Italian White Bread, 6"	487
SUBS - CHICKEN BREAST	
9 Grain Honey Oat Bread, 6"	319
9 Grain Wheat Bread, 6"	304
with Salad, Hearty Italian Bread, 6"	306
with Salad, Italian Herb & Cheese Bread, 6"	338
with Salad, Italian White Bread, 6"	293
SUBS - CHICKEN PIZZIOLA	
with Salad, 9 Grain Honey Oat Bread, 6"	455
with Salad, 9 Grain Wheat Bread, 6"	440
with Salad, Hearty Italian Bread, 6"	442
with Salad, Italian Herb & Cheese Bread, 6"	474
with Salad, Italian White Bread, 6"	429
SUBS - CHICKEN TERIYAKI	
with Salad, 9 Grain Honey Oat Bread, 6"	319
with Salad, 9 Grain Wheat Bread, 6"	320
with Salad, Hearty Italian Bread, 6"	306
with Salad, Italian Herb & Cheese Bread, 6"	338
with Salad, Italian White Bread, 6"	293
SUBS - CHICKEN TIKKA	
with Salad, 9 Grain Honey Oat Bread, 6"	323
with Salad, 9 Grain Wheat Bread, 6"	309
with Salad, Hearty Italian Bread, 6"	310
with Salad, Italian Herb & Cheese Bread, 6"	342

SUBWAY	KCAL
SUBS - CHICKEN TIKKA	
with Salad, Italian White Bread, 6"	297
SUBS - CHICKEN, BBQ, PIZZA	
with Salad, 9 Grain Honey Oat Bread, 6"	364
with Salad, 9 Grain Wheat Bread, 6"	349
with Salad, Hearty Italian Bread, 6"	351
with Salad, Italian Herb & Cheese Bread, 6"	382
with Salad, Italian White Bread, 6"	338
SUBS - CHICKEN, CHIPOTLE MELT	
with Salad, 9 Grain Wheat Bread, 6"	436
with Salad, Italian White Bread, 6"	429
SUBS - CHICKEN, NACHO SALSA	
Hearty Italian Bread, Savers Menu, 6"	503
SUBS - EGG & CHEESE	
9 Grain Honey Oat Bread, Breakfast, 6"	258
9 Grain Wheat Bread, Breakfast, 6"	299
Hearty Italian Bread, Breakfast, 6"	245
Italian Herb & Cheese Bread, Breakfast, 6"	277
Italian White Bread, Breakfast, 6"	232
SUBS - HAM SALAD	
9 Grain Honey Oat Bread, 6"	305
9 Grain Wheat Bread, 6"	291
9 Grain Wheat Bread, Kids Pak, 4"	182
Hearty Italian Bread, 6"	292
Italian Herb & Cheese Bread, 6"	324
Italian White Bread, 6"	279
Italian White Bread, Kids Pak, 4"	182
SUBS - ITALIAN BMT	
Ultimate Cheesy Garlic Bread, 6"	720
with Salad, 9 Grain Honey Oat Bread, 6"	426
with Salad, 9 Grain Wheat Bread, 6"	412
with Salad, Hearty Italian Bread, 6"	414
with Salad, Italian Herb & Cheese Bread, 6"	445
with Salad, Italian White Bread, 6"	401
SUBS - ITALIAN, SPICY	
with Salad, 9 Grain Honey Oat Bread, 6"	495
with Salad, 9 Grain Wheat Bread, 6"	481
with Salad, Hearty Italian Bread, 6"	483
with Salad, Italian Herb & Cheese Bread, 6"	514
with Salad, Italian White Bread, 6"	470
SUBS - MARGHERITA PIZZA	
Hearty Italian, Savers Menu	359
SUBS - MEAT FEAST	
Italian Herbs & Cheese Bread, Savers Menu, 6"	450
SUBS - MEGA MELT	
9 Grain Honey Oat Bread, Breakfast, 6"	471
9 Grain Wheat Bread, Breakfast, 6"	512
Hearty Italian Bread, Breakfast, 6"	458
Italian Herb & Cheese Bread, Breakfast, 6"	490
Italian White Bread, Breakfast, 6"	445
SUBS - PEPPERONI PIZZA, SPICY	
with Salad, 9 Grain Honey Oat Bread, 6"	357
with Salad, 9 Grain Wheat Bread, 6"	343

SUBWAY	KCAL
SUBS - PEPPERONI PIZZA, SPICY	
with Salad, Hearty Italian Bread, 6"	344
with Salad, Italian Herb & Cheese Bread, 6"	376
with Salad, Italian White Bread, 6"	331
SUBS - SAUSAGE	
9 Grain Honey Oat Bread, Breakfast, 6"	394
9 Grain Wheat Bread, Breakfast, 6"	380
Hearty Italian Bread, Breakfast, 6"	382
Italian Herb & Cheese Bread, Breakfast, 6"	413
Italian White Bread, Breakfast, 6"	369
SUBS - SAUSAGE, EGG & CHEESE	
Standard, 6"	498
SUBS - STEAK & CHEESE	
with Salad, 9 Grain Honey Oat Bread, 6"	367
with Salad, 9 Grain Wheat Bread, 6"	353
with Salad, Hearty Italian Bread, 6"	354
with Salad, Italian Herb & Cheese Bread, 6"	386
with Salad, Italian White Bread, 6"	341
SUBS - SUBWAY MELT WITH CHEESE	
& Salad, 9 Grain Honey Oat Bread, 6"	384
& Salad, 9 Grain Wheat Bread, 6"	369
& Salad, Hearty Italian Bread, 6"	371
& Salad, Italian Herb & Cheese Bread, 6"	402
& Salad, Italian White Bread, 6"	358
SUBS - TIGER PIG	
Standard	423
SUBS - TUNA	
Standard, 6"	360
SUBS - TURKEY & HAM	
with Salad, 9 Grain Honey Oat Bread, 6"	307
with Salad, 9 Grain Wheat Bread, 6"	293
with Salad, Hearty Italian Bread, 6"	294
with Salad, Italian Herb & Cheese Bread, 6"	326
with Salad, Italian White Bread, 6"	281
SUBS - TURKEY BREAST	
with Salad, 9 Grain Honey Oat Bread, 6"	290
with Salad, 9 Grain Wheat Bread, 6"	276
with Salad, 9 Grain Wheat Bread, Kids Pak, 4"	184
with Salad, Hearty Italian Bread, 6"	277
with Salad, Italian Herb & Cheese Bread, 6"	309
with Salad, Italian White Bread, 6"	264
with Salad, Italian White Bread, Kids Pak, 4"	180
SUBS - TURKEY BREAST SUBSTACK	
Standard, 6"	350
SUBS - VEGAN	
with Salad, 9 Grain Honey Oat Bread, 6"	234
with Salad, 9 Grain Wheat Bread, 6"	371
with Salad, Hearty Italian Bread, 6"	221
with Salad, Italian Herb & Cheese Bread, 6"	252
with Salad, Italian White Bread, 6"	208
SUBS - VEGGIE DELITE	
with Salad, 9 Grain Honey Oat Bread, 6"	234
with Salad, 9 Grain Wheat Bread, 6"	219

SUBWAY

	KCAL
SUBS - VEGGIE DELITE	
with Salad, 9 Grain Wheat Bread, Kids Pak, 4"	147
with Salad, Hearty Italian Bread, 6"	221
with Salad, Italian Herb & Cheese Bread, 6"	252
with Salad, Italian White Bread, 6"	208
with Salad, Italian White Bread, Kids Pak, 4"	142
SUBS - VEGGIE PATTY	
with Salad, 9 Grain Wheat Bread, 6"	381
with Salad, Italian White Bread, 6"	373
SUBS - VEGGIE SUPREME PIZZA	
with Salad, 9 Grain Honey Oat Bread, 6"	251
with Salad, 9 Grain Wheat Bread, 6"	237
with Salad, Hearty Italian Bread, 6"	239
with Salad, Italian Herb & Cheese Bread, 6"	270
with Salad, Italian White Bread, 6"	226
TUNA	
Portion	135
TURKEY	
Breast, & Ham, Portion	72
Breast, Portion	56
VEGETARIAN	
Veggie Patty, Portion	160
WRAP	
Chicken, BBQ, & Bacon, Tomato Basil Wrap	553
Chicken, Caesar, Rotisserie-Style	596
Chicken, Pizziola, Standard	457
Sausage, Omelette, & Cheese, Standard	482
Sausage, Poached Egg, & Cheese, Standard	498
Sausage, Standard	408
Steak, Chipotle, & Cheese, Tomato Basil Wrap	660
Tuna, Standard	375
Turkey, & Bacon, with Guacamole	554
Vegan, with Garlic Aioli, Tomato Basil Wrap	729

TABLE TABLE

	KCAL
BACON	
Back, Cooked, Breakfast	49
BAGEL	
Cinnamon, & Raisin, Breakfast	293
BEANS	
Baked, in Tomato Sauce, Breakfast	91
BEEF	
Roast, Dinner, Kids Menu	671
Steak, Rib-eye, 10oz	1033
Steak, Rump, 8oz, with Chips	835
Steak, Rump, 8oz, with Salad	550
Steak, Rump, 8oz, with Skinny Fries, Value Menu	675
Steak, Sirloin, 8oz, & Prawns, King, Surf & Turf	1108
Steak, Sirloin, 8oz, with Chips	847
Steak, Sirloin, 8oz, with Salad	563
Roast, Topside, Dinner	1398
BLACK PUDDING	
Slice, Breakfast	122
BREAD	
Garlic, Flatbread, Side	306
Garlic, Flatbread, with BBQ Dip	492
Garlic, Flatbread, with Cheese, Side	456
Garlic, Flatbread, with Tomato Dip	496
Garlic, Side, Kids Menu	109
Garlic, Starter, Kids Menu	112
BROCCOLI	
Tenderstem, Side	139
BROWNIES	
Chocolate, Triple	666
Chocolate, Warm, Value Menu	523
BUBBLE & SQUEAK	
Breakfast	169
BURGERS	
Beef, with Chips, Kids Menu	619
Chicken, & Avocado	1121
Chicken, with Jacket Potato, & Beans	453
Lamb, & Feta	1015
Mac & Cheese	1380
Mac & Cheese, Value Menu	822
Sloppy Joe	1073
Steak, with Cheese, & Bacon, Double Stack	1308
Steak, with Cheese, Double Stack	1245
Steak, with Cheese, Value Menu	952
Surf & Turf	1471
BUTTER	
Salted, Portion, Breakfast	48
CAKE	
Chocolate, Fudge, Sensation	810
Lemon, Drizzle	144
CAULIFLOWER CHEESE	
Sunday Roast	283
CHEESE	
Camembert, Baked, Starter	622

	KCAL
TABLE TABLE	
CHEESECAKE	
Baked	551
Strawberry, Mini	223
CHICKEN	
Breast, Pancetta, Wrapped, & Mozzarella Stuffed	947
Breast, Topped, Bacon & Cheese, with Chips	747
Breast, Topped, Bacon & Cheese, with Jacket Potato	760
Escalope	1357
Forestiere	713
Goujons, Buttermilk, & Rosemary, Starter	407
Half, Roast, Dinner	1458
Paprika, Value Menu	525
Poppin, with Chips, & Beans, Kids Menu	394
Roast, Kids Menu	581
Wings, BBQ, Starter	304
CHIPS	
Side, Kids Menu	181
Side	363
COD	
Bites, Breaded, Kids Menu	507
CORN	
Cob, Side, Kids Menu	79
CROISSANT	
Breakfast	161
CRUMBLE	
Apple, Bramley, & Blackberry	633
CRUMPETS	
Sourdough, Breakfast	91
CURRY	
Chicken, Kids Menu	444
Chicken, Makhani	934
DOUGHNUTS	
Mini, Kids Menu	203
DRIED FRUIT MIX	
Breakfast	308
EGGS	
Boiled, Single, Breakfast	82
Fried, Single, Breakfast	108
Poached, Single, Breakfast	79
Scrambled, Breakfast	269
FISH & CHIPS	
Battered, with Peas, Value Menu	909
Haddock, Hand Battered, with Peas, Value Menu	1087
FRIES	
Dirty, Side	516
Halloumi, Side	586
Skinny Cut, Side	328
Sweet Potato, Side	290
Tiger, Side	353
FRUIT MIX	
Berry, Breakfast	23
FRUIT SALAD	
Breakfast	49

	KCAL
TABLE TABLE	
FRUIT SALAD	
Kids Menu	49
GAMMON	
Steak, with Chips, & Egg, Value Menu	769
Steak, with Chips, & Eggs	877
Steak, with Chips, & Pineapple	953
Steak, with Chips, & Pineapple, Value Menu	699
Steak, with Chips, Egg, & Pineapple	807
Steak, with Jacket Potato, & Eggs	890
Steak, with Jacket Potato, & Pineapple	751
Steak, with Jacket Potato, Egg, & Pineapple	820
HADDOCK	
Beer Battered, & Chips, with Mushy Peas	1125
Beer Battered, & Chips, with Peas	1087
HAM	
Egg, & Chips, Dayime Value Menu	857
HASH BROWNS	
Single, Breakfast	94
HONEY	
Breakfast	65
ICE CREAM	
Dairy, with Caramel Sauce	277
Dairy, with Chocolate Sauce	276
Dairy, with Raspberry Sauce	273
Vanilla, with Caramel Sauce, Kids Menu	199
Vanilla, with Chocolate Sauce, Kids Menu	199
Vanilla, with Raspberry Sauce, Kids Menu	197
JAM	
Strawberry, Breakfast	33
LAMB	
Rump	631
LASAGNE	
Beef, & Pork, Value Menu	577
Beef, Luxury	949
Sweet Potato, & Feta	704
Sweet Potato, & Feta, Value Menu	608
MEATBALLS	
Chicken, Kids Menu	177
MIXED GRILL	
Table Table	1205
Table Table, with Rump Steak, 8oz	1355
MUFFIN	
Blueberry, Breakfast	114
MUSHROOMS	
Breaded, Garlic & Herb	314
with Butter, Breakfast	161
NACHOS	
Loaded, Sharing	1175
Loaded, Starter	614
OMELETTE	
Breakfast	404
ONION RINGS	
Battered, Beer, Side	210

	KCAL
TABLE TABLE	
PAIN AU CHOCOLAT	
Mini, Breakfast	172
PAIN AU RAISIN	
Mini, Breakfast	128
PANCAKE	
Kids Menu	218
Reduced Sugar, Breakfast	96
PASTA	
Penne, Tomato Sauce, Kids Menu	359
Tomato, with Chicken Meatballs	525
PATE	
Chicken, & Pork, Starter	392
PAVLOVA	
Mixed Berry	137
PEAS	
Side, Kids Menu	47
PIE	
Apple, Caramel, with Custard, Value Menu	475
Beef, & Doom Bar	1175
Chicken, & Mushroom	1121
Chicken, & Chorizo	551
Chicken, & Ham, Value Menu	1061
Cottage, Luxury	710
Fake, & Ale, Vegan, Sunday Roast	1708
Fake, & Ale, Vegan	837
Fish, Luxury	765
PLATTER	
Fish & Chip Shop	1240
Sharing	2102
Sharing, with Chicken Wings	2285
PORK	
Roast, Kids Menu	761
PORK DINNER	
Loin, Roast	1508
POTATOES	
Dippers, with Cheese, & Bacon, Starter	401
Jacket, Mini, Side, Kids Menu	155
Jacket, with Cheese, & Beans, Value Menu	758
Mashed, Side, Kids Menu	131
PRAWN COCKTAIL	
Classic, Starter	462
PUDDING	
Chocolate, Fondant, Warm	578
Sticky Toffee	720
RIBS	
Whole Rack, & Smoky Paprika Chicken	1380
Ā,½ Rack, & Smoky Paprika Chicken	988
RICE	
Brown, Side, Kids Menu	192
SALAD	
Bacon, & Blue Cheese	387
Chicken, Grilled	233
Halloumi, Grilled	360

	KCAL
TABLE TABLE	
SALAD	
Mixed, Side, Kids Menu	23
Mixed, Side	39
SANDWICH	
Chicken, & Bacon, Club, Open, Value Menu	835
SAUCE	
Bearnaise	122
Diane	73
Peppercorn, Creamy	29
SAUSAGE	
Breakfast	114
Quorn*, Breakfast	78
SAUSAGE & MASH	
Bangers, Kids Menu	402
Vegetarian, Bangers, Kids Menu	354
SCAMPI	
Breaded, & Chips, with Mushy Peas	828
Breaded, & Chips, with Peas	790
SORBET	
Coconut	233
SOUP	
Broccoli	255
Carrot, & Coriander	261
Leek, & Potato	312
Mushroom, Cream Of	291
SPAGHETTI BOLOGNAISE	
Kids Menu	322
SPREAD	
Sunflower, Portion, Breakfast	43
SQUID	
Calamari, with Sweet Chilli, Starter	438
SUNDAE	
Chocolate, Churros	748
Chocolate, with Kit Kat	526
Chocolate Browne, Mini, Value Menu	277
Funny Face, Kids Menu	196
SYRUP	
Maple, Breakfastr	62
TART	
Lemon	450
TOAST	
GF, Breakfast	84
Malted, Breakfast	92
White, Breakfast	92
TOMATOES	
Half, Breakfast	9
TORTE	
Chocolate, Greek Yoghurt, Mini	295
VEGETABLES	
Green, Side	112
Sticks, Side, Kids Menu	26
Sticks, Starter, Kids Menu	48

TABLE TABLE

	KCAL
YOGHURT	
Greek Style	87
Strawberry, Frozen, Kids Menu	142
Strawberry, Kids Menu	115
Strawberry	115
Vanilla	96

THE REAL GREEK FOOD COMPANY LTD

	KCAL
ASPARAGUS	
Grilled, Hot Meze	140
CHEESE	
Halloumi, Grilled, Hot Meze	151
Halloumi, Skewers, Hot Meze	118
Halloumi, Skewers, Kids Menu	118
CHICK PEAS	
Revithia, Cold Meze	286
CHICKEN	
Skewers, Hot Meze	177
Skewers, Kids Menu	88
CHIPS	
Side	528
COD	
Salt, Hot Meze	346
CRUDITES	
Cold Meze	37
DESSERT	
Watermelon, Sweet & Salty	124
Yoghurt, Greek with Raspberries	223
DIP	
Aioli, Parsley	176
Dip, Selection	589
Mayonnaise, Lemon, Preserved	279
Melitzanasalata, Cold Meze	236
Relish, Chilli, Smoked	42
Relish, Sun-Dried Tomato & Roast Red Pepper	92
DOLMADES	
Cold Meze	254
FLATBREAD	
Greek, Cold Meze	615
Greek, with Olive & Dukkah, Nibbles	538
HOUMOUS	
Cold Meze	298
LAMB	
Cutlets, Hot Meze	881
Kefte, Hot Meze	344
Skewers, Hot Meze	255
NUTS	
Mixed, Athenian, Nibbles	479
OCTOPUS	
Grilled, Hot Meze	447
OLIVES	
Nibbles	317
PARCELS	
Tiropitakia, Filo Pastry, Hot Meze	416
PORK	
Skewers, Hot Meze	281
POTATOES	
New, in Olive Oil & Lemon Juice, Hot Meze	293
RICE	
Saffron, Hot Meze	406

THE REAL GREEK FOOD COMPANY LTD	KCAL
SALAD	
Cos	42
Tabouleh, Cold Meze	117
Watermelon, Mint & Feta, Cold Meze	102
SARDINES	
Grilled, Hot Meze	619
SOUVLAKI	
Lamb, Kefte	730
Lamb	607
Pork	633
Souvlaki, Halloumi & Vegetable	451
SQUID	
Kalamari, Grilled, Hot Meze	286
TARAMASALATA	
Cold Meze	913
TZATZIKI	
Cold Meze	163

TIM HORTONS	KCAL
BAGEL	
Breakfast Sandwich, Grilled, with Bacon	321
Breakfast Sandwich, Grilled, with Sausage	402
Cinnamon Raisin, with Butter	324
Cinnamon Raisin, with Cream Cheese	357
Everything, with Butter	312
Everything, with Cream Cheese	345
Plain, with Butter	301
Plain, with Cream Cheese	334
BARS	
Rocky Road, Traybake	380
Shortbread, Caramel, Traybake	349
BREAKFAST CEREAL	
Porridge	237
Porridge, with Mixed Berries	246
BURGERS	
Veggie, Moving Mountains	514
CAKE	
Chocolate, & Hazelnut	600
CHICKEN	
Tenders, 3	236
Tenders, 5	394
Tenders, Timmies Minis	158
COFFEE	
Cappuccino, Iced, Large	399
Cappuccino, Iced, Medium	305
Cappuccino, Iced, Small	211
Cappuccino, Large	140
Cappuccino, Iced, Light, Large	202
Cappuccino, Iced, Light, Medium	152
Cappuccino, Iced, Light, Small	101
Cappuccino, Medium	110
Cappuccino, Small	75
Cappuccino, Iced, Supreme, Large	490
Cappuccino, Iced, Supreme, Medium	395
Cappuccino, Iced, Small	302
Cappuccino, Iced, with Caramel, Large	616
Cappuccino, Iced, with Caramel, Medium	479
Cappuccino, Iced, with Caramel, Small	344
Cappuccino, Iced, with Chocolate Syrup, Large	604
Cappuccino, Iced, with Chocolate Syrup, Medium	472
Cappuccino, Iced, with Chocolate Syrup, Small	340
Cappuccino, Iced, with Oreo, Large	566
Cappuccino, Iced, Supreme, with Oreo, Medium	444
Cappuccino, Iced, Supreme, with Oreo, Small	322
Dark Roast, Large	5
Dark Roast, Medium	4
Decaf, Large	5
Decaf, Medium	4
Decaf, Small	3
Espresso, Single	1
Flat White, Medium	121
Latte, Chai, Large	270

TIM HORTONS	KCAL
COFFEE	
Latte, Chai, Medium	214
Latte, Chai, Small	158
Latte, Chocolate, Large	279
Latte, Chocolate, Medium	210
Latte, Chocolate, Small	137
Latte, Iced, Large	134
Latte, Iced, Medium	99
Latte, Iced, Small	65
Latte, Large	164
Latte, Medium	134
Latte, Small	99
Latte, Vanilla, French, Large	384
Latte, Vanilla, French, Medium	329
Latte, Vanilla, French, Small	274
Mocha, Large	378
Mocha, Medium	324
Mocha, Small	270
Original Blend, Large	5
Original, Medium	4
Original Blend, Small	3
Dark Roast, Small	3
COOKIES	
Chocolate, Chunk, Double	232
Chocolate, Chunk, Triple	239
Chocolate, Chunk, White	239
CROISSANT	
Single	231
DOUGHNUTS	
Apple, Fritter	319
Apple, Fritter, Timbit	41
Boston Cream	239
Chocolate, Birthday Cake, Timbit	94
Chocolate, Dip	234
Chocolate, Doughnut	287
Chocolate, Filled, Timbit	64
Chocolate, Glazed, Timbit	80
Glazed, Old Fashioned	298
Honey, Dip, Timbit	48
Honey Cruller	260
Honey Cruller, Timbit	60
Maple, Canadian	242
Maple, Dip	233
Maple, Moose	313
Strawberry, Filled, Timbit	54
Strawberry, Vanilla	270
Valentines	289
Vanilla, Dip	276
HASH BROWNS	
Portion	79
HOT CHOCOLATE	
Frozen, Large	539
Frozen, Medium	391

TIM HORTONS	KCAL
HOT CHOCOLATE	
Frozen, Small	254
Large	377
Medium	323
Small	269
White, Frozen, Large	619
White, Frozen, Medium	466
White, Frozen, Small	332
White, Praline, Frozen, Large	579
White, Praline, Frozen, Medium	402
White, Praline, Frozen, Small	342
JUICE DRINK	
Mango, & Passionfruit, Fruit Cooler, Large	263
Mango, & Passionfruit, Fruit Cooler, Medium	198
Mango, & Passionfruit, Fruit Cooler, Small	136
Raspberry, Fruit Cooler, Large	255
Raspberry, Fruit Cooler, Medium	185
Raspberry, Fruit Cooler, Small	136
LEMONADE	
Frozen	178
Original, Large	260
Original, Medium	200
Original, Small	120
MILK	
Whole, Timmies Minis	365
MUFFIN	
Bacon, Double, Egg, & Cheese	346
Bacon, Egg, & Cheese	301
Bacon	198
Blueberry	366
Chocolate, Chip	452
Chocolate, Lava	456
Egg, & Cheese	257
Sausage, Double, Egg, & Cheese	507
Sausage, Egg, & Cheese	382
Sausage	225
Sausage, Vegetarian, Egg, & Cheese	416
PANCAKE	
Bacon, & Maple, Meal	505
Bacon, & Maple	426
Chocolate, & Hazelnut	577
Maple, Caramel, & White Chocolate	481
Maple Syrup, Meal	447
Maple Syrup	368
Nutella, Meal	467
Nutella	388
Red Berry, & White Chocolate	407
PANINI	
Chicken, & Mozzarella	506
Meatball	608
Mozzarella, & Tomato	431
POTATO WEDGES	
Portion	260

TIM HORTONS	KCAL
ROLL	
Bacon	587
SANDWICH	
Chicken, Crispy	590
Ham, Timmies Minis	136
Tuna, Timmies Minis	160
SMOOTHIE	
Strawberry, Banana, Large	332
Strawberry, Banana, Medium	249
Strawberry, Banana, Small	175
SOUP	
Tomato, & Basil, Vegan	110
TEA	
Freshly Brewed, Large	0
Freshly Brewed, Medium	0
Freshly Brewed, Small	0
Speciality, Large	0
Speciality, Medium	0
Speciality, Small	0
TEACAKES	
Toasted	265
TOAST	
Plain	218
with Butter	325
with Jam	266
TOASTIE	
Cheese, & Bacon, Melt	559
Cheese, & Ham, Melt	339
Cheese, Grilled, Melt	487
Cheese, Melt, Timmies Minis	158
Ham, & Cheese, Melt, Timmies Minis	190
Ham, Melt, Timmies Minis	156
Tuna, & Cheese, Melt	380
WRAP	
Breakfast, Big	743
Breakfast, Big, Vegetarian, Moving Mountains	725
Breakfast, Original	589
Breakfast, Vegetarian, Moving Mountains	572
Chicken, Crispy, & Bacon	645
Chicken, Crispy	460
Chicken, Grilled, & Bacon	525
Chicken, Grilled	340
Chicken, Timmies Minis	251
Meatball	449
Tuna	340
Vegan, Moving Mountains	365
Veggie, Chipotle, Moving Mountains	367
YOGHURT	
& Granola, Rachels	227

TOBY CARVERY	KCAL
BAKE	
Leek, Crumble, Carvery	103
Potato, & Carrot, Carvery	121
Potato, & Leek, Carvery	120
Potato, & Parsnip, Carvery	145
Potato, & Squash, Carvery	123
Tomato, Crumble, Carvery	118
BEANS	
Baked, Breakfast	77
Baked, Side, Kids Menu	76
Green, Carvery	44
Romano, Carvery	63
BEEF	
Deck Veg Garnish	65
Roast, Carvery	274
BREAD	
Brown, Sandwich Choice	405
Ciabatta, Sanwich Choice	311
Ciabatta, with Lurpak	337
Garlic, Ciabatta	363
Garlic, Ciabatta, with Cheese	488
Garlic, Kids Menu	182
White, Bap, Sandwich Choice	342
White, Sandwich Choice	438
Wholemeal, Bap, Sandwich Choice	264
BREAKFAST	
Kids, Vegetarian	1330
Toby Carvery	1838
Toby Carvery, Vegetarian	1330
BREAKFAST CEREAL	
Porridge, Breakfast	243
BROCCOLI	
Carvery	51
BROWNIES	
Chocolate, Pieces, Mini	352
BUBBLE & SQUEAK	
Carvery	88
BURGERS	
Chicken, Kids Menu	340
CABBAGE	
Red, Carvery	63
Seasonal, Carvery	241
CAKE	
Birthday	587
Black Forest Square	863
Chocolate, Fudge	567
Mousse, Chocolate, & Orange	319
Salted Caramel, Sticky, Giant	869
CARROTS	
Carvery	31
CAULIFLOWER CHEESE	
Carvery	55

TOBY CARVERY	KCAL
CHEESE	
Camembert, Baked, for Two	897
CHEESECAKE	
Vanilla, Baked	772
CHICKEN	
Nuggets, Kids Menu	190
Strips, Southern Fried, Spicy, with BBQ Sauce	302
CHICKEN DINNER	
Baby's, Heinz, Kids Menu	123
CHOCOLATE	
Flake, Extra	44
COOKIES	
Chocolate Chip, Sundae Topping	256
CORN	
Cob, Mini, Carvery	51
COURGETTE	
Lemon & Thyme, Roasted, Carvery	39
CREAM	
Whipped, for Desserts	148
CRUMBLE	
Apple, Blackberry, & Redcurrant, Mini	285
Apple, Blackberry, & Redcurrant	402
CUSTARD	
for Desserts	90
Soya, Vegan, for Desserts	81
DESSERT	
Eton Mess	2315
DUMPLINGS	
in Onion Gravy, Carvery	469
EGGS	
Fried, Free Range, Breakfast	157
Scrambled, Breakfast	181
FRUIT COMPOTE	
Apple, with Cinnamon, Porridge Topping	33
Toffee, Apple, & Banana, Porridge Topping	82
GAMMON	
Deck Veg Garnish	57
Pomegranate Glaze, Carvery	196
GATEAU	
Black Forest	863
GRAVY	
Breakfast	54
Classic, Carvery	23
Vegan, Carvery	36
Vegetarian, Carvery	317
HASH	
Potato, Cheese, & Onion, Breakfast	102
HASH BROWNS	
Breakfast	166
HOUMOUS	
with Veg, & Bread	474
with Veg, Vegan	374

TOBY CARVERY	KCAL
ICE CREAM	
for Desserts	105
Kids Menu	176
No Sauce	209
ICE LOLLY	
Pip Organic, Kids Menu	20
LAMB	
Deck Veg Garnish	215
Roast, Carvery	214
LEEKS	
Carvery	30
MACARONI CHEESE	
Carvery	99
Kids Menu	150
MARSHMALLOWS	
Sundae Topping	50
MASH	
Colcannon, Carvery	92
MUSHROOMS	
Garlic	251
Roasted, Breakfast	461
MUSTARD	
English, Carvery	194
Wholegrain, Carvery	213
ONIONS	
in Gravy, Carvery	61
PARCELS	
Broccoli, & Brie	492
PARSNIP	
Honey Roast, Carvery	162
PASTA	
Tomato, & Meatballs, Kids Menu	316
PEAS	
Carvery	82
PETIT POIS	
Ala Creme, Carvery	97
PIE	
Allotment	352
Apple	246
Mushroom, & Ale, Roast	761
PLATTER	
Taster	1708
Tobys Ultimate, Sharing	2734
Vegetarian, Sharing	1950
PORK	
Deck Veg Garnish	78
Roast, Apple & Sage Glaze, Carvery	230
PORK CRACKLING	
Cravery	669
POTATOES	
Mashed, Carvery	103
Mashed, Cheesy, Carvery	149
Roast, Beef Dripping, Carvery	111

	KCAL
TOBY CARVERY	
POTATOES	
Roast, Bowl, Side	229
Roast, Carvery	94
Roast, Loaded	350
PRAWN COCKTAIL	
King, with Bread	417
King, with Wholemeal Bread, Mini, Kids Menu	300
PUDDING	
Arctic Roll, with Whipped Cream	418
Three Little	1226
SALAD	
House, Small	107
House	107
Topping, Cheddar Cheese	311
Topping, Prawns	387
SANDWICH FILLING	
Beef, Mushroom, & Chutney, Add Bread	912
Cheese, & Chutney, Add Bread	304
Gammon, Camembert, & Cranberry, Add Bread	894
Hunters Gammon, Add Bread	643
Pork, Roast, Add Bread	521
Prawn, King, Add Bread	332
Turkey, Roast, Club, add Bread	497
SAUCE	
Apple, Carvery	103
Bread, Carvery	443
Chocolate, Belgian	58
Cranberry, Carvery	148
Horseradish, Carvery	178
Lemon, Sicillian	55
Mint, Carvery	124
Parsley, Carvery	467
Strawberry	57
Toffee, Devon Cream	64
SAUSAGE	
& Giant Yorkshire Pudding, Kids Menu	327
Pigs, In Blankets, Mini	531
Pigs in Blankets, Apple & Sage Glazed, Sharer	494
Pigs in Blankets, Pomegranate Glazed, Sharer	487
Pigs in Blankets, Glazed, Sharer	587
Pigs in Blankets, Maple Glazed, Sharer	517
Pork, British, Breakfast	217
Quorn, Breakfast	128
Quorn*, & Giant Yorkshire Pudding, Kids Menu	292
SAUSAGE ROLL	
Squashage, Salad Topping	507
Vegan, with Gravy	542
SEA BASS	
Steamed	362
SORBET	
Trio	453
SOUP	
Small, Side	58

	KCAL
TOBY CARVERY	
SOUP	
Tomato, with Wholemeal Bread, Kids Menu	226
SPINACH	
Creamed, Carvery	41
SPONGE	
Apricot, with Custard	405
Cherry, with Custard	398
Rhubarb, with Custard	410
Rolo Toffee, with Custard	509
Strawberry, with Custard	407
Treacle	526
SPROUTS	
Carvery	65
STRAWBERRIES	
& Cream	200
& Ice Cream	164
STUFFING	
Sage, & Cranberry, Carvery	340
Sage, & Onion, Carvery	204
SUNDAE	
Banoffee	955
Chocolate Heaven, Kids Menu	364
Cookie Dough	473
Honeycomb Dream	397
Ice Cream, Make Your Own, Kids Menu	158
SUNDAE TOPPING	
Banana, Make Your Own, Kids Menu	72
Chocolate Chip Cookie, Make Your Own, Kids Menu	256
Fruit Salad Crunch, Make Your Own, Kids Menu	40
Honeycomb Pieces, Make Your Own, Kids Menu	59
Marshmallows, Make Your Own, Kids Menu	50
Meringue, Make Your Own, Kids Menu	25
Strawberries, Make Your Own, Kids Menu	20
SWEDE	
Carvery	188
SWEETS	
Bear Yo Yo's, Strawberry, Kids Menu	56
TOAD IN THE HOLE	
Veggie	1091
TOAST	
White, Breakfast	451
TOMATOES	
Plum, Breakfast	15
TURKEY	
Deck Veg Garnish	88
Roast, Carvery	118
VEGETABLES	
Greens, Leek, Cabbage, & Peas, Carvery	64
Sticks, Side, Kids Menu	25
Sticks, wih Houmous Dip, Kids Menu	201
WAFERS	
Extra	8

TOBY CARVERY	KCAL
YORKSHIRE PUDDING	
& Gravy, Side	168
Breakfast	381
Carvery	224
Sandwich Choice	328
Stuffed, Beef	313

VINTAGE INNS	KCAL
BAKE - SLOW ROASTED TOMATO	
& Almond, with Roast Potatoes, & Veg	1170
BEANS	
Baked, Side, Childrens	80
BEEF - STEAK SIRLOIN, 8OZ	
Triple Cooked Chips, Onions Rings, Roasted Tomato	966
BEEF - STEAK, FILLET, 7OZ	
Triple Cooked Chips, Onion Rings, Roasted Tomato	798
BEEF - STEAK, RIBEYE, 10OZ	
Triple Cooked Chips, Onion Rings, Roasted Tomato	963
BEEF - STEAK, RUMP, 8OZ	
Triple Cooked Chips, Onion Rings, Roasted Tomato	927
BEEF BOURGUIGNON	
Porcini, with Mash, Carrots, & Dumplings	432
BEEF DINNER, SIRLOIN	
Yorkshire Pudding, Roast Potatoes, Veg, & Gravy	1598
BEEF DINNER, TRIO	
Turkey, & Pork, Roast Potatoes, Veg, & Gravy	1379
BITES	
Black Pudding	417
Black Pudding, Yorkshire	367
Yorkshire Pudding	299
BREAD	
Garlic, Side, Childrens	373
BREAD & BUTTER PUDDING	
Marmalade, with Custard	642
BROWNIES - CHOCOLATE	
Belgian, Chocolate Sauce, & Irish Liqueur Ice Cream	832
with Vanilla Ice Cream, Childrens	553
BURGERS	
Beef, Chargrilled, Dirty	1324
Beef, Chargrilled, with Mayo, Relish, & Onion Rings	734
Beef, no Sides, Children's	173
Beef, Prime, Dirty	933
Beef, Prime, with Mayo, Relish, & Onion Rings	343
Beef, Wagyu, with Salsa, Mayo, & Onion Rings	1460
Chicken, no Sides, Childrens	328
Chickpea, & Aubergine, Spiced	447
Plant Based, Moving Mountanis, with Side Salad	601
CAULIFLOWER	
Roasted, Spiced, with Couscous, & Coconut Sauce	1104
CAULIFLOWER CHEESE	
Portion	222
CHEESE	
Camembert, Garlic & Rosemary, Baked	1035
Cheeseboard, with Biscuits, Grapes, & Chutney	1122
CHEESECAKE	
Blackcurrant, & Prosecco	471
Caramel, Biscuit, Vegan, with Banana	777
Vanilla, Baked	414
CHICKEN	
Hunters, with Bacon, & Tomato Sauce, & Chips	1478
Hunters, with Gammon, Chips, & BBq Sauce	1430

VINTAGE INNS	KCAL
CHICKEN	
Wings, Southern Fried	599
CHIPS	
Side, Childrens	698
Triple Cooked	499
COD	
Battered, Fillet, no Sides, Childrens	290
Loin, & Chorizo Roasted Potatoes	572
Loin, & Tomatoes, Heirloom	330
CREME BRULEE	
Apricot, with Biscuits	416
CRUMBLE	
Winter Fruit, Spiced, with Custard	557
Winter Fruit, Spiced, with Soya Custard	572
DESSERT	
Eton Mess	372
FISH & CHIPS - COD, BATTERED	
Chips, Mushy Peas, & Tartare Sauce, Lunch Bites	963
Chips, Mushy Peas, & Tartare Sauce	1330
FISH CAKES - LOBSTER	
with Bouillabaisse, Broccoli, & Potatoes, Lunch Bites	441
with Bouillabaisse, Broccoli, & Potatoes	602
FLATBREAD - GARLIC BUTTER	
with Cheese, Stonebaked, Sharers & Grazing	864
FRIES	
Skin On, Side, Childrens	539
Sweet Potato, Side, Childrens	293
Sweet Potato	377
GAMMON	
Steak, 4oz, with Eggs, & Chips, Lunch Bites	765
Steak, 8oz, with Eggs, & Chips	1262
ICE CREAM	
Chocolate, Childrens	355
Chocolate, Double	315
Irish Cream Liqueur	255
Vanilla, Childrens	278
Vanilla Pod	122
ICE LOLLY	
Tropical Fruit, Childrens	20
JELLY	
Peach, Childrens	144
KEBAB	
Lamb Kofta, with Tzatziki, & Dressed Slaw, Starter	340
LAMB - DINNER, RUMP	
Yorkshire Pudding, Roast Potatoes, Veg, & Gravy	1758
LAMB - DUO	
Rump, & Shepherd's Pie, Veg, & Red Wine Jus	1204
LAMB - RACK	
Roasted, with Veg, & Spiced Potatoes	1142
LASAGNE	
Beef, & Red Wine	583
Beef. no Sides. Children's	349

VINTAGE INNS	KCAL
MUSHROOMS - GARLIC, BAKED	
& Cheese, Steak Add On	109
& Cheddar Sauce, with Rustic Bread, Starter	296
OLIVES	
Mixed, Marinated in Garlic & Red Pepper	184
ONION RINGS	
Homemade	86
PASTA	
Tomato, Childrens	238
PATE	
Duo, with Rustic Bread, Starter	432
PEAS	
Side, Childrens	45
PIE - APPLE, BRAMLEY	
with Custard, & Vanilla Pod Ice Cream	754
PIE - CHICKEN & MUSHROOM	
with Mash, Roasted Carrots, & Veg	942
PIE - LEMON MERINGUE	
Portion	393
PIE - STEAK & ALE	
with Mash, Seasonal Veg, & a Jug of Gravy	1004
PIZZA	
Chicken, Spicy Cajun, Stonebaked	1288
Four Cheese, Stonebaked	1209
Margherita, Childrens	577
Margherita, Stonebaked	963
Meat Feast, Stonebaked	1404
Vegetable, Roasted, with Pesto, Stonebaked	1134
PLATTER	
Mezze, Sharers & Grazing	1293
Pudding, Tasting	2391
Sticky, Sharers & Grazing	2200
PORK - BELLY, ROAST	
Yorkshire Pudding, Roast Potatoes, Veg, & Gravy	1703
PORK - BELLY, SLOW COOKED	
with Mash, Crackling & Veg	1365
POTATOES	
Baby, Side, Childrens	77
Mashed, Side, Children's	141
Roast	482
PRAWN COCKTAIL	
with Lobster, with Rustic Bread, Starter	751
PRAWNS	
Garlic, Steak Add On	209
Tempura, with Rice Cracker, & Soy, Lime & Chilli Dip	475
PUDDING	
Sticky Toffee, with Butterscotch Sauce, & Custard	356
RIBS	
Pork, Caramelised Sticky, with Mango Salsa	466
RICE	
Sunshine, Side, Childrens	190
RISOTTO	
Mushroom, Wild	1045

VINTAGE INNS	KCAL
RISOTTO	
Mushroom, Wild, with Chicken	1243
Mushroom, Wild, with Halloumi	1443
Mushroom, Wild, with Salmon	1871
Seafood, with Roasted Tomatoes	1097
ROLLS	
Squashsage & Mushroom, Vegan	409
SALAD	
Super Green	135
SALAD - CAESAR	
with Chicken, & Garlic Flatbread	1201
with Garlic Flatbread	710
with Halloumi, & Garlic Flatbread	1050
with Salmon, & Garlic Flatbread	1141
SALAD - DUCK	
Aromatic	337
SALAD - SIDE	
Childrens	46
SALAD - WHEATBERRY, APPLE & CRANBERRY	
Main	1223
with Chicken, Lunch Bites	1212
with Chicken	1459
with Halloumi, Lunch Bites	1064
with Halloumi	1311
with Lamb Koftas, Lunch Bites	890
with Lamb Koftas	1137
with Salmon, Lunch Bites	1078
with Salmon	1753
SALMON	
Pesto Crusted, & Mascarpone, Broccoli, Butter Sauce	1107
SANDWICH	
Beef, Brisket, on Sourdough, no Chips	729
Beef, Roast, on a Rustic Roll, no Chips	1086
Chicken, & Camembert, Hot, on Foccacia, no Chips	769
Fish Finger, Cod, on a Rustic Roll, no Chips	578
Ham, & Cheddar, Melt, on Sourdough, no Chips	733
SAUCE	
Bearnaise, Steak Sauce	210
Beef Dripping, Steak Sauce	162
Peppercorn, Steak Sauce	46
SAUSAGE	
Pork, with Gravy, no Sides, Childrens	278
SCALLOPS	
Extra	47
Black Pudding, Minted Pea Puree, Bacon, Starter	731
SEA BASS	
with Pancetta Veloute, Broccoli, & Mash	754
SOUP	
Broccoli, & Stilton	213
Pea, Mint, & Ham	302
Pea & Mint	204
SQUID - CALAMARI	
Salt, Pepper, Chorizo, & Chipotle Chilli Mayo, Starter	476

VINTAGE INNS	KCAL
STUFFING	
Lemon & Thyme, Bacon Wrapped, Extra	385
TART	
Carrot, & Apricot Chutney, & Salad, & Baby Potatoes	1078
TURKEY DINNER	
Yorkshire Pudding, Roast Potatoes, Veg, & Gravy	1408
VEGETABLES	
Skewer, no Sides, Childrens	83
Sticks, Side, Childrens	38
WRAP	
Jackfruit, Smoky, with Side Salad, Vegan	233
Jackfruit, Smoky, without Chips	215
YORKSHIRE PUDDING	
Extra	99
Roast Potatoes, Veg, & Gravy, No Meat, Childrens	660
Roast Potatoes, Veg, & Gravy, No Meat	660

	KCAL
WAGAMAMA	
BANANA	
Katsu, with Salted Caramel Ice Cream	247
BEANS	
Edamame, with Chilli	255
Edamame, with Salt	247
BEEF	
Teriyaki, & Rice, Donburi	882
BROCCOLI	
& Bok Choi, Wok-Fried, Greens	177
BUNS	
Beef, Korean BBQ, & Red Onion, Steamed, Hirata	306
Mushroom, Mixed, Steamed, Hirata	338
Pork, Belly, & Panko Apple, Steamed, Hirata	391
CAKE	
Chocolate, Caramel, Smoked, with Vanilla Ice Cream	518
Chocolate Orange, with Miso Caramel Ice Cream	567
CAULIFLOWER	
Bang Bang	472
CHEESECAKE	
Salted Caramel	383
White Chocolate, & Matcha	510
White Chocolate, & Ginger	449
CHICKEN	
Grilled, Katsu, Naked	607
Grilled, Katsu, with Amai Sauce, Mini, Kids Menu	402
Grilled, Katsu, with Curry Sauce, Mini, Kids Menu	426
Katsu, with Amai Sauce, Mini, Kids Menu	453
Katsu, with Curry Sauce, Mini, Kids Menu	477
Skewers, Teriyaki, Yakitori	266
Teriyaki, & Rice, Donburi	778
CHILLI	
Side	2
CURRY - FIRECRACKER	
Chicken, & White Rice	1185
Prawn, & White Rice	1067
CURRY - KATSU	
Chicken & Sticky Rice	1076
Chicken Hot, & Sticky Rice	1140
Yasai & Sticky Rice	1107
Yasai Hot, & Sticky Rice	1170
CURRY - RAISUKAREE	
Chicken, & White Rice	1123
Prawn, & White Rice	1035
CURRY - VEGATSU	
Hot, Seitan, Panko Crusted, with Sticky Rice	1173
Seitan, Panko Crusted, with Sticky Rice	1110
CURRY - YASAI, VEGETABLE	
& Sticky Rice, Katsu, Amai Sauce, Mini, Kids Menu	369
& Sticky Rice, Katsu, Curry Sauce, Mini, Kids Menu	393
DUCK	
Grilled, Teriyaki, with Rice, Donburi	1395
DUMPLINGS	
Chicken, Steamed, Gyoza	223

	KCAL
WAGAMAMA	
DUMPLINGS	
Duck, Fried, Gyoza	373
Pork, Pulled, Steamed, Gyoza	231
Prawn, Fried, Gyoza	231
Yasai, Steamed, Gyoza	221
EGGS	
Tea Stained, Side	95
FISH - BITES	
Crispy, with Amai Sauce, Mini, Kids Menu	565
Crispy, with Curry Sauce, Mini, Kids Menu	588
ICE CREAM	
Chocolate, & Orange Blossom	294
Coconut, Reika	432
Coffee, Vietnamese	337
Guava, Pink, & Passion Fruit	166
Miso Caramel	419
Strawberry, & Yuzu	325
Vanilla, Pod, Kids Menu	136
ICE LOLLY	
Blackcurrant, & Apple, Little Ko Pop	30
Mango, & Apple, Little Ko Pop	34
JUICE	
Apple, & Orange, Mini, Kids Menu	87
Apple, Mini, Kids Menu	68
Blueberry, Spice	164
High-Five	211
Nourish-Mint	155
Orange	110
Positive	234
Power	170
Tropical	152
Up-Beet	150
KIMCHI	
Side	15
LEMONADE	
Cloudy	0
NOODLES	
Chicken, Grilled, Mini, KIds	450
Fish, Grilled, Mini, KIds	380
Plain, Side	398
NOODLES - RAMEN	
Beef, Brisket, Tantanmen	703
Beef, Steak, Sirloin, Chilli	6800
Chicken, Grilled, Chilli	605
Chicken, Grilled, Mini, Kids Menu	400
Chicken, Grilled	499
Cod, Miso Glazed	668
Pork, Belly, Shirodashi	725
Prawn, Chilli,& Kimchee	532
Tofu, & Vegetable, Rice Noodles, Mini, Kids Menu	306
Tofu, & Vegetable, Thin Noodles, Mini, Kids Menu	328
Tofu, & Vegetable, Udon Noodles, Mini, Kids Menu	954
Tofu, Kare Burosu, Ramen	604

WAGAMAMA	KCAL
NOODLES - TEPPANYAKI	
Beef, Steak, Sirloin, Teriyaki, Soba	900
Chicken, & Prawn, Pad-Thai	801
Chicken, & Prawn, Yaki Soba	824
Chicken, & Prawn, Yaki Udon	650
Chicken, Ginger, Udon	680
Cod, Mokutan Soba	830
Salmon, Teriyaki, Soba	883
Tofu, & Vegetable, Yasai, Pad-Thai	849
Vegetable, Yasai Yaki Soba, Teppanyaki	790
NOODLES - YAKI SOBA	
Chicken, Mini, Kids Menu	410
Tofu, & Vegetable, Rice Noodles, Mini, Kids Menu	338
Tofu, & Vegetable, Thin Noodles, Mini, Kids Menu	402
Tofu, & Vegetable, Udon Noodles, Mini, Kids Menu	259
PICKLE	
Japanese, Side	4
PRAWNS	
Ebi Katsu, Crispy, Fried, with Chilli Garlic Sauce	281
Skewers, Lollipop, Kushiyaki	140
RICE	
Brown, Side	501
Steamed, Side	480
Sticky, Side	492
SORBET	
Pink Guava, & Passion Fruit	166
SOUP	
Miso, & Japanese Pickles, Side	35
SQUID	
Balls, Tama	344
STIR FRY	
Avant Gard'n, Vegan	567
Chicken, Cha Han, Mini, Kids	403
Chicken, Shu's 'Shiok', with Coconut Rice	570
Tofu, Cha Han, Yasai, Mini, Kids	395
Tofu, Cha Han, Yasai, Vegan, Mini, Kids	352
TART	
Yuzu, & Lemon	305
TEA	
Ginger & Lemongrass	0
Green	0
Jasmine, Flowering	0
Mint, Fresh	0
Peach, Iced	0
TUNA	
Steak,Nuoc Cham, Seared	468
VEGETABLES	
Tempura	384

WIMPY	KCAL
BACON	
Slice	65
BEANS	
Baked, Heinz, Extra	69
BREAKFAST	
All Day	832
Country	359
Hashbrown	396
Sunrise	340
The Great Wimpy	758
BROWNIES	
Chocolate	639
BURGERS	
Bender, in a Bun, with Cheese	527
Fish Finger	577
Hamburger	392
Kingsize	823
Mega	789
BURGERS - BEAN	
Spicy, & Slaw, Stack, Vegetarian	673
Spicy, Vegetarian	557
BURGERS - CHEESEBURGER	
Double	647
Original	433
Junior, with Beans, Kids	477
Junior, with Chips, Kids	601
Junior, with Salad, Kids	422
BURGERS - CHICKEN	
Fillet, Firecracker Sauce	498
Fillet, with BBQ Sauce	503
Fillet, with Wimpy Mayo	527
Gourmet	510
BURGERS - HALFPOUNDER	
Original	876
with Bacon & Cheese	861
BURGERS - JUNIOR	
with Beans, Kids	436
with Chips, Kids	560
with Salad, Kids	381
BURGERS - QUARTERPOUNDER	
Club	736
Patty Only	264
Smoky BBQ	693
with Cheese, Original	613
with Mushroom	646
with Bacon & Cheese	597
BURGERS - QUORN	
Southern Fried, Spicy, Vegetarian	506
CHEESE	
Mozzarella, Melts, 6	390
Slices, Extras	41
CHICKEN	
Platter, Gourmet	645

	KCAL
WIMPY	
CHICKEN	
Strips, & Chips	685
Strips, with Beans, Kids	310
Strips, with Chips, Kids	433
Strips, with Salad, Kids	254
Wings, Coated, with BBQ Sauce	477
Wings, Coated, with Firecracker Sauce	466
CHIPS	
Large	333
Reg	267
Sweet Potato, Large	340
Sweet Potato, Reg	269
CHOCOLATE	
Flake, for Sundae	45
COFFEE - AMERICANO	
Black, Large	5
Black, Reg	3
with Milk, Large	26
with Milk, Reg	16
COFFEE - CAPPUCCINO	
Large	109
Reg	81
COFFEE - ESPRESSO	
Large	5
Reg	3
COFFEE - LATTE	
Large	139
Reg	111
COFFEE - MOCHA	
Large	248
Reg	183
COFFEE - SHOT	
Extra	3
COLA	
Pepsi, Diet, Kids	2
Pepsi, Diet, Large	3
Pepsi, Diet, Reg	2
Pepsi, Large	181
Pepsi, Max, Kids	1
Pepsi, Max, Large	2
Pepsi, Max, Reg	2
Pepsi, Reg	143
COLESLAW	
Extra	171
CREAM	
Extra, for Desserts	70
Extra, for Drinks	39
DESSERT	
Brown Derby with Dairy Ice Cream	436
DRESSING	
Caesar	219
French	60
Wimpy Mayo	199

	KCAL
WIMPY	
EGGS	
Fried, Extra	90
Fried, on Toast, White	458
Scrambled, Extra	65
Scrambled, on Toast, White	409
FISH	
Bites, with Beans, Kids	255
Bites, with Chips, Kids	379
Bites, with Salad, Kids	200
FISH & CHIPS	
Cod	705
GRILLS	
International	1024
Wimpy	803
HASH BROWNS	
Extra	98
HOT CHOCOLATE	
without Cream, Large	281
without Cream, Reg	224
ICE CREAM	
Extra	95
ICE CREAM FLOAT	
7 Up	99
Pepsi, Diet	96
Pepsi	183
Pepsi Max	96
Tango Orange	97
JAM	
Extra	48
JELLY	
Orange, Pot, Kids	3
Strawberry, Pot, Kids	5
JUICE	
Apple, Kids	122
Apple, Large	206
Apple, Reg	163
Orange, Kids	120
Orange, Large	202
Orange, Reg	160
LEMONADE	
7 Up, Free, Kids	5
7 Up, Free, Large	9
7 Up, Free, Reg	7
MARMALADE	
Extra	49
MILK	
Kids	125
Large	211
Reg	167
MILK SHAKE - BANANA	
Thick, Kids	187
Thick, Large	300
Thick, Reg	244

	KCAL
WIMPY	
MILK SHAKE - CHOCO TOFFEE POPCORN	
Thick, Reg	425
MILK SHAKE - CHOCOLATE	
Thick, Kids	189
Thick, Large	303
Thick, Reg	246
MILK SHAKE - CHOCOLATE PEPPERMINT	
Thick, Reg	365
MILK SHAKE - LIME	
Thick, Kids	152
Thick, Large	243
Thick, Reg	197
MILK SHAKE - STRAWBERRY	
Thick, Kids	187
Thick, Large	299
Thick, Reg	243
MILK SHAKE - VANILLA	
Thick, Kids	151
Thick, Large	241
Thick, Reg	196
MUFFIN	
Bacon, & Egg	347
Bacon, & Hasbrown	445
Hashbrown	380
Sausage, & Egg	380
Sausage, & Hashbrown	478
MUSHROOMS	
Extra	110
ONION RINGS	
8	317
CheesO, 4	481
PANCAKE	
& Ice Cream, no Toppings, Kids	178
& Ice Cream, no Toppings	344
PEAS	
Extras	86
PEPPER	
Jalapeno, Burger Extras	1
POTATO FILLING	
Bacon	65
Beans, Baked, Heinz	79
Cheese, Grated	189
Coleslaw	194
Mushrooms	137
POTATOES	
Baked, Jacket, Half, with Beans, Kids	297
Baked, Jacket, Half, with Cheese, Kids	347
Baked, Jacket, Half, with Chips, Kids	421
Baked, Jacket, Half, with Salad, Kids	241
Baked, Jacket, Plain, with Butter	516
Jacket, with Butter, & Salad, add Fillings Seperately	523
SALAD	
Chicken, Breaded, no Dressing	360

	KCAL
WIMPY	
SALAD	
Chicken, Gourmet, no Dressing	317
Junior, Side, Kids	8
Mixed, Side	67
Quorn, Southern Fried, Spicy, no Dressing	320
SAUCE	
BBQ	41
Chocolate, for Sundae	81
Firecracker	29
Ketchup	29
Mango, for Sundae	25
Maple Flavoured, for Sundae	86
Special	114
Strawberry, for Sundae	80
Summer Fruits, for Sundae	38
Toffee Fudge, for Sundae	91
Mayo	100
SAUSAGE	
Bender, with Egg & Chips, Grill	628
Patty, Extra	98
Pork, Bender	271
Pork, Breakfast	130
with Beans, Kids	322
with Chips, Kids	446
with Egg & Chips, Grill	615
with Salad, Kids	267
SMOOTHIE	
Mango, Iced	181
Summer Fruits, Iced	274
SQUASH	
Apple, & Blackcurrant, Kids	4
Orange, Kids	3
SUNDAE	
Brownie	591
Ice Cream, No Toppings, Kids	95
Ice Cream, No Toppings	159
Knickerbocker Glory	372
TANGO*	
Orange, Free, Kids	3
Orange, Free, Large	4
Orange, Free, Reg	3
TEA	
Black, Large	1
Black, Reg	1
Herbal, Large	3
Herbal, Reg	2
with Milk, Large	22
with Milk, Reg	14
TEACAKES	
Toasted, with Butter	295
TOAST	
White, with Butter	279

	KCAL
WIMPY	
TOASTIE	
Cheese, & Red Onion, White	391
Cheese, & Tomato, White	386
Cheese, with Beans, White, Kids	400
Cheese, with Chips, White, Kids	521
Cheese, with Salad, White, Kids	345
Chicken, BBQ, White	523
Ham, & Cheese, White	436
TOPPING	
Flake, Crushed, for Drinks	45
Fruit Cocktail, for Sundae	18
Fudge, Pieces, Mini	40
Marshmallows, Mini, for Drinks	32
Marshmallows, Mini, for Sundae	32
Strawberries, for Sundae	10
TORTE	
Apple, no Toppings	245
VEGETABLES	
Sticks, Carrot, & Cucumber, Kids	24
WAFFLES	
Eskimo, no Toppings	663

	KCAL
YO! SUSHI	
AUBERGINE	
Fried, in Garlic, Ginger, Sesame, & Soy, Harusame	108
BEANS	
Edamame, Side	134
BEEF	
Tataki	96
BEEF TERIYAKI	
Large	940
Standard	329
BROCCOLI	
Tenderstem, & Sesame	135
BROWNIES	
Chocolate	363
BURGERS	
Chicken, Katsu	476
Chicken, Teriyaki	286
Mushroom, Teriyaki	228
CAULIFLOWER	
Pepper, Spicy	146
CHEESECAKE	
Japanese	195
CHICKEN	
Fried, Japanese	382
Fried, Korean	386
CHICKEN TERIYAKI	
Large	837
Standard	272
DESSERT	
Mochi, Chocolate	236
Mochi, Strawberry Cheesecake	188
Platter	605
DOUGH BALLS	
Takoyaki	276
YO! SUSHI	
DUMPLINGS - GYOZA	
Chicken, 5	206
Chicken	140
Prawn, 5	220
Prawn	148
Vegetable, 5	193
Vegetable	132
FRIES	
YO!	400
FRUIT	
Fresh, Plate	61
KATSU	
Chicken, Curry, with Rice, Large	936
Chicken, Curry, with Rice	522
Chicken	225
Prawn, Curry, with Rice, Large	757
Prawn, Curry, with Rice	432
Prawn	173
Pumpkin, Curry, with Rice, Large	789

	KCAL
YO! SUSHI	
KATSU	
Pumpkin, Curry, with Rice	434
Pumpkin	152
Tofu, Curry, with Rice, Large	794
Tofu, Curry, with Rice	451
Tofu	154
MOUSSE	
Chocolate, Pot	246
NOODLES	
Side	187
NOODLES - RAMEN	
Chicken, Curry, Large	758
Chicken, Curry	416
Seafood, Spicy, Large	466
Seafood, Spicy	269
Shitake, Large	377
Shitake	225
NOODLES - YAKISOBA	
Chicken	264
Vegetable	202
PAK CHOI	
& Garlic, Stir Fried	86
PANCAKE	
Dorayaki	130
RICE	
Brown, Side	198
Chicken, Fried	347
Salmon, Fried	348
Vegetable, Fried	343
White, Side	303
SALAD	
Chicken, & Tangerine	148
Leaf, Side	35
SEAWEED	
Kaiso	175
SHRIMP	
Popcorn	355
SOUP	
Miso	53
SQUID	
Pepper, Spicy	207
SUSHI	
Aubergine, Glazed, Nigiri	74
Avocado, Maki	204
Avocado, Nigiri	110
Beef, Seared, Nigiri	108
Chicken, & Avocado, Roll, Platter	656
Chicken, & Avocado, Roll	215
Chicken, Katsu, Spicy, Roll, Platter	423
Chicken, Katsu, Spicy, Roll	145
Cucumber, Maki	150
Duck, Aromatic, Roll	218
Mixed, Maki, Plate	196

Useful Resources

Weight Loss
Weight Loss Resources is home to the UK's largest calorie and nutrition database along with diaries, tools and expert advice for weight loss and health.
Tel: 01733 345592 Email: helpteam@weightlossresources.co.uk
Website: www.weightlossresources.co.uk

Products to Help You Keep Track
From food diaries to weight graphs and calorie counted recipe books visit the wlr shop.
Tel: 01733 345592 Email: helpteam@weightlossresources.co.uk
Website: www.weightlossresources.co.uk/shop

Dietary Advice
The British Dietetic Association has helpful food fact leaflets and information on how to contact a registered dietitian.
Tel: 0121 200 8080 Email: info@bda.uk.com
Website: www.bda.uk.com

Healthy Eating
The British Nutrition Foundation has lots of in depth scientifically based nutritional information, knowledge and advice on healthy eating for all ages.
Tel: 0207 7557 7930 Email: postbox@nutrition.org.uk
Website: www.nutrition.org.uk

Healthy Heart
The British Heart Foundation provides advice and information for all on all heart aspects from being healthy, to living with heart conditions, research and fundraising.
Tel: 0207 554 000 Email: via their website
Website: www.bhf.org.uk

Cancer Research
Cancer Research UK is the leading UK charity dedicated to research, education and fundraising for all forms of cancer.
Tel: 0300 123 1022 Email: via their website
Website: www.cancerresearchuk.org

Diabetes Advice

Diabetes UK is the leading charity working for people with diabetes. Their mission is to improve the lives of people with diabetes and to work towards a future without diabetes

Tel : 0345 123 2399 Email: info@diabetes.org.uk

Website: www.diabetes.org.uk

Beating Bowel Cancer

Beating Bowel Cancer is a leading UK charity for bowel cancer patients, working to raise awareness of symptoms, promote early diagnosis and encourage open access to treatment choice for those affected by bowel cancer.Tel: 08450 719301 Email: nurse@beatingbowelcancer.org

Website: www.beatingbowelcancer.org

Safety and Standards

The Food Standards Agency is an independent watchdog, set up to protect the public's health and consumer interests in relation to food.

Tel: 0207 276 8829 Email: helpline@foodstandards.gsi.gov.uk

Website: www.food.gov.uk

Feedback

If you have any comments or suggestions about The Calorie, Carb & Fat Bible, or would like further information on Weight Loss Resources, please call, email, or write to us:

Tel:	01733 345592
Email:	helpteam@weightlossresources.co.uk
Address:	Rebecca Walton, Weight Loss Resources Ltd, 2C Flag Business Exchange, Vicarage Farm Road, Peterborough, PE1 5TX.

Reviews for The Calorie Carb & Fat Bible

'What a brilliant book. I know I'll be sinking my teeth into it.'
GMTV Nutritionist Amanda Ursell, BSc RD

'To help you make low-cal choices everyday, invest in a copy.'
ZEST magazine

'There is no doubt that the food listings are extremely helpful for anyone wishing to control their calorie intake in order to lose pounds or maintain a healthy weight.'
Women's Fitness magazine

'Useful if you don't want to exclude any overall food groups.'
Easy Living magazine

'Quite simply an astonishing achievement by the authors.'
Evening Post, Nottingham

'The book gives you all the basic information so you can work out your daily calorie needs.'
Woman magazine

'This is a welcome resource in view of the 'national epidemic of obesity.'

Bryony Philip, Bowel Cancer UK

'The authors seem to understand the problems of slimming.'

Dr John Campion

'Jam-packed with info on dieting, and full to bursting point with the calorie, carbohydrate and fat values of thousands of different foods, it's the perfect weight loss tool.'

Evening Express, Aberdeen

'Excellent resource tool - used by myself in my role as a Practice Nurse.'

Pam Boal, Sunderland

'I recently bought your book called the Calorie, Carb & Fat Bible and would love to tell you what a brilliant book it is. I have recently started a weight management programme and I honestly don't know where I'd be without your book. It has helped me a lot and given me some really good advice.'

Rachel Mitchell

About Weight Loss Resources

If you want to lose weight in a healthy, sustainable way, you'll find all the tools and support you need at wlr. Available on your phone, tablet, or PC.

HERE'S THE HIGHLIGHTS:

- Track calories: how many you need, how many you've consumed and burned, and how many you have left
- New Visual Food Diary, a more relaxed way to track. Enables you to reflect on choices and gain insights about your relationship with food
- The best kept online UK food database
- 1000s of recipes and meal ideas that you can add to your online diary and adapt to suit yourself
- Create and calorie count your own recipes and diet plans
- Set a weight loss goal, see how many calories you need to get there, and the date you can expect to reach it
- Fantastic support from our knowledgeable Helpteam, available 7 days a week